The ICU Book

THIRD EDITION

Paul L. Marino, **MD, PhD, FCCM**

Physician-in-Chief
Saint Vincent's Midtown Hospital
New York, New York

Clinical Associate Professor
New York Medical College
Valhalla, New York

With contributions from
Kenneth M. Sutin, MD, FCCM

Department of Anesthesiology
Bellevue Hospital Center

Associate Professor of Anesthesiology & Surgery
New York University School of Medicine
New York, New York

Illustrations by Patricia Gast

To Daniel Joseph Marino,
My 18-year-old son.
No longer a boy,
And not yet a man,
But always terrific.

I would especially commend the physician who, in acute diseases, by which the bulk of mankind are cutoff, conducts the treatment better than others.

—HIPPOCRATES

Preface to Third Edition

The third edition of *The ICU Book* marks its 15th year as a fundamental sourcebook in critical care. This edition continues the original intent to provide a generic textbook that presents fundamental concepts and patient care practices that can be used in any intensive care unit, regardless of the specialty focus of the unit. Highly specialized areas, such as obstetrical emergencies, thermal injury, and neurocritical care, are left to more qualified authors and their specialty textbooks.

Most of the chapters in this edition have been completely rewritten (including 198 new illustrations and 178 new tables), and there are two new chapters on infection control in the ICU (Chapter 3) and disorders of temperature regulation (Chapter 38). Most chapters also include a final section (called A Final Word) that contains an important take-home message from the chapter. The references have been extensively updated, with emphasis on recent reviews and clinical practice guidelines.

The ICU Book has been unique in that it reflects the voice of one author. This edition welcomes the voice of another, Dr. Kenneth Sutin, who added his expertise to the final 13 chapters of the book. Ken and I are old friends who share the same view of critical care medicine, and his contributions add a robust quality to the material without changing the basic personality of the work.

Preface to First Edition

In recent years, the trend has been away from a unified approach to critical illness, as the specialty of critical care becomes a hyphenated attachment for other specialties to use as a territorial signpost. The landlord system has created a disorganized array of intensive care units (10 different varieties at last count), each acting with little communion. However, the daily concerns in each intensive care unit are remarkably similar because serious illness has no landlord. The purpose of *The ICU Book* is to present this common ground in critical care and to focus on the fundamental principles of critical illness rather than the specific interests for each intensive care unit. As the title indicates, this is a 'generic' text for all intensive care units, regardless of the name on the door.

The present text differs from others in the field in that it is neither panoramic in scope nor overly indulgent in any one area. Much of the information originates from a decade of practice in intensive care units, the last three years in both a Medical ICU and a Surgical ICU. Daily rounds with both surgical and medical housestaff have provided the foundation for the concept of generic critical care that is the theme of this book.

As indicated in the chapter headings, this text is problem-oriented rather than disease-oriented, and each problem is presented through the eyes of the ICU physician. Instead of a chapter on GI bleeding, there is a chapter of the principles of volume resuscitation and two others on resuscitation fluids. This mimics the actual role of the ICU physician in GI bleeding, which is to manage the hemorrhage. The other features of the problem such as locating the bleeding site, are the tasks of other specialists. This is how the ICU operates and this is the specialty of critical care. Highly specialized topics such as burns, head trauma, and obstetric emergencies are not covered in this text. These are distinct subspecialties with their own texts and their own experts, and devoting a few pages to each would merely complete and outline rather than instruct.

The emphasis on fundamentals in *The ICU Book* is meant not only as a foundation for patient care but also to develop a strong base in clinical problem solving for any area of medicine. There is a tendency to rush past the basics in the stampede to finish formal training, and this leads to empiricism and irrational practice habits. Why a fever should or should not be treated, or whether a blood pressure cuff provides accurate readings, are questions that must be dissected carefully in the early stages of training, to develop the reasoning skills needed to be effective in clinical problems solving. This inquisitive stare must replace the knee-jerk approach to clinical problems if medicine is to advance. *The ICU Book* helps to develop this stare.

Wisely or not, the use of a single author was guided by the desire to present a uniform view. Much of the information is accompanied by published works listed at the end of each chapter and anecdotal tales are held to a minimum. Within an endeavor such as this, several shortcomings are inevitable, some omissions are likely and bias may occasionally replace sound judgment. The hope is that these deficiencies are few.

Acknowledgments

Acknowledgements are few but well deserved. First to Patricia Gast, the illustrator for this edition, who was involved in every facet of this work, and who added an energy and intelligence that goes well beyond the contributions of medical illustrators. Also to Tanya Lazar and Nicole Dernoski, my editors, for understanding the enormous time committment required to complete a work of this kind. And finally to the members of the executive and medical staff of my hospital, as well as my personal staff, who allowed me the time and intellectual space to complete this work unencumbered by the daily (and sometimes hourly) tasks involved in keeping the doors of a hospital open.

Contents

SECTION VI
Critical Care Cardiology

SECTION VII
Acute Respiratory Failure

SECTION VIII
Mechanical Ventilation

SECTION IX
Acid-Base Disorders

SECTION X
Renal and Electrolyte Disorders

SECTION XI
Transfusion Practices in Critical Care

SECTION XII
Disorders of Body Temperature

SECTION XIII
Inflammation and Infection in the ICU

SECTION XIV
Nutrition and Metabolism

SECTION XV
Critical Care Neurology

SECTION XVI
Toxic Ingestions

SECTION XVII
Appendices

BASIC SCIENCE REVIEW

The first step in applying the scientific method consists in being curious about the world.

LINUS PAULING

Chapter 1

CIRCULATORY BLOOD FLOW

When is a piece of matter said to be alive? When it goes on "doing something," moving, exchanging material with its environment.

Erwin Schrodinger

The human organism has an estimated 100 trillion cells that must go on exchanging material with the external environment to stay alive. This exchange is made possible by a circulatory system that uses a muscular pump (the heart), an exchange fluid (blood), and a network of conduits (blood vessels). Each day, the human heart pumps about 8,000 liters of blood through a vascular network that stretches more than 60,000 miles (more than twice the circumference of the Earth!) to maintain cellular exchange (1).

This chapter describes the forces responsible for the flow of blood though the human circulatory system. The first half is devoted to the determinants of cardiac output, and the second half describes the forces that influence peripheral blood flow. Most of the concepts in this chapter are old friends from the physiology classroom.

CARDIAC OUTPUT

Circulatory flow originates in the muscular contractions of the heart. Since blood is an incompressible fluid that flows through a closed hydraulic loop, the volume of blood ejected by the left side of the heart must equal the volume of blood returning to the right side of the heart (over a given time period). This conservation of mass (volume) in a closed hydraulic system is known as the *principle of continuity* (2), and it indicates that the stroke output of the heart is the principal determinant of circulatory blood flow. The forces that govern cardiac stroke output are identified in Table 1.1.

TABLE 1.1 The Forces that Determine Cardiac Stroke Output

Force	Definition	Clinical Parameters
Preload	The load imposed on resting muscle that stretches the muscle to a new length	End-diastolic pressure
Contractility	The velocity of muscle contraction when muscle load is fixed	Cardiac stroke volume when preload and afterload are constant
Afterload	The total load that must be moved by a muscle when it contracts	Pulmonary and systemic vascular resistances

Preload

If one end of a muscle fiber is suspended from a rigid strut and a weight is attached to the other free end, the added weight will stretch the muscle to a new length. The added weight in this situation represents a force called the *preload*, which is a force imposed on a resting muscle (prior to the onset of muscle contraction) that stretches the muscle to a new length. According to the length–tension relationship of muscle, an increase in the length of a resting (unstimulated) muscle will increase the force of contraction when the muscle is stimulated to contract. Therefore **the preload force acts to augment the force of muscle contraction**.

In the intact heart, the stretch imposed on the cardiac muscle prior to the onset of muscle contraction is a function of the volume in the ventricles at the end of diastole. Therefore the end-diastolic volume of the ventricles is the preload force of the intact heart (3).

Preload and Systolic Performance

The pressure-volume curves in Figure 1.1 show the influence of diastolic volume on the systolic performance of the heart. As the ventricle fills during diastole, there is an increase in both diastolic and systolic pressures. The increase in diastolic pressure is a reflection of the passive stretch imposed on the ventricle, while the difference between diastolic and systolic pressures is a reflection of the strength of ventricular contraction. Note that as diastolic volume increases, there is an increase in the difference between diastolic and systolic pressures, indicating that the strength of ventricular contraction is increasing. The importance of preload in augmenting cardiac contraction was discovered independently by Otto Frank (a German engineer) and Ernest Starling (a British physiologist), and their discovery is commonly referred to as the *Frank-Starling relationship of the heart* (3). This relationship can be stated as follows: **In the normal heart, diastolic volume is the principal force that governs the strength of ventricular contraction** (3).

Clinical Monitoring

In the clinical setting, the relationship between preload and systolic performance is monitored with *ventricular function curves* like the ones

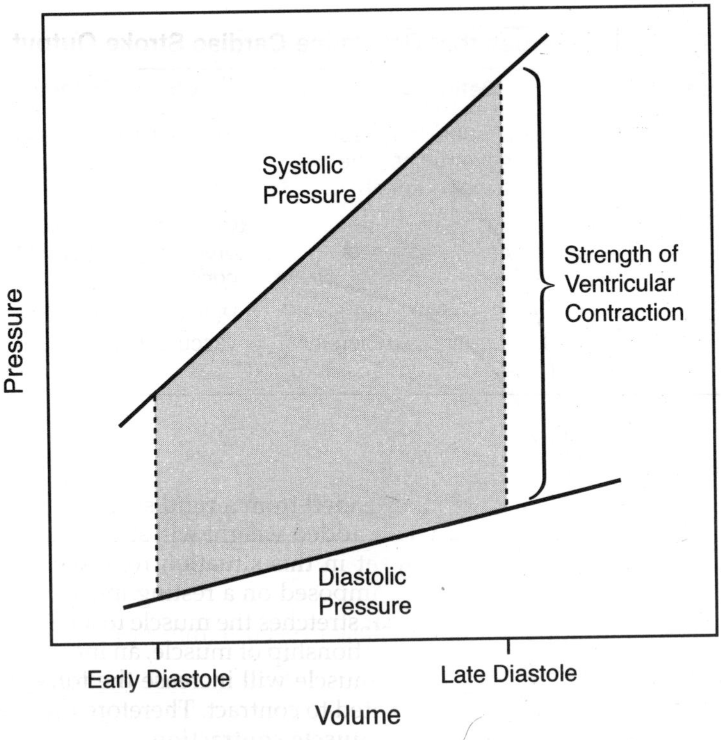

FIGURE 1.1 Pressure-volume curves showing the influence of diastolic volume on the strength of ventricular contraction.

shown in Figure 1.2. End-diastolic pressure (EDP) is used as the clinical measure of preload because end-diastolic volume is not easily measured (the measurement of EDP is described in Chapter 10). The normal ventricular function curve has a steep ascent, indicating that changes in preload have a marked influence on systolic performance in the normal heart (i.e., the Frank-Starling relationship). When myocardial contractility is reduced, there is a decrease in the slope of the curve, resulting in an increase in end-diastolic pressure and a decrease in stroke volume. This is the hemodynamic pattern seen in patients with heart failure.

Ventricular function curves are used frequently in the intensive care unit (ICU) to evaluate patients who are hemodynamically unstable. However, these curves can be misleading. The major problem is that conditions other than myocardial contractility can influence the slope of these curves. These conditions (i.e., ventricular compliance and ventricular afterload) are described next.

Preload and Ventricular Compliance

The stretch imposed on cardiac muscle is determined not only by the volume of blood in the ventricles, but also by the tendency of the ventricular wall to distend or stretch in response to ventricular filling.

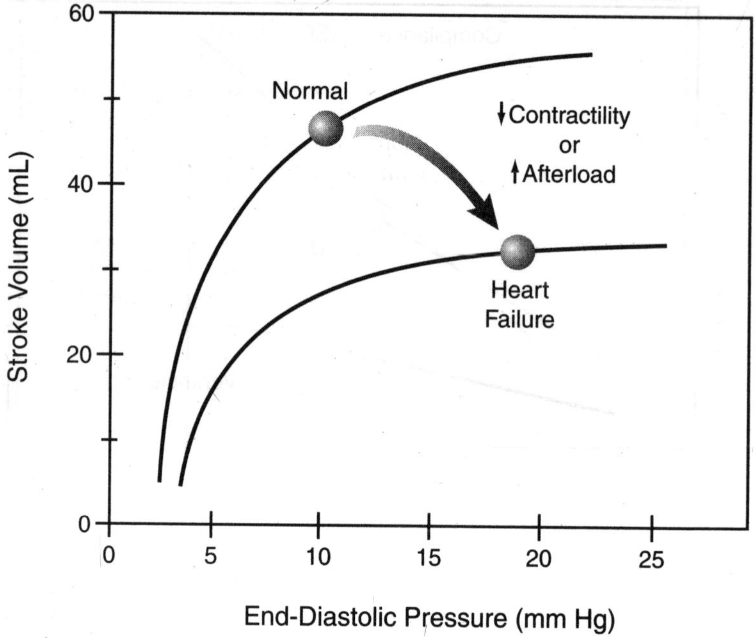

FIGURE 1.2 Ventricular function curves used to describe the relationship between preload (end-diastolic pressure) and systolic performance (stroke volume).

The distensibility of the ventricles is referred to as *compliance* and can be derived using the following relationship between changes in end-diastolic pressure (EDP) and end-diastolic volume (EDV) (5):

$$\text{Compliance} = \Delta\text{EDV}/\Delta\text{EDP} \tag{1.1}$$

The pressure-volume curves in Figure 1.3 illustrate the influence of ventricular compliance on the relationship between ΔEDP and ΔEDV. As compliance decreases (i.e., as the ventricle becomes stiff), the slope of the curve decreases, resulting in a decrease in EDV at any given EDP. In this situation, the EDP will overestimate the actual preload (EDV). This illustrates how changes in ventricular compliance will influence the reliability of EDP as a reflection of preload. The following statements highlight the importance of ventricular compliance in the interpretation of the EDP measurement.

1. End-diastolic pressure is an accurate reflection of preload only when ventricular compliance is normal.
2. Changes in end-diastolic pressure accurately reflect changes in preload only when ventricular compliance is constant.

Several conditions can produce a decrease in ventricular compliance. The most common are left ventricular hypertrophy and ischemic heart

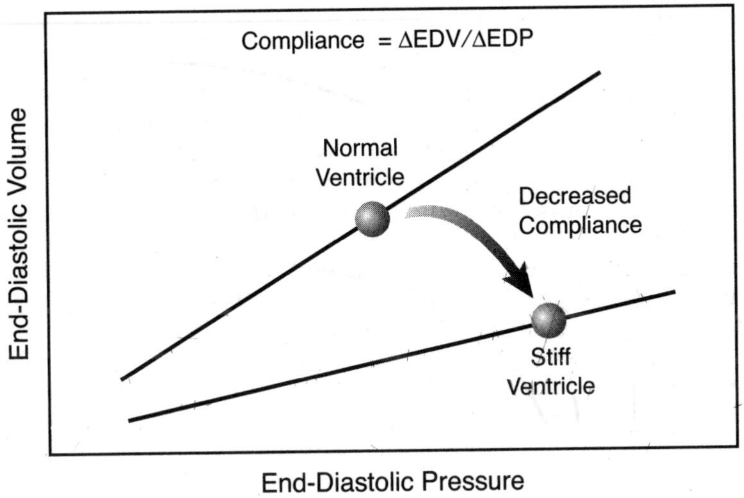

FIGURE 1.3 Diastolic pressure-volume curves in the normal and noncompliant (stiff) ventricle.

disease. Since these conditions are also commonplace in ICU patients, the reliability of the EDP measurement is a frequent concern.

Diastolic Heart Failure

As ventricular compliance begins to decrease (e.g., in the early stages of ventricular hypertrophy), the EDP rises, but the EDV remains unchanged. The increase in EDP reduces the pressure gradient for venous inflow into the heart, and this eventually leads to a decrease in EDV and a resultant decrease in cardiac output (via the Frank-Starling mechanism). This condition is depicted by the point on the lower graph in Figure 1.3, and is called *diastolic heart failure* (6). Systolic function (contractile strength) is preserved in this type of heart failure.

Diastolic heart failure should be distinguished from conventional (systolic) heart failure because the management of the two conditions differs markedly. For example, since ventricular filling volumes are reduced in diastolic heart failure, diuretic therapy can be counterproductive. Unfortunately, it is not possible to distinguish between the two types of heart failure when the EDP is used as a measure of preload because the EDP is elevated in both conditions. The ventricular function curves in Figure 1.3 illustrate this problem. The point on the lower curve identifies a condition where EDP is elevated and stroke volume is reduced. This condition is often assumed to represent heart failure due to systolic dysfunction, but diastolic dysfunction would also produce the same changes. This inability to distinguish between systolic and diastolic heart failure is one of the major shortcomings of ventricular function curves. (See Chapter 14 for a more detailed discussion of systolic and diastolic heart failure.)

Afterload

When a weight is attached to one end of a contracting muscle, the force of muscle contraction must overcome the opposing force of the weight before the muscle begins to shorten. The weight in this situation represents a force called the *afterload*, which is defined as the load imposed on a muscle *after* the onset of muscle contraction. Unlike the preload force, which facilitates muscle contraction, **the afterload force opposes muscle contraction** (i.e., as the afterload increases, the muscle must develop more tension to move the load). In the intact heart, **the afterload force is equivalent to the peak tension developed across the wall of the ventricles during systole** (3).

The determinants of ventricular wall tension (afterload) were derived from observations on soap bubbles made by the Marquis de Laplace in 1820. His observations are expressed in the Law of Laplace, which states that the tension (T) in a thin-walled sphere is directly related to the chamber pressure (P) and radius (r) of the sphere: $T = Pr$. When the LaPlace relationship is applied to the heart, T represents the peak systolic transmural wall tension of the ventricle, P represents the transmural pressure across the ventricle at the end of systole, and r represents the chamber radius at the end of diastole (5).

The forces that contribute to ventricular afterload can be identified using the components of the Laplace relationship, as shown in Figure 1.4. There are three major contributing forces: pleural pressure, arterial impedance, and end-diastolic volume (preload). Preload is a component of afterload because it is a volume load that must be moved by the ventricle during systole.

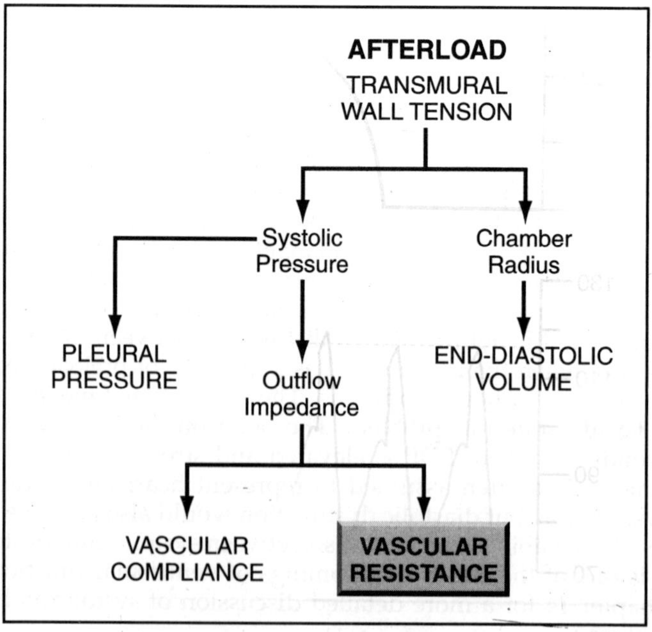

FIGURE 1.4 The forces that contribute to ventricular afterload.

Pleural Pressure

Since afterload is a transmural force, it is determined in part by the pleural pressure on the outer surface of the heart. Negative pleural pressures will increase transmural pressure and increase ventricular afterload, while positive pleural pressures will have the opposite effect. Negative pressures surrounding the heart can impede ventricular emptying by opposing the inward displacement of the ventricular wall during systole (7,8). This effect is responsible for the transient decrease in systolic blood pressure (reflecting a decrease in cardiac stroke volume) that normally occurs during the inspiratory phase of spontaneous breathing. When the inspiratory drop in systolic pressure is greater than 15 mm Hg, the condition is called "pulsus paradoxus" (which is a misnomer, since the response is not paradoxical, but is an exaggeration of the normal response).

Positive pleural pressures can promote ventricular emptying by facilitating the inward movement of the ventricular wall during systole (7,9). This effect is illustrated in Figure 1.5. The tracings in this figure show the effect of positive-pressure mechanical ventilation on the arterial blood pressure. When intrathoracic pressure rises during a positive-pressure breath, there is a transient rise in systolic blood pressure (reflecting an increase in the stroke volume output of the heart). This response indicates that positive intrathoracic pressure can provide

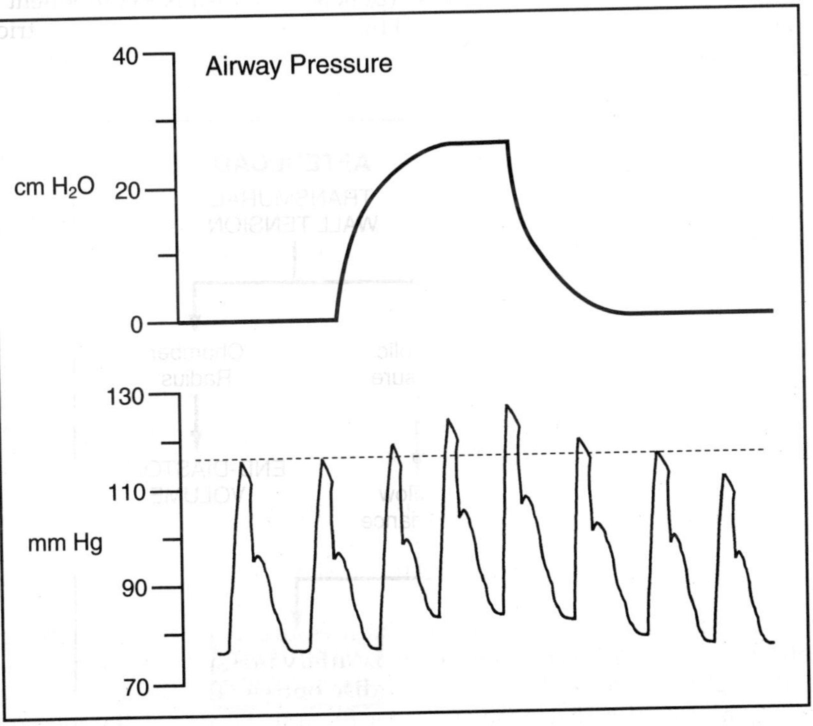

FIGURE 1.5 Respiratory variations in blood pressure during positive-pressure mechanical ventilation.

cardiac support by "unloading" the left ventricle. Although this effect is probably of minor significance, positive-pressure mechanical ventilation has been proposed as a possible therapeutic modality in patients with cardiogenic shock (10). The hemodynamic effects of mechanical ventilation are discussed in more detail in Chapter 24.

Impedance

The principal determinant of ventricular afterload is a hydraulic force known as *impedance* that opposes phasic changes in pressure and flow. This force is most prominent in the large arteries close to the heart, where it acts to oppose the pulsatile output of the ventricles. **Aortic impedance is the major afterload force for the left ventricle**, and pulmonary artery impedance serves the same role for the right ventricle. Impedance is influenced by two other forces: (a) a force that opposes the rate of change in flow, known as *compliance*, and (b) a force that opposes steady flow, called *resistance*. Arterial compliance is expressed primarily in the large, elastic arteries, where it plays a major role in determining vascular impedance. Arterial resistance is expressed primarily in the smaller peripheral arteries, where the flow is steady and nonpulsatile. Since resistance is a force that opposes nonpulsatile flow, while impedance opposes pulsatile flow, **arterial resistance may play a minor role in the impedance to ventricular emptying**. Arterial resistance can, however, influence pressure and flow events in the large, proximal arteries (where impedance is prominent) because it acts as a downstream resistance for these arteries.

Vascular impedance and compliance are complex, dynamic forces that are not easily measured (12,13). Vascular resistance, however, can be calculated as described next.

Vascular Resistance

The resistance (R) to flow in a hydraulic circuit is expressed by the relationship between the pressure gradient across the circuit (ΔP) and the rate of flow (Q) through the circuit:

$$R = \Delta P/Q \tag{1.2}$$

Applying this relationship to the systemic and pulmonary circulations yields the following equations for systemic vascular resistance (SVR) and pulmonary vascular resistance (PVR):

$$SVR = SAP - RAP/CO \tag{1.3}$$

$$PVR = PAP - LAP/CO \tag{1.4}$$

SAP is the mean systemic arterial pressure, RAP is the mean right atrial pressure, PAP is mean pulmonary artery pressure, LAP is the mean left atrial pressure, and CO is the cardiac output. The SAP is measured with an arterial catheter (see Chapter 8), and the rest of the measurements are obtained with a pulmonary artery catheter (see Chapter 9).

Clinical Monitoring

There are no accurate measures of ventricular afterload in the clinical setting. The SVR and PVR are used as clinical measures of afterload, but they are unreliable (14,15). There are two problems with the use of vascular resistance calculations as a reflection of ventricular afterload. First, arterial resistance may contribute little to ventricular afterload because it is a force that opposes nonpulsatile flow, while afterload (impedance) is a force that opposes pulsatile flow. Second, the SVR and PVR are measures of total vascular resistance (arterial and venous), which is even less likely to contribute to ventricular afterload than arterial resistance. These limitations have led to the recommendation that PVR and SVR be abandoned as clinical measures of afterload (15).

Since afterload can influence the slope of ventricular function curves (see Figure 1.2), changes in the slope of these curves are used as indirect evidence of changes in afterload. However, other forces, such as ventricular compliance and myocardial contractility, can also influence the slope of ventricular function curves, so unless these other forces are held constant, a change in the slope of a ventricular function curve cannot be used as evidence of a change in afterload.

Contractility

The contraction of striated muscle is attributed to interactions between contractile proteins arranged in parallel rows in the sarcomere. The number of bridges formed between adjacent rows of contractile elements determines the contractile state or *contractility* of the muscle fiber. The contractile state of a muscle is reflected by the force and velocity of muscle contraction when loading conditions (i.e., preload and afterload) are held constant (3). The standard measure of contractility is the acceleration rate of ventricular pressure (dP/dt) during isovolumic contraction (the time from the onset of systole to the opening of the aortic valve, when preload and afterload are constant). This can be measured during cardiac catheterization.

Clinical Monitoring

There are no reliable measures of myocardial contractility in the clinical setting. The relationship between end-diastolic pressure and stroke volume (see Figure 1.2) is often used as a reflection of contractility; however, other conditions (i.e., ventricular compliance and afterload) can influence this relationship. There are echocardiography techniques for evaluating contractility (15,16), but these are very specialized and not used routinely.

PERIPHERAL BLOOD FLOW

As mentioned in the introduction to this chapter, there are over 60,000 miles of blood vessels in the human body! Even if this estimate is off by 10,000 or 20,000 miles, it still points to the incomprehensible vastness of the human circulatory system. The remainder of this chapter will describe the forces that govern flow through this vast network of blood vessels.

A Note of Caution: The forces that govern peripheral blood flow are derived from observations on idealized hydraulic circuits where the flow is steady and laminar (streamlined), and the conducting tubes are rigid. These conditions bear little resemblance to the human circulatory system, where the flow is often pulsatile and turbulent, and the blood vessels are compressible and not rigid. Because of these differences, the description of blood flow that follows should be viewed as a very schematic representation of what really happens in the circulatory system.

Flow in Rigid Tubes

Steady flow (Q) through a hollow, rigid tube is proportional to the pressure gradient along the length of the tube (ΔP), and the constant of proportionality is the hydraulic resistance to flow (R):

$$Q = \Delta P \times 1/R \tag{1.5}$$

The resistance to flow in small tubes was described independently by a German physiologist (G. Hagen) and a French physician (J. Poisseuille). They found that resistance to flow is a function of the inner radius of the tube (r), the length of the tube (L), and the viscosity of the fluid (μ). Their observations are expressed in the following equation, known as the Hagen-Poisseuille equation (18):

$$Q = \Delta P \times (\pi r^4/8\mu L) \tag{1.6}$$

The final term in the equation is the reciprocal of resistance (1/R), so resistance can be described as

$$R = 8\mu L/\pi r^4 \tag{1.7}$$

The Hagen-Poisseuille equation is illustrated in Figure 1.6. Note that flow varies according to the fourth power of the inner radius of the tube. This means that **a two-fold increase in the radius of the tube will result in a sixteen-fold increase in flow**: $(2r)^4 = 16r$. The other components of resistance (i.e., tube length and fluid viscosity) exert a much smaller influence on flow.

Since the Hagen-Poisseuille equation describes steady flow through rigid tubes, it may not accurately describe the behavior of the circulatory system (where flow is not steady and the tubes are not rigid). However, there are several useful applications of this equation. In Chapter 6, it will be used to describe flow through vascular catheters (see Figure 6.1). In Chapter 12, it will be used to describe the flow characteristics of different resuscitation fluids, and in Chapter 36, it will be used to describe the hemodynamic effects of anemia and blood transfusions.

Flow in Tubes of Varying Diameter

As blood moves away from the heart and encounters vessels of decreasing diameter, the resistance to flow should increase and the flow should decrease. This is not possible because (according to the principle of

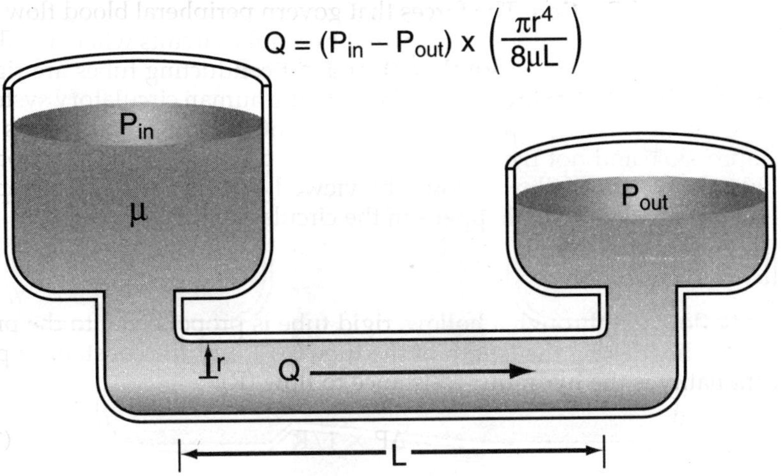

FIGURE 1.6 The forces that influence steady flow in rigid tubes. Q = flow rate, P_{in} = inlet pressure, P_{out} = outlet pressure, μ = viscosity, r = inner radius, L = length.

continuity) blood flow must be the same at all points along the circulatory system. This discrepancy can be resolved by considering the influence of tube narrowing on flow velocity. For a rigid tube of varying diameter, the velocity of flow (v) at any point along the tube is directly proportional to the bulk flow (Q), and inversely proportional to the cross-sectional area of the tube: $v = Q/A$ (2). Rearranging terms (and using $A = \pi r^2$) yields the following:

$$Q = v \times (\pi r^2) \tag{1.8}$$

This shows that bulk flow can remain unchanged when a tube narrows if there is an appropriate increase in the velocity of flow. This is how the nozzle on a garden hose works and is how blood flow remains constant as the blood vessels narrow.

Flow in Compressible Tubes

Flow through compressible tubes (like blood vessels) is influenced by the external pressure surrounding the tube. This is illustrated in Figure 1.7, which shows a compressible tube running through a fluid reservoir. The height of the fluid in the reservoir can be adjusted to vary the external pressure on the tube. When there is no fluid in the reservoir and the external pressure is zero, the driving force for flow through the tube will be the pressure gradient between the two ends of the tube ($P_{in} - P_{out}$). When the reservoir fills and the external pressure exceeds the lowest pressure in the tube ($P_{ext} > P_{out}$), the tube will be compressed. In this situation, the driving force for flow is the pressure gradient between the inlet pressure and the external pressure ($P_{in} - P_{ext}$). Therefore **when a tube is compressed by external pressure, the driving force for flow is independent of the pressure gradient along the tube** (20).

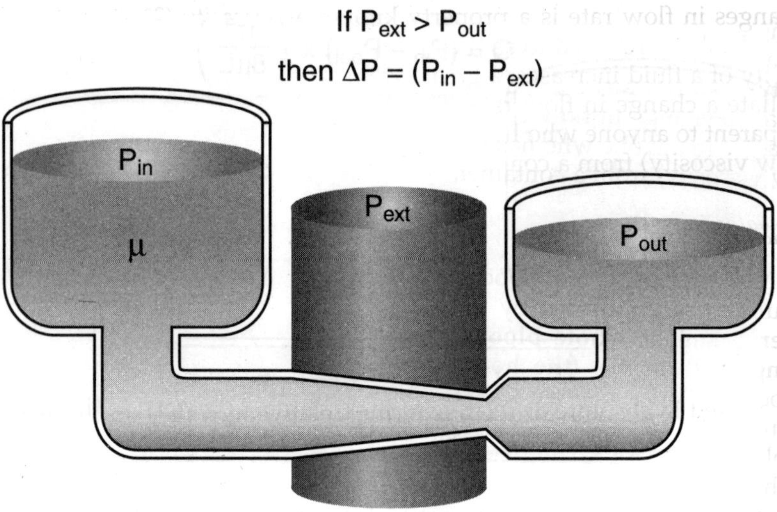

FIGURE 1.7 The influence of external pressure on flow through compressible tubes. P_{in} = inlet pressure, P_{out} = outlet pressure, P_{ext} = external pressure.

The Pulmonary Circulation

Vascular compression has been demonstrated in the cerebral, pulmonary, and systemic circulations. It can be particularly prominent in the pulmonary circulation during positive-pressure mechanical ventilation, when alveolar pressure exceeds the hydrostatic pressure in the pulmonary capillaries (20). When this occurs, the driving force for flow through the lungs is no longer the pressure gradient from the main pulmonary arteries to the left atrium (PAP − LAP), but instead is the pressure difference between the pulmonary artery pressure and the alveolar pressure (PAP − Palv). This change in driving pressure not only contributes to a reduction in pulmonary blood flow, but it also affects the pulmonary vascular resistance (PVR) calculation as follows:

$$\text{Normal: PVR} = \text{PAP} - \text{LAP/CO} \quad (1.9)$$

$$\text{When Palv} > \text{LAP:} \quad \text{PVR} = \text{PAP} - \text{Palv/CO} \quad (1.10)$$

Vascular compression in the lungs is discussed again in Chapter 10 (the measurement of vascular pressures in the thorax) and in Chapter 24 (the hemodynamic effects of mechanical ventilation).

Blood Viscosity

A solid will resist being deformed (changing shape), while a fluid will deform continuously (flow) but will resist changes in the rate of deformation (i.e., changes in flow rate) (21). The resistance of a fluid to changes in flow rate is a property known as *viscosity* (21–23). Viscosity has also been referred to as the "gooiness" of a fluid (21). When the viscosity of a fluid increases, a greater force must be applied to the fluid to initiate a change in flow rate. The influence of viscosity on flow rate is apparent to anyone who has poured molasses (high viscosity) and water (low viscosity) from a container.

Hematocrit

The viscosity of whole blood is almost entirely due to cross-linking of circulating erythrocytes by plasma fibrinogen (22,23). **The principal determinant of whole blood viscosity is the concentration of circulating erythrocytes (the hematocrit).** The influence of hematocrit on blood viscosity is shown in Table 1.2. Note that blood viscosity can be expressed in absolute or relative terms (relative to water). In the absence of blood cells (zero hematocrit), the viscosity of blood (plasma) is only slightly higher than that of water. This is not surprising, since plasma is 92% water. At a normal hematocrit (45%), blood viscosity is three times the viscosity of plasma. Thus plasma flows much more easily than whole blood, and anemic blood flows much more easily than normal blood. The influence of hematocrit on blood viscosity is the single most important factor that determines the hemodynamic effects of anemia and blood transfusions (see later).

Shear Thinning

The viscosity of some fluids varies inversely with a change in flow velocity (21,23). Blood is one of these fluids. (Another is ketchup, which is thick and difficult to get out of the bottle, but once it starts to flow, it thins out and flows more easily.) Since the velocity of blood flow increases as the blood vessels narrow, the viscosity of blood will also decrease as the

TABLE 1.2 Blood Viscosity as a Function of Hematocrit

	Viscosity*	
Hematocrit	**Relative**	**Absolute**
0	1.4	
10	1.8	1.2
20	2.1	1.5
30	2.8	1.8
40	3.7	2.3
50	4.8	2.9
60	5.8	3.8
70	8.2	5.3

*Absolute viscosity expressed in centipoise (cP).
Data from Documenta Geigy Scientific Tables. 7th ed. Basel: Documenta Geigy, 1966:557–558.

blood moves into the small blood vessels in the periphery. The decrease in viscosity occurs because the velocity of plasma increases more than the velocity of erythrocytes, so the relative plasma volume increases in small blood vessels. This process is called *shear thinning* (shear is a tangential force that influences flow rate), and it facilitates flow through small vessels. It becomes evident in blood vessels with diameters less than 0.3 mm (24).

Hemodynamic Effects

The Hagen-Poisseuille equation indicates that blood flow is inversely related to blood viscosity, and further that blood flow will change in proportion to a change in viscosity (i.e., if blood viscosity is doubled, blood flow will be halved) (22). The effect of changes in blood viscosity on blood flow is shown in Figure 1.8. In this case, changes in hematocrit are used to represent changes in blood viscosity. The data in this graph is from a patient with polycythemia who was treated with a combination of phlebotomy and fluid infusion (isovolemic hemodilution) to achieve a therapeutic reduction in hematocrit and blood viscosity. The progressive decrease in hematocrit is associated with a steady rise in cardiac output, and the change in cardiac output is far greater than the change in hematocrit. The disproportionate increase in cardiac output is more than expected from the Hagen-Poisseuille equation and may be due in part

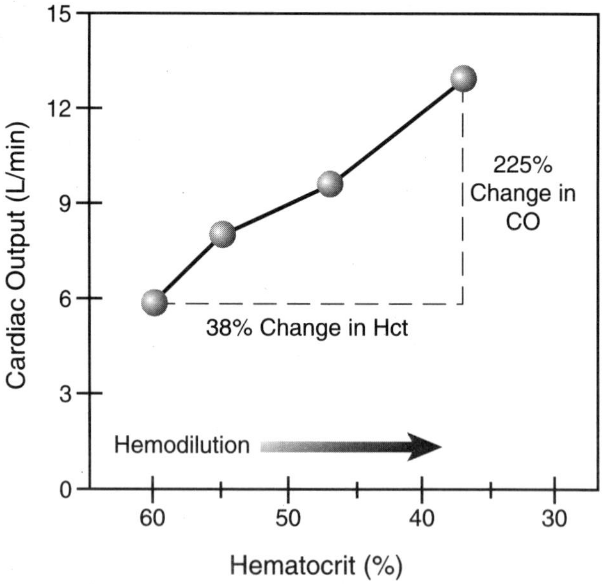

FIGURE 1.8 The influence of progressive hemodilution on cardiac output in a patient with polycythemia. CO = cardiac output. (From LeVeen HH, Ip M, Ahmed N, et al. Lowering blood viscosity to overcome vascular resistance. Surg Gynecol Obstet 1980;150:139.)

to the fact that blood viscosity varies inversely with flow rate. That is, as viscosity decreases and flow rate increases, the increase in flow rate will cause a further reduction in viscosity, which will then lead to a further increase in flow rate, and so on. This process would then magnify the influence of blood viscosity on blood flow. Whether or not this is the case, the graph in Figure 1.8 demonstrates that changes in hematocrit have a profound influence on circulatory blood flow. This topic is presented in more detail in Chapter 36.

Clinical Monitoring

Viscosity can be measured with an instrument called (what else?) a viscometer. This device has two parallel plates: one fixed and one that can move over the surface of the fixed plate. A fluid sample is placed between the two plates, and a force is applied to move the moveable plate. The force needed to move the plate is proportional to the viscosity of the fluid between the plates. Viscosity is expressed as force per area (surface area of the plates). The units of measurement are the "poise" (or dyne · sec/cm^2) in the CGS system, and the "Pascal · second" (Pa · s) in the SI system. (A poise is one/tenth of a Pascal · second.) Viscosity is also expressed as the ratio of the test sample viscosity to the viscosity of water. This "relative viscosity" is easier to interpret.

Viscosity is rarely measured in the clinical setting. The main reason for this is the consensus view that *in vitro* viscosity measurements are unreliable because they do not take into account conditions in the circulatory system (like shear thinning) that influence viscosity (21–24). Monitoring changes in viscosity may be more useful than single measurements. For example, serial changes in blood viscosity could be used to monitor the effects of aggressive diuretic therapy (e.g., a rise in viscosity to abnormally high levels might trigger a reduction in diuretic dosage). The value of blood viscosity measurements is underappreciated at the present time.

REFERENCES

General Texts

Berne R, Levy M. Cardiovascular physiology, 8th ed. St. Louis: Mosby, 2001.

Guyton AC, Jones CE, Coleman TG. Circulatory physiology: cardiac output and its regulation, 2nd ed. Philadelphia: WB Saunders, 1973.

Nichols WW, O'Rourke M. McDonald's blood flow in arteries, 3rd ed. Baltimore: Williams & Wilkins, 1990.

Vogel S. Vital circuits. New York: Oxford University Press, 1992.

Warltier DC. Ventricular function. Baltimore: Williams & Wilkins, 1995.

Cardiac Output

1. Vogel S. Vital circuits. New York: Oxford University Press, 1992:1–17.
2. Vogel S. Life in moving fluids. Princeton: Princeton University Press, 1981: 25–28.

3. Opie LH. Mechanisms of cardiac contraction and relaxation. In: Braunwald E, Zipes DP, Libby P, eds. Heart disease: a textbook of cardiovascular medicine, 6th ed. Philadelphia: WB Saunders, 2001:443–478.
4. Parmley WM, Talbot L. The heart as a pump. In: Berne RM, ed. Handbook of physiology: the cardiovascular system. Bethesda: American Physiological Society, 1979:429–460.
5. Gilbert JC, Glantz SA. Determinants of left ventricular filling and of the diastolic pressure-volume relation. Circ Res 1989;64:827–852.
6. Zile M, Baicu C, Gaasch W. Diastolic heart failure: abnormalities in active relaxation and passive stiffness of the left ventricle. N Engl J Med 2004;350: 1953–1959.
7. Pinsky MR. Cardiopulmonary interactions: the effects of negative and positive changes in pleural pressures on cardiac output. In: Dantzger DR, ed. Cardiopulmonary critical care, 2nd ed. Philadelphia: WB Saunders, 1991: 87–120.
8. Hausnecht N, Brin K, Weisfeldt M, et al. Effects of left ventricular loading by negative intrathoracic pressure in dogs. Circ Res 1988;62:620–631.
9. Magder S. Clinical usefulness of respiratory variations in blood pressure. Am J Respir Crit Care Med 2004;169:151–155.
10. Peters J. Mechanical ventilation with PEEP: a unique therapy for failing hearts. Intens Care Med 1999;25:778–780.
11. Nichols WW, O'Rourke MF. Input impedance as ventricular load. In: McDonald's blood flow in arteries, 3rd ed. Philadelphia: Lea & Febiger, 1990: 330–342.
12. Finkelstein SM, Collins R. Vascular impedance measurement. Progr Cardiovasc Dis 1982;24:401–418.
13. Laskey WK, Parker G, Ferrari VA, et al. Estimation of total systemic arterial compliance in humans. J Appl Physiol 1990;69:112–119.
14. Lang RM, Borrow KM, Neumann A, et al. Systemic vascular resistance: an unreliable index of left ventricular afterload. Circulation 1986;74:1114–1123.
15. Pinsky MR. Hemodynamic monitoring in the intensive care unit. Clin Chest Med 2003;24:549–560.
16. Bargiggia GS, Bertucci C, Recusani F, et al. A new method for estimating left ventricular dP/dt by continuous wave Doppler echocardiography: validation studies at cardiac catheterization. Circulation 1989;80:1287–1292.
17. Broka S, Dubois P, Jamart J, et al. Effects of acute decrease in afterload on accuracy of Doppler-derived left ventricular rate of pressure rise measurement in anesthetized patients. J Am Soc Echocardiogr 2001;14:1161–1165.

Peripheral Blood Flow

18. Chien S, Usami S, Skalak R. Blood flow in small tubes. In: Renkin EM, Michel CC, eds. Handbook of physiology, Section 2: the cardiovascular system. Vol IV: The microcirculation. Bethesda: American Physiological Society, 1984:217–249.
19. Little RC, Little WC. Physiology of the heart and circulation, 4th ed. Chicago: Year Book Publishers, 1989:219–236.
20. Gorback MS. Problems associated with the determination of pulmonary vascular resistance. J Clin Monit 1990;6:118–127.

21. Vogel S. Life in moving fluids. Princeton: Princeton University Press, 1981: 11–24.
22. Merrill EW. Rheology of blood. Physiol Rev 1969;49:863–888.
23. Lowe GOD. Blood rheology in vitro and in vivo. Baillieres Clin Hematol 1987;1:597.
24. Berne RM, Levy MN. Cardiovascular physiology, 8th ed. Philadelphia: Mosby, 1992:127–133.

Chapter 2

OXYGEN AND CARBON DIOXIDE TRANSPORT

Respiration is thus a process of combustion, in truth very slow, but otherwise exactly like that of charcoal.

Antoine Lavoisier

The business of aerobic metabolism is the combustion of nutrient fuels to release energy. This process consumes oxygen and generates carbon dioxide. The business of the circulatory system is to deliver the oxygen and nutrient fuels to the tissues of the body, and then to remove the carbon dioxide that is generated. The dual role of the circulatory system in transporting both oxygen and carbon dioxide is referred to as the *respiratory function of blood*. The business of this chapter is to describe how this respiratory function is carried out.

OXYGEN TRANSPORT

The transport of oxygen from the lungs to metabolizing tissues can be described by using four clinical parameters: (a) the concentration of oxygen in blood, (b) the delivery rate of oxygen in arterial blood, (c) the rate of oxygen uptake from capillary blood into the tissues, and (d) the fraction of oxygen in capillary blood that is taken up into the tissues. These four *oxygen transport parameters* are shown in Table 2.1, along with the equations used to derive each parameter. Thorough knowledge of these parameters is essential for the management of critically ill patients.

O_2 Content in Blood

Oxygen does not dissolve readily in water (1) and, since plasma is 93% water, a specialized oxygen-binding molecule (hemoglobin) is needed to

TABLE 2.1 Oxygen and Carbon Dioxide Transport Parameters

Parameter	Symbol	Equations
Arterial O_2 content	CaO_2	$1.34 \times Hb \times SaO_2$
Venous O_2 content	CvO_2	$1.34 \times Hb \times SvO_2$
O_2 Delivery	DO_2	$Q \times CaO_2$
O_2 Uptake	VO_2	$Q \times (CaO_2 - CvO_2)$
O_2 Extraction ratio	O_2ER	VO_2/DO_2
CO_2 Elimination	VCO_2	$Q \times (CvCO_2 - CaCO_2)$
Respiratory quotient	RQ	VCO_2/VO_2

Abbreviations: Hb = hemoglobin concentration in blood; SaO_2 and SvO_2 = oxygen saturation of hemoglobin (ratio of oxygenated hemoglobin to total hemoglobin) in arterial and mixed venous blood, respectively; Q = cardiac output; $CaCO_2$ = CO_2 content in arterial blood; $CvCO_2$ = CO_2 content in mixed venous blood.

facilitate the oxygenation of blood. The concentration of oxygen (O_2) in blood, also called the *O_2 content*, is the summed contribution of O_2 that is bound to hemoglobin and O_2 that is dissolved in plasma.

Hemoglobin-Bound O_2

The concentration of hemoglobin-bound O_2 (HbO_2) is determined by the variables in Equation 2.1 (2).

$$HbO_2 = 1.34 \times Hb \times SO_2 \qquad (2.1)$$

Hb is the hemoglobin concentration in blood (usually expressed in grams per deciliter, which is grams per 100 mL); 1.34 is the oxygen-binding capacity of hemoglobin (expressed in mL O_2 per gram of Hb); and SO_2 is the ratio of oxygenated hemoglobin to total hemoglobin in blood (SO_2 = HbO_2/total Hb), also called the *O_2 saturation of hemoglobin*. The HbO_2 is expressed in the same units as the Hb concentration (g/dL).

Equation 2.1 predicts that, when hemoglobin is fully saturated with O_2 (i.e., when the SO_2 = 1), each gram of hemoglobin will bind 1.34 mL oxygen. One gram of hemoglobin normally binds 1.39 mL oxygen, but a small fraction (3% to 5%) of circulating hemoglobin is present as methemoglobin and carboxyhemoglobin and, since these forms of Hb have a reduced O_2-binding capacity, the lower value of 1.34 mL/g is considered more representative of the O_2-binding capacity of the total hemoglobin pool (3).

Dissolved O_2

The concentration of dissolved oxygen in plasma is determined by the solubility of oxygen in water (plasma) and the partial pressure of oxygen (PO_2) in blood. The solubility of O_2 in water is temperature-dependent (solubility increases slightly as temperature decreases). At normal body temperature (37°C), 0.03 mL of O_2 will dissolve in one liter of water when the PO_2 is 1 mm Hg (4). This is expressed as a *solubility coefficient* of 0.03 mL/L/mm Hg (or 0.003 mL/100 mL/mm Hg). The concentration of

TABLE 2.2 Normal Levels of Oxygen in Arterial and Venous Blood*

Parameter	Arterial Blood	Venous Blood
PO_2	90 mm Hg	40 mm Hg
O_2 Saturation of Hb	0.98	0.73
Hb-bound O_2	197 mL/L	147 mL/L
Dissolved O_2	2.7 mL/L	1.2 mL/L
Total O_2 content	200 mL/L	148 mL/L
Blood volume†	1.25 L	3.75 L
Volume of O_2	250 mL	555 mL

*Values shown are for a body temperature of 37°C and a hemoglobin concentration of 15 g/dL (150 g/L) in blood.
†Volume estimates are based on a total blood volume (TBV) of 5 L, arterial blood volume of 0.25 × TBV, and venous blood volume of 0.75 × TBV.
Abbreviations: Hb, hemoglobin = PO_2, partial pressure of O_2.

dissolved O_2 (in mL/dL) (at normal body temperature) is then described by Equation 2.2.

$$\text{Dissolved } O_2 = 0.003 \times PO_2 \tag{2.2}$$

This equation reveals the limited solubility of oxygen in plasma. For example, if the PO_2 is 100 mm Hg, one liter of blood will contain only 3 mL of dissolved O_2.

Arterial O_2 Content (CaO_2)

The concentration of O_2 in arterial blood (CaO_2) can be defined by combining Equations 2.1 and 2.2, by using the SO_2 and PO_2 of arterial blood (SaO_2 and PaO_2).

$$CaO_2 = (1.34 \times Hb \times SaO_2) + (0.003 \times PaO_2) \tag{2.3}$$

The normal concentrations of bound, dissolved, and total O_2 in arterial blood are shown in Table 2.2. There are approximately 200 mL oxygen in each liter of arterial blood, and only 1.5% (3 mL) is dissolved in the plasma. The oxygen consumption of an average-sized adult at rest is 250 mL/min, which means that if we were forced to rely solely on the dissolved O_2 in plasma, a cardiac output of 89 L/min would be necessary to sustain aerobic metabolism. This emphasizes the importance of hemoglobin in the transport of oxygen.

Venous O_2 Content (CvO_2)

The concentration of O_2 in venous blood (CvO_2) can be calculated in the same fashion as the CaO_2, using the O_2 saturation and PO_2 in venous blood (SvO_2 and PvO_2).

$$CvO_2 = (1.34 \times Hb \times SvO_2) + (0.003 \times PvO_2) \tag{2.4}$$

The SvO_2 and PvO_2 are best measured in a pooled or "mixed venous" blood sample taken from the pulmonary artery (using a pulmonary artery catheter, as described in Chapter 9). As shown in Table 2.2, the normal SvO_2 is 73% (0.73), the normal PvO_2 is 40 mm Hg, and the normal CvO_2 is approximately 15 mL/dL (150 mL/L).

Simplified O_2 Content Equation

The concentration of dissolved O_2 in plasma is so small that it is usually eliminated from the O_2 content equation. The O_2 content of blood is then considered equivalent to the Hb-bound O_2 fraction (see Equation 2.1).

$$O_2 \text{ Content} \approx 1.34 \times \text{Hb} \times SO_2 \qquad (2.5)$$

Anemia versus Hypoxemia

Clinicians often use the arterial PO_2 (PaO_2) as an indication of how much oxygen is in the blood. However, as indicated in Equation 2.5, the hemoglobin concentration is the principal determinant of the oxygen content of blood. The comparative influence of hemoglobin and PaO_2 on the oxygen level in blood is shown in Figure 2.1. The graph in this figure shows the effect of proportional changes in hemoglobin concentration and PaO_2 on the oxygen content of arterial blood. A 50% reduction in hemoglobin (from 15 to 7.5 g/dL) is accompanied by an equivalent 50% reduction in CaO_2 (from 200 to 101 mL/L), while a similar 50% reduction in the PaO_2 (from 90 to 45 mm Hg) results in only an 18% decrease in CaO_2 (from 200 to 163 mL/L). This graph shows that anemia has a much more profound effect on blood oxygenation than hypoxemia. It should also serve as a reminder to avoid using the PaO_2 to assess arterial oxygenation. The PaO_2 should be used to evaluate the efficiency of gas exchange in the lungs (see Chapter 19).

The Paucity of O_2 in Blood

The total volume of O_2 in circulating blood can be calculated as the product of the blood volume and the O_2 concentration in blood. An estimate of the volume of O_2 in arterial and venous blood is shown in Table 2.2. The combined volume of O_2 in arterial and venous blood is a meager 805 mL. To appreciate what a limited volume this represents, consider that the whole-body O_2 consumption of an average-sized adult at rest is about 250 mL/min. This means that **the total volume of O_2 in blood is enough to sustain aerobic metabolism for only 3 to 4 minutes**. Thus if a patient stops breathing, you have only a precious few minutes to begin assisted breathing maneuvers before the oxygen stores in the blood are completely exhausted.

The limited quantity of O_2 in blood can also be demonstrated by considering the oxidative metabolism of glucose, which is described by the formula: $C_6H_{12}O_6 + 6\ O_2 \rightarrow 6\ CO_2 + 6\ H_2O$. This formula indicates that complete oxidation of one mole of glucose utilizes 6 moles of oxygen. To determine if the O_2 in blood is enough to metabolize the glucose in blood, it is necessary to express the amount of glucose and oxygen in blood in

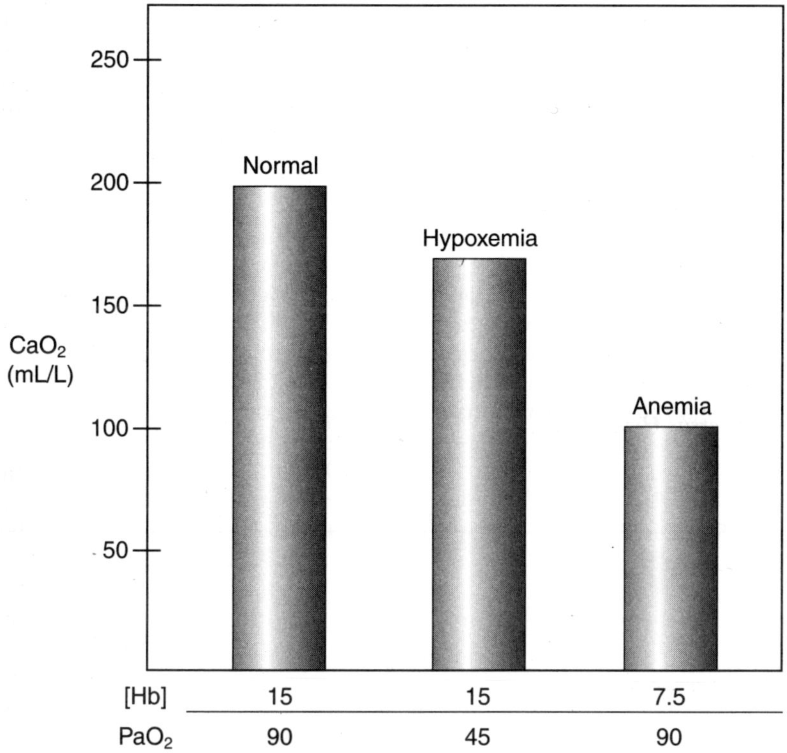

FIGURE 2.1 Graph showing the effects of equivalent (50%) reductions in hemoglobin concentration (Hb) and arterial PO_2 (PaO_2) on the oxygen concentration in arterial blood (CaO_2).

millimoles (mmol). (The values shown here are based on a blood glucose level of 90 mg/dL or 90/180 = 0.5 mmol/dL, a blood volume of 5 liters, and a total blood O_2 of 805 mL or 805/22.4 = 36.3 mmol):

Total glucose in blood	25 mmol
Total O_2 in blood	36.3 mmol
O_2 need of glucose metabolism	150 mmol

This shows that the O_2 in blood is only about 20% to 25% of the amount needed for the complete oxidative metabolism of the glucose in blood.

Why so Little O_2?

The obvious question is why an organism that requires oxygen for survival is designed to carry on metabolism in an oxygen-limited environment? The answer may be related to the toxic potential of oxygen. Oxygen is well known for its ability to produce lethal cell injury via the production of toxic metabolites (superoxide radical, hydrogen peroxide, and the hydroxyl radical), so **limiting the oxygen concentration in the vicinity of cells may be a mechanism for protecting cells from oxygen-induced cell injury.** The role of oxygen-induced injury (oxidant injury) in clinical disease is a very exciting and active area of study, and the bibliography at the end of this chapter includes a textbook (*Free Radicals in Biology and Medicine*) that is the best single source of information on this subject.

The Abundance of Hemoglobin

In contrast to the small volume of oxygen in blood, the total mass of circulating hemoglobin seems excessively large. If the normal serum Hb is 15 g/dL (150 g/L) and the normal blood volume is 5 liters (70 mL/kg), the total mass of circulating hemoglobin is 750 grams (0.75 kg) or 1.65 lbs. To demonstrate the enormous size of the blood hemoglobin pool, the illustration in Figure 2.2 compares the mass of hemoglobin to the normal

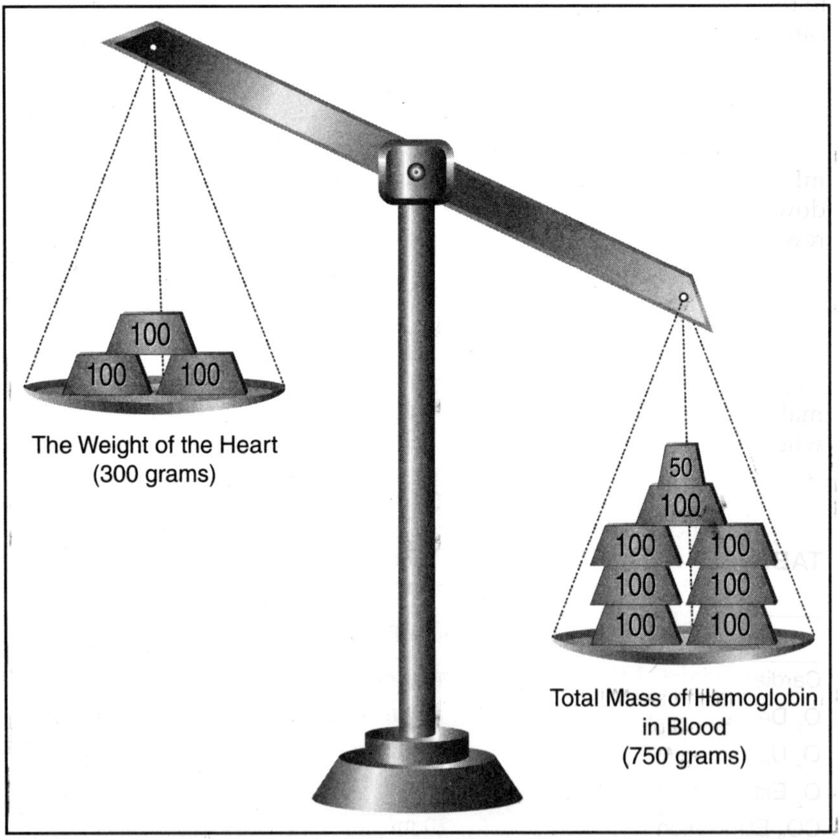

FIGURE 2.2 A balance scale demonstrating the excess weight of circulating hemoglobin when matched with the normal weight of the heart. The numbers on the small weights indicate the weight of each in grams.

weight of the heart. The heart weighs only 300 grams, so the pool of circulating hemoglobin is 2.5 times heavier than the heart! This means that every 60 seconds, the heart must move a mass that is more than twice its own weight through the circulatory system.

Is all this hemoglobin necessary? As shown later, when the extraction of oxygen from the systemic capillaries is maximal, 40% to 50% of the hemoglobin in venous blood remains fully saturated with oxygen. This means that **almost half of the circulating hemoglobin is not used to support aerobic metabolism**. What is the excess hemoglobin doing? Transporting carbon dioxide, as described later in the chapter.

Oxygen Delivery (DO_2)

The oxygen that enters the bloodstream in the lungs is carried to the vital organs by the cardiac output. The rate at which this occurs is called the *oxygen delivery* (DO_2). The DO_2 describes the volume of oxygen (in milliliters) that reaches the systemic capillaries each minute. It is equivalent to the product of the O_2 content in arterial blood (CaO_2) in mL/L and the cardiac output (Q) in L/min (2,5–7).

$$DO_2 = Q \times CaO_2 \times 10 \qquad (2.6)$$

(The multiplier of 10 is used to convert the CaO_2 from mL/dL to mL/L, so the DO_2 can be expressed in mL/min.) If the CaO_2 is broken down into its components ($1.34 \times Hb \times SaO_2$), Equation 2.6 can be rewritten as

$$DO_2 = Q \times 1.34 \times Hb \times SaO_2 \times 10 \qquad (2.7)$$

When a pulmonary artery catheter is used to measure cardiac output (see Chapter 9), the DO_2 can be calculated by using Equation 2.7. The normal DO_2 in adults at rest is 900–1,100 mL/min, or 500–600 mL/min/m^2 when adjusted for body size (see Table 2.3).

TABLE 2.3 Normal Ranges for Oxygen and Carbon Dioxide Transport Parameters

Parameter	Absolute Range	Size-Adjusted Range*
Cardiac output	5–6 L/min	2.4–4.0 L/min/m^2
O_2 Delivery	900–1,100 mL/min	520–600 mL/min/m^2
O_2 Uptake	200–270 mL/min	110–160 mL/min/m^2
O_2 Extraction ratio	0.20–0.30	
CO_2 Elimination	160–220 mL/min	90–130 mL/min/m^2
Respiratory quotient	0.75–0.85	

*Size-adjusted values are the absolute values divided by the patient's body surface area in square meters (m^2).

Oxygen Uptake (VO_2)

When blood reaches the systemic capillaries, oxygen dissociates from hemoglobin and moves into the tissues. The rate at which this occurs is called the *oxygen uptake* (VO_2). The VO_2 describes the volume of oxygen (in mL) that leaves the capillary blood and moves into the tissues each minute. Since oxygen is not stored in tissues, the VO_2 is also a measure of the *oxygen consumption* of the tissues. The VO_2 (in mL/min) can be calculated as the product of the cardiac output (Q) and the arteriovenous oxygen content difference ($CaO_2 - CvO_2$).

$$VO_2 = Q \times (CaO_2 - CvO_2) \times 10 \quad (2.8)$$

(The multiplier of 10 is included for the same reason as explained for the DO_2.) This method of deriving VO_2 is called the *reverse Fick method* because Equation 2.8 is a variation of the Fick equation (where cardiac output is the derived variable: $Q = VO_2/CaO_2 - CvO_2$) (8). Since the CaO_2 and CvO_2 share a common term ($1.34 \times Hb \times 10$), Equation 2.8 can be restated as

$$VO_2 = Q \times 13.4 \times Hb \times (SaO_2 - SvO_2) \quad (2.9)$$

This equation expresses VO_2 using variables that can be measured in clinical practice. The determinants of VO_2 in this equation are illustrated in Figure 2.3. The normal range for VO_2 in healthy adults at rest is 200–300 mL/min, or 110–160 mL/min/m^2 when adjusted for body size (see Table 2.3).

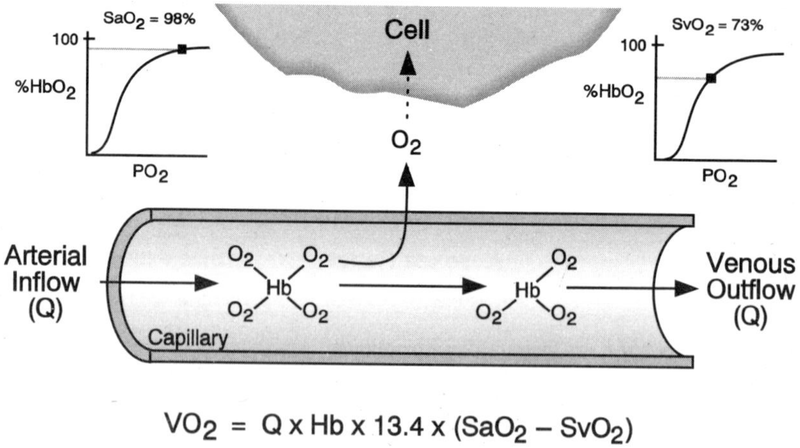

FIGURE 2.3 A schematic representation of the factors that determine the rate of oxygen uptake (VO_2) from the microcirculation. SaO_2 and SvO_2 = Oxygen saturation of hemoglobin in arterial and venous blood, respectively; PO_2 = partial pressure of oxygen; Hb = a hemoglobin molecule.

Fick vs Whole-Body VO_2

The VO_2 in the modified Fick equation is not equivalent to the whole-body VO_2 because it does not include the O_2 consumption of the lungs (8–10). Normally, the VO_2 of the lungs represents less than 5% of the whole-body VO_2 (9), but it can make up 20% of the whole-body VO_2 in patients with inflammatory conditions in the lungs (which are common in ICU patients) (10). This discrepancy can be important when VO_2 is used as an end-point of hemodynamic management (see Chapter 11) because an underestimate of whole-body VO_2 could lead to overaggressive management to augment the VO_2. Direct measurement of the VO_2 (described next) is a more accurate representation of the whole-body VO_2.

Direct Measurement of VO_2

The whole-body VO_2 can be measured directly by monitoring the rate of oxygen disappearance from the lungs. This can be accomplished with a specialized instrument equipped with an oxygen gas analyzer that is connected to the proximal airway (usually in intubated patients) to measure the O_2 concentration in inhaled and exhaled gas. The device records and displays the VO_2 as the product of minute ventilation (V_E) and the fractional concentration of oxygen in inhaled and exhaled gas (FIO_2 and FEO_2).

$$VO_2 = V_E \times (FIO_2 - FEO_2) \tag{2.10}$$

The direct measurement of VO_2 is more accurate than the calculated (Fick) VO_2 because it is a closer approximation to the whole-body VO_2. It has several other advantages over the Fick VO_2, and these are described in Chapter 11. The major shortcoming of the direct VO_2 measurement is the lack of availability of monitoring equipment in many ICUs, and the need for trained personnel to operate the equipment.

Oxygen-Extraction Ratio (O_2ER)

The fraction of the oxygen delivered to the capillaries that is taken up into the tissues is an index of the efficiency of oxygen transport. This is monitored with a parameter called the *oxygen extraction ratio* (O_2ER), which is the ratio of O_2 uptake to O_2 delivery.

$$O_2ER = VO_2/DO_2 \tag{2.11}$$

This ratio can be multiplied by 100 and expressed as a percentage. Since the VO_2 and DO_2 share common terms ($Q \times 1.34 \times Hb \times 10$), Equation 2.11 can be reduced to an equation with only two measured variables:

$$O_2ER = (SaO_2 - SvO_2)/SaO_2 \tag{2.12}$$

When the SaO_2 is close to 1.0 (which is usually the case), the O_2ER is roughly equivalent to the ($SaO_2 - SvO_2$) difference: $O_2ER \approx SaO_2 - SvO_2$.

The O_2ER is normally about 0.25 (range = 0.2–0.3), as shown in Table 2.3. This means that only 25% of the oxygen delivered to the systemic capillaries is taken up into the tissues. Although O_2 extraction is normally low, it is adjustable and can be increased when oxygen delivery is impaired. The adjustability of O_2 extraction is an important factor in the control of tissue oxygenation, as described next.

CONTROL OF OXYGEN UPTAKE

The oxygen transport system operates to maintain a constant flow of oxygen into the tissues (a constant VO_2) in the face of changes in oxygen supply (varying DO_2). This behavior is made possible by the ability of O_2 extraction to adjust to changes in O_2 delivery (11). The control system for VO_2 can be described by rearranging the O_2 extraction equation (Equation 2.11) to make VO_2 the dependent variable:

$$VO_2 = DO_2 \times O_2ER \qquad (2.13)$$

This equation shows that the VO_2 will remain constant if changes in O_2 delivery are accompanied by equivalent and reciprocal changes in O_2 extraction. However, if the O_2 extraction remains fixed, changes in DO_2 will be accompanied by equivalent changes in VO_2. The ability of O_2 extraction to adjust to changes in DO_2 therefore determines the ability to maintain a constant VO_2.

The DO_2–VO_2 Relationship

The normal relationship between O_2 delivery and O_2 uptake is shown in the graph in Figure 2.4 (11). As O_2 delivery (DO_2) begins to decrease below normal (as indicated by the arrowhead on the graph), the O_2 uptake (VO_2) initially remains constant, indicating that the O_2 extraction (O_2ER) is increasing as the DO_2 decreases. Further decreases in DO_2 eventually leads to a point where the VO_2 begins to decrease. The transition from a constant to a varying VO_2 occurs when the O_2 extraction increases to a maximum level of 50% to 60% (O_2ER = 0.5 to 0.6). Once the O_2ER is maximal, further decreases in DO_2 will result in equivalent decreases in VO_2 because the O_2ER is fixed and cannot increase further. When this occurs, the VO_2 is referred to as being *supply-dependent*, and the rate of aerobic metabolism is limited by the supply of oxygen. This condition is known as *dysoxia* (12). As aerobic metabolism (VO_2) begins to decrease, the oxidative production of high energy phosphates (ATP) begins to decline, resulting in impaired cell function and eventual cell death. The clinical expression of this process is *clinical shock* and progressive *multiorgan failure* (13).

The Critical DO_2

The DO_2 at which the VO_2 becomes supply-dependent is called the *critical oxygen delivery* (critical DO_2). It is the lowest DO_2 that is capable of

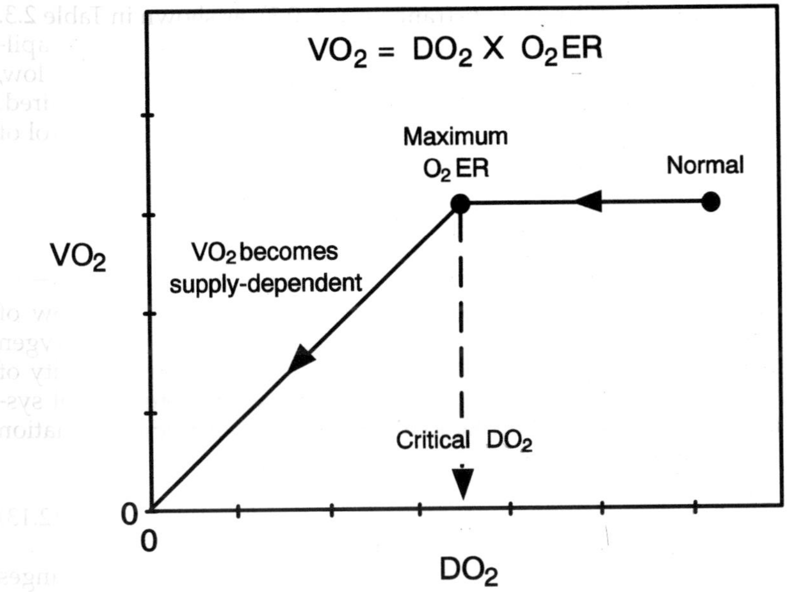

FIGURE 2.4 Graph showing the normal relationship between O_2 delivery (DO_2) and O_2 uptake (VO_2) when O_2 delivery is decreased progressively, as indicated by the *arrowheads*.

fully supporting aerobic metabolism and is identified by the bend in the DO_2–VO_2 curve (see Fig. 2.4). Despite the ability to identify the anaerobic threshold, the critical DO_2 has limited clinical value. First, the critical DO_2 has varied widely in studies of critically ill patients (11,13,14), and it is not possible to predict the critical DO_2 in any individual patient in the ICU. Second, the DO_2–VO_2 curve can be curvilinear (i.e., without a single transition point from constant to changing VO_2) (15), and in these cases, it is not possible to identify a critical DO_2.

The DO_2:VO_2 ratio may be a more useful parameter than the critical DO_2 for identifying (and avoiding) the anaerobic threshold. Maintaining a DO_2:VO_2 ratio of 4:1 or higher has been recommended as a management strategy to avoid the anaerobic threshold in critically ill patients (7).

CARBON DIOXIDE TRANSPORT

Carbon dioxide (CO_2) is the major end-product of oxidative metabolism, and because it readily hydrates to form carbonic acid, it can be a source of significant acidosis if allowed to accumulate. The importance of eliminating CO_2 from the body is apparent in the behavior of the ventilatory control system, which operates to maintain a constant PO_2 in arterial blood ($PaCO_2$). An increase in $PaCO_2$ of 5 mm Hg can result in a twofold increase in minute ventilation. To produce an equivalent increment in ventilation, the arterial PO_2 must drop to 55 mm Hg (16). The tendency for the ventilatory control system to pay attention to hypercapnia and ignore hypoxemia is intriguing because it suggests that the ventilatory system is more concerned with eliminating metabolic waste (CO_2) than promoting aerobic metabolism (by supplying oxygen).

The Hydration of CO_2

The total body CO_2 in adults is reported at 130 liters (17), which doesn't seem possible in light of the fact that the total body water of an adult averages only 40 to 45 liters. This dilemma can be explained by the tendency for CO_2 to enter into a chemical reaction with water and produce carbonic acid. The hydration of CO_2 and its transformation to carbonic acid is a continuous process, and this creates a perpetual gradient that drives CO_2 into solution. Since the CO_2 is continuously disappearing, the total volume of CO_2 in the solution could exceed the volume of the solution. If you have ever opened a bottle of warm champagne, you have witnessed how much CO_2 can be dissolved in a solution.

CO_2 Transport Scheme

The transport of CO_2 is a complex process that is shown in Figure 2.5. The centerpiece of CO_2 transport is the reaction of CO_2 with water. The first stage of this reaction involves the formation of carbonic acid. This is normally a slow reaction and takes about 40 seconds to complete (18). The reaction speeds up considerably in the presence of the enzyme carbonic anhydrase and takes less than 10 milliseconds (msec) to complete (18). Carbonic anhydrase is confined to the red cell and is not present in

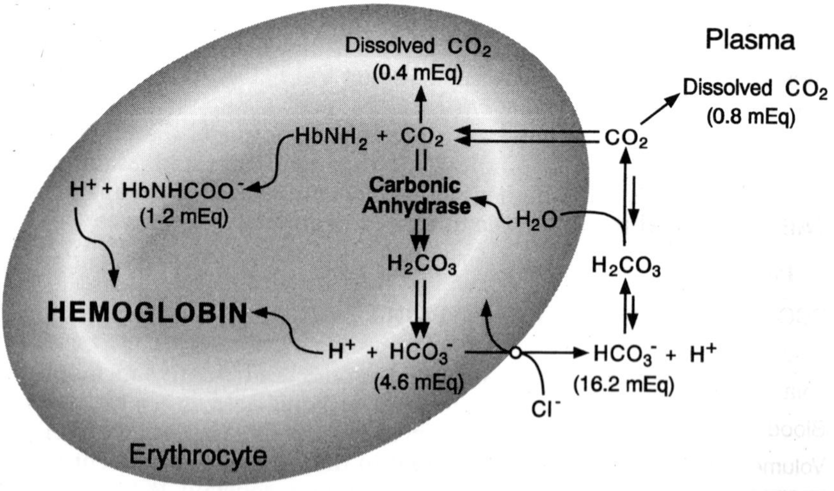

FIGURE 2.5 The chemical reactions involved in CO_2 transport. Values in parentheses indicate the amount of each component normally present in 1 L of venous blood. The *double arrows* indicate favored pathways.

plasma. Thus CO_2 is rapidly hydrated only in the red blood cell, and this creates a pressure gradient that drives CO_2 into the cell.

Carbonic acid dissociates instantaneously to produce hydrogen and bicarbonate ions. A large fraction of the bicarbonate generated in the red cell is pumped back into the plasma in exchange for chloride. The hydrogen ion generated in the red cell is buffered by the hemoglobin. In this way, the CO_2 that enters the red cell is dismantled and the parts stored (hemoglobin) or discarded (bicarbonate) to create room for more CO_2 to enter the red cell. These processes create a sink to accommodate large volumes of CO_2 in the red cell.

A small fraction of CO_2 in the red cell reacts with free amino groups on hemoglobin to produce carbamic acid, which dissociates to form carbamino residues (HbNHCOO) and hydrogen ions. This reaction provides another opportunity for hemoglobin to act as a buffer.

CO_2 Content of Blood

The different measures of CO_2 in blood are listed in Table 2.4. Like oxygen, CO_2 is present in a dissolved form, and the concentration of dissolved CO_2 is determined as the product of the PCO_2 and the solubility coefficient for CO_2 in water (i.e., 0.69 mL/L/mm Hg at 37°C) (19). The dissolved CO_2 content in arterial and venous blood is shown in Table 2.4 (20). Like oxygen, the dissolved CO_2 is only a small fraction of the total CO_2 content of blood.

The total content of CO_2 in blood is the summed contribution of several components, including the dissolved CO_2 and bicarbonate concentrations in plasma and erythrocytes, and the carbamino CO_2 content in erythrocytes. The normal values for each of these components in venous blood are shown in Figure 2.5. If these values are summed, the total CO_2 content is 23 mEq/L, with 17 mEq/L in plasma and 6 mEq/L in the red cell. The preponderance of CO_2 in plasma is deceiving because most of the plasma component is in the form of bicarbonate that has been expelled from the red blood cell.

TABLE 2.4 Normal Levels of CO_2 in Arterial and Venous Blood*

Parameter	Arterial Blood	Venous Blood
PCO_2	40 mm Hg	45 mm Hg
Dissolved CO_2	27 mL/L	29 mL/L
Total CO_2 content	490 mL/L	530 mL/L
Blood volume†	1.25 L	3.75 L
Volume of CO_2	613 mL	1,988 mL

*Values shown are for a body temperature of 37°C.
†Volume estimates are based on a total blood volume (TBV) of 5 L, arterial blood volume of 0.25 × TBV, and venous blood volume of 0.75 × TBV.
Abbreviations: PCO_2= partial pressure of CO_2.

TABLE 2.5 Buffering Capacity of Blood Proteins

	Hemoglobin	Plasma Proteins
Inherent buffer capacity	0.18 mEq H^+/g	0.11 mEq H^+/g
Concentration in blood	150 g/L	38.5 g/L
Total buffer capacity	27.5 mEq H^+/L	4.2 mEq H^+/L

Because CO_2 readily dissociates into ions (hydrogen and bicarbonate), the concentration of CO_2 is often expressed in ion equivalents (mEq/L), as in Figure 2.5. Conversion to units of volume (mL/L or mL/dL) is possible because one mole of CO_2 will occupy a volume of 22.3 liters. Therefore:

$$CO_2\ (mL/L) = CO_2\ (mEq/L \times 22.3)$$

Table 2.4 includes the CO_2 content of blood expressed in volume units (20). Note that the total volume of CO_2 in blood (about 2.6 liters) is more than 3 times the volume of O_2 in blood (805 mL).

Hemoglobin As a Buffer

Figure 2.5 shows that hemoglobin plays a central role in CO_2 transport by acting as a buffer for the hydrogen ions generated by the hydration of CO_2 in the red blood cell. The buffering capacity of hemoglobin is shown in Table 2.5 (21). Note that the total buffering capacity of hemoglobin is six times greater than the combined buffering capacity of all the plasma proteins.

The buffering actions of hemoglobin are attributed to imidazole groups that are found on the 38 histidine residues in the molecule. These imidazole groups have a dissociation constant with a pK of 7.0, so they will act as effective buffers in the pH range from 6 to 8 (buffers are effective within one pH unit on either side of the pK) (20). In contrast, the carbonic acid–bicarbonate buffer system has a pK of 6.1, so this buffer system will be effective in the pH range from 5.1 to 7.1. Comparing the buffer ranges of hemoglobin and bicarbonate shows that **hemoglobin is a more effective buffer than bicarbonate in the pH range encountered clinically** (pH 7 to 8)! This aspect of hemoglobin function deserves more attention.

Why the Excess Hemoglobin?

As described earlier, the mass of hemoglobin in blood is far greater than needed to transport oxygen, and considering the role played by hemoglobin in CO_2 transport, it is likely that the excess hemoglobin is needed for CO_2 transport. Considering the large volume of CO_2 in blood (see Table 2.4), it is easier to understand why there is so much hemoglobin in blood.

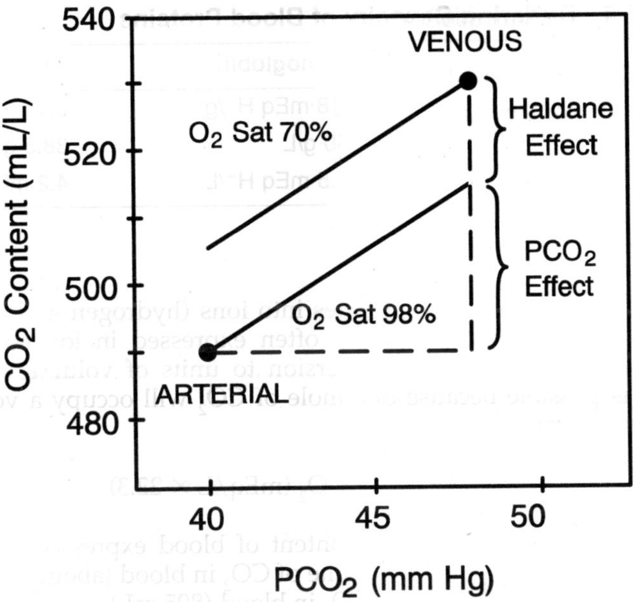

FIGURE 2.6 Carbon dioxide dissociation curves for arterial blood (O_2 Sat = 98%) and venous blood (O_2 Sat = 70%). The two points indicate the CO_2 content of arterial and venous blood. The brackets show the relative contributions of hemoglobin desaturation (Haldane effect) and metabolic CO_2 production (PCO_2 effect) to the increase in CO_2 content that occurs from arterial to venous blood. (From Forster RE II, DuBois A, Briscoe WA, et al. The lung, 3rd ed. Chicago: Yearbook Medical Publishers, 1986:238.)

The Haldane Effect

Hemoglobin has a greater buffer capacity when it is in the desaturated form, and blood that is fully desaturated can bind an additional 60 mL/L of carbon dioxide. The increase in CO_2 content that results from oxyhemoglobin desaturation is known as the *Haldane effect*. The CO_2 dissociation curves in Figure 2.6 show that the Haldane effect plays an important role in the uptake of CO_2 by venous blood. The two points on the graph show that the CO_2 content in venous blood is 40 mL/L higher than in arterial blood. The brackets indicate that about 60% of the increased CO_2 content in venous blood is due to an increase in PCO_2, while 40% is due to oxyhemoglobin desaturation. Thus, the Haldane effect is responsible for almost half of the rise in CO_2 content in venous blood. This is another example of the important role played by hemoglobin in CO_2 transport.

CO_2 Elimination (VCO_2)

The dissociation of CO_2 that occurs during transport in venous blood is reversed when the blood reaches the lungs. The reconstituted CO_2 is then eliminated through the lungs. The elimination of CO_2 (VCO_2) can

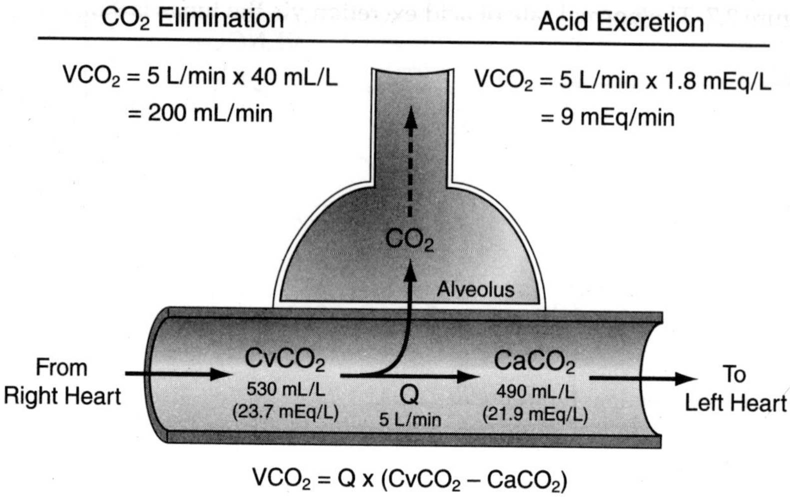

FIGURE 2.7 A schematic representation of the factors that contribute to CO_2 elimination through the lungs (VCO_2). The VCO_2 is expressed as gas flow (mL/min) and as acid excretion (mEq/min). Q = cardiac output; $CaCO_2$ = arterial CO_2 content; $CvCO_2$ = venous CO_2 content.

be described by using an equation that is similar in form to the VO_2 equation (Equation 2.8).

$$VCO_2 = Q \times (CvCO_2 - CaCO_2) \tag{2.14}$$

$CvCO_2$ and $CaCO_2$ represent the CO_2 content in venous and arterial blood, respectively (note that the arterial and venous components are reversed when compared with the VO_2 equation). The determination of VCO_2 by using the variables in Equation 2.14 is shown in Figure 2.7.

Unfortunately, there are no simple derivative equations for CO_2 content in blood, so the VCO_2 is usually measured directly. As shown in Table 2.3, the normal VCO_2 in adults is 160–220 mL/min, or 90–130 mL/ min/m^2 when adjusted for body size. The VCO_2 is normally about 80% of the VO_2, so the VCO_2/VO_2 ratio is normally 0.8. The VCO_2/VO_2 ratio, which is called the *respiratory quotient* (RQ), is used to identify the predominant type of nutrient substrate (i.e., protein, fat, or carbohydrate) being metabolized. Chapter 45 contains more information on the RQ.

VCO_2 as Acid Excretion

Carbon dioxide is essentially an acid because of its tendency to dissociate and form carbonic acid. Thus when the CO_2 content is expressed in ion equivalents (mEq/L), the VCO_2 (mEq/min) can be used to describe the rate of volatile acid excretion through the lungs. This is shown in

Figure 2.7. The normal rate of acid excretion via the lungs is 9 mEq/min, or 12,960 mEq in 24 hours. Since the kidneys excrete only 40 to 80 mEq of acid every 24 hours (20), the principal organ of acid excretion in the body is the lungs, not the kidneys.

REFERENCES

General Works

Halliwell B, Gutteridge JMC. Free radicals in biology and medicine, 3rd ed. New York: Oxford University Press, 1999.

Edwards JD, Shoemaker WC, Vincent J-L, eds. Oxygen transport: principles and practice. London: WB Saunders, 1993.

Zander R, Mertzlufft F, eds. The oxygen status of arterial blood. Basel: Karger, 1991.

Oxygen Content in Blood

1. Pauling L. General chemistry, 3rd ed. Mineola, NY: Dover Publications, 1988:215.
2. Little RA, Edwards JD. Applied physiology. In: Edwards JD, Shoemaker WC, Vincent JL, eds. Oxygen transport: principles and practice. London: WB Saunders, 1993:21–40.
3. Zander R. Calculation of oxygen concentration. In: Zander R, Mertzlufft F, eds. The oxygen status of arterial blood. Basel: Karger, 1991:203–209.
4. Christoforides C, Laasberg L, Hedley-Whyte J. Effect of temperature on solubility of O_2 in plasma. J Appl Physiol 1969;26:56–60.

Oxygen Delivery and Oxygen Uptake

5. Hameed SM, Aird WC, Cohn SM. Oxygen delivery. Crit Care Med 2003; 31(suppl):S658–S667.
6. Little RA, Edwards JD. Applied physiology. In: Edwards JD, Shoemaker WC, Vincent J-L, eds. Oxygen transport: principles and practice. London, WB Saunders, 1993:21–40.
7. Bartlett RH. Oxygen kinetics: integrating hemodynamic, respiratory, and metabolic physiology. In: Critical care physiology. Boston: Little, Brown, 1996:1–23.
8. Ledingham IM, Naguib M. Overview: evolution of the concept from Fick to the present day. In: Edwards JD, Shoemaker WC, Vincent J-L, eds. Oxygen transport: principles and practice. London: WB Saunders, 1993:3–20.
9. Nunn JF. Nonrespiratory functions of the lung. In: Nunn JF, ed. Applied respiratory physiology. London: Butterworths 1993:306–317.
10. Jolliet P, Thorens JB, Nicod L, et al. Relationship between pulmonary oxygen consumption, lung inflammation, and calculated venous admixture in patients with acute lung injury. Intens Care Med 1996;22:277–285.
11. Leach RM, Treacher DF. The relationship between oxygen delivery and consumption. Dis Mon 1994;30:301–368.

12. Connett RJ, Honig CR, Gayeski TEJ, et al. Defining hypoxia: a systems view of VO_2, glycolysis, energetics, and intracellular PO_2. J Appl Physiol 1990;68: 833–842.
13. Shoemaker WC. Oxygen transport and oxygen metabolism in shock and critical illness. Crit Care Clin 1996;12:939–969.
14. Ronco J, Fenwick J, Tweedale M, et al. Identification of the critical oxygen delivery for anaerobic metabolism in critically ill septic and nonseptic humans. JAMA 1993;270:1724–1730.
15. Lebarsky DA, Smith LR, Sladen RN, et al. Defining the relationship of oxygen delivery and consumption: use of biological system models. J Surg Res 1995;58:503–508.

Carbon Dioxide Transport

16. Lambertson CJ. Carbon dioxide and respiration in acid-base homeostasis. Anesthesiology 1960;21:642–651.
17. Henneberg S, Soderberg D, Groth T, et al. Carbon dioxide production during mechanical ventilation. Crit Care Med 1987;15:8–13.
18. Brahm J. The red cell anion-transport system: kinetics and physiologic implications. In: Gunn R, Parker C, eds. Cell physiology of blood. New York: Rockefeller Press, 1988:142–150.
19. Nunn RF. Nunn's applied respiratory physiology, 4th ed. Oxford: Butterworth-Heinemann, 1993:220.
20. Forster RE II, DuBois A, Briscoe WA, et al. The lung, 3rd ed. Chicago: Yearbook Medical Publishers, 1986:223–247.
21. Comroe JH Jr. Physiology of respiration, 2nd ed. Chicago: Year Book, 1974: 201–210.

Section II

PREVENTIVE PRACTICES IN THE CRITICALLY ILL

We . . . repeatedly enlarge our instrumentalities without improving our purpose.

WILL DURANT

Chapter 3

INFECTION CONTROL IN THE ICU

Laymen always associate bacteria, microbes, and germs with disease.

John Postgate, Microbes and Man

Microbial organisms (microbes) make up about 90% of the living matter on this planet. They're all around us: in the air we breathe, the food we eat, and the water we drink. They're on our skin, under our fingernails, in our nose and mouth, and armies of them congregate in our intestinal tract. Are these organisms the nasty little "germs" that are eager to invade the human body to conquer and destroy, as they are so often portrayed, or are they peace-loving creatures that mean us no harm? More the latter, it seems. Most microbes have nothing to gain by invading the human body (I'll exclude viruses here), but they have much to lose because they can be killed by the inflammatory response. It seems then that survival would dictate that microorganisms avoid the interior of the human body, not invade it.

For more than a century, medicine has viewed the microbial world as an enemy that should be destroyed, and the practices described in this chapter are an expression of that belief. These practices are collectively known as "infection control," and they are designed to prevent the spread of microorganisms from one person to another, or from one site to another on the same person. Most of the information in this chapter is taken from clinical practice guidelines published by the Centers for Disease Control and Prevention (CDC) and other expert agencies, and these are listed in the bibliography at the end of the chapter (1–7). As you will see, some infection control practices are rational, and some are ritual, but all are an essential part of daily life in the ICU.

SKIN HYGIENE

The surface of the skin is home to several species of bacteria and fungi, some of them attached to the underlying squamous cells of the skin (resident flora), and some of them are unattached and easily removed (transient flora) (3,4,8). Because most microbes are aquatic in nature and thrive in a moist environment, the microflora on the skin tend to congregate in moist regions like the groin and axilla. Contact surfaces like the skin on the hands can also be densely populated with microorganisms, and this microflora is a principal concern in infection control because it can be transmitted to others. An example of the organisms that populate the hands of ICU personnel is shown in Table 3.1. The most frequent isolate is *Staphylococcus epidermidis* (a coagulase-negative staphylococcus), followed by gram-negative enteric organisms and *Candida* species (3,4,8,9). Eradicating microbes on the hands of hospital personnel is one of the holy crusades of infection control.

Cleaning vs Decontamination

Plain soaps are detergents that can disperse particulate and organic matter, but they lack antimicrobial activity. Cleaning the skin with plain soap and water will remove dirt, soil, and organic matter from the skin, but will not eradicate the microbes on the skin. Scrubbing the skin with soap and water can remove transient (unattached) organisms, but the attached (resident) microorganisms are left in place. The removal of microbes from the skin, known as decontamination, requires the application of agents that have antimicrobial activity. Antimicrobial agents that are used to decontaminate the skin are called *antiseptics*, while those used to decontaminate inanimate objects are called *disinfectants*.

TABLE 3.1 Organisms Isolated from the Hands of ICU Personnel

Organism	% Total Cultures
Gram-positive cocci	
Staph. epidermidis	100%
Staph. aureus (MSSA)	7%
Gram-negative Bacilli	21%
Acinetobacter spp.	
Klebsiella spp.	
Enterobacter spp.	
Pseudomonas spp.	
Serratia spp.	
Yeasts and fungi	16%
Candida spp.	

MSSA, methicillin-sensitive *Staph. aureus.*
From Larson EL, Rackoff WR, Weiman M, et al. Assessment of two hand-hygiene regimens for intensive care unit personnel. Crit Care Med, 2001;29:944.

TABLE 3.2 Commonly Used Antiseptic Agents

Antiseptic Agent	Advantages	Disadvantages
Alcohols	Rapid onset of action	Little residual activity
	Broad spectrum of activity	Aqueous solutions can cause skin dryness.
Iodophors	Broad spectrum of activity	Slow onset of action
		Prolonged contact can irritate the skin
Chlorhexidine	Good residual activity	Relatively narrow spectrum of activity
		An ocular irritant

From References 3, 4, and 8.

Antiseptic Agents

The popular antiseptic agents in the United States are the alcohols (ethanol, propanol, and isopropyl alcohol), iodophors (slow-release iodine preparations), and chlorhexidine. (Hexachlorophene, once the most popular antiseptic agent in the U.S., is no longer recommended because of its limited spectrum of activity.) The relative advantages and disadvantages of each antiseptic agent are summarized in Table 3.2.

Alcohols

The alcohols have excellent germicidal activity against gram-positive and gram-negative bacteria (including multidrug-resistant bacteria), various fungi (including *Candida* spp.), and viruses such as human immunodeficiency virus (HIV), hepatitis B virus (HBV), and hepatitis C virus (HCV) (3,4,8). Alcohol solutions containing 60% to 95% alcohol are most effective. Alcohols have a rapid onset of action but little persistent (residual) activity. They are less effective in the presence of dirt and organic matter, and are not recommended for use when the skin is visibly dirty or soiled with body fluids (e.g., blood) (4). Repeated use of aqueous (water-based) alcohol solutions can lead to drying and irritation of the skin, but these adverse effects are virtually eliminated when a waterless alcohol gel is used (4,8,9). Alcohol-impregnated towelettes are available but have limited amounts of alcohol and are no more effective in removing skin microbes than plain soap and water (4).

Iodophors

Iodine is germicidal and has a broad spectrum of activity similar to the alcohols, but it is irritating to the skin and soft tissues. Skin irritation is reduced when a carrier molecule is used to release iodine slowly. Preparations that contain iodine and a carrier molecule are called iodophors, and the most popular iodophor in the United States is povidone-iodine (Betadine). Since the active ingredient in iodophors (iodine) is released slowly, *iodophors must be left in contact with the skin for a few minutes to achieve maximal efficacy*. However, prolonged contact with iodine can be irritating, so iodophors should be wiped from the skin after drying (3). Persistent (residual) activity is inconsistent after iodophors are wiped from the skin. Iodophors are neutralized by organic matter (3,4,9), so skin that is soiled with blood and body fluids should be cleaned before applying an iodophor. Povidone-iodine is usually provided as an aqueous solution, but alcohol-based solutions of povidone-iodine are available and may be more effective (10).

Chlorhexidine

Chlorhexidine gluconate is a germicidal agent that is equally effective against gram-positive bacteria as the alcohols and iodophors, but is less effective against gram-negative bacilli and fungi. Its onset of action is slower than the alcohols but faster than the iodophors. The major advantage of chlorhexidine over the other antiseptic agents is its prolonged activity, which can last for six hours or longer (4). This is demonstrated in Figure 3.1. The residual activity is reduced by soaps and hand creams (4). Chlorhexidine is available in aqueous solutions ranging in strength from 0.5% to 4.0%. The 4% solution is most effective, but repeated use can

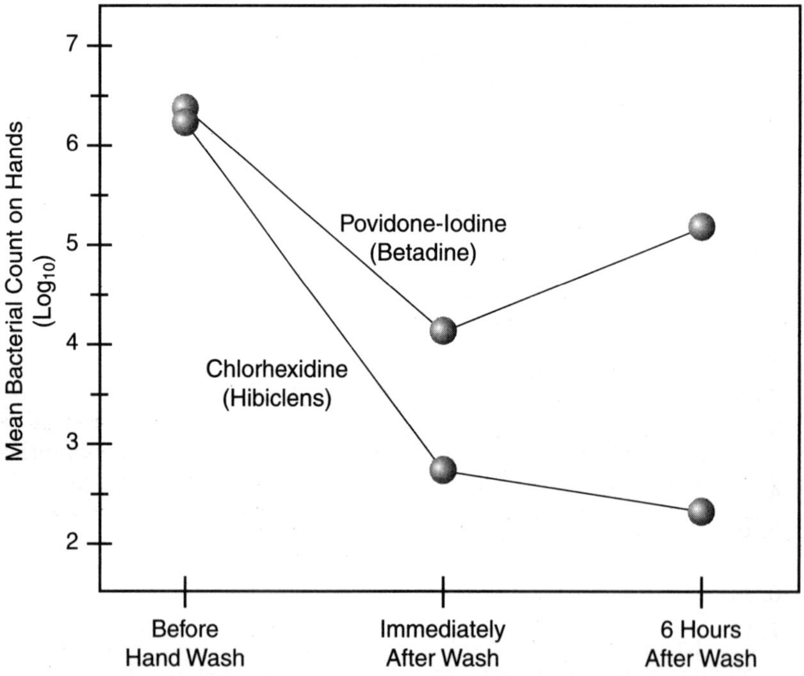

FIGURE 3.1 Comparative effects of a 6-minute hand scrub with 0.75% povidone-iodine (Betadine) and 4% chlorhexidine gluconate (Hibiclens) on microbial growth on the hands. Bacterial counts are expressed as log base 10 values. (From Peterson AF, Rosenberg A, Alatary SD, et al. Comparative evaluation of surgical scrub preparations. Surg Gynecol Obstet 1978;146:63*.)

cause skin irritation and dermatitis (4). Chlorhexidine is also an ocular irritant (4), and care should be taken to avoid contact with the eyes.

Spore-Forming Organisms

None of the antiseptic agents described here is an effective sporicidal agent that can prevent the spread of spore-forming bacteria like *Clostridium difficile* and *Bacillus anthracis* (4). Gloves are needed whenever contact with these organisms is possible.

Handwashing

Handwashing (a nebulous term that can include cleaning, antisepsis, or both) has been described as " . . .the single most important measure to reduce the risks of transmitting organisms from one person to another or from one site to another on the same patient" (ref. 2, updated guidelines). The recommendations for handwashing issued by the Centers for Disease Control are shown in Table 3.3. Note that an antiseptic solution rather than plain soap and water is recommended for most instances of handwashing, and that a waterless alcohol gel is recommended if the hands are not visibly soiled (remember that alcohol is much less effective in the presence of organic matter). The preference for alcohol gel is based

TABLE 3.3 Recommendations for Hand Hygiene

I. Handwashing with soap (plain or antiseptic) and water is recommended:
   1. When hands are visibly dirty or contaminated with proteinaceous material or are visibly soiled with blood or other body fluids
   2. Before eating
   3. After leaving a restroom

II. Handwashing with an antiseptic preparation[a] is recommended:
   1. Before direct contact with patients
   2. After contact with a patient's skin (intact or nonintact)
   3. After contact with body fluids, secretions, excretions, mucous membranes, wound dressings, and contaminated items
   4. Before donning sterile gloves to insert central intravascular catheters
   5. Before inserting urinary catheters, peripheral venous catheters, or other invasive devices that do not require a surgical procedure
   6. After removing gloves
   7. When moving from a contaminated body site to a clean body site during patient care
   8. After contact with inanimate objects in the immediate vicinity of the patient

From References 2, 4, and 8.

[a]A waterless alcohol gel is recommended if the hands are not visibly soiled. Otherwise, an antiseptic soap-and-water wash is recommended.

on evidence that alcohol-containing products are superior to povidone-iodine or chlorhexidine solutions for reducing bacterial counts on the hands (4) and evidence that alcohol gels cause less skin irritation than antimicrobial soaps or aqueous antiseptic solutions (4,9).

Compliance

Despite the accolades showered on the practice of handwashing, surveys of ICU personnel reveal a consistent pattern of poor compliance with published guidelines for handwashing. Compliance rates are well below 50% in most surveys, and physicians are consistently the worst offenders (3,4,8,9). There are several reasons for this observation, and one of them is evident in Table 3.3: i.e., there are simply too many indications for handwashing. Anyone who has taken care of patients in an ICU will realize that full compliance with the recommendations in Table 3.3, particularly the recommendation that handwashing be performed before and after every patient contact, is neither practical, affordable, nor achievable on a consistent basis.

Technique

Handwashing can be performed with plain soap or a variety of antiseptic preparations (soaps, aqueous solutions, or waterless gels). In general, alcohol-based products are more effective in reducing bacterial counts on the hands than are antiseptic soaps containing povidone-iodine or chlorhexidine (4). Whenever a soap (plain or antiseptic) is used, the wash should begin by wetting the hands with tap water. The soap should be applied to the palms of the hands and then rubbed over the entire surface of the hands for at least 30 seconds (4,8). Special attention should be given to the subungual areas under the fingernails, where microbes are usually most concentrated (3,4). The soap is then removed by rinsing with water, and the hands dried with a disposable towel. Hot water is not recommended for handwashing (4) because it is not more effective in removing organisms from the skin than warm or cold water (11) and can be irritating to the skin. Using a disposable towel to dry the hands is equivalent to forced air drying (12) but is favored because it is quicker and more convenient.

When a waterless alcohol gel is used, the hands should be cleaned first if necessary (remember that alcohol does not work well in the presence of organic matter), and the gel should be rubbed into the hands until they are dry. Repeated application of gels can leave the hands with a greasy feeling, and a periodic soap and water wash is sometimes preferred to remove any residual gel from the hands.

PROTECTIVE BARRIERS

Protective barriers like gloves, gowns, masks, and eye shields provide a physical impediment to the transmission of infectious agents. The principal role of these barriers is to protect hospital staff from infectious agents

TABLE 3.4 Recommendations for Glove Use in the ICU

I. Sterile gloves
1. Recommended for the following procedures
   A. Central venous catheterization
   B. Peripherally inserted central catheters (PICC)
   C. Artherial catheterization
   D. Placement of drainage catheters in a closed space (pleural, pericardial, or peritoneal cavities)
   E. Insertion of epidural catheters (for analgesia) or intraventricular catheters (for intracranial pressure monitoring

II. Nonsterile gloves
1. Should be used for contact with any moist body substance—blood, body fluids, secretions, excretions, nonintact skin, and mucous membranes. Clean (unsoiled) gloves should be used for contact with nonintact skin and mucous membranes
2. Can be used for insertion of peripheral venous catheters as long as the gloved hands do not touch the catheter

III. General recommendations
1. Gloves should be changed between tasks and procedures on the same patient if there has been contact with material that may be infectious
2. Gloves should be removed immediately after use, before contact with noncontaminated objects in the environment, and before going to another patient

From References 2, 6, and 13.

that can be transmitted by blood and body fluids, such as the human immunodeficiency virus (HIV) and hepatitis B and C viruses.

Gloves

Rubber gloves were popularized in this country in the late nineteenth century by William Halstead, the first (and enigmatic) Chief of the Surgery at Johns Hopkins Hospital, who covered only his palms and three fingers with the gloves because they were heavy and impaired the sense of touch. Today, sterile rubber gloves are the second skin of the operating surgeon. In the ICU, sterile gloves are used primarily for placing catheters in the bloodstream (see Table 3.4).

In the 1980s (a century after the introduction of surgical gloves), the use of nonsterile gloves was popularized by the discovery that HIV is transmitted in blood and body fluids. This discovery prompted a policy known as Universal Precautions (1), which considered all patients as possible sources of HIV. An updated policy known as Standard Precautions (2,13) contains the current recommendations for nonsterile gloves, and these are shown in Table 3.4. Nonsterile gloves should be used for any contact with a moist body substance, which includes blood, body fluids, secretions, excretions, nonintact skin, and mucous membranes. Note also in Table 3.4 that nonsterile gloves are considered safe for insertion of peripheral venous catheters as long as a "no touch" technique is used (i.e., as long as the gloved hands are not permitted to touch the catheter) (6).

Handwashing and Gloves

As indicated in Table 3.3, handwashing is recommended before donning gloves and again after they are removed. This recommendation is based on two concerns. The first is the fear that gloves can leak or tear and thereby allow microbial transmission between the hands of the healthcare worker and the patient. The second concern is the potential for moisture buildup on the hands during prolonged glove use, which would favor microbial growth on the hands while the gloves are on. Both of these are valid concerns for invasive surgical procedures, where glove use is prolonged and soiling of gloves is prominent. However, the significance of these concerns in a nonsurgical setting like the ICU (where glove use is not prolonged and soiling of gloves is usually not prominent) is less certain.

The graph in Figure 3.2 provides some interesting observations about the need for antiseptic handwashing when gloves are used. The data in this graph is from a study involving two groups of ICU nurses: one group performed an antiseptic hand wash with 4% chlorhexidine before donning sterile gloves, while the other group did not wash their hands before donning gloves (14). Hand cultures were then obtained before, during, and after short-term glove use. The two graphs in Figure 3.2 show that microbial growth on the gloved hands was minimal in both groups, indicating that the pre-glove antiseptic handwash did not influence the infectious risk to patients from the gloved hands. The graphs also show that microbial activity on the hands was reduced in both groups after the gloves were removed. Thus, microbial proliferation on the hands is not a concern during short-term glove use. These results suggest that handwashing before and after short-term glove use in a nonsurgical setting like the ICU may be unnecessary.

Latex Allergy

The dramatic increase in the use of rubber gloves over the last two decades has created a problem with latex hypersensitivity in hospital workers. Latex is a natural rubber product that is used in over 40,000 household and medical products, including gloves, face masks, blood pressure cuffs, and catheters (15). Repeated exposure to latex can promote hypersensitivity reactions that can be evident clinically as either contact dermatitis (urticaria or eczema), anaphylaxis, rhinoconjunctivitis, or asthma (16,17). Latex hypersensitivity is reported in 10% to 20% of hospital workers, compared to 1% of the general population (16). For unclear reasons, patients with spina bifida have the highest risk of latex allergy, with as many as 40% of the population having this condition (18).

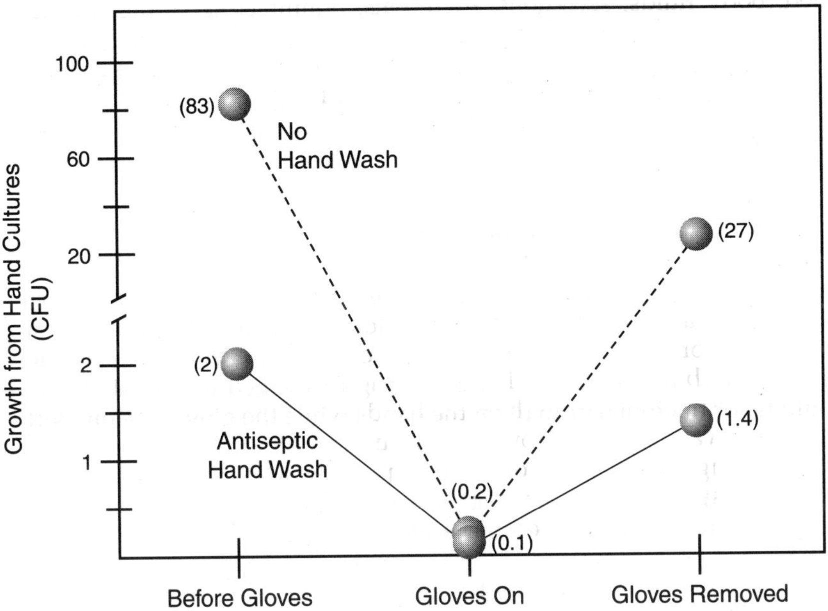

FIGURE 3.2 Influence of pre-glove handwashing with an antiseptic agent (4% chlorhexidine) on hand cultures obtained during and after the use of sterile gloves. CFU = Colony-forming units 48 hours after the fingers of both hands were pressed directly on culture plates. The numbers in parentheses correspond to the values on the vertical axis of the graph. Note the break in the vertical axis and the different scales above and below the break. (From Rossoff LJ, Borenstein M, Isenberg HD. Is hand washing really needed in an intensive care unit? Crit Care Med 1995;23:1211, with permission.)

DIAGNOSIS. The diagnosis of latex allergy can be elusive. One problem is the nonspecific manifestations of disease. Another problem is the fact that *symptoms of latex allergy can appear without direct physical contact with latex*. This is often the case with the rhinoconjunctivitis and asthma, which are triggered by airborne latex particles. A history of symptoms confined to the workplace should create suspicion for latex allergy. The clinical manifestations of latex allergy often coincide with exposure to latex, so hospital workers with symptomatic latex allergy often display these symptoms while in the hospital and are symptom-free at home.

There are two tests for latex hypersensitivity (19). One is a skin test, and the other is an assay for latex-specific immunoglobulin E levels in the bloodstream. Both have shortcomings. There is no standardized extract for the skin test (allergists have to make their own extract by pulverizing latex gloves!), so results are operator-dependent. The assay for latex-specific IgE in blood is currently the favored test, but the sensitivity can be low (19). If confronted with a case of possible latex allergy, you should contact the clinical laboratory in your hospital and ask about the availability and reliability of these tests in your region.

TREATMENT. The treatment of latex allergy is symptom-driven and nonspecific. Removing latex from the patient's immediate environment is the best strategy, but this may not be possible because latex is ubiquitous in the hospital environment (it is even found on tongue depressors!). The hospital should provide substitutes for latex products (e.g., vinyl gloves) when necessary.

Masks and Other Barriers

As was the case with nonsterile gloves, the use of other barriers like masks, eye shields, face shields, and gowns increased markedly after the discovery that HIV is transmitted in blood and body fluids. These barriers are currently recommended for all procedures or patient care activities that are likely to generate splashes of blood, body fluids, secretions, or excretions (2,14). Nonsterile gowns are adequate, and gowns coated with a plastic covering are the least impervious to blood and body fluids (20). Soiled gowns and other barriers should be removed and discarded as soon as possible, and before going to another patient (14).

Types of Masks

There are two types of face masks: surgical masks and respirators. Surgical masks were introduced to prevent contamination of the operative field during surgical procedures. In the past 2 decades, they have been adopted as a means of protecting healthcare workers from inhalation of airborne infectious agents. There is no evidence that surgical masks are effective in preventing infection (23), yet they continue to be used without question.

Respirators are devices that protect the wearer from inhaling a dangerous substance (23). The different types of respirators include particulate respirators (block particulate matter), gas mask respirators (filter or clean chemical gases in the air), and the Self-Contained Breathing Apparatus (equipped with its own air tank), which is used by firefighters. Particulate respirators are used to block inhalation of airborne pathogens, particularly the tubercle bacillus that causes pulmonary tuberculosis. The respirator currently recommended for this purpose is called an N95 respirator (22,23). The "N" indicates that the mask will block non–oil-based or aqueous aerosols (the type that transmits the tubercle bacillus), and the "95" indicates the mask will block 95% of the intended particles (a requirement for a respirator mask to be judged effective) (23).

Types of Airborne Illness

Infectious organisms that are capable of airborne transmission are divided into two categories: those greater than 5 microns ($>5\mu$) in diameter, and those that are 5 microns or less ($\leq 5\mu$) in diameter. The organisms and airborne illnesses in each category are shown in Figure 3.3 (2). In each of these illnesses, airborne infectious particles are produced by coughing or sneezing (one cough or sneeze can produce 3,000 airborne

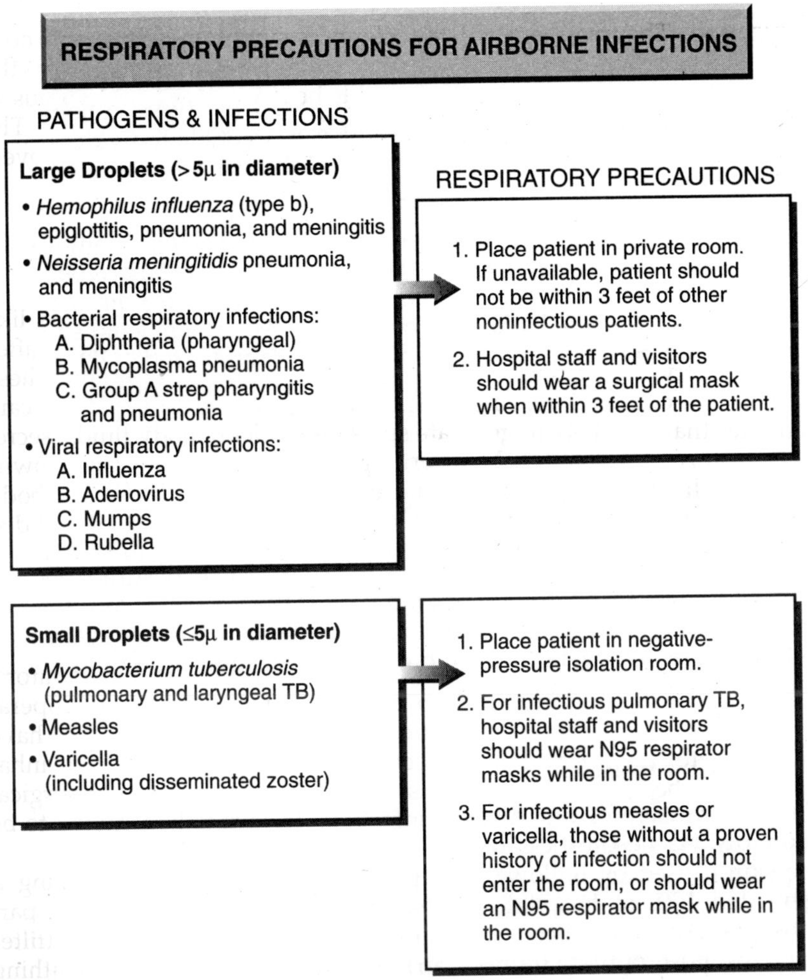

FIGURE 3.3 Infection control precautions for diseases that can spread via the airborne route. (From Reference 2.)

particles) or procedures such as airways suctioning and bronchoscopy. The airborne particles can be inhaled or can impact on nonintact skin, or on the mucosa in the nose or mouth.

Infectious particles >5μ in diameter usually travel no farther than 3 feet through the air, and to block transmission of these particles, a surgical mask is recommended (despite lack of proven efficacy!) when hospital staff or visitors are within 3 feet of the patient (2,21). The smaller (≤5μ in diameter) infectious particles can travel long distances in the air, and to prevent transmission of these particles, patients should be isolated in private rooms that are maintained at a negative pressure relative to the surrounding areas. For patients with infectious tuberculosis (pulmonary or laryngeal), all hospital staff and visitors should wear an N95 respirator mask while in the room (2,22). For patients in the infectious stages of rubeola (measles) and varicella (chickenpox or herpes zoster), individuals with no prior history of these infections who are also pregnant, immunocompromised, or otherwise debilitated by disease should not be allowed in the patient's room. For other susceptible individuals who must enter the room (i.e., hospital workers), an N95 respirator mask should be worn at all times while in the room.

ATYPICAL PULMONARY TB. It is important to distinguish infections caused by *Mycobacterium tuberculosis* from those caused by atypical mycobacteria (e.g., *Mycobacterium avium* complex) when determining the need for respiratory protection. Unlike the behavior of *M. z*, there is no evidence for person-to-person transmission of atypical mycobacteria (22), so special respiratory precautions (isolation and masks) are not required for patients with atypical pulmonary tuberculosis (2).

BLOOD-BORNE PATHOGENS

The greatest infectious risk you face in the ICU is exposure to blood-borne pathogens like HIV, hepatitis B virus (HBV), and hepatitis C virus (HCV). This section will describe the occupational risks associated with each of these pathogens and the preventive measures used to minimize these risks.

Needlestick Injuries

The transmission of blood-borne infections to hospital workers occurs primarily via needlestick injuries (i.e., accidental puncture wounds of the skin caused by hollow needles and suture needles). Each year, an estimated 10% of hospital workers sustain a needlestick injury (24). Most of these injuries occur in nurses, but the risk is also high in medical students, postgraduate trainees, and staff surgeons. As many as 70% of residents and medical students report a needlestick injury during their training (the incidence is highest in surgical residents) (25), and a survey in one hospital revealed that 60% of the staff surgeons experienced a needlestick injury at some time in their careers (26). The activities most often associated with needlestick injuries outside the operating room involve recapping and disposal of used needles (24).

Safety Devices

The problem of needlestick injuries came to the attention of the United States Congress in the year 2000, and as a result, Congress passed the Needlestick Safety and Prevention Act that mandates the use of "safety-engineered" needles in all American health care facilities. The illustration in Figure 3.4 shows a simple safety device designed to eliminate the risk of needlestick injuries. The needle is equipped with a rigid, plastic housing that is attached by a hinge joint to the hub of the needle. The protective housing is normally positioned away from the needle so it

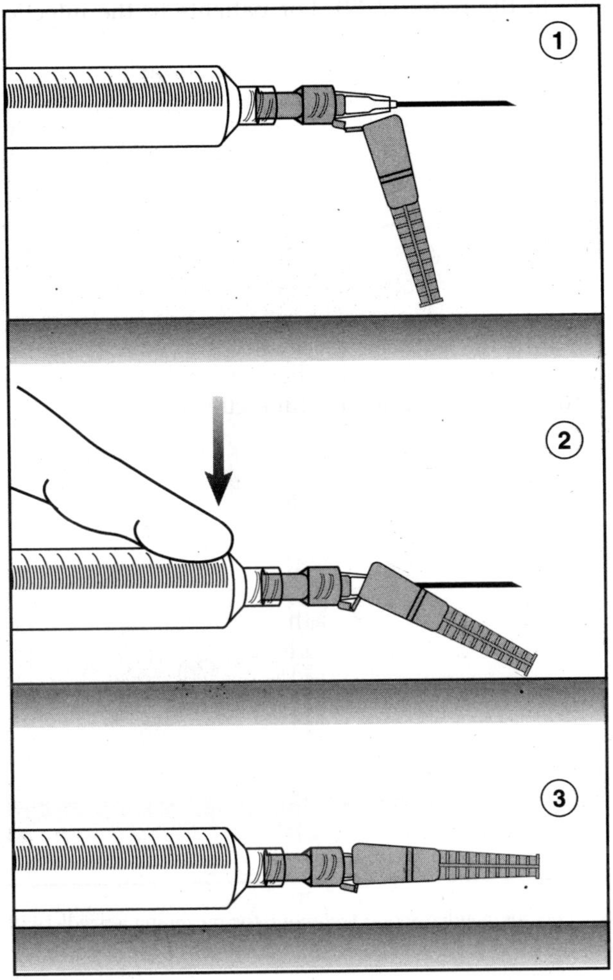

FIGURE 3.4 Safety device to prevent needlestick injuries from recapping and disposal of used needles.

does not interfere with needle use. When the needle is no longer needed, it is locked into the protective housing by holding the housing against a rigid structure and moving the needle about the hinge joint (like closing a door) until it snaps in place in the housing. The needle stays attached to the syringe during this procedure, and the hands never touch the needle. The protected needle and attached syringe are then placed in a puncture-proof "sharps container" for eventual disposal.

One-Handed Recapping Technique

Once the needle is locked in its protective housing, it is not possible to remove it for further use. In situations where a needle has multiple uses (e.g., filling a syringe with a drug preparation and later injecting the drug

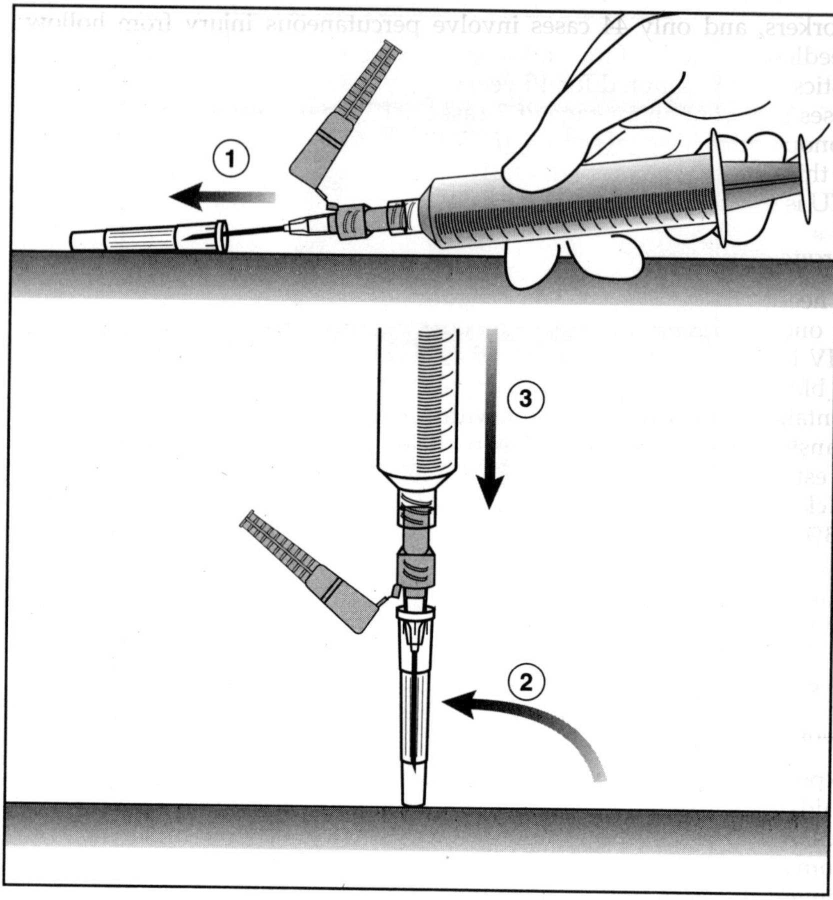

FIGURE 3.5 The one-handed scoop technique for recapping a needle without the risk of a needlestick injury.

in several increments), the needle can be rendered harmless between uses by recapping it with the one-handed "scoop technique" shown in Figure 3.5. With the needle cap resting on a horizontal surface, the needle is advanced into the needle cap. Using the tip of the needle cap as a fulcrum, the needle and cap are then lifted vertically until they are perpendicular to the horizontal surface. The needle is then pushed into the cap until it locks in place. The hands are never in a position to permit an accidental needle puncture.

Human Immunodeficiency Virus (HIV)

The spread of HIV to hospital staff, although universally feared, is not a common event. As of June, 2000, there have been a total of 56 cases of HIV seroconversion in healthcare workers that can be definitely linked to HIV exposure in the workplace. Some of these cases involve laboratory workers, and only 44 cases involve percutaneous injury from hollow needles (the mode of transmission expected in ICUs) (24). Since HIV statistics were monitored for 15 years up to the year 2000, the 44 pertinent cases represent an average of 3 cases per year of HIV transmission in a nonoperative hospital setting. If all these cases occurred in the 6,000 ICUs in this country, the average yearly occurrence of HIV transmission in the ICU is one case for every 2,000 ICUs. Not much of a risk.

Percutaneous Exposures

A needlestick puncture with a hollow needle will transfer an average of one microliter (10^{-6} L) of blood (27). During the viremic stages of HIV infection, there are as many as 5 infectious particles per microliter of blood (28). Therefore puncture of the skin with a hollow needle that contains blood from a patient with active HIV infection is expected to transfer at least a few infectious particles. Fortunately, this is not enough to establish HIV infection in the recipient in most cases. **A single needlestick injury with blood from an HIV-infected patient carries an average 0.3% risk of HIV seroconversion** (5,24). This means that for every 1,000 needlestick injuries with HIV-infected blood, there will be an average of 3 cases of effective HIV transmission. The likelihood of HIV transmission is greater than 0.3% in the following circumstances: a deep skin puncture, visible blood on the needle, and injury from a needle that was placed in an artery or vein of the source patient (29).

Mucous Membrane Exposures

Exposure of mucous membranes and nonintact skin to infectious body fluids carries much less risk of HIV transmission than needlestick injuries. **A single exposure of broken skin or mucous membranes to blood from an HIV-infected patient carries an average 0.09% risk of HIV seroconversion** (5,24). This means that for every 1,000 mucous membrane exposures to contaminated blood, there will be one (0.9) case of HIV transmission. (A one-in-a-thousand risk!)

Postexposure Management

When a member of the ICU staff experiences a possible exposure to HIV from a needlestick injury or blood splash to the face, the appropriate steps to take are determined by the presence or absence of HIV anti-bodies in the blood of the source patient. If the HIV antibody status of the source patient is unknown, you should (with permission) perform a rapid HIV-antibody test on a blood sample from the source patient. This is done at the bedside (by an appropriately trained member of the staff), and the results are available in 10 to 15 minutes. The results of this test can be used to guide initial management decisions, but a positive result must be confirmed by another test such as a Western blot or immunofluorescent antibody assay. The recommendations for possible HIV exposure based on the HIV status of the source patient are outlined in Table 3.5 (5).

The major decision following possible HIV transmission is whether or not to begin prophylactic therapy with antiretroviral agents in the exposed individual. If HIV infection is proven or suspected in the

TABLE 3.5 Postexposure Prophylaxis for HIV Infection

Indications for Each Type of Postexposure Drug Regimen		
No Drugs	**Two Drugs[a]**	**Three Drugs[b]**
1. When source is HIV-negative	1. When source is HIV-positive but asymptomatic	1. When source is HIV-positive and symptomatic
2. When HIV status of source is not known but HIV is unlikely[c]	2. When HIV status of source is not known but HIV is likely.[c]	2. When source is HIV-positive and asymptomatic but exposure is severe[e]
3. When source is not known but HIV is unlikely[d]	3. When source is not known but HIV is likely[d]	

From Reference 5.

[a] The recommended two-drug regimen is zidovudine (200 mg TID) plus lamivudine (150 mg BID) for 4 weeks. The two agents are available together as COMBIVIR.

[b] Add one of the following drugs to the two-drug regimen: efavirenz (600 mg at bedtime), indinavir (800 mg every 8 hr, between meals), or nelfinavir (2.5 g daily in 2 or 3 divided doses, with meals).

[c] When the HIV status of the source is unknown, the likelihood of HIV is based on the presence or absence of risk factors.

[d] When the source is unknown, the likelihood of HIV is based on the prevalence of HIV in the population served.

[e] Severe exposure is defined as deep injury, needle soiled with blood from source patient, and exposure from needle inserted into artery or vein of source patient.

source patient, prophylactic therapy with at least 2 antiretroviral agents is started and continued for 4 weeks (or until there is convincing evidence for the absence of HIV infection in the source patient). A popular two-drug regimen is the combination of zidovudine (200 mg TID) and lamovudine (150 mg daily). These two drugs are available in a combination tablet (COMBIVIR, GlaxoSmithKline), each containing 150 mg lamovudine and 300 mg zidovudine. A third antiretroviral agent is added if there is evidence for symptomatic or advanced HIV infection in the source patient, or if the HIV exposure is severe (i.e., deep needlestick injury, injury from a needle soiled with infectious blood, or injury from a needle that was placed in an artery or vein of an HIV-infected patient) (29). The agents that can be added to the two-drug regimen are included at the bottom of Table 3.5.

It is important to emphasize that the current recommendations for prophylaxis with antiretroviral agents are empiric, and not based on proven efficacy. Even if antiretroviral therapy is completely effective in preventing HIV transmission, an average of 330 patients who have been exposed to HIV-infected blood would have to be treated to prevent one case of HIV transmission. Considering that the prophylactic regimens of antiretroviral drug therapy are poorly tolerated (one of every three subjects given antiretroviral drugs for postexposure prophylaxis will stop taking the drugs because of troublesome side effects) (5), the risks of antiretroviral drug prophylaxis may outweigh the overall benefit in many subjects, particularly when HIV infection in the source patient is not proven.

POSTEXPOSURE SURVEILLANCE. Antibody responses to acute or primary HIV infection can take 4 to 6 weeks to become evident. Therefore anyone with documented exposure to HIV infection should have serial tests for HIV antibodies at 6 weeks, 3 months, and 6 months after the exposure (5). More prolonged testing is not warranted unless the exposed person develops symptoms compatible with HIV infection.

POSTEXPOSURE HOTLINE. The National Clinicians' Postexposure Prophylaxis Hotline (PEP line) is a resource for anyone with questions about postexposure prophylaxis for HIV infection. The toll-free number is 888-448-4911.

Hepatitis B Virus

The blood-borne hepatitis B virus (HBV) is much more transmission-prone than HIV. One microliter (10^{-6} L) of blood from a patient with HBV-induced acute hepatitis can have as many as one million infectious particles, whereas, as just mentioned, a similar volume of blood from a patient with active HIV infection will have only 5 or fewer infectious particles (28). Fortunately, there is a vaccine that can provide immunity against HBV infection.

Hepatitis B Vaccination

Vaccination against hepatitis B is recommended for anyone who has contact with blood, body fluids, and sharp instruments (5), which is virtually everyone who works in an ICU. The only contraindication to the vaccine is a prior history of anaphylaxis from baker's yeast (5). The vaccination involves 3 doses and should proceed as follows (5):

1. The first 2 doses (given by deep IM injection) are given 4 weeks apart, and the third dose is administered 5 months after the second dose.
2. If the vaccination series is interrupted after the first dose, the whole sequence is not repeated. If the second dose was missed, it is given as soon as possible, and the third dose is administered at least 2 months later. If the third dose was missed, it is administered as soon as possible, and the vaccination series is considered completed.

The hepatitis B vaccine produces immunity by stimulating production of an antibody to the hepatitis B surface antigen (anti-HBs). The primary vaccination series is not always successful in providing immunity, so the following evaluation is recommended (5).

3. One to two months after the vaccination is completed, the serum anti-HBs level should be measured. Immunity is indicated by an anti-HBs level that is $\geq$10 mIU/mL. If the anti-HBs is $<$10 mIU/mL, the 3-dose vaccination series should be repeated.

Nonresponders have a 30% to 50% chance of responding to the second vaccination series (5). If there is no response after the second vaccination (i.e., if the anti-HBs is still below 10 mIU/mL), then the subject is classified as a nonresponder and receives no further vaccination attempts. Nonresponders have the same risk for acquiring HBV as those who have never received the vaccine. Responders do not require a booster dose of the vaccine, even though antibody levels wane with time (5).

Postexposure Risks and Management

The risk of acquiring HBV is determined by the vaccination history of the individual at risk. For those who are vaccinated and have responded appropriately, there is virtually no risk of acquiring HBV infection. For unvaccinated (or nonresponsive) individuals who have been exposed to infectious blood via needlestick injuries, the risk of developing serologic evidence of HBV infection is as high as 60%, and the risk of developing clinical hepatitis is as high as 30% (5).

The management strategies following possible exposure to HBV are outlined in Table 3.6 (5). These strategies are guided by the vaccination status of the exposed individual and the presence or absence of the hepatitis B surface antigen (HBsAg) in the blood of the source patient. For exposed individuals who have completed the HBV vaccination and have documented evidence of immunity, no treatment is necessary following exposure. For all others (i.e., unvaccinated, vaccinated but not immune, and vaccinated with unknown immunity), the management is based on the likelihood of HBV infection in the source patient. If HBV infection in the source patient is proven (by the presence of HBsAg in the blood) or suspected (by the presence of risk factors for HBV or a high prevalence of HBV infection in the source population), the treatment usually involves an intramuscular dose of hepatitis B immune globulin (0.06 mL/kg) and initiation of the HBV vaccine series.

Hepatitis C Virus

Hepatitis C virus (HCV) is a blood-borne pathogen of some concern because HCV infection leads to chronic hepatitis in about 70% of cases (7). Fortunately, HCV transmission in the hospital setting is uncommon. The prevalence of anti-HCV antibodies in the blood of hospital personnel is only 1% to 2% (7), which is no different than the general population. Following after needlestick injuries with HCV-infected blood, the average risk of acquiring HCV is only 1.8% (5). Transmission from mucous membrane exposure is rare, and there are no documented cases of HCV transmission through nonintact skin.

There is no effective prophylaxis for HCV following exposure to infected blood. Both immunoglobulin therapy and antiviral agents such as interferon have been ineffective in preventing HCV infection following exposure to blood (7). In addition, there is currently no vaccine for HCV. When hospital workers are exposed to HCV, they should be counseled about the risks associated with HCV infection, particularly the risk for chronic liver disease. For those with documented exposure

TABLE 3.6 Postexposure Management for Hepatitis B Virus (HBV)

Vaccination Status of Exposed Person	Management Based on HBsAg Status of Source Patient		
	HBsAg Positive	HBsAg Negative	HBsAg Unknown
Not vaccinated	HBIG × 1[a] & start HBV vaccination	Start HBV vaccination	Start HBV vaccination
Vaccinated and Immune[b]	No treatment	No treatment	No treatment
Not immune[c]	HBIG × 1[a] & start HBV revaccination or HBIG × 2[d]	No treatment	If source is high risk for HBV, treat as if source is HBsAg positive
Immunity unknown	Measure anti-HBs level in exposed person 1. If immune,[b] no treatment 2. If not immune,[c] HBIG × 1[c] and vaccine booster	No treatment	Measure anti-HBs level in exposed person 1. If immune,[b] no treatment. 2. If not immune,[c] vaccine booster & recheck titer in 1–2 mo

From Reference 5.
HBsAg = hepatitis B surface antigen; Anti-HBs = serum antibody to hepatitis B surface antigen.
[a] HBIG × 1 = hepatitis B immune globulin in one intramuscular dose of 0.06 mL/kg.
[b] Immunity is defined as postvaccination level of ≥10 mIU/mL for the serum antibody to hepatitis B surface antigen (anti-HBs).
[c] Nonimmunity is defined as a postvaccination level of <10 mIU/mL for the serum antibody to hepatitis B surface antigen (anti-HBs).
[d] HBIG × 2 = hepatitis B immune globulin in two intramuscular doses of 0.06 mIU/mL each. This regimen is usually reserved for those without immunity after two vaccination courses.

to HCV-infected blood via needlestick injuries, serial determinations of anti-HCV antibodies is recommended for 6 months (7).

REFERENCES

Clinical Practice Guidelines

1. Centers for Disease Control and Prevention. Perspectives in disease prevention and health promotion update: universal precautions for prevention of transmission of human immunodeficiency virus, hepatitis B virus, and other bloodborne pathogens in health-care settings. MMWR 1988;37:377–388.
2. Garner JS, Hospital Infection Control Practices Advisory Committee. Guideline for isolation precautions in hospitals. Am J Infect Control 1996; 24:24–52. (Available at http://www.cdc.gov/ncidod/hip/ISOLAT/Isolat.

htm) Updated guidelines available at www.cdc.gov/ncidod/hip/ISOLAT/isopart2.htm
3. Larson EL, Rackoff WR, Weiman M, et al. APIC guideline for hand antisepsis in health-care settings. Am J Infect Control 1995;23:251–269. (Available in pdf format at www.apic.org/pdf/gdhandws.pdf)
4. Centers for Disease Control and Prevention. Guidelines for hand hygiene in health-care settings: recommendations of the Healthcare Infection Control Practices Advisory Committee and the HICPAC/SHEA/APIC/IDSA Hand Hygiene Task Force. MMWR 2002;51(No. RR-16):1–45. (Available in pdf format at www.cdc.gov/mmwr/PDF/RR/RR5116.pdf)
5. Centers for Disease Control and Prevention. Updated U.S. Public Health Service guidelines for the management of occupational exposures to HBV, HCV, and HIV and recommendations for postexposure prophylaxis. MMWR 2001;50(No. RR-11):1–52. (Available at www.cdc.gov/NIOSH/bbppg.html)
6. Centers for Disease Control and Prevention. Guidelines for the prevention of intravascular catheter-related infections. MMWR 2002;51(No. RR-10):1–29. (Available in pdf format at www.cdc.gov/mmwr/pdf/RR/RR5110.pdf)
7. Centers for Disease Control and Prevention. Immunization of health-care workers: recommendations of the Advisory Committee on Immunization Practices (ACIP) and the Hospital Infection Control Practices Advisory Committee (HICPAC). MMWR 1997;46(RR-18):1–42. (Available at www.cdc.gov/hip/publications/ACIP-list.htm)

Skin Hygiene

8. Katz JD. Hand washing and hand disinfection: more than your mother taught you. Anesthesiol Clin North Am 2004;22:457–471.
9. Larson EL, Aiello AE, Bastyr J, et al. Assessment of two hand hygiene regimens for intensive care unit personnel. Crit Care Med 2001;29:944–951.
10. Parienti J-J, du Cheyron D, Ramakers M, et al. Alcoholic povidone-iodine to prevent central venous catheter colonization: a randomized unit-crossover study. Crit Care Med 2004;32:708–713.
11. Laestadius JG, Dimberg L. Hot water for handwashing—where is the proof? J Occup Environ Med 2005;47:434–435.
12. Gustafson DR, Vetter EA, Larson DR, et al. Effects of 4 hand-drying methods for removing bacteria from washed hands: a randomized trial. Mayo Clin Proc 2000;75:705–708.

Protective Barriers

13. Division of Healthcare Quality Promotion, National Center for Infectious Diseases, Centers for Disease Control and Prevention. Standard precautions: excerpted from guideline for isolation precautions in hospitals. Accessed at www.cdc.gov/ncidod /hip/ ISOLAT/ std _prec_excerpt.htm
14. Rossoff LJ, Borenstein M, Isenberg HD. Is handwashing really needed in an intensive care unit? Crit Care Med 1995;25:1211–1216.
15. Nakamura CT, Ferdman RM, Keens TG, et al. Latex allergy in children on home mechanical ventilation. Chest 200;118:1000–1003.
16. Charous L, Charous MA. Is occupational latex allergy causing your patient's asthma? J Respir Dis 2002;23:250–256.

17. Guin JD. Clinical presentation of patients sensitive to natural rubber latex. Dermatitis 2004;4:192–196.
18. Food and Drug Administration. Allergic reactions to latex-containing medical devices. Publication #MDA91-1, March 29, 1991. Bethesda: FDA,1991.
19. Hamilton RG, Peterson EL, Ownby DR. Clinical and laboratory-based methods in the diagnosis of natural rubber latex allergy. J Allergy Clin Immunol 2002;110(suppl 2):S47–S56.
20. Smith JW, Nichols RL. Barrier efficiency of surgical gowns. Arch Surg 1991; 126:756–763.
21. Division of Healthcare Quality Promotion, National Center for Infectious Diseases, Centers for Disease Control and Prevention. Droplet precautions: excerpted from guideline for isolation precautions in hospitals. Accessed at www.cdc.gov/ncidod /hip/ ISOLAT/ droplet _prec_excerpt.htm
22. Division of Healthcare Quality Promotion, National Center for Infectious Diseases, Centers for Disease Control and Prevention. Airborne precautions: excerpted from guideline for isolation precautions in hospitals. Accessed at www.cdc.gov/ncidod /hip/ ISOLAT/ airborne _prec_excerpt.htm
23. Fennelly KP. Personal respiratory protection against *Mycobacterium* tuberculosis. Clin Chest Med 1997;18:1–17.

Blood-Borne Pathogens

24. National Institute for Occupational Safety and Health. Preventing needlestick injuries in health care settings. DHHS (NIOSH) Publication No. 2000–108, 1999. Bethesda: NIOSH, 1999. (Available at www.cdc.gov/niosh/pdfs/2000-108.pdf)
25. Radechi S, Abbott A, Eloi L. Occupational human immunodeficiency virus exposure among residents and medical students. Arch Intern Med 2000;160: 3107–3100.
26. Berguer R, Heller PJ. Preventing sharps injuries in the operating room. J Am Coll Surg 2004;199:462–467.
27. Berry AJ, Greene ES. The risk of needlestick injuries and needlestick-transmitted diseases in the practice of anesthesiology. Anesthesiology 1992;77:1007–1021.
28. Moran GJ. Emergency department management of blood and body fluid exposures. Ann Emerg Med 2000;35:47 62.
29. Cardo DM, Culver DH, Ciesielski CA, et al. A case-control study of HIV seroconversion in healthcare workers after percutaneous exposure. N Engl J Med 1997;337:1485–1490.

Chapter 4

ALIMENTARY PROPHYLAXIS

We are told the most fantastic biological tales. For example, that it is dangerous to have acid in your stomach.

J.B.S. Haldane (1939)

The last chapter demonstrated that standard infection control practices are designed to prevent microbial invasion from the skin. However, the skin is not the only body surface that can be breached by microbes. The alimentary tract, which extends from the mouth to the rectum, is outside the body (like the hole in a donut), and the mucosa that lines the alimentary canal serves as a barrier to microbial invasion, just like the skin. However, unlike the skin, which is multilayered and covered with a keratinized surface, the mucosa of the alimentary tract is a single cell layer that is only 0.1 mm thick. Facing this thin barrier in most regions of the gastrointestinal (GI) tract is a population of microbes that far outnumbers the microflora on the skin. **In fact, the number of bacteria in just one gram of stool** (10 to 100 billion) **is greater than the number of people on Earth** (6.5 billion in 2005). Considering the thin mucosa and the hordes of microbes in the GI tract, it seems that the real threat of microbial invasion comes from the bowel, not the skin.

This chapter will introduce you to the importance of the oral cavity and the bowel as sources of infection in critically ill patients, and what can be done to prevent infections from these sites. A section is included on stress-related injury to the gastric mucosa (stress ulcers), and the preventive measures that limit troublesome bleeding from these lesions.

MICROBIAL INVASION FROM THE BOWEL

Microbial organisms are aquatic creatures that require a watery environment to thrive, and the moist environment in the mouth and GI tract is ideal for microbial proliferation. There are 400 to 500 different species of bacteria and fungi in the adult alimentary tract (1,2) with an estimated

TABLE 4.1 Microbial Density in the Alimentary Tract

Segment	Population Density*
Oral cavity	10^5–10^6
Stomach	$<10^3$
Distal small bowel	10^7–10^9
Rectum	10^{10}–10^{12}

*Colony-forming units (CFUs) per gram or mL of luminal contents.
From Simon GL, Gorbach SL. Intestinal microflora. Med Clin North Am 1982;66:557.

total mass of 2 kg (about 4½ pounds) (3). The protective mechanisms that help to prevent this army of microbes from gaining access to the interior of the body are described next.

Protective Mechanisms

There are three levels of protection from microbial invasion in the alimentary tract. The first level of protection takes place in the lumen of the upper gastrointestinal (GI) tract, where the antimicrobial actions of gastric acid help to eradicate microorganisms that are swallowed in food and saliva. This is demonstrated in Table 4.1, which shows a marked decrease in microbial density in the stomach compared to the oral cavity. The second level of protection occurs at the bowel wall, where the mucosal lining of the GI tract acts as a physical barrier that blocks the movement of microbes across the bowel wall. The third level of protection takes place on the extraluminal side of the bowel wall, where the reticuloendothelial system traps and destroys microbes that breach the mucosal barrier. Roughly two-thirds of the reticuloendothelial system in the body is located in the abdomen (4), which suggests that microbial invasion across the bowel wall may be a frequent occurrence.

Gastric Acid

Gastric acid is often misperceived as a digestive aid. An acid environment in the stomach can facilitate the absorption of iron and calcium, but patients with achlorhydria (inability to acidify gastric secretions) are not troubled by malabsorption (5). So what is the function of gastric acid? It seems to be an antimicrobial defense mechanism, as described next.

ANTISEPTIC ACTIONS. Most microorganisms do not survive in an acid environment, as demonstrated in Figure 4.1. In this case, the common enteric organism *Escherichia coli* is completely eradicated in one hour when the pH of the growth medium is reduced from 5 to 3 pH units. The antimicrobial effects of an acid environment was appreciated by Sir Joseph Lister, the father of antiseptic practices in medicine, who used carbolic acid as the first antiseptic agent for the skin. Another use of acid as a microbe killer is the method of food preservation known as *pickling*, which used vinegar, a weak acid, to preserve food.

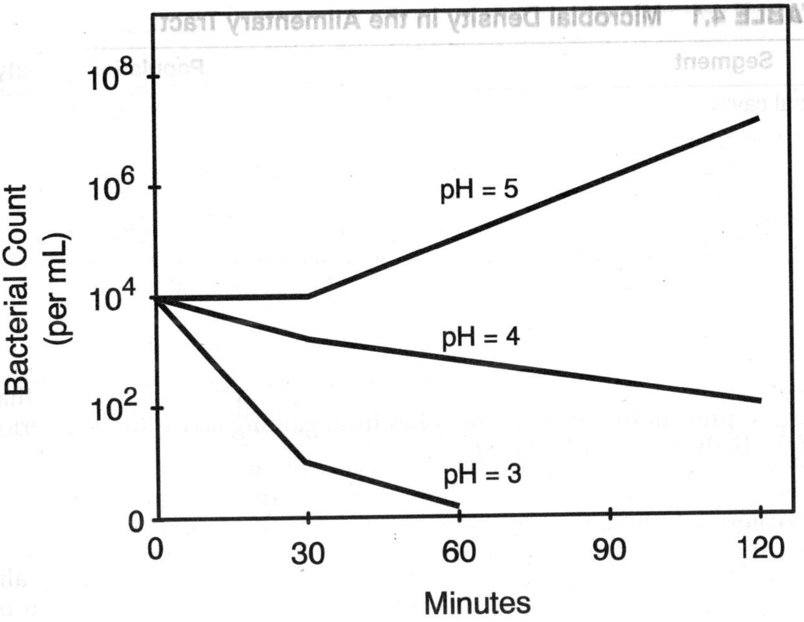

FIGURE 4.1 The influence of pH on the growth of *Escherichia coli*. (From Gianella RA, Broitman SA, Zarncheck N. Gastric acid barrier to ingested microorganisms in man: studies in vivo and in vitro. Gut 1972;13:251.)

In light of the antimicrobial activity of acid, it is likely that **gastric acid serves as an endogenous antiseptic agent that eradicates microorganisms swallowed in saliva and food.** The eradication of microbes swallowed in saliva would explain why gastric acid secretion is a continuous process that does not require food ingestion. However, the importance of this function is unclear because the microbes that populate the mouth are mostly harmless saprophytes. The eradication of microbes in ingested food may be a more important role for gastric acid. This would explain why drug-induced inhibition of gastric acid production is associated with recurrent *Salmonella* enteritis (6) and why achlorhydria is associated with an increased risk of bacterial gastroenteritis (5–7). Food processing techniques might not completely eradicate microbes, and gastric acid could then serve as our own built-in method of disinfecting the food we eat.

The Acid Phobia

Gastric acid has a long-standing reputation of being a corrosive agent that can eat through an unprotected stomach wall and "burn a hole in your stomach." However, as stated in the introductory quote by J.B.S. Haldane (a popular science writer in the early twentieth century), the perceived dangers of gastric acid are more fantasy than fact. An acid environment can be corrosive for certain inorganic compounds like metals and enamel, but acid is not destructive for organic matter. If you have ever spilled orange juice (pH=3) or lime juice (pH=2) on your hands, you have experienced the non-destructive nature of acidity in the organic world. In fact, as mentioned in the last section, the pickling process uses an acid (vinegar) to *preserve* organic matter (food).

The perception of gastric acid as a destructive force is a direct result of the traditional notion that gastric acid is the principal cause of peptic ulcer disease. However, recent evidence indicates that local infection with *Helicobacter pylori* is responsible for most cases of peptic ulcer disease.

Predisposing Conditions

A defect in any of the protective mechanisms just described will promote the movement of organisms across the bowel wall and into the systemic circulation. This process is called *translocation* (8), and it is considered an important source of septicemia in critically ill patients (see Chapter 42). The illustration in Figure 4.2 shows three conditions that will promote translocation: microbial overgrowth in the bowel lumen, disruption of the mucosal barrier, and defective clearance by the lymphatic system.

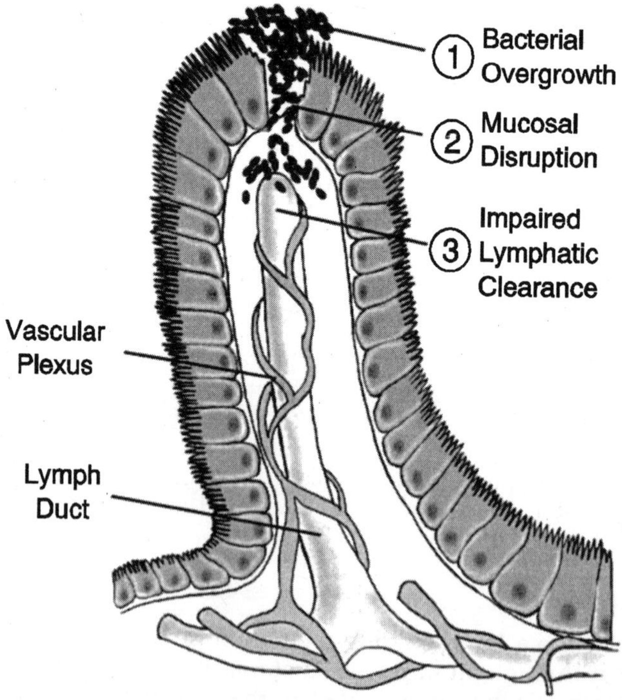

FIGURE 4.2 The triple threat of translocation. This diagram of an intestinal microvillus shows three conditions that predispose to bloodstream invasion by enteric microorganisms.

Reduced Gastric Acidity

Loss of the normal antiseptic actions of gastric acid will result in bacterial overgrowth in the stomach, and this can be a prelude to several types of infections, including infectious gastroenteritis (as described previously), pneumonia from aspiration of infectious gastric contents into the lungs (9,10), and septicemia from bacterial translocation across the bowel wall (11). The risk of bacterial overgrowth and its consequences is reason to avoid the use of drugs that inhibit gastric acid secretion, if possible.

STRESS-RELATED MUCOSAL INJURY

Stress-related mucosal injury is a term used to describe erosions in the gastric mucosa that occur in almost all patients with acute, life-threatening illness (12,13). These erosions can be superficial and confined to the mucosa, or they can bore deeper and extend into the submucosa (see Figure 4.3). The deeper lesions are called *stress ulcers*.

Pathogenesis

The mucosal lining of the GI tract is normally shed and replaced every 2 to 3 days. When nutrient blood flow is inadequate to support the replacement process, the surface of the bowel becomes denuded, creating superficial erosions. The actions of gastric acid may serve to aggravate this condition, but **the principal cause of stress-related mucosal injury is impaired blood flow, not gastric acidity** (13). This is an important distinction when considering a rational approach to preventing this condition, as described later.

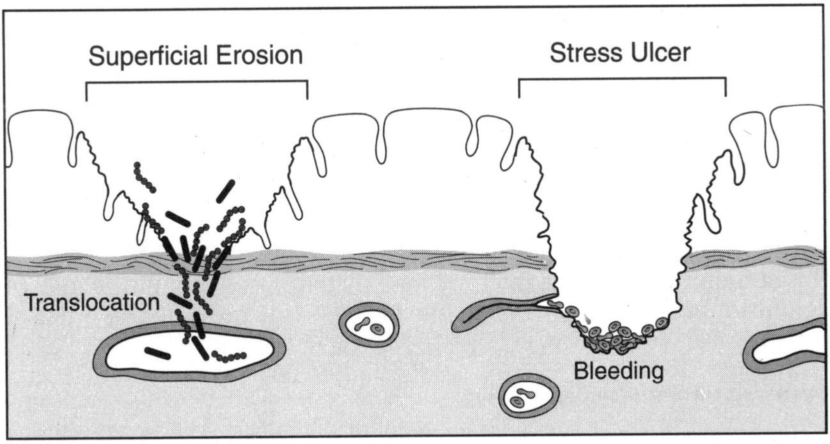

FIGURE 4.3 The different types of gastric erosions that develop in critically ill patients.

Clinical Consequences

Erosions in the gastric mucosa can be demonstrated in as many as 75% to 100% of patients within 24 hours of admission to the ICU (14). Fortunately, these lesions are often clinically silent. The disruption of the gastric mucosa can, however, promote bleeding from surface vessels, and can also promote microbial translocation across the gastric mucosa. Clinical studies of gastric erosions have focused exclusively on the risk of GI bleeding. Without prophylactic measures to prevent bleeding (see later), clinically apparent GI bleeding can occur in as many as 25% of ICU patients (14), while clinically significant bleeding (i.e., causes a significant drop in blood pressure or requires transfusion) occurs in only 1% to 5% of ICU patients (14,15). The low incidence of clinically significant bleeding is explained by the superficial location of most gastric erosions, which disrupts only small capillaries.

High-Risk Conditions

Since most patients have gastric erosions after just one day in the ICU, the concern in the individual patient is the risk of developing complications from these lesions. The conditions listed below are associated with an increased risk of clinically significant bleeding from gastric erosions (12,15).

1. Mechanical ventilation for longer than 48 hours
2. Coagulopathy (i.e., platelets <50,000, INR >1.5, or PTT >2 × control)
3. Hypotension
4. Severe sepsis
5. Multisystem trauma
6. Severe head injury
7. Burns involving >30% of body surface area
8. Renal failure or hepatic failure

Only two of these conditions have proven to be independent risk factors for significant bleeding: mechanical ventilation for longer than 48 hours, and coagulopathy (15). For the other conditions, at least two must be present to consider the patient high-risk for bleeding. These high-risk conditions also serve as indicators for prophylactic therapy to prevent GI bleeding from gastric erosions.

Preventive Strategies

This section describes the interventions that are used to limit the risk of significant bleeding from gastric erosions. Each is presented in order of (my personal) preference.

Preserving Gastric Blood Flow

Because impaired blood flow is the culprit in most cases of stress-related mucosal injury, preserving gastric blood flow should be the best preventive measure. Unfortunately, there are no readily-available methods for monitoring gastric blood flow in the clinical setting. Sublingual capnometry, which is a technique that measures the PCO_2 in the tissue on the underside of the tongue, is a promising method for detecting significant decreases in gastric blood flow at the bedside (16), but the experience with this methodology is currently limited. The best strategy for now is to maintain systemic blood flow and oxygen transport using standard markers (e.g., blood lactate levels) or invasive parameters (e.g., oxygen delivery, oxygen uptake) if available. The bedside methods for monitoring the adequacy of tissue perfusion (including sublingual capnometry) are described in Chapter 11.

Enteral Nutrition

Enteral tube feedings exert a trophic effect on the bowel mucosa that helps to maintain the structural and functional integrity of the bowel mucosa (17). Both of these effects should provide protection against the development of stress-related gastric erosions. Clinical studies in burn patients (18) and patients receiving mechanical ventilation (19) have shown that enteral tube feedings are effective in preventing overt bleeding from the GI tract. Although more clinical studies are needed, **enteral tube feedings can be considered adequate prophylaxis for stress-related gastric hemorrhage unless there is some other condition that raises special concern for GI bleeding,** such as a coagulopathy, a prior history of bleeding from gastritis or peptic ulcer disease, or active peptic ulcer disease.

Pharmacologic Strategies

There are two pharmacologic approaches to prevent bleeding from gastric erosions. One approach uses an agent that provides local protection to the gastric mucosa (cytoprotection), and the other approach uses drugs that block the production of gastric acid (reduced acidity). The drugs involved in both of these approaches are shown in Table 4.2 (antacids have fallen out of favor and are not included here). There has been a

TABLE 4.2 Drugs Used for Prophylaxis of Stress Ulcer Bleeding

Agent	Type	Route	Dose Recommendations
Sucralfate	Cytoprotective agent	NG tube	1. 1 g every 6 hr 2. Watch for drug interactions
Famotidine	H_2 Blocker	IV	1. 20 mg every 12 hr 2. Adjust dose in renal insufficiency
Ranitidine	H_2 Blocker	IV	1. 50 mg every 8 hr 2. Adjust dose in renal insufficiency
Pantoprazol	Proton-pump inhibitor	IV	1. 40 mg daily as a single dose

long-standing debate over which pharmacologic approach is the best, and much of this debate concerns the role of gastric acid as a defense against infections of bowel origin (see later).

Sucralfate

Sucralfate is an aluminum salt of sucrose sulfate that forms a protective covering on the gastric mucosa and helps to preserve the structural and functional integrity of the mucosa (20). Part of this effect may be due to local stimulation of prostaglandin production, which helps to preserve gastric blood flow. The pH of gastric secretions is not altered by sucralfate. The drug is given orally or via nasogastric tube in the dosage shown in Table 4.2, and it is the least expensive of the prophylactic drug regimens.

Sucralfate is effective in reducing overt bleeding from gastric erosions in critically ill patients (21). Its efficacy in preventing clinically significant bleeding is not well studied. Several studies have compared sucralfate with drugs that reduce gastric acidity, and these will be described later.

INTERACTIONS. Sucralfate can bind to a number of drugs in the bowel lumen and reduce their absorption. The most important of these are listed below (22).

Warfarin (Coumadin)	Ranitidine
Digoxin	Quinidine
Fluoroquinolones	Thyroxine
Ketoconazole	Tetracycline
Phenytoin	Theophylline

To avoid potential interactions in the bowel, these drugs should be given at least 2 hours before sucralfate. The aluminum in sucralfate can also bind phosphate in the bowel, but hypophosphatemia is only rarely reported in association with sucralfate therapy (23). Nevertheless, sucralfate is not advised for patients with persistent or severe hypophosphatemia. Despite its aluminum content, sucralfate does not elevate plasma aluminum levels with prolonged use (24).

Histamine Type-2 Receptor Antagonists

Inhibition of gastric acid secretion with histamine type-2 receptor antagonists (H_2 blockers) is currently the most popular method of stress ulcer prophylaxis (25). Cimetidine, the original drug in this class, has fallen out of favor because of frequent drug interactions, and has been replaced in popularity by famotidine (Pepcid) and ranitidine (Zantac). Both these drugs are given intravenously in the dosing regimens shown in Table 4.2. Continuous infusion of H_2 blockers is the most effective method of maintaining gastric acid inhibition (26); however, intermittent dosing is currently the favored regimen for stress ulcer prophylaxis. Famotidine is longer lasting than ranitidine [i.e., a single 20 mg intravenous dose of famotidine will inhibit gastric acid for 10–12 hours (27), while a single 50 mg intravenous dose of ranitidine inhibits gastric acid for 6–8 hrs (28)].

DOSE ADJUSTMENTS. Intravenous doses of famotidine and ranitidine are largely excreted unchanged in the urine, and accumulation of these drugs in renal insufficiency can produce a neurotoxic condition characterized by confusion, agitation, and even seizures (27,28). Therefore, the dose of these drugs should be reduced in renal insufficiency. (See the Appendix at the end of the book for drug dosing guidelines in renal insufficiency.)

BENEFITS VERSUS RISKS. Clinical studies have shown that H_2 blockers can reduce the incidence of clinically significant bleeding from gastric erosions (21). However, as expected from gastric acid inhibition, H_2 blocker therapy has been associated with an increased risk of infection (6,7,9–11), most notably pneumonia in ICU patients (10). Therefore, the benefits of H_2 blockers in preventing bleeding must be weighed against the risks associated with bacterial overgrowth in the stomach. More on this in the next section.

Sulcrafate versus H_2 Receptor Antagonists

Several clinical trials have evaluated the relative effects of sucralfate (cytoprotection) and H_2 blockers (reduced acidity) in critically ill patients (29,30). The results of the most recent clinical trial are shown in Figure 4.4 (29). This study involved 1,200 ventilator-dependent patients in 16 ICUs who were randomized to receive sucralfate (1 gram every 6 hours) or

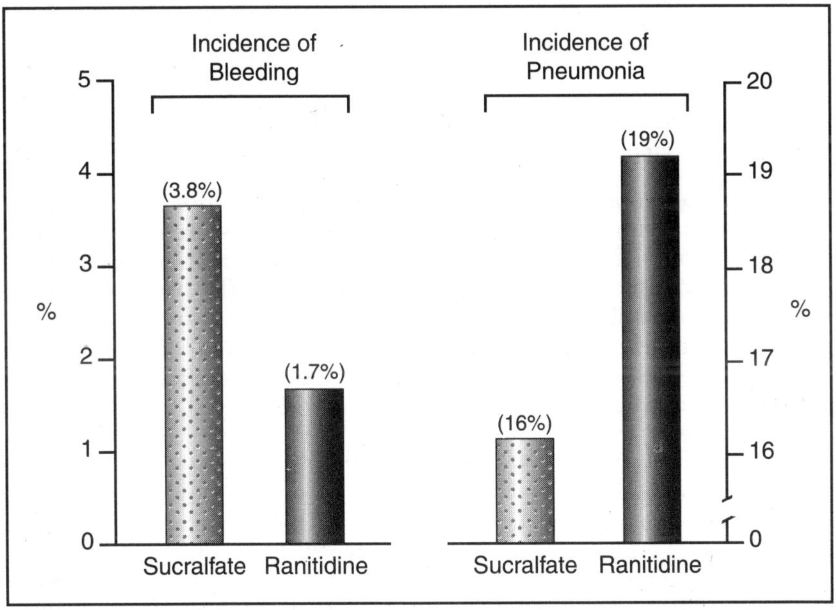

FIGURE 4.4 A comparison of the effects of stress ulcer prophylaxis with sucralfate and ranitidine on the incidence of clinically significant bleeding and hospital-acquired pneumonia in ventilator-dependent patients. (From Cook D, Laine LA, Guyatt GH, et al. A comparison of sucralfate and ranitidine for the prevention of upper gastrointestinal bleeding in patients requiring mechanical ventilation. N Engl J Med 1998;338:791.)

ranitidine (50 mg every 6 hours, adjusted for renal insufficiency). The results show that clinically significant bleeding occurred more frequently in the patients receiving sucralfate (the absolute difference was 2.1%), while hospital-acquired pneumonia occurred more frequently in the patients receiving ranitidine (the absolute difference was 2.9%). Although the pneumonia difference was not statistically significant in this study, a combined analysis of 8 other studies comparing sucralfate and ranitidine shows a significantly greater incidence of pneumonia with ranitidine (30).

The results in Figure 4.4 show that ranitidine is superior to sucralfate for the prevention of bleeding from gastric erosions, while sucralfate is superior to ranitidine for the prevention of pneumonia. So which is preferred: fewer bleeding episodes or fewer pneumonias? The answer can't be based on survival benefit because the mortality in sucralfate- and ranitidine-treated patients is the same (30). One consideration that may be important is the relative incidence of GI bleeding versus pneumonia in ICU patients. As indicated in Figure 4.3, pneumonia occurs much more frequently than GI bleeding, which means that fewer patients would have to be treated with sucralfate to see a benefit (i.e., fewer pneumonias) as compared to ranitidine. Therefore sucralfate may offer an advantage over ranitidine simply because it reduces the risk of the disorder with the greatest risk.

Which approach is preferred by critical care specialists? A recent survey showed that H_2 blockers are used much more frequently than sucralfate for stress ulcer prophylaxis in the ICU (25). However, the major reason for this preference was drug availability rather than clinical efficacy (25).

Proton Pump Inhibitors

Proton Pump Inhibitors (PPIs) block gastric acid secretion by binding to the membrane pump responsible for hydrogen ion secretion by gastric parietal cells (31). These drugs are actually prodrugs, and must be converted to the active form within gastric parietal cells (31). Once activated, PPIs bind irreversibly to the membrane pump and produce complete inhibition of gastric acid secretion. These drugs are much more effective in reducing gastric acidity than H_2 blockers, and unlike H_2 blockers, they do not produce tolerance with prolonged use (31).

PPIs have replaced H_2 blockers as the agents of choice for the treatment of gastroesophageal reflux and peptic ulcer disease. They have also been recommended to prevent stress ulcer bleeding in ICU patients, and the lack of tolerance to PPIs has been proposed as an advantage over H_2 blockers (31). Intragastric administration of PPIs can be problematic because these agents are inactivated by acid. Enteric coated granules of omeprazole (Prilosec) and lansoprazole (Prevacid) have been mixed in 8.4% sodium bicarbonate solutions and given via nasogastric tube (32), but this regimen is time consuming to prepare, and the bioavailability may be inconsistent (31). Pantoprazole (Protonix) is available for intravenous use (31,33), but there is no experience with this formulation in stress ulcer prophylaxis.

Given the low frequency of bleeding from gastric erosions and the effectiveness of other prophylactic measures, the use of PPIs for stress ulcer prophylaxis seems unnecessary. Furthermore, the potency of PPIs in raising gastric pH will create even greater risks from bacterial overgrowth in the bowel than the H_2 blockers.

Occult Blood Testing

Testing for occult blood in gastric aspirates is not necessary for evaluating the efficacy of stress ulcer prophylaxis. Nasogastric aspirates almost always contain occult blood in the presence of gastric erosions (34), and because few of these cases progress to clinically significant bleeding, the presence of occult blood in nasogastric aspirates has no predictive value for assessing the risk of significant bleeding. For those who insist on monitoring occult blood in gastric aspirates, guaiac and Hemoccult tests are not appropriate because they give false-positive and false-negative results when the test fluid has a pH less than 4 (35). The Gastroccult test (Smith, Kline Laboratories) is not influenced by pH (35) and is the more appropriate test for occult blood in gastric aspirates.

DECONTAMINATION OF THE ALIMENTARY TRACT

The microorganisms that normally inhabit the oral cavity and GI tract seem to live in peaceful coexistence with us. However, in the presence of severe or chronic illness, the alimentary tract becomes populated by more pathogenic organisms capable of causing invasive infections. This section describes two methods for combating this pathogenic colonization. Both methods haven proven effective in reducing the incidence of hospital-acquired infections in the ICU.

Oral Decontamination

The aspiration of mouth secretions into the upper airways is believed to be the inciting event in most cases of hospital-acquired pneumonia. An average of 1 billion (10^9) microorganisms are present in each milliliter of saliva (36), so **aspiration of one microliter (10^{-3} mL) of saliva will introduce about one million (10^6) microbes into the airways**. Fortunately, the microbes that normally inhabit the mouth are harmless saprophytes (e.g., lactobacillus and α-hemolytic streptococci) that show little tendency to produce invasive infection. Critically ill patients are not as fortunate, as described next.

Colonization of the Oral Cavity

The oral cavity in hospitalized patients is often colonized with pathogenic organisms, most notably aerobic gram-negative bacilli like *Pseudomonas aeruginosa* (37). The change in microflora is not environmentally driven, but is directly related to the severity of illness in each patient. This is demonstrated in Figure 4.5. Note that healthy subjects were not colonized

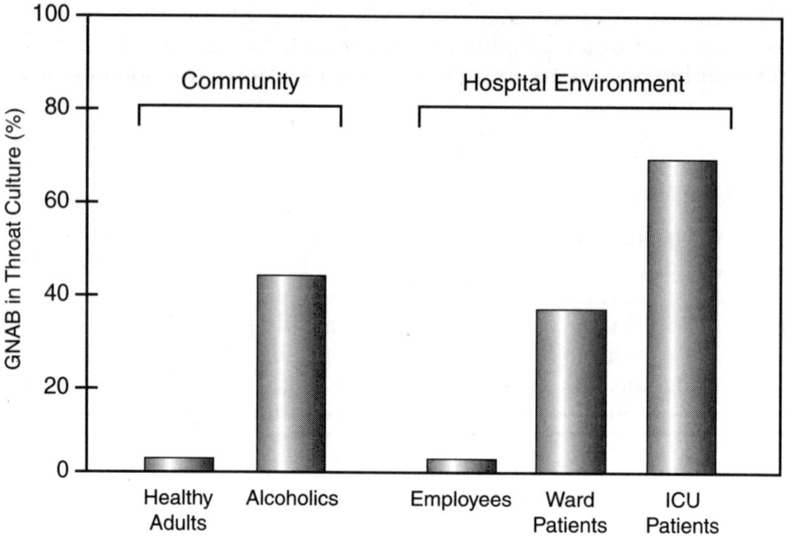

FIGURE 4.5 Colonization of the oral cavity with gram-negative aerobic bacilli (*GNAB*) in different groups of subjects. (From Johanson WG, Pierce AK, Sanford JP. Changing pharyngeal bacterial flora of hospitalized patients. N Engl J Med 1969;281:1137.)

with aerobic gram-negative bacilli, regardless of the time spent in the hospital environment. This highlights the importance of host-specific factors in the microbial colonization of body surfaces.

BACTERIAL ADHERENCE. The host-specific factor in colonization of body surfaces is the tendency for bacteria to adhere to underlying cells. Colonization is not merely a result of microbial proliferation; it requires that microbes adhere to the underlying surface. Epithelial cells on body surfaces have specialized receptor proteins that can bind to adhesion proteins (called *adhesins*) on the surface of bacteria. In healthy subjects, epithelial cells in the mouth express receptors that bind harmless organisms (e.g., lactobacillus), but in seriously ill patients, the epithelial cells bind organisms that are more pathogenic. This change in bacterial adherence is a prelude to hospital-acquired infections. Bacterial adherence is an exciting field of study because manipulation of epithelial cell receptors could be used to prevent (colonization and) infection in seriously ill patients (38).

Oral Decontamination Regimen

Colonization of the oral mucosa with aerobic gram-negative bacilli can be viewed as a prelude to pneumonia because gram-negative aerobic organisms are the most common isolates in nosocomial pneumonia (see Chapter 41). This is the basis for a decontamination regimen that uses nonabsorbable antibiotics applied locally in the mouth. One regimen that has proven successful in ICU patients is shown on the next page (39,40):

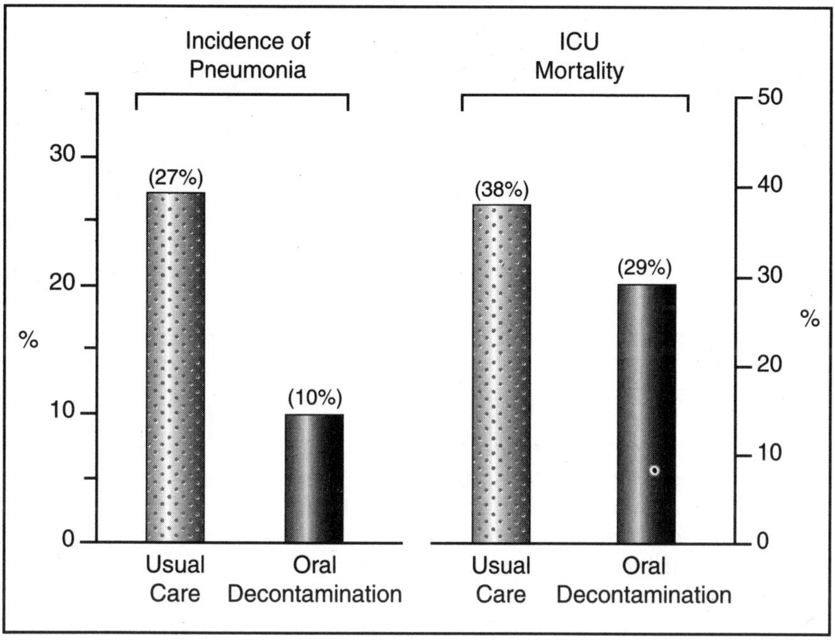

FIGURE 4.6 The effects of oral decontamination on the incidence of pneumonia and the mortality rate in a group of ventilator-dependent ICU patients. (From Bergmans C, Bonten M, Gaillard C, et al. Prevention of ventilator-associated pneumonia by oral decontamination. Am J Respir Crit Care Med 2001;164:382–388.)

Preparation: Have the pharmacy prepare a mixture of 2% gentamicin, 2% colistin, and 2% vancomycin as a paste.

Regimen: Apply paste to the buccal mucosa with a gloved finger every 6 hours until the patient is extubated.

This regimen will eradicate most aerobic bacteria and *Candida* species from the mouth in about one week. The clinical impact of this regimen on the incidence of pneumonia in the ICU is demonstrated in Figure 4.6. This data is from a study of ventilator-dependent patients (39), and oral decontamination reduced the incidence of pneumonia (from 27% to 10%) and the mortality rate (from 38% to 29%) in these patients. This represents a 60% reduction in acquired pneumonias and a 23% reduction in death rate that can be attributed to oral decontamination. A more recent study using the same decontamination regimen showed similar reductions in the incidence of pneumonia (40). Prolonged use of this locally applied antibiotic regimen has not resulted in the emergence of antibiotic-resistant organisms (39,40).

INDICATIONS. The success of oral decontamination in reducing the incidence of nosocomial pneumonia has prompted the Centers for Disease Control (CDC) to include a recommendation for oral decontamination in their updated guidelines on preventing pneumonia in health-care

TABLE 4.3 Conditions in the ICU that Might Benefit from Decontamination of the Alimentary Tract

Oral Decontamination	Selective Digestive Decontamination
1. Ventilator dependence for longer than 1 wk	1. After liver transplantation
2. Severely impaired lung function from any condition	2. Severe burn injuries
3. Increased risk of pulmonary aspiration from any condition	3. Recurrent septicemia of unknown origin
4. Recurrent pneumonia in the ICU	4. Neutropenia in the ICU that lasts 1 wk
	5. Postgastrectomy patients with a prolonged ICU stay

settings (41). Table 4.3 lists the conditions in the ICU that might benefit from oral decontamination. The patients who are best suited for this intervention are ventilator-dependent patients with severe respiratory impairment, because the chances of developing a pneumonia in the ICU is highest in these patients, and they are the least likely to tolerate the added insult of a lung infection.

Selective Digestive Decontamination

Selective digestive decontamination (SDD) is a more extensive version of oral decontamination that includes the entire alimentary tract. An example of a successful SDD regimen is shown below (42):

Oral cavity: A paste containing 2% polymyxin, 2% tobramycin, and 2% amphotericin is applied to the inside of the mouth with a gloved finger every 6 hours.

GI tract: A 10 mL solution containing 100 mg polymyxin E, 80 mg tobramycin, and 500 mg amphotericin is given via a nasogastric tube every 6 hours.

Systemic: Intravenous cefuroxime, 1.5 grams every 8 hours, for the first four days of therapy.

This regimen uses nonabsorbable antibiotics in the mouth and GI tract, and it will eradicate most gram-negative aerobic bacteria and yeasts after one week. The intravenous antibiotic provides systemic protection until the bowel regimen is fully effective at one week. Some SDD regimens do not include an intravenous antibiotic, but they are less successful (see later). The oral and GI components of SDD are continued until the patient is well enough to be discharged from the ICU. SDD is selective because it does not eliminate the normal inhabitants of the bowel. Preserving the normal microflora in the bowel is considered an important factor in preventing colonization with opportunistic pathogens.

The influence of SDD on the incidence of ICU-acquired infections is shown in Figure 4.7 (42). In this study, all three infections (pneumonia, urinary tract infections, and septicemia from vascular catheters) were

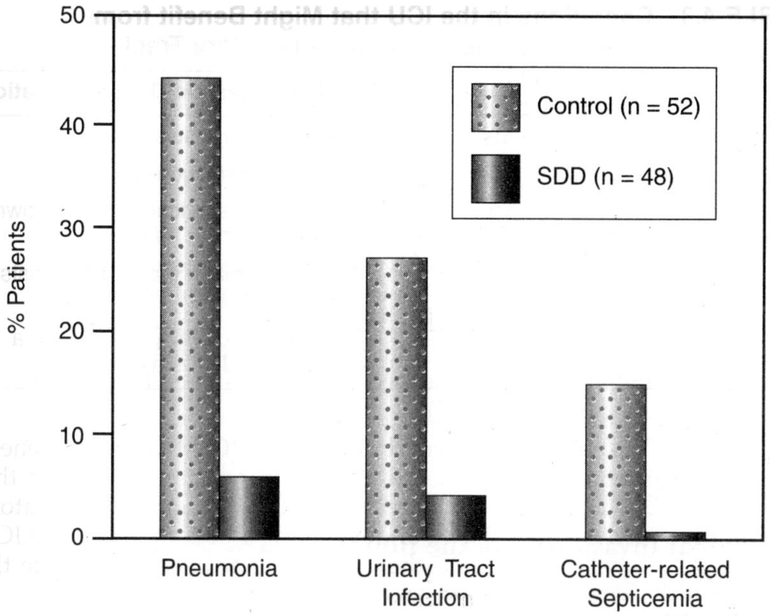

FIGURE 4.7 The effects of selective digestive decontamination (SDD) on the incidence of hospital-acquired infections in ICU patients. (From Ulrich C, Harinck-de Weerd JE, Bakker NC, et al. Intensive Care Med 1989;15:424.)

significantly less frequent in patients who received SDD. Similar results were reported in 10 other clinical trials of SDD, which showed a combined 40% relative reduction in the frequency of acquired infections in the ICU (43).

The Never-Ending Debate

Despite over 20 years of experience with SDD and numerous reports of its efficacy as an infection control measure, there is a continuing debate over the merits of this practice. Two concerns fuel this debate: the impact of SDD on mortality, and the possible emergence of antibiotic-resistant organisms. As for mortality, most of the early studies of SDD showed no reduction in mortality despite the decreased rate of infections. However, a recent large-scale study involving almost 1,000 ICU patients showed a relative 35% reduction in mortality in patients who received SDD (44). The recent study used an intravenous antibiotic for the first few days of treatment, while many of the early SDD regimens did not include an intravenous antibiotic, and this may explain the improved results of the most recent study.

As for the fear of antibiotic resistance, there is no evidence to support this fear (45). The debate over the merits of SDD seems to overlook one simple fact: the goal of SDD is to reduce hospital-acquired infections, and it achieves this goal consistently. Therefore, SDD must be considered an effective method of infection control in the ICU. The observation that lower incidences of hospital-acquired infections are not accompanied by a lower mortality is a separate issue and should not detract from the success of SDD in reducing acquired infections in the ICU. In fact, the notion that every therapy in the ICU has to save lives to be considered worthwhile is both unfocused and unreasonable.

Indications for SDD

The conditions that are most likely to benefit from SDD are listed in Table 4.3. SDD seems best suited for burn patients (because the incidence of translocation is particularly high in these patients) and following liver transplantation (because SDD reduces the risk of translocation, and this can counteract the diminished ability of the newly transplanted liver to clear organisms that have escaped the bowel lumen and entered the venous outflow from the bowel).

REFERENCES

Microbial Invasion from the Bowel

1. Simon GL, Gorbach SL. Intestinal microflora. Med Clin North Am 1982;66: 557–574.
2. Borriello SP. Microbial flora of the gastrointestinal tract. In: Microbial metabolism in the digestive tract. Boca Raton, FL: CRC Press, 1989:2–19.
3. Bengmark S. Gut microbial ecology in critical illness: is there a role for prebiotics, probiotics, and synbiotics? Curr Opin Crit Care 2002;8:145–151.
4. Langkamp-Henken B, Glezer JA, Kudsk KA. Immunologic structure and function of the gastrointestinal tract. Nutr Clin Pract 1992;7:100–108.
5. Howden CW, Hunt RH. Relationship between gastric secretion and infection. Gut 1987;28:96–107.
6. Wingate DL. Acid reduction and recurrent enteritis. Lancet 1990;335:222.
7. Cook GC. Infective gastroenteritis and its relationship to reduced acidity. Scand J Gastroenterol 1985;20(suppl 111):17–21.
8. Alexander JW, Boyce ST, Babcock GF, et al. The process of microbial translocation. Ann Surg 1990;212:496–510.
9. Cook DJ, Laine LA, Guyatt GH, et al. Nosocomial pneumonia and the role of gastric pH. Chest 1991;100:7–13.
10. Laheij R, Sturkenboom M, Hassing R-J, et al. Risk of community-acquired pneumonia and use of gastric acid-suppressive drugs. JAMA 2004;292:1955–1960.
11. Garvey BM, McCambley JA, Tuxen DV. Effects of gastric alkalization on bacterial colonization in critically ill patients. Crit Care Med 1989;17:211–216.

Stress-related Mucosal Injury

12. Steinberg KP. Stress-related mucosal disease in the critically ill patient: risk factors and strategies to prevent stress-related bleeding in the intensive care unit. Crit Care Med 2002;30(suppl):S362–S364.
13. Fennerty MB. Pathophysiology of the upper gastrointestinal tract in the critically ill patient: rationale for the therapeutic benefits of acid suppression. Crit Care Med 2002;30(suppl):S351–S355.

14. Muthu GM, Mutlu EA, Factor P. GI complications in patients receiving mechanical ventilation. Chest 2001;119:1222–1241.
15. Cook DJ, Fuller MB, Guyatt GH. Risk factors for gastrointestinal bleeding in critically ill patients. N Engl J Med 1994;330:377–381.
16. Marik PE. Sublingual capnography. a clinical validation study. Chest 2001; 120:923–927.
17. Kompan L, Kremzar B, Gadzijev E, et al. Effects of enteral nutrition on intestinal permeability and the development of multiple organ failure after multiple injury. Intensive Care Med 1999;25:157–161.
18. Raff T, Germann G, Hartmann B. The value of early enteral nutrition in the prophylaxis of stress ulceration in the severely burned patient. Burns 1997; 23:313–318.
19. Pingleton SK, Hadzima SK. Enteral alimentation and gastrointestinal bleeding in mechanically ventilated patients. Crit Care Med 1983;11:13–16.
20. McCarthy DM. Sucralfate. N Engl J Med 1990;325:1016–1025.
21. Cook DJ, Reeve BK, Guyatt GH. Stress ulcer prophylaxis in critically ill patients. JAMA 1996;275:308–314.
22. McEvoy GK, ed. AHFS drug information. Bethesda, MD: American Society of Health System Pharmacists, 1995:2021–2065.
23. Miller SJ, Simpson J. Medication–nutrient interactions: hypophosphatemia associated with sucralfate in the intensive care unit. Nutr Clin Pract 1991;6: 199–201.
24. Tryba M, Kurz-Muller K, Donner B. Plasma aluminum concentrations in long-term mechanically ventilated patients receiving stress ulcer prophylaxis with sucralfate. Crit Care Med 1994;22:1769–1773.
25. Daley RJ, Rebuck JA, Welage LS, et al. Prevention of stress ulceration: current trends in critical care. Crit Care Med 2004;32:2008–2013.
26. Morris DL, Markham SJ, Beechey A, et al. Ranitidine-bolus or infusion prophylaxis for stress ulcer. Crit Care Med 1988;16:229–232.
27. Famotidine. Mosby's Drug Consult. Mosby, 2005. Accessed at www.mdconsult.com on June 26, 2005.
28. Ranitidine. Mosby's Drug Consult. Mosby, 2005. Accessed at www.mdconsult.com. on June 26, 2005.
29. Cook D, Guyatt G, Marshall J, et al. A comparison of sucralfate and ranitidine for the prevention of upper gastrointestinal bleeding in patients requiring mechanical ventilation. N Engl J Med 1998;338:791–797.
30. Messori A, Trippoli S, Vaiani M, et al. Bleeding and pneumonia in intensive care patients given ranitidine and sucralfate for prevention of stress ulcer: meta-analysis of randomised controlled trials. Br Med J 2000;321:1–7.
31. Pisegna JR. Pharmacology of acid suppression in the hospital setting: focus on proton pump inhibition. Crit Care Med 2002;30(suppl):S356–S361.
32. Sharma VK, Vasudeva R, Howden CW. Simplified lansoprazole suspension: a liquid formulation of lansoprazole effectively suppresses intragastric acidity when administered through a gastrostomy. Am J Gastroenterol 1999;94: 1813–1817.
33. Morgan D. Intravenous proton pump inhibitors in the critical care setting. Crit Care Med 2002; 30(suppl):S369–S372.
34. Maier RV, Mitchell D, Gentiello L. Optimal therapy for stress gastritis. Ann Surg 1994;220:353–363.

35. Rosenthal P, Thompson J, Singh M. Detection of occult blood in gastric juice. J Clin Gastroenterol 1984;6:119.

Decontamination of the Alimentary Tract

36. Higuchi JH, Johanson WG. Colonization and bronchopulmonary infection. Clin Chest Med 1982;3:133–142.
37. Estes RJ, Meduri GU. The pathogenesis of ventilator-associated pneumonia, I: mechanisms of bacterial transcolonization and airway inoculation. Intensive Care Med 1995;21:365–383.
38. Rendell PM, Seger A, Rodrigues J, et al. Glycodendriproteins: a synthetic glycoprotein mimic enzyme with branched sugar-display potently inhibits bacterial aggregation. J Am Chem Soc 2004. Web-based journal accessed on June 26, 2005 at pubs.acs.org/cen/ news/8215/8215notw1.html
39. Bergmans C, Bonten M, Gaillard C, et al. Prevention of ventilator-associated pneumonia by oral decontamination. Am J Respir Crit Care Med 2001;164: 382–388.
40. van Nieuwenhoven CA, Buskens E, Bergmans DC, et al. Oral decontamination is cost-saving in the prevention of ventilator associated pneumonia in intensive care units. Crit Care Med 2004;32:126–130.
41. Centers for Disease Control and Prevention. Guidelines for preventing healthcare-associated pneumonia, 2003: recommendations of CDC and the Healthcare Infection Control Practices Advisory Committee. MMWR 2004; 53:1–40. Also available at http://www.cdc.gov/mmwr/PDF/rr/rr5303.pdf (Accessed June 19, 2005).
42. Stoutenbeek CP, van Saene HKF, Miranda DR, et al. The effect of selective decontamination of the digestive tract on colonization and infection rate in multiple trauma patients. Intensive Care Med 1984;10:185–192.
43. D'Amico R, Pifferi S, Leonetti C, et al. Effectiveness of antibiotic prophylaxis in critically ill adult patients: a systematic review of randomised controlled trials. Br Med J 1998;316:1275–1285.
44. de Jonge E, Schultz MJ, Spanjaard L, et al. Effects of selective decontamination of digestive tract on mortality and acquisition of resistant bacteria in intensive care: a randomized controlled trial. Lancet 2003;362:1011–1016.
45. Krueger WA, Unertl KE. Selective decontamination of the digestive tract. Curr Opin Crit Care 2002;8:139–144.

Chapter 5

VENOUS THROMBO-EMBOLISM

Two words best characterize the mortality and morbidity due to venous thromboembolism in the United States: substantial and unacceptable.

Kenneth M. Moser, MD

The threat of venous thrombosis and acute pulmonary embolism (i.e., venous thromboembolism) is a daily concern in the ICU. Several conditions promote venous thrombosis in ICU patients (1–4). These thrombi usually form in proximal leg veins and are often clinically silent, becoming evident only when a portion of the thrombus breaks loose and travels to the lungs to become a pulmonary embolus. This progression from silent thrombosis in the legs to acute pulmonary embolism is believed to be responsible for 10% of all hospital deaths (5) and, because it is possible to prevent thrombus formation in the legs (3,5–7), deaths from pulmonary emboli are considered preventable. In fact, pulmonary embolism is one of the leading causes of preventable deaths in hospitalized patients (5).

The principal goal in the approach to venous thromboembolism is to prevent unnecessary deaths from pulmonary embolism. This is best accomplished by preventing thrombus formation (thromboprophylaxis) in proximal leg veins. The importance of thromboprophylaxis in preventing unnecessary hospital deaths has been emphasized by the Agency for Healthcare Research and Quality, who issued a report stating that **prophylaxis for venous thromboembolism is the single most important measure for ensuring patient safety in hospitalized patients** (8).

This chapter presents the current practices for preventing venous thromboembolism in hospitalized patients. Sections also are included on the diagnostic and therapeutic approaches to suspected or documented thromboembolism. Some useful clinical practice guidelines (5–7) are included in the bibliography at the end of the chapter.

PATIENTS AT RISK

There are several factors that promote venous thromboembolism (VTE) in hospitalized patients, and the major ones are listed in Table 5.1 (1–3). These risk factors are responsible for the prevalence of VTE in the clinical groupings shown in Figure 5.1. (The high prevalence of VTE in this figure is an exaggeration of the problem because these rates include asymptomatic cases of VTE that may have no clinical consequence). VTE is most prevalent in three clinical conditions: major surgery (particularly if it is cancer-related or involves the hip or knee), acute stroke, and major trauma (especially spinal cord injury).

Major Surgery

Autopsy studies of surgery patients who die in the hospital reveal pulmonary emboli in up to 30% of cases, and about 30% of these emboli are the direct cause of death (9). There are several factors that predispose to VTE after major surgery, but the most important are vascular injury (in orthopedic procedures) and a generalized hypercoagulable state caused by thromboplastin release during surgery. Patient-specific factors (e.g., increasing age over 40, prior history of VTE) add further to the risk of postoperative VTE.

TABLE 5.1 Risk Factors for Venous Thromboembolism in Hospitalized Patients

Surgery
Major surgery: abdominal, gynecologic, urologic, orthopedic, neurosurgery, cancer-related surgery
Trauma
Multisystem trauma, spinal cord injury, spinal fracture, fractures of the hip and pelvis
Malignancy
Any malgnancy, overt or covert, local or metastatic. Risk higher during chemotherapy and radiotherapy
Acute medical illness
Stroke, acute myocardial infarction, heart failure, neuromuscular weakness syndromes (e.g., Guillain-Barre)
Patient-specific factors
History of thromboembolism, obesity, increasing age older than 40, hypercoagulable state (e.g., estrogen therapy)
ICU-related factors
Prolonged mechanical ventilation, neuromuscular paralysis (drug-induced), central venous catheters, severe sepsis, consumptive coagulopathy, heparin-induced thrombocytopenia

From References 2, 3 and 5.

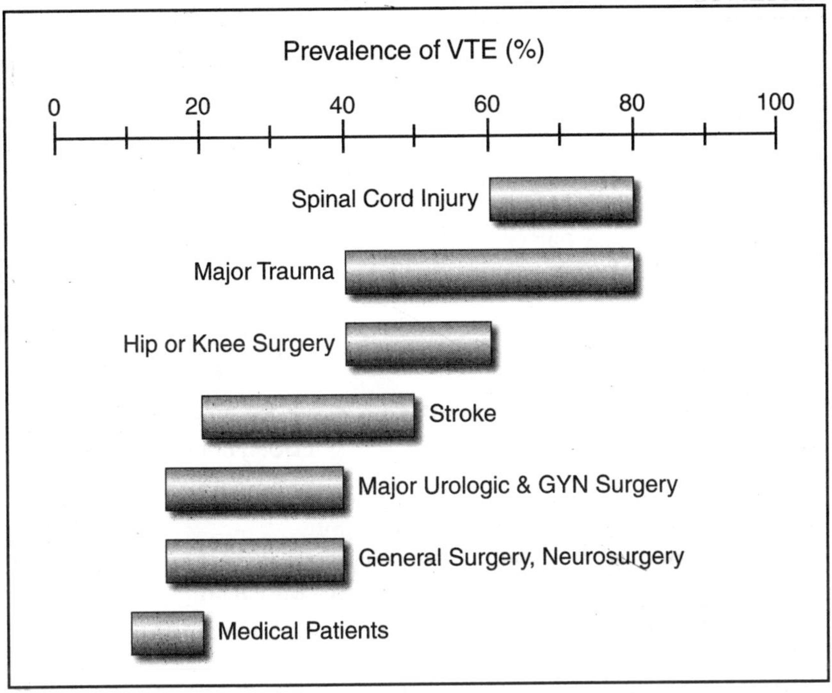

FIGURE 5.1 The prevalence of thromboembolism in different groups of hospitalized patients. From Geerts WH, Pineo GF, Heit JA, et al. Prevention of venous thromboembolism: the Seventh ACCP Conference on Antithrombotic and Thrombolytic Therapy. Chest 2004;126:338S.

General Surgery

The risk of VTE after general surgery is determined by 3 factors: the type of procedure (e.g., major vs. minor procedure, cancer-related surgery), the age of the patient, and the presence of other patient-specific risk factors (e.g., malignancy, obesity, prior history of VTE) (3,5). These factors are combined in the risk stratification system shown in Table 5.2. The lowest risk of VTE occurs after minor procedures performed on young patients (<40 years of age) who have no other risk factors for VTE. No special preventive measures are required in these patients (5). The highest risk of VTE occurs after major surgery in older patients (>40 years of age) who have one or more risk factors for VTE. The effective methods of thromboprophylaxis for these patients are shown in Table 5.2 and will be described later in the chapter.

Orthopedic Surgery

The highest incidence of postoperative VTE (40 to 60%) occurs after major orthopedic procedures involving the hip and knee. Table 5.3 shows the high-risk procedures and the recommended methods of

TABLE 5.2 Thromboprophylaxis for General Surgery

Risk Categories‡	Recommended Prophylaxis†
I. *Low risk*	
Minor surgery + age <40 yr and no other risk factors	Early mobilization only
II. *Moderate risk*	
Major surgery + age <40 yr and no other risk factors	$LDUH_1$ or $LMWH_1$: First dose 2 hr before surgery
III. *High risk*	
Major surgery + age >40 yr or other risk factors	$LDUH_2$ or $LMWH_2$: First dose 2 hr before surgery
IV. *Highest risk*	
Major surgery + age >40 yr and other risk factors	$LDUH_2$ or $LMWH_2$ as above plus mechanical aid

Prophylaxis Regimens

$LDUH_1$: Unfractionated heparin, 5,000 units SC every 12 hr

$LDUH_2$: Unfractionated heparin, 5,000 units SC every 8 hr

$LMWH_1$: Enoxaparin, 40 mg SC once daily, or dalteparin, 2,500 units SC once daily

$LMWH_2$: Enoxaparin, 30 mg SC every 12 hr, or dalteparin, 5,000 units SC once daily

Mechanical aid: graded compression stockings or intermittent pneumatic compression

‡Minor surgery: performed under local or spinal anesthesia and lasts <30 min; major surgery: performed under general anesthesia and lasts >30 min; other risk factors: cancer, obesity, history of thromboembolism, estrogen Rx or other hypercoagulable state.
LDUH: low-dose unfractionated heparin; LMWH: low-molecular-weight heparin; GCS: graded compression stockings; IPC: intermittent pneumatic compression, SC: subcutaneous.
†Adapted from Reference 5.

thromboprophylaxis. Arthroscopy alone does not carry a high risk of VTE and does not require thromboprophylaxis (5).

Other Surgeries

The other types of major surgery that have a moderate-to-high risk of VTE are listed in Table 5.4. Missing from this list are **laparoscopy, vascular surgery, and closed urologic procedures** (e.g., transurethral prostatectomy). These procedures **have a low risk of VTE**, and thromboprophylaxis is not required unless the patient has one or more of the risk factors for VTE in Table 5.1 (5).

Major Trauma

Major trauma shares the same predisposing factors for VTE as major surgery (which is a form of controlled trauma) (2,3,5). Victims of major

TABLE 5.3 Thromboprophylaxis for Hip and Knee Surgery

Procedures

Elective hip and knee arthroplasty, hip fracture surgery

Drug regimens

Use any of the following:

1. LMWH: Enoxaparin, 30 mg SC every 12 hr, or dalteparin, 2,500 units SC as first dose, then 5,000 units SC once daily. Give first dose 12–24 hr before surgery or 6 hr after surgery.
2. Fondaparinux, 2.5 mg SC once daily. First dose 6–8 hr after surgery (may be the preferred regimen for hip fracture surgery).
3. Adjusted-dose warfarin to achieve INR of 2.0 to 3.0. Give first dose the evening before surgery.

Duration

A. For elective hip and knee surgery, prophylaxis should continue for 10 days after surgery.

B. For hip fracture surgery, prophylaxis should continue for 28 to 35 days after surgery.

LMWH: low-molecular-weight heparin; SC: subcutaneous.
Adapted from Reference 5.

trauma have a greater than 50% chance of developing VTE while hospitalized, and pulmonary embolism is the leading cause of death in those who survive the first week (5). The trauma conditions with the highest risk of VTE are spinal cord injuries, spinal fractures, and fractures of the pelvis (3,5).

Acute Medical Illness

Patients with acute medical illnesses (other than stroke) have a much lower risk of developing VTE than their comrades in the surgery and trauma wards (see Figure 5.1). Despite the relatively low incidence of VTE in medical patients, autopsy studies show that **a majority of deaths due to pulmonary embolism occur in medical patients** (10). This tendency for VTE to be life threatening in medical patients is reason not to overlook the importance of thromboprophylaxis in this patient population.

The ICU Patient

The typical ICU patient has several risk factors for VTE. Some are present on admission (e.g., advanced age, malignancy, major surgery, and major trauma), and some are acquired while in the ICU (e.g., prolonged mechanical ventilation, central venous catheters). Because of this multitude of risk factors, most patients who stay in the ICU more than a few days are considered candidates for thromboprophylaxis. Unfortunately, as many as one of every four ICU patients will continue to have evidence

TABLE 5.4 Thromboprophylaxis for Other Clinical Conditions

Clinical Situation	Recommended Prophylaxis
1. Major trauma	1. $LMWH_2$ or leg compression (IPC)
2. Spinal cord injury	2. $LMWH_2$ plus leg compression
3. Intracranial surgery	3. Leg compression (IPC)
4. Gynecologic surgery	
a. Benign disease	4a. $LDUH_1$
b. Malignancy	4b. $LDUH_2$ or $LMWH_2$
5. Urologic surgery	
a. Closed procedures	5a. Early mobilization only
b. Open procedures	5b. $LDUH_1$ or leg compression (IPC)
6. High-risk medical illness	6. $LDUH_1$ or $LMWH_1$

Prophylaxis Regimens

$LDUH_1$: Unfractionated heparin, 5,000 units SC every 12 hr

$LDUH_2$: Unfractionated heparin, 5,000 units SC every 8 hr

$LMWH_1$: Enoxaparin, 40 mg SC once daily, or dalteparin, 2,500 units SC once daily

$LMWH_2$: Enoxaparin, 30 mg SC every 12 hr, or dalteparin, 5,000 units SC once daily

Leg-compression methods: graded compression stockings (GCS) or intermittent pneumatic compression (IPC)

LDUH: low-dose unfractionated heparin; LMWH: low-molecular-weight heparin; SC: subcutaneous.
From Reference 5.

of deep vein thrombosis (usually asymptomatic) despite appropriate thromboprophylaxis (11,12).

METHODS OF THROMBOPROPHYLAXIS

A number of interventions have proven effective in reducing the incidence of thromboembolism in hospitalized patients (3–6). These include both mechanical and pharmacologic methods of thromboprophylaxis.

External Leg Compression

There are two external compression devices for the legs: graded compression stockings and intermittent pneumatic compression pumps. These devices can be used as an adjunct to anticoagulant prophylaxis or as a replacement for anticoagulant prophylaxis in patients who are bleeding or have a high risk of bleeding.

Graded Compression Stockings

Graded compression stockings (also known as thromboembolism deterrent or TED stockings) are designed to create 18 mm Hg external pressure at the ankles and 8 mm Hg external pressure in the thigh (13). The resulting 10 mm Hg pressure gradient acts as a driving force for venous outflow from the legs. These stockings have been shown to reduce the incidence of VTE when used alone after abdominal surgery and neurosurgery (14,15). However, this is considered the least effective method of thromboprophylaxis, and it is almost never used alone in patients with a moderate or high risk of VTE.

Intermittent Pneumatic Compression

Intermittent pneumatic compression (IPC) pumps are inflatable bladders that are wrapped around the lower leg. When inflated, they create 35 mm Hg external compression at the ankle and 20 mm Hg external compression at the thigh (13). These devices also create a pumping action by inflating and deflating at regular intervals, and this acts to further augment venous flow. Intermittent pneumatic compression is considered more effective than graded compression stockings for thromboprophylaxis (5), and this method can be used alone for selected patients who are not suitable for anticoagulant prophylaxis because of bleeding. This method is particularly popular after intracranial surgery (Table 5.4) and in trauma victims who are at risk for bleeding.

Low-Dose Unfractionated Heparin

The standard heparin preparation is a heterogeneous collection of mucopolysaccharide molecules that can vary in size by a factor of 10 or more. The anticoagulant activity is dependent on the size of the heparin molecule (smaller molecules have greater anticoagulant activity), so the variable size of the molecules in the standard or *unfractionated* heparin (UFH) preparation means that these preparations will have variable anticoagulant activity. In general, only one third or fewer of the molecules have anticoagulant activity (6,7).

Rationale for Low-Dose Heparin

Heparin is an indirect-acting drug that must bind to a cofactor (antithrombin III or AT) to produce its effect. The heparin-AT complex is capable of inactivating several coagulation factors, including factors IIa (thrombin), IXa, Xa, XIa, and XIIa (6). The inactivation of factor II_a (antithrombin effect) is a sensitive reaction and occurs at heparin doses far below those needed to inactivate the other coagulation factors (6). This means that **small doses of heparin can inhibit thrombus formation** (antithrombin effect), **without producing full anticoagulation** (because the other coagulation factors are unaffected). This is the basis for the effect of low-dose heparin in preventing venous thrombosis in high-risk hospitalized patients.

The heparin-AT complex also binds to platelet factor 4, and some patients develop a heparin-induced antibody that can cross-react with this platelet binding site to produce platelet clumping and subsequent thrombocytopenia. This is the mechanism for heparin-induced thrombocytopenia, and it can be triggered by low-dose heparin as well as therapeutic-dose heparin (4,6). (See Chapter 37 for more information on heparin-induced thrombocytopenia.)

Dosing Regimen

The regimen for low-dose unfractionated heparin (LDUH) is **5,000 Units given by subcutaneous injection twice or three times daily**. More frequent (3 times daily) dosing is recommended for higher risk conditions (see the $LDUH_2$ regimen in Tables 5.2 and 5.4). When LDUH is used for surgical prophylaxis, the first dose should be given 2 hours before the procedure. Pre-surgical dosing is recommended because thrombosis can begin during the procedure, and allowing time for the thrombus to grow will reduce the anticoagulant effect of heparin. Postoperative prophylaxis is continued for 7 to 10 days, or until the patient is fully ambulatory. Monitoring laboratory tests of coagulation is not necessary.

Who Benefits

Low-dose unfractionated heparin (LDUH) provides effective thromboprophylaxis for high-risk medical conditions and most non-orthopedic surgical procedures (see Tables 5.2 and 5.4) (3,5). It does not provide optimal prophylaxis for major trauma (including spinal cord injury) and for orthopedic surgery involving the hip and knee. These conditions benefit more from a special preparation of heparin described next.

Low-Molecular-Weight Heparin

The variable-sized heparin molecules in unfractionated heparin can be cleaved enzymatically to produce smaller molecules of more uniform size. Because smaller heparin molecules have more anticoagulant activity, the resultant **low-molecular-weight heparin (LMWH) is more potent and has more uniform anticoagulant activity than UFH**. LMWH has several potential advantages over unfractionated heparin, including less frequent dosing, a lower risk of both bleeding and heparin-induced thrombocytopenia, and no need for routine anticoagulant monitoring with full anticoagulant dosing (this is described later in the chapter) (4,6). The disadvantage of LMWH is the cost: LMWH can be 10 times more costly (per day) than unfractionated heparin (16–18).

Who Benefits

LMWH is more effective than unfractionated heparin for orthopedic procedures involving the hip and knee, and for major trauma, including spinal cord injury (5).

Low-Dose Regimens

There are currently seven LMWH preparations available for clinical use, but only two have been studied extensively for thromboprophylaxis:

enoxaparin (Lovenox) and **dalteparin** (Fragmin). Enoxaparin was the first LMWH approved for use in the United States (in 1993), and the clinical experience with this drug is the most extensive.

The recommended doses of enoxaparin and dalteparin for thromboprophylaxis are shown in Tables 5.2–5.4 (see $LMWH_1$ and $LMWH_2$). Both drugs are given by subcutaneous injection. **Enoxaparin is given once daily (40 mg) for moderate-risk conditions, and twice daily (30 mg in each dose) for high-risk conditions** (3–6,17). Dalteparin is given once daily in a dose of 2,500 units for moderate-risk conditions and 5,000 units for high-risk conditions (3–6,18).

TIMING. For non-orthopedic surgery, the first dose of each drug (30 mg for enoxaparin, 2,500 U for dalteparin) should be given 2 hrs before surgery (5). For orthopedic procedures, the first dose of each drug has traditionally been given 12–24 hours before surgery. However, preoperative drug administration can increase bleeding in orthopedic procedures and may offer no added protection, so **preoperative dosing may be abandoned in favor of starting prophylaxis 6 hours after surgery** (waiting longer reduces efficacy) (19).

SPINAL ANESTHESIA. The use of **LMWH in conjunction with spinal anesthesia for orthopedic surgery can result in a spinal hematoma and paralysis** (17–19). When spinal anesthesia is used for an orthopedic procedure, the first dose of LMWH should be delayed until 12 to 24 hours after surgery (19), or adjusted-dose warfarin should be used for thromboprophylaxis.

RENAL FAILURE. LMWHs are excreted primarily by the kidneys, although the extent of renal clearance differs for individual agents. For patients with renal failure, the prophylactic dose of enoxaparin should be decreased from 30 mg twice daily to 40 mg once daily for high-risk patients (5). No dose adjustment is recommended for dalteparin (18).

Adjusted-Dose Warfarin

Systemic anticoagulation with warfarin (Coumadin; Bristol-Meyers Squibb) is a popular method of prophylaxis for major orthopedic surgery. There are two benefits with warfarin: the preoperative dose does not create a bleeding tendency during surgery because of the delayed onset of action with vitamin K antagonists, and warfarin can be continued after discharge if prolonged prophylaxis is required (see later). The disadvantages of warfarin prophylaxis include a multitude of drug interactions (20), the need to monitor laboratory tests of coagulation, and difficulty adjusting doses to the desired effect because of the delayed onset of action.

Dosing Regimen

The initial dose of warfarin is 10 mg orally, given the evening before surgery. This is followed by a daily dose of 2.5 mg, starting the evening after surgery. The dosage is then adjusted to achieve a prothrombin time with an international normalized ratio (INR) of 2 to 3 (5). This is usually not reached until at least the third postoperative day.

Who Benefits

Adjusted-dose warfarin is one of three effective regimens for major orthopedic procedures involving the hip and knee (see Table 5.3) (5). It is the most popular prophylactic regimen for hip replacement surgery in North America, despite evidence that LMWH is more effective (5). Warfarin may be preferred in patients who require prolonged prophylaxis after hospital discharge (see later) because of the convenience of oral dosing.

Fondaparinux

Fondaparinux (Arixtra; GlaxoSmithKline) is a synthetic anticoagulant that selectively inhibits coagulation factor Xa. Like heparin, it must bind to antithrombin III to exert its anticoagulant effect but, unlike heparin, it only inhibits the activity of factor Xa. The benefits of fondaparinux are a predictable anticoagulant effect (thus obviating the need for laboratory monitoring) and the absence of a heparin-like, immune-mediated thrombocytopenia (4,21).

Dosing Regimen

The prophylactic dose of fondaparinux is **2.5 mg given once daily as a subcutaneous injection.** When used for surgical prophylaxis, the first dose should be given 6 to 8 hours after surgery (if given sooner, there's an increased risk of bleeding) (5). The drug is cleared by the kidney, and, when creatinine clearance is <30 mL/min, drug accumulation and bleeding can occur (21). Therefore the drug is **contraindicated in patients with severe renal impairment** (creatinine clearance <30 mL/min) (22). It also is **contraindicated in patients who weigh <50 kg** because of a marked increase in bleeding in these patients (22).

Who Benefits

Fondaparinux is as effective as LMWH for thromboprophylaxis after major orthopedic surgery involving the hip and knee (5). The only advantage of fondaparinux over LMWH is the absent risk of heparin-induced thrombocytopenia.

Duration of Prophylaxis

Following major orthopedic procedures involving the hip and knee, there is an increase in symptomatic VTE after prophylaxis is terminated and patients are discharged from the hospital, and symptomatic VTE is the most common cause of readmission after hip replacement surgery (5). These observations prompted the following recommendations: 1) thromboprophylaxis should be continued for at least 10 days following major orthopedic surgery, even if patients are discharged before this time (5), and 2) **following hip surgery, patients with additional risk factors for VTE** (e.g., malignancy, advanced age, prior history of VTE), **should receive prophylaxis for a total of 28 to 35 days** (5). Post-discharge thromboprophylaxis can be achieved with usual prophylactic doses of warfarin, LMWH, or fondaparinux (the latter two agents require subcutaneous injections, which may be a problem in some outpatients).

DIAGNOSTIC APPROACH TO THROMBOEMBOLISM

As mentioned earlier, thrombosis in the deep veins of the legs is often clinically silent, and becomes evident only when a pulmonary embolus occurs. Therefore, the diagnostic evaluation of symptomatic thromboembolism usually involves cases of suspected acute pulmonary embolism.

The Clinical Evaluation

The clinical presentation of acute pulmonary embolism is non-specific, and there are **no clinical or laboratory findings that will confirm or exclude the diagnosis of pulmonary embolism** (23). The predictive value of clinical and laboratory findings in acute pulmonary embolism is shown in Table 5.5. Note that none of the findings provides more than a 50% chance of identifying pulmonary embolism when present, and none is able to absolutely exclude the presence of pulmonary embolism when absent (a normal test must have a predictive value of 98% or greater to reliably exclude the diagnosis). Note also that hypoxemia has a negative predictive value of 70%, which means that 30% of patients with acute pulmonary embolism are not hypoxemic. Although not included in

TABLE 5.5 Clinical and Laboratory Findings in Patients with Suspected Pulmonary Embolism

Findings	Positive Predictive Value	Negative Predictive Value
Dyspnea	37%	75%
Tachycardia	47%	86%
Tachypnea	48%	75%
Pleuritic chest pain	39%	71%
Hemoptysis	32%	67%
Hypoxemia	34%	70%
Elevated plasma D-dimer[a]	27%	92%
Increased dead-space ventilation[b]	36%	92%

Positive predictive value: the percentage of patients with the findings who had a pulmonary embolus. It expresses the likelihood that a pulmonary embolus is present when the finding is present; negative predictive value: the percentage of patients without the finding who did not have a pulmonary embolus. It expresses the likelihood that a pulmonary embolus is not present when the finding is also not present.

[a]From Reference 26.

[b]From Reference 27. Other data from Reference 23.

Table 5.5, a normal alveolar–arterial PO_2 gradient likewise does not exclude the presence of acute pulmonary embolism (24).

Plasma D-Dimer Levels

Cross-linked fibrin monomers, also called *fibrin D-dimers* or simply *D-dimers*, are products of clot lysis and are expected to be elevated in the setting of active thrombosis. Although popular in the emergency department, plasma D-dimer assays have little value in the evaluation of thromboembolism in the ICU. The problem is the multitude of other conditions that can elevate plasma D-dimer levels, including sepsis, malignancy, pregnancy, heart failure, renal failure, and advanced age (25). As a result, **a majority (up to 80%) of ICU patients have elevated plasma D-dimer levels in the absence of venous thromboembolism** (26). This is reflected in the poor positive predictive value shown in Table 5.5.

Plasma D-dimer levels may be more valuable for excluding the diagnosis of venous thromboembolism. In ICU patients, the negative predictive value of a normal plasma D-dimer level is 92% (see Table 5.5), which means that when the plasma D-dimer level is not elevated, 92% of the patients will not have venous thromboembolism. However, since only a small percentage of ICU patients have normal plasma D-dimer levels, the value of a normal test result is limited.

Alveolar Dead Space

The cardiopulmonary consequences of pulmonary emboli include a decrease in pulmonary blood flow leading to an increase in alveolar dead space ventilation (see Chapter 19 for a description of dead space ventilation). In patients who present to the emergency room with suspected pulmonary embolism, **a normal dead space measurement (i.e., < 15% of total ventilation) has a high predictive value for excluding the diagnosis of pulmonary embolism** (see the negative predictive value of 92% in Table 5.5) (27). Adding a normal plasma D-dimer level to a normal dead space measurement adds further to the predictive power for excluding pulmonary embolism (27).

The value of the dead space measurement has not been studied in ICU patients. Most patients in the ICU are expected to have elevated dead space ventilation (from cardiopulmonary disease), so a normal measurement might be too infrequent to be useful. Monitoring for *changes* in dead space ventilation (which is easily done in ventilator-dependent patients) might be more useful for evaluating patients who develop respiratory distress while in the ICU.

Venous Ultrasound

Because the clinical evaluation of suspected pulmonary embolism will not confirm or exclude the diagnosis, specialized tests are required. These tests are included in the flow diagram in Figure 5.2.

Since most pulmonary emboli originate from thrombosis in proximal leg veins (28), the evaluation of suspected pulmonary embolism

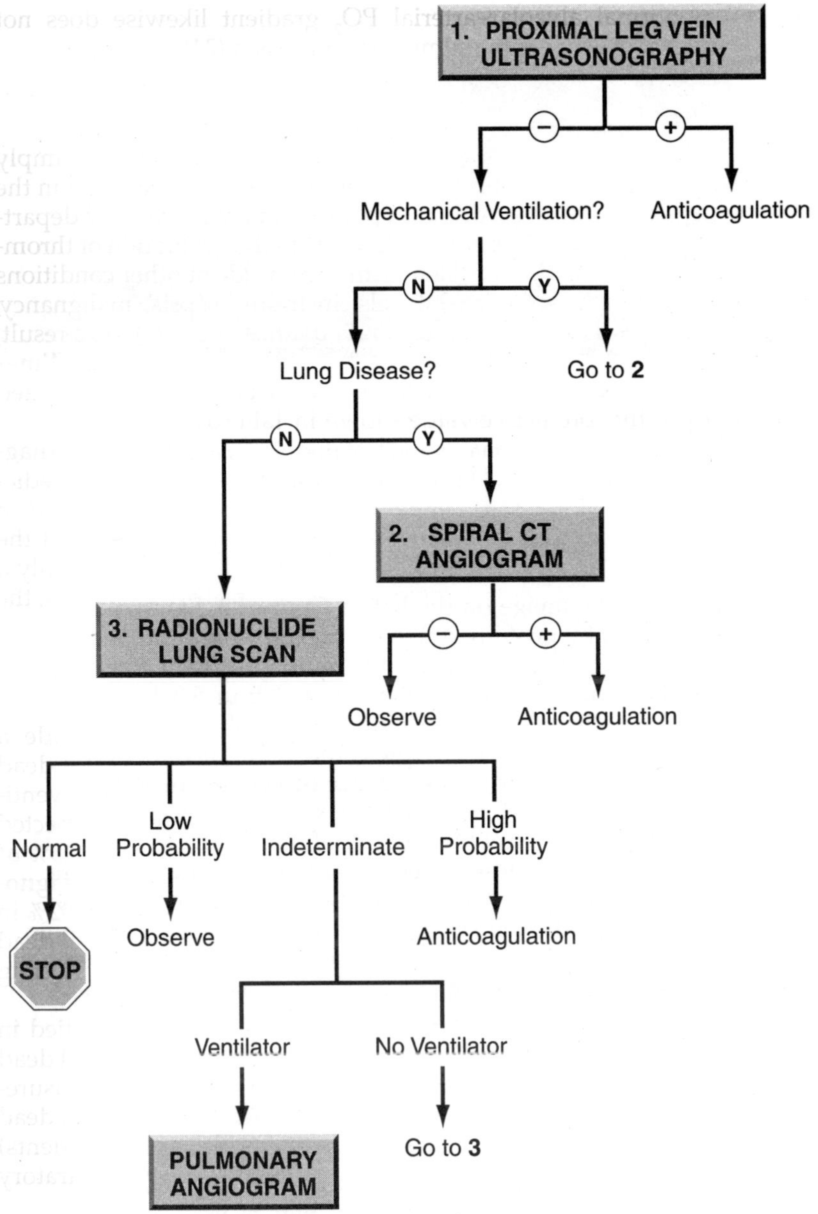

FIGURE 5.2 Flow diagram for the evaluation of suspected pulmonary embolism.

often begins with an ultrasound evaluation of the femoral veins. Two complementary techniques are combined for the ultrasound detection of venous thrombosis. One of these techniques is *compression ultrasound*. This method uses two-dimensional brightness modulation (B-mode) ultrasound to obtain a cross-sectional view of the femoral artery and

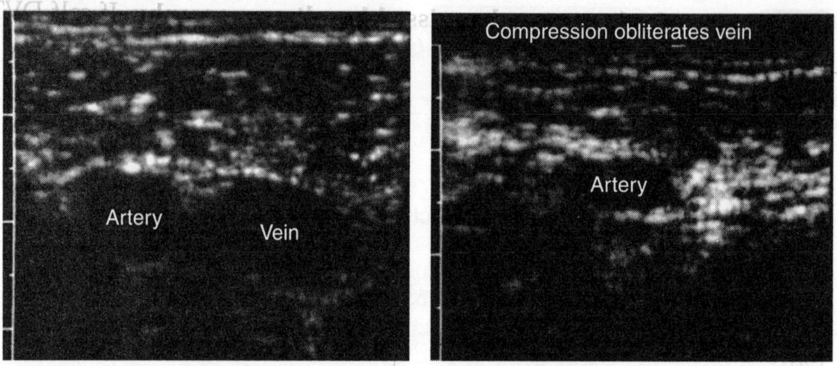

FIGURE 5.3 Ultrasound images showing a transverse view of the femoral artery and vein (image on the left) and obliteration of the femoral vein by compression of the overlying skin (image on the right). (From Cronan J, Murphy T. A comprehensive review of vascular ultrasound for intensivists. J Intensive Care Med 1993;8:188, with permission.) Images digitally retouched.

vein, as shown in the image on the left in Figure 5.3. External compression is then applied by pushing down on the ultrasound probe to indent the skin. This will normally compress the underlying vein and obliterate its lumen, as shown in the image on the right in Figure 5.3. When a vein is filled with blood clots (which are usually not visualized by ultrasound), external compression does not compress the vein. Therefore **an incompressible vein is used as indirect evidence of venous thrombosis** (29).

The other technique is *Doppler ultrasound,* which relies on the well-known Doppler shift to detect the velocity of blood flow in vessels. Flow velocity can be recorded audibly (the faster the flow, the higher the frequency of the Doppler signal) or by color changes (faster flows cause a shift from the blue to the red spectrum of light). Doppler ultrasound is valuable for distinguishing arteries from veins and can also detect sluggish flow in veins (a possible sign of partial occlusion by thrombi). The combination of compression and Doppler ultrasound is known as *duplex ultrasound.*

Accuracy

For the detection of deep vain thrombosis (DVT) in the thigh (proximal DVT), duplex ultrasound has a sensitivity of 95% to 100% a specificity of 97 to 100%, a positive predictive value as high as 97%, and a negative predictive value as high as 98% (29). These numbers show that duplex ultrasound is highly accurate and reliable for the detection of proximal DVT in the legs.

Unlike its performance for proximal DVT, duplex ultrasound does not perform well for the detection of venous thrombosis below the knee (calf DVT). For the detection of calf DVT, ultrasound has a sensitivity of only 33% to 70% (2). This means that **as many as two-thirds of cases of**

DVT below the knees can be missed by ultrasonography. If calf DVT is suspected because of symptoms (pain, swelling, etc.) and ultrasound is unrevealing, one option is to follow with serial ultrasound examinations (as long as the thrombus does not propagate to above the knee, there is little risk of pulmonary embolism), and the other is to perform contrast venography.

Leg DVT and Pulmonary Embolism

Despite the consensus view that most pulmonary emboli originate from proximal DVT in the legs, as many as 30% of patients with acute pulmonary embolism show no evidence of venous thrombosis in the legs (30). As a result, **a negative evaluation for proximal DVT in the legs does not exclude the diagnosis of acute pulmonary embolus**. When the search for leg vein thrombosis is unrevealing and the clinical suspicion of pulmonary embolism is high, the next step in the evaluation is either spiral computed tomography (CT) or a radionuclide lung scan. As shown in Figure 5.2, the procedure that is most appropriate is determined by the presence of mechanical ventilation and the presence of lung disease.

Radionuclide Lung Scan

Ventilation-perfusion lung scans are widely used in the evaluation of suspected pulmonary embolism, but they secure the diagnosis in only about 25% to 30% of cases (31). The problem is that the presence of lung disease (particularly infiltrative disease) will produce an abnormal scan in about 90% of cases (31). Lung scans are most helpful in patients with no underlying lung disease (which, unfortunately, excludes most ICU patients). If the decision is made to proceed with a lung scan, the results can be used as follows (31):

A *normal* lung scan excludes the presence of a (clinically important) pulmonary embolus, whereas a high-probability lung scan carries a 90% probability that a pulmonary embolus is present.

A *low-probability* lung scan does not reliably exclude the presence of a pulmonary embolism. However, when combined with a negative ultrasound evaluation of the legs, a low-probability scan is sufficient reason to stop the diagnostic workup and observe the patient.

An *intermediate-probability* or *indeterminate* lung scan has no value in predicting the presence or absence of a pulmonary embolus. In this situation, the options include spiral CT angiography (see next) or conventional pulmonary angiography.

Spiral CT Angiography

Spiral (helical) computed tomography (spiral CT) is a technique where the detector is rotated around the patient to produce a volumetric two-dimensional view of the lungs (32). (This differs from conventional CT,

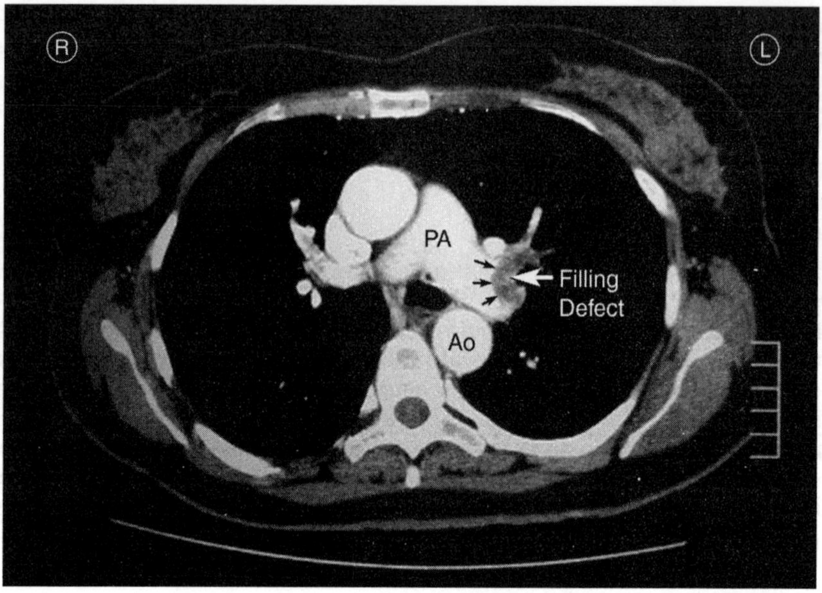

FIGURE 5.4 Spiral CT angiogram showing a pulmonary embolus (filling defect) in the left main pulmonary artery. PA = pulmonary artery; AO = aorta. Image digitally retouched.

where the detector is moved in increments along the thorax to create two-dimensional "slices" of the lungs.) This procedure is completed in about 30 seconds. There must be no lung motion during the procedure, which means that **patients must be able to breath-hold for 30 seconds** to perform a spiral CT scan (32). This excludes patients who are ventilator-dependent or are unable to follow commands. Spiral CT has been performed on a few ventilator-dependent patients using continuous positive airways pressure (CPAP) combined with heavy sedation to inhibit chest wall movements (33), but the safety and reliability of this approach has not been validated in large numbers of patients.

When spiral CT is combined with peripheral injection of a contrast agent, the central pulmonary arteries can be visualized. A pulmonary embolus appears as a filling defect, as shown in Figure 5.4. Spiral CT angiography is best suited for detecting clots in the main pulmonary arteries, where the sensitivity and specificity are 93% and 97%, respectively (34). Unfortunately, as many as 70% of emboli in smaller, subsegmental vessels can be missed with this technique (34). However, the importance of detecting smaller, subsegmental emboli is questionable because withholding anticoagulant therapy based on a negative CT scan does not seem to adversely affect clinical outcomes (35).

Spiral CT is gaining popularity in the evaluation of suspected pulmonary embolism. It is most valuable in patients who have lung disease (see Figure 5.2), because lung scans are often non-diagnostic in these patients. Its value in the ICU is limited by the difficulty of performing the procedure in ventilator-dependent patients.

Pulmonary Angiography

Pulmonary angiography, still considered the most accurate method for detecting pulmonary emboli, is performed in fewer than 15% of cases of suspected pulmonary embolism (36). Considering the array of other diagnostic modalities, the low rate of pulmonary angiography seems justified.

ANTITHROMBOTIC THERAPY

Anticoagulation

The initial treatment of thromboembolism that is not life-threatening is anticoagulation with heparin.

Unfractionated Heparin

The standard treatment of both deep vein thrombosis and acute pulmonary embolism is unfractionated heparin (UFH) given by continuous intravenous infusion using weight-based dosing, as shown in Table 5.6. These guidelines have been derived from patients weighing less than 130 kg (37). For body weights in excess of 130 kg, the guidelines in Table 5.6 can result in excessive anticoagulation (38), so it is important to monitor anticoagulation carefully in these patients.

TABLE 5.6 Weight-based Heparin Dosing Regimen

1. Prepare heparin infusion by adding 20,000 IU heparin to 500 mL diluent (40 IU/mL).
2. Give initial bolus dose of 80 IU/kg and follow with continuous infusion of 18 IU/kg/hr. (Use actual body weight.)
3. Check PTT 6 hr after start of infusion, and adjust heparin dose as indicated below.

PTT (sec)	PTT Ratio	Bolus Dose	Continuous Infusion
<35	<1.2	80 IU/kg	Increase by 4 IU/kg/hr
35–45	1.2–1.5	40 IU/kg	Increase by 2 IU/kg/hr
46–70	1.5–2.3	—	—
71–90	2.3–3.0	—	Decrease by 2 IU/kg/hr
>90	>3	—	Stop infusion for 1 hr then decrease by 3 IU/kg/hr

4. Check PTT 6 hr after each dose adjustment. When in the desired range (46–70 sec), monitor daily.

From Raschke RA, Reilly BM, Guidoy JR, et al. The weight-based heparin dosing nomogram compared with the "standard care" nomogram. Ann Intern Med 1993;119:874.

Low-Molecular-Weight Heparin

Low-molecular-weight heparin (LMWH) is an effective alternative to UFH for treatment of deep vein thrombosis and acute pulmonary embolism (7). The therapeutic dose of a standard LMWH preparation is:

Enoxaparin, 1 mg/kg by subcutaneous injection every 12 h

As mentioned earlier, LMWH is cleared by the kidneys, and dose adjustments are necessary in patients with renal impairment (see Chapter 17 for these dose adjustments). In patients with renal failure and thromboembolism who require heparin, UFH is recommended over LMWH (7).

LMWH offers several advantages over UFH, including simplified dosing, no need to monitor anticoagulant activity (see below), and the ability to treat outpatients (which could help to reduce hospital admissions for deep vein thrombosis). For these reasons, LMWH is slowly replacing UFH for the initial management of thromboembolism.

Monitoring Anticoagulation

As mentioned earlier in the chapter, the anticoagulation produced by a given dose of UFH can vary, primarily because of the variable size of the heparin molecules in UFH. As a result, laboratory tests of anticoagulant activity must be monitored to determine the anticoagulant response to UFH. The activated partial thromboplastin time (aPTT) can be used for this purpose because it is a reflection of coagulation factor IIa activity, and one of the prominent effects of UFH is inhibition of factor IIa (antithrombin effect). The aPTT cannot be used to monitor anticoagulation with LMWH because LMWH acts primarily to inhibit factor Xa, and the aPTT is not a reflection of factor Xa activity. Since LMWH produces a more predictable level of anticoagulation than heparin, monitoring laboratory tests of anticoagulation is usually not necessary with LMWH. If needed, the anticoagulant response to LMWH can be assessed by measuring factor Xa activity (7).

Warfarin Anticoagulation

For patients with a reversible cause of venous thromboembolism (e.g., major surgery), oral anticoagulation with **warfarin (Coumadin) can be started on the first day of heparin therapy**. When the prothrombin time reaches an international normalized ratio (INR) of 2 to 3, the heparin can be discontinued. (See reference 39 for a description of the INR.) Oral anticoagulation with coumadin is continued for at least 3 months (7). Patients with cancer-related or recurrent VTE require longer periods of anticoagulation (see reference 7 for more information on long-term anticoagulant therapy).

Thrombolytic Therapy

Thrombolytic therapy is usually reserved for life-threatening cases of pulmonary embolism accompanied by hemodynamic instability (7,40).

Some also recommend thrombolytic therapy for hemodynamically stable patients with right ventricular dysfunction (41) and for cardiac arrest (42), although the benefits of lytic therapy in these situations is unclear (7,42). The major problem with thrombolytic therapy is bleeding: there is a 12% incidence of major hemorrhage (40) and a 1% incidence of intracranial hemorrhage (7,40). Although the presence of risk factors for bleeding is usually a contraindication to thrombolytic therapy, in the setting of a life-threatening condition, the risk of withholding lytic therapy (i.e., death) can sometimes outweigh the risk of bleeding.

All thrombolytic agents are considered equally effective (7,40), and systemic drug administration is favored over local infusion into the pulmonary arteries because of bleeding at the catheter insertion site (7). The two drug regimens shown below are designed to achieve rapid clot lysis.

Alteplase: 0.6 mg/kg over 15 minutes.
Reteplase: 10 Units by bolus injection, and repeat in 30 minutes.

The usual alteplase dose is 100 mg infused over 2 hours, but the alteplase regimen shown here achieves the same degree of clot lysis in a shorter period of time (43). Reteplase is not currently approved for treatment of thromboembolism in this country, but the bolus administration of this drug is well-suited for rapid clot dissolution (44). For more information on the use of thrombolytic agents, see Chapter 17.

Inferior Vena Cava Filters

Meshlike filter devices can be placed in the inferior vena cava to trap thrombi that break loose from leg veins and prevent them from traveling to the lungs. These devices can be used in any of the conditions listed below.

Indications

A. Patient has proximal deep vein thrombosis in the legs and has one of the following conditions:
   1. A contraindication to anticoagulation
   2. Pulmonary embolization during full anticoagulation
   3. A free-floating thrombus (i.e., the leading edge of the thrombus is not adherent to the vessel wall).
   4. Poor cardiopulmonary reserve and unlikely to tolerate a pulmonary embolus.

B. Patient does NOT have proximal deep vein thrombosis in the legs but has one of the following conditions:
   1. Requires long-term prophylaxis of pulmonary embolism (e.g., patients with a history of recurrent pulmonary embolism)
   2. Has a high risk of thromboembolism and a high risk of hemorrhage from anticoagulant drugs (e.g., trauma victims)

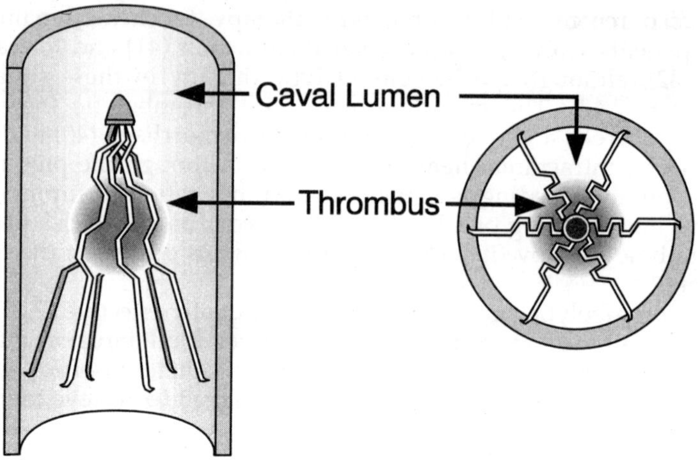

FIGURE 5.5 The Greenfield filter. The elongated shape allows the filter to trap thrombi without compromising the cross-sectional area of the vena cava.

About 80% of inferior vena cava (IVC) filters are placed in patients who have deep vein thrombosis in the legs combined with one of the conditions listed in section A (45).

The Greenfield Filter

The most widely used IVC filter in the United States is the Greenfield filter (Boston Scientific, Glen Allen, VA), shown in Figure 5.5. The major advantage of this filter is its elongated, conical shape, which allows the basket to fill with thrombi to 75% of its capacity without compromising the cross-sectional area of the vena cava. This limits the risk for vena cava obstruction and troublesome leg edema, which plagued earlier models of IVC filters.

Insertion

IVC filters are inserted percutaneously, usually through the internal jugular vein or femoral vein, and are placed below the renal veins, if possible. Suprarenal placement is occasionally necessary when the thrombus extends to the level of the renal veins, but this does not impair venous drainage from the kidneys. Although usually inserted in the radiology department, IVC filters can be placed at the bedside, thereby eliminating the risks and manpower involved in patient transport (46).

IVC filters have proven both safe and effective, which explains why their use has increased 25-fold over the last two decades (45). The incidence of post-insertion pulmonary embolism is about 5% (47), and major complications (e.g., migration of the filter) are reported in less than 1% of patients (47). Despite their intravascular location, IVC filters rarely become infected in the face of septicemia (for unclear reasons).

REFERENCES

Reviews

1. Rocha AT, Tapson VF. Venous thromboembolism in the intensive care unit. Clin Chest Med 2003;24:103–122.
2. Heit JA. Risk factors for venous thromboembolism. Clin Chest Med 2003;24: 1–12.
3. Bick RL, Haas S. Thromboprophylaxis and thrombosis in medical, surgical, trauma, and obstetric/gynecologic patients. Hematol Oncol Clin North Am 2003;17:217–258.
4. Bick RL, Frenkel EP, Walenga J, et al. Unfractionated heparin, low molecular weight heparins, and pentasaccharide: basic mechanism of actions, pharmacology and clinical use. Hematol Oncol Clin North Am 2005;19:1–51.

Clinical Practice Guidelines

5. Geerts WH, Pineo GF, Heit JA, et al. Prevention of venous thromboembolism: the Seventh ACCP Conference on Antithrombotic and Thrombolytic Therapy. Chest 2004;126(suppl):338S–400S (794 citations!)
6. Hirsch J, Raschke R. Heparin and low-molecular-weight heparin: the Seventh ACCP Conference on Antithrombotic and Thrombolytic Therapy. Chest 2004;126:(suppl)188S–203S.
7. Buller HR, Agnelli G, Hull RD, et al. Antithrombotic therapy for venous thromboembolic disease: the Seventh ACCP Conference on Antithrombotic and Thrombolytic Therapy. Chest 2004;126(suppl):401S–428S.

Thromboprophylaxis

8. Shojania KG, Duncan BW, McDonald KM, et al., eds. Making health care safer: a critical analysis of patient safety practices. Evidence report/technology assessment No. 43. AHRQ Publication No. 01-E058. Rockville, MD: Agency for Healthcare Research and Quality, July, 2001.
9. Linblad B, Eriksson A, Bergqvist D. Autopsy-verified pulmonary embolism in a surgical department: analysis of the period from 1951 to 1988. Br J Surg 1991;78:849–852.
10. Ageno W, Turpie AGG. What's new for DVT prophylaxis for the medically ill. Dis Mon 2005;51:194–199.
11. Cook D, Crowther M, Meade M, et al. Deep vein thrombosis in medical-surgical critically ill patients: prevalence, incidence, and risk factors. Crit Care Med 2005;33:1565–1571.
12. Ibrahim E, Iregui M, Prentice D, et al. Deep vein thrombosis during prolonged mechanical ventilation despite prophylaxis. Crit Care Med 2002;30: 771–774.
13. Goldhaber SZ, Marpurgo M, for the WHO/ISFC Task Force on Pulmonary Embolism. Diagnosis, treatment and prevention of pulmonary embolism. JAMA 1992;268:1727–1733.
14. Wells PS, Lensing AW, Hirsh J. Graduated compression stockings in the prevention of postoperative venous thromboembolism: a meta-analysis. Arch Intern Med 1994;154:67–72.

15. Turpie AG, Hirsch J, Gent M, et al. Prevention of deep vein thrombosis in potential neurosurgical patients. Arch Intern Med 1989;149:679–681.
16. Heparin. Mosby Drug Consult 2005. Accessed at www.mdconsult.com on July 4, 2005.
17. Enoxaparin. Mosby Drug Consult 2005. Accessed at www.mdconsult.com on July 4, 2005.
18. Dalteparin. Mosby Drug Consult 2005. Accessed at www.mdconsult.com on July 4, 2005.
19. Raskob G, Hirsch J. Controversies in timing of first dose of anticoagulant prophylaxis against venous thromboembolism after major orthopedic surgery. Chest 2003;124(suppl):379S–385S.
20. Ansell J, Hirsh J, Poller L, et al. The pharmacology and management of the vitamin K antagonists: the Seventh ACCP Conference on Antithrombotic and Thrombolytic Therapy. Chest 2004;126(suppl):204S–233S.
21. Bauer KA. New pentasaccharides for prophylaxis of deep vein thrombosis: pharmacology. Chest 2003;124(suppl):364S–370S.
22. Fondaparinux. Mosby's Drug Consult 2005. Accessed at www.mdconsult.com on July 6, 2005.

Diagnostic Approach

23. Hoellerich VL, Wigton RS. Diagnosing pulmonary embolism using clinical findings. Arch Intern Med 1986;146:1699–1704.
24. Stein PD, Goldhaber SZ, Henry JW. Alveolar–arterial oxygen gradient in the assessment of acute pulmonary embolism. Chest 1995;107:139–143.
25. Kelly J, Rudd A, Lewis RR, et al. Plasma D-dimers in the diagnosis of venous thromboembolism. Arch Intern Med 2002;162:747–756.
26. Kollef MH, Zahid M, Eisenberg PR. Predictive value of a rapid semiquantitative D-dimer assay in critically ill patients with suspected thromboembolism. Crit Care Med 2000;28:414–420.
27. Kline JA, Israel EG, Michelson EA, et al. Diagnostic accuracy of a bedside D-dimer assay and alveolar dead space measurement for rapid exclusion of pulmonary embolism. JAMA 2001;285:761–768.
28. Moser KM. Is embolic risk conditioned by location of deep vein thrombosis? Ann Intern Med 1981;94:439–444.
29. Tracey JA, Edlow JA. Ultrasound diagnosis of deep venous thrombosis. Emerg Med Clin North Am 2004;22:775–796.
30. Hull RD, Hirsh J, Carter CJ, et al. Pulmonary angiography, ventilation lung scanning, and venography for clinically suspected pulmonary embolism with abnormal perfusion scans. Ann Intern Med 1983;98:891–899.
31. The PIOPED Investigators. Value of the ventilation/perfusion scan in acute pulmonary embolism: results of the Prospective Investigation of Pulmonary Embolism Diagnosis (PIOPED). JAMA 1990;263:2753–2759.
32. Remy-Jardin M, Remy J, Wattinine L, et al. Central pulmonary thromboembolism: diagnosis with spiral volumetric CT with the single-breath-hold technique: comparison with pulmonary angiography. Radiology 1992;185:381–387.
33. Kaplan AE, Frankenthaler ML, Schneider RF, et al. A strategy to avoid respiratory motion artifact in mechanically ventilated patients undergoing helical chest computed tomography angiography. Crit Care Med 2001;29:1292.

34. Mullins MD, Becker DM, Hagspeil KD, et al. The role of spiral volumetric computed tomography in the diagnosis of pulmonary embolism. Arch Intern Med 2000;160:293–298.
35. Quiroz R, Kucher N, Zou KH, et al. Clinical validity of a negative computed tomography scan in patients with suspected pulmonary embolism. JAMA 2005;293:2012–2017.
36. Wolfe TR, Hartsell SC. Pulmonary embolism: making sense of the diagnostic evaluation. Ann Emerg Med 2001;37:504–514.

Antithrombotic Therapy

37. Raschke RA, Reilly BM, Guidry JR, et al. The weight-based heparin dosing nomogram compared with a "standard care" nomogram. Ann Intern Med 1993;119:874–881.
38. Holliday DM, Watling SM, Yanos J. Heparin dosing in the morbidly obese patient. Ann Pharmacother 1994;28:1110–1111.
39. Le DT, Weibert RT, Sevilla BK, et al. The international normalized ratio (INR) for monitoring warfarin therapy: reliability and relation to other monitoring methods. Ann Intern Med 1994;120:552–558.

Thrombolytic Therapy

40. Wood KE. Major pulmonary embolism. Chest 2002;121:877–905.
41. Comeraota AJ. The role of fibrinolytic therapy in the treatment of venous thromboembolism. Dis Mon 2005;51:124–134.
42. Bailen MR, Cuarda JAR, de Hoyos EA. Thrombolysis during cardiopulmonary resuscitation in fulminant pulmonary embolism: a review. Crit Care Med 2001;29:2211–2219.
43. Goldhaber SZ, Agnelli G, Levine MN. Reduced dose bolus alteplase vs conventional alteplase infusion for pulmonary embolism thrombolysis: an international multicenter randomized trial: the Bolus Alteplase Pulmonary Embolism Group. Chest 1994;106:718–724.
44. Tebbe U, Graf A, Kamke W, et al. Hemodynamic effects of double bolus reteplase versus alteplase infusion in massive pulmonary embolism. Am Heart J 1999;138:39–44.

Vena Cava Filters

45. Stein PD, Kayali F, Olson RE. Twenty-one year trends in the use of inferior vena cava filters. Arch Intern Med 2004;164:1541–1545.
46. Sing RF, Cicci CK, Smith CH, et al. Bedside insertion of inferior vena cava filters in the intensive care unit. J Trauma 1999;47:1104–1107.
47. Athanasoulis CA, Kaufman JA, Halpern EF, et al. Inferior vena cava filters: review of 26-year single-center clinical experience. Radiology 2000;216:54–66.

Section III

VASCULAR ACCESS

He who works with his hands is a laborer. He who works with his head and his hands is a craftsman.

St. Francis of Assisi

Chapter 6

ESTABLISHING VENOUS ACCESS

Establishing and maintaining access to the vascular system is one of the seminal tasks in critical care. This chapter presents some practical guidelines for the insertion of vascular catheters, and the next chapter describes the considerations involved in maintaining vascular access. The emphasis in this chapter is not the technique of catheter insertion (which must be mastered at the bedside) but the information that will allow you to make appropriate decisions about vascular cannulation in the individual patient (e.g., selecting the appropriate catheter and insertion site). The goal here is to follow the advice of Saint Francis of Assissi and teach you the craft of vascular cannulation.

PREPARING FOR VASCULAR CANNULATION

Hospital Staff

Anyone who inserts a vascular catheter must follow standard infection control practices in preparation for catheter insertion. Handwashing with an antimicrobial soap or gel is recommended for all vascular catheter insertions, including those involving small peripheral veins (1,2). (Handwashing is described in detail in Chapter 3.) The hands should be decontaminated before donning gloves and again after the gloves are removed. Sterile gloves are recommended for insertion of central venous catheters and arterial catheters (1), while **nonsterile disposable gloves can be used for cannulation of peripheral veins** as long as the gloved hands do not touch the catheter (2). Full barrier precautions using masks, gowns, and sterile drapes are recommended for insertion of central venous catheters, including peripherally-inserted central catheters (PICCs) (1).

Catheter Insertion Site

The skin around the catheter insertion site should be decontaminated with an antiseptic agent (see Chapter 3 for information on antiseptic agents). The Centers for Disease Control (CDC) recommends chlorhexidine because of its residual antimicrobial activity, which can last for 6 hours after one application (see Figure 3.1) (2). The clinical significance of this is, however, unproven, and other antiseptic agents like povidone-iodine (Betadine) and 70% alcohol are also acceptable (1). Remember that **chlorhexidine and povidone-iodine should be allowed to dry on the skin and not wiped off** to maximize their antibacterial effects (1).

VASCULAR CATHETERS

Vascular catheters are made of polymers impregnated with barium or tungsten salts to enhance radiopacity. Catheters designed for short-term cannulation (days) are usually made of polyurethane, a synthetic polymer known for its strength, durability, and moisture resistance. Catheters designed for prolonged use (weeks to months) are made of a silicone polymer that is more flexible and less thrombogenic than polyurethane. Because of their flexibility, silicone catheters must be inserted over a semi-rigid guidewire or through a surgically-created subcutaneous tunnel.

Catheter Size

The size of vascular catheters is expressed in terms of the outside diameter of the catheter. Two units of measurement are used to describe catheter size: a metric-based French size and a wire-based gauge size. The French size is a series of whole numbers that increases from zero in increments of 0.33 millimeters (e.g., a size 5 French catheter will have an outside diameter of $5 \times 0.33 = 1.65$ mm). The gauge size was introduced for solid wires and is an expression of how many wires can be placed side-by-side in a given space. The gauge size varies inversely with the diameter of the wire (or catheter). However, there is no simple relationship between gauge size and other units of measurement, and a table of reference values like Table 6.1 is needed.

Determinants of Flow Rate

The influence of catheter size on flow through the catheter is defined by the Hagen-Poiseuille equation, which is presented in detail in Chapter 1 (see Figure 1.6).

$$Q = \Delta P(\pi r^4/8\mu L) \tag{6.1}$$

Steady flow (Q) in a catheter is directly related to the pressure gradient along the catheter (ΔP) and the fourth power of the radius of the catheter (r^4) and is inversely related to the length of the catheter (L) and the viscosity of the fluid (μ). The principal determinant of flow in this equation is the radius of the catheter. The relationship between catheter diameter and flow rate is demonstrated in Figure 6.1. The data in this graph pertain to the gravity flow of blood through a catheter of constant length but varying diameter (3). As demonstrated, a given change in

TABLE 6.1 Catheter Size Chart

French Size	Gauge	Inner Diameter	Outer Diameter
1	27	0.007 in or 0.1 mm	0.016 in or 0.4 mm
2	23	0.012 in or 0.3 mm	0.025 in or 0.6 mm
3	20	0.020 in or 0.5 mm	0.037 in or 0.9 mm
4	18	0.025 in or 0.6 mm	0.047 in or 1.2 mm
5	16	0.030 in or 0.7 mm	0.065 in or 1.7 mm
7	13	0.050 in or 1.3 mm	0.095 in or 2.4 mm
9	11	0.062 in or 1.6 mm	1.25 in or 3.2 mm

Accessed at www.norfolkaccess.com/Catheters.html on 7/4/2005.

diameter resulted in a proportionately greater change in flow, reflecting the dependence of flow on a power function of catheter radius.

The relationships in the Hagen-Poiseuille equation indicate that **short catheters with large diameters are most appropriate for rapid infusion rates**. Furthermore, catheter diameter takes precedence over

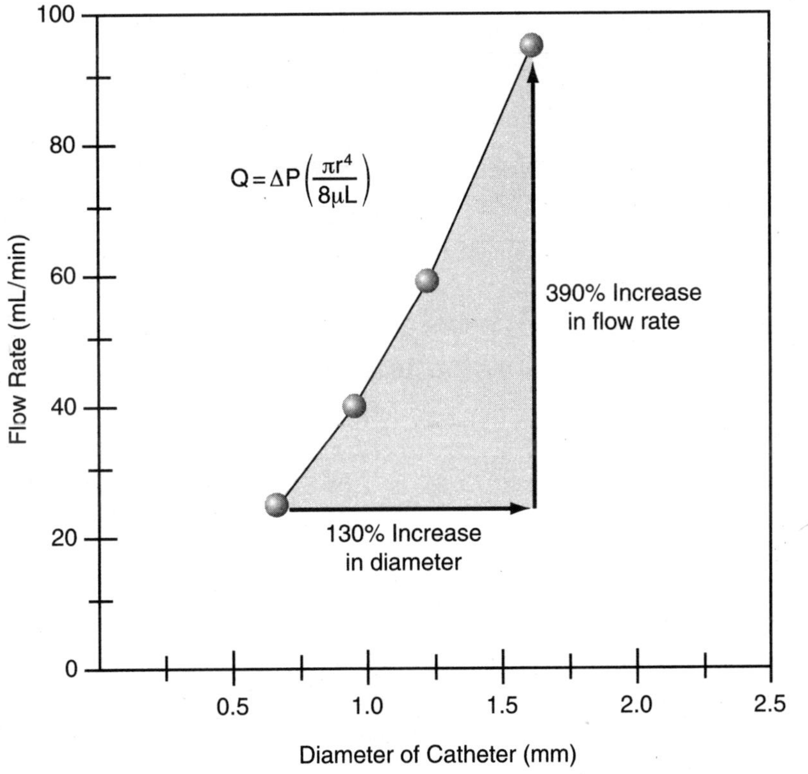

FIGURE 6.1 Relationship between flow rate and outside diameter of a catheter. (From de la Roche M, Gauthier L. Rapid transfusion of packed red blood cells: effects of dilution, pressure, and catheter size. Ann Emerg Med 1993;22:1551.)

catheter length when rapid infusions are needed. The performance of different sized catheters for volume resuscitation is described in more detail in Chapter 12.

Peripheral Venous Catheters

Catheters that are designed for cannulation of peripheral veins are typically short (usually 5 cm, or 2 inches in length) and about 18 to 22 gauge in diameter (see Table 6.2). These catheters are usually inserted using a catheter-over-needle device like the one shown in Figure 6.2. The catheter fits snugly over the needle, and has a tapered end to minimize damage to the catheter tip and soft tissues during insertion. The needle has a clear hub, called a flash chamber, which fills with blood when the tip of the needle enters the lumen of a blood vessel. The cap on the needle should be removed before insertion to facilitate the movement of blood into the flash chamber. When the tip of the needle enters the blood vessel (and blood fills the flash chamber), the catheter is advanced over the needle and into the lumen of the vessel.

Central Venous Catheters

The term *central venous catheter* refers to a catheter that is designed for cannulation of the subclavian vein, the internal jugular vein, or the

TABLE 6.2 Different Types of Vascular Catheters

Type of Catheter	Sizes	Lengths
Peripheral venous catheter	18 ga	5 cm, 7 cm
	22 ga	4 cm, 5 cm
Central venous catheter		
Single lumen	16 ga, 18 ga	15 cm, 12 cm
	20 ga	8 cm
Double lumen (18, 18 ga)	7.5 Fr	15 cm, 20 cm, 25 cm
Triple lumen (18, 18, 16 ga)	7 Fr	15 cm, 20 cm, 25 cm
Peripherally inserted central catheter (PICC)	3 Fr	50 cm
	4 & 5 Fr	60 cm
Hemodialysis catheter	16 Fr	26 cm
Introducer catheter	9 Fr	10 cm, 13 cm
Radial artery catheter	20 ga, 21 ga	5 cm, 2.5 cm, 5 cm
Femoral artery catheter	18 ga, 20 ga	12 cm, 8 cm

Catheter dimensions listed here are from one manufacturer (Cook Critical Care, Bloomington, IN) and may differ from those of other manufacturers.
Fr: French unit (one French unit = 0.33 mm): ga: gauge unit.

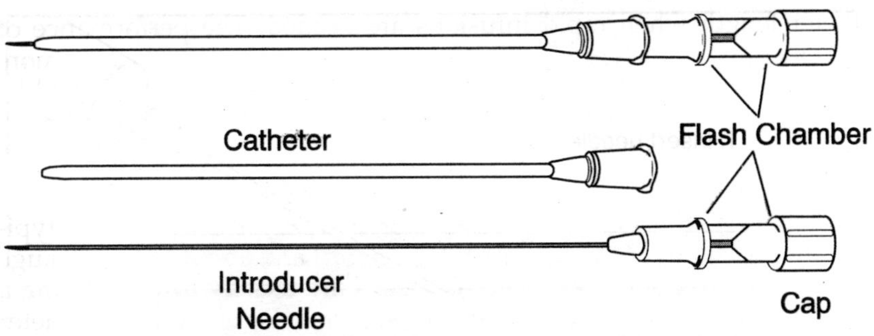

FIGURE 6.2 A catheter-over-needle device used to cannulate peripheral veins.

femoral vein. As indicated in Table 6.2, these catheters are much longer than the catheters used to cannulate peripheral veins and are typically 15 to 25 cm (6 to 10 inches) in length. They also are available with two or three separate infusion channels, which is advantageous when multiple medications are required.

Seldinger Technique

Central venous catheters are placed by threading the catheter over a guidewire (a technique introduced in the early 1950s and called the *Seldinger technique* after its founder). This technique is illustrated in Figure 6.3. A small-bore needle (usually 20 gauge) is used to probe for the target vessel. When the tip of the needle enters the vessel, a long, thin wire with a flexible tip is passed through the needle and into the vessel lumen. The needle is then removed, and a catheter is advanced over the guidewire and into the blood vessel. When cannulating deep vessels, a rigid dilator catheter is first threaded over the guidewire to create a tract that facilitates insertion of the vascular catheter.

Introducer Catheters

The first catheter inserted in the large, central veins is usually a large-bore introducer catheter like the one shown in Figure 6.4 (see Table 6.2 for the dimensions of an introducer catheter). Once in place, these catheters are fixed to the skin with a single suture. A central venous catheter can then be threaded through the introducer catheter and advanced to the desired tip location. Introducer catheters allow central venous catheters to be inserted and removed repeatedly without a new venipuncture. A side-arm infusion port on the catheter provides an additional infusion line and also allows the introducer catheter to be used as a stand-alone infusion device (a rubber membrane on the hub of the catheter provides an effective seal when fluids are infusing through the side-arm port of the catheter). The large diameter of introducer catheters (9 French) makes them particularly valuable when rapid infusion rates are necessary (e.g., in hemorrhagic shock).

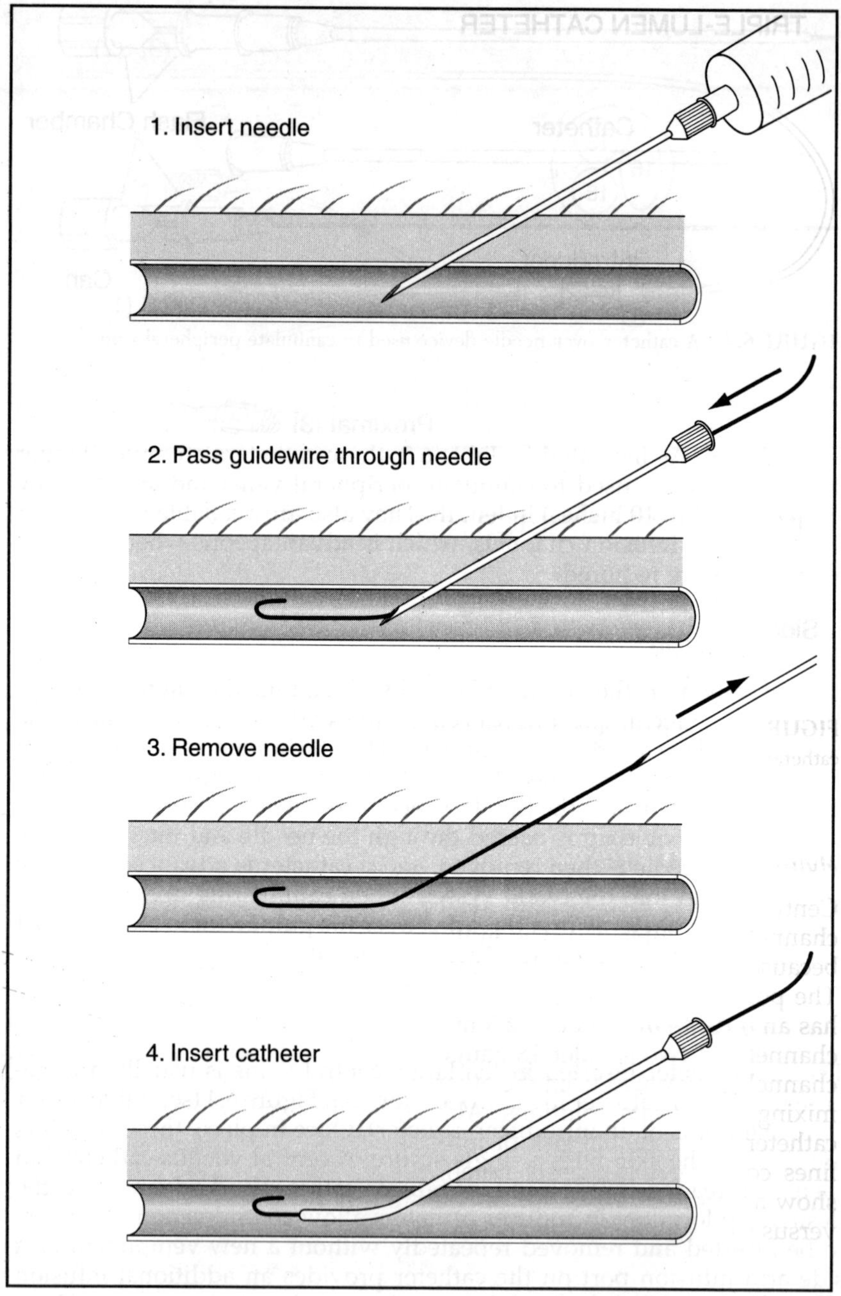

FIGURE 6.3 The steps involved in guidewire-assisted cannulation of blood vessels (the Seldinger technique).

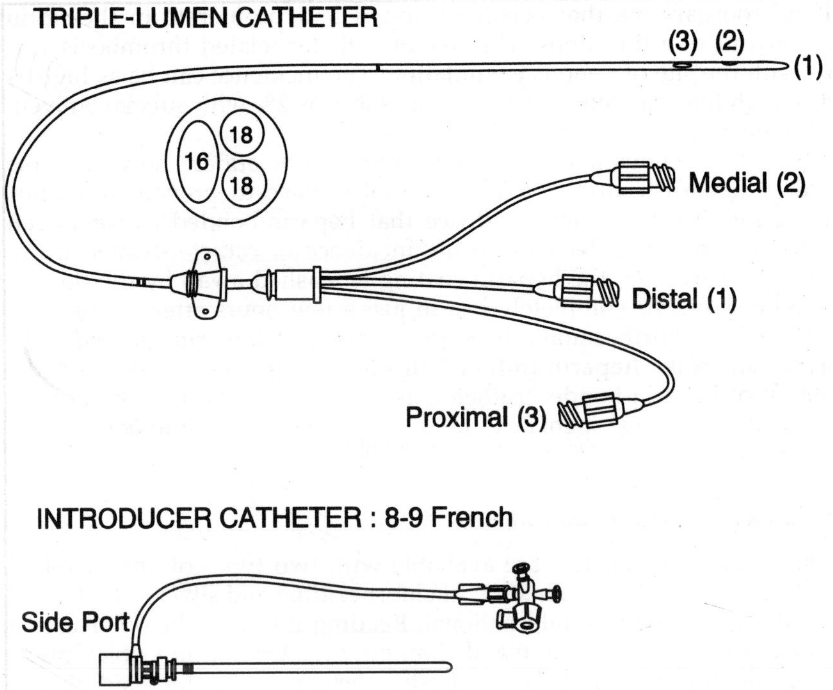

FIGURE 6.4 A triple-lumen central venous catheter and a large-bore introducer catheter.

Multilumen Catheters

Central venous catheters are available with one, two, or three infusion channels (see Table 6.2). The multilumen catheters are the most popular because they allow multiple infusions through a single venipuncture site. The popular triple-lumen catheter is shown in Figure 6.4. This catheter has an outside diameter of 2.3 mm (7 French) and houses one 16 gauge channel and two smaller 18 gauge channels. The distal opening of each channel is separated from the others by at least one centimeter to prevent mixing of infusate solutions. Although each channel of a multilumen catheter is a potential risk of infection (through breaks in the infusion lines connected to each channel), several clinical trials have failed to show a higher incidence of catheter-related infections with multilumen versus single lumen catheters (4).

Heparin-Bonded Catheters

The intravascular portion of a central venous catheter can serve as a nidus for thrombus formation, and this can be a prelude to thrombotic occlusion of the involved blood vessel as well as catheter-related septicemia. The link between thrombosis and infection may be the result of microorganisms that become trapped and proliferate in the fibrin meshwork of a thrombus. The risk of catheter-related thrombosis varies with the site of venous cannulation. The incidence can be as high as 20% with femoral vein catheters and as low as 2% with subclavian vein catheters (5).

Central venous and pulmonary artery catheters are now available with a heparin coating on the external surface to prevent thrombus formation. There is some evidence that heparin-bonded catheters can cause a small (2%) decrease in the incidence of catheter-related infections (6). However, the heparin coating is washed away by the flow of blood and can be completely lost in just a few hours after the catheter is placed (5). Furthermore, there are reports that **heparin-bonded catheters can cause heparin-induced thrombocytopenia** (7). Because the benefit of heparin-bonded catheters is small, while the risk of heparin-induced thrombocytopenia can be serious, it seems wise to avoid these catheters.

Antimicrobial-Impregnated Catheters

Central venous catheters are available with two types of antimicrobial coating: one uses a combination of chlorhexidine and silver sulfadiazine (available from Arrow International, Reading PA), and the other uses a combination of minocycline and rifampin (available from Cook Critical Care, Bloomington, IN). The earliest catheters used chlorhexidine and silver sulfadiazine on the outer catheter surface, and only 2 of 9 studies evaluating these catheters showed a significant reduction in catheter-related septicemia (6). A single multicenter study comparing both types of antimicrobial catheters showed superior results with the minocycline-rifampin catheters (1,8). These catheters have antimicrobial bonding on both (outer and inner) surfaces, and also show antimicrobial activity for up to 4 weeks, compared to one week for the chlorhexidine-silver sulfadiazine catheters (9). At the present time, it seems the minocycline-rifampin catheters are preferable, although newer chlorhexidine-silver sulfadiazine catheters are now available with antimicrobial bonding on both catheter surfaces.

Antimicrobial-impregnated catheters should be considered if the rate of catheter-related septicemia in your ICU is higher than the national average (which is 3.8 to 5.3 infections per 1,000 catheter-days in medical-surgical ICUs) (1). They should also be considered in neutropenic patients and burn patients.

Peripherally Inserted Central Catheters

Long catheters (50 to 60 cm in length) can be inserted in the basilic vein or cephalic vein in the arm and advanced into the superior vena cava (see Figure 6.5) (10,11). These *peripherally inserted central catheters* (PICCs) offer one advantage over cannulation of the more centrally located subclavian and internal jugular veins: i.e., there is no risk of pneumothorax. PICCs are made of soft silicone rubber, and a guidewire is required to insert these catheters. PICC insertion is described briefly in the next section.

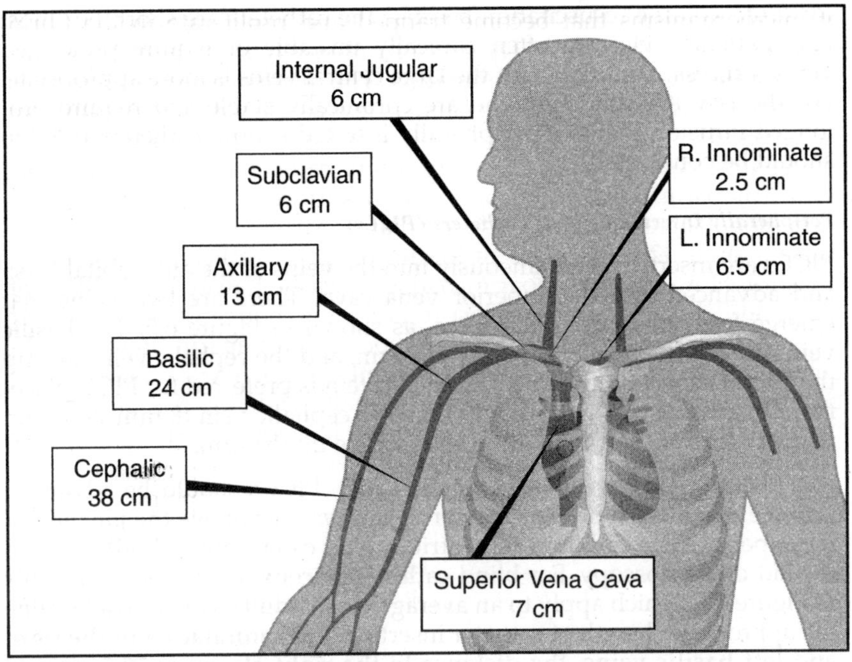

FIGURE 6.5 The length of venous segments involved in the insertion of peripherally inserted central catheters (PICCs) and central venous (i.e., subclavian and internal jugular vein) catheters. The circle in the third anterior intercostal space marks the junction of the superior vena cava and right atrium.

VENOUS ACCESS SITES

The following is a brief description of the common sites used for percutaneous cannulation of the venous system, including the advantages and disadvantages of each site, and the surface landmarks used to locate each target vessel.

The Upper Extremity

Cannulation of peripheral veins provides rapid and safe access to the systemic circulation. As mentioned earlier, the catheters used to cannulate peripheral veins are typically narrow (18 to 22 gauge) and short (5 cm or 2 inches) and are inserted using a catheter-over-needle device like the one in Figure 6.2. These **peripheral venous catheters should be replaced every 3 to 4 days** (using a new venipuncture) to limit the risk of phlebitis (1). The arms are preferred over the legs because of the higher incidence of venous thrombosis in the legs (1).

Comment

Cannulation of peripheral veins is best suited for rapid, short-term venous access (e.g., in the emergency department) and is advantageous for acute volume resuscitation because the catheters are short. For most ICU patients, who are often clinically unstable or require prolonged venous access, cannulation of the large central veins is more appropriate. For the few ICU patients who are chronically stable and require prolonged infusion therapy, peripherally inserted central catheters (PICCs) should be considered.

Peripherally Inserted Central Catheters (PICCs)

PICCs are inserted percutaneously into the veins of the antecubital fossa and advanced into the superior vena cava. There are two veins that emerge from the antecubital fossa, as shown in Figure 6.5. The basilic vein runs up the medial aspect of the arm, and the cephalic vein runs up the lateral aspect of the arm. The basilic vein is preferred for PICC placement because it is slightly larger than the cephalic vein (8 mm vs. 6 mm in diameter), and it runs a straighter course up the arm.

POSITIONING THE CATHETERS. Once inserted, PICCs should be advanced into the lower third of the superior vena cava, just above the junction of the superior vena cava and right atrium. This can be done blindly or with the aid of fluoroscopy. For blind catheter placement, the measurements in Figure 6.5 (which apply to an average-sized adult) will help determine the appropriate length of catheter insertion. **For cannulation of the right and left basilic veins, the distance to the right atrium is 52.5 cm and 56.5 cm, respectively.** For cannulation of the right and left cephalic veins, the distance to the right atrium is 53.5 cm and 57.5 cm, respectively. These approximate measurements can be used to guide catheter placement, or a direct measurement can be made of the distance from the antecubital fossa to the right third intercostal space in individual patients. Without fluoroscopic guidance, malposition of PICCs is common (10,11).

Comment

PICCs can be left in place for 30 days or longer without an increased risk of catheter-related septicemia when compared with central venous catheters (10,11). However, thrombotic obstruction of these catheters can be problematic because of their narrow bore, and mechanical phlebitis can be a problem because of their long length (10). The only advantage of PICCs over central venous catheters is the absence of any risk of pneumothorax. However, as you will see, the risk of pneumothorax from central venous catheters is minimal if the procedure is performed by experienced personnel.

Overall, PICCs offer few advantages over central venous catheters. They can be used for long-term (30 days or longer) infusion therapy in clinically stable patients, but they have no role in the care of acutely ill or unstable patients.

The Subclavian Vein

The subclavian vein is well suited for cannulation because it is a large vessel (with a diameter of 20 mm) that runs a fixed course. The major

TABLE 6.3 Adverse Effects of Large-Vein Cannulation*

	Complication Rates		
Adverse Effect	Subclavian Vein	Internal Jugular Vein	Femoral Vein
Arterial puncture	1%–15%	3%	9%†
Major Bleeding	2%	1%	1%
Occlusive Thrombosis	1%	0	6%†
Pneumothorax	1%–3%	1%	—
Systemic sepsis	1%–4%	0–8%	2%–5%

*Combined data from References 16–18. Rates shown here are rounded to the nearest whole number.
†Indicates a rate that is significantly different from the others.

concern with subclavian vein cannulation is the risk of pneumothorax, but, as demonstrated in Table 6.3 (12–14), this is not a common occurrence. Major bleeding is also uncommon, and the presence of a coagulopathy does not increase the risk of bleeding. In fact, **the presence of a coagulation disorder is not a contraindication to placement of central venous catheters** (15–17). Based on the information in Table 6.3, subclavian vein catheterization is a reasonably safe procedure when performed by experienced personnel.

Anatomy

The subclavian vein is a continuation of the axillary vein as it passes over the first rib (see Figure 6.5). It runs most of its course along the underside of the clavicle, and at some points is only 5 mm above the apical pleura of the lungs. The underside of the vein sits on the anterior scalene muscle, with the subclavian artery situated just deep to the muscle. Since the artery lies deep to the vein, avoiding deep penetration by the probe needle will limit the risk of subclavian artery puncture. The subclavian vein continues to the thoracic inlet, where it joins the internal jugular vein to form the innominate vein. The convergence of the right and left innominate veins forms the superior vena cava.

The average distance from cannulation sites in the subclavian (and internal jugular) vein to the right atrium can be inferred from the vein lengths in Figure 6.5. The average distance is 14.5 cm and 18.5 cm for right-sided and left-sided cannulations, respectively. Therefore to avoid placing catheters in the right side of the heart (which creates a risk of cardiac perforation), **catheters used for subclavian and internal jugular vein cannulation should be no longer than 15 cm in length** (18).

Locating the Vessel

The insertion points on the skin for subclavian vein cannulation are shown in Figure 6.6. To locate the subclavian vein, identify the sternocleidomastoid muscle, which is the large muscle that runs down the neck

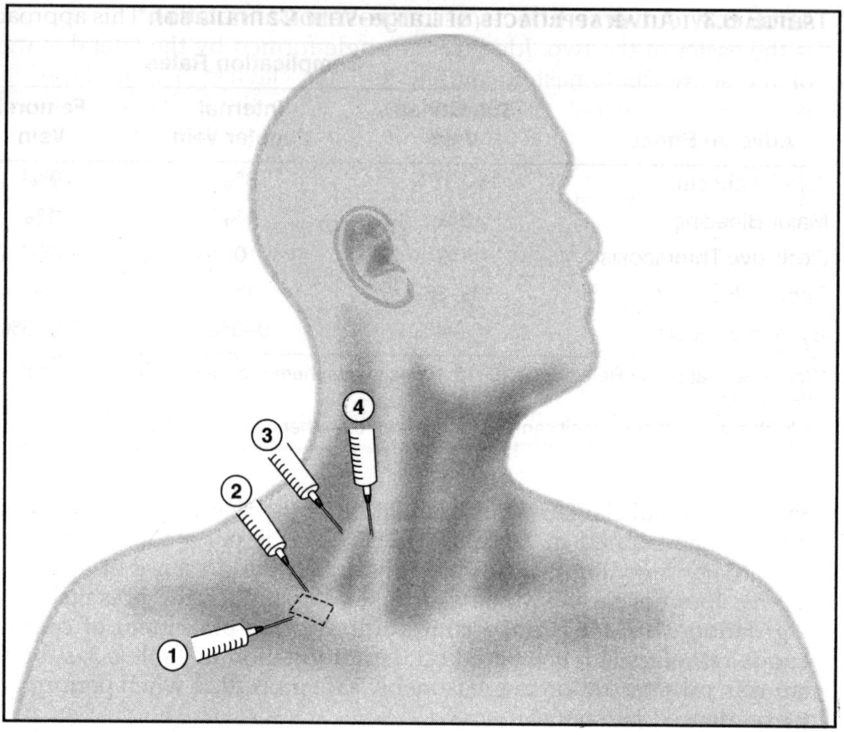

FIGURE 6.6 The points of entry and appropriate orientation of probe needles for cannulation of the subclavian vein (points 1 and 2) and internal jugular vein (points 3 and 4).

on either side of the midline. This muscle splits into a medial portion that inserts on the sternum and a lateral portion that inserts on the clavicle. Identify the lateral head of the muscle (by palpation if necessary), and note where the muscle inserts onto the clavicle. The subclavian vein lies just underneath the clavicle at this point. Mark the area of the clavicle that overlies the vein, as shown in Figure 6.6. The vein can be entered at this point from above or below the clavicle.

INFRACLAVICULAR APPROACH (NEEDLE POSITION 1 IN FIG. 6.6). The probe needle should enter the skin just below the clavicle and at the lateral boundary of the site marked on the clavicle. The bevel of the needle should be pointed upward (toward the ceiling) during insertion, and the needle should be advanced under the marked area on the clavicle. The needle will puncture the vein within a few centimeters of the surface. When the vein is entered, the bevel of the needle should be rotated to 3 o'clock so the guidewire threads in the direction of the superior vena cava. A common mistake made by the unexperienced is inserting the needle at the bend in the clavicle, which places the needle too far from the target vessel (probe needles are only a few inches in length, and might not reach the vein if the skin puncture is removed from the vein).

SUPRACLAVICULAR APPROACH (NEEDLE POSITION 2 IN FIG. 6.6). This approach is the easier of the two. Identify the angle formed by the lateral margin of the sternocleidomastoid muscle and the clavicle. The probe needle is inserted so that it bisects this angle. Keep the bevel of the needle facing upward, and direct the needle under the clavicle in the direction of the opposite nipple. The vein should be entered at a distance of 1 to 2 cm from the skin surface (the subclavian vein is more superficial in the supraclavicular approach). When the vein is entered, turn the bevel of the needle to 9 o'clock so the guidewire threads in the direction of the superior vena cava.

Comment

The subclavian vein should be preferred for central venous cannulation because of the ease of insertion, the low complication rate, and the high degree of patient acceptance once the catheter is in place. The fear of pneumothorax is not justified, at least when experienced personnel are performing the procedure. Avoiding deep penetration of the probe needle should limit the risk of subclavian artery puncture and pneumothorax.

The Internal Jugular Vein

Cannulation of the internal jugular vein was popularized because of the assumption that this procedure, which is performed at the base of the neck, should eliminate the risk of pneumothorax. However, this is not the case, as demonstrated in Table 6.3. In fact, the incidence of pneumothorax is almost the same following cannulation of the internal jugular vein and subclavian vein. How can a puncture at the base of the neck cause a pneumothorax? Aside from poor technique, it is possible that the cupola of the lung protrudes into the base of the neck as a result of the high tidal volumes used during mechanical ventilation. In addition to the occasional pneumothorax, cannulation of the internal jugular vein has other disadvantages, such as carotid artery puncture and poor patient acceptance due to limitations in neck mobility.

Anatomy

The internal jugular vein is located under the sternocleidomastoid muscle in the neck and runs obliquely down the neck on a line from the pinna of the ear to the sternoclavicular joint. Turning the head to the opposite side will straighten the course of the vein. Near the base of the neck, the internal jugular vein lies just lateral to the carotid artery in the carotid sheath, and this position creates the risk of carotid artery puncture.

Locating the Vessel

The right internal jugular vein is preferred because the vessels run a straighter course to the right atrium. This is particularly advantageous for placing temporary transvenous pacemakers and to ensure adequate flow through hemodialysis catheters. The vein can be entered from an anterior or posterior approach.

THE ANTERIOR APPROACH (NEEDLE POSITION 4 IN FIG. 6.6). For the anterior approach, the operator must first identify a triangular area at the base of the neck created by the separation of the two heads of the sternocleidomastoid muscle. The carotid artery pulse is then palpated with the fingers of the left hand (for a right-sided approach), and the artery is retracted toward the midline. The probe needle is then inserted at the apex of the triangle with the bevel facing up, and the needle is advanced toward the ipsilateral nipple, at a 45° angle with the skin surface. If the vein is not entered by a depth of 5 cm, the needle is drawn back and advanced again in a more lateral direction. Two failed attempts should warrant abandoning this approach for the posterior approach.

THE POSTERIOR APPROACH (NEEDLE POSITION 3 IN FIG. 6.6). The insertion site for this approach is 1 centimeter superior to the point where the external jugular vein crosses over the lateral edge of the sternocleidomastoid muscle. The probe needle is inserted with the bevel positioned at 3 o'clock. The needle is advanced along the underbelly of the muscle in a direction pointing to the suprasternal notch. The internal jugular vein should be encountered 5 to 6 cm from the skin surface (19). The vein runs just lateral to the carotid artery in this region and can act as a shield for the carotid artery as long as the advancing needle is kept in the same plane as the internal jugular vein.

CAROTID ARTERY PUNCTURE. If the carotid artery has been punctured with a probing needle (as suggested by the return of pulsating bright red blood through the needle), the needle should be removed and pressure applied to the site for at least 5 minutes (double the compression time for patients with a coagulopathy). No further attempts should be made to cannulate the internal jugular vein on either side, to avoid puncture of both carotid arteries. **If a catheter has been mistakenly placed in the carotid artery, do not remove the catheter** because this could provoke serious hemorrhage. In this situation, get a vascular surgeon pronto.

Comment

The internal jugular vein offers no advantages over the subclavian vein other than the occasional benefit for pacemaker catheters and hemodialysis catheters because of the straight course from the right internal jugular vein to the heart. The disadvantages of internal jugular vein cannulation (i.e., carotid artery puncture and poor patient acceptance) make this approach less desirable than subclavian vein cannulation.

The Femoral Vein

The femoral vein is the largest, easiest, and most problematic vein to cannulate. The problems with femoral vein cannulation include the risk for femoral artery puncture and a high rate of venous thrombosis (see Table 6.3). The risk of thrombosis may be overstated because most cases are clinically silent and without consequence (20). Earlier studies suggested a higher rate of infection with femoral vein catheters, but more recent observations (see Table 6.3) show no increase in infectious risk (14).

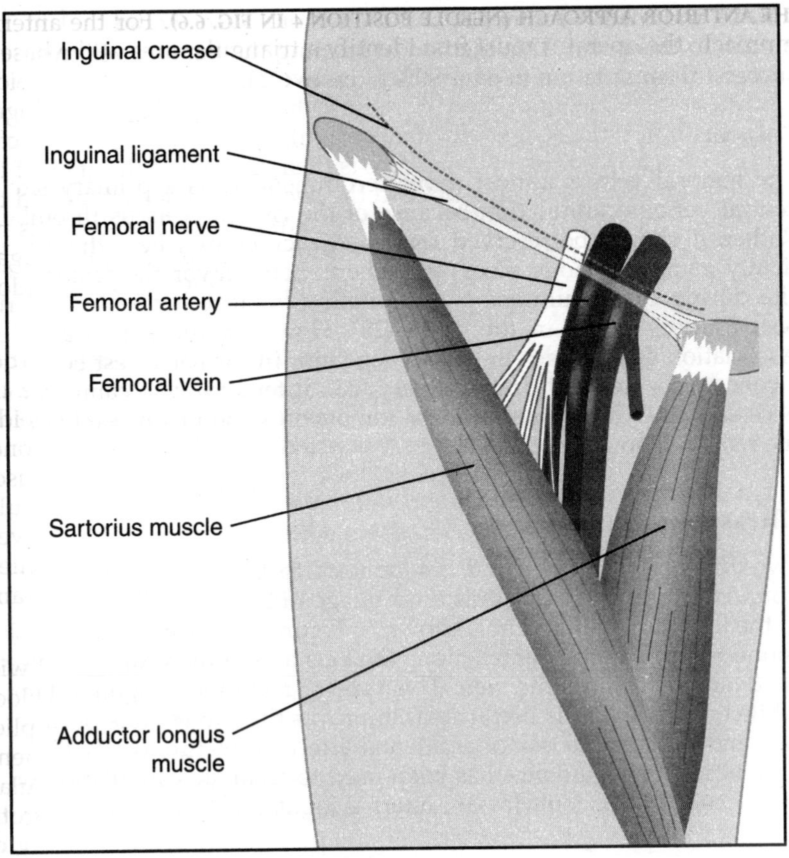

FIGURE 6.7 The anatomy of the femoral triangle.

Anatomy

The femoral vein is the main conduit for venous drainage from the legs. In the proximal one-third of the thigh, the femoral vein runs next to the femoral artery. Both vessels are located in the medial portion of the femoral triangle (see Figure 6.7), with the femoral vein running just medial to the femoral artery. These blood vessels are within a few centimeters of the skin at the inguinal crease.

Locating the Vessel

The femoral vein can be located by palpating the femoral artery pulse just below the inguinal crease. The probe needle should be inserted (bevel up) 1 to 2 cm medial to the palpated pulse. The vein should be entered at a depth of 2 to 4 cm from the skin. If the femoral artery pulse is not palpable, draw an imaginary line from the anterior superior iliac crest to the pubic tubercle, and divide the line into three equal segments. The femoral artery should be just underneath the junction between the middle and medial segments, and the femoral vein should be 1 to 2 cm medial to this point. This method of locating the femoral vein results in successful cannulation in over 90% of cases (21).

Comment

The femoral vein is almost never recommended as a primary site for central venous cannulation because of the risk for venous thrombosis. Rather, it should be reserved for emergency cases where there is difficulty gaining venous access elsewhere. Some favor the femoral vein site during cardiopulmonary resuscitation because it does not disrupt resuscitation efforts in the chest (22). However, the American Heart Association discourages the use of leg veins in cardiac arrest because of a concern for delayed drug delivery (23). If femoral vein cannulation is necessary, the catheters should be removed as soon as possible to limit the risk of venous thrombosis.

Ultrasound Guidance

Two-dimensional ultrasound can be used to facilitate venous cannulation. An example of an ultrasound image obtained during cannulation of the internal jugular vein is shown in Figure 6.8. In this case, the ultrasound transducer is oriented along the long axis of the vein as the needle is advanced towards the vein. This type of real-time imaging (obtained while the procedure is performed) improves the success rate of cannulation and reduces the risk of accidental arterial puncture (22,24,25). Real-time ultrasound guidance has been used to facilitate cannulation of the large central veins (subclavian, internal jugular, and femoral veins) and

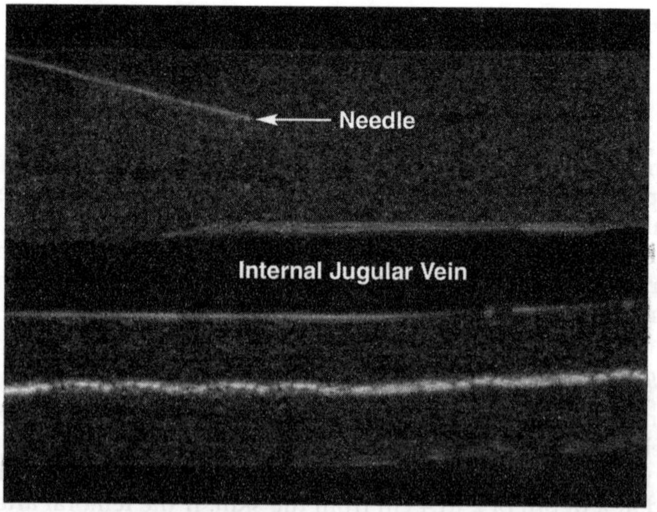

FIGURE 6.8 Real-time ultrasound visualization of a needle being advanced toward the internal jugular vein. (From Abboud PAC, Kendall JL. Ultrasound guidance for vascular access. Emerg Med Clin North Am 2004;22:749.) Image is digitally retouched.

smaller peripheral veins in the arm (22,24–26). Most of the reported experience has been with the internal jugular vein, which is easy to visualize.

Comment

Ultrasound guidance for venous cannulation is expensive, time-consuming, and requires an experienced operator. As a result, this method is not used routinely but is reserved for situations where attempted central venous cannulation using anatomical landmarks has failed. Failed venous cannulation is most likely to occur when physicians with limited experience are attempting emergency venous cannulation, such as during cardiopulmonary resuscitation (27,28). Unfortunately, this situation is not well suited for the use of ultrasound because of the time required and the need for experienced personnel. Therefore ultrasound is rarely a useful adjunct for venous cannulation.

IMMEDIATE CONCERNS

Venous Air Embolism

Air entry into the venous circulation is one of the most feared complications of central venous cannulation in the chest. Fortunately, this complication can be prevented with attention to the measures described in the next section.

Preventive Measures

When the tip of a venous catheter is advanced into the thorax, the negative intrathoracic pressures generated during spontaneous breathing can draw air into the venous circulation through an open catheter and produce a venous air embolism. A pressure gradient of only 4 mm Hg along a 14-gauge catheter can entrain air at a rate of 90 mL/second and produce a fatal air embolus in one second (29). This highlights the importance of keeping the venous pressure higher than the atmospheric pressure to prevent venous air embolism. This is facilitated by placing the patient in the Trendelenburg position with the head 15° below the horizontal plane. Remember that the **Trendelenburg position does not prevent venous air entry** because patients still generate negative intrathoracic pressures while in the Trendelenburg position. When changing connections in a central venous line, a temporary positive pressure can be created by having the patient hum audibly. This not only produces a positive intrathoracic pressure but allows clinicians to hear when the intrathoracic pressure is positive. In ventilator-dependent patients, the nurse or respiratory therapist should initiate a mechanical lung inflation when changing connections.

Clinical Presentation

The usual presentation is acute onset of dyspnea that occurs during the procedure. Hypotension and cardiac arrest can develop rapidly. Air can pass across a patent foramen ovale and obstruct the cerebral circulation, producing an acute ischemic stroke. A characteristic "mill wheel" murmur can be heard over the right heart, but this murmur may be fleeting.

Therapeutic Maneuvers

If a venous air embolism is suspected, a syringe should be attached to the hub of the catheter immediately (to prevent any further air entry), and you should attempt to aspirate air through the indwelling catheter. The patient can also be placed with the left side down, which presumably keeps air in the right side of the heart. In dire circumstances, a needle can be inserted through the anterior chest wall and into the right ventricle to aspirate the air. (This is accomplished by inserting a long needle in the fourth intercostal space just to the right of the sternum and advancing the needle under the sternum at a 45 degree angle until there is blood return.) Unfortunately, in severe cases of venous air embolism, the mortality is high despite any of the suggested therapeutic maneuvers.

Pneumothorax

Pneumothorax is a feared complication of subclavian vein cannulation but can also occur with jugular vein cannulation (2,30). The risk of pneumothorax is one of the principal reasons that postinsertion chest x-rays are recommended after central venous cannulation (or attempts). Postinsertion chest x-rays should be obtained in the upright position and during expiration, if possible. **Films obtained during expiration will facilitate the detection of a small pneumothorax** because expiration decreases the volume of air in the lungs but not the volume of air in the pleural space. Thus during expiration, the volume of air in the pleural space is a larger fraction of the total volume of the hemithorax, thereby magnifying the radiographic appearance of the pneumothorax (31).

Upright films are not always possible in ICU patients. When supine films are necessary, remember that **pleural air does not collect at the apex of the lung when the patient is in the supine position** (32,33). In this situation, pleural air tends to collect in the subpulmonic recess and along the anteromedial border of the mediastinum (see Chapter 26), which are the highest points in the thorax in the supine position.

Delayed Pneumothorax

A catheter-induced pneumothorax may not be radiographically evident until 24 to 48 hours after catheter insertion (31,33), which means that **the absence of a pneumothorax on an immediate postinsertion chest film does not absolutely exclude the possibility of a catheter-induced pneumothorax.** This is an important consideration only in patients who develop dyspnea or progressive hypoxemia in the first few days after central venous cannulation. For patients who remain asymptomatic after a central venous catheter is inserted, serial chest x-rays are not justified.

Catheter Tip Position

A properly placed subclavian or internal jugular vein catheter should run parallel to the shadow of the superior vena cava, and the tip of the

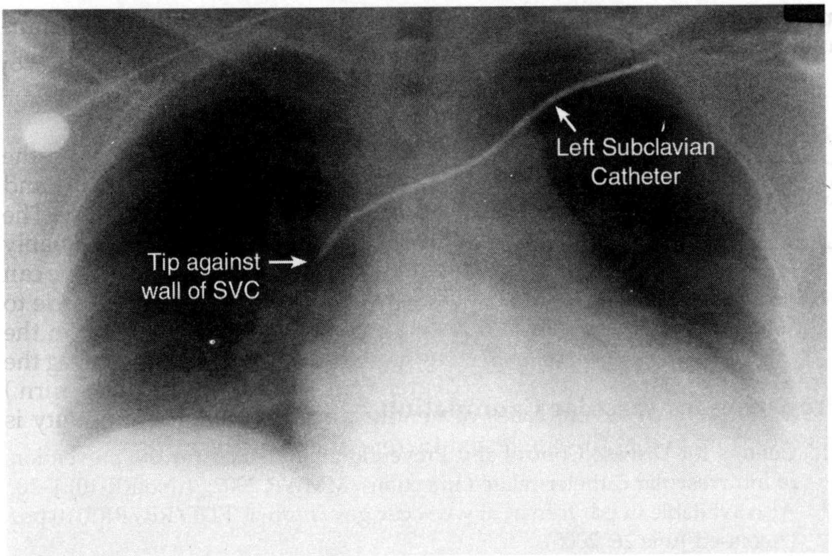

FIGURE 6.9 Left subclavian catheter in a position to perforate the superior vena cava. (Image of catheter digitally enhanced.)

catheter should be at or slightly above the third anterior intercostal space (see Figure 6.5). The following catheter malpositions warrant corrective measures.

Tip Against the Wall of the Vena Cava

Catheters inserted from the left side must make an acute turn downward when they enter the superior vena cava from the left innominate vein. Catheters that do not make this turn can end up in a position like the one shown in Figure 6.9. The tip of this catheter is pointed directly at the lateral wall of the superior vena cava and can perforate the vessel (see Figure 7.1). Catheters in this position should either be withdrawn into the innominate vein or advanced further down the superior vena cava.

Tip in the Right Atrium

A catheter tip that extends below the third right anterior intercostal space is likely to be in the right side of the heart. These catheters are considered a risk for cardiac perforation (31). However, cardiac perforation is rare (35), even though over half of central venous catheters may be misplaced in the right atrium (35). Despite the low risk for cardiac perforation, placement of catheters in the right side of the heart should be avoided. This is best accomplished by using central venous catheters that are no longer than 15 cm in length, as mentioned earlier. If a catheter tip extends below the third anterior intercostal space, the catheter should be withdrawn until the tip is in the appropriate position. If the anterior portion of the third rib cannot be visualized, keep the catheter tip at or above the tracheal carina (i.e., the division of the trachea into the right and left main-stem bronchi).

REFERENCES

General Texts

Latto IP, Ng WS, Jones PL, et al. Percutaneous central venous and arterial catheterization, 3rd ed. Philadelphia: WB Saunders, 2000.

Wilson SE. Vascular access: principles and practice, 3rd ed. St. Louis: Mosby, 1996.

Preparing for Vascular Cannulation

1. Centers for Disease Control and Prevention. Guidelines for the prevention of intravascular catheter-related infections. MMWR 2002;51(No.RR-10):1–30. Also available in pdf format at www.cdc,gov/mmwr/PDF/RR/RR5110.pdf (Accessed June 26, 2005).
2. Centers for Disease Control and Prevention. Guidelines for hand hygiene in health-care settings: recommendations of the Healthcare Infection Control Practices Advisory Committee and the HICPAC/SHEA/APIC/IDSA Hand Hygiene Task Force. MMWR 2002;51 (No.RR-16):1–45. Also available in pdf format at www.cdc.gov/mmwr/PDF/RR/ RR5116.pdf (Accessed April 10, 2005).

Vascular Catheters

3. de la Roche MRP, Gauthier L. Rapid transfusion of packed red blood cells: effects of dilution, pressure, and catheter size. Ann Emerg Med 1993;22: 1551–1555.
4. McGee DC, Gould MK. Preventing complications of central venous catheterization. N Engl J Med 2003;348:1123–1133.
5. Jacobs BR. Central venous catheter occlusion and thrombosis. Crit Care Clin 2003;19:489–514.
6. Marin MG, Lee JC, Skurnick JH. Prevention of nosocomial bloodstream infections: effectiveness of antimicrobial-impregnated and heparin-bonded central venous catheters. Crit Care Med 2000;28:3332–3338.
7. Laster JL, Nichols WK, Silver D. Thrombocytopenia associated with heparin-coated catheters in patients with heparin-associated antiplatelet antibodies. Arch Intern Med 1989;149:2285–2287.
8. Darouche RO, Raad II, Heard SO, et al. A comparison of antimicrobial-impregnated central venous catheters. N Engl J Med 1999;340:1–8.
9. Hanna H, Darouche R, Raad I. New approaches for prevention of intravascular catheter-related infections. Infect Med 2001;18:38–48.
10. Ng P, Ault M, Ellrodt AG, et al. Peripherally inserted central catheters in general medicine. Mayo Clin Proc 1997;72:225–233.
11. Heffner JE. A guide to the management of peripherally inserted central catheters. J Crit Illness 2000;15:165–169.

Vascular Access Sites

12. Merrer J, DeJonghe B, Golliot F, et al. Complications of femoral and subclavian venous catheterization in critically ill patients. JAMA 2001;286:700–707.
13. Ruesch S, Walder B, Tramer M. Complications of central venous catheters: internal jugular versus subclavian access: a systematic review. Crit Care Med 2002;30:454–460.
14. Deshpande K, Hatem C, Ulrich H, et al. The incidence of infectious complications of central venous catheters at the subclavian, internal jugular, and femoral sites in an intensive care unit population. Crit Care Med 2005;33: 13–20.
15. Foster PF, Moore LR, Sankary HN, et al. Central venous catheterization in patients with coagulopathy. Arch Surg 1992;127:273–275.
16. Fisher NC, Mutimer DJ. Central venous cannulation in patients with liver disease and coagulopathy: a prospective audit. Intensive Care Med 1999;25: 481–485.
17. Doerfler M, Kaufman B, Goldenberg A. Central venous catheter placement in patients with disorders of hemostasis. Chest 1996;110:185–188.
18. McGee WT, Ackerman BL, Rouben LR, et al. Accurate placement of central venous catheters: a prospective, randomized, multicenter trial. Crit Care Med 1993;21:1118–1123.
19. Seneff MG. Central venous catheterization. A comprehensive review. Intensive Care Med 1987;2:163–175, 218–232.
20. Joynt GM, Kew J, Gomersall CD, et al. Deep venous thrombosis caused by femoral venous catheters in critically ill adult patients. Chest 2000;117: 178–183.
21. Getzen LC, Pollack EW. Short-term femoral vein catheterization. Am J Surg 1979;138:875–877.
22. Hilty WM, Hudson PA, Levitt MA, et al. Real-time ultrasound-guided femoral vein catheterization during cardiopulmonary resuscitation. Ann Emerg Med 1997;29:311–316.
23. Cummins RO, ed. ACLS provider manual. Dallas, TX: American Heart Association, 2001:38–39.

Ultrasound Guidance

24. Abboud PAC, Kendall JL. Ultrasound guidance for vascular access. Emerg Med Clin North Am 2004;22:749–773.
25. Hind D, Calvert N, Mcwilliams R, et al. Ultrasonic locating devices for central venous cannulation: a meta-analysis. Br Med J 2003;327:361–367.
26. Keyes LA, Frazee BW, Snoey ER, et al. Ultrasound-guided brachial and basilic vein cannulation in emergency department patients with difficult venous access. Ann Emerg Med 1999;34:711–714.
27. Bo-Lin GW, Andersen DJ, Andersen KC, et al. Percutaneous central venous catheterization performed by medical house officers: a prospective study. Cathet Cardiovasc Diagn 1982;8:23–29.
28. Emerman CI, Bellon EM, Lukens TW, et al. A prospective study of femoral versus subclavian vein catheterization during cardiac arrest. Ann Emerg Med 1990;19:26–30.

Immediate Concerns

29. Muth CM, Shank ES. Gas embolism. N Engl J Med 2000;342:476–482.
30. Sladen A. Complications of invasive hemodynamic monitoring in the intensive care unit. Curr Probl Surg 1988;25:69–145.
31. FDA Task Force. Precautions necessary with central venous catheters. FDA Drug Bull 1989;15–16.
32. Marino PL. Delayed pneumothorax: a complication of subclavian vein catheterization. J Parenter Enteral Nutr 1985;9:232.
33. Tocino IM, Miller MH, Fairfax WR. Distribution of pneumothorax in the supine and semirecumbent critically ill adult. Am J Radiol 1985;144: 901–905.
34. Collin GR, Clarke LE. Delayed pneumothorax: a complication of central venous catheterization. Surg Rounds 1994;17:589–594.
35. McGee WT, Ackerman BL, Rouben LR, et al. Accurate placement of central venous catheters: a prospective, randomized, multicenter trial. Crit Care Med 1993;21:1118–1123.

Chapter 7

THE INDWELLING VASCULAR CATHETER

This chapter is a continuation of Chapter 6 and describes the routine care and adverse consequences of indwelling vascular catheters. Many of the recommendations in this chapter are taken from the clinical practice guidelines and reviews listed in the bibliography at the end of the chapter (1–4).

ROUTINE CATHETER CARE

The following practices are designed to prevent or limit complications of indwelling vascular catheters.

Protective Dressings

Catheter insertion sites on the skin are covered at all times as a standard antiseptic measure. Although sterile gauze is adequate (1), catheter insertion sites are often covered with costly adhesive dressings made of transparent, semipermeable polyurethane membranes (5–7). These dressings (e.g., Opsite, Tegaderm) partially block the escape of water vapor from the underlying skin and create a moist environment that is considered beneficial for wound healing. Although they allow inspection of the underlying catheter insertion site, **occlusive polyurethane dressings do not reduce the incidence of catheter colonization or infection when compared to sterile gauze dressings** (1,5–7). In fact, occlusive dressings can *increase* the risk of infection (5,6) because the enhanced moisture they create provides a favorable environment for the growth of microorganisms.

Because of the added cost and minimal benefit provided by occlusive polyurethane dressings, **sterile gauze should be the preferred dressing for most catheter insertion sites**. Adhesive polyurethane dressings can be reserved for catheter insertion sites that are close to a source of infectious secretions (e.g., internal jugular vein insertion sites that are close to a tracheostomy).

Antimicrobial Ointment

Antimicrobial ointments or gels are often applied to the insertion site of central venous catheters. These ointments are applied when the catheter is inserted and then re-applied each time the dressings are changed (which is usually every 48 hours). However, this practice does not reduce the incidence of catheter-related infections (3), and it can promote the development of antibiotic-resistant organisms (8). Therefore, it is wise to **avoid the use of topical antimicrobial ointments** on catheter insertion sites (1,3).

Replacing Catheters

Peripheral Venous Catheters

The risk with peripheral vein cannulation is phlebitis (from the catheter or infusate), not septicemia. The incidence of phlebitis increases significantly after peripheral vein catheters are left in place longer than 72 hours (1), but the incidence does not change from 72 to 96 hours (9). Therefore, replacement of peripheral vein catheters (using a new venipuncture site) is recommended every 72 to 96 hours (1).

Central Venous Catheters

Septicemia from central venous catheters begins to appear after catheters have been in place for 3 days (1,10). This observation led to the common practice of replacing vascular catheters every few days to reduce the risk of infection. However, replacing vascular catheters at regular intervals, using either guidewire exchange or a new venipuncture site, does not reduce the incidence of catheter-related infections (11) and may actually increase the risk of complications (both mechanical and infectious) (12). This latter point deserves emphasis because there is a 7% complication rate associated with replacement of central venous catheters (3). The lack of benefit combined with the added risk is the reason that **routine replacement of indwelling vascular catheters is not recommended** (1,3,4).

Indications for Catheter Replacement

Vascular catheters should be replaced in the following situations:

When there is purulent drainage from the catheter insertion site. Erythema around the insertion site of a central venous catheter is not absolute evidence of infection (13) and is not an indication for catheter replacement.

When a percutaneously inserted vascular catheter is suspected as a source of systemic sepsis and the patient has a prosthetic valve, is immunocompromised, or has severe sepsis or septic shock.
When a catheter has been placed emergently, without strict aseptic technique, and it can be replaced safely.
When a femoral vein catheter has been in place longer than 48 hours and it can be replaced safely. This will limit the risk of venous thrombosis from femoral vein catheters (see Table 6.3).

Flushing Catheters

Vascular catheters are flushed at regular intervals to prevent thrombotic obstruction, although this may not be necessary for peripheral catheters used for intermittent infusions (14). The standard flush solution is heparinized saline (with heparin concentrations ranging from 10 to 1,000 units/mL) (1,15). Catheter lumens that are used only intermittently are capped and filled with heparinized saline when idle. (The term *heparin lock* is used to describe this process because the cap that seals the catheter creates a partial vacuum that holds the flush solution in place.) Arterial catheters are flushed continuously at a rate of 3 mL/hour using a pressurized bag to drive the flush solution through the catheter (16).

Alternatives to Heparin

The use of heparin in catheter flush solutions has two disadvantages: the cost of the heparin (which can be substantial if you consider all the catheter flushes that are performed each day in a hospital), and the risk of heparin-induced thrombocytopenia (see Chapter 37). These disadvantages can be eliminated by using heparin-free flush solutions (see Table 7.1). **Saline alone is as effective as heparinized saline for flushing venous catheters** (15). This is not the case for arterial catheters (16), but 1.4% sodium citrate is a suitable alternative to heparinized saline for flushing arterial catheters (17).

TABLE 7.1 Alternatives to Heparinized Flushes

Vascular Device	Alternate Flush Technique	Indications
Central and peripheral venous catheters	Flush with 0.9% sodium chloride, using the same volume (1–5 mL) and time interval (every 8–12 hr) used with heparin (14)	Standard protocol for all venous catheters
Peripheral venous catheters	Flush with 0.9% sodium chloride (1–5 mL) only after drug administration (16)	Standard protocol for peripheral catheters
Arterial catheters	Flush with 1.4% sodium citrate,using a continuous-flow technique (17)	Heparin-induced thrombocytopenia

MECHANICAL COMPLICATIONS

The mechanical complications of indwelling catheters can be classified as occlusive (e.g., catheter or vascular occlusion) or erosive (e.g., vascular or cardiac perforation). The following are the more common or preventable mechanical complications.

Catheter Occlusion

Sources of catheter occlusion include sharp angles or kinks and localized indentations along the catheter (usually created during insertion), thrombosis (from backwash of blood into the catheter), insoluble precipitates in the infusates (from medications or inorganic salts), or lipid residues (from total parenteral nutrition). **Thrombosis is the most common cause of catheter obstruction**, and thrombotic occlusion is the most common complication of indwelling central venous catheters (4). Insoluble precipitates can be the result of drugs that have limited solubility in water (e.g., barbiturates, diazepam, digoxin, phenytoin, and trimethoprim–sulfa) or anion–cation complexes (e.g., calcium phosphate and heparin–aminoglycoside complexes) precipitated by an acid or alkaline pH (18,19).

Signs of catheter occlusion include limited flow (partial occlusion), cessation of infusate (forward) flow but able to withdraw blood (partial occlusion), and total cessation of flow in both directions (complete occlusion).

Restoring Patency

Every effort should be made to relieve catheter occlusion and avoid replacing the catheter. Replacement over a guidewire is not advised because the guidewire can dislodge an obstructing mass and create an embolus, so a new venipuncture site is required to replace obstructed catheters.

THROMBOTIC OCCLUSION. Since thrombosis is the most common cause of catheter occlusion, the initial attempt to restore patency should involve the local instillation of a thrombolytic agent. Table 7.2 shows a regimen using alteplase (recombinant tissue plasminogen activator) that has proven 90% effective in restoring patency in partially and completely occluded vascular catheters (19–21). The total thrombolytic dose in this regimen (up to 4 mg) is too small to cause systemic thrombolysis, even if the entire dose is reaches the systemic circulation (19).

Non-Thrombotic Occlusion

Dilute acid will promote the solubility of calcium phosphate precipitates and some medications, and catheter occlusion refractory to thrombolytic agents will occasionally respond to instillation of 0.1N hydrochloric acid (22). If lipid residues are suspected as a cause of catheter occlusion (i.e., in patients receiving concentrated lipid infusions as part of a parenteral nutrition regimen), instillation of 70% ethanol (2 mL) can restore catheter patency (19).

TABLE 7.2 A Protocol for Restoring Patency in Occluded Vascular Catheters

Drug: Alteplase (recombinant tissue plasminogen activator)

Preparation: Reconstitute 50 mg vial of alteplase with 50 mL sterile water for a drug concentration of 1 mg/mL. Prepare 2 mL aliquots and freeze until needed.

Regimen:

1. Thaw two aliquots (2 mL each) of drug solution. (Drug must be used within 8 hr after thawing).
2. Draw 2 mL of drug solution (2 mg) into a 5 mL syringe and attach to hub of the occluded catheter.
3. Inject as much volume as possible (≤2 mL) into the lumen of the catheter and then cap the hub of the catheter.
4. Leave the drug solution in the catheter lumen for 2 hr (dwell time).
5. Attempt to flush the catheter with a saline solution. DO NOT use a tuberculin syringe to flush occluded catheters (the high velocities generated by these syringes can fracture the hub of a catheter).
6. If the catheter is still obstructed, repeat steps 1 up to 4.
7. If the catheter remains obstructed, consider using 0.1N HCL (2 mL) for drug or calcium phosphate precipitates, or 70% ethanol (2 mL) if lipid residues are suspected. Otherwise, replace the catheter.

From References 19–22.

Venous Thrombosis

Thrombus formation around the catheter can occasionally extend to cause thrombotic obstruction of the surrounding vein. The following types of venous thrombosis can originate from an indwelling vascular catheter.

Upper Extremity Thrombosis

Clinically apparent thrombosis of the subclavian vein occurs in about 1% of patients with subclavian vein catheters (see Table 6.3). The hallmark of subclavian vein thrombosis is unilateral arm swelling on the side of the catheter insertion (23). Symptomatic pulmonary embolism can occur, but the reported incidence varies from zero to 17% (23,24). On occasion, the thrombus can extend proximally into the superior vena cava (23), but complete occlusion of the superior vena cava with the resultant *superior vena cava syndrome* (swelling of neck and face, etc.) is rare (25).

Doppler ultrasound is often used to evaluate possible subclavian vein thrombosis, but the sensitivity and specificity of this test can be as low as 56% and 69%, respectively (26). Contrast venography is the gold standard but is rarely performed.

If a subclavian vein thrombosis is confirmed, the catheter should be removed. Systemic anticoagulation with heparin is a popular (but not standard) therapy for catheter-induced subclavian vein thrombosis

(23,24), but the efficacy of this treatment is unproven, and there are no guidelines regarding duration of treatment or the need for continued anticoagulation with coumadin.

Lower Extremity Thrombosis

As mentioned in the last chapter, the risk of venous thrombosis is higher with femoral catheters than subclavian or internal jugular vein catheters (see Table 6.3), and this is why the femoral vein is almost never used as a primary site for central venous cannulation. The diagnosis and treatment of deep vein thrombosis in the legs is described in detail in Chapter 5 and will not be repeated here.

Vascular Perforation

Catheter-induced perforations of the superior vena cava and right atrium are uncommon but avoidable complications of central venous cannulation, as described at the end of Chapter 6. Attention to proper catheter position is the most important measure for preventing perforation.

Superior Vena Cava Perforation

Perforation of the superior vena cava is most often caused by left-sided central venous catheters that cross the mediastinum and enter the superior vena cava but do not make the acute turn downward toward the heart (see Figures 6.9 and 7.1) (27). This complication has also been reported after guidewire exchange of left-sided catheters (28). Perforation can occur at any time in the life span of an indwelling catheter. Most occur in the first 7 days after catheter insertion, but perforations have been reported up to 2 months after catheter placement (27). The clinical symptoms (substernal chest pain, cough, and dyspnea) are nonspecific, and suspicion is usually raised by the sudden appearance of mediastinal widening or a pleural effusion on a chest x-ray (see Figure 7.1). The pleural effusions represent leakage of the infusion fluid, and they can be unilateral (right- or left-sided) or bilateral. **The unexpected appearance of a pleural effusion in a patient with a central venous catheter should always raise suspicion of superior vena cava perforation.**

DIAGNOSIS. Thoracentesis is required to confirm that the pleural fluid is similar in composition to the infusion fluid. Pleural fluid glucose levels are useful if the infusion fluid is a glucose-rich parenteral nutrition formula. The diagnosis can be confirmed by injecting radiocontrast dye through the catheter: the presence of dye in the mediastinum confirms the perforation.

MANAGEMENT. When vena cava perforation is first suspected, the infusion should be stopped immediately. If the diagnosis is confirmed, the catheter should be removed immediately (this does not provoke mediastinal bleeding) (27). Antibiotic therapy is not necessary (27) unless there

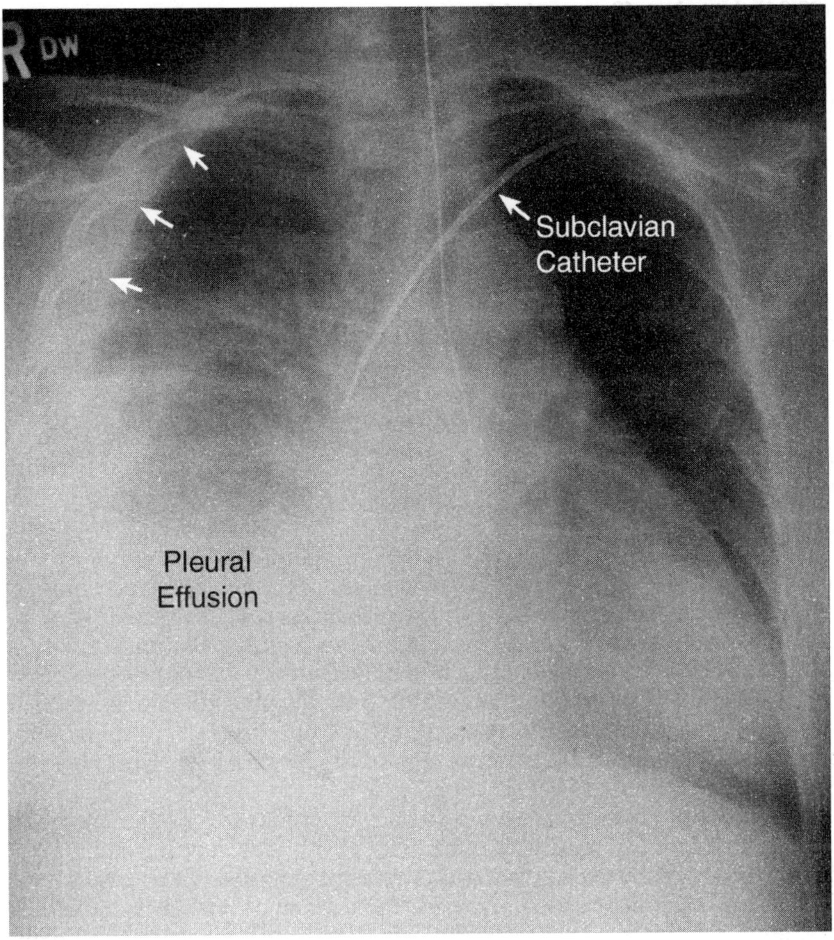

FIGURE 7.1 Chest x-ray of a patient with a superior vena cava perforation from a left-sided subclavian catheter (which is positioned like the one in Figure 6.9). [Image courtesy of Dr. John E. Heffner (from Reference 27)].

is evidence of infection in the pleural fluid. If the pleural effusion is a glucose-rich parenteral nutrition formula, it is wise to drain the effusion because the high glucose concentration provides a favorable medium for microbial proliferation.

Cardiac Tamponade

Cardiac perforation from a catheter misplaced in the right heart chambers is a rare but life-threatening complication of central venous cannulation. Perforation can lead to rapidly progressive cardiac tamponade and sudden cardiovascular collapse (29), and the diagnosis can be overlooked in the commotion of cardiopulmonary resuscitation. Immediate pericardiocentesis is necessary to confirm the diagnosis (the fluid will have the same composition as the infusate) and to relieve the tamponade. Emergency thoracotomy may be necessary if there is a large tear in the wall of the heart. Repositioning catheters that extend below the right third anterior intercostal space (which marks the junction of the superior vena cava with the right atrium) should prevent this life-threatening complication.

INFECTIOUS COMPLICATIONS

Hospital-acquired (nosocomial) bloodstream infections occur 2 to 7 times more often in ICU patients than in other hospitalized patients (30), and indwelling vascular catheters are responsible for over half of these bloodstream infections (31). Catheter-related bloodstream infections add to the morbidity and mortality of the ICU stay (32).

Pathogenesis

Biofilms

Most microorganisms are not free-living but exist in protected colonies called *biofilms* that are found on moist environmental surfaces (the slippery material that covers rocks in a stream is a biofilm). Biofilm formation takes place in two stages: the attachment of the microbe to the object, and the production of an extracellular matrix (called a glycocalyx or *slime*) that surrounds the microbes and protects them from adverse environmental conditions. The protected environment of the biofilm allows microbes to thrive and proliferate (33).

Biofilms can also form on the surface of implanted medical devices, including urinary and vascular catheters (34). The biofilms that form on vascular catheters can shield the encased microbes from circulating antibiotics, and **antibiotic concentrations must be 100 to 1,000 times greater to eradicate bacteria in biofilms than to kill free-flowing bacteria** (2). *Staphylococcus epidermidis*, which is the organism most frequently involved in catheter-related bloodstream infections, shows a propensity for adhering to polymer surfaces and producing a protective biofilm (see Figure 7.2) (35).

Understanding the behavior of biofilms has important implications for the prevention and management of infections arising from medical devices. For example, hydrogen peroxide has been shown to disrupt biofilms (36), and it is possible that such "biocides" will prove much more effective in eradicating catheter-related infections than conventional antimicrobial therapy. Biofilms deserve much more attention if we are to develop a more effective approach to infections involving indwelling medical devices.

Sources of Infection

The common sources of infection involving indwelling vascular catheters are shown in Figure 7.3. Each source is described below by using the corresponding numbers in Figure 7.3.

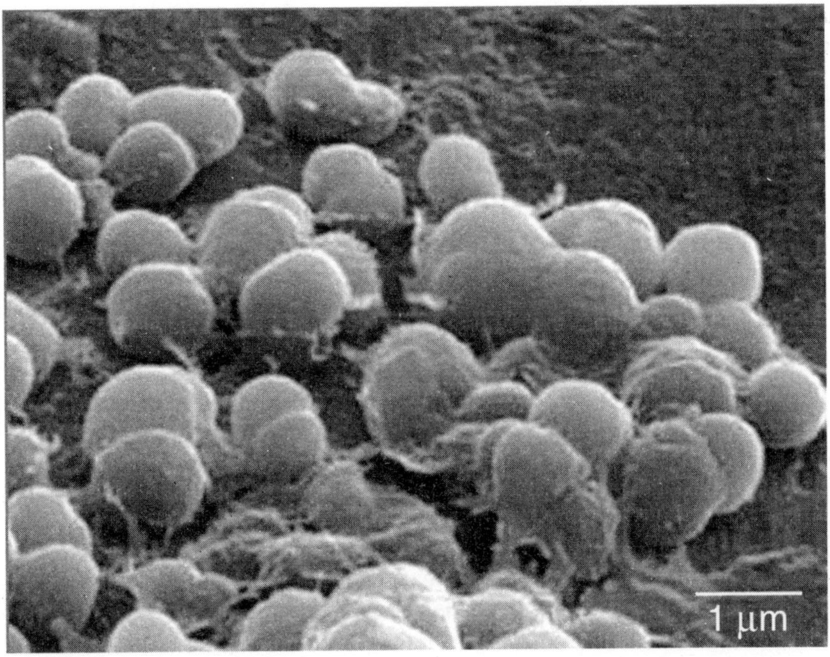

FIGURE 7.2 Electron micrograph of a biofilm formed by *Staphylococcus epidermidis*. The large, rounded tufts represent bacteria that are encased in an extracellular matrix. (Image courtesy of Jeanne M. Van Briesen, and Vanessa Dorn Briesen, Department of Biomedical Engineering Carnegie Mellon University.)

1. Microbes can gain access to the internal lumen of vascular catheters through break points in the infusion system, such as stopcocks and catheter hubs. This may be a prominent route of infection for long-term catheters inserted through a subcutaneous tunnel (2).

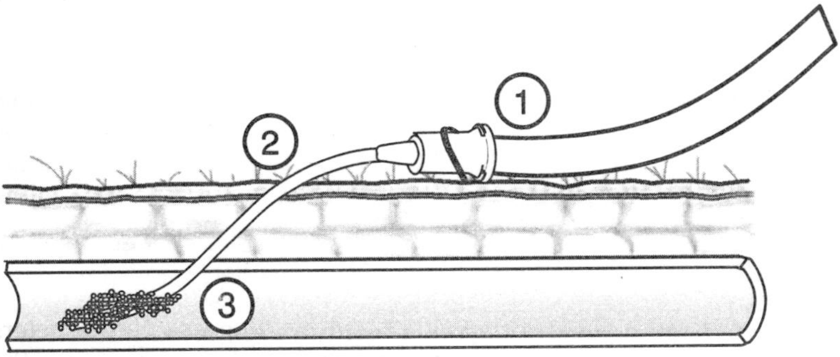

FIGURE 7.3 The sources of infection involving vascular catheters.

2. Microbes on the skin can migrate along the subcutaneous tract created by indwelling catheters. This is considered the principal route of infection for percutaneous (non-tunneled) catheters (2).
3. Microorganisms in circulating blood can attach directly to indwelling vascular catheters or can become trapped in the fibrin meshwork that surrounds indwelling catheters.

Definitions

The Centers for Disease Control and Prevention has identified the following infectious complications of indwelling vascular catheters (2).

Catheter colonization is characterized by significant growth of a microorganism on the catheter (the criteria for significant growth are presented later in the chapter) but no growth in blood cultures.

Exit-site infection is present when there is drainage from the catheter insertion site that grows a microorganism on culture. Blood cultures may be positive or negative.

Catheter-related septicemia is present when a blood culture taken from a site other than the catheter grows a microorganism and the same microorganism is isolated in significant numbers from the catheter or from blood withdrawn through the catheter.

Clinical Features

Catheter colonization is asymptomatic, while catheter-related septicemia is usually accompanied by non-specific signs of systemic inflammation (i.e., fever, leukocytosis, etc.). The diagnosis of catheter-related septicemia is not possible on clinical grounds (2). Purulent drainage from the catheter insertion site is uncommon and could indicate exit-site infection without septicemia, and the presence or absence of inflammation around the insertion site has no predictive value for the presence of absence of bloodstream infection (2,13). Catheter-related septicemia is usually suspected when a patient with a vascular catheter in place for longer than 48 hours has an unexplained fever. Confirmation requires identification of the same organism in blood and on the catheter.

Culture Methods

The following culture methods are useful for the diagnosis of catheter-related septicemia.

Quantitative Blood Cultures

This method requires two blood specimens (see Table 7.3): One specimen is withdrawn through the indwelling vascular catheter, and the other is drawn from a peripheral vein. The blood is processed by lysing the cells to release intracellular organisms then adding broth to the supernatant (Isolator System, Dupont, Wilmington, DE). This mixture is placed on an

TABLE 7.3 Diagnosis of Catheter-Related Septicemia using Quantitative Blood Cultures

Specimens: 10 mL blood withdrawn through the indwelling catheter and 10 mL blood drawn from a peripheral vein. Place blood specimens in evacuator culture tubes (e.g., Isolator System, Dupont Co.). DO NOT place blood specimens in routine culture bottles.

Criteria for catheter-related septicemia:

The same species of organism must be isolated from both blood specimens, and condition A or B must be satisfied

A. Blood from the catheter grows ≥100 colony-forming units per mL (CFU/mL)

B. Colony count from catheter blood is ≥5 times greater than colony count from peripheral blood

Test performance: Sensitivity = 40%–50%

Comment: This method does not require removal of the indwelling catheter, but it has a low sensitivity because it does not detect infections arising from the outer surface of the catheter

All information in this table is taken from the clinical practice guideline in Reference 2.

agar plate and allowed to incubate for 24 hours. Growth is measured as the number of colony-forming units per milliliter (CFU/mL).

The criteria for the diagnosis of catheter-related septicemia are shown in Table 7.3. The same organism must be isolated from both blood samples (catheter and peripheral vein), *and* the colony count in blood from the catheter must be 100 CFU/mL or higher, or the colony count in catheter blood must be 5- to 10-fold higher than in peripheral blood (2). The comparative growth in a case of catheter-related septicemia is shown in Figure 7.4.

ADVANTAGES AND DISADVANTAGES. The major advantage of this culture method is that it obviates replacement of indwelling catheters. The major disadvantage is the inability to detect infections arising from the outer surface of the catheter, which may explain the low sensitivity (40 to 50%) of this method for detecting catheter-related septicemia (2).

Catheter Tip Cultures

The intravascular segment of the catheter can be cultured by removing the catheter and (using sterile technique) severing a 5 cm (2 inch) segment from the distal tip of the catheter. This is placed in a sterile culturette tube for transport to the microbiology laboratory. The following two culture methods are available (see Table 7.4).

SEMIQUANTITATIVE (ROLL-PLATE) CULTURE. The severed catheter segment is rolled directly over the surface of a blood agar plate, and the plate is incubated for 24 hours. Growth is measured as the number of colony-forming units (CFUs) on the agar plate after 24 hours, and **significant growth is defined as ≥ 15 CFUs per catheter tip** (2). This is the standard

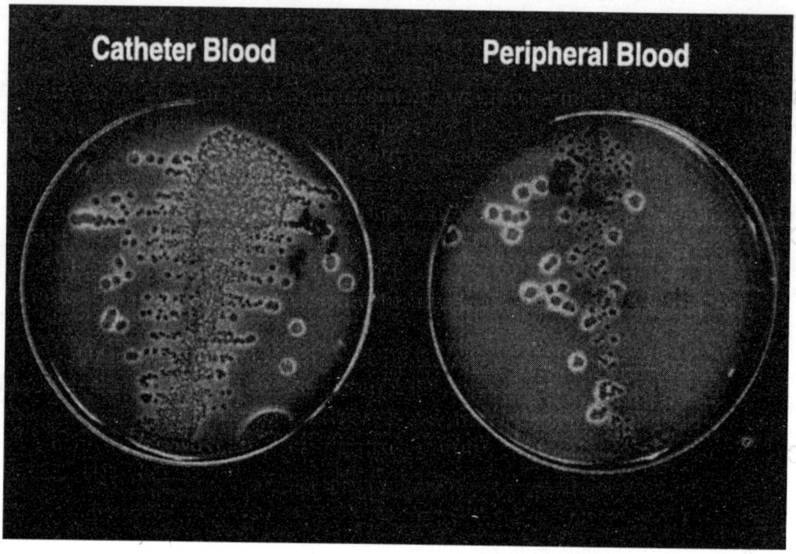

FIGURE 7.4 Comparative growth of quantitative blood cultures from a case of catheter-related septicemia. Blood withdrawn through a central venous catheter (*Catheter Blood*) shows markedly greater growth than does blood taken from a peripheral vein (*Peripheral Blood*). (From Curtas S, Tramposch K. Culture methods to evaluate central venous catheter sepsis. Nutr Clin Pract 1991;6:43.)

method of culturing catheter tips, but it does not detect infections arising from the inner surface of the catheter.

QUANTITATIVE CULTURE. The catheter tip is placed in culture broth and vigorously stirred to release attached organisms. The broth is then subjected to serial dilutions and is placed on a blood agar plate. **Significant growth is identified as ≥ 100 CFUs per catheter tip** at 24 hours (2). This method can detect infections arising from both surfaces of a catheter, which explains why it has a higher sensitivity than the semiquantitative (roll plate) method for detecting catheter-related infections (see Table 7.4).

Which Method is Preferred?

The choice of culture method is dictated in part by the desirability of replacing the catheter. **The quantitative blood culture method is preferred when replacement of indwelling catheters is not desirable.** This situation arises when catheter replacement might not be necessary (e.g., for patients with isolated fever), when catheter replacement is not easily accomplished (i.e., for tunneled catheters, which must be surgically replaced), and when venous access is limited (e.g., chronic hemodialysis patients). Since over half of vascular catheters removed for suspected infection are sterile when cultured (2), the use of paired quantitative blood cultures will limit unnecessary catheter removal.

TABLE 7.4 Diagnosis of Catheter-related Septicemia using Catheter-Tip Cultures

Specimens:

1. The distal 5 cm of the catheter is severed and placed in a sterile culturette tube
2. One set of blood cultures is drawn from a peripheral vein

Culture methods:

Semiquantitative culture: The catheter tip is rolled across the surface of a blood agar plate, and the number of colony-forming units (CFUs) is recorded after 24 hr

Quantitative culture: The catheter tip is agitated in culture broth, and the broth is placed on a blood agar plate. Growth is recorded as the number of colony-forming units (CFUs) after 24 hr

Criteria for catheter-related septicemia:

The same species of organism must be isolated from the catheter tip and blood, and growth from the catheter tip should reveal the following:

A. Semiquantitative culture: ≥15 CFU

B. Quantitative culture: ≥100 CFU

Test performance: Sensitivity of 60% for semiquantitative cultures and 80% for quantitative cultures

Comment: Semiquantitative cultures will miss infections arising from the inner surface of the catheter. Quantitative cultures are more sensitive for detecting catheter-related infections

All information in this table is taken from the clinical practice guideline in Reference 2.

Whenever catheter replacement is indicated (see earlier in the chapter), cultures of the catheter tip are essential. **For catheter tip cultures, the quantitative method is preferred to the semiquantitative (roll-plate) method** (2) because it can detect infection on both surfaces of the catheter and has a higher sensitivity for detecting catheter-related septicemia.

The Microbial Spectrum

A survey of 112 medical ICUs in the United States revealed the following microbial spectrum in primary hospital-acquired bacteremias (most caused by indwelling catheters) (37): coagulase-negative staphylococci, mostly *Staphylococcus epidermidis* (36%), enterococci (16%), gram-negative aerobic bacilli (*Pseudomonas aeruginosa, Klebsiella pneumoniae, E coli,* etc.) (16%), *Staphylococcus aureus* (13%), *Candida* species (11%), and other organisms (8%). About half of the infections involve staphylococci, and half involve organisms usually found in the bowel, including *Candida* organisms. This microbial spectrum is important to consider when selecting empiric antimicrobial therapy.

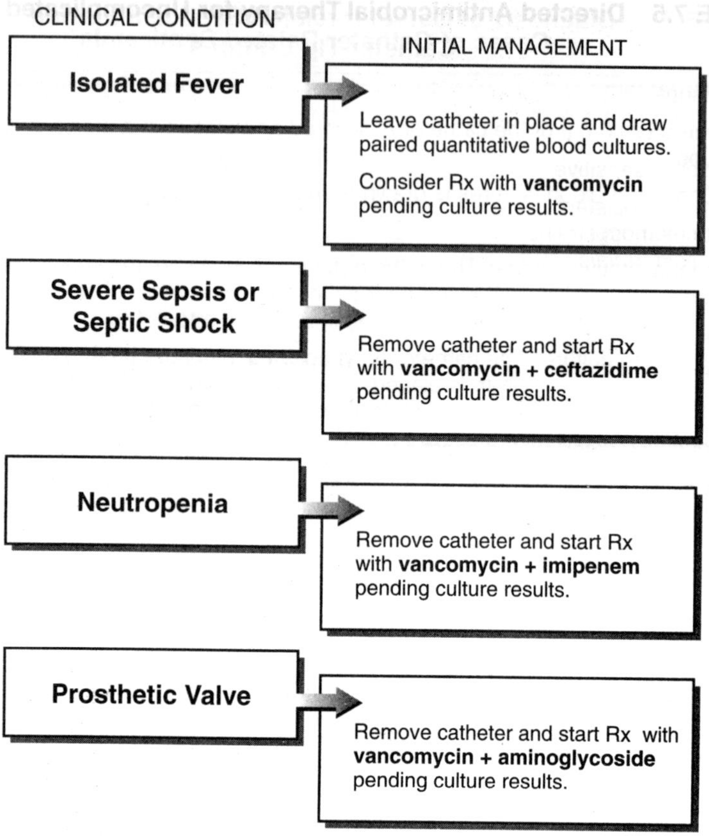

FIGURE 7.5 Recommendations for the initial management of suspected catheter-related septicemia. (From References 2 and 38.)

Management

The initial management of suspected catheter-related septicemia can be conducted as shown in Figure 7.5. In patients with isolated fever and no other signs of infection, catheters can be kept in place while performing paired, quantitative blood cultures. This approach is supported by studies showing that **up to 70% of catheters removed for suspected catheter-related septicemia prove to be sterile** (2). Removal of catheters is usually recommended for patients with the following: purulent drainage from the insertion site, severe sepsis, septic shock, neutropenia, or a prosthetic valve (2).

Empiric Antibiotic Therapy

Empiric antibiotic therapy is recommended for most patients with suspected catheter-related septicemia (2). Despite concern about vancomycin

TABLE 7.5 Directed Antimicrobial Therapy for Uncomplicated Cases of Catheter-Related Septicemia

Organism	Effective Antibiotics
Staphylococci	
Methicillin-sensitive	Nafcillin or oxacillin (2 g every 4 hr)
Methicillin-resistant (includes most strains of *S. epidermidis*)	Vancomycin (1 g every 12 hr)
Enterococci	
Ampicillin-sensitive	Ampicillin (2 g every 4–6 hr)
Ampicillin-resistant	Vancomycin (1 g every 12 hr)
Vancomycin-resistant	Linezolid (600 mg every 12 hr)
Gram-negative bacilli	Imipenem (500 mg every 6 hr) or
E. coli	Meropenem (1 g every 8 hr)
Klebsiella spp	
Enterobacter spp	For *P. aeruginosa*, some prefer Ceftazidime (2 g every 8 hr) or an Antipseudomonal penicillin
P. aeruginosa	
Candida organisms	Fluconazole (6 mg/kg/day) or Capsofungin (70 mg load, then 50 mg daily)
	Amphotericin B (0.7 mg/kg/day) is reserved for severe infections

Antibiotic recommendations from References 2 and 39.

resistance, this antibiotic is well-suited for suspected catheter-related infections because it is active against *Staph. epidermidis*, *Staph. aureus* (including methicillin-resistant strains), and most strains of enterococci (which together are responsible for over 50% of catheter-related infections). Gram-negative coverage with ceftazidime or cefepime (for antipseudomonal activity) can be added for patients with severe sepsis (i.e., sepsis plus dysfunction in 2 or more major organs) or septic shock, and for patients with neutropenia (neutrophil count $<500/mm^3$), a carbapenem (imipenem or meropenem) can be added to vancomycin (2,38). For patients with a prosthetic valve, an aminoglycoside should be added to vancomycin (the two agents can be synergistic for *Staph. epidermidis* endocarditis). The dosage of these antibiotics is shown in Table 7.5.

Directed Antibiotic Therapy

If the culture results confirm a catheter-related septicemia, directed antibiotic therapy can proceed using the antibiotics in Table 7.5 (2,39). For uncomplicated cases of catheter-related septicemia, 10 to 14 days of antibiotics is recommended, but only 5 to 7 days is sufficient for most cases of *Staph. epidermidis* septicemia (2). Antifungal therapy for candidemia should continue for 14 days after blood cultures become sterile or signs of sepsis resolve (39). Catheters that have been left in place should be removed if cultures confirm the presence of catheter-related septicemia (2). There are two situations where catheters can be left in place if the patient shows a favorable response to antimicrobial therapy: when catheter removal is not easily accomplished (e.g., tunneled catheters), and when the responsible organism is *Staphlococcus epidermidis*. However, relapse after systemic antimicrobial therapy is higher when catheters have been left in place (40), and this relapse is less likely when *antibiotic lock therapy* is used (see next).

Antibiotic Lock Therapy

Antibiotic lock therapy involves the instillation of concentrated antibiotic solutions (usually 1 to 5 mg/mL) into the lumen of an infected catheter and leaving the solution in place for hours to days (2). This treatment is recommended only for infected catheters that have not been removed, and only when a lumen of the catheter is not used continuously for infusion therapy. It is best suited for tunneled catheters that have been in place for longer than 2 weeks, because these catheters are likely to have an intraluminal source of infection (2). The recommended duration of therapy is 2 weeks (2). This approach has had only limited success when *Candida* species are responsible for the infection (2).

Persistent Sepsis

Continued signs of sepsis after a few days of antibiotic therapy can signal the following conditions.

Suppurative Thrombosis

Thrombosis surrounding the catheter tip is a common finding in catheter-related septicemia (4), and if the thrombus becomes infected, it can transform into an intravascular abscess. When this occurs, there is persistent septicemia despite catheter removal and appropriate antimicrobial therapy. Purulent drainage from the catheter insertion site may or may not be evident (2), and thrombotic occlusion of the great central veins can result in ipsilateral arm swelling. Septic emboli in the lungs has also been reported in this condition (2). Catheter removal is mandatory in cases of suppurative thrombosis. Surgical incision and drainage is often required if peripheral vessels are involved. In the large central veins, antimicrobial therapy combined with heparin anticoagulation can produce satisfactory results in 50% of cases (41).

Endocarditis

Persistent septicemia despite antimicrobial therapy and catheter removal can also be a sign of infective endocarditis. Vascular catheters are the most common cause of nosocomial endocarditis, and *Staph. aureus* is the most common offending organism (2). Because of the risk of endocarditis, **all**

cases of *Staph. aureus* bacteremia should be evaluated for endocarditis (2). Transesophageal ultrasound is the procedure of choice. If vegetations are evident on ultrasound, 4 to 6 weeks of antimicrobial therapy is warranted (2).

Disseminated Candidiasis

Persistent candidemia or persistent sepsis despite broad spectrum antimicrobial therapy can be a sign of invasive candidiasis (42). The most common cause of this condition is vascular catheters, and patients at risk include those with abdominal surgery, burns, organ transplantation, human immunodeficiency virus infection, and those receiving cancer chemotherapy, long-term steroids, or broad-spectrum antimicrobial therapy (42). The diagnosis can be missed in over 50% of cases because blood cultures are often negative (43). Suspicion of this condition is often prompted by colonization of multiple sites with *Candida* organisms (e.g., urine, sputum, wounds, vascular catheters).

Clinical markers of disseminated candidiasis include candiduria in the absence of an indwelling urethral catheter and endophthalmitis. Heavy colonization of the urine in high-risk patients, even in the presence of an indwelling Foley catheter, can be used as an indication to initiate empiric antifungal therapy (44). Endophthalmitis can occur in up to one-third of patients with disseminated candidiasis (43) and can lead to permanent blindness. Because the consequences of this condition can be serious, **all patients with persistent candidemia should have a detailed eye exam** (43).

The standard treatment for invasive candidiasis is amphotericin B (0.7 mg/kg/day), which is now available in a special lipid formulation (liposomal amphotericin B, 3 mg/kg/day) that produces less toxicity. The newer antifungal agent capsofungin (70 mg loading dose, followed by 50 mg/day) has proven as effective as amphotericin for invasive candidiasis (45) and may become the preferred agent in this condition because of its safety profile. Unfortunately, satisfactory outcomes are achieved in only 60 to 70% of cases of invasive candidiasis despite our best efforts (45).

REFERENCES

Practice Guidelines

1. Centers for Disease Control and Prevention. Guidelines for the prevention of intravascular catheter-related infections. MMWR 2002;51(no. RR-10:1–30. Also available at www.cdc,gov/mmwr/PDF/RR/RR5110.pdf (Accessed on June 26, 2005).
2. Mermel LA, Farr BM, Sherertz RJ, et al. Guidelines for the management of intravascular catheter-related infections. Clin Infect Dis 2001;32:1249–1272. Also available at www.sccm.org/professional_resources/guidelines/table_of_contents/index.asp (accessed on June 26, 2005).

Reviews

3. McGee DC, Gould MK. Preventing complications of central venous catheterization. N Engl J Med 2003;348:1123–1133.
4. Jacobs BR. Central venous catheter occlusion and thrombosis. Crit Care Clin 2003;19:489–514.

Protective Dressings

5. Hoffman KK, Weber DJ, Samsa GP, et al. Transparent polyurethane film as intravenous catheter dressing: a meta-analysis of infection risks. JAMA 1992;267:2072–2076.
6. Maki DG, Stolz SS, Wheeler S, et al. A prospective, randomized trial of gauze and two polyurethane dressings for site care of pulmonary artery catheters: implications for catheter management. Crit Care Med 1994;22:1729–1737.
7. Marshall DA, Mertz PA, Eaglestein WH. Occlusive dressings. Arch Surg 1990;125:1136–1139.

Antimicrobial Ointments

8. Zakrzewska-Bode A, Muytjens HL, Liem KD, et al. Muciprocin resistance in coagulase-negative staphylococci after topical prophylaxis for the reduction of colonization of central venous catheters. J Hosp Infect 1995;31:189–193.

Replacing Catheters

9. Lai KK. Safety of prolonging peripheral cannula and IV tubing use from 72 hours to 96 hours. Am J Infect Control 1998;26:66–70.
10. Ullman RF, Guerivich I, Schoch PE, et al. Colonization and bacteremia related to duration of triple-lumen intravascular catheter placement. Am J Infect Control 1990;18:201–207.
11. Cook D, Randolph A, Kernerman P, et al. Central venous replacement strategies: a systematic review of the literature. Crit Care Med 1997;25:1417–1424.
12. Cobb DK, High KP, Sawyer RP, et al. A controlled trial of scheduled replacement of central venous and pulmonary artery catheters. N Engl J Med 1992;327:1062–1068.
13. Safdar N, Maki D. Inflammation at the insertion site is not predictive of catheter-related bloodstream infection with short-term, noncuffed central venous catheters. Crit Care Med 2002;30:2632–2635.

Catheter Flushes

14. Walsh DA, Mellor JA. Why flush peripheral intravenous cannulae used for intermittent intravenous injection? Br J Clin Pract 1991;45:31–32.
15. Peterson FY, Kirchhoff KT. Analysis of research about heparinized versus non-heparinized intravascular lines. Heart Lung 1991;20:631–642.
16. American Association of Critical Care Nurses. Evaluation of the effects of heparinized and nonheparinized flush solutions on the patency of arterial pressure monitoring lines: the AACN Thunder Project. Am J Crit Care 1993;2:3–15.

17. Branson PK, McCoy RA, Phillips BA, et al. Efficacy of 1.4% sodium citrate in maintaining arterial catheter patency in patients in a medical ICU. Chest 1993;103:882–885.

Mechanical Complications

18. Trissel LA. Drug stability and compatibility issues in drug delivery. Cancer Bull 1990;42:393–398.
19. Calis KA, ed. Pharmacy update: Drug Information Service, National Institutes of Health. Bethesda, MD:1999 (Accessed at www.cc.nih.gov/phar/updates/.99nov-dec.html on August 5, 2005).
20. Davis SN, Vermeulen L, Banton J, et al. Activity and dosage of alteplase dilution for clearing occlusions of vascular-access devices. Am J Health Syst Pharm 2000;57:1039–1045.
21. Zacharias JM. Alteplase versus urokinase for occluded hemodialysis catheters. Ann Pharmacother 2003;37:27–33.
22. Shulman RJ, Reed T, Pitre D, et al. Use of hydrochloric acid to clear obstructed central venous catheters. J Parent Enteral Nutr 1988;12:509–510.
23. Mustafa S, Stein P, Patel K, et al. Upper extremity deep venous thrombosis. Chest 2003;123:1953–1956.
24. Hingorani A, Ascher E, Hanson J, et al. Upper extremity versus lower extremity deep venous thrombosis. Am J Surg 1997;174:214–217.
25. Otten TR, Stein PD, Patel KC, et al. Thromboembolus disease involving the superior vena cava and brachiocephalic veins. Chest 2003;123:809–812.
26. Mustafa BO, Rathbun SW, Whitsett TL, et al. Sensitivity and specificity of ultrasonography in the diagnosis of upper extremity deep venous thrombosis: a systematic review. Arch Intern Med 2002;162:401–404.
27. Heffner JE. A 49-year-old man with tachypnea and a rapidly enlarging pleural effusion. J Crit Illness 1994;9:101–109.
28. Armstrong CW, Mayhall CG. Contralateral hydrothorax following subclavian catheter replacement using a guidewire. Chest 1983;84:231–233.
29. Long R, Kassum D, Donen N, et al. Cardiac tamponade complicating central venous catheterization for total parenteral nutrition: a review. J Crit Care 1987;2:39–44.

Infectious Complications

30. Pittet D, Tarara D, Wenzel RP. Nosocomial bloodstream infection in critically ill patients. JAMA 1994;271:1598–1601.
31. Edgeworth J, Treacher D, Eykyn S. A 25-year study of nosocomial bacteremia in an adult intensive care unit. Crit Care Med 1999;27:1421–1428.
32. Laupland KB, Zygun DA, Davies D, et al. Population-based assessment of intensive care unit-acquired bloodstream infection in adults: incidence, risk factors, and associated mortality rate. Crit Care Med 2002;30:2462–2467.
33. O'Toole G, Kaplan HB, Kolter R. Biofilm formation as microbial development. Annu Rev Microbiol 2000;54:49–79.
34. Chenoweth CE. Biofilms and catheter-associated urinary tract infections. Infect Dis Clin North Am 2003;17:411–432.

35. von Eiff C, Peters G, Heilman C. Pathogenesis of infections due to coagulase-negative staphylococci. Lancet Infect Dis 2002;2:677–685.
36. Biofilm: Disinfecting biofilms using hydrogen peroxide/silver based bioside. Available at www.accepta.com/Industry_Water_Treatment/Biofilm_biocide.asp (Accessed 8/07/2005).
37. Richards M, Edwards J, Culver D, et al. Nosocomial infections in medical intensive care units in the United States. Crit Care Med 1999;27:887–892.
38. Hughes WT, Armstrong D, Bodey GP, et al. 2002 guidelines for the use of antimicrobial agents in neutropenic patients with cancer. Clin Infect Dis 2002;34:730–751.
39. Pappas PG, Rex JH, Sobel JD, et al. Guidelines for treatment of candidiasis. Clin Infect Dis 2004;38:161–189.
40. Raad I, Davis S, Khan A, et al. Impact of central venous catheter removal on the recurrence of catheter-related coagulase-negative staphylococcal bacteremia. Infect Control Hosp Epidemiol 1992;154:808–816.
41. Verghese A, Widrich WC, Arbeit RD. Central venous septic thrombophlebitis: the role of antimicrobial therapy. Medicine 1985;64:394–400.
42. Ostrosky-Zeichner L, Rex JH, Bennett J, et al. Deeply invasive candidiasis. Infect Dis Clin North Am 2002;16:821–835.
43. Calandra T. Candida infections in the intensive care unit. Curr Opin Crit Care 1997;3:335–341.
44. British Society for Antimicrobial Chemotherapy Working Party. Management of deep *Candida* infection in surgical and intensive care unit patients. Intensive Care Med 1994;20:522–528.
45. Mora-Duarte J, Betts R, Rotstein C, et al. Comparison of capsofungin and amphotericin B for invasive candidiasis. N Engl J Med 2002;347:2020–2029.

Section **IV**

HEMODYNAMIC MONITORING

Not everything that counts can be counted. And not everything that can be counted counts.

ALBERT EINSTEIN

Chapter 8

ARTERIAL BLOOD PRESSURE

It should be clearly recognized that arterial pressure cannot be measured with precision by means of sphygmomanometers.

American Heart Association, Committee for Arterial Pressure Recording, 1951

The arterial blood pressure is one of the most popular measurements in modern medicine. However, as emphasized in the introductory quote made *over a half century ago,* the standard method of recording arterial pressure with an inflatable cuff (sphygmomanometer) is not expected to produce accurate results. The imprecision of the indirect blood pressure measurement (which makes one wonder about the diagnosis of hypertension) can be corrected by cannulating a peripheral artery and recording direct intra-arterial pressures. This is a common method of recording arterial blood pressure in the ICU, but direct arterial blood pressure measurements can (like their indirect counterparts) be misleading.

This chapter provides a brief description of both indirect and direct methods of arterial blood pressure recording and highlights the important shortcomings of each method.

INDIRECT MEASUREMENTS

The indirect method of measuring blood pressure that is used today was first introduced in Italy in 1896 (by an Italian physician named Riva-Rocci) and was brought to this country at the turn of the century by the famed neurosurgeon, Dr. Harvey Cushing. This method employs a device called a *sphygmomanometer* (*sphygmos* is a Greek term for pulse, and a manometer measures pressure), which consists of an inflatable bladder covered by a cloth sleeve and a gauge or column to measure pressure. The cloth sleeve is wrapped around the arm or leg in an area that overlies a major artery, and the bladder in the sleeve is inflated until it reaches a pressure that should compress the underlying artery. The bladder is then slowly deflated, allowing the compressed artery to open,

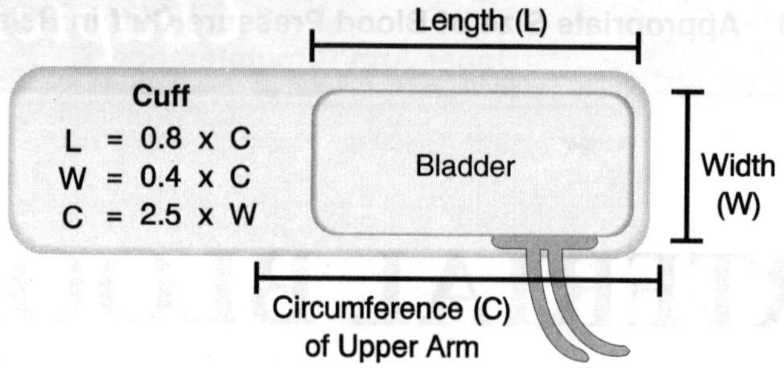

FIGURE 8.1 Optimal dimensions of the cuff bladder for accurate blood pressure readings. The width (*W*) and length (*L*) of the bladder are expressed in relation to the circumference (*C*) of the upper arm.

and the arterial pressure is determined by recording either the sounds (auscultation method) or the vascular pulsations (oscillometric method) that are generated as the artery opens.

Influence of Bladder Size

The sounds or vibrations created by the opening of the artery are more reproducible when the artery is compressed uniformly for a short distance. Therefore to ensure a reliable blood pressure recording, the inflatable bladder in the blood pressure cuff should produce a uniform compression of the underlying artery. This is determined by the size of the inflatable bladder relative to the size of the limb being compressed. Figure 8.1 shows the optimal dimensions of the cuff bladder for indirect measurements of brachial artery pressure. The length of the bladder should be at least 80% of the circumference of the upper arm (measured midway between the shoulder and elbow), and **the width of the bladder should be at least 40% of the upper arm circumference** (1). If the bladder is too small for the size of the arm, the pressure measurements will be falsely elevated (1–5).

Miscuffing

Miscuffing is the term used to describe **the use of inappropriately sized cuffs** for the blood pressure measurement (1). This **is considered the most common source of errors in the blood pressure measurement**, so it deserves some attention. Table 8.1 shows the appropriate cuff sizes for upper arm circumferences ranging from 22 cm (about 9 inches) to 52 cm (about 21 inches). Since this information is not always available when measuring blood pressures, a simple bedside method of determining appropriate cuff size is described next.

Bedside Assessment of Cuff Size

Before wrapping the cuff around the arm, align the cuff so that the long axis is parallel to the long axis of the arm. Then turn the cuff over so the bladder on the underside is facing you, and wrap the cuff lengthwise around the upper arm. The bladder (width) should encircle half of the upper arm

TABLE 8.1 Appropriate Size of Blood Pressure Cuff in Relation to Upper Arm Circumference

Upper Arm Circumference	Blood Pressure Cuff	
	Size	Dimensions
22 to 26 cm	Small adult	12 × 24 cm
27 to 34 cm	Adult	16 × 30 cm
35 to 44 cm	Large adult	16 × 36 cm
45 to 52 cm	Adult thigh	16 × 42 cm

From Reference 1.

(circumference). If the bladder encircles less than half of the upper arm, the cuff is too small, and the blood pressure measurement may be spuriously high. If the cuff encircles most of the upper arm and seems too big for the arm, no change in cuff size is necessary (i.e., a cuff that is larger than needed will not produce spurious pressure recordings) (1).

Auscultatory Method

The standard method of measuring blood pressure involves manual inflation of an arm cuff placed over the brachial artery. The cuff is then gradually deflated, and the pressure is determined by sounds (called Korotkoff sounds) that are generated when the artery begins to open.

The Korotkoff Sounds

The Korotkoff sounds are very low frequency sounds (25 to 50 Hz) and are just above the normal threshold for human hearing, which is 16 Hz (6). Human speech is generally in the frequency range of 120 to 250 Hz, and the human ear detects sounds optimally when they have frequencies of 2,000 to 3,000 Hz. (6). What this means is the room should be quiet when listening for Korotkoff sounds (because you will hear people talking more easily than you hear these sounds), and even then, the sounds will be faint to the human ear.

Stethoscope Head

The bell-shaped head of a stethoscope is a low frequency transducer, while the flat, diaphragm-shaped head is designed to detect high frequency sounds. Therefore to optimize detection of the low-frequency Korotkoff sounds, the **bell-shaped head of the stethoscope should be used to measure blood pressure** (1). This is often neglected, and some stethoscopes are manufactured without a bell-shaped head!

Low Flow States

Because Korotkoff sounds are generated by blood flow, **low flow states can** diminish the intensity of these sounds. When this occurs, the sounds may not be heard at first (i.e., at the systolic pressure), and this will **result in falsely low recordings for the systolic blood pressure**. The tendency

TABLE 8.2 Discrepancy Between Direct and Indirect Blood Pressure Measurements in Shock

Systolic BP Difference (Direct BP—Cuff BP)	% Patients
0–10 mm Hg	0
11–20 mm Hg	28
21–30 mm Hg	22
>30 mm Hg	50

From Cohn JN. Blood pressure measurement in shock. JAMA 1967; 119:118.

to underestimate the systolic blood pressure in low flow states is shown in Table 8.2. This is from a study comparing direct and indirect measurements of systolic blood pressure in patients with a low flow state and hypotension (3). In half of the patients, the indirect auscultatory method underestimated the actual systolic blood pressure by more than 30 mm Hg. According to the American Association for Medical Instrumentation, indirect pressure measurements should be within 5 mm Hg of directly recorded pressures to be considered accurate (4). Using this criterion, there was not a single pressure recording with the auscultatory method that could be considered accurate. Observations like these are the reason that direct blood pressure measurements are preferred in hemodynamically compromised patients.

Oscillometric Method

The oscillometric method uses the principle of plethysmography to detect pulsatile pressure changes (oscillations) in an underlying artery. When an inflated cuff is placed over an artery, the pulsatile pressure changes in the artery will be transmitted to the inflated cuff, producing similar changes in cuff pressure. The periodic changes in cuff pressure (i.e., oscillations) are then processed electronically to derive a value for the mean, systolic, and diastolic blood pressures (5).

Performance

Oscillometric devices first appeared in the mid 1970s and since then have gained widespread acceptance for monitoring blood pressure in operating rooms, ICUs, and emergency rooms. However, **the accuracy of oscillometric blood pressure measurements is disturbingly low**. This is demonstrated in Figure 8.2, which shows a comparison of directly measured systolic pressures with oscillometric measurements in patients undergoing major surgery. The dark line is the line of unity (where the measurements using both techniques would be identical) and the area bounded by the lighter lines (which are 5 mm Hg on either side of unity) is the zone of acceptable accuracy for oscillometric pressure measurements. Note that most of the oscillometric measurements (closed squares) fall outside the zone of acceptable accuracy, indicating that a majority of the oscillometric measurements in this study were inaccurate.

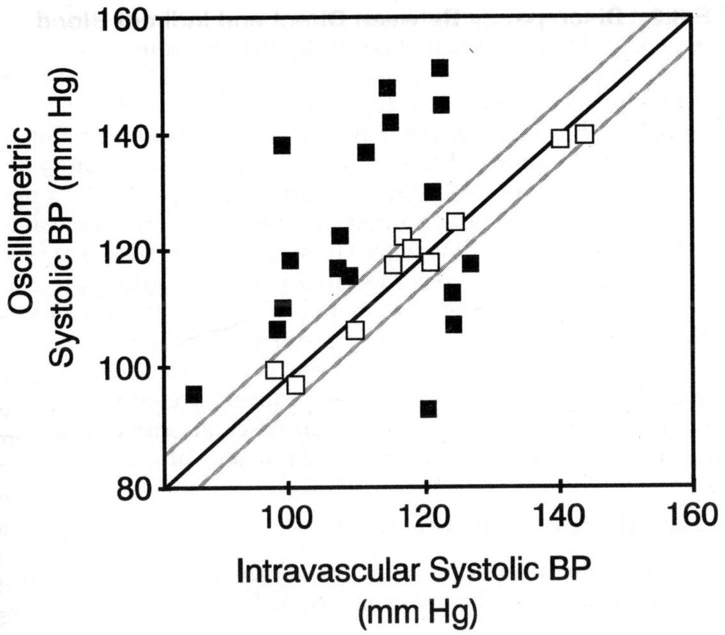

FIGURE 8.2 Comparison of direct (open squares) and oscillometric (closed squares) measurements of systolic pressure in the brachial artery. (From Gravlee GP, Brockschmidt JK. Accuracy of four indirect methods of blood pressure measurement, with hemodynamic correlations. J Clin Monit 1990;6:284–298.)

Other studies in ICU patients have shown that **oscillometric measurements are consistently lower than direct blood pressure measurements** (6,7). Some of this discrepancy is due to "miscuffing" (6,7), so attention to proper cuff sizes is important for oscillometric measurements, as it is for auscultatory measurements. However, until accuracy and reliability improve, **oscillometric blood pressure measurements should not be regarded as an adequate substitute for direct blood pressure measurements** in the ICU.

DIRECT MEASUREMENTS

Direct recording of intravascular pressures is recommended for all patients in the ICU who are hemodynamically unstable or are at risk for hemodynamic instability. Unfortunately, direct arterial pressure recordings have their own shortcomings, and some of these will be described in the remainder of the chapter.

Pressure Versus Flow

The distinction between pressure and flow is important to recognize because there is a tendency to equate pressure and flow in certain situations. This is most evident in the popularity of pressor or vasoconstrictor agents in the management of clinical shock. In this setting, an increase in blood pressure is often assumed to indicate an increase in systemic blood flow, but the opposite effect (a decrease in flow) is also possible.

One of the important distinctions between pressure and flow is the transmission of pressure and flow waves through the circulatory system. Ejection of the stroke volume from the heart is accompanied by a pressure wave and a flow wave. Under normal conditions, the pressure wave travels 20 times faster than the flow wave (10 m/second versus 0.5 m/second), and thus the pulse pressure recorded in a peripheral artery precedes the corresponding stroke volume by a matter of seconds (8). When vascular impedance (i.e., compliance and resistance) is increased, the velocity of the pressure wave is increased, while the velocity of the flow wave is decreased. (When vascular impedance is reduced, pressure can be diminished while flow is enhanced.) Thus **when vascular impedance is abnormal, the arterial pressure is not a reliable index of blood flow**.

The Arterial Pressure Waveform

The contour of the arterial pressure waveform changes as the pressure wave moves away from the proximal aorta. This is shown in Figure 8.3.

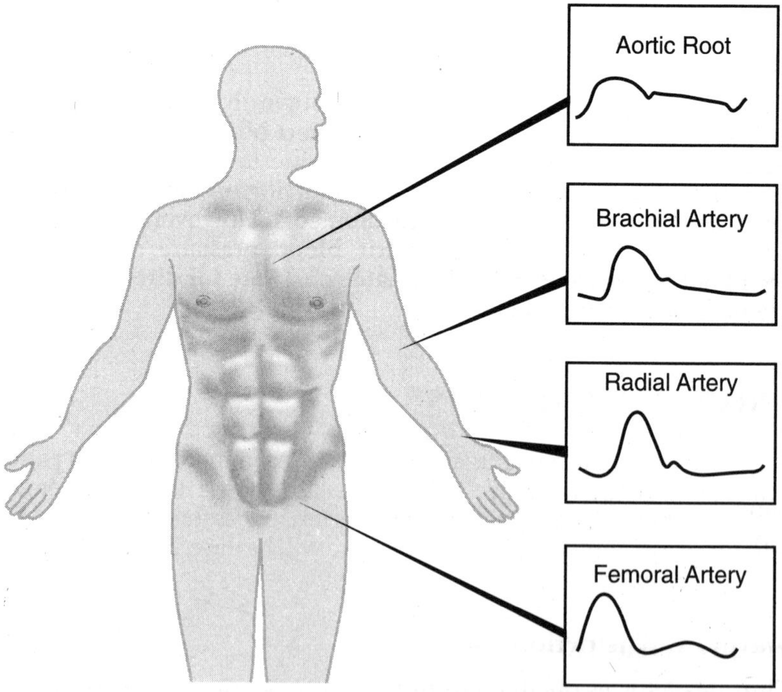

FIGURE 8.3 Arterial pressure waveforms at designated points in the arterial circulation.

Note that **as the pressure wave moves toward the periphery, the systolic pressure gradually increases,** and the systolic portion of the waveform narrows. The systolic pressure can increase as much as 20 mm Hg from the proximal aorta to the radial or femoral arteries. This increase in peak systolic pressure is offset by the narrowing of the systolic pressure wave, so that **the mean arterial pressure remains unchanged**. Therefore, the mean arterial pressure is a more accurate measure of central aortic pressure.

Systolic Amplification

The increase in systolic pressure in peripheral arteries is the result of pressure waves that are reflected back from the periphery (9). These reflected waves originate from vascular bifurcations and from narrowed blood vessels. As the pressure wave moves peripherally, wave reflections become more prominent, and the reflected waves add to the systolic pressure wave and amplify the systolic pressure. **Amplification of the systolic pressure is particularly prominent when the arteries are noncompliant,** causing reflected waves to bounce back faster. This is the mechanism for systolic hypertension in the elderly (9). Because a large proportion of patients in the ICU are elderly, systolic pressure amplification is probably commonplace in the ICU.

RECORDING ARTIFACTS

Fluid-filled recording systems can produce artifacts that further distort the arterial pressure waveform. Failure to recognize recording system artifacts can lead to errors in interpretation.

Resonant Systems

Vascular pressures are recorded by fluid-filled plastic tubes that connect the arterial catheters to the pressure transducers. This fluid-filled system can oscillate spontaneously, and the oscillations can distort the arterial pressure waveform (10,11).

The performance of a resonant system is defined by the resonant frequency and the damping factor of the system. The resonant frequency is the inherent frequency of oscillations produced in the system when it is disturbed. When the frequency of an incoming signal approaches the resonant frequency of the system, the resident oscillations add to the incoming signal and amplify it. This type of system is called an underdamped system. The damping factor is a measure of the tendency for the system to attenuate the incoming signal. A resonant system with a high damping factor is called an overdamped system.

Waveform Distortion

Three waveforms obtained from different recording systems are shown in Figure 8.4. The waveform in panel *A*, with the rounded peak and

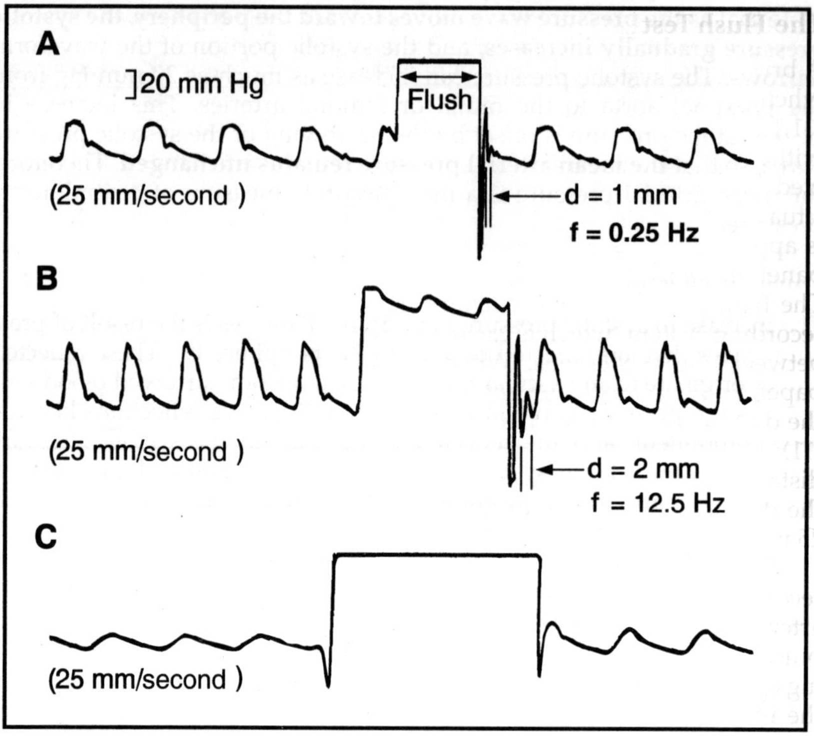

FIGURE 8.4 The rapid flush test. A, Normal test. B, Underdamped system. C, Overdamped system.

the dicrotic notch, is the normal waveform expected from a recording system with no distortion. The waveform in panel *B,* with the sharp systolic peak, is from an underdamped recording system. The recording systems used in clinical practice are naturally underdamped, and these systems can amplify the systolic pressure by as much as 25 mm Hg (12). The systolic amplification can be minimized by limiting the length of the connector tubing between the catheter and the pressure transducer.

The waveform in panel C of Figure 8.4 shows an attenuated systolic peak with a gradual upslope and downslope and a narrow pulse pressure. This waveform is from an overdamped system. Overdamping reduces the gain of the system and is sometimes the result of air bubbles trapped in the connector tubing or in the dome of the pressure transducer. Flushing the hydraulic system to evacuate air bubbles should improve an overdamped signal.

Unfortunately, it is not always possible to identify underdamped and overdamped systems using the arterial pressure waveform. The test described in the next section can help in this regard.

The Flush Test

A brief flush to the catheter-tubing system can be applied to determine whether the recording system is distorting the pressure waveform (11,13). Most commercially available transducer systems are equipped with a one-way valve that can be used to deliver a flush from a pressurized source. Figure 8.4 shows the results of a flush test in three different situations. In each case, the pressure increases abruptly when the flush is applied. However, the response at the end of the flush differs in each panel. In panel *A*, the flush is followed by a few oscillating waveforms. The frequency of these oscillations is the resonant frequency (f) of the recording system, which is calculated as the reciprocal of the time period between the oscillations. When using standard strip-chart recording paper divided into 1 mm segments, f can be determined by measuring the distance between oscillations and dividing this into the paper speed (11); that is, f (in Hz) = paper speed (in mm/second) divided by the distance between oscillations (in mm). In the example shown in panel *A*, the distance (d) between oscillations is 1.0 mm, and the paper speed is 25 mm/second, so $f = 25$ Hz (25 mm/second divided by 1.0 mm).

Signal distortion is minimal when the resonant frequency of the recording system is five times greater than the major frequency in the arterial pressure waveform. Because the major frequency in the arterial pulse is approximately 5 Hz (14), the resonant frequency of the recording system in panel *A* (25 Hz) is five times greater than the frequency in the incoming waveform, and the system will not distort the incoming waveform.

The flush test in panel *B* of Figure 8.4 reveals a resonant frequency of 12.5 Hz ($f = 25/2$). This is too close to the frequency of arterial pressure waveforms, so this system will distort the incoming signal and produce systolic amplification.

The flush test shown in panel C of Figure 8.4 does not produce any oscillations. This indicates that the system is overdamped, and this system will produce a spuriously low pressure recording. When an overdamped system is discovered, the system should be flushed thoroughly (including all stopcocks in the system) to release any trapped air bubbles. If this does not correct the problem, the arterial catheter should be repositioned or changed.

Mean Arterial Pressure

The **mean arterial pressure** has two features that make it **superior to the systolic pressure for arterial pressure monitoring**. First, the mean pressure is the true driving pressure for peripheral blood flow. Second, the mean pressure does not change as the pressure waveform moves distally, nor is it altered by distortions generated by recording systems (10).

The mean arterial pressure can be measured or estimated. Most electronic pressure monitoring devices can measure mean arterial pressure by integrating the area under the pressure waveform and dividing this by the duration of the cardiac cycle. The electronic measurement is preferred to the estimated mean pressure, which is derived as the diastolic pressure plus one-third of the pulse pressure. This formula is based on the assumption that diastole represents two-thirds of the cardiac cycle, which corresponds to a heart rate of 60 beats/minute. Therefore heart rates faster than 60 beats/minute, which are common in critically ill patients, lead to errors in the estimated mean arterial pressure.

Cardiopulmonary Bypass

In most circumstances, the mean pressures in the aorta, radial artery, and femoral artery are within 3 mm Hg of each other. However, in patients undergoing cardiopulmonary bypass surgery, the mean radial artery pressure can be significantly (more than 5 mm Hg) lower than the mean pressures in the aorta and femoral artery (15). This condition may be caused by a selective decrease in vascular resistance in the hand, because compression of the wrist often abolishes the pressure difference. An increase in radial artery pressure of at least 5 mm Hg when the wrist is compressed (distal to the radial artery catheter) suggests a discrepancy between radial artery pressure and pressures in other regions of the circulation (16).

A FINAL WORD

> *I would venture to guess that, of all the procedures done in clinical medicine that have important consequences, measurement of blood pressure is likely the one that is done most haphazardly.*
>
> *Norman Kaplan, M.D.*

There are an estimated 50 million people in the United States with the diagnosis of hypertension (17). This represents about 25% of the adult population (210 million) and indicates that hypertension is the number one health problem in this country. Hypertension is clearly an enormous health burden, and the source of this burden is a single diagnostic test: the (indirect) blood pressure measurement. Yet, as indicated by the hypertension expert Dr. Norman Kaplan, this measurement receives little attention and is usually performed haphazardly. This means that **a diagnostic test that is performed poorly (i.e., the blood pressure measurement) is responsible for the number one health problem in this country**. The implications are obvious.

The consequences of an improperly performed blood pressure measurement are illustrated in the following scenario. About 180 million adults (85% of the adult population) have their blood pressured measured each year. If an improperly performed measurement results in a falsely elevated blood pressure reading in just 1% of these subjects, 1.8 million new cases of (erroneously diagnosed) hypertension would be created each year. This might explain why there are *so* many people with hypertension in this country.

Regardless of whether you are working in the ICU or elsewhere, it is imperative that you learn all you can about the indirect blood pressure measurement to obtain the most accurate readings possible. You owe this to your patients and to our overburdened healthcare system.

REFERENCES

Indirect Measurements

1. Pickering TG, Hall JE, Appel LJ, et al. Recommendations for blood pressure measurement in humans and experimental animals, part 1: blood pressure measurement in humans: a statement for professionals from the Subcommittee of Professional and Public Education of the AHA Council on HBP. Circulation 2005;111:697–716.
2. Ellestad MH. Reliability of blood pressure recordings. Am J Cardiol 1989;63: 983–985.
3. Cohn JN. Blood pressure measurement in shock. JAMA 1967;199:118–122.
4. Davis RF. Clinical comparison of automated auscultatory and oscillometric and catheter-transducer measurements of arterial pressure. J Clin Monit 1985;1:114–119.
5. Ramsey M. Blood pressure monitoring: automated oscillometric devices. J Clin Monit 1991;7:56–67.
6. Bur A, Hirschl M, Herkner H, et al. Accuracy of oscillometric blood pressure measurement according to the relation between cuff size and upper-arm circumference in critically ill patients. Crit Care Med 2000;28:371–376.
7. Bur A, Herkner H, Vleck M, et al. Factors influencing the accuracy of oscillometric blood pressure measurements in critically ill patients. Crit Care Med 2003;31:793–799.

Direct Measurements

8. Darovic GO, Vanriper S. Arterial pressure recording. In: Darovic GO, ed. Hemodynamic monitoring, 2nd ed. Philadelphia: WB Saunders, 1995:177–210.
9. Nichols WW, O'Rourke MF. McDonald's blood flow in arteries, 3rd ed. Philadelphia: Lea & Febiger, 1990:251–269.
10. Gardner RM. Direct blood pressure measurement dynamic response requirements. Anesthesiology 1981;54:227–236.
11. Darovic GO, Vanriper S, Vanriper J. Fluid-filled monitoring systems. In: Darovic GO, ed. Hemodynamic monitoring, 2nd ed. Philadelphia: WB Saunders, 1995:149–175.
12. Rothe CF, Kim KC. Measuring systolic arterial blood pressure. Crit Care Med 1980;8:683–689.
13. Kleinman B, Powell S, Kumar P, et al. The fast flush test measures the dynamic response of the entire blood pressure monitoring system. Anesthesiology 1992;77:1215–1220.
14. Bruner JMR, Krewis LJ, Kunsman JM, et al. Comparison of direct and indirect methods of measuring arterial blood pressure. Med Instr 1981;15:11–21.
15. Rich GF, Lubanski RE Jr, McLoughlin TM. Differences between aortic and radial artery pressure associated with cardiopulmonary bypass. Anesthesiology 1992;77:63–66.
16. Pauca AL, Wallenhaupt SL, Kon ND. Reliability of the radial arterial pressure during anesthesia. Chest 1994;105:69–75.

Chapter 9

THE PULMONARY ARTERY CATHETER

A searchlight cannot be used effectively without a fairly thorough knowledge of the territory to be searched.

Fergus Macartney, FRCP

The birth of critical care as a specialty is largely the result of two innovations: positive-pressure mechanical ventilation and the pulmonary artery catheter. The latter device is notable for the multitude of physiologic parameters that can be measured at the bedside. Prior to the introduction of the pulmonary artery catheter, the bedside evaluation of cardiovascular function was essentially a "black box" approach that relied on indirect, qualitative markers provided by sounds (e.g., pulmonary rales, cardiac gallops, cuff-based blood pressures), visual cues (e.g., edema, skin color), and tactile cues (e.g., pulse, skin temperature). The pulmonary artery catheter improved dramatically on this approach, allowing physicians to measure quantitative physiologic parameters at the bedside and to apply the basic principles of cardiovascular physiology to the bedside management of patients with cardiovascular disorders.

This chapter describes the multitude of parameters that can be measured with pulmonary artery catheters (1–5). Most of these parameters are described in detail in Chapters 1 and 2, so it may help to review these chapters before proceeding further.

CAVEAT. The value of the pulmonary artery catheter is not determined solely by the measurements it allows but is also dependent on the clinician's ability to understand the measurements and how they are obtained. This deserves mention because surveys indicate that **physicians have an inadequate understanding of the measurements provided by pulmonary artery catheters** (6,7).

CATHETER DESIGN

The balloon-flotation pulmonary artery (PA) catheter was conceived by Dr. Jeremy Swan, who was Chief of Cardiology at Cedars-Sinai Hospital when the following experience occurred.

> In the fall of 1967, I had occasion to take my (then young) children to the beach in Santa Monica. It was a hot Saturday, and the sailboats on the water were becalmed. However, about half-a-mile offshore, I noted a boat with a large spinnaker well set and moving through the water at a reasonable velocity. The idea then came to put a sail or parachute on the end of a highly flexible catheter and thereby increase the frequency of passage of the device into the pulmonary artery (1).

Three years later (in 1970), Dr. Swan introduced a PA catheter that was equipped with a small inflatable balloon at its tip. When inflated, the balloon acted like a sail to allow the flow of venous blood to carry the catheter through the right side of the heart and out into one of the pulmonary arteries. This "balloon flotation" principle allows a right-heart catheterization to be performed at the bedside, without fluoroscopic guidance.

Basic Features

The basic features of a PA catheter are shown in Figure 9.1. The catheter is 110 cm long and has an outside diameter of 2.3 mm (7 French). There are two internal channels: One runs the entire length of the catheter and opens at the tip of the catheter (the PA lumen), and the other ends 30 cm from the catheter tip, which should place it in the right atrium (the RA lumen). The tip of the catheter is equipped with a small (1.5 mL capacity) inflatable balloon. When fully inflated, the balloon creates a recess for the tip of the catheter that prevents the tip from coming into contact with (and damaging) vessel walls as the catheter is advanced. The catheter also has a small thermistor (i.e., a transducer device that senses changes in temperature) that is located 4 cm from the catheter tip. The thermistor can measure the flow of a cold fluid that is injected through the proximal port of the catheter, and this flow rate is equivalent to the cardiac output. This is the *thermodilution method* of measuring cardiac output and will be described in more detail later in the chapter.

Additional Accessories

Other accessories that are available on specially-designed PA catheters include:

- An extra channel that opens 14 cm from the catheter tip that can be used to thread temporary pacemaker leads into the right ventricle (8)
- A fiberoptic system that allows continuous monitoring of mixed venous oxygen saturation (9)
- A rapid-response thermistor that can measure the ejection fraction of the right ventricle (10)

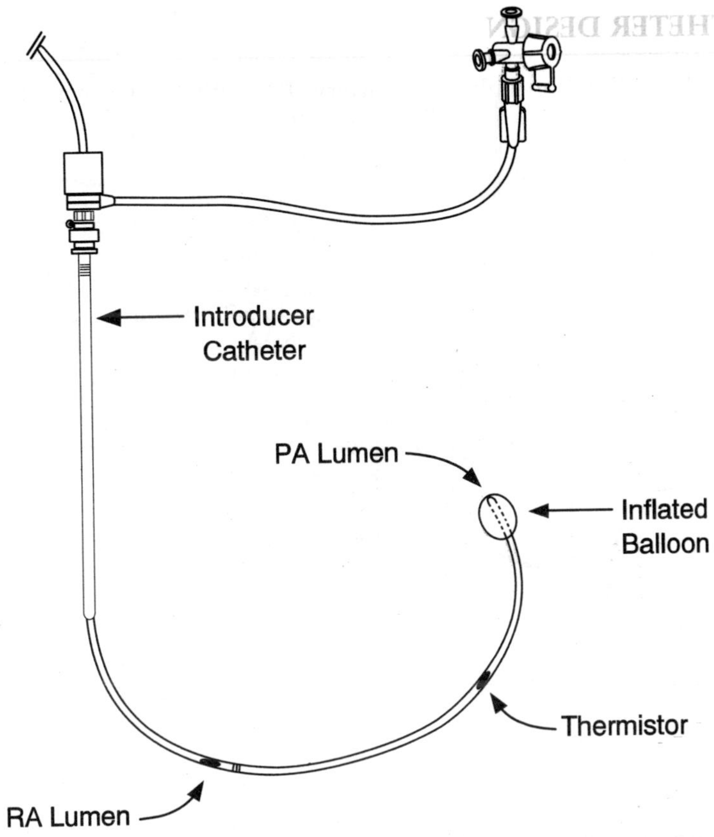

FIGURE 9.1 The basic features of a pulmonary artery (PA) catheter. Note that the PA catheter has been threaded through a large-bore introducer catheter that has a side-arm infusion port.

A thermal filament that generates low-energy heat pulses and allows continuous thermodilution measurement of the cardiac output (11)

With such a large variety of accessories, the PA catheter is the Swiss Army knife of the critical care specialist.

CATHETER INSERTION

The PA catheter is inserted into the subclavian or internal jugular veins. A large-bore introducer catheter is inserted first (see Figure 6.4), and the PA catheter is then passed through the introducer catheter. Just before the PA catheter is inserted, the distal (PA) lumen is attached to a pressure transducer, and the pressure is monitored continuously during insertion. When the PA catheter is passed through the introducer catheter and enters the superior vena cava, a venous pressure waveform appears. When this occurs, the balloon is inflated with 1.5 mL of air, and the

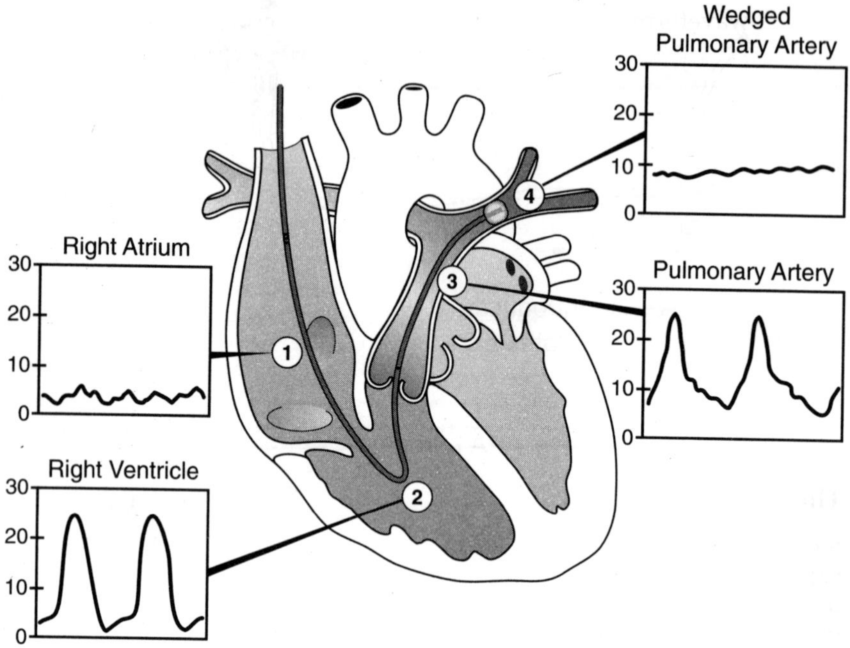

FIGURE 9.2 The pressure waveforms at different points along the normal course of a pulmonary artery catheter. These waveforms are used to identify the location of the catheter tip as it is advanced.

catheter is advanced with the balloon inflated. The location of the catheter tip is determined by the pressure tracings recorded from the distal (PA) lumen, as shown in Figure 9.2.

1. The superior vena cava pressure is identified by a venous pressure waveform, which appears as small amplitude oscillations. This pressure remains unchanged after the catheter tip is advanced into the right atrium. The normal pressure in the superior vena cava and right atrium is 1 to 6 mm Hg.
2. When the catheter tip is advanced across the tricuspid valve and into the right ventricle, a pulsatile waveform appears. The peak (systolic) pressure is a function of the strength of right ventricular contraction, and the lowest (diastolic) pressure is equivalent to the right-atrial pressure. The systolic pressure in the right ventricle is normally 15 to 30 mm Hg.
3. When the catheter moves across the pulmonic valve and into a main pulmonary artery, the pressure waveform shows a sudden rise in diastolic pressure with no change in the systolic pressure. The rise in diastolic pressure is caused by resistance to flow in the pulmonary circulation. The pulmonary artery diastolic pressure is normally 6 to 12 mm Hg.
4. As the catheter is advanced along the pulmonary artery, the pulsatile waveform disappears, leaving a venous-type pressure

waveform at the same level as the pulmonary artery diastolic pressure. This is the pulmonary artery occlusion pressure, also called the *pulmonary capillary wedge pressure* (PCWP), or simply the *wedge pressure*. This pressure is obtained in the absence of flow between the catheter tip and the left atrium and is a reflection of the venous pressure in the left side of the heart (i.e., left atrial pressure and left-ventricular diastolic pressure). The wedge pressure is equivalent to the pulmonary artery diastolic pressure.

5. When the wedge pressure tracing appears, the catheter is left in place (not advanced further), and the balloon is deflated. The pulsatile pulmonary artery pressure should reappear when the balloon is deflated. If this occurs, the PA catheter should be secured in place (usually with a single suture that anchors the catheter to the skin), and the balloon should be left deflated.

The Balloon

Sustained periods of balloon inflation creates a risk of pulmonary artery rupture or pulmonary infarction, so the balloon should be deflated at all times while the catheter is in place. Balloon inflation is reserved only for measurements of the wedge pressure. When obtaining a wedge pressure, do not fully inflate the balloon with 1.5 mL air all at once (catheters often migrate into smaller pulmonary arteries, and a fully inflated balloon could result in vessel rupture). The balloon should be slowly inflated until a wedge pressure tracing is obtained. Once a satisfactory wedge pressure is recorded, the balloon should be fully deflated. (Detaching the syringe from the balloon injection port will help prevent undetected balloon inflation while the catheter is in place.)

Troubleshooting

The following are some common problems encountered during advancement of a PA catheter.

Catheter Will Not Advance into the Right Ventricle

Most catheters should enter the right ventricle after they are advanced a distance of 20 to 25 cm (see Figure 6.5). Difficulty advancing a catheter into the right ventricle (which can occur with tricuspid regurgitation or right heart failure) can sometimes be corrected by filling the balloon with sterile saline instead of air (12) and positioning the patient with the left side down. The fluid adds weight to the balloon, and with the left side down, the balloon can fall into the right ventricle. When the right ventricle is entered, the saline should be removed and replaced with air.

Catheter Will Not Advance into the Pulmonary Artery

Catheters can become coiled in the right ventricle and fail to enter the pulmonary circulation. This problem is sometimes corrected by withdrawing the catheter into the superior vena cava and re-advancing the catheter using a slow, continuous motion (allowing the venous flow to carry the catheter into the pulmonary circulation) and avoiding rapid thrusts. This problem can persist in patients with pulmonary hypertension.

Arrhythmias

Atrial and ventricular arrhythmias can appear in over half of PA catheter placements (13), but they are almost always benign and self-limited and require no treatment. Complete heart block that appears during catheter placement should prompt immediate withdrawal of the catheter and, if necessary, a brief period of transthoracic pacing. Prolonged heart block could indicate injury to the AV node, and might require transvenous pacing.

Unable to Obtain a Wedge Pressure

In about 25% of PA catheter placements, the pulsatile PA pressure never disappears despite maximum advancement of the catheter in the pulmonary circulation. This can be the result of nonuniform balloon inflation, but in most cases, the phenomenon is unexplained. If this occurs, the pulmonary artery diastolic pressure can be used as a substitute for the pulmonary capillary wedge pressure (in the absence of pulmonary hypertension, the two pressures should be equivalent).

THERMODILUTION CARDIAC OUTPUT

The addition of a thermistor to the PA catheter increased the monitoring capacity of the catheter from 2 parameters (i.e., central venous pressure and wedge pressure) to over 10 parameters (see Tables 9.1 and 9.2).

TABLE 9.1 Cardiovascular Parameters

Parameter	Abbreviation	Normal Range
Central venous pressure	CVP	1–6 mm Hg
Pulmonary capillary wedge pressure	PCWP	6–12 mm Hg
Cardiac index	CI	2.4–4 L/min/m^2
Stroke volume index	SVI	40–70 mL/beat/m^2
Left-ventricular stroke work index	LVSWI	40–60 g · m/m^2
Right-ventricular:		
Stroke work index	RVSWI	4–8 g · m/m^2
Ejection fraction	RVEF	46–50%
End-diastolic volume	RVEDV	80–150 mL/m^2
Systemic vascular resistance index	SVRI	1,600–2,400 dynes · sec^1 · cm^5/m^2
Pulmonary vascular resistance index	PVRI	200–400 dynes · sec^1 · cm^5/m^2

TABLE 9.2 Oxygen-Transport Parameters

Parameter	Symbol	Normal Range
Mixed venous oxygen saturation	SvO_2	70–75%
Oxygen delivery	DO_2	520–570 mL/min/m^2
Oxygen uptake	VO_2	110–160 mL/min/m^2
Oxygen-extraction ratio	O_2ER	20%–30%

The Method

Thermodilution is an indicator-dilution method of measuring blood flow, and is based on the premise that when an indicator substance is added to circulating blood, the rate of blood flow is inversely proportional to the change in concentration of the indicator over time (14,15). The indicator substance in this case is not a dye but a fluid with a different temperature than blood.

The thermodilution method is illustrated in Figure 9.3. A dextrose or saline solution that is colder than blood is injected through the proximal port of the catheter in the right atrium. The cold fluid mixes with blood in the right heart chambers, and the cooled blood is ejected into the pulmonary artery and flows past the thermistor on the distal end of the catheter. The thermistor records the change in blood temperature with time and sends this information to an electronic instrument that records and displays a temperature–time curve. The area under this curve is inversely proportional to the rate of blood flow in the pulmonary artery. In the absence of intracardiac shunts, this flow rate is equivalent to the (average) cardiac output.

Thermodilution Curves

Examples of thermodilution curves are shown in Figure 9.4. The low cardiac output curve (upper panel) has a gradual rise and fall, whereas the high output curve (middle panel) has a rapid rise, an abbreviated peak, and a steep downslope. Note that the area under the low cardiac output curve is greater than the area under the high output curve; that is, the area under the curves is inversely related to the flow rate. Electronic cardiac monitors integrate the area under the temperature–time curves and provide a digital display of the calculated cardiac output.

Technical Considerations

The indicator solution can be cooled in ice or injected at room temperature, and the volume of injectate is either 5 mL or 10 mL. In general, higher-volume, lower-temperature injectates produce the highest signal-to-noise ratios and thus the most accurate measurements (16). However, room temperature injectates (which require less preparation than iced injectates) produce reliable measurements in most critically ill patients (17,18). When the indicator fluid is injected at room temperature, the large (10 mL) injection volume produces the most reliable results.

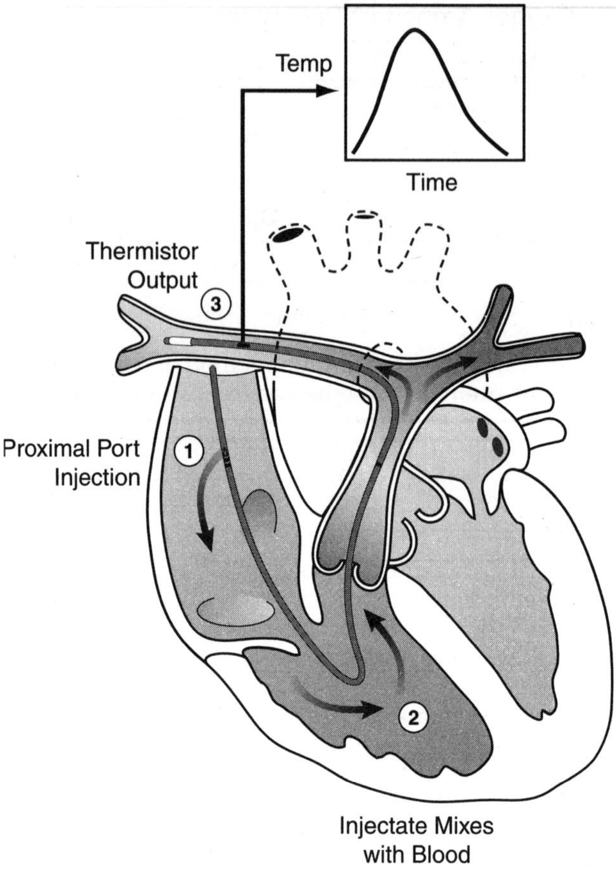

FIGURE 9.3 The thermodilution method of measuring cardiac output.

Serial measurements are recommended for each cardiac output determination. Three measurements are sufficient if they differ by 10% or less, and the cardiac output is taken as the average of all measurements. Serial measurements that differ by more than 10% are considered unreliable (19).

Variability

Thermodilution cardiac output can vary by as much as 10% without any apparent change in the clinical condition of the patient (20). This means that a baseline cardiac output of 5 L/min can vary from 4.5 to 5.5 L/min without the change being clinically significant. **A change in thermodilution cardiac output must exceed 10% to be considered clinically significant.**

Other Considerations

The following clinical conditions can affect the accuracy of thermodilution cardiac output measurements.

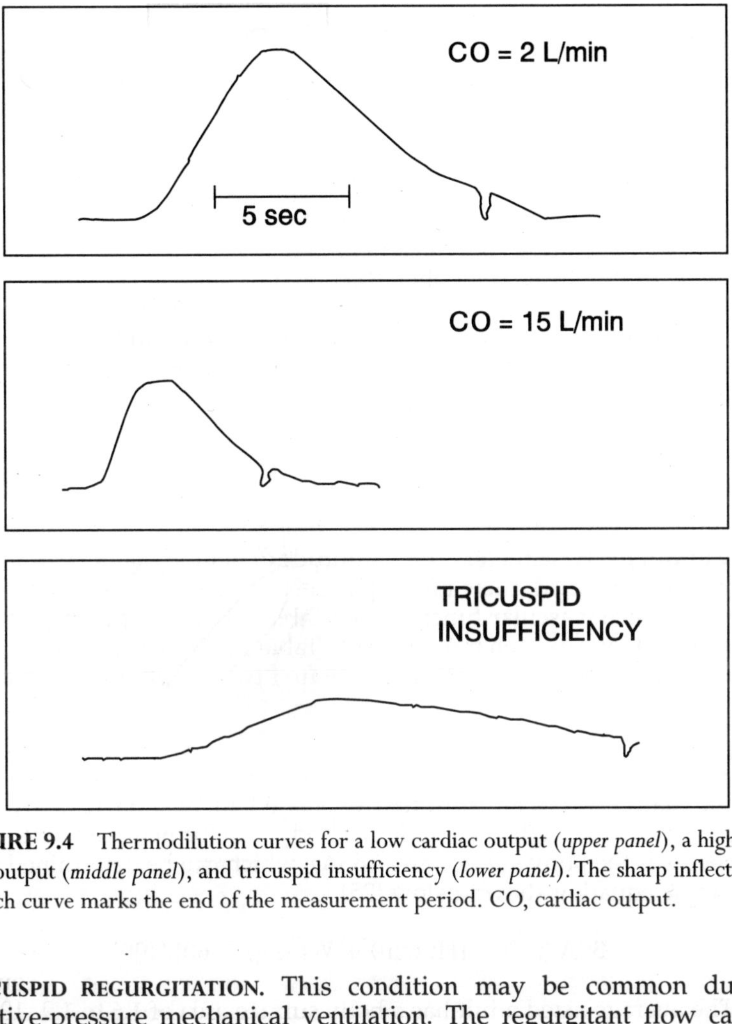

FIGURE 9.4 Thermodilution curves for a low cardiac output (*upper panel*), a high cardiac output (*middle panel*), and tricuspid insufficiency (*lower panel*). The sharp inflection in each curve marks the end of the measurement period. CO, cardiac output.

TRICUSPID REGURGITATION. This condition may be common during positive-pressure mechanical ventilation. The regurgitant flow causes the indicator fluid to be recycled, producing a prolonged, low-amplitude thermodilution curve similar to the low-output curve in the bottom frame of Figure 9.4. This results in a falsely low thermodilution cardiac output (21).

INTRACARDIAC SHUNTS. Intracardiac shunts produce falsely high thermodilution cardiac output measurements. In right-to-left shunts, a portion of the cold indicator fluid passes through the shunt, thereby creating an abbreviated thermodilution curve (similar to the abbreviated high-output curve). In left-to-right shunts, the thermodilution curve is abbreviated because the shunted blood increases the blood volume in the right heart chambers, and this dilutes the indicator solution that is injected.

Continuous Cardiac Output

The thermodilution method has been adapted to allow automatic, minute-by-minute measurements of cardiac output without the tedium of intermittent bolus injections of indicator fluid (22). This method uses a specialized PA catheter (Baxter Edwards Critical Care, Irvine, CA) equipped with a 10-cm thermal filament located 15 to 25 cm from the catheter tip. The filament generates low-energy heat pulses that are transmitted to the surrounding blood. The resulting change in blood temperature is then used to generate a thermodilution curve. This method records an average cardiac output over successive 3-minute time intervals.

The continuous thermodilution method provides reliable measurements of cardiac output in critically ill patients (23), and it is more accurate than the intermittent bolus-injection thermodilution method (24). Because **the continuous method of monitoring cardiac output is less time consuming and more accurate than the intermittent bolus-injection method**, this method should be preferred for cardiac output determinations in the ICU.

HEMODYNAMIC PARAMETERS

The value of the PA catheter is the multitude of hemodynamic parameters that can be generated: there are 10 parameters used to describe different aspects of cardiovascular function (see Table 9.1), and 4 parameters that describe systemic oxygen transport (see Table 9.2). A detailed description of these parameters can be found in the first two chapters of this book.

Body Size

Hemodynamic variables are often expressed in relation to body size. Instead of mass (weight), the index of body size for hemodynamic measurements is the body surface area (BSA), which can be determined with the simple equation shown below (25).

$$\text{BSA (m}^2\text{)} = [\text{Ht (cm)} + \text{Wt (kg)} - 60]/100 \tag{9.1}$$

The average-sized adult has a body surface area of 1.6 to 1.9 m^2.

Cardiovascular Parameters

The parameters used to evaluate cardiovascular function are shown in Table 9.1. Size-adjusted parameters (expressed in relation to body surface area) are identified by the term *index*.

Central Venous Pressure

When the PA catheter is properly placed, the proximal port of the catheter should be situated in the right atrium, and the pressure recorded from this port should be the right atrial pressure. As mentioned previously, the pressure in the right atrium is the same as the pressure in the superior vena cava, and these pressures are collectively called the *central venous pressure* (CVP). In the absence of tricuspid valve dysfunction, the

CVP should be equivalent to the right atrial pressure (RAP) and the right-ventricular end-diastolic pressure (RVEDP).

$$CVP = RAP = RVEDP \tag{9.2}$$

Pulmonary Capillary Wedge Pressure

The measurement of the pulmonary capillary wedge pressure (PCWP) is described earlier in the chapter (and the next chapter is devoted almost exclusively to this measurement). The PCWP is measured when there is no flow between the catheter tip and the left atrium (because the balloon on the PA catheter tip is inflated), so the PCWP will be the same as the left-atrial pressure (LAP). When the mitral valve is normal, the LAP should be equivalent to the left-ventricular end-diastolic pressure (LVEDP).

$$PCWP = LAP = LVEDP \tag{9.3}$$

Cardiac Index

The thermodilution cardiac output is usually corrected for body size as shown below. The size-corrected cardiac output is called the *cardiac index* (CI).

$$CI = CO/BSA \tag{9.4}$$

Stroke Volume

The stroke volume is the volume of blood ejected by the ventricles during systole. It is derived as the cardiac output divided by the heart rate (HR). When cardiac index (CI) is used, the parameter is called the stroke volume index (SVI).

$$SVI = CI/HR \tag{9.5}$$

Right-Ventricular Ejection Fraction

The ejection fraction is the fraction of the ventricular volume that is ejected during systole and is equivalent to the ratio of the stroke volume and the ventricular end-diastolic volume. This parameter provides an indication of the strength of ventricular contraction during systole. The ejection fraction of the right ventricle (RVEF) is the ratio of the stroke volume (SV) to the right-ventricular end-diastolic volume (RVEDV).

$$RVEF = SV/RVEDV \tag{9.6}$$

As mentioned earlier, the right ventricular ejection fraction can be measured with a specialized PA catheter that is equipped with a rapid-response thermistor (see Reference 10 for a description of this technique).

Right-Ventricular End-Diastolic Volume

Ventricular end-diastolic volume is the true measure of ventricular preload (see Chapter 1). The end-diastolic volume of the right ventricle can be determined when the RVEF is measured using the specialized PA catheter mentioned above. The equation below is derived by rearranging the terms in Equation 9.6.

$$RVEDV = SV/RVEF \tag{9.7}$$

Left-Ventricular Stroke Work Index

Left-ventricular stroke work (LVSW) is the work performed by the ventricle to eject the stroke volume. Stroke work is a function of the systolic pressure load (afterload minus preload), which is equivalent to the mean arterial pressure minus the wedge pressure (MAP − PCWP) and the stroke volume (SV). The equation below is corrected for body size (so LVSW becomes LVSWI), and the factor 0.0136 converts pressure and volume to units of work.

$$LVSWI = (MAP - PCWP) \times SVI\ (\times\ 0.0136) \tag{9.8}$$

Right-Ventricular Stroke Work Index

The right-ventricular stroke work (RVSW) is the work needed to move the stroke volume across the pulmonary circulation. It is derived as the systolic pressure load of the right ventricle, which is equivalent to the mean pulmonary artery pressure minus the CVP (PAP − CVP), and the stroke volume (SV). The equation below is corrected for body size and includes the same unit correction factor as in Equation 9.8.

$$RVSWI = (PAP - CVP) \times SVI\ (\times\ 0.0136) \tag{9.9}$$

Systemic Vascular Resistance Index

The systemic vascular resistance (SVR) is the vascular resistance across the systemic circulation. It is directly proportional to the pressure gradient from the aorta to the right atrium (MAP − CVP) and is inversely related to blood flow (CI). The equation below is corrected for body size, and the factor of 80 is necessary to convert units.

$$SVRI = (MAP - RAP) \times 80/CI \tag{9.10}$$

Pulmonary Vascular Resistance Index

The pulmonary vascular resistance index (PVR) is directly proportional to the pressure gradient across the entire lungs, from the pulmonary artery (PAP) to the left atrium (LAP). Because the wedge pressure (PCWP) is equivalent to the LAP, the pressure gradient across the lungs can be expressed as (PAP − PCWP). The PVR can then be derived using Equation 9.11, which is corrected for body size. As in Equation 9.10, the factor of 80 is used to convert units.

$$PVRI = (PAP - PCWP) \times 80/CI \tag{9.11}$$

Oxygen-Transport Parameters

The transport of oxygen from the lungs to the systemic organs is described using the parameters in Table 9.2. These parameters are described in detail in Chapter 2 and are presented only briefly here.

Oxygen Delivery

The rate of oxygen transport in arterial blood is called the *oxygen delivery* (DO_2) and is a function of the cardiac output and the oxygen concentration in arterial blood. The determinants of DO_2 are shown in Equation 9.12. This equation is explained in Chapter 2.

$$DO_2 = CI \times 13.4 \times Hb \times SaO_2 \tag{9.12}$$

Mixed Venous Oxygen Saturation

The oxygen saturation of hemoglobin in pulmonary artery (mixed venous) blood (SvO_2)can be monitored continuously with a specialized PA catheter, or it can be measured *in vitro* with a blood sample obtained from the distal port of the PA catheter. (See Chapter 20 for a description of how O_2 saturation of hemoglobin is measured.) The SvO_2 is used as an indirect marker of systemic blood flow. A decrease in cardiac output is accompanied by an increase in O_2 extraction from the capillaries, and this will decrease the SvO_2. Therefore a decrease in SvO_2 can signal a decrease in cardiac output. If O_2 extraction is fixed and does not vary with changes in blood flow (which can happen in sepsis), the SvO_2 is unreliable as an index of blood flow.

Oxygen Uptake

Oxygen uptake (VO_2), also called oxygen consumption, is the rate at which oxygen is taken up from the systemic capillaries into the tissues. The determinants of VO_2 are shown in Equation 9.13. This equation is explained in detail in Chapter 2.

$$VO_2 = CI \times 13.4 \times Hb \times (SaO_2 - SvO_2) \tag{9.13}$$

Oxygen-Extraction Ratio

The oxygen extraction ratio (O_2ER) is the fractional uptake of oxygen from the systemic microcirculation and is equivalent to the ratio of O_2 uptake to O_2 delivery. Multiplying the ratio by 100 expresses it as a percent.

$$O_2ER = VO_2/DO_2\ (\times 100) \tag{9.14}$$

HEMODYNAMIC SUBSETS

The parameters just described can be organized into groups or subsets that are tailored to specific problems. Some examples of hemodynamic subsets are presented below.

Hypotension

The mean arterial pressure is a function of the cardiac output and the systemic vascular resistance: MAP = CI × SVRI. The cardiac output, in turn, depends on the venous return. If the CVP is used as an index of venous return, there are three variables that can be used to describe any patient with hypotension: CVP, CI, and SVRI. This 3-variable subset is used below to describe the three classic forms of hypotension.

Hypovolemic	Cardiogenic	Vasogenic
Low CVP	High CVP	Low CVP
Low CI	Low CI	High CI
High SVRI	High SVRI	Low SVRI

These three hemodynamic parameters can be used to identify the hemodynamic problem in any patient with hypotension. For example, suppose a patient with hypotension has a low CVP, a normal CI, and a low SVRI. This pattern is closest to the vascular dysfunction (vasogenic) category shown above, except that the CI is normal instead of high. Therefore the hemodynamic problem in this patient is a combination of vascular dysfunction and cardiac dysfunction. There are 3^3 or 27 possible combinations of these 3 variables (CVP, CI, SVRI), and each of these combinations identifies a distinct hemodynamic problem. Therefore this hemodynamic subset of 3 variables will identify the hemodynamic problem in any patient with hypotension.

Clinical Shock

The three-variable hemodynamic subset just presented will identify a hemodynamic problem but not the consequences of the problem on tissue oxygenation. The addition of the oxygen uptake (VO_2) will correct this shortcoming and can help identify a state of clinical shock. Clinical shock can be defined as a condition where tissue oxygenation is inadequate for the needs of aerobic metabolism. Since a VO_2 that is below normal can be used as indirect evidence of oxygen-limited aerobic metabolism, a subnormal VO_2 can be used as indirect evidence of clinical shock. The following example shows how the VO_2 can add to the evaluation of a patient with a low output state.

Heart Failure	Cardiogenic Shock
High CVP	High CVP
Low CI	Low CI
High SVRI	High SVRI
Normal VO_2	Low VO_2

Without the VO_2 measurement in the above profiles, it is impossible to differentiate a low-output state from cardiogenic shock. This illustrates how oxygen transport monitoring can be used to determine the consequences of hemodynamic abnormalities on peripheral oxygenation. The uses and limitations of oxygen transport monitoring are described in more detail in Chapter 11.

A FINAL WORD

The PA catheter has been maligned in recent years because of clinical studies showing that mortality is not reduced (26) and can be higher (27) in patients who have PA catheters. As a result of these studies, use of the PA catheter in the western world has dropped about 10% in the past few years (28), and the most zealous critics of the catheter have called for a moratorium on its use.

There are two fundamental problems in the criticism of the PA catheter based on mortality data. The first is the simple fact that **the PA catheter is a monitoring device, not a therapy.** If a PA catheter is placed to evaluate a problem, and it uncovers a disorder that is untreatable and fatal (e.g., cardiogenic shock), the problem is not the catheter, it is the lack of effective therapy. **Mortality rates should be used to evaluate therapies, not measurements.**

The second problem is the seemingly prevalent notion that everything we do in the ICU must save lives to be of value. Mortality should not be the dominant outcome measure in ICUs because there are too many variables that can influence mortality in critically ill patients, and also because mortality is an eventual outcome in all patients admitted to the ICU. Management decisions should be based on the scientific rationale for an intervention—those who expect their management decisions to consistently save lives are doomed to failure.

REFERENCES

Reviews

1. Swan HJ. The pulmonary artery catheter. Dis Mon 1991;37:473–543.
2. Pinsky MR. Hemodynamic monitoring in the intensive care unit. Clin Chest Med 2003;24:549–560.
3. American Society of Anesthesiologists Task Force on Pulmonary Artery Catheterization. Practice guidelines for pulmonary artery catheterization: an updated report by the American Society of Anesthesiologists Task Force on Pulmonary Artery Catheterization. Anesthesiology 2003;99:988–1014.
4. Silvestry FE. Swan-Ganz catheterization: interpretation of tracings. UpToDate Online, Version 13.2. (Accessed on August 28, 2005).
5. Cruz K, Franklin C. The pulmonary artery catheter: uses and controversies. Crit Care Clin 2001;17:271–291.

Selected References

6. Iberti TJ, Fischer EP, Liebowitz AB, et al. A multicenter study of physicians' knowledge of the pulmonary artery catheter. JAMA 1990;264:2928–2932.

7. Gnaegi A, Feihl F, Perret C. Intensive care physicians' insufficient knowledge of right heart catheterization at the bedside: time to act? Crit Care Med 1997;25:213–220.
8. Halpern N, Feld H, Oropello JM, et al. The technique of inserting an RV port PA catheter and pacing probe. J Crit Illn 1991;6:1153–1159.
9. Armaganidis A, Dhainaut JF, Billard JL, et al. Accuracy assessment for three fiberoptic pulmonary artery catheters for SvO_2 monitoring. Intensive Care Med 1994;20:484–488.
10. Vincent JL, Thirion M, Brimioulle S, et al. Thermodilution measurement of right ventricular ejection fraction with a modified pulmonary artery catheter. Intensive Care Med 1986;12:33–38.
11. Yelderman M, Ramsay MA, Quinn MD, et al. Continuous thermodilution cardiac output measurement in intensive care unit patients. J Cardiothorac Vasc Anesth 1992;6:270–274.
12. Venus B, Mathru M. A maneuver for bedside pulmonary artery catheterization in patients with right heart failure. Chest 1982;82:803–804.
13. Jacobson B. Medicine and clinical engineering. Englewood Cliffs, NJ: Prentice Hall, 1977:388.
14. Gardner PE. Cardiac output: theory, technique, and troubleshooting. Crit Care Nurs Clin North Am 1989;1:577–587.
15. Daily EK, Schroeder JS. Cardiac output measurements. In: Techniques in bedside hemodynamic monitoring, 5th ed. St. Louis: CV Mosby, 1994: 173–194.
16. Renner LE, Morton MJ, Sakuma GY. Indicator amount, temperature, and intrinsic cardiac output affect thermodilution cardiac output accuracy and reproducibility. Crit Care Med 1993;21:586–597.
17. Nelson LD, Anderson HB. Patient selection for iced versus room temperature injectate for thermodilution cardiac output determinations. Crit Care Med 1985;13:182–184.
18. Pearl RG, Rosenthal MH, Nielson L, et al. Effect of injectate volume and temperature on thermodilution cardiac output determinations. Anesthesiology 1986;64:798–801.
19. Nadeau S, Noble WH. Limitations of cardiac output measurement by thermodilution. Can J Anesth 1986;33:780–784.
20. Sasse SA, Chen PA, Berry RB, et al. Variability of cardiac output over time in medical intensive care unit patients. Chest 1994;22:225–232.
21. Konishi T, Nakamura Y, Morii I, et al. Comparison of thermodilution and Fick methods for measurement of cardiac output in tricuspid regurgitation. Am J Cardiol 1992;70:538–540.
22. Yelderman M, Ramsay MA, Quinn MD, et al. Continuous thermodilution cardiac output measurement in intensive care unit patients. J Cardiothorac Vasc Anesth 1992;6:270–274.
23. Boldt J, Menges T, Wollbruck M, et al. Is continuous cardiac output measurement using thermodilution reliable in the critically ill patient? Crit Care Med 1994;22:1913–1918.
24. Mihaljevic T, vonSegesser LK, Tonz M, et al. Continuous versus bolus thermodilution cardiac output measurements: a comparative study. Crit Care Med 1995;23:944–949.
25. Mattar JA. A simple calculation to estimate body surface area in adults and its correlation with the Dubois formula. Crit Care Med 1989;17:846–847.

26. Yu DT, Platt R, Lamken PN, et al. Relationship of pulmonary artery catheter use to mortality and resource utilization in patients with severe sepsis. Crit Care Med 2003;31:2734–2741.
27. Connors AF, Speroff T, Dawson NV, et al. The effectiveness of right heart catheterization in the initial care of critically ill patients. JAMA 1996;276:889–897.
28. Pinsky MR, Vincent J-L. Let us use the pulmonary artery catheter correctly and only when we need it. Crit Care Med 2005;33:1119–1122.

Chapter 10

CENTRAL VENOUS PRESSURE AND WEDGE PRESSURE

It is what we think we know already that often prevents us from learning.

Claude Bernard

The central venous pressure (CVP) and pulmonary artery occlusion (wedge) pressure, which are clinical measures of right and left ventricular filling pressures, respectively (1–3), have been popularized as hemodynamic measures because of the *Frank-Starling relationship of the heart,* which identifies ventricular filling volume (preload) as the major determinant of cardiac stroke output (see Figure 1.1). Unfortunately, the CVP and pulmonary artery wedge pressure share two major shortcomings: they are often misleading as measures of ventricular preload (4), and the pressure waveforms are often misinterpreted (5–7). Attention to the information in this chapter will help reduce errors in the interpretation of these measurements.

SOURCES OF VARIABILITY

Body Position

The zero reference point for venous pressures in the thorax is a point on the external thorax where the fourth intercostal space intersects the mid-axillary line (i.e., the line midway between the anterior and posterior axillary folds). This point (called the phlebostatic axis) corresponds to the position of the right and left atrium when the patient is in the supine position. It is not a valid reference point in the lateral position, which means that central venous and pulmonary artery wedge pressures should not be recorded when patients are placed in lateral positions (8).

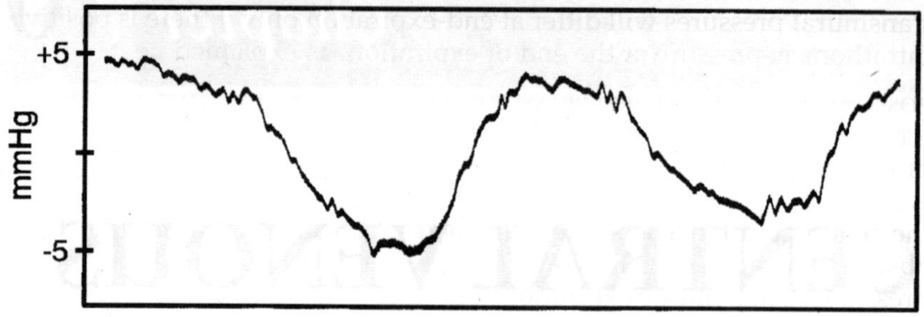

FIGURE 10.1 Respiratory variations in central venous pressure. The transmural pressure can remain constant throughout the respiratory cycle despite the variations in intravascular pressure.

Changes in Thoracic Pressure

The pressure recorded with a vascular cannula is the intravascular pressure [i.e., the pressure in the vessel lumen relative to atmospheric (zero) pressure]. However, the physiologically important vascular pressure (i.e., the one that determines distention of the ventricles and the rate of edema formation) is the *transmural pressure* (i.e., the difference between the intravascular and extravascular pressures). The intravascular pressure is an accurate reflection of the transmural pressure only when the extravascular pressure is zero (atmospheric pressure).

When vascular pressures are recorded in the thorax, changes in thoracic pressure can be transmitted across the wall of blood vessels, resulting in a discrepancy between intravascular and transmural pressures. This is illustrated by the respiratory variations in the CVP tracing shown in Figure 10.1. The intravascular pressure changes in this tracing are caused by respiratory variations in intrathoracic pressure that are transmitted into the lumen of the superior vena cava. In this situation, the transmural pressure (i.e., the cardiac filling pressure) may be constant despite the phasic changes in intravascular pressure. (It is not possible to determine how much of the change in thoracic pressure is transmitted into the blood vessel in an individual patient, and thus it is not possible to determine whether transmural pressure is absolutely constant.) Thus **respiratory variation in intravascular pressures in the thorax is not an indication that the transmural pressure (the cardiac filling pressure) is also changing** (9).

End-Expiration

Intravascular pressures will be equivalent to transmural pressures when the extravascular pressure is zero. In healthy subjects breathing at normal rates, this occurs at the end of expiration, when intrathoracic (extravascular) pressure returns to atmospheric or zero pressure. Therefore **intravascular pressures should be measured at the end of expiration**, when they are equivalent to the transmural pressure (1,9). Intravascular and transmural pressures will differ at end-expiration only if there is positive intrathoracic pressure at the end of expiration, as explained next.

POSITIVE END-EXPIRATORY PRESSURE (PEEP). There are two situations, where the intrathoracic pressure is above atmospheric pressure at the end of expiration. In one situation, positive end-expiratory pressure (PEEP) is applied during mechanical ventilation to prevent alveolar collapse. In the other situation, incomplete alveolar emptying (e.g., due to airflow obstruction) does not allow alveolar pressure to return to atmospheric pressure at the end of expiration. These two conditions are referred to as *extrinsic PEEP* (see Chapter 25) and *intrinsic PEEP* (see Chapter 26), respectively. In both conditions of PEEP, intravascular pressures measured at the end of expiration will exceed the transmural pressure.

When external PEEP is applied, intravascular pressures should be measured at end-expiration when the patient is briefly disconnected from the ventilator (10). In the presence of intrinsic PEEP, accurate recording of intravascular pressures can be difficult (11). See Chapter 26 for a description of how the CVP and wedge pressure can be corrected in the presence of intrinsic PEEP.

Pressure Monitors

If the bedside monitors in the ICU have oscilloscope display screens with horizontal grids, the CVP and wedge pressures should be measured directly from the pressure tracings on the screen. This provides more accurate measurements than pressures that are digitally displayed (12). Most ICU monitors have a digital display that includes systolic, diastolic, and mean pressures; each measured over successive 4-second time intervals (the time for one sweep across the oscilloscope screen). The systolic pressure is the highest pressure, the diastolic pressure is the lowest pressure, and the mean pressure is the integrated area under the pressure wave in each time period. **During spontaneous breathing, the pressure at the end of expiration is the highest pressure (i.e., systolic pressure), and during positive-pressure mechanical ventilation, the end-expiratory pressure is the lowest pressure (i.e., diastolic pressure).** Therefore systolic pressure should be used as the end-expiratory vascular pressure in patients who are breathing spontaneously, whereas diastolic pressure should be used in patients receiving positive-pressure mechanical ventilation. The **mean pressure should never be used** as a reflection of transmural pressure when there are respiratory variations in intravascular pressure (9).

Units of Measurement

Most intravascular pressures are measured with electronic transducers that record the pressure in millimeters of mercury (mm Hg). Water-filled manometers that record pressure in cm H_2O are occasionally used to measure CVP (13). Because mercury is 13.6 times more dense than water, pressures measured in cm H_2O can be divided by $13.6 \times 1/10 = 1.36$ to be expressed in mm Hg (the factor 1/10 converts cm to mm;) i.e.,

pressure in cm $H_2O \div 1.36 =$ pressure in mm Hg. A table of conversions for these units is included in Appendix 1.

Spontaneous Variations

Like any physiologic variable, vascular pressures in the thorax can vary spontaneously, without a change in the clinical condition of the patient. The spontaneous variation in wedge pressure is 4 mm Hg or less in 60% of patients, but it can be as high as 7 mm Hg in any individual patient (14). In general, **a change in CVP or wedge pressure of less than 4 mm Hg should not be considered a clinically significant change.**

PULMONARY ARTERY WEDGE PRESSURE

Few pressures in the ICU are misinterpreted as frequently, and as consistently, as pulmonary capillary wedge pressure (5–7,15). Probably the most important feature of the wedge pressure is what it is *not:*

Wedge pressure is *not* left-ventricular preload.
Wedge pressure is *not* the pulmonary capillary hydrostatic pressure.
Wedge pressure is *not* a reliable measure for differentiating cardiogenic from noncardiogenic pulmonary edema.

These limitations are explained in the description of the wedge pressure that follows.

Wedge Pressure Tracing

When the pulmonary artery catheter is properly positioned, inflation of the balloon at the tip of the catheter causes the pulsatile pressure to disappear. This is demonstrated in Figure 10.2. The nonpulsatile or "wedged" pressure is equivalent to the pulmonary artery diastolic pressure, and represents the pressure in the venous side of the pulmonary circulation. The magnified section of the wedge pressure in Figure 10.2 shows the individual components of the pressure: the a wave is produced by left atrial contraction, the c wave is produced by closure of the mitral valve during isometric contraction of the left ventricle, and the v wave is produced by systolic contraction of the left ventricle against a closed mitral valve. These components (which are also present in the central venous pressure tracing) are often not distinguishable in a normal wedge pressure tracing, but they can become evident in conditions where one component is magnified (e.g., mitral regurgitation produces large v waves, which can be identified in a wedge pressure tracing).

Principle of the Wedge Pressure

The wedge pressure is a measure of the filling pressure in the left side of the heart, and the basis for this is shown in Figure 10.3 (13). Inflation of the balloon at the tip of pulmonary aretery catheter creates a static column of blood between the catheter tip and the left atrium. In this

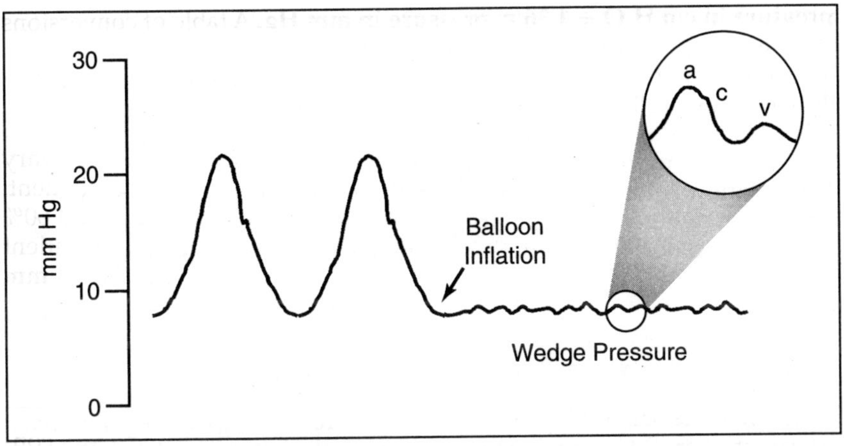

FIGURE 10.2 Pressure tracing showing the transition from a pulsatile pulmonary artery pressure to a balloon occlusion (wedge) pressure. The magnified area shows the components of the wedge pressure: a wave (atrial contraction), c wave (mitral valve closure), and v wave (ventricular contraction).

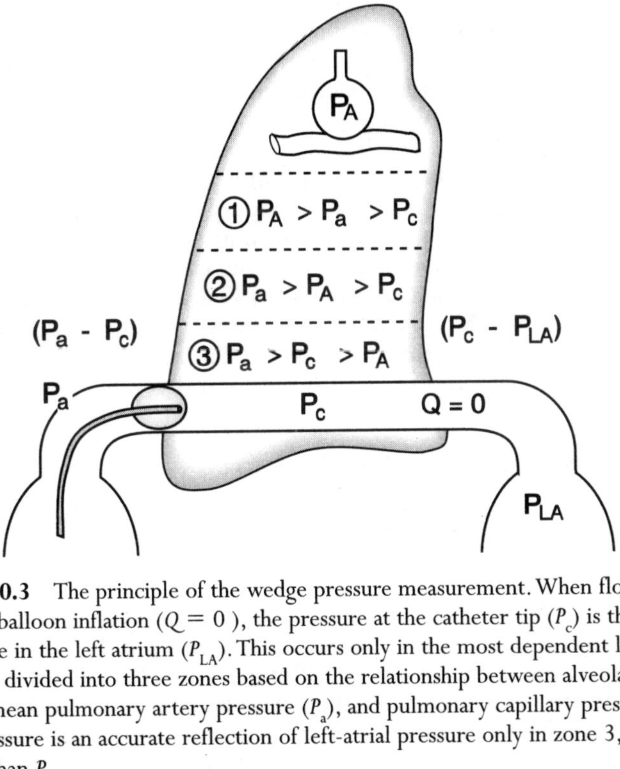

FIGURE 10.3 The principle of the wedge pressure measurement. When flow ceases because of balloon inflation ($Q = 0$), the pressure at the catheter tip (P_c) is the same as the pressure in the left atrium (P_{LA}). This occurs only in the most dependent lung zone. The lung is divided into three zones based on the relationship between alveolar pressure (P_A), mean pulmonary artery pressure (P_a), and pulmonary capillary pressure (P_c). Wedge pressure is an accurate reflection of left-atrial pressure only in zone 3, where P_c is greater than P_A.

situation, the pressure at the tip of the pulmonary artery catheter is the same as the pressure in the left atrium. This can be demonstrated using the simple hydraulic relationship $Q = \Delta P/R$, which indicates that steady flow in a tube (Q) is directly proportional to the pressure drop along the tube (ΔP) and is inversely proportional to the resistance to flow in the tube (R). Rearranging terms yields the following relationship: $\Delta P = Q \times R$. This relation is expressed below for the venous side of the pulmonary circulation, where P_c is capillary pressure, P_{LA} is left-atrial pressure, Q is pulmonary blood flow, and R_v is pulmonary venous resistance.

$$P_c - P_{LA} = Q \times R_v \tag{10.1}$$

if $Q = 0$, $P_c - P_{LA} = 0$, and $P_c = P_{LA}$

Thus when the balloon is inflated, the pressure at the tip of the pulmonary artery catheter (P_c) is equal to the pressure in the left atrium (P_{LA}). Because left-atrial pressure is normally the same as the left-ventricular end-diastolic pressure (LVEDP), the pulmonary capillary wedge pressure can be used as a measure of left-ventricular filling pressure. What the wedge pressure *actually* measures is the focus of the remainder of this chapter.

Wedge Pressure as Preload

The wedge pressure is often used as a reflection of left-ventricular filling during diastole (i.e., ventricular preload). In Chapter 1, preload was defined as the force that stretches a muscle at rest, and the preload for the intact ventricle was identified as end-diastolic volume (EDV). However, the pulmonary capillary wedge pressure (like the CVP) is a measure of end-diastolic pressure, and end-diastolic pressure may not be an accurate reflection of preload (EDV). The graph in Figure 10.4 shows the relationship between pulmonary capillary wedge pressure and left-ventricular end-diastolic volume in a group of normal subjects (4). Note the poor correlation between the two measurements ($r = 0.04$). In fact, only 7 of the 12 wedge pressure measurements (58%) are within the normal range (shaded area). This shows that **the pulmonary artery wedge pressure is not an accurate reflection of left-ventricular preload** (4,16). Similar results have also been reported with the central venous pressure (4).

Wedge Pressure as Left-Atrial Pressure

The following conditions can influence the accuracy of the wedge pressure as a measure of left-atrial pressure.

Lung Zones

If the pressure in the surrounding alveoli exceeds capillary (venous) pressure, the pressure at the tip of the pulmonary artery catheter may reflect the alveolar pressure rather than the left-atrial pressure. This is illustrated in Figure 10.3. The lung in this figure is divided into three zones based on the relationship between alveolar pressure and the pressures in the

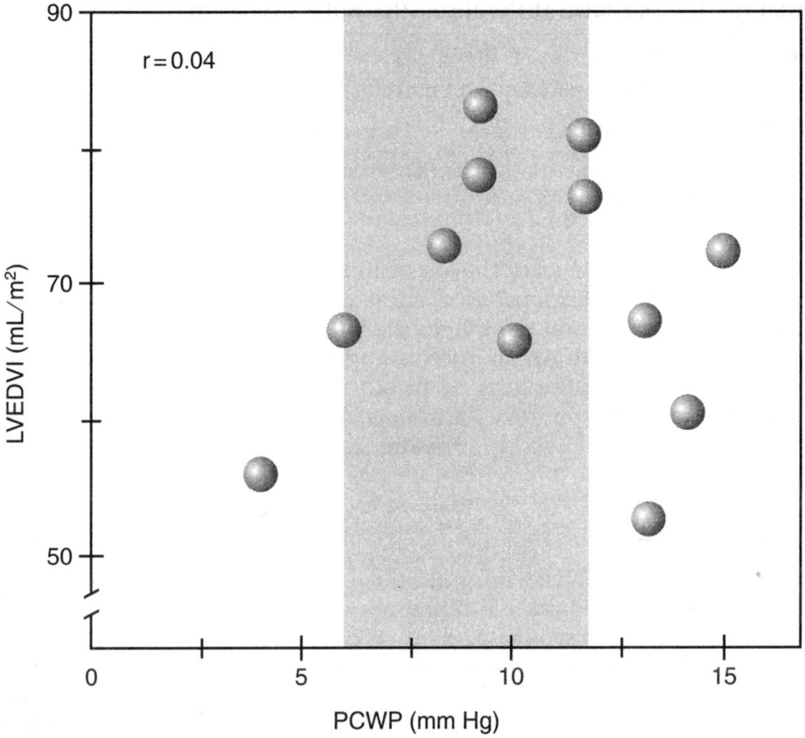

FIGURE 10.4 The relationship between the pulmonary capillary wedge pressure (PCWP) and the left-ventricular end-diastolic volume index (LVEDVI) in 12 normal subjects. The *shaded area* represents the normal range for PCWP, and the r value is the correlation coefficient. (From Kumar A, Anel R, Bunnell E, et al. Pulmonary artery occlusion pressure and central venous pressure fail to predict ventricular filling volume, cardiac performance, or the response to volume infusion in normal subjects. Crit Care Med 2004;32:691.)

pulmonary circulation (1,3). The most dependent lung zone (zone 3) is the only region where capillary (venous) pressure exceeds alveolar pressure. Therefore, wedge pressure is a reflection of left-atrial pressure only when the tip of the pulmonary artery catheter is located in zone 3 of the lung.

Catheter-tip Position

Although the lung zones shown in Figure 10.3 are based on physiologic rather than anatomic criteria, the lung regions below the left atrium are considered to be in lung zone 3 (1,3). Therefore **the tip of the pulmonary artery catheter should be positioned below the level of the left atrium** to ensure that the wedge pressure is measuring left-atrial pressure. Because of the higher blood flow in dependent lung regions, most pulmonary artery catheters are advanced into lung regions below the level of the left atrium. However, as many as 30% of PA catheters are positioned with

TABLE 10.1 Criteria for Wedge Pressure Validation

Wedge PO_2 − Arterial $PO_2 \geq 19$ mm Hg
Arterial PCO_2 − Wedge $PCO_2 \geq 11$ mm Hg
Wedge pH − Arterial pH ≥ 0.008

From Morris AH, Chapman RH, Gardner RM. Frequency of wedge pressure errors in the ICU. Crit Care Med 1985; 13:705–708, with permission.

their tips above the level of the left atrium (3). When patients are supine, routine portable (anteroposterior) chest x-rays cannot be used to identify the catheter-tip position relative to the left atrium. Rather, a lateral view of the chest is needed. An alternative approach is to assume that catheter tips are in zone 3 of the lung in all but the following conditions: when there are marked respiratory variations in the wedge pressure and when PEEP is applied and wedge pressure increases by 50% or more of the applied PEEP (3).

Wedged Blood Gases

As many as 50% of the nonpulsatile pressures produced by balloon inflation represent damped pulmonary artery pressures rather than pulmonary capillary wedge pressures (17). Aspiration of blood from the catheter tip during balloon inflation can be used to identify a true wedge (capillary) pressure using the three criteria shown in Table 10.1. Although this is a cumbersome practice that is not used routinely, it seems justified when making important diagnostic and therapeutic decisions based on the wedge pressure measurement.

Wedge Pressure as Left-Ventricular End-Diastolic Pressure

Even when wedge pressure is an accurate reflection of left-atrial pressure, there may be a discrepancy between left-atrial pressure and left-ventricular end-diastolic pressure (LVEDP). This can occur under the following conditions (3).

Aortic insufficiency: LVEDP can be higher than PCWP because the mitral valve closes prematurely while retrograde flow continues to fill the ventricle.

Noncompliant ventricle: Atrial contraction against a stiff ventricle produces a rapid rise in end-diastolic pressure that closes the mitral valve prematurely. The result is a PCWP that is lower than the LVEDP.

Respiratory failure: PCWP can exceed LVEDP in patients with pulmonary disease. The presumed mechanism is constriction of small veins in lung regions that are hypoxic (18).

Wedge Pressure as Capillary Hydrostatic Pressure

The wedge pressure is often assumed to be a measure of hydrostatic pressure in the pulmonary capillaries. The problem with this assumption is the fact that the wedge pressure is measured in the absence of blood flow. **When the balloon is deflated and blood flow resumes, the pressure in the pulmonary capillaries will remain the same as the left-atrial (wedge) pressure only if the resistance to flow in the pulmonary veins is negligible**. This is expressed below, where P_c is capillary hydrostatic pressure, R_v is the hydraulic resistance in the pulmonary veins, Q is blood flow, and wedge pressure (PCWP) is substituted for left-atrial pressure.

$$P_c - \text{PCWP} = Q \times R_v \tag{10.2}$$

If $R_v = 0$, $P_c - \text{PCWP} = 0$, and $P_c = \text{PCWP}$.

Pulmonary Venous Resistance

Unlike the systemic veins, the pulmonary veins contribute a significant fraction to the total vascular resistance across the lungs. (This is a reflection more of a low resistance in the pulmonary arteries than of a high resistance in the pulmonary veins.) As shown in Figure 10.5, 40% of the pressure drop across the pulmonary circulation occurs on the venous side of the circulation, which means that **the pulmonary veins contribute 40% of the total resistance in the pulmonary circulation** (19). Although this is derived from animal studies, the contribution in humans is probably similar in magnitude.

The contribution of the hydraulic resistance in the pulmonary veins may be even greater in critically ill patients because several conditions that are common in ICU patients can promote pulmonary venoconstriction. These conditions include hypoxemia, endotoxemia, and the acute respiratory distress syndrome (18,20). These conditions further magnify differences between wedge pressure and capillary hydrostatic pressure, as demonstrated below.

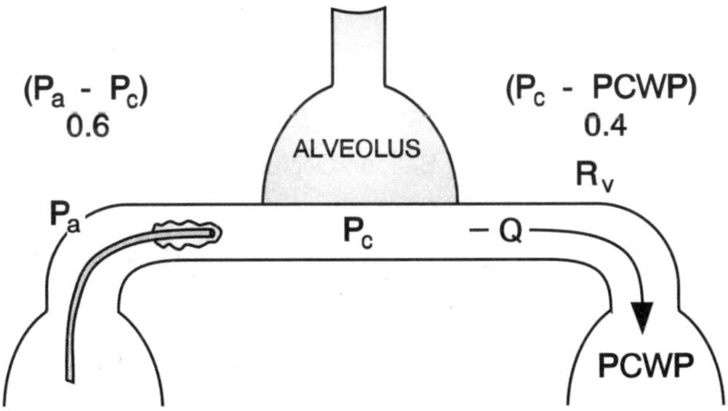

FIGURE 10.5. The distinction between capillary hydrostatic pressure (P_c) and wedge pressure (PCWP). When the balloon is deflated and flow (Q) resumes, P_c and PCWP are equivalent only when the hydraulic resistance in the pulmonary veins (R_v) is negligible. P_a = pulmonary artery pressure. If the pulmonary venous resistance (R_v) is greater than zero, the capillary hydrostatic pressure (P_c) will be higher than the wedge pressure.

Wedge–Hydrostatic Pressure Conversion

Equation 10.3 can be used to convert wedge pressure (PCWP) to pulmonary capillary hydrostatic pressure (P_c). This conversion is based on the assumption that the pressure drop from the pulmonary capillaries to the left atrium ($P_c - P_{LA}$) represents 40% of the pressure drop from the pulmonary arteries to the left atrium ($P_a - P_{LA}$). Substituting wedge pressure for left-atrial pressure (i.e., P_{LA} = PCWP) yields the following relationship:

$$P_c - \text{PCWP} = 0.4\,(P_a - \text{PCWP})$$

$$P_c = \text{PCWP} + 0.4\,(P_a - \text{PCWP}) \qquad (10.3)$$

For a normal (mean) pulmonary artery pressure of 15 mm Hg and a wedge pressure of 10 mm Hg, this relationship predicts the following:

$$\text{Normal lung: } P_c = 10 + 0.4 \times (15 - 10) \qquad (10.4)$$

P_c = 12 mm Hg, P_c − PCWP = 2 mm Hg.

Thus in the normal lung, wedge pressure is equivalent to capillary hydrostatic pressure. However, in the presence of pulmonary venoconstriction and pulmonary hypertension (e.g., in acute respiratory distress syndrome), there can be a considerable difference between wedge pressure and capillary hydrostatic pressure. The example below is based on a mean PA pressure of 30 mm Hg and a venous resistance that is 60% of the total pulmonary vascular resistance.

$$\text{ARDS: } P_c = 10 + 0.6 \times (30 - 10) \qquad (10.5)$$

P_c = 22 mm Hg, P_c − PCWP = 12 mm Hg.

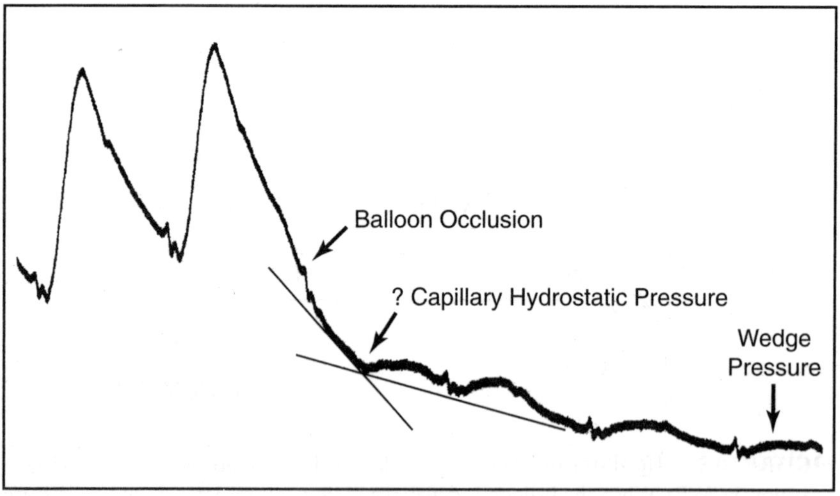

FIGURE 10.6 Pulmonary artery pressure tracing showing a rapid and slow component after balloon occlusion. The inflection point may represent the capillary hydrostatic pressure, which is higher than the wedge pressure.

Unfortunately, pulmonary venous resistance cannot be measured in critically ill patients, and this limits the accuracy of the wedge pressure as a measure of capillary hydrostatic pressure.

Occlusion Pressure Profile

The transition from pulsatile pulmonary artery pressure to nonpulsatile wedge pressure in Figure 10.6 shows an initial rapid phase followed by a slower, more gradual pressure change. The initial rapid phase may represent the pressure drop across the pulmonary arteries, while the slower phase may represent the pressure drop across the pulmonary veins. If this is the case, the inflection point marking the transition from the rapid to the slow phase represents the capillary hydrostatic pressure. Unfortunately, inflection points are often not recognizable following balloon occlusion (21,22).

A FINAL WORD

Despite their popularity, the central venous pressure and pulmonary artery wedge pressure provide limited and often misleading information about intravascular volume, cardiac filling volumes, and capillary hydrostatic pressure. What this means is that **these pressures should not be used (at least in isolation) to determine if a patient is dehydrated or fluid overloaded** (23), and the wedge pressure should not be used to diagnose hydrostatic pulmonary edema. The pulmonary artery catheter provides much more important measurements, particularly cardiac output and systemic oxygen transport variables, and these, together with other methods of assessing tissue oxygenation (see next chapter) make the CVP and wedge pressures outdated measures that are not necessary in the hemodynamic assessment of critically ill patients.

REFERENCES

Reviews

1. Leatherman JW, Marini JJ. Pulmonary artery catheterization: interpretation of pressure recordings. In: Tobin MJ, ed. Principles and practice of intensive care monitoring. New York: McGraw-Hill, 1998:821–837.
2. Pinsky MR. Hemodynamic monitoring in the intensive care unit. Clin Chest Med 2003;24:549–560.
3. O'Quin R, Marini JJ. Pulmonary artery occlusion pressure: clinical physiology, measurement, and interpretation. Am Rev Respir Dis 1983;128:319–326.

Selected References

4. Kumar A, Anel R, Bunnell E, et al. Pulmonary artery occlusion pressure and central venous pressure fail to predict ventricular filling volume, cardiac performance, or the response to volume infusion in normal subjects. Crit Care Med 2004;32:691–699.

5. Jacka MJ, Cohen MM, To T, et al. Pulmonary artery occlusion pressure estimation: how confident are anesthesiologists? Crit Care Med 2002;30:1197–1203.
6. Nadeau S, Noble WH. Misinterpretation of pressure measurements from the pulmonary artery catheter. Can Anesth Soc J 1986;33:352–363.
7. Komandina KH, Schenk DA, LaVeau P, et al. Interobserver variability in the interpretation of pulmonary artery catheter pressure tracings. Chest 1991;100:1647–1654.
8. Kee LL, Simonson JS, Stotts NA, et al. Echocardiographic determination of valid zero reference levels in supine and lateral positions. Am J Crit Care 1993;2:72–80.
9. Schmitt EA, Brantigen CO. Common artifacts of pulmonary artery and pulmonary artery wedge pressures: recognition and management. J Clin Monit 1986;2:44–52.
10. Pinsky M, Vincent J-L, De Smet J-M. Estimating left ventricular filling pressure during positive end-expiratory pressure in humans. Am Rev Respir Dis 1991;143:25–31.
11. Teboul J-L, Pinsky MR, Mercat A, et al. Estimating cardiac filling pressure in mechanically ventilated patients with hyperinflation. Crit Care Med 2000;28:3631–3636.
12. Dobbin K, Wallace S, Ahlberg J, et al. Pulmonary artery pressure measurement in patients with elevated pressures: effect of backrest elevation and method of measurement. Am J Crit Care 1992;2:61–69.
13. Halck S, Walther-Larsen S, Sanchez R. Reliability of central venous pressure measured by water column. Crit Care Med 1990;18:461–462.
14. Nemens EJ, Woods SL. Normal fluctuations in pulmonary artery and pulmonary capillary wedge pressures in acutely ill patients. Heart Lung 1982;11:393–398.
15. Morris AH, Chapman RH, Gardner RM. Frequency of wedge pressure errors in the ICU. Crit Care Med 1985;13:705–708.
16. Diebel LN, Wilson RF, Tagett MG, et al. End-diastolic volume: a better indicator of preload in the critically ill. Arch Surg 1992;127:817–822.
17. Morris AH, Chapman RH. Wedge pressure confirmation by aspiration of pulmonary capillary blood. Crit Care Med 1985;13:756–759.
18. Tracey WR, Hamilton JT, Craig ID, et al. Effect of endothelial injury on the responses of isolated guinea pig pulmonary venules to reduced oxygen tension. J Appl Physiol 1989;67:2147–2153.
19. Michel RP, Hakim TS, Chang HK. Pulmonary arterial and venous pressures measured with small catheters. J Appl Physiol 1984;57:309–314.
20. Kloess T, Birkenhauer U, Kottler B. Pulmonary pressure–flow relationship and peripheral oxygen supply in ARDS due to bacterial sepsis. Second Vienna Shock Forum, 1989:175–180.
21. Cope DK, Grimbert F, Downey JM, et al. Pulmonary capillary pressure: a review. Crit Care Med 1992;20:1043–1056.
22. Gilbert E, Hakim TS. Derivation of pulmonary capillary pressure from arterial occlusion in intact conditions. Crit Care Med 1994;22:986–993.
23. Leibowitz AB. More reliable determination of central venous and pulmonary artery occlusion pressures: does it matter? Crit Care Med 2005;33:243–244.

Chapter 11

TISSUE OXYGENATION

People say life can't exist without air, but it does under water; in fact, it started in the sea.

Richard Feynman

The management of critically ill patients has one universal goal: to maintain adequate levels of tissue oxygenation and sustain aerobic metabolism. However, much of what is done in the name of aerobic support is based on traditional beliefs rather than documented need because there is no direct measure of tissue oxygenation. This chapter describes some indirect measures of tissue oxygenation used by critical care specialists.

TISSUE OXYGEN BALANCE

The adequacy of tissue oxygenation is determined by the balance between the oxygen delivered into the tissues and oxygen required to sustain aerobic metabolism. This balance is illustrated in Figure 11.1. The VO_2 is the rate of oxygen delivery into the tissues, and the MRO_2 is the metabolic requirement for oxygen. When the VO_2 is equivalent to the MRO_2, glucose is completely oxidized to yield 36 ATP molecules (673 kcal) per mole glucose. When VO_2 cannot match MRO_2, some of the glucose is diverted to form lactate, with an energy yield of 2 ATP (47 kcal) molecules per mole glucose. Thus an inadequate supply of oxygen limits the energy yield from substrate metabolism. **The condition in which metabolic energy production is limited by the supply or utilization of oxygen is called *dysoxia* (1), and the clinical expression of this condition is known as *shock*.** Dysoxia can be the result of an inadequate supply of oxygen, as occurs in hypovolemic shock and cardiogenic shock, or it can be caused by a defect in mitochondrial oxygen utilization, as occurs in septic shock. Monitoring the VO_2 can help to identify the tissue dysoxia that results from an inadequate supply of oxygen (2), as described next.

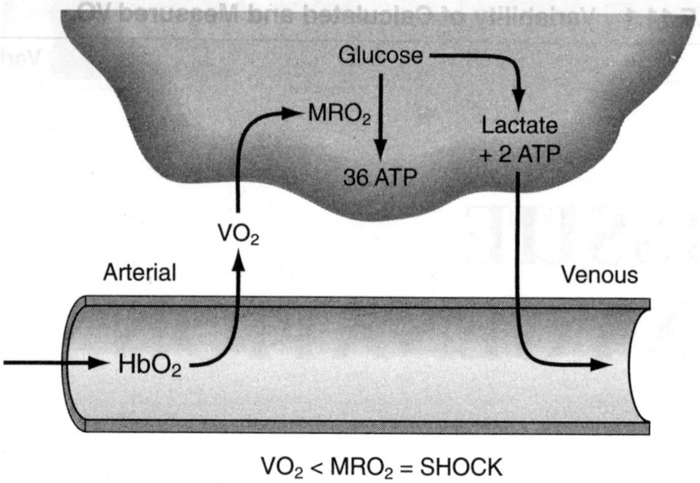

FIGURE 11.1 Illustration showing the relationship between oxygen uptake into tissues (VO_2) and the metabolic requirement for oxygen (MRO_2). When the VO_2 is equivalent to the MRO_2, oxidative metabolism proceeds unimpeded. Shock is defined as the condition in which the VO_2 is unable to match the MRO_2.

OXYGEN UPTAKE

The rate of oxygen uptake from the systemic capillaries (VO_2) is a measure of oxygen availability in the tissues, as just described. Because oxygen is not stored in tissues, the VO_2 is also a measure of tissue oxygen consumption.

Calculated Versus Measured VO_2

The VO_2 can be calculated by using a modification of the Fick equation (Equation 11.1), or it can be measured directly as the rate of oxygen disappearance from the lungs. Each of these methods is described in Chapter 2. The directly measured VO_2 is more accurate and more reliable than the calculated VO_2 , as described next.

$$VT_2 = Q \times (CaT_2 - CvT_2) \qquad (11.1)$$

Whole-Body VO_2

The calculated VO_2 is not a measure of whole-body VO_2 because it does not include the VO_2 of the lungs. This distinction is of little importance in healthy subjects because the VO_2 of the lungs is normally less than 5% of the whole-body VO_2 (3). However, in patients with inflammation in the lungs (e.g., from pneumonia or acute respiratory distress syndrome), the VO_2 of the lungs can be 20% of the whole-body VO_2 (4). Therefore **when lung inflammation is present, the calculated VO_2 will underestimate the whole-body VO_2 by as much as 20%**. This is one reason to **avoid using the calculated VO_2** if possible **in patients with inflammatory**

TABLE 11.1 Variability of Calculated and Measured VO_2

Parameter	Variability
Thermodilution cardiac output	±10%
Hemoglobin concentration	±2%
% Oxyhemoglobin saturation	±2%
Oxygen content of blood	±4%
CaO_2–CvO_2	±8%
Calculated VO_2	±18%
Measured VO_2	±5%

From References 5–7.

conditions in the lungs. As you will learn a little later, the VO_2 determined by either method (i.e., calculated or measured) may not be a worthwhile measure in patients with widespread inflammation.

Variability

Another shortcoming of the calculated VO_2 is its variability. The equation used to derive VO_2 includes four separate measurements (cardiac output, hemoglobin concentration in blood, and the percent oxyhemoglobin saturation in arterial and mixed venous blood), and each has its own inherent variability. These are shown in Table 11.1 (5–7). The variability of the calculated VO_2 is 18%, which is equivalent to the summed variability of its components (see Equation 11.1). As a result of this variability, **the calculated VO_2 must change by at least 18 or 20% for the change to be considered significant**. The measured VO_2 has a variability of less than 5% (6,7) and thus is much more reliable than the calculated VO_2.

Availability

The calculated VO_2 is readily available in patients who have an indwelling pulmonary artery catheter (used to measure cardiac output and the percent oxyhemoglobin saturation in mixed venous blood). The directly measured VO_2, on the other hand, requires specialized equipment (i.e., a device such as a metabolic cart that is equipped with an oxygen sensor) and trained personnel to operate the equipment. For this reason, the measured VO_2 is not readily available, at least on a 24-hour basis, in most ICUs.

Using the VO_2

The VO_2 can be used to identify a global (whole-body) state of tissue dysoxia due to impaired tissue oxygenation, as described in the next section.

VO_2 Deficit

An abnormally low VO_2 (less than 100 mL/min/m^2) can be the result of hypometabolism or tissue dysoxia due to impaired tissue oxygenation.

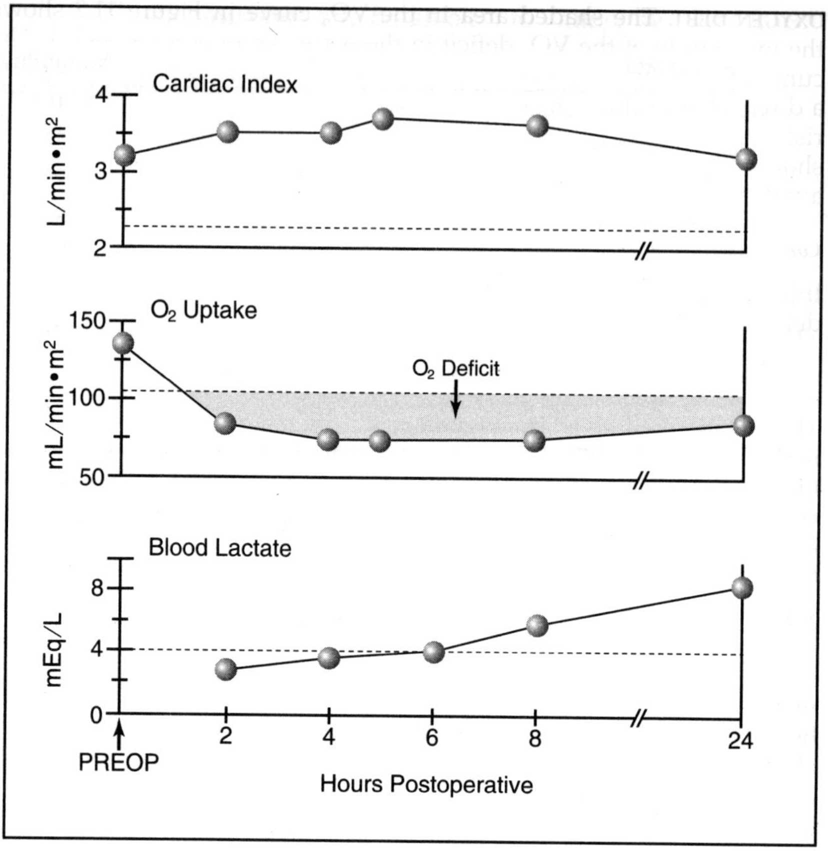

FIGURE 11.2 Serial measurements of cardiac index, systemic oxygen uptake, and blood lactate levels in a patient who underwent abdominal aortic aneurysm repair. The *dotted lines* indicate the lower limits of normal for each measurement. The *shaded area* represents the oxygen debt.

Because hypometabolism is uncommon in critically ill patients, **a VO_2 that is below the normal range (below 100 mL/minute/m²) can be used as evidence of impaired tissue oxygenation**. An example of this is shown in Figure 11.2. The measurements in this figure are from a patient who underwent an abdominal aortic aneurysm repair. The first set of postoperative measurements (at 2 hours following surgery) show a normal cardiac index and blood lactate level along with an abnormally low VO_2. The low VO_2 persists, and the blood lactate level begins to rise, steadily, reaching 9 mEq/L at 24 hours after surgery. The abnormally low VO_2 is evidence of a generalized oxygen deficit, as confirmed by the eventual rise in blood lactate levels. Monitoring the VO_2 in this case therefore provided early evidence of impaired tissue oxygenation. Note that the cardiac index remains in the normal range despite the evidence of impaired tissue oxygenation. This illustrates the nonvalue of cardiac output monitoring in the assessment of tissue oxygenation.

OXYGEN DEBT. The shaded area in the VO_2 curve in Figure 11.2 shows the magnitude of the VO_2 deficit in the early postoperative period. The cumulative deficit is called the *oxygen debt*. Clinical studies have shown a direct relationship between the magnitude of the oxygen debt and the risk of multiorgan failure and death (8,9). This indicates that VO_2 deficits should be corrected, if possible, to prevent progressive organ injury and avoid a fatal outcome.

Correcting VO_2 Deficits

Interventions designed to correct a VO_2 deficit can be identified using the determinants of VO_2 in the equation shown below.

$$VT_2 = Q \times 13.4 \times Hb \times (SaT_2 - SvT_2) \qquad (11.2)$$

This equation is derived from Equation 11.1 by removing the common term in the O_2 content (CaO_2 and CvO_2) equations (see Chapter 2). This equation identifies **three determinants of VO_2: cardiac output (Q), hemoglobin concentration in blood (Hb), and the difference in oxyhemoglobin saturation between arterial and venous blood ($SaO_2 - SvO_2$)**. The following interventions are designed to augment each of these determinants.

AUGMENT CARDIAC OUTPUT. If the cardiac output is low (i.e., cardiac index < 2.4 L/min/m^2), the next step is to measure the ventricular filling pressure [i.e., the central venous pressure (CVP) or the pulmonary capillary wedge pressure (PCWP)]. If the CVP is below 4 mm Hg or the PCWP is below 6 mm Hg, volume resuscitation is indicated until the CVP rises to about 10 mm Hg, or the PCWP rises to about 15 mm Hg (these values are slightly above the normal range for each pressure). If the ventricular filling pressures are normal or elevated, the cardiac output should be normalized by using dobutamine (a positive inotropic agent described in Chapter 16).

CORRECT ANEMIA. If the hemoglobin is below 7 g/dL, consider blood transfusion. This approach is problematic in low output states because an increase in hematocrit will increase blood viscosity, and this can decrease the cardiac output (see Figure 1.8).

CORRECT HYPOXEMIA. If the arterial oxyhemoglobin saturation (SaO_2) is below 90%, the concentration of inhaled oxygen should be increased until the SaO_2 rises above 90%.

This approach is designed to correct VT_2 deficits in patients with impaired tissue oxygenation due to hypovolemic shock or cardiogenic shock. It may not be appropriate for patients with septic shock, where tissue dysoxia may be the result of a defect in oxygen utilization rather than oxygen availability, as explained next.

The VO_2 in Sepsis

The VO_2 may not be an appropriate parameter to monitor in patients with severe sepsis or septic shock because the VO_2 may not reflect the rate of aerobic metabolism in sepsis. Activation of neutrophils and macrophages is accompanied by a marked increase in cellular oxygen consumption,

TABLE 11.2 Oxygen-Transport Variables, Blood Lactate, and Survival in Septic Shock

Measurement	Survivors	Nonsurvivors	Difference
Cardiac index (L/min/m^2)	3.8	3.9	+2.6%
Oxygen uptake (mL/min/m^2)	173	164	−5.2%
Arterial lactate (mmol/L)	2.6	7.7	+296%

Measurements in nonsurvivors are the last ones before death.
From Reference 23.

called the *respiratory burst*. The oxygen consumed in this process is used to generate toxic oxygen intermediates (e.g., superoxide radical and hydrogen peroxide) that are released as part of the inflammatory process (10). This oxygen consumption contributes to the VO_2 measurement but is unrelated to aerobic metabolism. This means that in sepsis, there is a *non-metabolic* VO_2, which is the contribution of the respiratory burst in phagocytes, that adds to the metabolic VO_2, or the rate of aerobic metabolism.

As just described, **in patients with severe sepsis or a systemic inflammatory condition, the measured VO_2 is not a true reflection of aerobic metabolism (i.e., the metabolic VO_2).** The measured VT_2 is expected to overestimate the metabolic VT_2 in sepsis by an amount that is equivalent to the non-metabolic VT_2 in phagocytes. The magnitude of the non-metabolic VT_2 in sepsis is unknown, but it may be considerable (11).

The non-value of the measured VT_2 in sepsis is demonstrated in Table 11.2. In this study of patients with septic shock, the VT_2 was slightly above the normal range (100 to 160 mL/min/m^2) in both survivors and nonsurvivors. However, the metabolic VT_2 should be lower than normal (reflecting anaerobic metabolism) in patients with shock, especially in patients who do not survive. The higher-than-expected VO_2 in Table 11.2 may then be a reflection of the added contribution of the non-metabolic VT_2 in activated phagocytes. In fact, **the elevated VO_2 that is often observed in sepsis may not represent true hypermetabolism but may be a reflection of the added O_2 consumption in activated phagocytes.**

Tissue Oxygenation in Sepsis

The graph in Figure 11.3 shows the PO_2 recorded with an oxygen electrode placed in a forearm muscle in a group of healthy subjects and a group of patients with severe sepsis (12). Note that the tissue PO_2 is *increased* in the septic patients, indicating that **tissue oxygenation is not impaired in sepsis**. Similar results have been reported in the bowel mucosa of animals injected with endotoxin (13). Despite the improved tissue oxygenation, aerobic metabolism is challenged in sepsis because there is an apparent defect in oxygen utilization in mitochondria (14). Nevertheless, because tissue oxygen levels are not impaired in sepsis, **therapy designed to improve tissue oxygenation does not seem warranted in patients with severe sepsis or septic shock.**

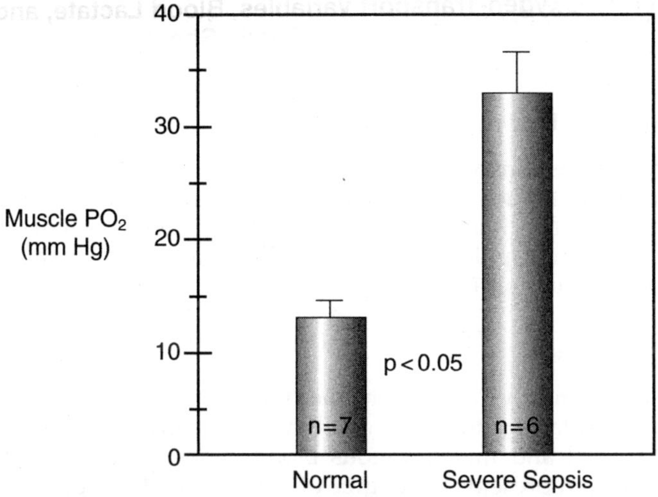

FIGURE 11.3 Tissue PO_2 (mean) recorded in the forearm muscles of 6 healthy volunteers and 7 patients with severe sepsis. *Crossbars* represent the standard error of the mean. (From Sair M, Etherington PJ, Winlove CP, et al. Tissue oxygenation and perfusion in patients with systemic sepsis. Crit Care Med 2001;29:1343.)

Clinical Outcomes

The value of the oxygen transport variables (i.e., oxygen delivery and oxygen uptake) as therapeutic end-points in critically ill patients is a matter of considerable debate. Some studies show improved outcomes with this approach (15), whereas others do not (16). One source of confusion may be the fact that many of these studies included septic patients (16), who are not expected to have impaired tissue oxygen levels and are not expected to improve with interventions designed to promote tissue oxygenation.

Summary

To summarize, **an abnormally low VO_2 (less than 100 mL/min/m²) can be a marker of impaired tissue oxygenation, but only in patients who are free of sepsis or systemic inflammation** (see Chapter 40 for a description of the sepsis and inflammatory syndromes). Furthermore, management designed to improve tissue oxygenation may not be appropriate in sepsis because tissue oxygenation does not seem to be impaired in this condition.

VENOUS O_2 SATURATION

The oxygen saturation of hemoglobin in mixed venous (pulmonary artery) blood can be used to evaluate the balance between systemic oxygen delivery and systemic oxygen uptake. This concept is described in Chapter 2 (see the section, Control of Oxygen Uptake) and is briefly reviewed here.

Control of O_2 Uptake

The oxygen transport system operates to maintain a constant rate of oxygen uptake into tissues (VO_2) in the face of variations in systemic oxygen delivery (DO_2). This is accomplished by varying the oxygen desaturation of hemoglobin in capillary blood as the DO_2 varies. This relationship is expressed in Equation 11.3.

$$VT_2 = DT_2 \times (SaT_2 - SvT_2) \tag{11.3}$$

The SaT_2 and SvT_2 represent the oxygen saturation of hemoglobin (i.e., the percentage of total hemoglobin that is fully saturated with oxygen) in arterial and mixed venous blood, respectively. The difference (SaT_2 − SvT_2) represents the degree of oxygen desaturation of hemoglobin as it passes through the capillaries, also known as the *oxygen extraction* from hemoglobin in capillary blood.

The graph in Figure 11.4 shows the relationship between O_2 delivery (DT_2), O_2 uptake (VT_2), and O_2 extraction (SaT_2 − SvT_2) when O_2 delivery is progressively decreased. The normal SaT_2 and SvT_2 are 95%

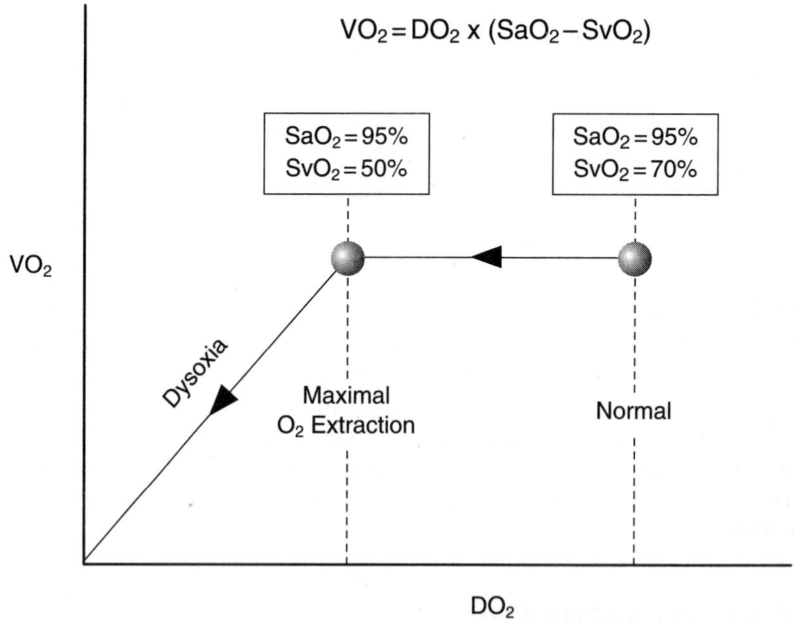

FIGURE 11.4 The relationship between systemic oxygen delivery (DO_2), systemic oxygen uptake (VO_2), and oxygen extraction ($SaO_2 - SvO_2$) in capillary blood. SaO_2 and SvO_2 represent the oxygenated hemoglobin expressed as a percentage of total hemoglobin in arterial and mixed venous (pulmonary artery) blood, respectively.

and 70%, respectively, indicating a normal O_2 extraction of 25%. This means that 25% of the hemoglobin molecules desaturate as they pass through the capillaries. As the DO_2 begins to decrease below normal, the VO_2 remains constant, indicating that the O_2 extraction is increasing. At the point where O_2 extraction is maximal, the SaO_2 is unchanged at 95%, but the SvO_2 has decreased to 50%. The maximum O_2 extraction is thus 45%, or almost twice normal. When O_2 extraction reaches its maximum level, further decreases in DO_2 are accompanied by similar decreases in VO_2. This condition of delivery-dependent VO_2 is a sign of tissue dysoxia (i.e., oxygen-limited aerobic energy production).

Using the SvO_2

According to the relationships shown in Figure 11.4, monitoring the SvO_2 can provide the following information.

1. A decrease in SvO_2 below 70% indicates that systemic O_2 delivery is impaired. The possible sources of impaired O_2 delivery are identified by the determinants of DO_2 in Equation 11.4 (which is described in more detail in Chapter 2). A decrease in DO_2 can be the result of a low cardiac output (Q), anemia (Hb), or hypoxemia (SaO_2).

$$DO_2 = Q \times 13.4 \times Hb \times SaT_2 \tag{11.4}$$

2. A decrease in SvO_2 to 50% indicates a global state of tissue dysoxia or impending dysoxia.

The SvO_2 measurement requires a pulmonary artery (PA) catheter (described in Chapter 9) because blood from the pulmonary artery is considered to be a mix of venous blood from all tissue beds (hence the term "mixed" venous blood). The measurement is usually performed on a blood sample taken from the distal lumen of the PA catheter. There is also a specialized PA catheter that is capable of performing continuous *in vivo* measurements of the SvO_2 in pulmonary artery blood. The methodology for the measurement of O_2 saturation in blood (which is called *oximetry*) is described in detail in Chapter 20.

Variability

Continuous monitoring of SvO_2 with specialized pulmonary artery catheters has revealed **a spontaneous variation that averages 5% but can be as high as 20%** (17). In general, a greater than 5% change in SvO_2 that persists for longer than 10 minutes is considered a significant change (18).

Central Venous O_2 Saturation

For patients who do not have a pulmonary artery catheter, blood from the superior vena cava (drawn through a central venous catheter) has been recommended as a suitable alternative to mixed venous (pulmonary artery) blood for the measurement of O_2 saturation (19). The agreement between *central venous O_2 saturation* ($ScvO_2$) and mixed venous O_2 saturation (SvO_2) is reasonable (within 5%) if multiple measurements are averaged, but single measurements of $ScvO_2$ can differ from SvO_2 by as much as 10% (absolute difference) (20). Therefore multiple measurements of $ScvO_2$ are recommended before making diagnostic and therapeutic decisions based on the measurement.

The $ScvT_2$ is gaining popularity as a surrogate measure of mixed venous O_2 saturation because it obviates the cost and morbidity associated with pulmonary artery catheters. Recent guidelines for the early management of patients with severe sepsis and septic shock includes an $ScvT_2$ of greater than 70% as a therapeutic end-point (19).

LACTATE LEVELS IN BLOOD

As indicated in Figure 11.1, lactate accumulation in tissues and blood is an expected consequence of dysoxia (21). Monitoring blood lactate levels is the most widely used method of evaluating tissue oxygen balance and detecting global (whole-body) tissue dysoxia. Lactate can be measured in whole blood or plasma (22), and concentrations above 2 mEq/L are considered abnormal. Increasing the threshold to 4 mEq/L may be more appropriate for predicting survival (22).

Blood Lactate and Survival

As demonstrated in Figure 11.2, lactate accumulation in blood can be a delayed finding in patients with impaired tissue oxygenation. However, once elevated, blood lactate levels show a direct correlation with mortality in patients with circulatory shock. This is demonstrated in Figure 11.5. Note that most patients survive when the blood lactate concentration is below 2 mmol/L, while most patients do not survive when the blood lactate level approaches 10 mmol/L. In patients with circulatory shock (e.g., hypotension, oliguria, etc.), the likelihood of a fatal outcome is 60% when the blood lactate is above 2 mmol/L, and 80% when the blood lactate exceeds 4 mmol/L (22).

In patients with septic shock, an elevated blood lactate level is more predictive of a fatal outcome than the oxygen transport variables. This is demonstrated in Table 11.2 (23). Neither cardiac output nor systemic oxygen uptake (VT_2) differs significantly in survivors and nonsurvivors, whereas the lactate levels are three times higher in patients with a fatal outcome.

Other Sources of Lactate

Unfortunately, lactate accumulation in blood is not specific for global tissue dysoxia. Other causes of hyperlactatemia include hepatic insufficiency (which impairs lactate clearance from the blood), thiamine deficiency (which inhibits pyruvate dehydrogenase activity and blocks pyruvate entry

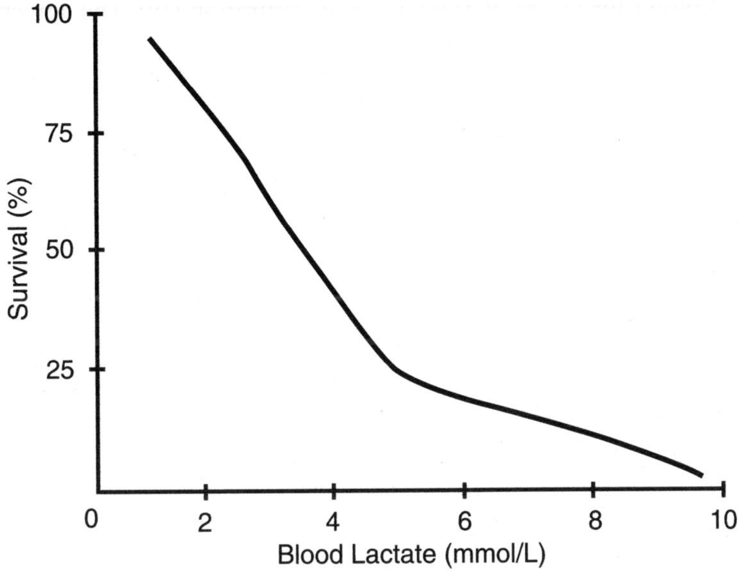

FIGURE 11.5 The relationship between blood lactate and survival in patients with circulatory shock. [From Weil MH, Afifi AA. Experimental and clinical studies on lactate and pyruvate as indicators of the severity of acute circulatory failure (shock). Circulation 1970;16:989.]

into mitochondria), severe sepsis (same mechanism as thiamine deficiency, as described below), and intracellular alkalosis (which stimulates glycolysis) (21,24). For more information on these disorders, see Chapter 29.

Sepsis

Lactate accumulation in sepsis may not be the result of tissue oxygen deprivation. The culprit may be endotoxin, which blocks the actions of the pyruvate dehydrogenase enzyme that moves pyruvate into mitochondria. Pyruvate is allowed to accumulate in the cell cytoplasm, where it is converted to lactate. The ability of endotoxin to promote lactate formation is shown in the graph in Figure 11.6 (25). In this animal study, a one-hour infusion of endotoxin was associated with a progressive rise in blood lactate. The animals were then given dichloroacetate, a substance that activates pyruvate dehydrogenase in the presence of oxygen. This causes a progressive decline in lactate levels to normal, indicating that pyruvate dehydrogenase was activated and oxygen was present in cells to permit activation. Finally, when the animals were subjected to hypoxemia by breathing a low-oxygen gas mixture, blood lactate levels failed to rise. These findings suggest that **impaired tissue oxygenation is not the source of blood lactate accumulation in sepsis**.

The combination of elevated tissue oxygen levels (Fig. 11.3) and lactate accumulation in sepsis is consistent with the notion that dysoxia in sepsis may be the result of a defect in the cellular utilization of oxygen.

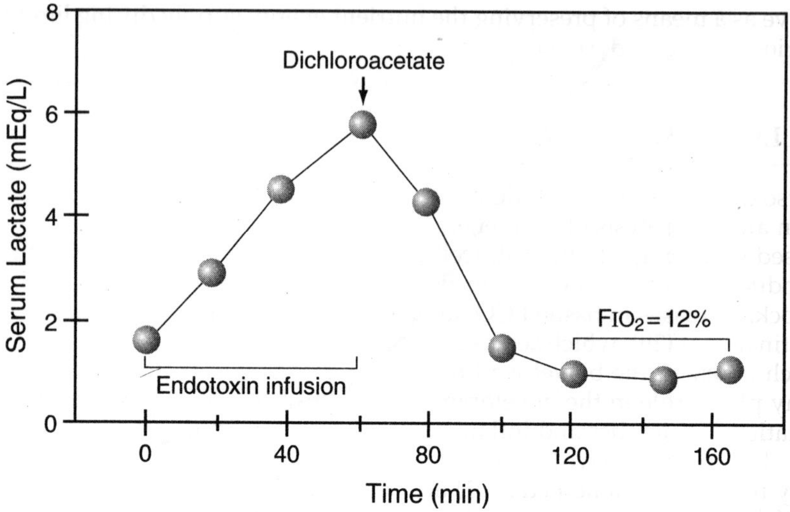

FIGURE 11.6 Influence of endotoxin, dichloroacetate, and hypoxic challenge on arterial lactate levels. Response to dichloroacetate indicates that endotoxin-associated lactic acidosis is not caused by anaerobic conditions. (From Curtis SE, Cain SM. Regional and systemic oxygen delivery/uptake relations and lactate flux in hyperdynamic, endotoxin-treated dogs. Am Rev Respir Dis 1992;145:348–354.)

Lactate as a Fuel

One feature of lactate that is often overlooked is its ability to serve as an oxidative fuel. The energy yield from the oxidation of both glucose and lactate is shown in Table 11.3. The energy yield from glucose oxidation is twice that of lactate, but each mole of glucose produces 2 moles of lactate. Therefore the energy yield from glucose metabolism is about the same when glucose is directly oxidized and when glucose is converted to lactate and the lactate is oxidized.

Lactate can serve as an oxidative fuel in several organs, including the heart, brain, liver, and skeletal muscle (26,27). If the lactate generated by tissue dysoxia can undergo oxidation in these organs at a later time, when aerobic metabolism is restored, then the energy yield of glucose oxidation will be preserved. In this context, lactate production could

TABLE 11.3 Lactate as an Oxidative Fuel

Substrate	Molecular Weight	Heat of Combustion	Caloric Value
Glucose	180	673 kcal/mole	3.74 kcal/g
Lactate	90	326 kcal/mole	3.62 kcal/g

$$\text{Glucose} \xrightarrow{\text{Oxidation}} 673\ \text{kcal}$$
$$\downarrow$$
$$\text{(2) Lactate} \xrightarrow{\text{Oxidation}} 652\ \text{kcal}$$

From Lehninger AL. Bioenergetics. New York: WA Benjamin, 1965:16, with permission.

serve as a means of preserving the nutrient energy supply during limited periods of tissue dysoxia.

ALIMENTARY TRACT HYPERCARBIA

Dysoxia promotes intracellular acidosis from enhanced lactate production and hydrolysis of high energy phosphate compounds. Bicarbonate-based buffering of this intracellular acidosis leads to enhanced CO_2 production and an increase in tissue PCO_2 (28). In cases of circulatory shock, increases in tissue PCO_2 are prominent in the wall of the gastrointestinal tract (29), which seems particularly vulnerable to ischemic injury. Such injury in the bowel wall may occur early in circulatory shock and may play a role in the development of multiple organ failure (via translocation of microbes and inflammatory cytokines) (30).

Two methods have been developed to detect hypercarbia in the alimentary tract: gastric tonometry (31) and sublingual capnometry (32). Despite initial enthusiasm for these methods, neither has gained widespread acceptance, and sublingual capnometry is not currently available. The reader is directed to references 31 and 32 for information on these methods.

A FINAL WORD

There are three take-home messages in this chapter. First, it is not possible to reliably assess tissue oxygenation in the clinical setting, and thus all interventions aimed at promoting tissue oxygenation are performed without justification and without a measurable end-point. Second, tissue oxygen levels are apparently not depressed in patients who are septic or have systemic inflammation, and thus efforts to promote tissue oxygenation are not warranted in these patients. And finally, the consensus view that tissue oxygenation is an important determinant of viability in critically ill patients is without proof.

REFERENCES

Tissue Oxygen Balance

1. Connett RJ, Honig CR, Gayeski TEJ, et al. Defining hypoxia: a systems view of VO_2, glycolysis, energetics, and intracellular PO_2. J Appl Physiol 1990;68: 833–842.
2. Shoemaker WC, Kram HB, Appel PL. Therapy of shock based on pathophysiology, monitoring, and outcome prediction. Crit Care Med 1990;18(suppl): S19–S25.

Oxygen Uptake

3. Nunn JF. Nonrespiratory functions of the lung. In: Nunn JF, ed. Applied respiratory physiology. London: Butterworth, 1993:306–317.

4. Jolliet P, Thorens JB, Nicod L, et al. Relationship between pulmonary oxygen consumption, lung inflammation, and calculated venous admixture in patients with acute lung injury. Intensive Care Med 1996;22:277–285.
5. Sasse SA, Chen PA, Berry RB, et al. Variability of cardiac output over time in medical intensive care unit patients. Chest 1994;22:225–232.
6. Bartlett RH, Dechert RE. Oxygen kinetics: pitfalls in clinical research. J Crit Care 1990;5:77–80.
7. Schneeweiss B, Druml W, Graninger W, et al. Assessment of oxygen-consumption by use of reverse Fick-principle and indirect calorimetry in critically ill patients. Clin Nutr 1989;8:89–93.
8. Dunham CM, Seigel JH, Weireter L, et al. Oxygen debt and metabolic acidemia as quantitative predictors of mortality and the severity of the ischemic insult in hemorrhagic shock. Crit Care Med 1991;19:231–243.
9. Shoemaker WC, Appel PL, Krom HB. Role of oxygen debt in the development of organ failure, sepsis, and death in high-risk surgical patients. Chest 1992;102:208–215.
10. Hurst JK, Barrette WC, Jr. Leukocyte activation and microbicidal oxidative toxins. Crit Rev Biochem Mol Biol 1989;24:271–328.
11. Jolliet P, Thorens JB, Nicod L, et al. Relationship between pulmonary oxygen consumption, lung inflammation, and calculated venous admixture in patients with acute lung injury. Intensive Care Med 1996;22:277–285.
12. Sair M, Etherington PJ, Winlove CP, et al. Tissue oxygenation and perfusion in patients with systemic sepsis. Crit Care Med 2001;29:1343–1349.
13. VanderMeer TJ, Wang H, Fink MP. Endotoxemia causes ileal mucosal acidosis in the absence of mucosal hypoxia in a normodynamic porcine model of septic shock. Crit Care Med 1995;23:1217–1226.
14. Fink MP. Impaired cellular use of oxygen in critically ill patients. J Crit Illness 2001;16(suppl):S28–S32.
15. Kern JW, Shoemaker WC. Meta-analysis of hemodynamic optimization in high-risk patients. Crit Care Med 2002;30:1686–1692.
16. Alia I, Esteban A, Gordo F, et al. A randomized and controlled trial of the effect of treatment aimed at maximizing oxygen delivery in patients with severe sepsis and septic shock. Chest 1999;115:453–461.

Venous O_2 Saturation

17. Noll ML, Fountain RL, Duncan CA, et al. Fluctuations in mixed venous oxygen saturation in critically ill medical patients: a pilot study. Am J Crit Care 1992;3:102–106.
18. Krafft P, Stelzer H, Heismay M, et al. Mixed venous oxygen saturation in critically ill septic shock patients. Chest 1993;103:900–906.
19. Dellinger RP, Carlet JM, Masur H, et al. Surviving sepsis campaign guidelines for management of severe sepsis and septic shock. Crit Care Med 2004; 32:858–873.
20. Dueck MH, Kilmek M, Appenrodt S, et al. Trends but not individual values of central venous oxygen saturation agree with mixed venous oxygen saturation during varying hemodynamic conditions. Anesthesiology 2005;103: 249–257.

Lactate Levels in Blood

21. Duke T. Dysoxia and lactate. Arch Dis Child 1999;81:343–350.
22. Aduen J, Bernstein WK, Khastgir T, et al. The use and clinical importance of a substrate-specific electrode for rapid determination of blood lactate concentrations. JAMA 1994;272:1678–1685.
23. Bakker J, Coffernils M, Leon M, et al. Blood lactate levels are superior to oxygen-derived variables in predicting outcome in septic shock. Chest 1991;99: 956–962.
24. Mizock BA, Falk JL. Lactic acidosis in critical illness. Crit Care Med 1992;20: 80–93.
25. Curtis SE, Cain SM. Regional and systemic oxygen delivery/uptake relations and lactate flux in hyperdynamic, endotoxin-treated dogs. Am Rev Respir Dis 1992;145:348–354.
26. Brooks GA. Lactate production under fully aerobic conditions: the lactate shuttle during rest and exercise. Fed Proc 1986;45:2924–2929.
27. Maran A, Cranston I, Lomas J, et al. Protection by lactate of cerebral function during hypoglycemia. Lancet 1994;343:16–20.

Tissue PCO_2

28. Sato Y, Weil MH, Tang W. Tissue hypercarbic acidosis as a marker of acute circulatory failure (shock). Chest 1998;114:263–274.
29. Tang W, Weil MH, Sun S, et al. Gastric intramural PCO_2 as a monitor of perfusion failure during hemorrhagic and anaphylactic shock. J Appl Physiol 1994;76:572–577.
30. Fiddian-Green RG. Studies in splanchnic ischemia and multiple organ failure. In: Marston A, Bulkley GB, Fiddian-Green RG, et al., eds. Splanchnic ischemia and multiple organ failure. St. Louis: CV Mosby, 1989:349–364.
31. Hameed SM, Cohn SM. Gastric tonometry: the role of mucosal pH measurement in the management of trauma. Chest 2003;123(suppl):475S–481S.
32. Weil MH, Nakagawa Y, Tang W, et al. Sublingual capnometry: a new noninvasive measurement for diagnosis and quantitation of severity of circulatory shock. Crit Care Med 1999;27:1225–1229.

Section V

DISORDERS OF CIRCULATORY FLOW

Movement is the cause of all life.

LEONARDO DA VINCI

Chapter 12

HEMORRHAGE AND HYPOVOLEMIA

The dominant concern in the bleeding patient is the intolerance of the circulatory system to acute blood loss. The circulatory system operates with a small volume and a volume-responsive pump. This seems to be an energy efficient design, but the system falters when blood volume is not maintained. While most internal organs can lose more than 50% of their functional mass before organ failure is apparent, loss of only 30 to 40% of the blood volume can result in life-threatening circulatory failure. This intolerance of the circulatory system to blood loss means that **time is the enemy of the bleeding patient**.

This chapter describes the evaluation and early management of acute blood loss (1,2), and the next chapter describes the variety and use of asanguinous resuscitation fluids. These two chapters will introduce you to the fluids you will live with in the ICU, including body fluids (blood and plasma), transfusion fluids (whole blood and erythrocyte concentrates), and infusion fluids (colloids and crystalloids).

BODY FLUIDS AND BLOOD LOSS

Fluids account for at least half of the body weight in healthy adults. The volume of total body fluid (in liters) is equivalent to 60% of lean body weight (in kilograms) in males, and 50% of lean body weight in females. In Table 12.1, these volumes are shown as 600 mL/kg for males and 500 mL/kg for females. A healthy adult male who weighs 80 kg (176 lbs) will then have $0.6 \times 80 = 48$ liters of total body fluid, and a healthy adult female who weighs 60 kg (132 lbs) will have $0.5 \times 60 = 30$ liters of total body fluid. Table 12.1 also contains weight-based estimates for blood volume (3): 66 mL/kg for males and 60 mL/kg for females. An 80 kg adult male will then have $0.066 \times 80 = 5.3$ liters of blood, and a 60 kg

TABLE 12.1 Body Fluid and Blood Volumes

Fluid	Men	Women
Total body fluid	600 mL/kg	500 mL/kg
Whole blood	66 mL/kg	60 mL/kg
Plasma	40 mL/kg	36 mL/kg
Erythrocytes	26 mL/kg	24 mL/kg

Values expressed for lean body weights.
American Association of Blood Banks Technical Manual. 10th ed. Arlington, VA: American Association of Blood Banks, 1990:650.

adult female will have $0.06 \times 60 = 3.6$ liters of blood. According to these estimates, **blood represents about 11 to 12% of the total body fluid.**

The graduated beakers in Figure 12.1 show a comparison of the volumes of total body fluid, blood, and the components of blood (plasma and red blood cells) for an 80 kg adult male. The beakers are drawn to scale (i.e., the small, 5 mL beakers are one-tenth the size of the large, 50 mL beaker) to help demonstrate that only a small portion of the total body fluid is in the vascular compartment (the small beaker). The limited volume in the bloodstream is a disadvantage during hemorrhage because loss of seemingly small volumes of blood can represent loss of a significant fraction of the blood volume.

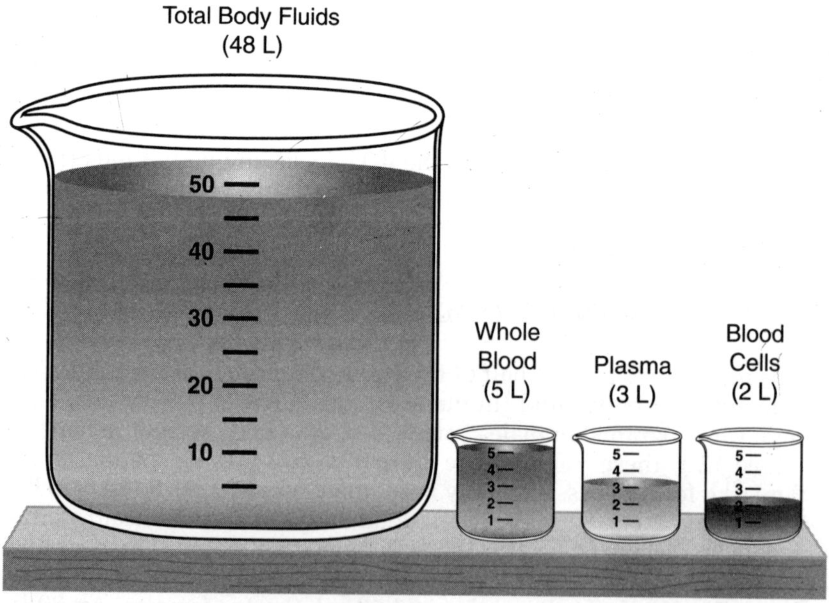

FIGURE 12.1 Scaled drawing comparing the volume of total body fluids and the volume of whole blood and its components in an adult male weighing 80 kg. The small beakers are one-tenth the size of the large beaker.

Compensatory Responses

The loss of blood triggers certain compensatory responses that help to maintain blood volume and tissue perfusion (4). The earliest response involves movement of interstitial fluid into the capillaries. This *transcapillary refill* can replenish about 15% of the blood volume, but it leaves an interstitial fluid deficit.

Acute blood loss also leads to activation of the renin–angiotensin–aldosterone system, resulting in sodium conservation by the kidneys. The retained sodium distributes uniformly in the extracellular fluid. Because interstitial fluid makes up about 2/3 of the extracellular fluid, the retained sodium helps to replenish the interstitial fluid deficit created by transcapillary refill. **The ability of sodium to replace interstitial fluid deficits, not blood volume deficits, is the reason that crystalloid fluids containing sodium chloride (saline fluids) gained early popularity as resuscitation fluids for acute blood loss** (5).

Within a few hours after the onset of hemorrhage, the bone marrow begins to increase production of red blood cells. This response develops slowly, and complete replacement of lost erythrocytes can take up to 2 months (4).

These compensatory responses can maintain an adequate blood volume in cases of mild blood loss (i.e., loss of <15% of the blood volume). When blood loss exceeds 15% of blood volume, volume replacement is usually necessary.

Progressive Blood Loss

The American College of Surgeons identifies four categories of acute blood loss based on the percent loss of blood volume (6).

Class I. Loss of 15% or less of the total blood volume. This degree of blood loss is usually fully compensated by transcapillary refill. Because blood volume is maintained, clinical findings are minimal or absent.

Class II. Loss of 15 to 30% of the blood volume. The clinical findings at this stage may include orthostatic changes in heart rate and blood pressure. However, these clinical findings are inconsistent (see later). Sympathetic vasoconstriction maintains blood pressure and perfusion of vital organs (7), but urine output can fall to 20 or 30 mL/hr, and splanchnic flow may also be compromised (8). Splanchnic hypoperfusion is a particular concern because it can lead to breakdown of the intestinal barrier and translocation of microbes and inflammatory cytokines, setting the stage for systemic inflammation and multiple organ failure (8). (See Chapters 4 and 40 for more information on this topic.)

Class III. Loss of 30 to 40% of the blood volume. This marks the onset of decompensated hypovolemic shock, where the vasoconstrictor response to hemorrhage is no longer able to sustain blood pressure and organ perfusion. The clinical consequences include hypotension and reduced urine output (usually 5 to 15 mL/hr).

Systemic vasoconstriction may be attenuated or lost at this stage (7), resulting in exaggerated hypotension.

Class IV. Loss of more than 40% of blood volume. Hypotension and oliguria are profound at this stage (urine output may be <5 mL/hr), and these changes may be irreversible.

CLINICAL EVALUATION

The clinical evaluation of the bleeding (or otherwise hypovolemic) patient is aimed at determining the magnitude of the blood volume deficit and the impact of this deficit on circulatory flow and organ viability. A variety of bedside, laboratory, and invasive techniques are available for this evaluation, and these are described briefly in this section.

Vital Signs

Resting tachycardia (>90 beats per minute) is often assumed to be a common occurrence in the hypovolemic patient, but **tachycardia in the supine position is absent in a majority of patients with moderate-to-severe blood loss** (see Table 12.2) (9). In fact, bradycardia may be more prevalent in acute blood loss (9). Hypotension (systolic blood pressure <90 mm Hg) in the supine position is also an insensitive marker of blood loss. This is shown in Table 12.2 (i.e., the sensitivity of supine hypotension is 50% or less in patients with either moderate or severe blood loss) (9). Hypotension usually appears in the advanced stages of hypovolemia, when the loss of blood exceeds 30% of the blood volume (6). The method used to measure blood pressure is an important consideration in the bleeding patient because, in low flow states, noninvasive measures of blood pressure often yield spuriously low values (see Chapter 8,

TABLE 12.2 Accuracy of Vital Signs in the Detection of Acute Blood Loss‡

Parameter	Range of Reported Sensitivities: Moderate Blood Loss (450–630 mL)	Range of Reported Sensitivities: Severe Blood Loss (630–1150 mL)
Supine tachycardia	0–42%	5–24%
Supine hypotension	0–50%	21–47%
Postural pulse increment* or postural dizziness	6–48%	91–100%
Postural hypotension†		
Age < 65 yrs	6–12%	Not known
Age ≥ 65 yrs	14–40%	Not known

*Increase in pulse rate ≥ 30 beats/min on standing.
†Decrease in systolic pressure > 20 mm Hg on standing.
‡The summed results of 9 clinical studies. From McGee S, et al. JAMA 1999; 281:1022.

Table 8.2). As a result, direct intraarterial recordings are recommended for monitoring blood pressure in the bleeding patient.

Orthostatic Vital Signs

Moving from the supine to the standing position causes a shift of 7 to 8 mL/kg of blood to the lower extremities (9). In healthy subjects, this change in body position is associated with a small increase in heart rate (about 10 beats/min) and a small decrease in systolic blood pressure (about 3 to 4 mm Hg) (9). These changes can be exaggerated in the hypovolemic patient, but this is not a consistent finding.

When recording postural changes in pulse rate and blood pressure, the patient should move from the supine to standing position (sitting instead of standing reduces the magnitude of change and the sensitivity of the test) and at least one minute should elapse in the standing position before the measurements are obtained (9). A significant postural (orthostatic) change is defined as any of the following: an increase in pulse rate of at least 30 beats/minute, a decrease in systolic pressure > 20 mm Hg, or dizziness on standing. The sensitivity of these postural changes for detecting hypovolemia is shown in Table 12.2. The only tests with a sensitivity high enough to be of any value are postural dizziness and postural increments in heart rate in severe blood loss (defined in Table 12.1 as loss of 630 to 1,150 mL of blood). The information in Table 12.1 indicates that **orthostatic vital signs have limited value in the evaluation of hypovolemia**.

The Hematocrit

The use of the hematocrit (and hemoglobin concentration in blood) to determine the extent of acute blood loss is both common and inappropriate. The following statement from the Advanced Trauma Life Support Course deserves emphasis. **"Use of the hematocrit to estimate acute blood loss is unreliable and inappropriate"** (6). Changes in hematocrit show a poor correlation with blood volume deficits and erythrocyte deficits in acute hemorrhage (10), and the reason for this discrepancy is demonstrated in Figure 12.2. Acute blood loss involves the loss of whole blood, with proportional decreases in the volume of plasma and erythrocytes. As a result, the hematocrit will not change significantly in the early period after acute blood loss. In the absence of volume resuscitation, the hematocrit will eventually decrease because hypovolemia activates the renin-angiotensin-aldosterone system, leading to renal conservation of sodium and water and expansion of the plasma volume. This process begins 8 to 12 hours after acute blood loss and can take a few days to become fully established.

Resuscitation Fluids & Hematocrit

Decreases in hematocrit in the early hours after acute hemorrhage is usually the result of volume resuscitation rather than ongoing blood loss. The influence of different resuscitation fluids on the hematocrit is demonstrated in Figure 12.2. Infusion of saline (0.9% sodium chloride)

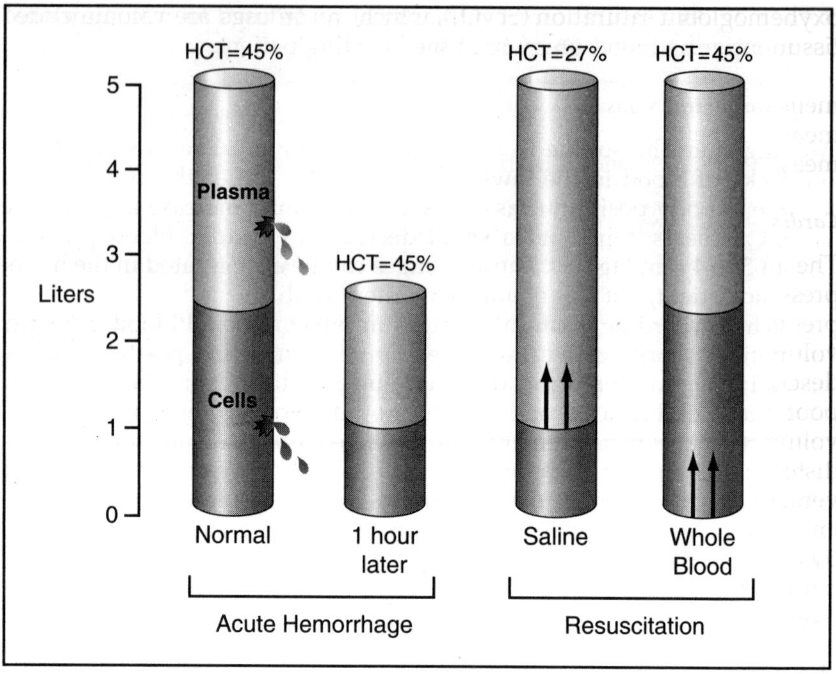

FIGURE 12.2 Influence of acute hemorrhage and type of resuscitation fluid on blood volume and hematocrit. Each vertical column shows the contribution of plasma and red blood cells to the blood volume, and the corresponding hematocrit is shown above the columns.

increases the plasma volume selectively and thereby decreases the hematocrit without affecting the volume of red blood cells. All cell-free resuscitation fluids have a similar dilutional effect on the hematocrit (11). Figure 12.2 also shows the effect of resuscitation with whole blood: in this case, the erythrocyte and plasma volumes are increased proportionately, without a change in hematocrit. Thus Figure 12.2 clearly shows that, **in the early hours after acute hemorrhage, the hematocrit is a reflection of the resuscitation effort** (the type of infusion fluid and the volume infused), **not the severity of blood loss**. The change in hematocrit produced by each type of resuscitation fluid is shown below.

Resuscitation Fluid	**Expected Change in Hematocrit**
Asanguinous fluids	Decrease
Whole blood	No change
Packed red cells	Increase

Invasive Hemodynamic Measures

Central venous catheters are inserted routinely in hypovolemic patients, and these catheters allow the measurement of pressure in the superior vena cava, which is equivalent to the filling pressure of the right side of the heart. These catheters also permit the measurement of central venous oxyhemoglobin saturation ($ScvO_2$), which can be used to evaluate global tissue oxygen balance (see Chapter 11).

Pulmonary artery catheters may be inserted to guide the management of hemodynamically unstable patients, and these catheters allow measurement of cardiac output and systemic oxygen transport. (The measurements provided by this catheter are described in Chapter 9.)

Cardiac Filling Pressures

The popular notion that cardiac filling pressures (the central venous pressure for the right heart, and the pulmonary artery occlusion [wedge] pressure for the left heart) provide an accurate representation of blood volume status is not supported by experimental studies (12–14). As described in Chapter 10 and demonstrated in Figure 10.4, there is a poor correlation between ventricular filling pressures and ventricular volumes (13). This discrepancy is caused by the influence of ventricular distensibility (compliance) on cardiac filling pressures (i.e., a decrease in ventricular distensibility will result in higher cardiac filling pressures at any given ventricular volume). In fact, hypovolemia can be accompanied by a decrease in ventricular distensibility (presumably as a result of sympathetic activation) (15), which means that **cardiac filling pressures will overestimate the intravascular volume status in hypovolemic patients**.

The cardiac filling pressures can provide *qualitative* information about the general state of intravascular volume, but only when the measurements are very high (e.g., CVP >15 mm Hg) or very low (e.g., CVP = 0–1 mm Hg). Intermediate-range measurements are not interpretable.

Oxygen Transport Parameters

Monitoring oxygen transport parameters permits identification of patients with hypovolemic shock. This is illustrated in Figure 12.3. Progressive hypovolemia causes a steady decline in systemic O_2 delivery (DO_2), but in the early stages of hypovolemia, systemic O_2 uptake (VO_2) remains unchanged. This condition (where VO_2 remains constant despite reductions in blood volume) is known as *compensated hypovolemia,* and it is characterized by an increase in O_2 extraction from capillary blood to compensate for the decrease in O_2 delivery. When O_2 extraction reaches its maximum level of about 50% (which means that 50% of the hemoglobin molecules release their oxygen in the capillaries), VO_2 begins to decrease in response to decreases in DO_2. The point where the VO_2 (O_2 consumption) begins to decline is the onset of anaerobic metabolism and *hypovolemic shock.* (The O_2 transport parameters are described in detail in Chapter 2.)

According to the relationships in Figure 12.3, compensated hypovolemia is identified by a normal VO_2 (>100 mL/min/m^2) and an O_2 extraction that is less than 50%, while hypovolemic shock is identified by an abnormally low VO_2 (<100 mL/min/m^2) and an O_2 extraction that is 50%.

Acid-Base Parameters

Two measures of acid-base balance can provide information about the adequacy of tissue oxygenation: arterial base deficit and arterial lactate concentration. Both are used as markers of impaired tissue oxygenation.

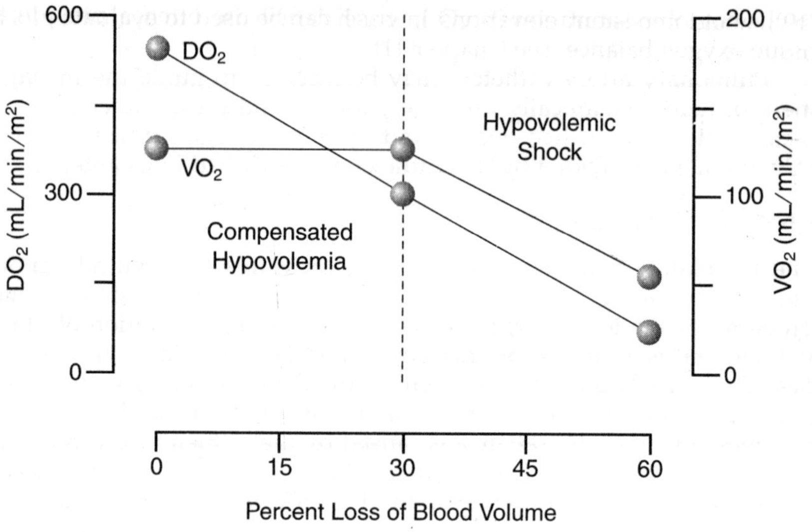

FIGURE 12.3 The effects of progressive hypovolemia on systemic oxygen delivery (DO_2) and oxygen uptake (VO_2). The point where O_2 uptake begins to decrease marks the onset of hypovolemic shock.

Arterial Base Deficit

The base deficit is the amount (in millimoles) of base needed to titrate one liter of whole blood to a pH of 7.40 (at temperature of 37°C and PCO_2 = 40 mm Hg). Because base deficit is measured when the PCO_2 is normal, it was introduced as a more specific marker of non-respiratory acid-base disturbances than serum bicarbonate (16). In the injured or bleeding patient, an elevated base deficit is a marker of global tissue acidosis from impaired oxygenation (17).

One advantage of the base deficit is its availability. Most blood gas analyzers determine the base deficit routinely using a PCO_2/HCO_3 nomogram, and the results are included in the blood gas report. The base deficit (BD) can also be calculated using the equation below (18), where BD is base deficit in mmol/L, Hb is the hemoglobin concentration in blood, and HCO_3 is the serum bicarbonate concentration.

$$\begin{aligned} BD = {} & [(1 - 0.014\ \text{Hb}) \times HCO_3] - 24 \\ & + [(9.5 + 1.63\ \text{Hb}) \times (\text{pH} - 7.4)] \end{aligned} \tag{12.1}$$

The normal range for base deficit is +2 to −2 mmol/L. Abnormal elevations in base deficit are classified as mild (−2 to −5 mmol/L), moderate (−6 to −14 mmol/L), and severe (<−15 mmol/L).

Clinical studies in trauma patients have shown a direct correlation between the magnitude of increase in base deficit at presentation and the extent of blood loss (19). Correction of the base deficit within hours after volume replacement is associated with a favorable outcome

(19), while persistent elevations in base deficit are often a prelude to multiorgan failure.

Arterial Lactate Concentration

As described in Chapter 11, the lactate concentration in blood is a marker of impaired tissue oxygenation and a prognostic factor in circulatory shock (see Figure 11.5). Whole blood or serum lactate concentrations above 2 mEq/L are considered abnormal. When compared with the base deficit, blood lactate levels show a closer correlation with both the magnitude of blood loss (20) and the risk of death from hemorrhage (20,21). The predictive value of serum lactate is not confined to the time of initial assessment but also extends to the period of volume resuscitation. Persistent elevations in serum lactate despite volume resuscitation carry a poor prognosis (20,21).

BASICS OF VOLUME RESUSCITATION

The mortality in hypovolemic shock is directly related to the magnitude and duration of organ hypoperfusion (22), which means that prompt replacement of volume deficits is the hallmark of success for managing the hypovolemic patient. The following information will help to ensure prompt volume replacement and will also help to dispel some common misconceptions about volume resuscitation.

The Trendelenburg Position

Elevation of the pelvis above the horizontal plane in the supine position was introduced in the latter part of the 19th century as a method of facilitating surgical exposure of the pelvic organs. The originator was a surgeon named Friedrich Trendelenburg, who specialized in the surgical correction of vesicovaginal fistulas (23). The body position that now bears his name was later adopted during World War I as an antishock maneuver that presumably promotes venous return by shifting blood volume from the legs toward the heart. This maneuver continues to be popular today, despite evidence that it does not perform as expected (24–27).

Hemodynamic Effects

The hemodynamic effects of the Trendelenburg position (legs elevated and head below the horizontal plane) are shown in Table 12.3. The data in this table are from a study we performed on postoperative patients with indwelling pulmonary artery catheters who had evidence of severe hypovolemia (i.e., low cardiac filling pressures and hypotension) (24). The hemodynamic measurements were obtained in the supine position and then repeated after the patients were placed in a position with the legs elevated 45 degrees above the horizontal plane and the head placed 15 degrees below the horizontal plane. As shown in the table, the change in position was associated with significant increases in the mean arterial pressure, wedge (left-ventricular filling) pressure, and systemic vascular

TABLE 12.3 Hemodynamic Effects of the Trendelenburg Position in Hypovolemic ICU Patients

Parameter	Supine	Legs Up, Head Down	Change %	Change p	Change Effect
Mean arterial blood pressure (mm Hg)	64	71	11	<.001	↑
Wedge pressure (mm Hg)	4.6	7.2	57	<.001	↑
Cardiac index (L/min · m²)	2.1	1.9	9	NS	↔
Systemic vascular resistance (dyne · sec/cm⁵ · m²)	2347	2905	24	<.001	↑

Sing R et al. Ann Emerg Med 1994;23:564.

resistance, while the cardiac output remained the same. This lack of an effect on the cardiac output indicates that the **Trendelenburg position does *not* promote venous return to the heart**. The increase in the wedge pressure can be due to an increase in intrathoracic pressure (transmitted into the pulmonary capillaries) caused by cephalad displacement of the diaphragm during the body tilt. The increase in blood pressure during body tilt is likely due to systemic vasoconstriction (indicated by the rise in systemic vascular resistance). These observations are consistent with other studies in animals and humans (25–27).

Why the Trendelenburg Position Doesn't Work

The inability of the Trendelenburg position to augment cardiac output is likely explained by the high capacitance (distensibility) of the venous circulation. To augment cardiac output, the Trendelenburg position must increase the pressure gradient from peripheral to central veins, which would then increase venous blood flow. However, the venous system is a high-capacitance system designed to absorb pressure and act as a volume reservoir. When pressure is applied to a vein, the pressure is dissipated as the vein distends and increases its volume capacity. The distensibility of veins will thereby limit any increase in pressure gradient between peripheral and central veins. The venous system is more likely to transmit pressure when the veins are volume overloaded and less distensible. In other words, the Trendelenburg position is more likely to augment venous return during volume *overload*, not volume depletion.

In summary, the Trendelenburg position has (for a sound physiologic reason) not proven effective in promoting venous return or cardiac output in hypovolemia. As such, **this maneuver should be abandoned for the management of hypovolemia**. It remains axiomatic that the effective treatment for hypovolemia is volume replacement.

Central Versus Peripheral Vein Cannulation

There is a tendency to cannulate the large central veins for volume resuscitation because larger veins permit more rapid fluid infusions. However, **the rate of volume infusion is determined by the dimensions**

of the vascular catheter, not the size of the vein. The catheters used for central venous cannulation are 15 cm (about 6 inches) to 20 cm (about 8 inches) in length, whereas catheters used to cannulate peripheral veins are only 2 inches in length. The influence of catheter length on infusion rate is defined by the Hagen-Poiseuille equation, which is described in Chapters 1 and 6 (see Figure 1.6) and is shown below.

$$Q = \Delta P(\pi r^4/8\mu L) \tag{12.2}$$

According to this equation, steady flow (Q) through a catheter is directly related to the driving pressure (ΔP) for flow and the fourth power of the radius (r) of the catheter and is inversely related to the length (L) of the catheter and the viscosity (μ) of the infusate. This equation predicts that flow through longer central venous catheters will be much slower than flow through short peripheral venous catheters of equal diameter.

The influence of catheter length on infusion rate is demonstrated in Figure 12.4 (28). The fluid in this case is water, and the driving force for flow is the height of the fluid reservoir above the catheter. Using catheters of equal diameter (16 gauge), flow in the 2-inch catheter is about 30% higher than flow in the 5.5-inch catheter and is more than twice the flow rate in the 12-inch catheter. Therefore **for rapid volume resuscitation, cannulation of peripheral veins with short catheters is preferred to cannulation of large central veins with long catheters.**

Introducer Catheters

Volume resuscitation of trauma victims sometimes requires flow rates in excess of 5 L/min (29). Because flow increases with the fourth power

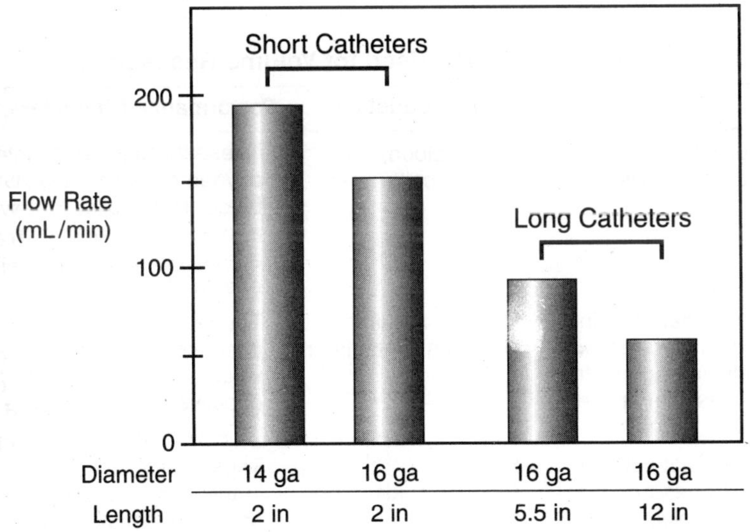

FIGURE 12.4 The influence of catheter dimensions on the gravity-driven infusion rate of water. Catheter dimensions are indicated below the horizontal axis of the graph. (From Mateer JR Thompson BM, Aprahamian C, et al. Rapid fluid resuscitation with central venous catheters. Ann Emerg Med 1983;12:149–152.)

of the radius of a catheter, very rapid flow rates are best achieved with large-bore catheters such as the *introducer catheters* described in Chapter 6 (see Figure 6.4). These catheters are 5 to 6 inches in length and are available in 8.5 French (2.7 mm outer diameter) and 9 French (3 mm outer diameter) sizes. They are normally inserted to facilitate placement and exchange of multilumen central venous catheters and pulmonary artery catheters, but they can be used as stand-alone infusion devices when rapid infusion rates are desirable.

Gravity-driven flow through introducer catheters can reach 15 mL/sec (using low viscosity, cell-free fluids), which is only slightly less than the flow through standard (3 mm diameter) intravenous tubing (18 mL/sec) (30). There is an additional side infusion port on the hub of introducer catheters (see Figure 6.4), but the flow capacity is only 25% of that in the catheter (30). Therefore when introducer catheters are used for rapid infusion, the side infusion port should be bypassed.

Flow Properties of Resuscitation Fluids

There are three types of resuscitation fluids (see Table 12.4): fluids that contain red blood cells (whole blood and erythrocyte concentrates or "packed" cells), fluids that contain large molecules with limited movement out of the bloodstream (called *colloid* fluids), and fluids that contain only electrolytes (sodium and chloride) and small molecules that move freely out of the bloodstream (called *crystalloid* fluids). The flow capabilities of these fluids are determined by their viscosity, as described in the Hagen-Poiseuille equation (Equation 12.2).

The infusion rates of the resuscitation fluids in Figure 12.5 are explained by differences in viscosity (31). The erythrocyte-containing

TABLE 12.4 Types of Fluids Used for Volume Resuscitation

Type of Fluid	Products	Performance Characteristics
1. Fluids that contain red blood cells.	Whole blood, Packed cells	These fluids increase the oxygen-carrying capacity of blood. Their ability to flow and augment cardiac output are limited by the viscosity effects of the cells.
2. Fluids that contain large molecules with restricted egress from the vascular space. Called *colloids*.	Plasma, Albumin, Dextrans, Hetastarch	These fluids preferentially increase intravascular volume, and are the most effective fluids for increasing cardiac output.
3. Fluids that contain electrolyes and other small molecules that move freely in the extracellular. space. Called *crystalloids*.	Saline, Ringer's fluids, Normosol	These fluids distribute evenly in the extracellular space, and preferentially increase interstitial fluid volume.

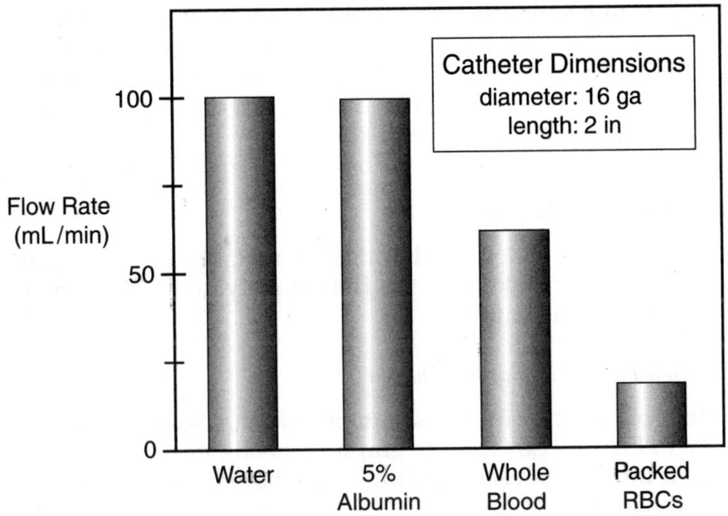

FIGURE 12.5 Comparative infusion rates of erythrocyte-containing and cell-free resuscitation fluids. Catheter size and driving pressure are the same for all fluids. (From Dula DJ, Muller A, Donovan JW, et al. Flow rate variance of commonly used IV infusion techniques. J Trauma 1981;21:480.)

fluids are the only resuscitation fluids with a viscosity greater than that of water, and the viscosity of these fluids is a function of the erythrocyte density or hematocrit (see Table 1.2 in Chapter 1). Therefore whole blood flows less rapidly than the cell-free fluids (water and 5% albumin), and densely packed erythrocytes (packed RBCs) have the slowest infusion rates. The sluggish flow of packed RBCs can be improved by increasing the driving pressure for flow with an inflatable cuff wrapped around the blood bag (which works like a blood pressure cuff). Adding saline to the infusion line (in equal volumes) will also improve infusion rates by decreasing the viscosity of the infusate.

A popular misconception is that colloid fluids, because of their large molecules, flow less rapidly than crystalloid fluids or water. However, viscosity is a function of cell density, so cell-free resuscitation fluids will have the same flow capabilities as water. This is demonstrated by the equivalent flow rates of water and 5% albumin in Figure 12.5.

RESUSCITATION STRATEGIES

The ultimate goal of volume replacement for acute blood loss is to maintain oxygen uptake (VO_2) into tissues and sustain aerobic metabolism (29). The strategies used to maintain VO_2 are identified by the determinants of VO_2 in Equation 12.3. (This equation is described in detail in Chapter 2.)

$$VO_2 = Q \times Hb \times 13.4 \times (SaO_2 - SvO_2) \qquad (12.3)$$

Acute blood loss affects two components of this equation: cardiac output (Q) and hemoglobin concentration in blood (Hb). Therefore promoting cardiac output and correcting hemoglobin deficits are the two goals of resuscitation for acute blood loss. Each of these goals involves a distinct strategy, as described next.

Promoting Cardiac Output

The consequences of a low cardiac output are far more threatening than the consequences of anemia, so **the first priority in the bleeding patient is to support cardiac output.**

Resuscitation Fluids and Cardiac Output

The ability of each type of resuscitation fluid to augment cardiac output is shown in Figure 12.6 (32). The graph in this figure shows the effects of a one-hour infusion of each fluid on the cardiac output. The infusion volume of whole blood (1 unit = 450 mL), packed cells (2 units = 500 mL), and dextran-40 (500 mL) is equivalent, while the infusion volume of lactated Ringer's (1 L) is twice that of the other fluids. The colloid fluid (dextran-40) is the most effective: on a volume-to-volume basis, the colloid fluid is about twice as effective as whole blood, six times more effective than packed cells, and eight times more effective than the crystalloid fluid (lactated Ringer's). The limited ability of blood (whole blood or

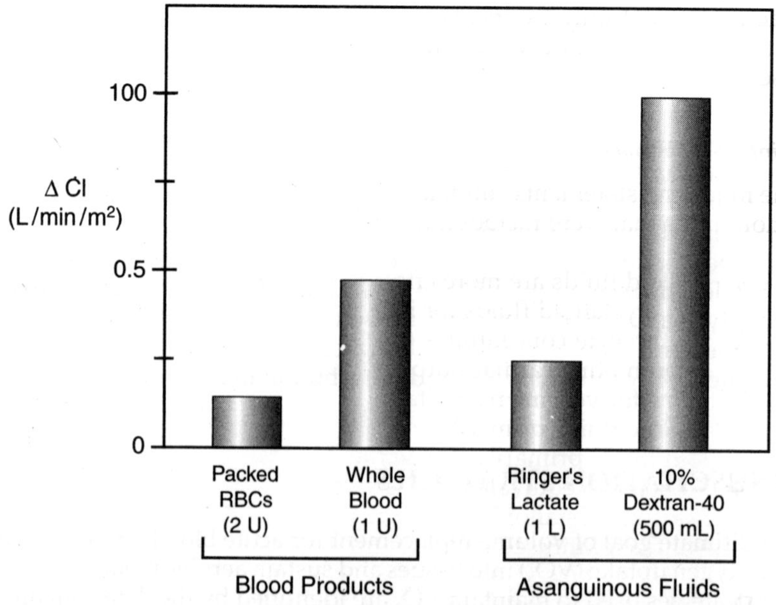

FIGURE 12.6 Effectiveness of different types of resuscitation fluids in augmenting cardiac output. (From Shoemaker WC. Relationship of oxygen transport patterns to the pathophysiology and therapy of shock states. Intensive Care Med 1987;13:230.)

packed cells) to augment cardiac output is due to the viscosity effects of erythrocytes.

If augmenting cardiac output is the first priority in the management of acute hemorrhage, then Figure 12.6 indicates that **blood is not the fluid of choice for early volume resuscitation in acute blood loss**. This is particularly the case with concentrated erythrocyte products (packed cells), which can actually *decrease* cardiac output (33).

Colloid and Crystalloid Fluids

The graph in Figure 12.6 shows a marked difference in the ability of colloid and crystalloid fluids to augment blood flow. This difference cannot be explained by viscosity, because both types of fluids are cell-free and have a viscosity equivalent to water. The difference is due to the differences in volume distribution. Crystalloid fluids are primarily sodium chloride solutions, and because sodium is distributed evenly in the extracellular fluid, crystalloid fluids will also distribute evenly in the extracellular fluid. Because plasma represents only 20% of the extracellular fluid, **only 20% of the infused volume of crystalloid fluids will remain in the vascular space and add to the plasma volume,** while the remaining 80% will add to the interstitial fluid volume. Colloid fluids, on the other hand, will add primarily to the plasma volume because the large molecules in colloid fluids do not readily escape from the vascular compartment. **As much as 75 or 80% of the infused volume of colloid fluids will remain in the vascular space and add to the plasma volume,** at least in the first few hours after infusion. The increase in plasma volume augments cardiac output not only by increasing ventricular preload (volume effect) but also by decreasing ventricular afterload (dilutional effect on blood viscosity).

Points to Remember

The following statements summarize the important points about resuscitation fluids that were included in this section (22,32,34–36).

1. Colloid fluids are more effective than whole blood, packed cells, and crystalloid fluids for increasing cardiac output.
2. Erythrocyte concentrates (packed cells) are relatively ineffective in promoting cardiac output, and thus they should never be used alone for volume resuscitation.
3. Colloid fluids primarily add to the plasma volume, while crystalloid fluids primarily add to the interstitial fluid volume.
4. To achieve equivalent effects on cardiac output, the volume of infused crystalloid fluid is at least three times greater than the volume of infused colloid fluid.

Despite the superiority of colloid fluids over crystalloid fluids for increasing plasma volume and promoting cardiac output, crystalloid fluids continue to be the more popular resuscitation fluid. This preference is due to the lack of documented survival benefit with colloid

TABLE 12.5 Estimating the Resuscitation Volume

Sequence of Determinations	Equations
1. Estimate normal blood volume (BV)	BV = 66 mL/kg (males) = 60 mL/kg (females)
2. Estimate % loss of blood volume	Class I: <15% Class II: 15–30% Class III: 30–40% Class IV: >40%
3. Calculate volume deficit (VD)	VD = BV × % loss BV
4. Determine resuscitation volume (RV)	RV = VD × 1.5 (colloids) = VD × 4 (crystalloids)

resuscitation (36). The next chapter (Chapter 13) expands further on the benefits and shortcomings of colloid and crystalloid fluids.

Estimating the Total Resuscitation Volume

The following stepwise approach is designed to obtain a rough estimate of the volume of each type of resuscitation fluid that is needed to fully restore cardiac output and organ perfusion. This approach is outlined in Table 12.5.

1. **Estimate the normal blood volume** using the weight-based estimates in Table 12.1 (60 mL/kg for females, 66 mL/kg for males). Remember to use lean body weight.
2. **Estimate the percent loss of blood volume** by assigning the patient to one of the four stages of progressive blood loss described earlier in the chapter. Then apply the following relationships: class I, <15% loss of blood volume; class II, 15–30% loss of blood volume; class III, 30–40% loss of blood volume class IV, >40% loss of blood volume.
3. **Calculate the volume deficit** using the estimated normal blood volume and the percent volume loss. (Volume deficit = normal blood volume × % volume loss)
4. **Determine the resuscitation volume for each type of fluid** by assuming that the increase in blood volume is 100% of the infused volume of whole blood, 50 to 75% of the infused volume of colloid fluids, and 20 to 25% of the infused volume of crystalloid fluids (34). The resuscitation volume for each type of fluid is then determined as the volume deficit divided by the percent retention of the infused fluid. For example, if the volume deficit is 2 L and the resuscitation fluid is a colloid, which is 50 to 75% retained in the vascular space, then the resuscitation volume is 2/0.75 = 3 L to 2/0.5 = 4 L.

Once the total replacement volume is determined, the rapidity of volume replacement can be determined using the clinical condition of the patient.

End-Points of Resuscitation

The goal of resuscitation in hemorrhagic shock is to restore three parameters: blood flow, oxygen transport, and tissue oxygenation. The parameters are defined by the end-points shown below.

1. Cardiac index = 3 L/min/m^2
2. Systemic oxygen delivery (DO_2) > 500 mL/min/m^2
3. Systemic oxygen uptake (VO_2) > 100 mL/min/m^2
4. Arterial lactate < 2 mmol/L or base deficit > −2 mmol/L

Unfortunately, it is not always possible to reach these end-points despite aggressive volume replacement, and the ability to reach the desired end points is a principal determinant of survival (1,20,21,32,37–39). This is demonstrated in Figure 12.7. The graph in this figure shows the effects of controlled hemorrhage and resuscitation on oxygen uptake (VO_2) in an animal model of hemorrhagic shock (20). Note that in the survivors, the VO_2 increases and returns to the baseline (pre-hemorrhage) level in response to resuscitation. In contrast, the VO_2 in the nonsurvivors shows no response to resuscitation and actually deteriorates further. Thus when hemorrhagic shock becomes refractory to volume resuscitation, the prognosis is bleak.

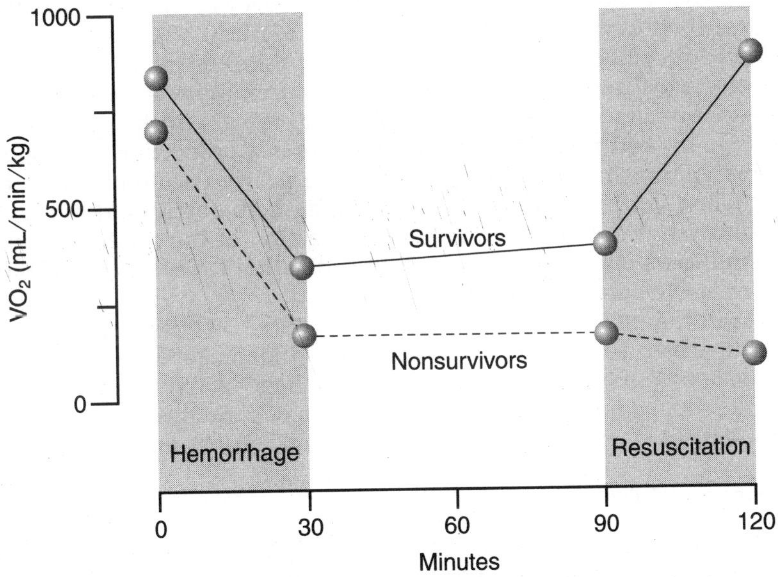

FIGURE 12.7 The effects of controlled hemorrhage and subsequent volume resuscitation on systemic oxygen uptake (VO_2) in an animal model of hemorrhagic shock. (From Moomey CB Jr, Melton SM, Croce MA, et al. Prognostic value of blood lactate, base deficit, and oxygen-derived variables in an LD_{50} model of penetrating trauma. Crit Care Med 1999;27:154.)

The time required to reach the desired end-points is another determinant of survival in hemorrhagic shock. One of the most predictive parameters in this regard is lactate clearance. In one study of trauma victims (39), there were no deaths when arterial lactate levels returned to normal within 24 hours, but when lactate levels remained elevated after 48 hours, 86% of the patients died. Rapid restoration of tissue perfusion is one of the most important goals in hemorrhagic shock because continued tissue hypoperfusion creates a time-dependent *oxygen debt*, and the greater the oxygen debt, the greater the risk of multiorgan failure and a fatal outcome.

Correcting Anemia

After volume deficits are replaced and cardiac output is restored, attention can be directed to correcting deficits in the oxygen carrying capacity of blood. The use of erythrocyte transfusions to correct normovolemic anemia is discussed in detail in Chapter 36. The presentation here will be limited to the most appropriate indication for blood transfusion (transfusion trigger) in normovolemic anemia.

Hematocrit: A Lousy Transfusion Trigger

There is no rational basis for the use of hematocrit (or hemoglobin concentration) as an indicator for blood transfusion because the hematocrit is not an accurate representation of the total erythrocyte volume in blood, and it provides no information about the adequacy of tissue oxygenation. As described earlier (and demonstrated in Figure 12.2), the hematocrit and erythrocyte volume will change in opposite directions when there is a selective change in plasma volume (e.g., from diuresis or infusion of asanguinous fluids), and the hematocrit will remain unchanged despite a change in erythrocyte volume when there is a proportional change in plasma volume and erythrocyte volume (e.g., from acute blood loss or transfusion with whole blood). **Because the hematocrit (and hemoglobin concentration) is not an accurate reflection of the erythrocyte volume in blood, it cannot be used as an indication for blood transfusion to increase the erythrocyte volume.**

Abandoning the hemoglobin and hematocrit as transfusion triggers was suggested over a decade ago, when guidelines on red blood cell transfusions published by the American College of Physicians included the following statement (40): "In the absence of patient risks, transfusion is not indicated, *independent of hemoglobin level*" (italics mine).

O_2 Extraction: A Better Transfusion Trigger

The ultimate goal of correcting anemia is to improve tissue oxygenation, so a measure of tissue oxygen balance could be used to determine the need for correcting anemia with erythrocyte transfusions. The oxygen extraction from systemic capillaries could be such a measure. As described earlier in the chapter, an increase in systemic O_2 extraction to 50% represents the maximum compensation for a decrease in O_2 delivery. Thus in the setting of anemia (which results in a decrease in systemic O_2

delivery), an O_2 extraction of 50% can be used as an indirect marker of tissue dysoxia or impending dysoxia (dysoxia is defined in Chapter 2 as a state of oxygen-limited metabolic energy production). Because the ultimate goal of erythrocyte transfusions is to correct or prevent tissue dysoxia, **an O_2 extraction of 50% can be used as an indication for transfusion of erythrocytes** (i.e., a transfusion trigger). This approach has been used in patients with coronary artery disease (41).

An approximate measure of systemic O_2 extraction can be obtained by measuring the oxyhemoglobin saturation in both arterial blood (SaO_2) and central venous blood ($ScvO_2$).

$$O_2 \text{ Extraction } (\%) = SaO_2 - ScvO_2$$

The SaO_2 can be monitored continuously with a pulse oximeter, and the $ScvO_2$ is measured in a blood sample taken from an indwelling central venous catheter.

Refractory Shock

Prolonged periods of hemorrhagic shock can produce an irreversible condition with severe hypotension that is refractory to volume expansion and pressor agents. Vasopressin has shown some promise in this condition, as described next.

Vasopressin

Some cases of hemorrhagic hypotension that are unresponsive to conventional vasopressor therapy have shown a favorable response to vasopressin infusion at a rate of 1 to 4 mU/kg/min (42). The mechanism for this vasopressin effect is not clear. Circulating levels of vasopressin are reduced in the late stages of hemorrhagic shock (42), and it is possible that vasopressin deficiency plays a role in the refractory hypotension that accompanies severe or prolonged hemorrhagic shock. Vasopressin infusions can also raise blood pressure and reduce vasopressor requirements in patients with severe septic shock (43).

A FINAL WORD

The nonsurgical approach to hemorrhage and hypovolemia has not changed significantly in the past 20 years, which is unfortunate. The following are some of the persistent problems and practices that need to change.

1. The evaluation of intravascular volume is so flawed it has been called a "comedy of errors" (44).
2. The hemoglobin and hematocrit continue to be used inappropriately as transfusion triggers.
3. The Trendelenburg position continues to be as popular as it is ineffective.
4. There is still no satisfactory end-point for the resuscitation effort.

REFERENCES

Clinical Practice Guidelines

1. Tisherman SA, Barie P, Bokhari F, et al. Clinical practice guideline: endpoints of resuscitation. Winston-Salem, NC: Eastern Association for Surgery of Trauma, 2003. Available at www.east.org/tpg/endpoints.pdf (accessed 10/1/05)
2. Martel M-J, the Clinical Practice Obstetrics Committee. Hemorrhagic shock. J Obstet Gynaecol Can 2002;24:504–511. Also available at www.sogc.org (accessed 10/1/05)

Body Fluids and Blood Loss

3. Walker RH, ed. Technical manual of the American Association of Blood Banks, 10th ed. Arlington, VA: American Association of Blood Banks, 1990:650.
4. Moore FD. Effects of hemorrhage on body composition. N Engl J Med 1965; 273:567–577.
5. Shires GT, Coln D, Carrico J, et al. Fluid therapy in hemorrhagic shock. Arch Surg 1964;88:688–693.
6. Committee on Trauma. Advanced trauma life support student manual. Chicago: American College of Surgeons, 1989:47–59.
7. Schadt JC, Ludbrook J. Hemodynamic and neurohumoral responses to acute hypovolemia in conscious animals. Am J Physiol 1991;260:H305–H318.
8. Fiddian-Green RG. Studies in splanchnic ischemia and multiple organ failure. In: Marston A, Bulkley GB, Fiddian-Green RG, et al., eds. Splanchnic ischemia and multiple organ failure. St. Louis: CV Mosby, 1989:349–364.

Clinical Evaluation

9. McGee S, Abernathy WB, Simel DL. Is this patient hypovolemic? JAMA 1999; 281:1022–1029.
10. Cordts PR, LaMorte WW, Fisher JB, et al. Poor predictive value of hematocrit and hemodynamic parameters for erythrocyte deficits after extensive vascular operations. Surg Gynecol Obstet 1992;175:243–248.
11. Stamler KD. Effect of crystalloid infusion on hematocrit in nonbleeding patients, with applications to clinical traumatology. Ann Emerg Med 1989;18: 747–749.
12. Shippy CR, Appel PL, Shoemaker WC. Reliability of clinical monitoring to assess blood volume in critically ill patients. Crit Care Med 1984;12:107–112.
13. Kumar A, Anel R, Bunnell E, et al. Pulmonary artery occlusion pressure and central venous pressure fail to predict ventricular filling volumes, cardiac performance, or the response to volume infusion in normal subjects. Crit Care Med 2004;32:691–699.
14. Michard F, Teboud J-L. Predicting fluid responsiveness in ICU patients. Chest 2002;121:2000–2008.
15. Walley KR, Cooper DJ. Diastolic stiffness impairs left ventricular function during hypovolemic shock in pigs. Am J Physiol 1991;260:H702–H712.
16. Severinghaus JW. Case for standard-base excess as the measure of nonrespiratory acid-base imbalance. J Clin Monit 1991;7:276–277.

17. Kincaid EH, Miller PR, Meredith JW, et al. Elevated arterial base deficit in trauma patients: a marker of impaired oxygen utilization. J Am Coll Surg 1998;187:384–392.
18. Landow L. Letter to the editor. J Trauma 1994;37:870–871.
19. Davis JW, Shackford SR, Mackersie RC, et al. Base deficit as a guide to volume resuscitation. J Trauma 1998;28:1464–1467.
20. Moomey CB Jr, Melton SM, Croce MA, et al. Prognostic value of blood lactate, base deficit, and oxygen-derived variables in an LD_{50} model of penetrating trauma. Crit Care Med 1999;27:154–161.
21. Husain FA, Martin MJ, Mullenix PS, et al. Serum lactate and base deficit as predictors of mortality and morbidity. Am J Surg 2003;185:485–491.

Basics of Volume Resuscitation

22. Falk JL, O'Brien JF, Kerr R. Fluid resuscitation in traumatic hemorrhagic shock. Crit Care Clin 1992;8:323–340.
23. Trendelenburg F. The elevated pelvic position for operations within the abdominal cavity. Med Classics 1940;4:964–968. [Translation of original manuscript.]
24. Sing R, O'Hara D, Sawyer MJ, et al. Trendelenburg position and oxygen transport in hypovolemic adults. Ann Emerg Med 1994;23:564–568.
25. Taylor J, Weil MH. Failure of Trendelenburg position to improve circulation during clinical shock. Surg Gynecol Obstet 1967;122:1005–1010.
26. Bivins HG, Knopp R, dos Santos PAL. Blood volume distribution in the Trendelenburg position. Ann Emerg Med 1985;14:641–643.
27. Gaffney FA, Bastian BC, Thal ER, et al. Passive leg raising does not produce a significant auto transfusion effect. J Trauma 1982;22:190–193.
28. Mateer JR, Thompson BM, Aprahamian C, et al. Rapid fluid resuscitation with central venous catheters. Ann Emerg Med 1983;12:149–152.
29. Buchman TG, Menker JB, Lipsett PA. Strategies for trauma resuscitation. Surg Gynecol Obstet 1991;172:8–12.
30. Hyman SA, Smith DW, England R, et al. Pulmonary artery catheter introducers: do the component parts affect flow rate? Anesth Analg 1991;73: 573–575.
31. Dula DJ, Muller A, Donovan JW. Flow rate of commonly used IV techniques. J Trauma 1981;21:480–482.

Resuscitation Strategies

32. Shoemaker WC. Relationship of oxygen transport patterns to the pathophysiology and therapy of shock states. Intensive Care Med 1987;213:230–243.
33. Marik PE, Sibbald WJ. Effect of stored-blood transfusion on oxygen delivery in patients with sepsis. JAMA 1993;269:3024–3029.
34. Imm A, Carlson RW. Fluid resuscitation in circulatory shock. Crit Care Clin 1993;9:313–333.
35. Domsky MF, Wilson RF. Hemodynamic resuscitation. Crit Care Clin 1993;9: 715–726.
36. Whinney RR, Cohn SM, Zacur SJ. Fluid resuscitation for trauma patients in the 21st century. Curr Opin Crit Care 2000;6:395–400.

37. Velmahos GC, Demetriades D, Shoemaker WC, et al. Endpoints of resuscitation of critically injured patients: normal or supranormal? Ann Surg 2000; 232:409–418.
38. Shoemaker WC, Fleming AW. Resuscitation of the trauma patient: restoration of hemodynamic functions using clinical algorithms. Ann Emerg Med 1986; 12:1437–1444.
39. Abramson D, Scalea TM, Hitchcock R, et al. Lactate clearance and survival following injury. J Trauma 1993;35:584–589.
40. American College of Physicians. Practice strategies for elective red blood cell transfusion. Ann Intern Med 1992;116:403–406.
41. Levy PS, Chavez RP, Crystal GJ, et al. Oxygen extraction ratio: a valid indicator of transfusion need in limited coronary vascular reserve. J Trauma 1992; 32:769–774.
42. Morales D, Madigan J, Cullinane S, et al. Reversal by vasopressin of intractable hypotension in the late phase of hemorrhagic shock. Circulation 1999; 100:226–229.
43. Patel B, Chittock DR, Russell JA, et al. Beneficial effects of short-term vasopressin infusion during severe septic shock. Anesthesiology 2002;96:576–582.
44. Marik PE. Assessment of intravascular volume: a comedy of errors. Crit Care Med 2001;29:1635.

Chapter 13

COLLOID AND CRYSTALLOID RESUSCITATION

In 1861, Thomas Graham's investigations on diffusion led him to classify substances as crystalloids or colloids based on their ability to diffuse through a parchment membrane. Crystalloids passed readily through the membrane, whereas colloids (from the Greek word for glue) did not. Intravenous fluids are similarly classified based on their ability to pass from intravascular to extravascular (interstitial) fluid compartments (see Figure 13.1). This chapter describes the comparative features of crystalloid and colloid fluids, both individually and as a group. These fluids are used every day in the care of hospitalized patients, so you must become familiar with the material in this chapter.

CRYSTALLOID FLUIDS

Crystalloid fluids are electrolyte solutions with small molecules that can diffuse freely throughout the extracellular space. The principal component of crystalloid fluids is the inorganic salt sodium chloride (NaCl). Sodium is the most abundant solute in the extracellular fluid, where it is distributed uniformly. Because 75 to 80% of the extracellular fluid is located in the interstitial space, a similar proportion of the total body sodium is in the interstitial fluids. Intravenously administered sodium follows the same distribution, so 75 to 80% of the volume of infused sodium chloride (saline) solutions will be distributed in the interstitial space. This means that **the predominant effect of volume resuscitation with crystalloid fluids is to expand the interstitial volume rather than the plasma volume**.

Volume Effects

The effects of crystalloid fluid resuscitation on plasma volume and interstitial fluid volume are shown in Figure 13.2. Infusion of one liter of 0.9% sodium chloride (isotonic saline) adds 275 mL to the plasma volume

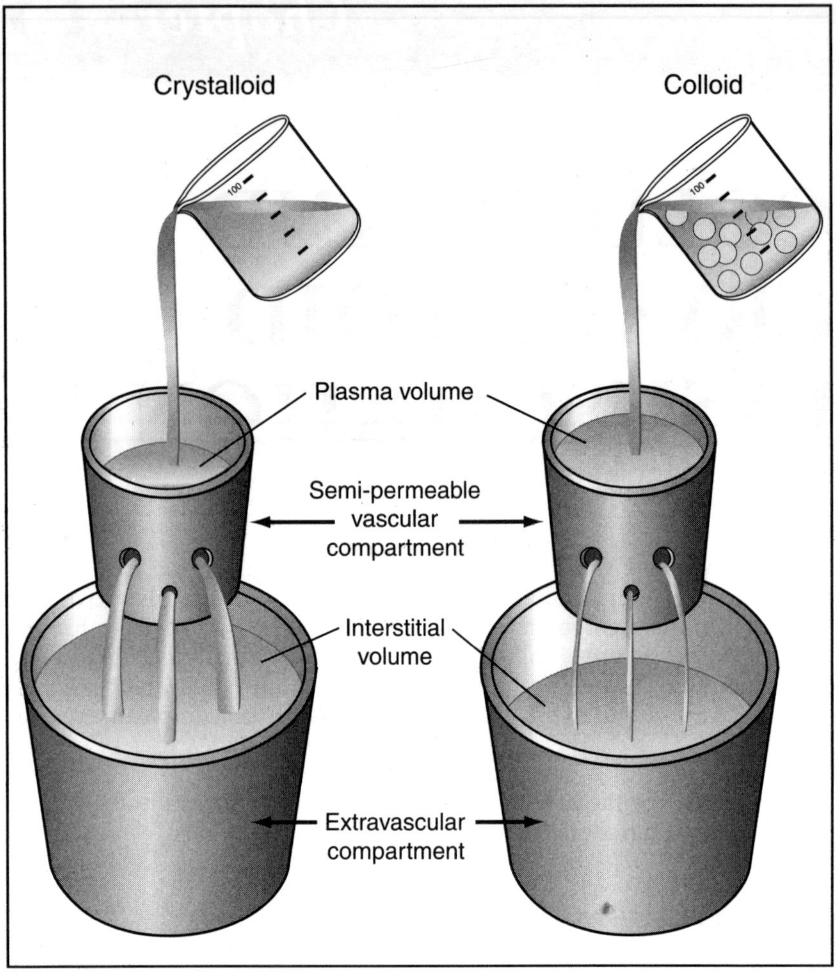

FIGURE 13.1 Illustration depicting the different tendencies of colloid and crystalloid fluids to flow out of the vascular space and into the interstitial space. The large spheres in the colloid fluid represent large molecules that do not pass readily through the semi-permeable barrier that separates the vascular and interstitial spaces. Note that the colloid fluid has a smaller stream flowing out of the vascular space.

and 825 mL to the interstitial volume (1). Note that the total volume expansion (1,100 mL) is slightly greater than the infused volume. This is the result of a fluid shift from intracellular to extracellular space, which occurs because 0.9% sodium chloride is slightly hypertonic to extracellular fluid. The comparative features of 0.9% sodium chloride and extracellular fluid (plasma) are shown in Table 13.1.

Isotonic Saline

The prototype crystalloid fluid is 0.9% sodium chloride (NaCl), also called isotonic saline or normal saline. The latter term is inappropriate

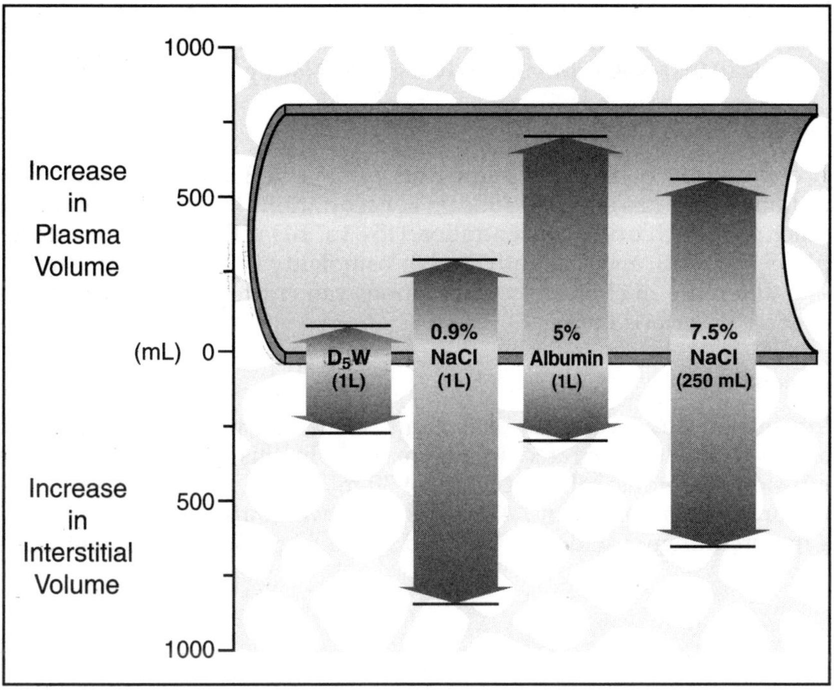

FIGURE 13.2 The effects of selected colloid and crystalloid fluids on the plasma volume and interstitial fluid volume. The volume of each fluid infused is shown in parentheses. (From Imm A, Carlson RW. Fluid resuscitation in circulatory shock. Crit Care Clin 1993;9:313.)

TABLE 13.1 Comparison of Plasma and Crystalloid Infusion Fluids

	mEq/L							
Fluid	**Na**	**Cl**	**K**	**Ca**	**Mg**	**Buffers**	**pH**	**Osmolality (mOsm/L)**
Plasma	140	103	4	5	2	Bicarb (25)	7.4	290
0.9% NaCl	154	154	—	—	—	—	5.7	308
7.5% NaCl[a]	1,283	1,283	—	—	—	—	5.7	2,567
Lactated Ringer's	130	109	4	3	—	Lactate (28)	6.4	273
Normosol Plasma-Lyte Isolyte[b]	140	98	5	—	3	Acetate (27) Gluconate (23)	7.4	295

[a]From Stapczynski JS et. al. Emerg Med Rep 1994:15:245.
[b]Isolyte also contains phosphate (1 mEq/L).

because a one-normal (1 N) NaCl solution contains 58 grams NaCl per liter (the combined molecular weights of sodium and chloride), whereas isotonic (0.9%) NaCl contains only 9 grams NaCl per liter.

Features

A comparison of isotonic saline and plasma in Table 13.1 shows that isotonic saline has a higher sodium concentration (154 vs. 140 mEq/L), a much higher chloride concentration (154 vs. 103 mEq/L), a much lower pH (5.7 vs. 7.4), and a slightly higher osmolality (308 vs. 290 mOsm/L). The difference in chloride concentrations can create an acid-base imbalance, as described next.

Disadvantages

Infusion of large volumes of isotonic saline can produce a **metabolic acidosis,** as demonstrated in Figure 13.3. In this case, intraoperative infusion of isotonic saline at a rate of 30 mL/kg/h was accompanied by a drop in serum pH from 7.41 to 7.28 after two hours (2). This acidosis is a **hyperchloremic acidosis** produced by the high chloride concentration

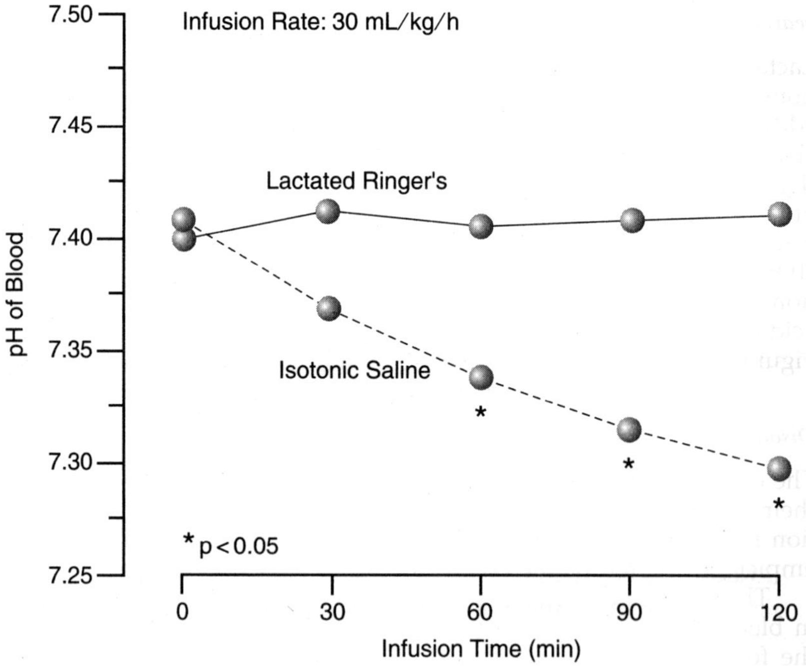

FIGURE 13.3 The effects of large-volume resuscitation with isotonic saline and lactated Ringer's solution on the pH of blood in patients undergoing elective surgery. Total volume infused after 2 hours was 5 to 6 liters for each fluid. (From Scheingraber S, Rehm M, Schmisch C, et al. Rapid saline infusion produces hyperchloremic acidosis in patients undergoing gynecologic surgery. Anesthesiology 1999;90:1265.)

in isotonic saline. Saline-induced acidosis occurs only after large volumes of isotonic saline are infused (e.g., during prolonged surgery), and it is usually has no adverse consequences (3). The major concern is differentiating this type of acidosis from lactic acidosis because the latter condition can be a marker of tissue ischemia (see Chapter 29 for the diagnostic approach to lactic acidosis).

Lactated Ringer's Solution

Sydney Ringer, a British physician who studied mechanisms of cardiac contraction, introduced a solution in 1880 that consisted of calcium and potassium in a sodium chloride diluent and was intended to promote the contraction of isolated frog hearts (4). This (Ringer's) solution slowly gained in popularity as an intravenous fluid, and, in the 1930s, an American pediatrician named Alexis Hartmann proposed the addition of sodium lactate to the solution to provide a buffer for the treatment of metabolic acidoses. This *lactated Ringer's solution*, also known as Hartmann's solution, eventually replaced the standard Ringer's solution for routine intravenous therapy. The composition of lactated Ringer's solution is shown in Table 13.1.

Features

Lactated Ringer's solution contains potassium and calcium in concentrations that approximate the free (ionized) concentrations in plasma. The addition of these cations requires a reduction in sodium concentration for electrical neutrality, so lactated Ringer's has a lower sodium concentration than either isotonic saline or plasma (see Table 13.1). The addition of lactate (28 mEq/L) similarly requires a reduction in chloride concentration, and the resultant chloride concentration in lactated Ringer's (109 mEq/L) is a close approximation of the plasma chloride concentration (103 mEq/L). This eliminates the risk of hyperchloremic metabolic acidosis with large-volume infusions of lactated Ringer's solution (see Figure 13.3).

Disadvantages

The calcium in Ringer's solutions can bind to certain drugs and reduce their effectiveness. Drugs that should not be infused with Ringer's solution for this reason include aminocaproic acid (Amicar), amphotericin, ampicillin, and thiopental (4).

The calcium in Ringer's can also bind to the citrated anticoagulant in blood products. This can inactivate the anticoagulant and promote the formation of clots in donor blood. For this reason, the American Association of Blood Banks has stated that **lactated Ringer's solution is contraindicated as a diluent for red blood cell transfusions** (5). However, clot formation in erythrocyte concentrates (packed RBCs) does not occur if the volume of Ringer's lactate does not exceed 50% of the volume of packed RBCs (6).

Serum Lactate Levels

The high concentration of lactate in lactated Ringer's solution (28 mEq/L) creates concern about the risk of spurious hyperlactatemia with large-volume infusions of the fluid. In healthy subjects, infusion of one liter of lactated Ringer's over one hour does not raise serum lactate levels (7). In critically ill patients, who may have impaired lactate clearance from circulatory shock or hepatic insufficiency, the effect of lactated Ringer's infusions on serum lactate levels is not known. However, if lactate clearance is zero, the addition of one liter of lactated Ringer's to a blood volume of 5 liters (which would require infusion of about 4 liters of fluid) would raise the serum lactate level by 4.6 mmol/L (7). Therefore **because only 25% of crystalloid fluids remain in the vascular compartment, lactated Ringer's infusions are not expected to have a considerable impact on serum lactate levels,** even in patients with impaired lactate clearance.

Blood samples obtained from intravenous catheters that are being used for lactated Ringer's infusions can yield spuriously high serum lactate determinations (8). Therefore in patients receiving lactated Ringer's infusions, blood samples for lactate measurements should be obtained from sites other than the infusion site.

Fluids with a Normal pH

Three crystalloid fluids contain both acetate and gluconate buffers to achieve a pH of 7.4 (see Table 13.1): Normosol (Abbott Labs), Isolyte (B. Braun Medical), and Plasma-Lyte (Baxter Healthcare). All three fluids contain potassium (5 mEq/L) and magnesium (3 mEq/L), while Isolyte also contains phosphate (1 mEq/L). These fluids are not commonly used as resuscitation fluids, but they may be preferred to saline for washing or diluting red blood cell preparations (9).

DEXTROSE SOLUTIONS

In the days before the introduction of enteral and parenteral nutrition, dextrose was added to intravenous fluids to provide calories. One gram of dextrose provides 3.4 kilocalories (kcal) when fully metabolized, so a 5% dextrose solution (50 grams dextrose per liter) provides 170 kcal per liter. Daily infusion of 3 liters of a 5% dextrose (D_5) solution will then provide about 500 kcal per day, which is enough nonprotein calories to limit the breakdown of endogenous proteins to meet daily caloric requirements. This *protein-sparing effect* is responsible for the early popularity of D_5 infusion fluids. However, with the advent of effective enteral and parenteral nutrition regimens, the popularity of D_5 infusion fluids is no longer justified.

Adverse Effects

Routine or aggressive use of dextrose-containing fluids can be harmful in a number of ways, as explained next.

Dextrose and Osmolality

The addition of dextrose to intravenous fluids increases osmolarity (50 g of dextrose adds 278 mOsm to an intravenous fluid). For a 5% dextrose-in-water solution (D_5W), the added dextrose brings the osmolality close to that of plasma. When dextrose is added to isotonic saline (D_5 normal saline), the infusion fluid becomes hypertonic to plasma (560 mOsm/L), and, if glucose utilization is impaired (as is common in critically ill patients), the hypertonic infusion creates an undesirable osmotic force that can promote cell dehydration.

5% Dextrose in Water (D_5W)

As shown in Figure 13.2, 5% dextrose in water (D_5W) is a relatively ineffective fluid for expanding the plasma volume. Less than 10% of the infused volume of D_5W remains in the vascular compartment. The total increase in extracellular fluid volume (plasma plus interstitial fluid) is much less than the infused volume of D_5W because 2/3 of the infused volume ends up inside cells. Therefore **the predominant effect of D_5W infusions is cellular swelling**.

Enhanced Lactate Production

In healthy subjects, only 5% of an infused glucose load will result in lactate formation, but in critically ill patients with tissue hypoperfusion, as much as 85% of glucose metabolism is diverted to lactate production (10). This latter effect is demonstrated in Figure 13.4. In this case, tissue hypoperfusion was induced by aortic clamping during abdominal aortic aneurysm surgery (11). Patients received intraoperative fluids to maintain normal cardiac filling pressures using either a Ringer's solution or a 5% dextrose solution. When the dextrose-containing fluid was infused, the serum lactate levels began to rise after the aorta was cross-clamped, and the increase in circulating lactate levels persisted throughout the remainder of the surgery. These results indicate that, **when circulatory flow is compromised, infusion of 5% dextrose solutions can result in metabolic acid production instead of metabolic energy production**.

Adverse Effects of Hyperglycemia

Hyperglycemia has several deleterious effects in critically ill patients, including immune suppression (12), increased risk of infection (13), aggravation of ischemic brain injury (14), and an increased mortality (13,15). The association between hyperglycemia and increased mortality is supported by studies showing that aggressive use of insulin to prevent hyperglycemia is associated with improved survival in ICU patients (13). The mechanism for the mortality-lowering effect of tight glycemic control is unclear at present.

About 20% of patients admitted to ICUs are diabetic (12), and as many as 90% of patients will develop hyperglycemia at some time during their ICU stay (13). Considering the high risk of hyperglycemia in ICU patients, and the numerous adverse consequences of hyperglycemia, infusion of dextrose-containing fluids should be avoided whenever

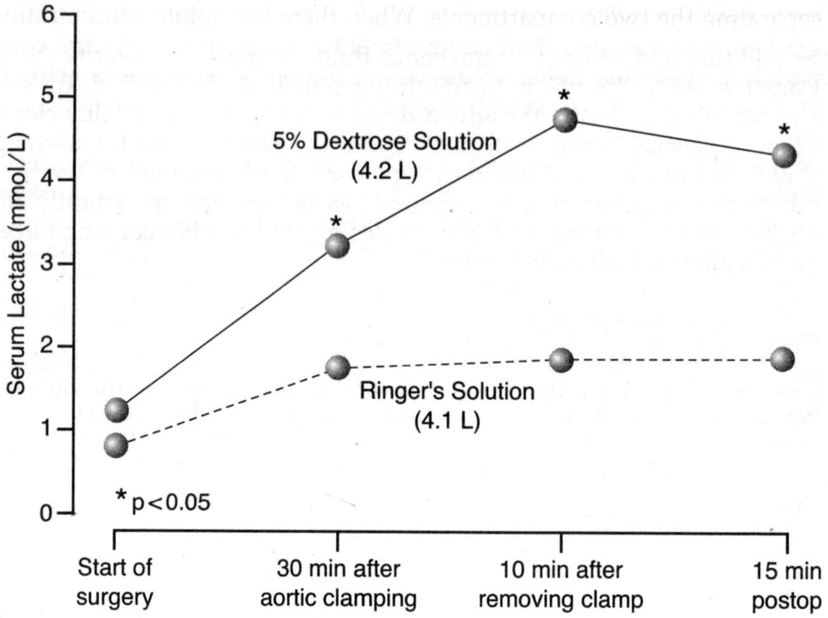

FIGURE 13.4 The effect of intravenous fluid therapy with and without dextrose on blood lactate levels in patients undergoing abdominal aortic aneurysm repair. Each point represents the mean lactate level in 10 study patients. The average infusion volume for each fluid is indicated in parentheses. (From Degoute CS, Ray MJ, Manchon M, et al. Intraoperative glucose infusion and blood lactate: endocrine metabolic relationships during abdominal aortic surgery. Anesthesiology 1989;17:355.)

possible. In fact, considering the overall potential for harm with dextrose infusions, it seems that **the routine use of 5% dextrose solutions should be abandoned in critically ill patients.**

COLLOID FLUIDS

Colloid fluids are more effective than crystalloid fluids for expanding the plasma volume because they contain large, poorly diffusible, solute molecules that create an osmotic pressure to keep water in the vascular space. A description of osmotic pressure and its influence on capillary fluid exchange is included next for those who need a brief review of the topic. This information will help to understand the behavior of colloid fluids.

Colloid Osmotic Pressure

The movement of water from one fluid compartment to another requires a difference in the concentration of solutes in the two compartments, and this requires a solute that does not diffuse readily through the barrier separating the two compartments. When there is a solute concentration gradient between two fluid compartments, water moves into the compartment with the higher solute concentration. (The water is actually moving down its own concentration gradient because the compartment with the higher solute concentration also has the lower concentration of free water). The movement of water into the compartment with the higher solute concentration creates an increase in pressure in the compartment, and this pressure increment is equivalent to the *osmotic pressure* in the compartment. Therefore osmotic pressure can be defined as the driving force for the movement of water into a fluid compartment.

Osmotic Pressure of Plasma

Plasma contains large proteins that do not diffuse readily across capillary walls, and these proteins (mostly albumin) create an osmotic pressure called the *colloid osmotic pressure* or oncotic pressure. In healthy subjects, **the colloid osmotic pressure of plasma is 25 mm Hg in the upright position and 20 mm Hg in the supine position**. The positional change in oncotic pressure is explained by changes in plasma volume. A change in body position from supine to standing can result in a 5 to 25% decrease in plasma volume (16) (presumably as a result of fluid losses from capillary blood in the lower extremities in response to gravitational increases in capillary hydrostatic pressure), and this can raise oncotic pressure by increasing plasma protein concentrations (hemoconcentration effect).

Capillary Fluid Exchange

The direction and rate of fluid exchange (Q) between capillary blood and interstitial fluid is determined, in part, by the balance between the hydrostatic pressure in the capillaries (P_c), which promotes the movement of fluid out of capillaries, and the colloid osmotic pressure of plasma (P_{osm}), which promotes the movement of fluid into capillaries.

$$Q \sim (P_c - P_{osm}) \qquad (13.1)$$

The direction of fluid flow is determined by which of the two pressures is highest. If P_c is greater than P_{osm}, fluid will flow from capillaries into the interstitial fluid, and if P_{osm} is greater than P_c, fluid will move from the interstitial fluid into the capillaries (in this condition, Q has a negative value). The rate of fluid flow is then determined by the magnitude of the difference between the two pressures. These relationships were identified over a century ago by the prolific British physiologist Ernest Starling, and the pressures P_c and P_{osm} are often referred to as the *Starling forces*. These forces will be used to explain the behavior of colloid fluids as plasma volume expanders.

Volume Effects

The effect of volume resuscitation with a colloid fluid is demonstrated in Figure 13.2. The colloid fluid in this case is a 5% albumin solution. Infusion of one liter of this solution results in a 700 mL increment in the

TABLE 13.2 Comparative Features of Colloid Fluids

Fluid	Average Molecular Wt (kilodaltons)	Oncotic Pressure (mm Hg)	ΔPlasma Volume / Infusate Volume	Duration of Effect
25% Albumin	69	70	4.0–5.0	16 hr
10% Dextran-40	26	40	1.0–1.5	6 hr
6% Hetastarch	450	30	1.0–1.3	10 hr
5% Albumin	69	20	0.7–1.3	16 hr

Data from References 17–20 and 28.

plasma volume and a 300 mL increment in the interstitial fluid volume. Thus 70% of the infused volume of this colloid fluid remains in the vascular space and adds to the plasma volume. Figure 13.2 also shows that infusion of an equivalent volume (one liter) of a crystalloid fluid (0.9% sodium chloride) results in a 250 mL increase in plasma volume and a 750 mL increase in interstitial fluid volume. Comparing the effects of the colloid and crystalloid fluid on the increment in plasma volume indicates that **colloid fluids are about three times more effective than crystalloid fluids for increasing plasma volume** (17–20).

Colloid Comparisons

Individual colloid fluids differ in their ability to augment the plasma volume, and this difference is a function of the colloid osmotic pressure of each fluid. This is demonstrated in Table 13.2. This table includes the commonly used colloid fluids in this country and shows the colloid osmotic pressure of each fluid (in mm Hg) and the increment in plasma volume produced by a given volume of each fluid. Note that fluids with higher colloid osmotic pressures produce greater increments in plasma volume. Note also that if a fluid has a colloid osmotic pressure greater than that of plasma (greater than 25 mm Hg), the increment in plasma volume can exceed the infusion volume of the fluid. This is most apparent with 25% albumin, which has a colloid osmotic pressure of 70 mm Hg (about 3 to 4 times greater than plasma), and produces an increment in plasma volume that is 3 to 4 times greater than the volume infused.

Albumin Solutions

Albumin is a versatile and abundant protein that is synthesized almost continuously by the liver (an average of 10 grams is produced daily). The average-sized adult has about 120 grams of albumin in plasma and another 160 grams in the interstitial fluid (21). Thus albumin is located primarily in the interstitial fluid, which is perplexing in light of the important role played by albumin in the plasma. Albumin is the principal transport protein in blood (see Table 13.3) and is also responsible for 75% of the colloid osmotic pressure in plasma (17,20,21). It also acts as a buffer (see Chapter 2), has significant antioxidant activity (22), and helps maintain

TABLE 13.3 Substances that are Transported by Albumin

Drugs	Others
Benzodiazepines	Adrenal hormones
Cephalosporins	Estrogen
Furosemide	Progesterone
NSAIDs	Testosterone
Phenytoin	Bilirubin
Quinidine	Fatty acids
Salicylates	Inflammatory mediators
Sulfonamides	Prostaglandins
Valproic acid	Metals
Warfarin	Copper
	Nickel
	Zinc

NSAID: nonsteroidal antiinflammatory drug.

blood fluidity by inhibiting platelet aggregation (21). What it does outside the bloodstream, where most of the albumin resides, is unknown.

Features

Albumin solutions are heat-treated preparations of human serum albumin that are available as a 5% solution (50 g/L) and a 25% solution (250 g/L) in an isotonic saline diluent. The 5% albumin solution has an albumin concentration of 5 g/dL and a colloid osmotic pressure of 20 mm Hg, both equivalent to plasma. Infusion of 5% albumin is performed using aliquots of 250 mL. About 70% of the infusate volume remains in the plasma for the first few hours post-infusion, but the increment in plasma volume dissipates rapidly thereafter, and the effect can be lost after just 12 hours (17,20).

The 25% albumin solution is a non-physiologic, hyperoncotic fluid that is given in aliquots of 50 mL or 100 mL. Following acute infusions of 25% albumin, plasma volume increases by 3 to 4 times the infusate volume. The effect is produced by fluid shifts from the interstitial space, so interstitial fluid volume is expected to decrease by equivalent amounts. Because the small volumes of 5% albumin solutions do not represent a significant sodium load, this solution is sometimes referred to as "salt-poor albumin."

It is important to emphasize that infusion of 25% albumin does not provide replacement of lost volume but merely shifts body fluid from one fluid compartment to another. Therefore **25% albumin should not be used as volume replacement therapy for patients with acute blood loss or dehydration**. This fluid should be reserved for the occasional patient with hypovolemia resulting from fluid shift into the interstitial space, which is usually the result of severe hypoalbuminemia.

Safety of Albumin Solutions

Albumin's reputation was sullied in 1998 when a clinical review was published claiming that one of every 17 patients who receive albumin infusions dies as a result of the fluid (23). This began a prolonged and passionate debate between albumin lovers and haters that continues to this day. However, the original claim that albumin is a lethal poison has not been corroborated in subsequent clinical reviews (24,25) or in a very large prospective, multicenter study of albumin and saline infusions that involved close to 7,000 patients (26). Thus the bulk of evidence indicates that albumin solutions are no more dangerous than any other colloid or crystalloid fluid. In fact, if adverse events are evaluated instead of deaths, the evidence indicates that albumin solutions are safer to use than crystalloid fluids (27). The influence of colloid and crystalloid fluids on clinical outcomes is discussed again later in the chapter.

Hetastarch

Hydroxyethyl starch (hetastarch) is a chemically modified starch polymer that is available as a 6% solution in isotonic saline. There are three types of hetastarch solution based on the average molecular weight (MW) of the starch molecules (28): high MW (450,000 daltons), medium MW (200,000 daltons), and low MW (70,000 daltons). High MW hetastarch is used exclusively in the United States, while in other countries, medium MW hetastarch is the popular fluid. High MW solutions have the greatest oncotic activity but also have the highest risk of certain adverse effects (see later).

Hetastarch elimination is a two-step process. First, circulating starch molecules undergo hydrolysis by amylase enzymes in blood. When the starch molecules are cleaved into small fragments (MW $<$ 50,000 daltons), they are cleared by the kidney. Clearance of hetastarch can take several weeks, but the oncotic activity is lost after one day.

Volume Effects

The performance of 6% hetastarch as a plasma volume expander is very similar to 5% albumin. The oncotic pressure (30 mm Hg) is higher than 5% albumin (20 mm Hg), and the increment in plasma volume can be slightly higher as well (see Table 13.2). The effect on plasma volume usually is lost by 24 hours (16,27).

Overall, **6% hetastarch is equivalent to 5% albumin as a plasma volume expander**. The major difference between these two fluids is cost (hetastarch is less costly) and the risk of altered hemostasis (which is greater with hetastarch).

Altered Hemostasis

The most celebrated side effect of hetastarch is a bleeding tendency caused by inhibition of factor VII and von Willebrand factor and impaired platelet adhesiveness (28,29). This effect is seen predominantly with high MW hetastarch, is less pronounced with medium MW hetastarch, and is absent with low MW hetastarch (29). The coagulation defects become pronounced when more than 1,500 mL hetastarch is infused within a 24 hr period (28). Overt bleeding is inconsistent, but it may be more frequent when hetastarch is used during cardiopulmonary bypass surgery. Despite lack of convincing evidence of harm, the Food and Drug Administration has issued a warning label to alert users of the bleeding risk from hetastarch in cardiopulmonary bypass surgery (30).

Troublesome bleeding from hetastarch can be minimized by limiting the infusion volume to less than 1,500 mL in 24 hours and by avoiding the use of hetastarch in patients with an underlying coagulopathy, particularly von Willebrand's disease. The use of hetastarch in cardiopulmonary bypass surgery should be left to the discretion of those who perform or are otherwise involved in bypass surgery on a daily basis.

Other Concerns

As mentioned earlier, hetastarch molecules are hydrolyzed by circulating amylases before they are cleared by the kidneys. The amylase enzymes attach to the hetastarch molecules, and this reduces amylase clearance by the kidneys. The result is an increase in serum amylase levels (2 to 3 times above normal) that represents **macroamylasemia** (28). Amylase levels return to normal within one week after the hetastarch is discontinued (29). The hyperamylasemia from hetastarch is not a deleterious side effect. The only adverse risk is misinterpretation of the elevated levels as a sign of acute pancreatitis, which could prompt unnecessary diagnostic and therapeutic interventions. Lipase levels are not elevated by hetastarch infusions (31), and this is an important consideration to avoid a misdiagnosis of acute pancreatitis.

Anaphylactic reactions to hetastarch are rare, occurring in 0.006% of infusions (28). Chronic administration of hetastarch can produce a troublesome pruritis that is difficult to treat. This is not an allergic reaction and is caused by extravascular starch deposits (27).

Hextend

Hextend is a 6% hetastarch solution with a buffered, multielectrolyte solution as a diluent instead of isotonic saline. This solution contains sodium (143 mEq/L), chloride (125 mEq/L), potassium (3 mEq/L), calcium (5 mEq/L), magnesium (0.9 mEq/L), lactate (28 mEq/L), and glucose (5 mM/L). Hextend has the same molecular weight and starch concentration as 6% hetastarch, so it is no surprise that it is equivalent to 6% hetastarch as a plasma volume expander.

Although the clinical experience is limited, Hextend offers no documented benefit over the other colloid resuscitation fluids. There is one study showing that Hextend infusions in an average volume of 1.6 liters had no detectable effect on blood coagulation during major surgery (32), but it is not possible to draw any conclusions based on this single study.

The Dextrans

The dextrans are glucose polymers produced by a bacterium (*Leuconostoc*) incubated in a sucrose medium. First introduced in the 1940s, these colloids are not popular (at least in the United States) because of the perceived risk of adverse reactions. The two most common dextran preparations are 10% dextran-40 and 6% dextran-70, each having a different average molecular weight (see Table 13.2). Both preparations use an isotonic saline diluent.

Features

Both dextran preparations have a colloid osmotic pressure of 40 mm Hg and cause a greater increase in plasma volume than either 5% albumin or 6% hetastarch (see Table 13.2). Dextran-70 may be preferred because the duration of action (12 hours) is longer than that of dextran-40 (6 hours) (17).

Disadvantages

Dextrans produce a dose-related bleeding tendency that involves impaired platelet aggregation, decreased levels of factor VIII and von Willebrand factor, and enhanced fibrinolysis (29,31). The hemostatic defects are minimized by limiting the daily dextran dose to 20 mL/kg.

Dextrans coat the surface of red blood cells and can interfere with the ability to cross-match blood. Red cell preparations must be washed to eliminate this problem. Dextrans also increase the erythrocyte sedimentation rate as a result of their interactions with red blood cells (31).

Dextrans have been implicated as a cause of acute renal failure (31,33). The proposed mechanism is a hyperoncotic state with reduced filtration pressure. However, this mechanism is unproven, and renal failure occurs only rarely in association with dextran infusions. Anaphylactic reactions, once common with dextrans, are now reported in only .032% of infusions (31).

THE COLLOID–CRYSTALLOID WARS

There is a long standing (and possibly eternal) debate concerning the type of fluid (crystalloid or colloid) that is most appropriate for volume resuscitation. Each fluid has its army of loyalists who passionately defend the merits of their fluid. The following are the issues involved in this debate.

Early Focus on Crystalloids

Early studies of acute blood loss in the 1960s produced two observations that led to the popularity of crystalloid fluids for volume resuscitation. The first observation was a human study showing that acute blood loss is accompanied by a shift of interstitial fluid into the bloodstream (transcapillary refill), leaving an *interstitial fluid deficit* (34). The second observation was an animal study showing that survival in hemorrhagic shock is improved if crystalloid fluid is added to reinfusion of the shed blood (35). The interpretation of these two observations, at that time, was that a major consequence of acute blood loss was an interstitial fluid deficit and that replenishing this deficit with a crystalloid fluid will reduce mortality.

Thus crystalloid fluids were popularized for volume resuscitation because of their ability to add volume to the interstitial fluids. Later studies using more sensitive measures of interstitial fluid revealed that the interstitial fluid deficit in acute blood loss is small and is unlikely to play a major role in determining the outcome from acute hemorrhage. This refuted the importance of filling the interstitial fluid compartment with crystalloids, yet the popularity of crystalloid fluids for volume resuscitation did not wane.

The Goal of Volume Resuscitation

The most convincing argument in favor of colloids for volume resuscitation is their superiority over crystalloid fluids for expanding the plasma volume. Colloid fluids will achieve a given increment in plasma volume with only one-quarter to one-third the volume required of crystalloid fluids. This is an important consideration in patients with brisk bleeding or severe hypovolemia, where rapid volume resuscitation is desirable.

The proponents of crystalloid resuscitation claim that crystalloids can achieve the same increment in plasma volume as colloids. This is certainly the case, but three to four times more volume is required with crystalloids than colloids to achieve this goal. This adds fluid to the interstitial space and can produce unwanted edema. In fact, as mentioned earlier (and demonstrated in Figure 13.2), **the principal effect of crystalloid infusions is to expand the interstitial fluid volume, not the plasma volume**. Since the goal of volume resuscitation is to support the intravascular volume, colloid fluids are the logical choice over crystalloid fluids.

Filling a Bucket

The following example illustrates the problem with using crystalloids to expand the plasma volume. Assume that you have two buckets, each representing the intravascular compartment, and each bucket is connected by a clamped hose to an overhanging reservoir that contains fluid. One reservoir contains a colloid fluid in the same volume as the bucket, and the other reservoir contains a crystalloid fluid in a volume that is three to four times greater than the colloid volume. Now release the clamp on each hose and empty the reservoirs: both buckets will fill with fluid, but most of the crystalloid fluid will spill over onto the floor. Now ask yourself which method is better suited for filling buckets: the colloid method, with the right amount of fluid and no spillage, or the crystalloid method, with too much fluid, most of which spills onto the floor.

Clinical Outcome

As mentioned earlier (see section on Safety of Albumin Solutions), the bulk of available evidence indicates that neither type of resuscitation fluid provides a survival benefit (24–26), while colloid (albumin-containing) fluids may cause fewer adverse events (27).

The Problem with Mortality Studies

There are two problems with the studies comparing mortality rates associated with colloid and crystalloid fluids. The first problem is that most studies included a diverse group of patients who could have died from a variety of illnesses, and there is no way of determining if an intravenous fluid was directly related to the cause of death. For example, a resuscitation fluid could restore a normal plasma volume, but the patient dies of pneumonia: in this case, the fluid should not be blamed for the death. The second problem is the assumption that an intervention must save lives to be considered beneficial. It seems that an intervention should be judged by whether it achieves its intended goal (e.g., a resuscitation fluid should be judged by how well it restores plasma volume); determining if that goal influences mortality is a separate question.

Expense

The biggest disadvantage of colloid resuscitation is the higher cost of colloid fluids. Table 13.4 shows a cost comparison for colloid and crystalloid fluids. Using equivalent volumes of 250 mL for colloid fluids and 1,000 mL for crystalloid fluids, the cost of colloid resuscitation is nine times higher (if hetastarch is used) to twenty-one times higher (if albumin is used) than volume resuscitation with crystalloid fluids.

A Suggestion

Most studies comparing colloid and crystalloid fluids have attempted to determine if one type of resuscitation fluid is better than the other for all critically ill patients. This seems unreasonable, considering the multitude

TABLE 13.4 Relative Cost of Intravenous Fluids

Fluid	Manufacturer	Unit size	AWP[a]
Crystalloid fluids			
Isotonic saline	Hospira	1,000 ml	$1.46
Lactated Ringer's	Hospira	1,000 ml	$1.48
Colloidal fluids			
5% Albumin	Bayer	250 ml	$30.63
25% Albumin	Bayer	50 ml	$30.63
6% Hetastarch	Abbott	500 ml	$27.63
6% Dextran-70	Hospira	500 ml	$14.96

[a]Average wholesale price listed in *2005 Redbook*. Montvale, NJ: Thomson PDR, 2005.

of clinical problems encountered in ICU patients. A more reasonable approach would be to determine if one type of fluid is more appropriate than the other for a given clinical condition (36). For example, patients with hypovolemia secondary to dehydration (where there is a uniform loss of extracellular fluid) might benefit more from a crystalloid fluid (which is expected to fill the extracellular space uniformly) than a colloid fluid, and patients with hypovolemia secondary to hypoalbuminemia (where there are fluid shifts from the intravascular to extravascular space) might benefit more from a colloid fluid (particularly 25% albumin) than a crystalloid fluid. **Tailoring the type of resuscitation fluid to the specific clinical condition seems a more logical approach than using the same type of fluid without exception for all ICU patients.**

HYPERTONIC RESUSCITATION

Volume resuscitation with hypertonic saline (7.5% NaCl) has received much attention as a method of small-volume resuscitation. A 7.5%

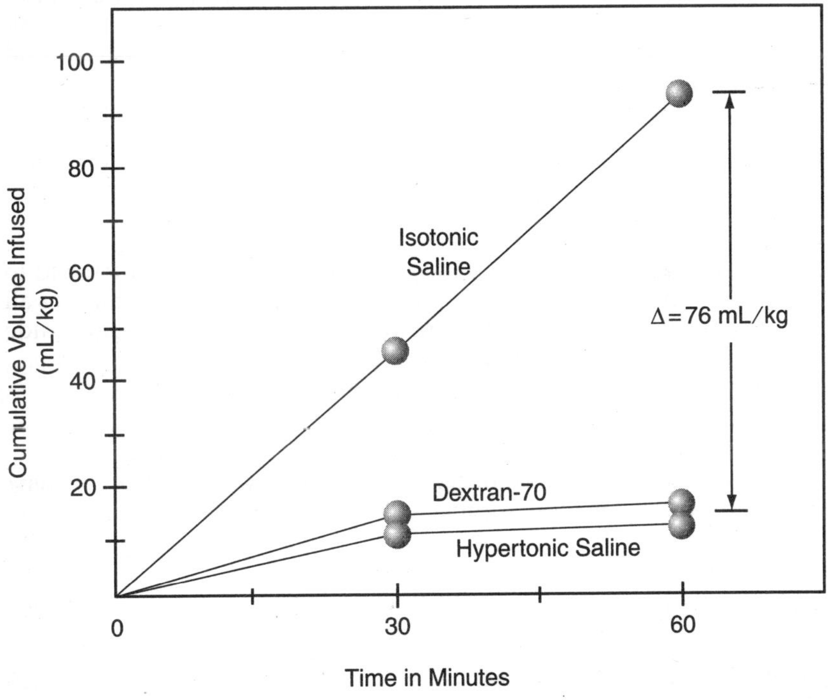

FIGURE 13.5 A comparison of the volume of three intravenous fluids needed to maintain a normal rate of aortic blood flow in an animal model of hemorrhagic shock. (From Chiara O, Pelosi P, Brazzi L, et al. Resuscitation from hemorrhagic shock: experimental model comparing normal saline, dextran, and hypertonic saline solutions. Crit Care Med 2003;31:1915.)

sodium chloride solution has an osmolality that is about 8.5 times greater than plasma (see Table 13.1). Figure 13.2 demonstrates that infusion of 250 mL of 7.5% NaCl will increase plasma volume by about twice the infused volume, indicating that hypertonic saline allows for volume resuscitation with relatively small volumes. Also note in Figure 13.2 that the total increase in extracellular fluid volume (1,235 mL) produced by 7.5% NaCl is about 5 times greater than the infused volume (250 mL). The additional volume comes from intracellular fluid that moves out of cells and into the extracellular space. This demonstrates one of the feared complications of hypertonic saline resuscitation: cell dehydration.

What Role?

The small volumes required with hypertonic saline resuscitation have been proposed as a possible benefit in the resuscitation of trauma victims with head injuries (to limit the severity of cerebral edema). However, the effective resuscitation volumes with hypertonic saline are similar to colloid resuscitation, as shown in Figure 13.5 (37), and a recent clinical study documented no advantage with hypertonic saline in the prehospital resuscitation of patients with traumatic head injury (38). At the present time, hypertonic saline is a resuscitation fluid without a clear indication.

A FINAL WORD

There is too much chatter about which type of resuscitation fluid (colloid or crystalloid) is most appropriate in critically ill patients because it is unlikely that one type of fluid is best for all patients. A more logical approach is to select the type of fluid that is best designed to correct a specific problem with fluid balance. For example, crystalloid fluids are designed to fill the extracellular space (interstitial space plus intravascular space) and would be appropriate for use in patients with dehydration (where there is a loss of interstitial fluid and intravascular fluid). Colloid fluids are designed to expand the plasma volume and are appropriate for patients with hypovolemia due to blood loss, while albumin-containing colloid fluids are appropriate for patients with hypovolemia associated with hypoalbuminemia. Tailoring fluid therapy to specific problems of fluid imbalance is the best approach to volume resuscitation in the ICU.

REFERENCES

Reviews

1. Alderson P, Schierhout G, Roberts I, et al. Colloid versus crystalloids for fluid resuscitation in critically ill patients: a systematic review of randomized trials. Cochrane Database Syst Rev 2000; Issue 3, Art. No. CD000567.
2. Choi PT, Yip G, Quinonez LG, et al. Crystalloids vs. colloids in fluid resuscitation: a systematic review. Crit Care Med 1999;27:200–210.

3. Whinney RR, Cohn SM, Zacur SJ. Fluid resuscitation for trauma patients in the 21st century. Curr Opin Crit Care 2000;6:396–400.
4. Bunn F, Alderson P, Hawkins V. Colloid solutions for fluid resuscitation. Cochrane Database Syst Rev 2001;:CD001319.

Crystalloid Fluids

1. Imm A, Carlson RW. Fluid resuscitation in circulatory shock. Crit Care Clin 1993;9:313–333.
2. Scheingraber S, Rehm M, Schmisch C, et al. Rapid saline infusion produces hyperchloremic acidosis in patients undergoing gynecologic surgery. Anesthesiology 1999;90:1265–1270.
3. Prough DS, Bidani A. Hyperchloremic metabolic acidosis is a predictable consequence of intraoperative infusion of 0.9% saline. Anesthesiology 1999;90:1247–1249.
4. Griffith CA. The family of Ringer's solutions. J Natl Intravenous Ther Assoc 1986;9:480–483.
5. American Association of Blood Banks. Technical manual, 10th ed. Arlington, VA: American Association of Blood Banks, 1990:368.
6. King WH, Patten ED, Bee DE. An *in vitro* evaluation of ionized calcium levels and clotting in red blood cells diluted with lactated Ringer's solution. Anesthesiology 1988;68:115–121.
7. Didwania A, Miller J, Kassel; D, et al. Effect of intravenous lactated Ringer's solution infusion on the circulating lactate concentration, part 3: result of a prospective, randomized, double-blind, placebo-controlled trial. Crit Care Med 1997;25:1851–1854.
8. Jackson EV Jr, Wiese J, Sigal B, et al. Effects of crystalloid solutions on circulating lactate concentrations, part 1: implications for the proper handling of blood specimens obtained from critically ill patients. Crit Care Med 1997;25: 1840–1846.
9. Halpern NA, Alicea M, Seabrook B, et al. [Q]olyte S, a physiologic multielectrolyte solution, is preferable to normal saline to wash cell saver salvaged blood: conclusions from a prospective, randomized study in a canine model. Crit Care Med 1997;12:2031–2038.

Dextrose Solutions

10. Gunther B, Jauch W, Hartl W, et al. Low-dose glucose infusion in patients who have undergone surgery. Arch Surg 1987;122:765–771.
11. DeGoute CS, Ray MJ, Manchon M, et al. Intraoperative glucose infusion and blood lactate: endocrine and metabolic relationships during abdominal aortic surgery. Anesthesiology 1989;71:355–361.
12. Turina M, Fry D, Polk HC Jr. Acute hyperglycemia and the innate immune system: clinical, cellular, and molecular aspects. Crit Care Med 2005;33:1624–1633.
13. Van Den Berghe G, Wouters P, Weekers F, et al. Intensive insulin therapy in critically ill patients. N Engl J Med 2001;345:1359–1367.
14. Sieber FE, Traystman RJ. Special issues: glucose and the brain. Crit Care Med 1992;20:104–114.

15. Finney SJ, Zekveld C, Elia A, et al. Glucose control and mortality in critically ill patients. JAMA 2003;290:2041–2047.

Colloid Fluids

16. Jacob G, Raj S, Ketch T, et al. Postural pseudoanemia: posture-dependent changes in hematocrit. Mayo Clin Proc 2005;80:611–614.
17. Griffel MI, Kaufman BS. Pharmacology of colloids and crystalloids. Crit Care Clin 1992;8:235–254.
18. Kaminski MV, Haase TJ. Albumin and colloid osmotic pressure: implications for fluid resuscitation. Crit Care Clin 1992;8:311–322.
19. Sutin KM, Ruskin KJ, Kaufman BS. Intravenous fluid therapy in neurologic injury. Crit Care Clin 1992;8:367–408.
20. Imm A, Carlson RW. Fluid resuscitation in circulatory shock. Crit Care Clin 1993;9:313–333.
21. Soni N, Margarson M.Albumin, where are we now? Curr Anesth Crit Care 2004;15:61–68.
22. Halliwell B. Albumin: an important extracellular antioxidant? Biochem Pharmacol 1988;37:569–571.
23. Cochrane Injuries Group Albumin Reviewers. Human albumin administration in critically ill patients: systematic review of randomized, controlled trials. Br Med J 1998;317:235–240.
24. Choi PT-L, Yip G, Quinonez LG, et al. Crystalloids vs. colloids in fluid resuscitation: a systematic review. Crit Care Med 1999;27:200–210.
25. Wilkes MN, Navickis RJ.Patient survival after human albumin administration: a meta-analysis of randomized, controlled trials. Ann Intern Med 2001;135: 149–164.
26. SAFE Study Investigators. A comparison of albumin and saline for fluid resuscitation in the intensive care unit. N Engl J Med 2004;350:2247–2256.
27. Vincent J-L, Navickis RJ, Wilkes MM. Morbidity in hospitalized patients receiving human serum albumin: a meta-analysis of randomized, controlled trials. Crit Care Med 2004;32:2029–2038.
28. Treib J, Baron JF, Grauer MT, et al. An international view of hydroxyethyl starches, Intensive Care Med 1999;25:258–268.
29. de Jonge E, Levi M. Effects of different plasma substitutes on blood coagulation: a comparative review. Crit Care Med 2001;29:1261–1267.
30. Haynes GR, Havidich JE, Payne KJ. Why the Food and Drug Administration changed the warning label for hetastarch. Anesthesiology 2004;101:560–561.
31. Nearman HS, Herman ML. Toxic effects of colloids in the intensive care unit. Crit Care Clin 1991;7:713–723.
32. Gan TJ. Hextend, a physiologically balanced plasma expander for large volume use in major surgery: a randomized phase III clinical trial. Anesth Analg 1999;88:992–998.
33. Drumi W, Polzleitner D, Laggner AN, et al. Dextran-40, acute renal failure, and elevated plasma oncotic pressure. N Engl J Med 1988;318:252–254.

Colloid–Crystalloid Wars

34. Moore FD. The effects of hemorrhage on body composition. N Engl J Med 1965;273:567–577.

35. Shires T, Carrico J, Lightfoot S. Fluid therapy in hemorrhagic shock. Arch Surg 1964;88:688–693.
36. Weil MH, Tang W. Albumin versus crystalloid solutions for the critically ill and injured [Editorial]. Crit Care Med 2004;32:2154–2155.

Hypertonic Resuscitation

37. Chiara O, Pelosi P, Brazzi L, et al. Resuscitation from hemorrhagic shock: experimental model comparing normal saline, dextran, and hypertonic saline solutions. Crit Care Med 2003;31:1915–1922.
38. Cooper DJ, Myles PS, McDermott FT, et al. Prehospital hypertonic saline resuscitation of patients with hypotension and severe traumatic brain injury. JAMA 2004;291:1350–1357.

Chapter 14

ACUTE HEART FAILURE SYNDROMES

There's no doubt that the proper functioning of our pipes and pumps does have an immediate urgency well beyond that of almost any of our other bits and pieces.

Steven Vogel (Vital Circuits, 1992)

Acute or decompensated heart failure is responsible for about 1 million hospital admissions each year in the United States (1), and it is the leading cause of hospital admissions for adults over the age of 65 (2). Heart failure is not a single entity but can be classified according to the side of the heart that is involved (right-sided vs. left-sided failure) or the portion of the cardiac cycle that is affected (diastolic vs. systolic failure). This chapter describes the diagnostic and therapeutic approach to each of these four heart failure syndromes using the principles of cardiac performance described in Chapter 1 (2–6). The approach to heart failure in this chapter is designed for the ICU: it is based on invasive hemodynamic measurements, rather than clinical symptoms and signs, and focuses on the mechanical problems of heart failure rather than the responsible diseases. The usual causes of heart failure are shown in Figure 14.1.

HEMODYNAMIC ALTERATIONS

The hemodynamic consequences of progressive left-sided heart failure are shown in Figure 14.2. (The measurements in this graph were obtained from a patient who had just undergone cardiopulmonary bypass surgery). The hemodynamic changes progress through three stages (the numbers below correspond to the circled numbers in Figure 14.2):

1. The earliest sign of ventricular dysfunction is an increase in cardiac filling pressures. The stroke volume is maintained, but at the expense of the elevated filling pressure.

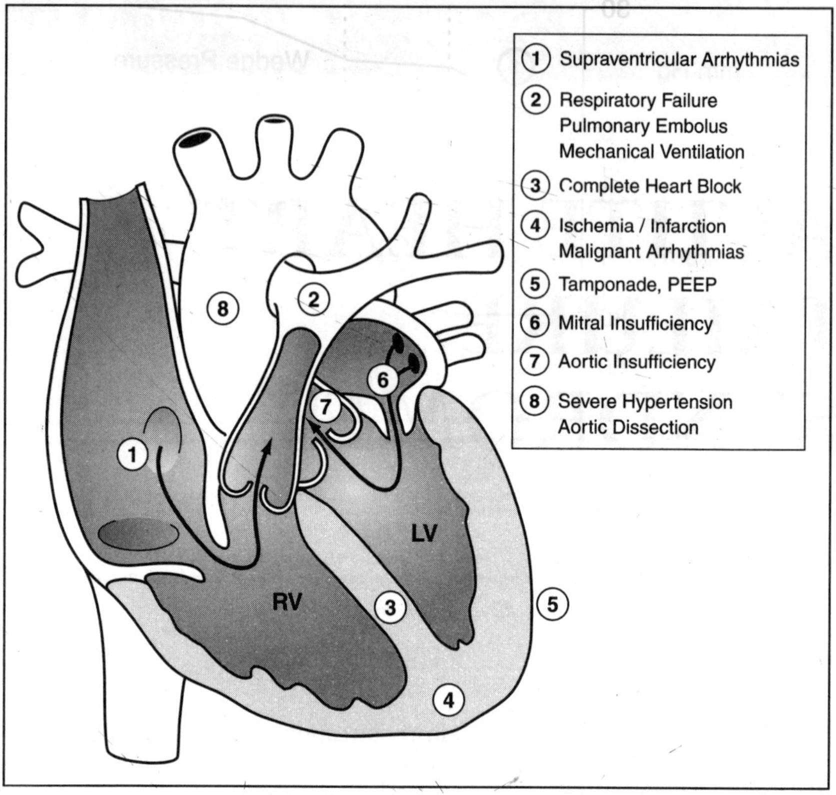

FIGURE 14.1 Common causes of acute heart failure, listed according to the anatomic region involved. *RV* = right ventricle; *LV* = left ventricle.

2. The next stage is marked by a decrease in stroke volume and an increase in heart rate. The tachycardia offsets the reduction in stroke volume, so the cardiac output remains unchanged.
3. The final stage is characterized by a decrease in cardiac output. The point at which the cardiac output begins to decline marks the transition from compensated to decompensated heart failure.

The serial hemodynamic changes shown in Figure 14.2 demonstrate that **cardiac output is impaired only in the more advanced stages of heart failure**; therefore a normal cardiac output is not necessarily a normal cardiac pump. Cardiac pump function should be evaluated using the relationship between ventricular filling pressure and stroke volume. This relationship is the basis for ventricular function curves, which are described in Chapter 1 (see Figure 1.2).

Systolic Versus Diastolic Failure

Heart failure is not synonymous with contractile failure because **systolic function is normal in 40 to 50% of newly-diagnosed cases of heart**

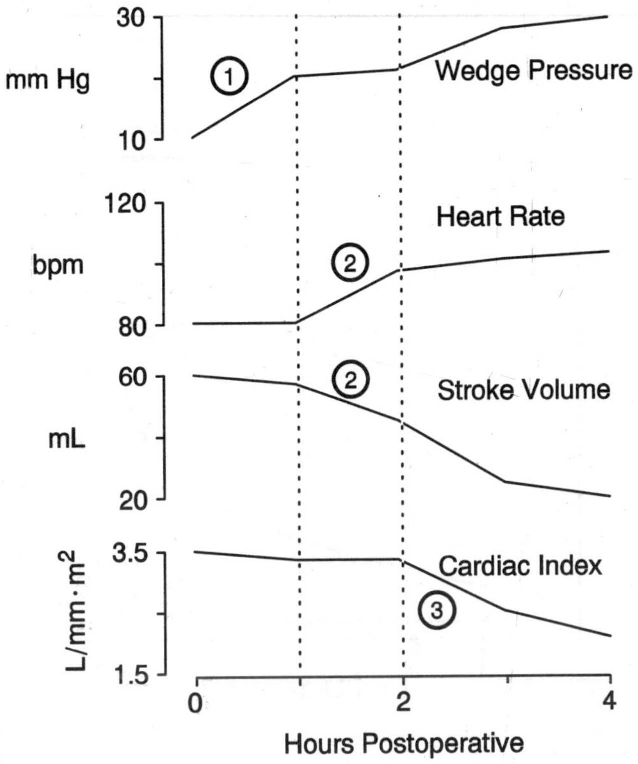

FIGURE 14.2 Hemodynamic effects of progressive left-sided heart failure in a post-operative patient.

failure (2). The problem in this condition is a combination of impaired ventricular relaxation and a decrease in passive ventricular distensibility, a disorder known as *diastolic heart failure* (6,7). In this type of heart failure, the decrease in cardiac output is due to inadequate ventricular filling, not impaired systolic contraction. Common causes of diastolic heart failure in ICU patients include ventricular hypertrophy, myocardial ischemia (stunned myocardium), and positive-pressure mechanical ventilation.

Diagnostic Difficulties

The usual method of evaluating cardiac pump function (by the relationship between ventricular filling pressure and stroke volume) will not distinguish between diastolic and systolic heart failure (7,8). This is illustrated in Figure 14.3. The curves in this figure are similar to the pressure–volume curves shown in Figures 1.2 and 1.3. The upper curves in the figure are ventricular function curves relating ventricular end-diastolic pressure and stroke volume. These curves indicate that heart failure is associated with an increase in end-diastolic pressure and a decrease in stroke volume. It is not possible, however, to determine if

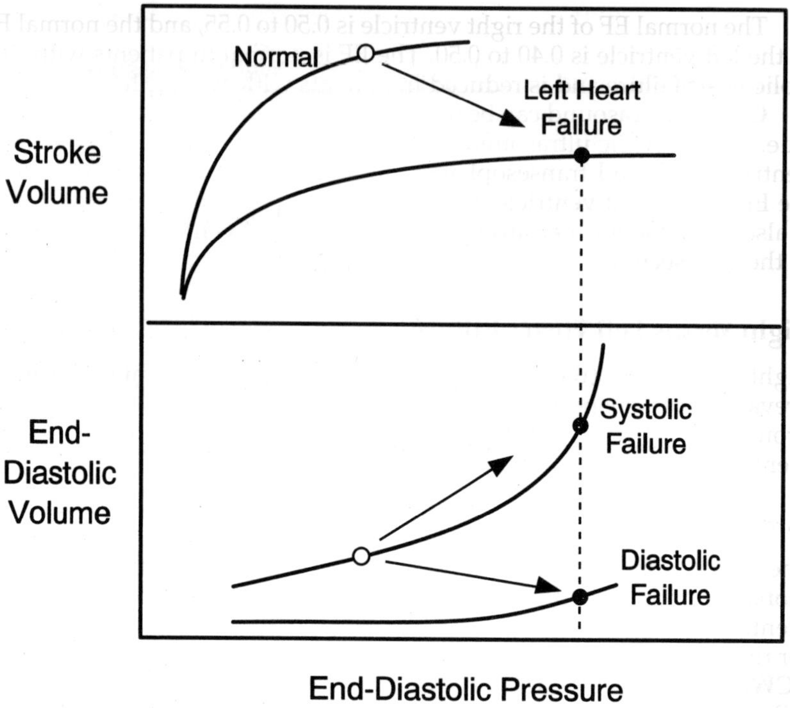

FIGURE 14.3 Graphs showing diastolic pressure volume curves in systolic and diastolic heart failure (lower curves) and ventricular function curves in heart failure (upper curves). The ventricular function curves, which are used to evaluate cardiac function in the clinical setting, are unable to distinguish between diastolic and systolic failure.

the heart failure is systolic or diastolic based on these measurements. The lower set of curves shows the pressure–volume relationships during diastole in the two types of heart failure. The end-diastolic pressure is increased in both types of heart failure, but the end-diastolic volume changes in different directions: it is increased in systolic heart failure and decreased in diastolic heart failure. Thus **the end-diastolic volume, not the end-diastolic pressure, is the hemodynamic measure that will distinguish diastolic from systolic heart failure**. There is a specialized pulmonary artery catheter that measures the end-diastolic volume of the right ventricle (see later), but otherwise this measurement is not readily available.

Ventricular Ejection Fraction

The measurement that is most often used to distinguish between diastolic and systolic heart failure is the ventricular *ejection fraction* (EF), which is a measure of the strength of ventricular contraction. The EF expresses the stroke volume (SV) as a fraction of the end-diastolic volume (EDV)

$$EF = SV/EDV \tag{14.1}$$

The normal EF of the right ventricle is 0.50 to 0.55, and the normal EF of the left ventricle is 0.40 to 0.50. The EF is normal in patients with diastolic heart failure and is reduced in patients with systolic heart failure.

Cardiac ultrasound can be used to measure ventricular EF at the bedside. Transthoracic ultrasound can be used to measure the EF of the left ventricle (6,7), and transesophageal ultrasound can be used to measure the EF of the right ventricle (8). A specialized pulmonary artery catheter is also available for measuring the EF of the right ventricle, as described in the next section.

Right Versus Left Heart Failure

Right heart failure (which is predominantly systolic heart failure) is more prevalent than suspected in ICU patients (9), and it may be particularly prominent in ventilator-dependent patients. The following measurements can prove useful in identifying right heart failure.

Cardiac Filling Pressures

The relationship between the central venous pressure (CVP) and the pulmonary capillary wedge pressure (PCWP) can sometimes be useful for identifying right heart failure. The following criteria have been proposed for right heart failure (10): **CVP > 15 mm Hg** and **CVP = PCWP** or **CVP > PCWP**. Unfortunately, at least one-third of patients with acute right heart failure do not satisfy these criteria (10). One problem is the insensitivity of the CVP; an increase in the CVP is seen only in the later stages of right heart failure. Contractile failure of the right ventricle results in an increase in end-diastolic volume, and only when the increase in volume of the right heart is impeded by the pericardium does the end-diastolic pressure (CVP) rise (9).

Another problem with the CVP–PCWP relationship for identifying right heart failure is the interaction between the right and left sides of the heart. This is shown in Figure 14.4. Both ventricles share the same septum, so enlargement of the right ventricle pushes the septum to the left and compromises the left-ventricular chamber. This interaction between right and left ventricles is called *interventricular interdependence*, and it can confuse the interpretation of ventricular filling pressures. In fact, as indicated by the diastolic pressures in Figure 14.4, **the hemodynamic changes in right heart failure can look much like the hemodynamic changes in pericardial tamponade** (9).

Thermodilution Ejection Fraction

A specialized pulmonary artery catheter is available that uses a fast-response thermistor to measure the ejection fraction (EF) of the right ventricle (11). Rapid-response thermistors can record the temperature changes associated with each cardiac cycle. This produces a thermodilution curve like the one shown in Figure 14.5. The change in temperature between each plateau on the curve is caused by dilution of the cold indicator fluid by venous blood that fills the ventricle during diastole. Because the volume that fills the ventricles during diastole is equivalent

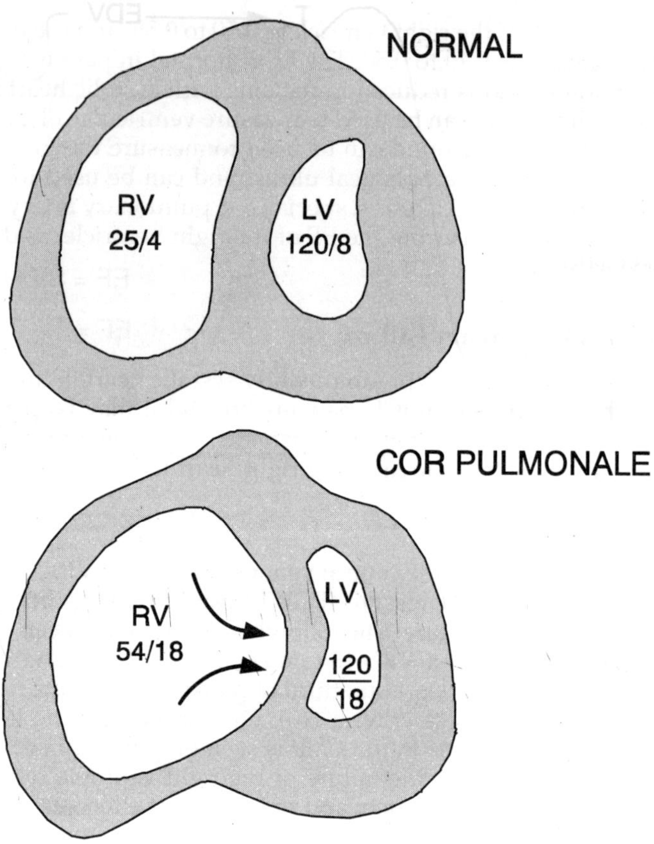

FIGURE 14.4 Interventricular interdependence: the mechanism whereby right heart failure can reduce diastolic filling of the left ventricle and increase the left-ventricular end-diastolic (wedge) pressure. *RV* = right ventricle; *LV* = left ventricle. The numbers in each chamber represent the systolic pressure as the numerator and the end-diastolic pressure as the denominator.

to the stroke volume, the temperature difference $T_1 - T_2$ is the thermal equivalent of the stroke volume (SV), and the temperature T_1 is thus a thermal marker of the end-diastolic volume (EDV). The ejection fraction is then equivalent to the ratio $T_1 - T_2/T_1$ (or SV/EDV). Once the EF is measured, the stroke volume can be measured in the usual fashion (as cardiac output divided by heart rate), and the EDV can be determined by rearranging Equation 14.1.

$$\text{EDV} = \text{SV}/\text{EF} \tag{14.2}$$

The normal right ventricular EF (RVEF) using thermodilution is 0.45 to 0.50, which is about 10% lower than the EF measured by radionuclide imaging (the gold standard). The normal right ventricular EDV (RVEDV) is 80 to 140 mL/m^2.

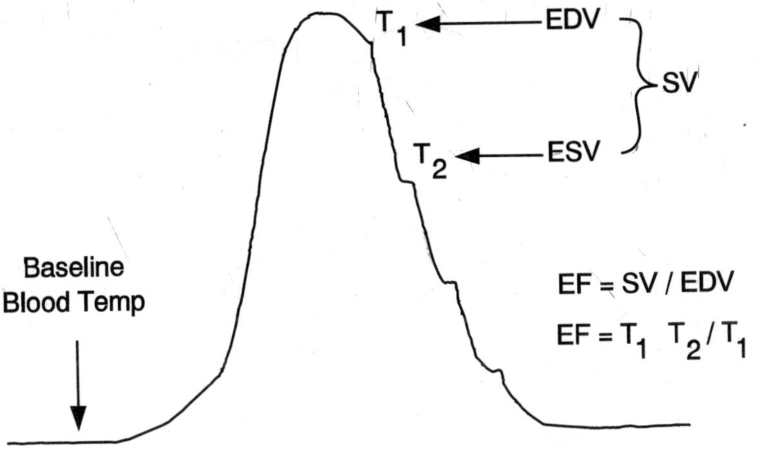

FIGURE 14.5 The thermodilution method of measuring the ejection fraction (*EF*) of the right ventricle using thermal equivalents for end-diastolic volume (*EDV*), end-systolic volume (*ESV*), and stroke volume (*SV*).

Since most cases of right heart failure represent systolic failure, the RVEF is expected to be less than 0.45, and the RVEDV is expected to be above 140 mL/m^2 in cases of right heart failure (12). The response of RVEDV to a fluid challenge may also be diagnostic: volume infusion is expected to increase the RVEDV in patients with right heart failure, while in other patients, the RVEDV is unchanged after a fluid challenge (13).

Echocardiography

Cardiac ultrasound can be useful at the bedside for differentiating right from left heart failure. Three findings typical of right heart failure are (a) an increase in right-ventricular chamber size, (b) segmental wall motion abnormalities on the right, and (c) paradoxical motion of the interventricular septum (10).

B-TYPE NATRIURETIC PEPTIDE

Brain-type (B-type) natriuretic peptide (BNP) is a neurohormone that is released by the ventricular myocardium in response to ventricular volume and pressure overload. Plasma levels of BNP increase in direct relation to increases in ventricular end-diastolic volume and end-diastolic pressure (both right-sided and left-sided), and the rise in BNP produces both vasodilatation and an increase in renal sodium excretion (14).

Diagnostic Value

The plasma BNP level has proven to be an important tool for the diagnosis of heart failure. In patients who present with dyspnea of unknown etiology, **a plasma BNP > 100 picograms/milliliter (pg/mL) can be used**

as evidence of heart failure as a cause of the dyspnea (diagnostic accuracy = 84%) (15). In fact, in patients who present to the emergency department with dyspnea of unknown etiology, the plasma BNP level (using a cutoff level of 100 pg/mL) is the single most accurate predictor of the presence or absence of heart failure (15). Rapid determination of plasma BNP levels is available at the bedside using a fluorescence immunoassay kit (Triage; Biosite Diagnostics, San Diego, CA) that allows for timely identification of acute heart failure in the emergency department (15).

Plasma BNP levels also show a direct correlation with the severity of heart failure (14,16) [i.e., plasma levels are higher in patients with more advanced stages of heart failure (see Table 14.1)]. This correlation indicates that plasma BNP levels may be useful for monitoring the clinical course of heart failure.

Other Contributing Factors

Plasma BNP levels are influenced by gender, age, and renal function. This is demonstrated in Table 14.1. Plasma BNP levels are about 50% higher in females than in males, and plasma levels increase with advancing age in both sexes (14). Renal insufficiency also increases plasma BNP levels (because BNP is cleared by the kidneys), but levels usually do not pass the 100 pg/mL threshold unless there is associated volume overload (see Table 14.1) (17).

TABLE 14.1 Plasma BNP Levels in Selected Conditions

Condition	Mean Plasma BNP (pg/mL)
Females—no CHF[a]	
Age 55–64	32
Age 75+	78
Males—no CHF[a]	
Age 55–64	20
Age 75+	48
Renal insufficiency[b]	
No volume overload	80
Volume overload	180
Heart failure[c]	
Mild	186
Moderate	791
Severe	2013

[a]From Reference 14.
[b]From Reference 17.
[c]From References 14,16.
Abbreviations: BNP = B-type natriuretic peptide, CHF = congestive heart failure, pg = picograms

What Role in the ICU?

Plasma BNP has been studied primarily in patients who present to emergency departments with possible heart failure. Few studies have been performed in ICU patients. One study of ICU patients with sepsis showed that plasma BNP levels were useful in identifying patients with cardiac dysfunction (18). However, it is unlikely that plasma BNP will replace more traditional methods of evaluating cardiac function in the ICU. Plasma BNP levels might prove useful for monitoring the effectiveness of treatment for heart failure in the ICU or to identify patients who develop fluid overload. Until further studies are conducted in the ICU, the plasma BNP assay will remain a tool for the emergency department.

MANAGEMENT STRATEGIES

The management of heart failure described here is meant for patients with advanced or decompensated heart failure, where the cardiac output is compromised (stage 3 in Figure 14.2). The approach here is specifically designed for ICU patients: it is based on invasive hemodynamic measurements rather than symptoms and uses only drugs that are given by continuous intravenous infusion (19–21). The hemodynamic drugs in this chapter are presented in detail in Chapter 16: the dose ranges and actions of each drug are shown in Table 14.2.

Left-Sided (Systolic) Heart Failure

The management of decompensated left-sided heart failure is traditionally designed for a systolic-type heart failure, even though some cases may involve diastolic failure. The recommendations here are based on three

TABLE 14.2 Drugs Used to Manage Acute, Decompensated Heart Failure in the ICU*

Drug	Dose Range	Principal Effect
Dobutamine	3–15 μg/kg/min	Positive inotropic effect and systemic vasodilatation
Dopamine	1–3 μg/kg/min	Renal vasodilatation and natriuresis
	3–10 μg/kg/min	Positive inotropic effect and systemic vasodilatation
	>10 μg/kg/min	Systemic vasoconstriction
Milrinone	50 μg/kg bolus, then 0.25–1 μg/kg/min	Positive inotropic effect, lusitropic effect, and systemic vasodilatation
Nitroglycerin	1–50 μg/min	Venous vasodilatation
	>50 μg/min	Arterial vasodilatation
Nitroprusside	0.3–2 μg/kg/min	Systemic vasodilatation

*Includes only drugs given by continuous intravenous infusion.

measurements: the pulmonary capillary wedge pressure (PCWP), the cardiac output (CO), and the arterial blood pressure (BP). Decompensated heart failure is associated with a high PCWP and a low CO, but the BP can vary. The management strategies that follow are based on the condition of the blood pressure (i.e., high, normal, or low).

High Blood Pressure

Decompensated heart failure with elevated blood pressure is a common scenario in the early period after cardiopulmonary bypass surgery (22).

Profile: High PCWP/Low CO/High BP
Treatment: Vasodilator therapy with nitroprusside or nitroglycerin. If the PCWP remains above 20 mm Hg, add diuretic therapy with furosemide.

Vasodilators like nitroprusside and nitroglycerin augment cardiac output by reducing ventricular afterload. The overall effect is a decrease in arterial blood pressure, an increase in cardiac output, and a decrease in ventricular filling pressure (20). Nitroprusside is a more effective vasodilator than nitroglycerin, but drug safety is a concern. The major **problem with nitroprusside is cyanide toxicity** (23), which is more common than suspected (see Chapter 16) and is particularly prevalent following cardiopulmonary bypass surgery. Nitroprusside is also **not advised in patients with ischemic heart disease** because the drug can produce a "coronary steal syndrome" (4).

Nitroglycerin is a safer alternative to nitroprusside. Low infusion rates (<50 μg/min) produce venous vasodilation (which can reduce cardiac output further), and dose rates in excess of 50 μg/min are usually required to produce effective arterial vasodilation. The **major drawback with nitroglycerin infusions is the development of tolerance**, which can appear after 16 to 24 hours of continuous drug administration (4). Vasodilator therapy with angiotensin-converting-enzyme (ACE) inhibitors, while beneficial in the long-term management of left heart failure, is not recommended for the acute management of decompensated left heart failure (4).

Diuretic therapy with furosemide is indicated only if vasodilator therapy does not reduce the wedge pressure to the desired level. The desired wedge pressure in left heart failure is the highest pressure that will augment cardiac output without producing pulmonary edema. This is shown in Figure 14.6 as the highest point on the lower (heart failure) curve that does not enter the shaded (pulmonary edema) region. **The desired or optimal wedge pressure in left heart failure is 18 to 20 mm Hg** (24). Therefore diuretic therapy is indicated only if the wedge pressure during vasodilator therapy remains above 20 mm Hg. The features of diuretic therapy for decompensated heart failure are described later.

Normal Blood Pressure

Decompensated heart failure with a normal blood pressure is the usual presentation of heart failure resulting from ischemic heart disease, acute myocarditis, and the advanced stages of chronic cardiomyopathy.

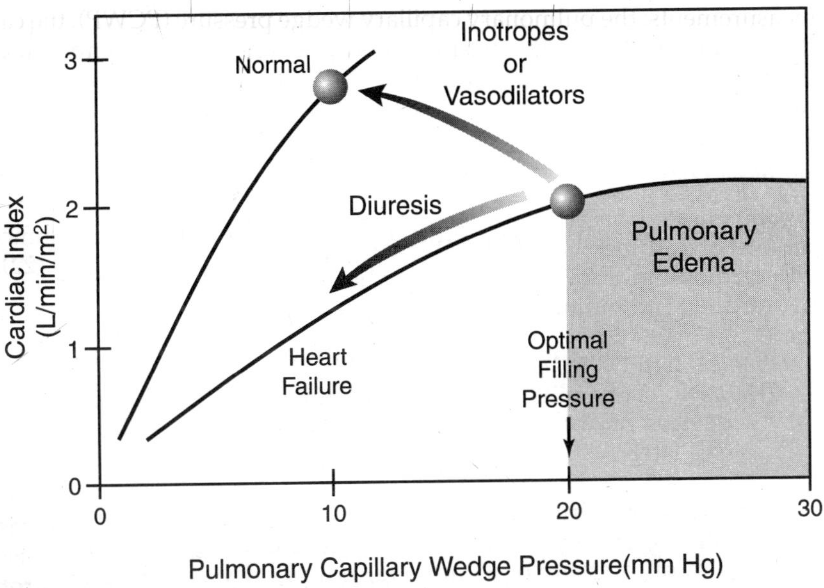

FIGURE 14.6 Ventricular function curves for the normal and failing left ventricle. Arrows show the expected changes associated with each type of drug therapy. The shaded area indicates the usual region where pulmonary edema becomes apparent.

Profile: High PCWP/Low CO/Normal BP

Treatment: Inodilator therapy with dobutamine or milrinone, or vasodilator therapy with nitroglycerin. If the PCWP does not decrease to <20 mm Hg, add diuretic therapy with furosemide.

Dobutamine and milrinone are called *inodilators* because they have both positive inotropic and vasodilator actions (19,21). Dobutamine is a β-receptor agonist, while milrinone is a phosphodiesterase inhibitor. Both drugs augment cardiac output and reduce ventricular filling pressures. Blood pressure is usually unaffected in the usual doses, but dobutamine can increase blood pressure, and milrinone can promote hypotension. **Dobutamine can increase myocardial O_2 consumption (19), and this effect can be counterproductive** in the ischemic myocardium (where oxygen supply is impaired) and in the failing myocardium (where O_2 consumption is already increased). Milrinone has no reported effect on myocardial O_2 consumption (19).

Because dobutamine can increase myocardial oxygen demands, vasodilator therapy (e.g., with nitroglycerin) has been recommended as a safer alternative to dobutamine, particularly in patients with ischemic heart disease (19,21). **Milrinone may also be preferred to dobutamine because of its lack of effect on myocardial O_2 consumption**. Milrinone is also preferred to dobutamine in patients receiving β-blocker drugs because its mechanism of action does not involve β-receptors.

Diuretic therapy in this condition is similar in principle to that described for hypertensive heart failure: it is reserved for cases where the wedge pressure remains above 20 mm Hg despite inodilator or vasodilator therapy.

Low Blood Pressure

Decompensated heart failure accompanied by hypotension is the *sine qua non* of cardiogenic shock. This condition is most often associated with cardiopulmonary bypass surgery, acute myocardial infarction, viral myocarditis, and pulmonary embolus (25).

Profile: High PCWP/Low CO/Low BP
Treatment: Dopamine in vasoconstrictor doses. Mechanical assist devices can be used as a temporary measure in selected cases (see later).

Hemodynamic drugs are notoriously unsuccessful in cardiogenic shock, with a mortality rate as high as 80% (24). Increasing blood pressure (to a mean pressure of 60 mm Hg) is a priority, and dopamine is a popular agent because it acts as a vasopressor in high doses (>10 μg/kg/min) and retains some positive inotropic actions associated with lower doses (5 to 10 μg/kg/min) (4,19,21). However, because low cardiac output states are accompanied by systemic vasoconstriction, drug-induced vasoconstriction can further aggravate tissue hypoperfusion. Dobutamine can be added to dopamine to further enhance cardiac output, but the combined effects of dopamine and dobutamine on promoting tachyarrhythmias and increasing myocardial O_2 consumption can be detrimental in the failing heart.

Mechanical cardiac support is indicated in the management of cardiogenic shock when myocardial function is expected to improve spontaneously (as occurs in the early period following cardiopulmonary bypass surgery) or when a corrective procedure (such as coronary angioplasty) is planned. This approach can reduce the mortality in cardiogenic shock to about 60%, although this is not a consistent finding (25). Mechanical assist devices are described later in the chapter.

The Role of Diuretic Therapy

Although diuretic therapy with furosemide has been a cornerstone of management for chronic heart failure, diuretics should be used cautiously in the management of acute, decompensated heart failure. The reason for caution is the observation that **intravenous furosemide often causes a decrease in cardiac output in patients with acute left heart failure** (26–30). This effect is the result of a decrease in venous return and an increase in systemic vascular resistance. The latter effect is due to the ability of furosemide to stimulate renin release and raise circulating levels of angiotensin, a vasoconstrictor (31).

There are two management goals in decompensated heart failure: (1) augment cardiac output (to promote tissue perfusion), and (2) reduce venous pressures (to eliminate the risk of edema formation). Vasodilator and inodilator drug therapy can achieve both goals, so these drugs should be used in the initial management of decompensated heart failure. Diuretic therapy with intravenous furosemide is indicated only when the first line drugs do not return the venous pressures to acceptable levels (i.e., a PCWP <20 mm Hg).

FUROSEMIDE BY CONTINUOUS INFUSION. Critically ill patients can have an attenuated response to furosemide (32). Several factors may be involved, including reduced drug transport by plasma proteins, reduced renal blood flow, and chloride depletion (furosemide acts by inhibiting chloride reabsorption in the Loop of Henle). Because the diuretic effect of furosemide is more closely related to its urinary excretion rate than to its plasma concentration (33), continuous infusion of the drug produces a more vigorous diuresis than bolus injection. The indications and dosage of continuous infusion furosemide are shown below.

Indication: Furosemide resistance (e.g., when 80 mg furosemide given as an IV bolus results in less than 2 liters of urine output in the ensuing 4 hours).

Dosage: Start with 100 mg furosemide as an IV bolus. Immediately follow with a continuous infusion of furosemide at 40 mg/hr. Double the dose rate every 12 hours if needed to achieve a urine output of at least 100 mL/h. The dose rate should not exceed a maximum of 169 mg/h (34).

NESIRITIDE. Nisiritide (Natrecor) is a recombinant human B-type natriuretic peptide that was introduced in 2001 for the treatment of decompensated heart failure. This agent is a systemic vasodilator that augments cardiac output by reducing ventricular afterload. The recommended dose regimen is shown below (36).

Dosage: Give initial intravenous bolus of 2 μg/kg and follow with a continuous infusion at 0.01 μg/kg/min. This dose rate can be increased 0.01 μg/kg/min every 3 hours to a maximum dose of 0.03 μg/kg/min (36).

Clinical studies indicate that nesiritide is an effective vasodilator but offers no advantage over other vasodilators such as nitroglycerin (36). In fact, there is concern about a report showing an increase in short-term (30 day) mortality attributed to nesiritide (37). This prompted the Food and Drug Administration to issue a warning (in the summer of 2005) about the possible dangers of nesiritide. At the present time, the clinical value of nesiritide is unproven.

Diastolic Heart Failure

The incidence of decompensated heart failure in the ICU that is purely diastolc in nature is not known, and it is likely that many cases of heart failure treated as systolic failure have some component of diastolic dysfunction. There is no general agreement about the optimal treatment of diastolic heart failure (7), but there are two recommendations that seem valid based on the distinguishing features of diastolic failure. First, because systolic function is normal in diastolic heart failure, **positive inotropic agents have no role in the treatment of diastolic heart failure**. Second, because ventricular filling is impaired in diastolic heart failure, **diuretic therapy can be counterproductive** and can further impair ventricular filling and cardiac output. Diuretic therapy does not play a major role in the management of acute, decompensated heart failure, and this deserves particular emphasis for diastolic-type heart failure.

Since most cases of diastolic failure are the result of hypertension-induced left ventricular hypertrophy, vasodilators have been a popular ingredient in treatment regimens for diastolic failure. Some vasodilator agents, such as nitroglycerin and milrinone, also have *lusitropic* actions that promote ventricular relaxation during diastole (7,21) and thus might be the preferred vasodilators for diastolic heart failure. Calcium channel blockers like verapamil are effective in diastolic failure caused by idiopathic hypertrophic cardiomyopathies (38), but these agents do not favorably improve diastolic function in other conditions that cause diastolic failure (39).

Right Heart Failure

Therapeutic strategies for right heart failure are similar in principle to those just described. The strategies below pertain only to primary right heart failure (e.g., following acute myocardial infarction) and not to right heart failure secondary to chronic obstructive lung disease. The PCWP and RVEDV are used as the focal points of management.

1. If PCWP is below 15 mm Hg, infuse volume until the PCWP or CVP increases by 5 mm Hg or either one reaches 20 mm Hg (10).
2. If the RVEDV is less than 140 mL/m^2, infuse volume until the RVEDV reaches 140 mL/m^2 (40).
3. If PCWP is above 15 mm Hg or the RVEDV is 140 mL/m^2 or higher, infuse dobutamine, beginning at a rate of 5 μg/kg/minute (41,42).
4. In the presence of AV dissociation or complete heart block, institute sequential A-V pacing and avoid ventricular pacing (10).

The response to volume infusion must be carefully monitored in right heart failure because aggressive volume infusion can overdistend the right ventricle and further reduce cardiac output through interventricular interdependence (see Figure 14.4).

Dobutamine is an effective agent in right heart failure (41,42). Nitroprusside has been used in right heart failure, but it is not as effective as dobutamine (42).

MECHANICAL CARDIAC SUPPORT

In selected cases of life-threatening cardiac pump failure that is refractory to hemodynamic drug support, mechanical devices can be used to generate blood flow and reduce the workload of the heart. There are two methods of providing mechanical cardiac support: intra-aortic balloon counterpulsation and circulatory support with specialized pumps called *ventricular-assist devices* that are placed in parallel with one or both ventricles.

Intra-Aortic Balloon Counterpulsation

Intra-aortic balloon counterpulsation was introduced in 1968 as a method of promoting coronary blood flow in patients with acute myocardial infarction complicated by cardiogenic shock (43). (The term *counterpulsation* is a misnomer for the process of providing pulsatile flow during diastole.) This technique uses a sausage-shaped polyurethane balloon that is attached to the distal end of a large-bore catheter. The catheter (with the balloon wrapped tightly around the distal end) is inserted percutaneously into the femoral artery in the groin and then advanced up the aorta until the tip lies just below the origin of the left subclavian artery. The balloon is available in various lengths to match body height. When properly placed, the balloon should extend from just below the left subclavian artery to just above the renal arteries. Correct balloon placement does not require fluoroscopy, which allows for timely placement of the device at the bedside.

Hemodynamic Effects

The intra-aortic balloon pump (IABP) uses helium, a low density gas, to inflate the balloon (inflation volume is generally 35 to 40 mL). Inflation begins at the onset of diastole, just after the aortic valve closes (the R wave on the ECG is a common trigger). The balloon is then deflated at the onset of ventricular systole, just before the aortic valve opens. This pattern of balloon inflation and deflation produces two changes in the aortic pressure waveform, as illustrated in Figure 14.7.

1. Inflation of the balloon increases the peak diastolic pressure and displaces blood toward the periphery. The increase in diastolic pressure increases the mean pressure in the aorta, which is the driving force for systemic blood flow. The increase in diastolic pressure should also augment coronary blood flow, because the bulk of coronary flow occurs during diastole. However, the IABP has been shown to increase coronary flow only in patients with hypotension (44).
2. Deflation of the balloon reduces the end-diastolic pressure, which reduces the impedance to flow when the aortic valve opens at the onset of systole. This decreases ventricular afterload and promotes ventricular stroke output.

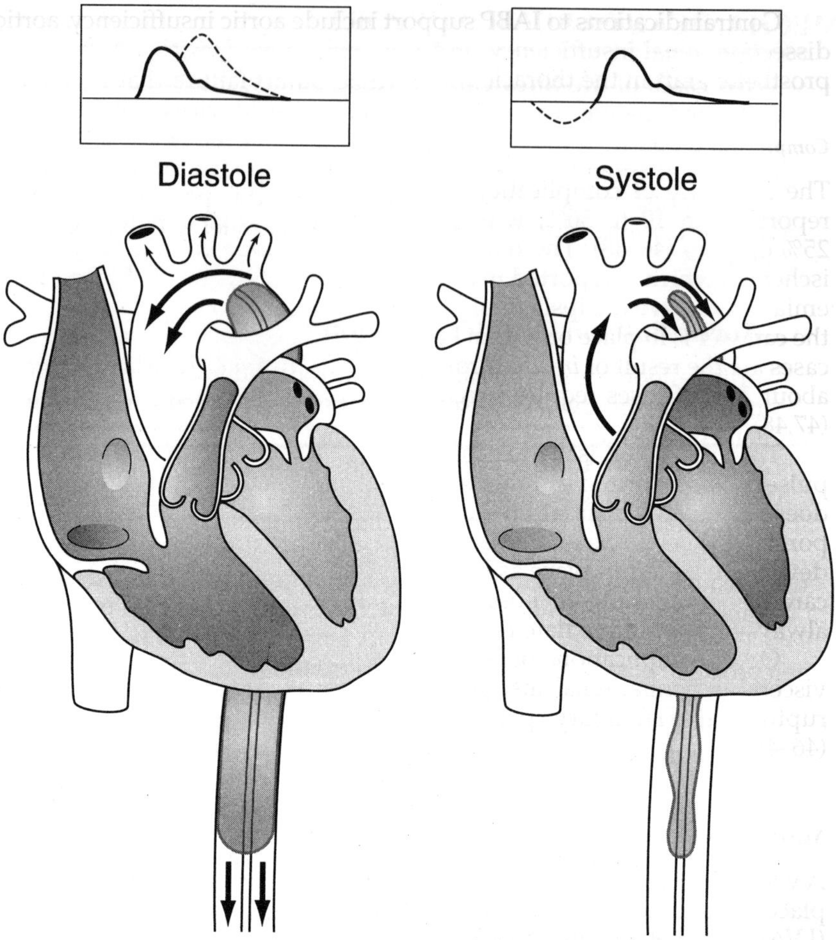

FIGURE 14.7 The effect of intra-aortic balloon counterpulsation on the aortic pressure waveform. The dotted lines indicate the change in aortic pressure produced by balloon inflation during diastole and balloon deflation just prior to systole. The arrows indicate the direction of blood flow.

The IABP thus promotes systemic blood flow in two ways: by increasing the driving pressure for systemic blood flow in the aorta and by reducing the impedance to ventricular ejection during systole.

Indications & Contraindications

In general, IABP support is indicated when cardiac pump failure is life-threatening and either pump function is expected to improve spontaneously, or a corrective procedure is planned. Most cases of IABP support are for cardiogenic shock following cardiopulmonary bypass surgery or acute myocardial infarction (45,46). Other indications include unstable angina, acute mitral insufficiency, and planned cardiac transplantation.

Contraindications to IABP support include aortic insufficiency, aortic dissection, renal insufficiency, and a recently-placed (within 12 months) prosthetic graft in the thoracic aorta (46).

Complications

The incidence of complications from IABP support varies in different reports from 10 to 50%, with serious complications reported in 5 to 25% of cases (46–48). The most common and feared complication is leg ischemia, which is reported in as many as 25% of cases (47,48). Leg ischemia can involve the ipsilateral or contralateral leg and can appear while the catheter is in place or within hours after the catheter is removed. Most cases are the result of *in-situ* thrombosis at the catheter insertion site, and about 75% of cases require surgical thrombectomy to restore limb flow (47,48).

The risk of leg ischemia mandates close monitoring of both distal pulses and sensorimotor function in both legs. Loss of distal pulses alone does not always mandate removal of the balloon catheter. If IABP support is life-sustaining and sensorimotor function in both legs is intact, the device can be left in place as long as sensorimotor function in the legs is carefully monitored (48). Loss of sensorimotor function in the legs should always prompt immediate removal of the device.

Other complications of IABP support include spinal cord ischemia, visceral ischemia, renal insufficiency, catheter-related infection, balloon rupture, arterial injury, peripheral neuropathy, and pseudoaneurysm (46–48).

Ventricular Assist Devices

A ventricular assist device (VAD) is a pump (usually nonpulsatile) that is placed in parallel with either the right ventricle (RVAD), the left ventricle (LVAD), or both ventricles (BiVAD) (49–51). The pump is adjusted to provide a total systemic flow of 2.0 to 3.0 L/min/m^2. The use of VADs is limited by the need for intraoperative placement: most are used for cardiogenic shock following cardiopulmonary bypass surgery. The duration of postoperative support is one to 4 days. Complications occur in over 50% of patients and most often include bleeding or systemic embolism. Most patients can never be weaned from pump support, but as many as one-third of patients progress and outlive the need for pump support (51). VADs are also used for long-term support (as long as one year) in cardiac transplant candidates, and newer devices can be used outside the hospital environment.

THE FUTURE

The treatment of acute, decompensated heart failure is basically the same today as it was 20 years ago. This is a concern because **none of the hemodynamic drugs used to treat acute heart failure has demonstrated the**

ability to alter the clinical course of the illness (52). The problem may be that the hemodynamic modulation of heart failure does not protect the myocardium from ongoing damage or decay. This concern has led to changes in the management of chronic heart failure, where the emphasis is shifting from the use of drugs that improve hemodynamic status (e.g., vasodilators) to the use of drugs that protect the myocardium from injury (e.g., β-blockers). A similar **focus on cardioprotection is now being recommended for the management of acute heart failure** (52).

Levosimendan

Levosimendan is an intravenous inodilator that augments cardiac output via positive inotropic and systemic vasodilator actions (53). This drug is unique because animal studies demonstrate its ability to protect the myocardium from ischemic injury (54). Furthermore, early clinical trials indicate that treatment of acute heart failure with levosimendan has a survival benefit (53). Levosimendan is not currently approved for clinical use in the United States, but this will be remedied quickly if the survival benefit in early clinical trials is corroborated.

A FINAL WORD

The approach to advanced or decompensated heart failure in the ICU is best guided by invasive hemodynamic measurements and by the type of heart failure involved (systolic, diastolic, left-sided, or right-sided failure). The following points deserve emphasis.

1. The combination of an increase in ventricular filling pressure and a decrease in cardiac output will identify decompensated heart failure but will not distinguish between systolic and diastolic heart failure.
2. The management of acute, decompensated heart failure should augment cardiac output and reduce ventricular filling pressures while producing little or no increase in myocardial O_2 consumption.
3. Diuretic therapy with intravenous furosemide can be counterproductive in acute, decompensated (low output) heart failure because cardiac output is often adversely affected. Diuretic therapy should not play a major role in the management of acute heart failure, particularly if the failure is due to diastolic dysfunction.
4. If cardiogenic shock is identified, mechanical cardiac support should be initiated as soon as possible, if indicated.

Remember that the current management of acute heart failure is designed to treat the hemodynamic consequences of heart failure and is not directed at the pathologic process in the myocardium. While this approach can achieve temporary hemodynamic improvement, it may not improve survival or otherwise alter the course of the cardiac pathology.

REFERENCES

Reviews

1. American Heart Association. Heart Disease and Stroke Statistics – 2005 Update. Dallas, TX: American Heart Association, 2005.
2. Nieminen MS, Harjola V-P. Definition and etiology of acute heart failure syndromes. Am J Cardiol 2005;96(Suppl):5G–10G.
3. Nohria A, Mielniczuk LM, Stevenson LW. Evaluation and monitoring of patients with acute heart failure syndromes. Am J Cardiol 2005;96(Suppl):32G–40G.
4. The Task Force on Acute Heart Failure of the European Society of Cardiology. Guidelines on the diagnosis and treatment of heart failure. European Society of Cardiology Web Site. Available at www.escardio.org.
5. Jain P, Massie BM, Gattis WA, et al. Current medical treatment for the exacerbation of chronic heart failure resulting in hospitalization. Am Heart J 2003;145:S3–S17.

Diastolic Heart Failure

6. Zile MR, Baicu CF, Gaasch WH. Diastolic heart failure – Abnormalities in active relaxation and passive stiffness of the left ventricle. New Engl J Med 2004;350:1953–1959.
7. Aurigemma GP, Gaasch WH. Diastolic heart failure. New Engl J Med 2004;351:1097–1015.
8. Numi Y, Haki M, Ishiguro Y, et al. Determination of right ventricular function by transesophageal echocardiography: impact of proximal right coronary artery stenosis. J Clin Anesthesia 2004;16:104–110.

Right Heart Failure

9. Hurford WE, Zapol WM. The right ventricle and critical illness: a review of anatomy, physiology, and clinical evaluation of its function. Intensive Care Med 1988;14:448–457.
10. Isner JM. Right ventricular myocardial infarction. JAMA 1988;259:712–718.
11. Vincent JL, Thirion M, Brimioulle S, et al. Thermodilution measurement of right ventricular ejection fraction with a modified pulmonary artery catheter. Intensive Care Med 1986;12:33–38.
12. Robotham JL, Takala M, Berman M, et al. Ejection fraction revisited. Anesthesiology 1991;74:172–183.
13. Boldt J, Kling D, Moosdorf R, Hempelmann G. Influence of acute volume loading on right ventricular function after cardiopulmonary bypass. Crit Care Med 1989;17:518–521.

B-Type Natriuretic Peptide

14. Maisel AS, Wanner EC. Measuring BNP levels in the diagnosis and treatment of CHF. J Crit Illness 2002;17:434–442.
15. Maisel AS, Krishnaswamy P, Nomak RM, et al. Rapid measurement of B-type natriuretic peptide in the emergency diagnosis of heart failure. New Engl J Med 2002;347:161–167.

16. Dao Q, Krishnaswamy P, Kazanegra R, et al. Utility of B-type natriuretic peptide (BNP) in the diagnosis of CHF in an urgent care setting. J Am Coll Cardiol 2001;37:379–385.
17. Takami Y, Horio T, Iwashima Y, et al. Diagnostic and prognostic value of plasma brain natriuretic peptide in non-dialysis-dependent CRF. Am J Kidney Dis 2004;44:420–428.
18. Charpentier J, Luyt C-E, Fulla Y, et al. Brain natriuretic peptide: a marker of myocardial dysfunction and prognosis during severe sepsis. Crit Care Med 2004;32:660–665.

Management Strategies

19. Bayram M, De Luca L, Massie B, Gheorghiade M. Reassessment of dobutamine, dopamine, and milrinone in the management of acute heart failure syndromes. Am J Cardiol 2005;96(Suppl):47G–58G.
20. Stough WG, O'Connor CM, Gheorghiade M. Overview of current noninodilator therapies for acute heart failure syndromes. Am J Cardiol 2005;96(Suppl): 41G–46G.
21. Chatterjee K, De Marco T. Role of nonglycosidic inotropic agents: indications, ethics, and limitations. Med Clin N Am 2003;87:391–418.
22. Flaherty JT, Magee PA, Gardner TL, et al. Comparison of intravenous nitroglycerin and sodium nitroprusside for treatment of acute hypertension developing after coronary artery bypass surgery. Circulation 1982;65:1072–1077.
23. Robin ED, McCauley R. Nitroprusside-related cyanide poisoning. Time (long past due) for urgent, effective interventions. Chest 1992;102:1842–1845.
24. Franciosa JA. Optimal left heart filling pressure during nitroprusside infusion for congestive heart failure. Am J Med 1983;74:457–464.
25. Samuels LE, Darze ES. Management of acute cardiogenic shock. Cardiol Clin 2003;21:43–49.
26. Davidson RM. Hemodynamic effects of furosemide in acute myocardial infarction. Circulation 1971;54(Suppl II):156.
27. Kiely J, Kelly DT, Taylor DR, Pitt B. The role of furosemide in the treatment of left ventricular dysfunction associated with acute myocardial infarction. Circulation 1973;58:581–587.
28. Mond H, Hunt D, Sloman G. Haemodynamic effects of frusemide in patients suspected of having acute myocardial infarction. Br Heart J 1974;36:44–53.
29. Nelson GIC, Ahuja RC, Silke B, et al. Haemodynamic advantages of isosorbide dinitrate over frusemide in acute heart failure following myocardial infarction. Lancet 1983a;i:730–733.
30. Nelson GIC, Ahula RC, Silke B, et al. Haemodynamic effects of frusemide and its influence on repetitive volume loading in acute myocardial infarction. Eur Heart J 1983b;4:706–711.
31. Francis GS, Siegel RM, Goldsmith SR, et al. Acute vasoconstrictor response to intravenous furosemide in patients with chronic congestive heart failure. Ann Intern Med 1986;103:1–6.
32. Brater DC. Resistance to loop diuretics: why it happens and what to do about it. Drugs 1985;30:427–443.
33. van Meyel JJM, Smits P, Russell FGM, et al. Diuretic efficiency of furosemide during continuous administration versus bolus injection in healthy volunteers. Clin Pharmacol Ther 1992;51:440–444.

34. Howard PA, Dunn MI. Aggressive diuresis for severe heart failure in the elderly. Chest 2001;119:807–810.
35. Aurigemma GP, Gaasch WH. Diastolic heart failure. New Engl J Med 2004; 351:1097–1105.
36. Vasodilation in the Management of Acute CHF (VMAC) Investigators. Intravenous nesiritide vs nitroglycerin for treatment of decompensated congestive heart failure. JAMA 2002;287:1531–1540.
37. Sackner-Bernstein JD, Kowalski M, Fox M, Aaronson K. Short-term risk of death after treatment with nesiritide for decompensated heart failure. JAMA 2005;293:1900–1905.
38. Tamborini G, Pepi M, Susini G, et al. Reversal of cardiogenic shock and severe mitral regurgitation through verapamil in hypertensive hypertrophic cardiomyopathy. Chest 1993;104:319–324.
39. Nishimura R, Schwartz RS, Holmes DR, Tajik J. Failure of calcium channel blockers to improve ventricular relaxation in humans. J Am Coll Cardiol 1993;21:182–188.
40. Reuse C, Vinvcent JL, Pinsky MR. Measurement of right ventricular volumes during fluid challenge. Chest 1990;98:1450–1454.
41. Vincent RL, Reuse C, Kahn RJ. Effects on right ventricular function of a change from dopamine to dobutamine in critically ill patients. Crit Care Med 1988;16:659–662.
42. Dell'Italia LJ, Starling MR, Blumhardt R, et al. Comparative effects of volume loading, dobutamine and nitroprusside in patients with predominant right ventricular infarction. Circulation 1986;72:1327–1335.

Mechanical Cardiac Support

43. Kantrowitz A, Tjonneland S, Freed PS, et al. Initial clinical experience with intraaortic balloon pumping in cardiogenic shock. JAMA 1968;203:113–118.
44. Williams DO, Korr KS, Gewirtz H, Most AS. The effect of intra-aortic balloon counterpulsation on regional myocardial blood flow and oxygen consumption in the presence of coronary artery stenosis with unstable angina. Circulation 1982;3:593–597.
45. Stevenson LW, Kormos RL. Mechanical cardiac support 2000: current applications and future trial design. J Am Coll Cardiol 2000;37:340–370.
46. Kantrowitz A, Cordona RR, Freed PS. Percutaneous intra-aortic balloon counterpulsation. Crit Care Clin 1992;8:819–837.
47. Baldyga AP. Complications of intra-aortic balloon pump therapy. In Maccioli GA, ed. Intra-aortic balloon pump therapy. Philadelphia: Williams & Wilkins, 1997, 127–162.
48. Mackenzie DJ, Wagner WH, Kulber DA, et al. Vascular complications of the intra- aortic balloon pump. Am J Surg 1992;164:517–521.
49. Bolno PB, Kresh Y. Physiologic and hemodynamic basis of ventricular assist devices. Cardiol Clin 2003;21:15–27.
50. Killen DA, Piehler JM, Borkon AM, et al. Bio-Medicus ventricular assist device for salvage of cardiac surgical patients. Ann Thorac Surg 1991;52:230–235.
51. Lee WA, Gillinov AM, Cameron DE, et al. Centrifugal ventricular assist device for support of the failing heart after cardiac surgery. Crit Care Med 1993;21:1186–1191.

The Future

52. Maytin M, Colucci WS. Cardioprotection: A new paradigm in the management of acute heart failure syndromes. Am J Cardiol 2005;96(Suppl):26G–31G.
53. Gheorghiade M, Teerlionk JR, Mebazaa A. Pharmacology of new agents for acute heart failure syndromes. Am J Cardiol 2005;96(Suppl):68G–73G.
54. Kersten JR, Montgomery MW, Pagel PL, Waltier DC. Levosimendan, a new positive inotropic drug, decreases myocardial infarct size via activation of K_{ATP} channels. Anesth Analg 2000;90:5–11.

Chapter 15

CARDIAC ARREST

Medicine cannot, except over a short period, increase the population of the world.

Bertrand Russell

In 1960, an article was published in the *Journal of the American Medical Association* that would eventually change the way we approach the dying process. The article, titled "Closed-Chest Cardiac Massage" (1), was the birth of what is known today as *cardiopulmonary resuscitation* (CPR). Despite being unsuccessful in a majority of attempts (see Figure 15.1) (2), CPR has grown to become a universally accepted practice. In fact, it is considered a human right and is withheld only upon request.

This chapter describes the mechanical and pharmacologic interventions involved in the management of cardiac arrest. Much of the information is taken from the most recent American Heart Association Guidelines for Cardiopulmonary Resuscitation, which are available on the Internet (see Reference 3).

BASIC LIFE SUPPORT

Basic life support has three components: achieving a patent airway, delivering periodic lung inflations, and promoting circulation with chest compressions. These components are often referred to as the *ABCs* of life support (*A*irway, *B*reathing, and *C*irculation).

Airway Patency

Tracheal intubation (which is considered a component of advanced life support) is the preferred method of maintaining a patent airway in unconscious patients with cardiac arrest. Prior to intubation, an oropharyngeal airway (an S-shaped device passed over the tongue and into the pharynx) can be used to keep the flaccid tongue from falling back and occluding the oropharynx. Delays to intubation should be minimized whenever possible.

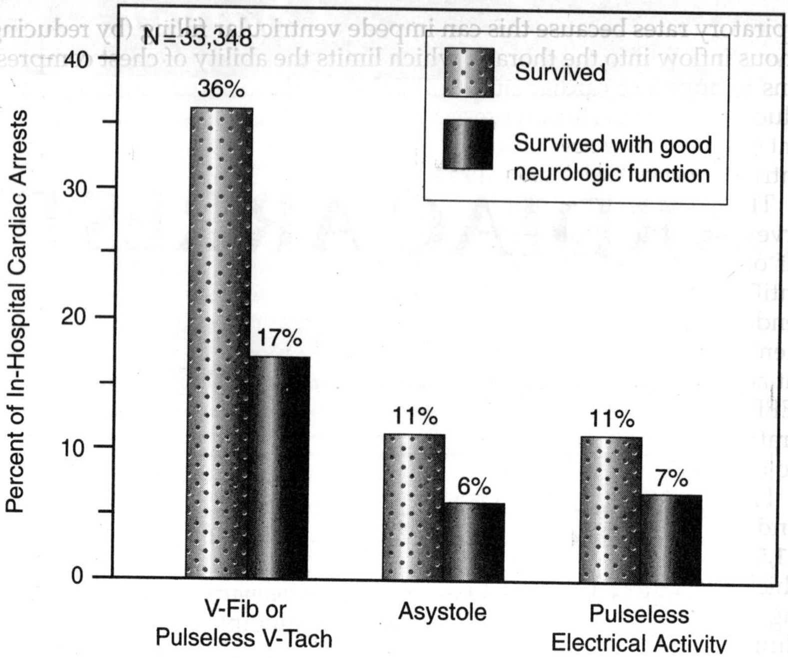

FIGURE 15.1 Outcomes of in-hospital cardiac arrest (grouped according to initial cardiac rhythm) reported by the National Registry of Cardiopulmonary Resuscitation, which includes 253 hospitals in the U.S. and Canada. N = total number of subjects included in the report; *V-Fib* = ventricular fibrillation, *V-Tach* = ventricular tachycardia. (From Reference 2.)

Ventilation

Lung inflations are usually delivered with a self-inflating bag that is connected at one end to a continuous flow of oxygen, and at the other end, to a face mask or endotracheal tube. The lungs are inflated by compressing the bag with one or both hands (one-way valves at each end of the bag ensure that the volume is directed to the patient). Following each lung inflation, the bag re-inflates spontaneously (in about one second). The current guidelines for CPR state that **the lungs should be inflated 8 to 10 times per minute without pausing for chest compressions, and the inflation volume should be delivered in one second** (4). This is a slower rate than previously recommended, for reasons described in the next section.

Avoiding Hyperventilation

One of the important discoveries about CPR in recent times is the tendency to over-ventilate patients during CPR and the negative impact of this practice on the success of CPR. The problem is the increase in positive intrathoracic pressure created by large tidal volumes and rapid respiratory rates because this can impede ventricular filling (by reducing venous inflow into the thorax), which limits the ability of chest compressions to augment cardiac output. High intrathoracic pressures can also reduce coronary perfusion pressure (4,5), which is an important determinant of outcome in cardiac arrest. These adverse circulatory effects could contribute to the low survival rates following CPR.

The use of high ventilatory rates is commonplace during CPR. In one survey, ventilatory rates above 20 breaths/min were recorded in over half of the cases of CPR (6), and in another survey, the average rate of ventilation during CPR was 30 breaths/min, which is 3 times the recommended rate (5). Such rapid rates are problematic because there is insufficient time for alveolar emptying after each lung inflation, and the air that accumulated in the lungs creates a positive end-expiratory pressure (PEEP) that adds further to the effects of positive-pressure ventilation on intrathoracic pressures. The PEEP created by rapid breathing, which is also called *intrinsic PEEP*, is described in more detail in Chapter 26.

High inflation volumes are also commonplace during CPR. **The standard ventilation bags used during CPR have a volume capacity of 1,600 mL** when fully inflated (7), and two-handed bag compression (which is standard during CPR) will expel most of this volume into the lungs, at least when the bag is connected to an endotracheal tube (some volume is lost when face masks are used because of the incomplete seal on the face). This is three times greater than the normal tidal volume in an average-sized adult (about 7 mL/kg, or 500 mL in a 70 kg subject). The current guidelines for CPR do not include a specific recommendation for the size of tidal volumes (prior guidelines recommended tidal volumes of 10 to 15 mL/kg, which is excessive), but volumes of 6 to 8 mL/kg seem reasonable. One-handed compression of standard size ventilation bags will expel a volume of about 800 mL (7), and this may be the appropriate method of lung inflation during CPR.

THE INSPIRATORY IMPEDANCE THRESHOLD DEVICE. A specialized valve has been developed that reduces the influence of positive-pressure lung inflations on intrathoracic pressure. When placed between the ventilation bag and the patient, this valve prevents positive pressure lung inflations from entering the thorax during the decompression phase of CPR (the time between chest compressions). This reduces mean intrathoracic pressures and should improve coronary and systemic blood flow during CPR. A small clinical trial using this *inspiratory impedance threshold device* has shown improved short-term survival in patients with pulseless electrical activity (8). Larger trials are underway.

In summary, hyperventilation is a common and potentially life-threatening problem during CPR. **To minimize the adverse circulatory effects of hyperventilation, avoid using lung inflation rates above 10 breaths/min,** and consider using smaller-volume bag compressions to limit tidal volumes. If the cardiac arrest occurs in a patient with an indwelling arterial catheter, you can observe the influence of different ventilatory rates and volumes on the blood pressure to determine if ventilation is adversely affecting systemic blood flow.

Chest Compressions

Chest compressions are performed by placing the heel of the dominant hand on the sternum in the center of the chest, with the non-dominant hand on top. The elbows should be locked so that both arms are kept straight, and the shoulders should be positioned directly above the point of contact. The sternum is then depressed at least 1.5 to 2 inches inward. When the compression is released, the sternum should be allowed to recoil completely before the next compression. **The recommended rate of chest compressions is at least 100 per minute (4), and each compression should be maintained for half of the total compression–release cycle.** With a lung inflation rate of 10 breaths/minute, the ratio of chest compressions to lung inflations is 10:1.

Although this sounds simple enough, maintaining a rate of 100 compressions per minute requires one compression every 0.6 seconds, which is not possible to perform accurately without a stop watch! In any event, allowing **full recoil of the chest wall after each compression is an important feature** because the decompression phase of CPR (the time between chest compressions) is the time when venous blood can return to the heart.

ADVANCED LIFE SUPPORT

Advanced life support (also called advanced cardiac life support, ACLS) includes a variety of interventions, including airway intubation, mechanical ventilation, defibrillation, and drugs given during cardiac arrest (9). The material in this section focuses on the use of defibrillation and cardiac arrest drugs to manage patients with pulseless cardiac arrest. This is summarized in Figure 15.2, which is taken from the most recent (2005) guidelines published by the American Heart Association (10).

Defibrillation

Direct-current (DC) cardioversion is the treatment of choice for ventricular tachycardia (V-tach) and ventricular fibrillation (V-fib), and it is the single most effective resuscitative measure for improving survival in cardiac arrest (see Figure 15.1). **The time elapsed from the cardiac arrest to the first electric shock is the most important factor in determining survival** (11,12). This is demonstrated in Figure 15.3. Note that 40% of patients survived when the first shock was delivered 5 minutes after the arrest, while only 10% of patients survived if defibrillation was delayed until 20 minutes after the arrest. These results emphasize the importance of avoiding delays in delivering the first electric shock.

Protocol

Some of the important recommendations for defibrillation are outlined in Table 15.1. The effective strength of electric shocks (which is expressed in units of energy, or joules) depends on the type of waveform delivered. Newer defibrillators deliver biphasic shocks, which are effective at lower

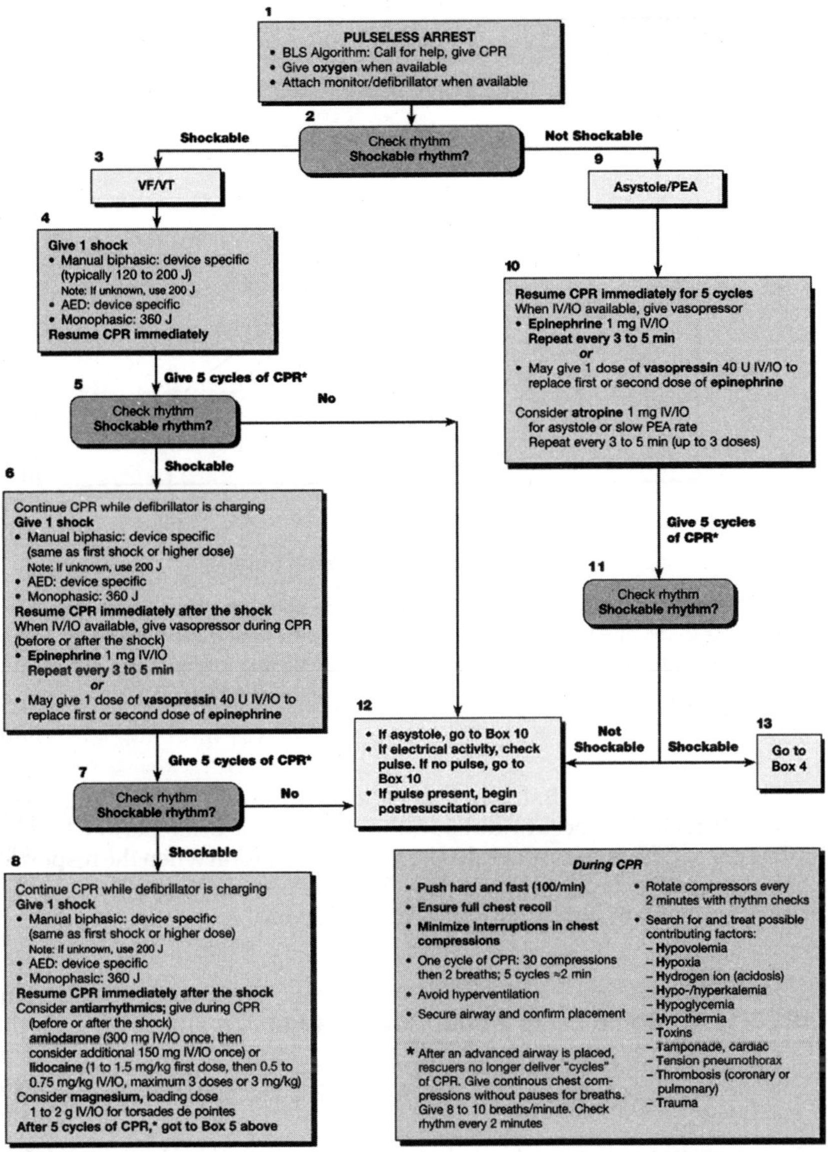

FIGURE 15.2 Algorithm for the management of pulseless cardiac arrest due to ventricular fibrillation (*VF*), ventricular tachycardia (*VT*), pulseless electrical activity (*PEA*), and ventricular asystole. From the 2005 American Heart Association Guidelines for CPR (see Reference 10).

energy levels than the monophasic shocks used by older defibrillators. **The recommended energy level for the first shock is 200 joules for biphasic shocks** (unless otherwise specified by the defibrillator manufacturer) **and 360 joules for monophasic shocks** (11).

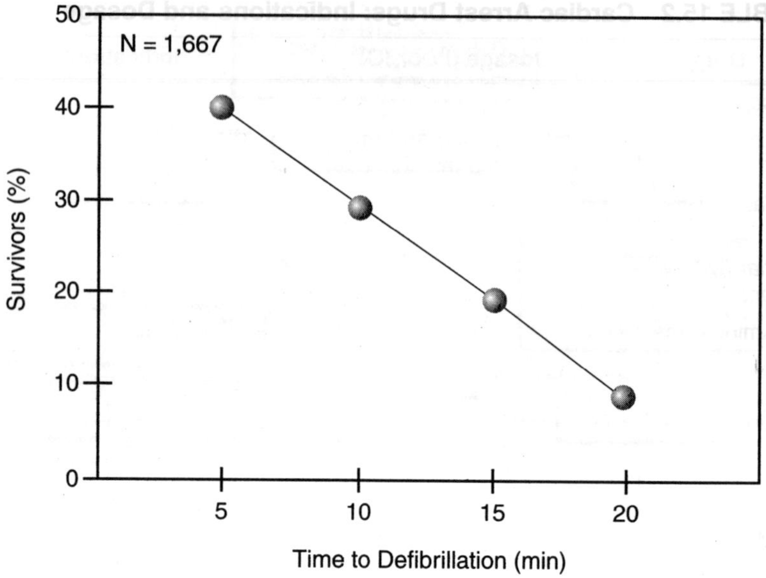

FIGURE 15.3 The relationship between survival rate and time elapsed from the cardiac arrest to the onset of defibrillation in patients with ventricular fibrillation. N = number of subjects studied. (From Larsen MP et al. Predicting survival from out-of-hospital cardiac arrest: a graphic model. Ann Emerg Med 1993;22:1652.)

The timing of the first shock depends on the setting. For pulseless V-fib or V-tach that occurs outside the hospital, a brief period (1.5 to 3 minutes) of CPR is recommended before defibrillation when the response interval is greater than 5 minutes (11). Otherwise (including all in-hospital arrests), immediate defibrillation is recommended.

TABLE 15.1 Some Facts About Defibrillation

1. If the cardiac arrest occurs outside the hospital and the response time is > 5 minutes, a brief period (1.5–3 min) of CPR is recommended prior to the first shock.
2. The recommended energy level of each shock is determined by the type of waveform.
   a) For biphasic waveforms, use 200 joules.
   b) For monophasic waveforms, use 360 joules.
3. There is no evidence that increasing the energy level in successive shocks is more effective than maintaining the energy level of the inititial shock.
4. Because delivering each shock requires an interrruption of CPR (which can be detrimental), a single-shock strategy may be preferable to the traditional triple-shock strategy.

From Reference 11.

TABLE 15.2 Cardiac Arrest Drugs: Indications and Dosage

Drug	Dosage (IV or IO)	Indications
Vasopressors:		
Epinephrine	1 mg first dose and repeat every 3 to 5 min if needed.	Asystole, PEA, and shock-resistant VF or VT.
Vasopressin	40 units as a single dose.	Can replace the first or second dose of epinephrine.
Antiarrhythmic agents		
Amiodarone	300 mg first dose, then 150 mg once if needed.	VF or pulseless VT that is refractory to defibrillation and vasopressors.
Lidocaine	1–1.5 mg/kg first dose, then 0.5–0.75 mg/kg to a total of 3 doses or 3 mg/kg.	Alternative to amiodarone.
Magnesium	1–2 g over 5 min	Pulseless polymorphic VT (torsades de pointes) with prolonged QT interval.
Atropine	1 mg first dose. Repeat every 3 to 5 min if needed to total of 3 doses.	Bradyarrhythmias, or as an adjunct to vasopressors for asystole and PEA.

From Reference 10.
Abbreviations: IV = intravenous, IO = intraosseous, VF = ventricular fibrillation, VT = ventricular tachycardia, PEA = pulseless electrical activity.

If the first shock is ineffective, two additional shocks can be attempted (don't forget to perform CPR between successive shocks). There is no evidence that increasing the energy levels in successive shocks is more effective than maintaining the energy level of the initial shock. If the second shock is unsuccessful, a vasopressor should be administered (see Table 15.2): either epinephrine (1 mg IV, repeated every 3 to 5 minutes) or vasopressin (40 units IV as a single dose) is recommended. If the V-fib or V-tach persists after the third shock, an antiarrhythmic agent should be administered: either amiodarone (300 mg IV, followed by 150 mg IV if needed) or lidocaine (1 to 1.5 mg/kg IV as first dose, followed by 0.5 to 0.75 mg/kg IV if needed up to a total dose of 3 mg/kg) is recommended. Because delivering each electric shock requires an interruption of CPR (which can be detrimental), **a single-shock strategy may be preferable to the traditional triple-shock strategy** (11).

Automated External Defibrillators

The introduction of the automated external defibrillator (AED) represents a significant advance in the use of DC cardioversion. The benefit of the AED is its ability to analyze a cardiac rhythm and determine if cardioversion is appropriate. When the two AED electrode pads are placed on the chest (one on the right anterior chest wall and the other on the left lateral chest wall), sensors in the pads act like precordial leads to record the cardiac rhythm. The AED analyzes the rhythm and then displays a prompt informing the operator if defibrillation is indicated (the operator does not see the cardiac rhythm). If defibrillation is indicated, the operator simply presses a button to deliver the shock. The machine automatically selects the strength of the pulse. After the shock is delivered, the machine will again analyze the cardiac rhythm and determine if a second shock is necessary. This sequence can continue until three shocks are delivered.

The benefit of the AED is the ability of untrained personnel (who are unable to interpret the cardiac rhythm) to initiate defibrillation (11). It also saves the time spent preparing to record the cardiac rhythm. These devices have been used primarily for cardiac arrests that occur outside the hospital, but they are also available in many hospitals as well. The ability to deliver rapid DC cardioversion should make AEDs popular in virtually all settings.

Drug Administration During CPR

Intravenous Sites

Peripheral veins are preferred to central veins for drug administration during CPR because cannulation of peripheral veins does not require interruption of CPR (10). Drugs given via peripheral veins should always be injected as a bolus, followed by a 20 mL bolus of an intravenous fluid (10). The extremity should be elevated for 10 to 20 seconds to facilitate drug delivery to the heart. If the initial drug injection is unsuccessful, central venous cannulation can be performed for subsequent drug administration. This latter maneuver reduces the transit time for drugs to reach the heart by 1 to 2 minutes (10).

Alternate Sites

When venous access is not readily available, drugs can be delivered by puncturing a marrow cavity (usually in the sternum) or by injection through an endotracheal tube. **The intraosseous route is preferred to the airway route** because drug absorption from the airways is erratic (10). However, the airway route seems favored by most critical care practitioners (probably because it is easier), at least in adults.

ENDOTRACHEAL DRUG ADMINISTRATION. The drugs that can be given via the endotracheal route are atropine, epinephrine, vasopressin, and lidocaine. **The endotracheal dose of each drug should be 2 to 2.5 times the recommended intravenous dose (10), and injection of the drug into the endotracheal tube is as effective as more distal injection into the airways** (9). All drugs injected into the airways should be diluted in 5 to 10 mL of water or isotonic saline. Water may be the preferred diluent because of enhanced drug absorption (9,10).

Vasopressor Drugs

One of the management goals in cardiac arrest is to promote systemic vasoconstriction and thereby direct blood flow to the coronary and cerebral circulations. Two vasopressor drugs are used for this purpose: epinephrine and vasopressin. As shown in Figure 15.2, vasopressor drugs are recommended for most cases of pulseless cardiac arrest, including those due to asystole, pulseless electrical activity, and V-fib or V-tach that persists after the initial defibrillation attempt. Despite the almost universal use of vasopressors in cardiac arrest, **there is no evidence that vasopressor drugs improve survival in cardiac arrest (10)**.

Epinephrine

Epinephrine (which is a β-receptor agonist in low doses and an α-receptor agonist in high doses) is the traditional vasopressor used in cardiac arrest. **The recommended intravenous dose of epinephrine is 1 mg (10 mL of a 1:10,000 solution), repeated every 3 to 5 minutes if necessary.** The recommended dose for endotracheal injection is 2 to 2.5 mg. Epinephrine is poorly absorbed from the airways, and the reduced serum concentration can produce predominant β-receptor stimulation and unwanted cardiac stimulation. For this reason, endotracheal injection of epinephrine is not advised (10).

Vasopressin

Vasopressin is a non-adrenergic vasoconstrictor that can be used as a single dose (40 units given as an intravenous bolus) to replace the first or second dose of epinephrine (see Figure 15.2). This strategy has two potential benefits: (1) vasopressin acts as a cerebral vasodilator, and (2) there is no risk of unwanted cardiac stimulation from epinephrine. However, several clinical trials have shown **no survival benefit when vasopressin is substituted for epinephrine** (13), and vasopressin causes coronary vasoconstriction (10), which is a reason to avoid its use. Vasopressin should be considered when the endotracheal route is used for drug delivery because epinephrine can cause unwanted cardiac stimulation when administered via this route.

Antiarrhythmic Agents

Amiodarone

Clinical studies involving adults with out-of-hospital cardiac arrests due to refractory V-fib have shown that a single dose of intravenous amiodarone given in the field improves survival to hospital admission when compared to placebo (14) or intravenous lidocaine (15). Unfortunately, amiodarone did not improve survival to hospital discharge in either study. **Despite having no long-term survival benefit, intravenous amiodarone is now recommended for cases of V-fib and pulseless V-tach that are refractory to defibrillation and vasopressor drugs** (10). The initial dose is 300 mg (intravenous or intraosseous), followed by a second dose of 150 mg if needed (the time between doses is not specified).

Amiodarone can produce hypotension and bradycardia (14), but these side effects have been minimized by a new aqueous formulation of amiodarone that does not contain vasoactive solvents (10).

Lidocaine

Intravenous lidocaine has been the traditional antiarrhythmic agent used for shock-resistant cases of V-fib and pulseless V-tach. However, because amiodarone seems to produce better results for short-term survival (15), **lidocaine is now recommended only as an alternative to amiodarone** (10). The recommended dosage of lidocaine is 1 to 1.5 mg/kg (intravenous or intraosseous) as an initial dose, then 0.5 to 0.75 mg/kg every 5 to 10 minutes if needed, to a maximum of 3 doses or 3 mg/kg. Despite its long history of use in cardiac arrest, lidocaine has no documented impact on survival (or any measure of clinical outcome) in cardiac arrest (10).

Magnesium

Intravenous magnesium is effective in terminating polymorphic V-tach (also called "*torsades de pointes*") when this arrhythmia is associated with a prolonged QT interval. For cardiac arrest associated with this rhythm, the magnesium dose (intravenous or intraosseous) is 1 to 2 grams infused over 5 minutes (10). The recognition and treatment of torsades de pointes is described in Chapter 18.

Atropine

Atropine is a well-known anticholinergic agent that is recommended as an adjunct to vasopressor therapy for cardiac arrest associated with asystole or pulseless electrical activity (see Figure 15.2). The intravenous dose is 1 mg, which can be repeated every 3 to 5 minutes to a total dose of 3 mg (which is the dose that produces complete vagal blockade) (10). The rationale for the use of atropine in this situation is the possibility that asystole or pulseless electrical activity could be precipitated by heightened vagal tone. The efficacy of atropine in these conditions is unproven.

MONITORING DURING CPR

The goal of the resuscitation effort is to restore adequate perfusion of the vital organs, particularly the heart and central nervous system. Unfortunately, it is not possible to directly measure blood flow (global or regional) during CPR, so surrogate measurements are used. These measurements, which are described below, are limited and sometimes misleading.

Arterial Pulse and Pressure

Despite their popularity, **the arterial pulse and pressure are not reliable markers of blood flow during CPR**. This is demonstrated by the pressure tracings in Figure 15.4. The tracings in this figure were recorded

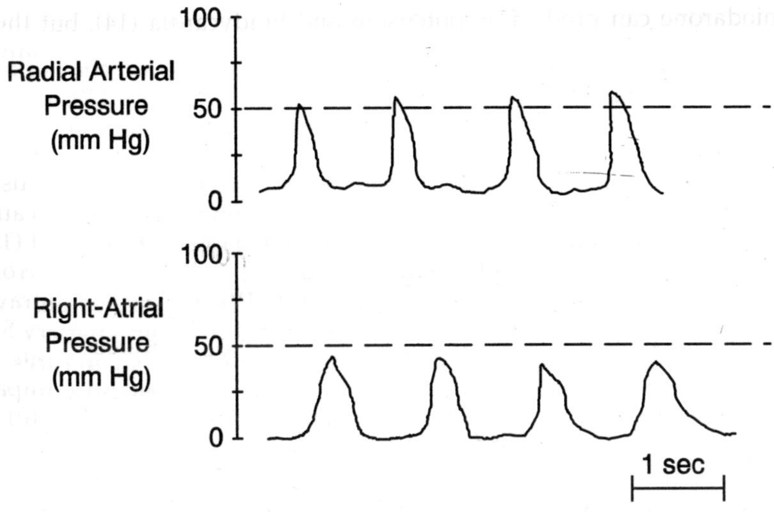

FIGURE 15.4 The influence of chest compressions on arterial and central venous (right atrial) pressure tracings in a patient with asystolic cardiac arrest. The chest compressions produce an arterial pressure wave, but the arterial and right atrial pressures are similar, so there is no pressure gradient to drive systemic blood flow.

from a patient who had an indwelling radial artery catheter and central venous catheter and had just been pronounced dead from asystolic cardiac arrest. The tracings show the effect of chest compressions on the arterial pressure and central venous (right atrial) pressure. If the arterial blood pressure is considered in isolation, the size of the pressure pulse (50 mm Hg systolic pressure) would be interpreted as indicating that the chest compressions were successful in promoting systemic blood flow. However, note that the central venous pressure is about the same as the arterial pressure, so there is no pressure gradient between the arterial and venous circuits, and thus there is no blood flow in the systemic circulation. (Remember from Chapter 1 that flow in a tube requires a pressure gradient along the tube). Therefore Figure 15.4 shows that it is possible to have an arterial pulse and blood pressure in the absence of peripheral blood flow during CPR.

Coronary Perfusion Pressure

The pressure gradient that drives coronary blood flow, which is called the coronary perfusion pressure (CPP) is the difference between the aortic diastolic pressure and the right-atrial pressure. Clinical studies have shown that **a CPP (15 mm Hg during CPR is associated with a successful outcome** (16,17). When CPR is performed on a patient with indwelling arterial and central venous catheters, the CPP can be estimated by using the peripheral arterial diastolic pressure as a substitute for the aortic diastolic pressure.

End-Tidal PCO_2

The excretion of carbon dioxide in exhaled gas is a direct function of pulmonary blood flow or cardiac output (see Chapter 2, Figure 2.7), and the partial pressure of CO_2 in end-expiratory gas (the end-tidal PCO_2) can be used as an indirect indicator of the cardiac output generated during CPR (16,18–20). The end-tidal PCO_2 is easily measured at the bedside using commercially-available infrared devices called capnometers that are connected to indwelling endotracheal tubes (see Chapter 20 for a detailed description of the end-tidal PCO_2 measurement).

An increase in end-tidal PCO_2 during CPR can serve as an indication that the resuscitation effort is successful in promoting cardiac output. This is consistent with clinical studies showing that **an increase in end-tidal PCO_2 during CPR is predictive of a successful outcome** (16,18–20). This is demonstrated in Figure 15.5, which shows the changes in end-tidal PCO_2 during CPR in survivors and nonsurvivors of cardiac arrest. As expected, the end-tidal PCO_2 is very low (indicating a low cardiac output) at the onset of CPR in both groups. In patients who survived, the end-tidal PCO_2 more than doubled (from 12 to 31 mm Hg) after 20 minutes of CPR, whereas in the patients who did not survive, the end-tidal PCO_2 decreased during CPR. This demonstrates the value of the end-tidal PCO_2 as a prognostic marker for CPR. A threshold of 10 mm Hg for end-tidal PCO_2 can be used to predict outcome (e.g., **when end-tidal PCO_2 does not rise above 10 mm Hg after 15 to 20 minutes of CPR, the resuscitative effort is unlikely to be successful).**

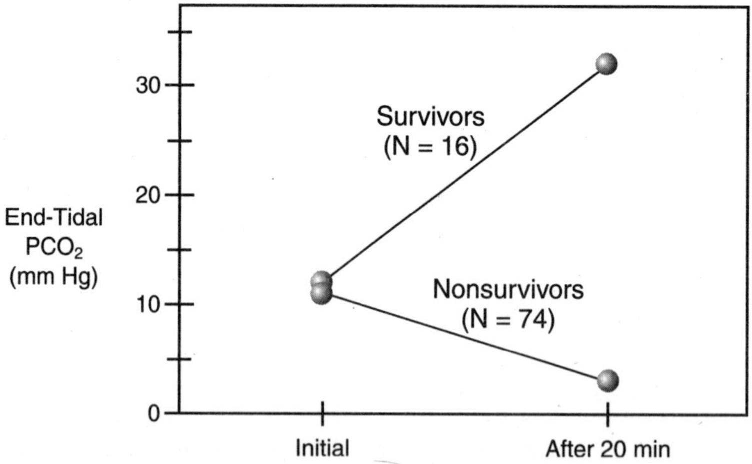

FIGURE 15.5 Changes in end-tidal PCO_2 during CPR in survivors and nonsurvivors of cardiac arrest due to pulseless electrical activity. Data points represent the mean end-tidal PCO_2 for each group. (From Wayne MA, Levine RL, Miller CC. Use of end-tidal carbon dioxide to predict outcome in prehospital cardiac arrest. Ann Emerg Med 1995;25:762–767.)

Venous Blood Gases

Clinical studies have shown that, during CPR, arterial blood gas analysis often reveals a respiratory alkalosis (indicating operator-induced hyperventilation), while venous blood gas analysis shows a metabolic acidosis (indicating systemic hypoperfusion) (21,22). Therefore venous blood gas analysis is more appropriate for evaluating tissue perfusion during CPR. Unfortunately, the time required to perform blood gas analysis limits the value of this test during CPR.

How Long to Resuscitate

There is little doubt that CPR is inappropriately prolonged in a significant percentage of resuscitative efforts. The problem with prolonged CPR is that survivors are often left with severe neurologic deficits. Identifying the appropriate time to discontinue CPR will achieve the optimal goal of CPR, which is to produce survivors who are able to interact with their surroundings and are capable of independent existence.

Ischemic Time and Neurologic Recovery

The risk of functional impairment in any of the major organs is directly related to the duration of the ischemic insult. The ischemic time following cardiac arrest includes the time from onset of the arrest to onset of CPR (arrest time) and the duration of the resuscitative effort (CPR time). The influence of these two time periods on neurologic recovery is shown in

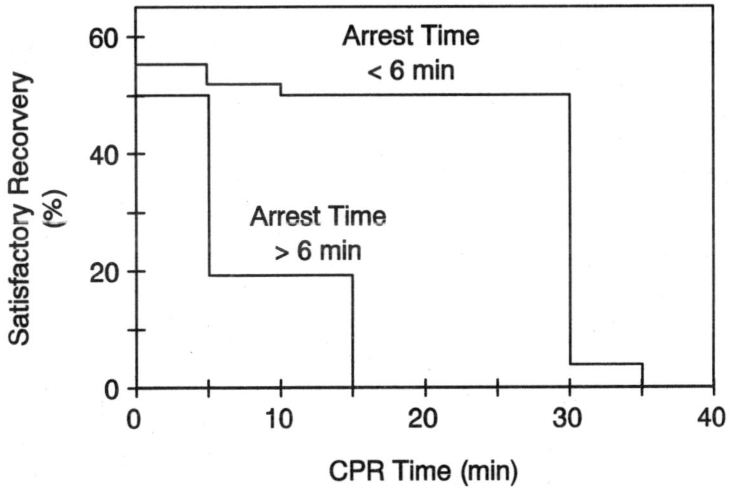

FIGURE 15.6 The incidence of satisfactory neurologic recovery as a function of the time from cardiac arrest to onset of CPR (arrest time), and the duration of the resuscitative effort (CPR time). (From Abramson NS, Safar P, Detre KM, et al. Neurologic recovery after cardiac arrest: effect of duration of ischemia. Crit Care Med 1985;13:930–931.)

Figure 15.6 (23). Note that when the arrest time is less than 6 minutes, at least half of the survivors had a satisfactory neurologic recovery when CPR was continued for as long as 30 minutes. However, if the arrest time exceeded 6 minutes, more than 15 minutes of CPR always produced neurologic impairment in the survivors. Thus if the goal of CPR is to produce functional survivors, then **CPR can be continued for 30 minutes if the time to onset of CPR is less than 6 minutes, but if there is a delay to onset of CPR longer than 6 minutes, CPR should be terminated after 15 minutes.**

POST-RESUSCITATION MANAGEMENT

The immediate goal of CPR is to restore spontaneous circulation, but this does not ensure a satisfactory recovery. This section describes some concerns in the post-resuscitation management that will help to optimize the recovery from cardiac arrest.

Avoiding Fever

Animal studies show that ischemic brain injury is aggravated by increased body temperature (24), and clinical studies show that increased body temperature after CPR is associated with an unfavorable neurologic outcome (25). These studies suggest that **it is wise to avoid increased body temperature following cardiac arrest**. The value of antipyretic therapy after CPR has not been studied, but fever reduction with acetaminophen (10 to 15 mg/kg per dose, 3 to 4 times a day) seems reasonable in patients with incomplete neurologic recovery after cardiac arrest. Acetaminophen must be given enterally and should not be given to patients with hepatic dysfunction. Cooling blankets are problematic because they can induce shivering (which is counterproductive) and can provoke vasospasm in diseased coronary arteries (26).

Therapeutic Hypothermia

Clinical studies have shown that **induced hypothermia can improve neurologic outcome in patients who remain comatose after successful resuscitation of out-of-hospital cardiac arrest due to V-fib or pulseless V-tach** (27,28). External cooling should be considered to improve neurologic function in patients who do not awaken after cardiac arrest, but there are strict eligibility criteria for this intervention. These are listed in Table 15.3, along with important features of the methodology. The hypothermia should be initiated as soon as possible after the resuscitation using an external cooling device. The target body temperature is 32°C to 34°C (89.6°F to 93.2°F), and this should be maintained for no less than 12 hours and no longer than 24 hours (27). Core body temperature can be monitored using tympanic temperatures or bladder temperatures. External cooling can provoke shivering, which is counterproductive because it increases body temperature. Therefore shivering should be suppressed by administering a neuromuscular blocker (e.g., atracurium).

TABLE 15.3 Induced Hypothermia after Cardiac Arrest

Eligible patients

Patients with out-of-hospital cardiac arrest due to VF or pulseless VT who remain comatose after successful resuscitation.

Inclusion criteria

All of the following criteria must be satisfied.

a) Cardiac arrest is cardiac in origin.

b) Body temperature is not reduced.

c) Patient is hemodynamically stable.

d) Patient is intubated and on a ventilator.

Methodology

1. Cooling should begin within 1–2 hr after CPR.
2. Use cooling blanket to achieve a body temperature of 32°C–34°C (89.6°F–93.2°F).
3. Use sedation and neuromuscular blockade to avoid shivering.
4. Watch for hyperkalemia and hyperglycemia during hypothermia.
5. Maintain hypothermia for 24 hr, and then allow passive rewarming.

The information in this table is taken from References 27 and 28.

Hypothermia is associated with hyperkalemia (usually mild and without clinical impact) and hyperglycemia (27), so attention to the serum potassium and glucose is warranted during hypothermia. Rewarming from hypothermia should be passive.

Therapeutic hypothermia, as indicated, has been adopted in many ICUs, but only a limited number of patients are eligible for this intervention by current criteria. In one study, only 8% of patients who survived cardiac arrest were suitable for treatment (27). Studies are needed to determine if the eligibility criteria for this intervention can be expanded.

Glycemic Control

Several clinical studies have documented that hyperglycemia following cardiac arrest is associated with a poor neurologic outcome (29,30). However, there are no studies to show that control of hyperglycemia after cardiac arrest improves neurologic outcome. Strict control of hyperglycemia is, however, associated with reduced morbidity and mortality in ICU patients (31). Based on these observations, the most recent American Heart Association Guidelines for CPR state that **strict control of blood glucose levels is a reasonable practice in the post-resuscitation period** (30). As an adjunct to this practice, **dextrose-containing intravenous solutions should be avoided** whenever possible. Remember that hypoglycemia can also be injurious to the central nervous system, so careful monitoring of blood glucose is necessary during aggressive management of hyperglycemia.

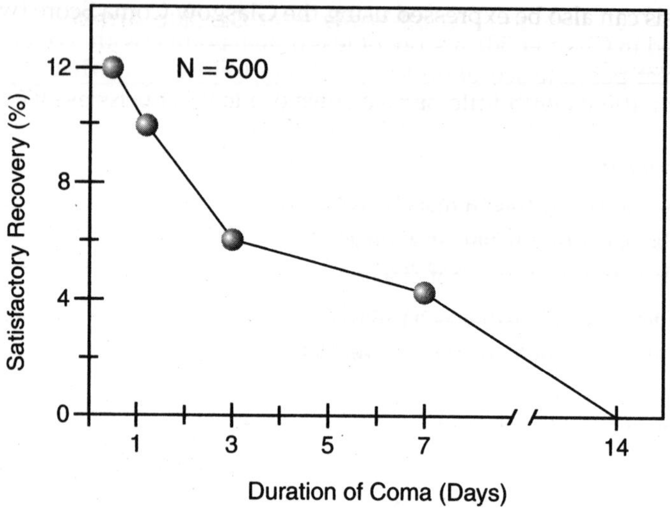

FIGURE 15.7 The relationship between the duration of non-traumatic coma and the incidence of favorable neurologic recovery. N = number of study subjects. (From Levy DE, Caronna JJ, Singer BH, et al. Prognosis in non-traumatic coma. Ann Intern Med 1981;94:293–301.)

Predicting Neurologic Recovery

In patients who do not awaken immediately after CPR, the single most important determination (for families as well as physicians) is the likelihood of neurologic recovery. The following are some prognostic factors that can help identify patients who are likely (and unlikely) to achieve a satisfactory neurologic recovery.

Duration of Coma

Failure to regain consciousness after CPR has prognostic significance if the coma persists for longer than 4 to 6 hours (32). The relation between prolonged coma and neurologic recovery is demonstrated in Figure 15.7 (32). The data in this graph are summarized in the following statements:

1. Only a small percentage of patients will recover fully if their coma persists for longer than 4 to 6 hours after cardiac arrest.
2. If a patient is not awake 24 hours after a cardiac arrest, there is only a 10% chance of satisfactory neurologic recovery. This is reduced to a 5% chance of recovery if the coma persists for 72 hours after CPR.
3. There is virtually no chance for a full neurologic recovery for a patient who is comatose 2 weeks after a cardiac arrest.

Although full neurologic recovery is unlikely for patients with coma 24 hours after cardiac arrest, most ICU physicians seem to use the 72 hour point of persistent coma to inform families of the poor prognosis.

Prognosis can also be expressed using the Glasgow Coma Score (which is described in Chapter 50): a score of less than 5 points (with 3 points being the lowest possible score) on the third day following cardiac arrest will identify patients with little or no chance of neurologic recovery (33).

Other Prognostic Signs

A review of 11 studies involving patients who did not awaken immediately after CPR identified four clinical signs that act as independent predictors of death or poor neurologic recovery (34). These are listed below.

1. No corneal reflex at 24 hours.
2. No pupillary light reflex at 24 hours.
3. No withdrawal to pain at 24 hours.
4. No motor response at 24 hours.

Note that each of these signs, if present, allows prediction of a poor outcome at 24 hours after cardiac arrest. Unfortunately, it is unlikely that these criteria will improve the disturbing tendency of physicians to avoid or delay the realization that a patient will never improve under their care.

A FINAL WORD

Despite its popularity, cardiopulmonary resuscitation is a failure as a resuscitative measure in most cases of cardiac arrest. The only practice that shows any evidence of success is timely defibrillation for ventricular fibrillation and pulseless ventricular tachycardia. When cardiac arrest is due to catastrophic pump failure (as occurs with asystole and pulseless electrical activity), the success rate of CPR is dismal. This is not unexpected, because chest compressions fail to generate adequate levels of systemic or regional blood flow, and cardiac arrest drugs add little to the resuscitative effort. Overall, CPR enjoys a popularity that far exceeds its efficacy.

Two caveats about CPR deserve mention. First, avoid hyperventilating patients during CPR, because this can impair the ability of chest compressions to generate blood flow. Also avoid prolonging CPR beyond a reasonable time period, because the goal of CPR is not just a functioning heart, but a functioning heart in a functioning person.

REFERENCES

Introduction

1. Kouwenhoven WB, Ing Jude JR, Knickerbocker GG. Closed chest cardiac massage. JAMA 1960;173:1064–1067.
2. Nadkarni VM, Laarkin GL, Peberdy MA, et al., for the National Registry of Cardiopulmonary Resuscitation Investigators. First documented rhythm and clinical outcome from in-hospital cardiac arrest among children and adults. JAMA 2006;295:50–57.

Guidelines

3. 2005 American Heart Association. Guidelines for cardiopulmonary resuscitation and emergency cardiovascular care. Circulation 2005;112(suppl 112). (Available online @ http://circ.ahajournals.org/content/vol112/24_suppl/)

Basic Life Support

4. 2005 American Heart Association. Guidelines for cardiopulmonary resuscitation and emergency cardiovascular care, Part 4: adult basic life support. Circulation 2005;112(suppl I):IV19–IV34. (Available online @ http://circ.ahajournals.org/content/vol112/24_suppl/)
5. Aufderheide TP, Lurie KG. Death by hyperventilation: a common and life-threatening problem during cardiopulmonary resuscitation. Crit Care Med 2004;32(suppl):S345–S351.
6. Abella BS, Alvarado JP, Mykelbust H, et al. Quality of cardiopulmonary resuscitation during in-hospital cardiac arrest. JAMA 2005;293:305–310.
7. Cummins RO, ed. ACLS provider manual. Dallas, TX: American Heart Association, 2001:25.
8. Aufderheide TP, Pirallo RG, Provo TA, et al. Clinical evaluation of an inspiratory impedance threshold device during standard cardiopulmonary resuscitation in patients with out-of-hospital cardiac arrest. Crit Care Med 2005;33:734–740.

Advanced Life Support

9. 2005 International consensus on cardiopulmonary resuscitation (CPR) and emergency cardiac care (ECC) science with treatment recommendations, Part 4: advanced life support. Circulation 2005;112(suppl I):III-25–III-54. (Available online @ http://circ.ahajournals.org/content/vol112/22_suppl/)
10. 2005 American Heart Association. Guidelines for cardiopulmonary resuscitation and emergency cardiovascular care: Part 7.2, management of cardiac arrest. Circulation 2005;112(suppl I):IV58–IV66. (Available online @ http://circ.ahajournals.org/content/vol112/ 24_suppl/)
11. 2005 American Heart Association. Guidelines for cardiopulmonary resuscitation and emergency cardiovascular care, Part 5: electrical therapies: automated external defibrillators, defibrillation, cardioversion, and pacing. Circulation 2005;112(suppl I):IV17–IV24. (Available online @ http://circ.ahajournals.org/content/vol112/ 24_suppl/)
12. Larsen MP, Eisenberg M, Cummins RO, et al. Predicting survival from out of hospital cardiac arrest: a graphic model. Ann Emerg Med 1993;22:1652–1658.
13. Aung K, Htay T. Vasopressin for cardiac arrest: a systematic review and meta-analysis. Arch Intern Med 2005;165:17–24.
14. Kudenchuk PJ, Cobb LA, Copass MK, et al. Amiodarone for out-of-hospital cardiac arrest due to ventricular fibrillation. N Engl J Med 1999;341:871–878.
15. Dorian P, Cass D, Schwartz B, et al. Amiodarone as compared to lidocaine for shock-resistant ventricular fibrillation. N Engl J Med 2002;346:884–890.

Monitoring During CPR

16. 2005 American Heart Association. Guidelines for cardiopulmonary resuscitation and emergency cardiovascular care, Part 7.4: monitoring and medications. Circulation 2005;112(suppl I):IV78–IV83. (Available online @ http://circ.ahajournals.org/content/vol112/ 24_suppl/)
17. Paradis NA, Martin GB, Rivers EP, et al. Coronary perfusion pressure and the return of spontaneous circulation in human cardiopulmonary resuscitation. JAMA 1990;263:1106–1113.
18. Falk JL, Rackow EC, Weil MH. End-tidal carbon dioxide concentration during cardiopulmonary resuscitation. N Engl J Med 1988;318:607–611.
19. Sanders AB, Kern KB, Otto CW, et al. End-tidal carbon dioxide monitoring during cardiopulmonary resuscitation. JAMA 1989;262:1347–1351.
20. Wayne MA, Levine RL, Miller CC. Use of end-tidal carbon dioxide to predict outcome in prehospital cardiac arrest. Ann Emerg Med 1995;25:762–767.
21. Weil MH, Rackow EC, Trevino R. Difference in acid–base state between venous and arterial blood during cardiopulmonary resuscitation. N Engl J Med 1986;315:153–156.
22. Steedman DJ, Robertson CE. Acid–base changes in arterial and central venous blood during cardiopulmonary resuscitation. Arch Emerg Med 1992; 9:169–176.
23. Abramson NS, Safar P, Detre KM, et al. Neurologic recovery after cardiac arrest: effect of duration of ischemia. Crit Care Med 1985;13:930–931.

Postresuscitation Management

24. Hickey RW, Kochanek PM, Ferimer H, et al. Induced hyperthermia exacerbates neurologic neuronal histologic damage after asphyxial cardiac arrest in rats. Crit Care Med 2003;31:531–535.
25. Zeiner A, Holzer M, Sterz F, et al. Hyperthermia after cardiac arrest is associated with an unfavorable neurologic outcome. Arch Intern Med 2001;161: 2007–2012.
26. Nobel EG, Gang P, Gordon JB, et al. Dilation of normal and constriction of atherosclerotic coronary arteries cause by the cold pressor test. Circulation 1987;77:43–52.
27. The Hypothermia after Cardiac Arrest Study Group. Mild therapeutic hypothermia to improve the neurologic outcome after cardiac arrest. N Engl J Med 2002;346:549–556.
28. Bernard SA, Gray TW, Buist MD, et al. Treatment of comatose survivors of out-of-hospital cardiac arrest with induced hypothermia. N Engl J Med 2002; 346:557-563.
29. Calle PA, Buylaert WA, Vanhaute OA. Glycemia in the post-resuscitation period: The Cerebral Resuscitation Study Group. Resuscitation 1989;17(suppl): S181–188.
30. 2005 American Heart Association. Guidelines for cardiopulmonary resuscitation and emergency cardiovascular care, Part 7.5: postresuscitation support. Circulation 2005;112(suppl I):IV84–IV88. (Available online @ http://circ.ahajournals.org/content/vol112/ 24_suppl/)
31. van der Berghe G, Wouters P, Weekers F, et al. Intensive insulin therapy in critically ill patients. N Engl J Med 2001;345:1359–1367.

32. Levy DE, Caronna JJ, Singer BH, et al. Predicting outcome from hypoxic-ischemic coma. JAMA 1985;253:1420–1426.
33. Edgren E, Hedstrand U, Kelsey S, et al. Assessment of neurologic prognosis in comatose survivors of cardiac arrest. Lancet 1994;343:1055–1059.
34. Booth CM, Boone RH, Tomlinson G, et al. Is this patient dead, vegetative, or severely neurologically impaired? Assessing outcome for comatose survivors of cardiac arrest. JAMA 2004;291:870–879.

Chapter 16

HEMODYNAMIC DRUG INFUSIONS

This chapter contains a brief description of five popular drugs given by continuous intravenous infusion to support the circulation. Each is listed below in order of presentation. Drugs marked by an asterisk have a dosage chart included in the chapter.

1. Dobutamine*
2. Dopamine*
3. Nitroglycerin*
4. Nitroprusside*
5. Norepinephrine

DRUG INFUSION RATES

Because the drugs in this chapter are given by continuous infusion, the recommended dose of each drug is expressed as a dose *rate*, either in micrograms per minute (μg/min) or micrograms per kilogram per minute (μg/kg/min). These drugs are first diluted in one of the common intravenous fluids, and the rate of infusion of these solutions is then set to achieve the desired dose rate. This is accomplished using the drug concentration in the infusate, as demonstrated in Table 16.1. In this case, the desired dose rate (R) is expressed in μg/min, and the drug concentration (C) in the infusate is expressed in μg/mL. The ratio R/C determines the infusion rate of the drug solution in mL/min. Drug infusions are often delivered in microdrops (1 mL = 60 microdrops) to improve the precision of drug dosing. To convert the infusion rate from mL/min to microdrops/minute requires a multiplier of 60 (mL/min × 60 = microdrops/min). The volumetric equivalent of microdrops/minute is mL/hr (i.e., microdrops/minute × 60/60 = mL/hr).

TABLE 16.1 Determining Drug Infusion Rates

If the desired dose rate = R μg/min and the drug concentration in the infusate = C μg/mL, then:

$$\text{Infusion rate} = \frac{R}{C}\ (\text{mL/min})$$

$$= \frac{R}{C} \times 60\ (\text{microdrops/min})$$

DOBUTAMINE

Dobutamine is a synthetic catecholamine that is used as a positive inotropic agent to increase cardiac stroke output in patients with severe, decompensated heart failure.

Actions

Dobutamine is a potent β_1-receptor agonist and a weak β_2-receptor agonist: the β_1 stimulation produces positive inotropic and chronotropic effects, and the β_2 stimulation produces peripheral vasodilatation (1–3). As demonstrated in Figure 16.1, dobutamine causes a dose-dependent increase in stroke volume (upper graph) accompanied by a decrease in cardiac filling pressures (lower graph). Heart rate may be increased or

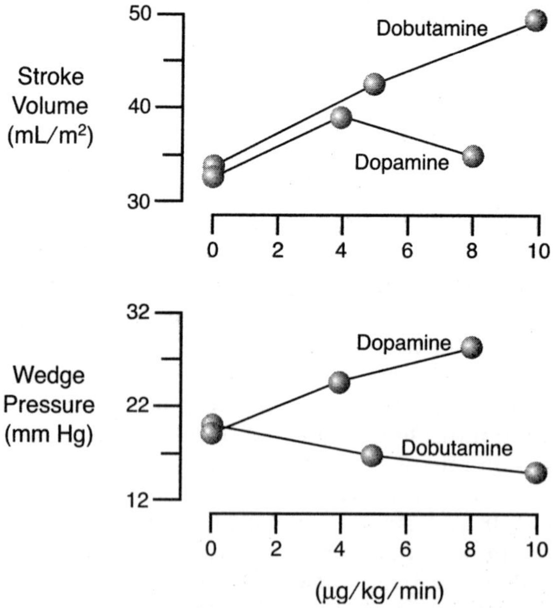

FIGURE 16.1 Effects of dobutamine and dopamine on cardiac performance in patients with severe heart failure. (From Leier CV, et al. Comparative systemic and regional hemodynamic effects of dopamine and dobutamine in patients with cardiomyopathic heart failure. Circulation 1978;58:466–475.)

decreased (the latter effect is due to reflex withdrawal of sympathetic tone in response to the increased cardiac output). The increase in cardiac stroke output is usually accompanied by a proportional decrease in systemic vascular resistance: as a result, the arterial blood pressure usually remains unchanged (1,3).

The cardiac stimulation produced by dobutamine is often accompanied by an increase in both cardiac work and myocardial O_2 consumption (2). These effects can be deleterious in heart failure because cardiac work and myocardial energy needs are already heightened in the failing myocardium (2).

Clinical Uses

Dobutamine is used primarily in patients with decompensated heart failure due to systolic dysfunction who also have a normal blood pressure. The drug is effective in both right-sided and left-sided heart failure. Because dobutamine does not usually raise the blood pressure, it is not recommended (at least as monotherapy) in patients with cardiogenic shock. The unfavorable effects of dobutamine on myocardial energetics have created a preference for vasodilator drug infusions (e.g., nitroglycerin) for the acute management of decompensated heart failure (2). (See Chapter 14 for more information on the management of heart failure.)

Dosage and Administration

A dobutamine dose chart is shown in Table 16.2. The drug is available in 250-mg vials and is infused in a concentration of 1 mg/mL. The usual dose range is 3 to 15 μg/kg/min (1), but doses as high as 200 μg/kg/min have been used safely (4). The response can be variable in critically ill patients (5), and elderly patients may show an attenuated response (6).

TABLE 16.2 Dobutamine Dosage Chart

Infusate: Premixed solutions of dobutamine in D_5W are available with drug concentrations of 0.5, 1, 2, and 4 mg/mL. The infusion chart below is for 1 mg/mL.

Usual dose: 3–15 μg/kg/min

	Body Weight (kg)						
Dose	40	50	60	70	80	90	100
(μg/kg/min)	Infusion Rate (mL/hr)						
2.5	6	8	9	11	12	14	15
5	12	15	18	21	24	27	30
7.5	18	23	27	32	36	41	45
10	24	30	36	42	48	54	60
12.5	30	38	45	53	60	68	75
15	36	45	54	63	72	81	90

Therapy should be driven by hemodynamic end-points and not by preselected dose rates.

Incompatibilities

An alkaline pH inactivates catecholamines such as dobutamine (1), and thus sodium bicarbonate or other alkaline solutions should not be administered with dobutamine.

Adverse Effects

The principal side effect of dobutamine is tachycardia and ventricular ectopic beats (1). The tachycardia is usually mild, and the ectopic beats are usually benign.

Contraindications

Dobutamine (like all positive inotropic agents) is contraindicated in patients with hypertrophic cardiomyopathy (1). It should also be avoided (if possible) in patients with a history of malignant ventricular tachyarrhythmias.

DOPAMINE

Dopamine is an endogenous catecholamine that serves as both a neurotransmitter and a precursor for norepinephrine synthesis. When given as an exogenous drug, dopamine activates a variety of receptors in a dose-dependent manner. This creates a variety of dose-dependent drug effects (7), as described next.

Actions

At low dose rates (≤3 μg/kg/min), dopamine selectively activates dopamine-specific receptors in the renal and splanchnic circulations, resulting in increased blood flow in these regions (2). Low-dose dopamine also directly affects renal tubular epithelial cells, causing an increase in urinary sodium excretion (natriuresis) that is independent of the changes in renal blood flow (8).

At intermediate dose rates (3 to 10 μg/kg/min), dopamine stimulates β-receptors in the heart and peripheral circulation, producing an increase in myocardial contractility, an increase in heart rate, and peripheral vasodilatation. The overall result is an increase in cardiac output. This effect is demonstrated in Figure 16.1 (upper graph). Note that the contractile response to dopamine is modest when compared to dobutamine.

At high dose rates (>10 μg/kg/min), dopamine produces a progressive activation of α-receptors in the systemic and pulmonary circulations, resulting in progressive pulmonary and systemic vasoconstriction. This vasopressor effect, by virtue of increasing ventricular afterload, counteracts the cardiac stimulation produced by intermediate-dose dopamine.

Figure 16.1 (upper graph) shows the loss in cardiac output augmentation that occurs when the dopamine dose is progressively increased.

The effects of dopamine on the pulmonary capillary wedge pressure are shown in Figure 16.1 (lower graph). There is a dose-dependent increase in the wedge pressure, which is independent of the changes in stroke volume. This effect may be the result of dopamine-induced vasoconstriction in pulmonary veins. This ability to constrict pulmonary veins makes the pulmonary capillary wedge pressure an unreliable measure of left-ventricular filling pressure during high-dose dopamine infusion. (See Chapter 10 for a detailed description of the pulmonary capillary wedge pressure.)

Clinical Uses

Dopamine is often used in situations where both cardiac stimulation and peripheral vasoconstriction are desired. The classic example of this is cardiogenic shock. Dopamine is also used to correct the hypotension in septic shock, but norepinephrine has become the preferred vasopressor in this condition (see later).

Low-dose dopamine is often used in an attempt to prevent or reverse acute renal failure. This is not appropriate. While low-dose dopamine does promote renal blood flow and urine output in healthy subjects, these effects are minimal or absent in patients with acute renal failure, particularly oliguric renal failure (8). As a result, low dose dopamine is NOT recommended for the prevention or reversal of acute renal failure in the ICU (8). (This topic is discussed again in Chapter 31.)

Dosage and Administration

A dose chart for dopamine is shown in Table 16.3. Commercial preparations of dopamine are concentrated drug solutions (containing 40 mg or 80 mg dopamine HCl per mL) provided in small-volume vials (5 mL or 10 mL). These preparations must be diluted to prevent intense vasoconstriction during drug infusion. In Table 16.3, the original dopamine solution is diluted 100-fold in isotonic saline to prepare the infusate. Dopamine infusions should always de delivered into large, central veins.

The dosing regimen for dopamine is weight-based, and dosing should be based on *ideal body weight*, not actual body weight (2,7). (For reasons that are unclear, the distinction between ideal and actual body weight is not mentioned for other hemodynamic drugs with weight-based dosing regimens.). As shown in Table 16.3, there are two recommended dose ranges for dopamine: 3 to 10 μg/kg/min is recommended for augmenting cardiac output, and > 10 μg/kg/min is recommended to increase the blood pressure. (Low-dose dopamine is not included in Table 16.3 because of the lack of efficacy mentioned previously.)

Incompatibilities

Like dobutamine, dopamine is inactivated by an alkaline pH, so alkaline fluids should not be infused along with dopamine.

TABLE 16.3 Dopamine Dosage Chart

Infusate: Use 10 mL vial containing 80 mg/mL dopamine HCL. Add to one liter of isotonic saline (final concentration = 800 μg/mL).

Dose rates: 3–10 μg/kg/min to augment cardiac output; > 10 μg/kg/min to increase blood pressure.

Dose (μg/kg/min)	Ideal Body Weight (kg) 40	50	60	70	80	90	100
	Infusion Rate (mL/hr)						
1	3	4	5	5	6	7	8
3	9	11	14	16	18	20	23
5	15	19	23	26	30	34	38
10	30	38	45	53	60	68	75
15	45	56	68	79	90	101	113
20	60	75	90	105	120	135	150

Adverse Effects

Tachyarrhythmias are the most common adverse effects of dopamine infusions. Sinus tachycardia is common (7) but rarely is severe enough to prompt a change in drug or dose rate. Malignant tachyarrhythmias (e.g., multifocal ventricular ectopics, ventricular tachycardia) can also occur but are uncommon.

The most feared complication of dopamine infusion is ischemic limb necrosis, which is usually caused by drug extravasation into perivascular tissues. Using large, central veins for dopamine infusions will prevent this complication. Extravasation of the drug through a peripheral vein can be treated with a local injection of phentolamine (5 to 10 mg in 15 mL saline) (7).

Other adverse effects of dopamine infusions include allergic reactions to the sulfite preservative used to prevent oxidative decomposition of dopamine (7), increased intraocular pressure (9), and delayed gastric emptying, which could predispose to nosocomial pneumonia (10).

NITROGLYCERIN

Nitroglycerin is an organic nitrate (glyceryl trinitrate) that relaxes vascular smooth muscle and produces a generalized vasodilation.

Actions

The actions of nitroglycerin on vascular smooth muscle are mediated by nitric oxide (11). This is illustrated in Figure 16.2. Nitroglycerin binds to the surface of endothelial cells and undergoes two reduction reactions to form

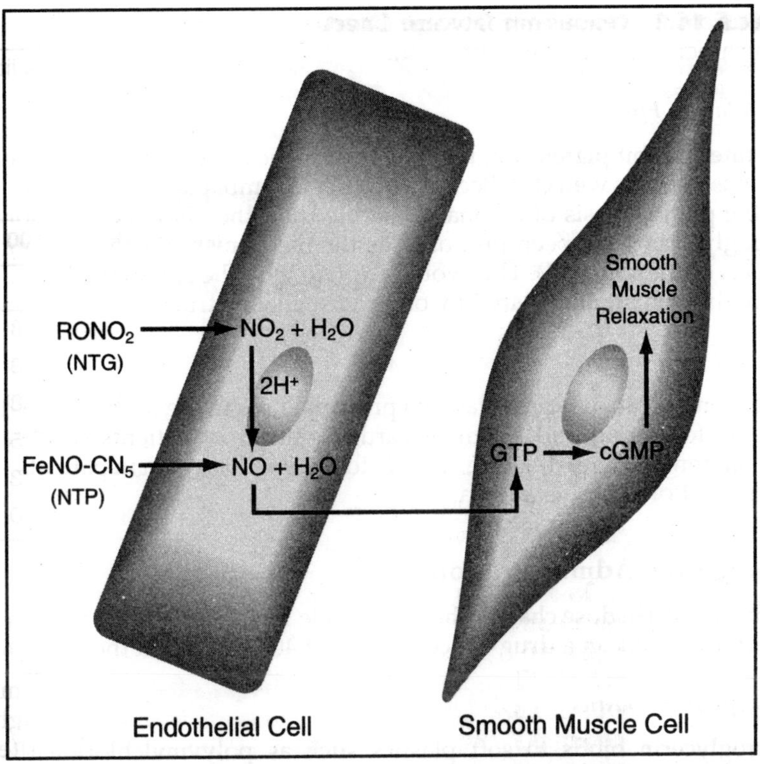

FIGURE 16.2 The biochemical mechanism for the vasodilator actions of nitroglycerin (NTG) and nitroprusside (NTP). Chemical symbols: nitroprusside ($Fe\text{-}NO\text{-}CN_5$), organic nitrate ($RONO_2$), inorganic nitrite (NO_2), nitric oxide (NO•), guanosine triphosphate (GTP), cyclic guanosine monophosphate (cGMP).

nitric oxide. The nitric oxide then moves out of the endothelial cells and into adjacent smooth muscle cells, where it produces muscle relaxation by promoting the formation of cyclic guanosine monophosphate (cGMP).

Vasodilator Effects

Nitroglycerin has a dose-dependent vasodilator effect involving arteries and veins in the systemic and pulmonary circulations (12,13). When the drug is given by continuous infusion, venous vasodilator effects are prominent at low dose rates (<40 μg/min), and arterial vasodilator effects predominate at high dose rates (> 200 μg/min). At intermediate dose rates (40 to 200 μg/min), a mixture of venous and arterial vasodilation occurs. At low dose rates, nitroglycerin produces a decrease in cardiac filling pressures (i.e., central venous pressure and wedge pressure) with little or no change in cardiac output. As the dose rate is increased through the intermediate dose range, the cardiac output begins to rise as a result of progressive arterial vasodilation. Further increases in the dose rate will eventually produce a drop in blood pressure. The hemodynamic effects of intravenous nitroglycerin have a rapid onset and short duration, which permits rapid dose titration.

Antiplatelet Effects

Nitrates inhibit platelet aggregation, and nitric oxide is believed to mediate this effect as well (14). Because platelet thrombi play an important role in the pathogenesis of coronary insufficiency, the antiplatelet actions of nitroglycerin have been proposed as the mechanism for the antianginal effects of the drug (14). This would explain why the antianginal effects of nitroglycerin are not shared by other vasodilator drugs.

Clinical Uses

Intravenous nitroglycerin has two principal uses in the ICU: (1) to reduce edema formation and augment cardiac output in patients with acute, decompensated heart failure, and (2) to relieve chest pain in patients with persistent or unstable angina.

Dosage and Administration

A nitroglycerin dose chart is shown in Table 16.4. The infusion rates in this chart are based on a drug concentration of 400 μg/mL in the infusate.

Adsorption to Plastics

Nitroglycerin binds to soft plastics such as polyvinylchloride (PVC), which is a common constituent in the plastic bags and tubing used for intravenous infusions. As much as 80% of the drug can be lost by

TABLE 16.4 Nitroglycerin Dosage Chart

Infusate: Add 50 mg or 100 mg nitroglycerin to 500 mL isotonic saline to achieve a drug concentration of 100 μg/mL or 200 μg/mL.

Dose rate: Start at 5 μg/min, and increase dose rate by 5 μg/min every 5 min to desired effect.

Caution: Do NOT use polyvinylchloride (PVC) infusion sets to prevent drug loss via adsorption to PVC. Use only glass bottles and polyethylene tubing.

Dose Rate (μg/min)	Infusion Rate (mL/hr)	
	100 μg/mL	200 μg/mL
5	3	—
10	6	3
20	9	6
40	24	18
80	48	36
160	96	72
320	—	96

adsorption to PVC in standard intravenous infusion systems (12). Nitroglycerin does not bind to glass or hard plastics like polyethylene (PET), so drug loss via adsorption can be eliminated by using glass bottles and PET tubing. Drug manufacturers often provide specialized infusion sets to prevent nitroglycerin loss via adsorption.

Drug Dosing

Nitroglycerin should be started at a dose rate of 5 to 10 μg/min. The rate is then increased in 5 μg/min increments every 5 minutes until the desired effect is achieved. The effective dose will vary in each patient, and the infusion should be guided by the selected end-point and not the infusion rate. However, the dose requirement should not exceed 400 μg/min in most patients. High dose requirements (e.g., > 350 μg/min) are often the result of drug loss via adsorption or nitrate tolerance (see below).

Contraindications

Nitroglycerin should not be used in patients who have taken a phosphodiesterase inhibitor for erectile dysfunction within the past 24 hours (longer for some preparations) because of the high risk of hypotension when these agents are combined.

Adverse Effects

Adverse Hemodynamic Effects

Nitroglycerin-induced increases in cerebral and pulmonary blood flow can be problematic. The increase in cerebral blood flow can lead to increased intracranial pressure and symptomatic intracranial hypertension (15). In patients with lung disease, the increase in pulmonary blood flow can be problematic when the increased flow occurs in lung regions that are poorly ventilated. This increases shunt fraction and can aggravate hypoxemia. This effect can be prominent when nitroglycerin is used in patients with acute respiratory distress syndrome (16).

The venodilating effects of nitroglycerin can promote hypotension in hypovolemic patients and in patients with acute right heart failure due to right ventricular infarction. In either of these conditions, aggressive volume loading is required prior to initiating a nitroglycerin infusion.

Methemoglobinemia

Nitroglycerin metabolism produces inorganic nitrites (see Fig. 16.2), and accumulation of nitrites can lead to oxidation of the heme-bound iron moieties in hemoglobin to create methemoglobin. Fortunately, clinically significant methemoglobinemia is not a common complication of nitroglycerin infusions, and occurs only at very high dose rates (15). (The diagnosis of methemoglobinemia is described in Chapter 20.)

Solvent Toxicity

Nitroglycerin does not readily dissolve in aqueous solutions, and nonpolar solvents such as ethanol and propylene glycol are required to keep the drug in solution. These solvents can accumulate during prolonged infusions. Both ethanol intoxication (17) and propylene glycol toxicity (18) have been reported as a result of nitroglycerin infusions. Propylene glycol toxicity may be more common than suspected because this solvent makes up 30 to 50% of some nitroglycerin preparations (15). Clinical manifestations include altered mental status, metabolic acidosis, and hemolysis. The propylene glycol level in blood is needed to confirm the diagnosis.

Nitrate Tolerance

Tolerance to the vasodilator and antiplatelet actions of nitroglycerin is a well-described phenomenon and can appear after only 24 hours of continuous drug administration (15). The underlying mechanism is unclear, but there is evidence that inactivation of nitric oxide by oxygen radicals may be involved (19). One study showed that concomitant use of hydralazine prevented nitrate tolerance (20), but the significance of this is unclear. The most effective measure for preventing or reversing nitrate tolerance is a daily drug-free interval of at least 6 hours (15).

NITROPRUSSIDE

Nitroprusside is a rapidly-acting vasodilator that is favored for the treatment of severe. life-threatening hypertension. The popularity of this drug is limited, however, by a significant risk of toxicity, as described later.

Actions

The vasodilator actions of nitroprusside, like those of nitroglycerin, are mediated by nitric oxide (11). The nitroprusside molecule, which is shown at the top of Figure 16.3, contains one nitrosyl group (NO). When nitroprusside enters the bloodstream, the nitrosyl group is released as nitric oxide, which then follows the pathway shown in Figure 16.2 to produce vasodilation.

Like nitroglycerin, nitroprusside dilates both arteries and veins, but it is less potent than nitroglycerin as a venodilator and more potent as an arterial vasodilator. The vascular responses are prompt and short lived, which allows for rapid dose titration. Vasodilator effects are often evident at low dose rates (0.5 μg/kg/min), but blood pressure reduction usually requires higher dose rates (≥1 μg/kg/min). Nitroprusside has variable effects on cardiac output in subjects with normal cardiac function (21), but it consistently improves cardiac output in patients with decompensated heart failure (21,22).

Clinical Uses

Nitroprusside is used to treat severe hypertension when rapid blood pressure control is desirable (e.g., hypertensive emergencies). It can also be used to treat decompensated heart failure (22) and is effective in treating severe heart failure due to aortic stenosis (23), where vasodilator therapy has traditionally been discouraged.

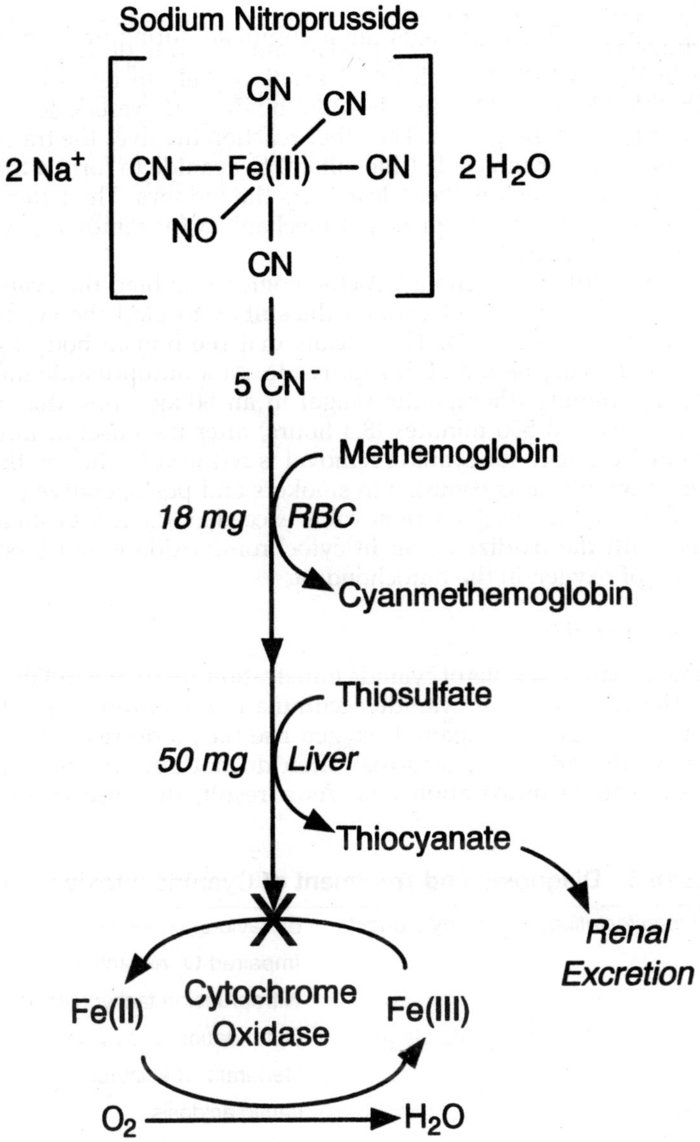

FIGURE 16.3 The fate of cyanide ions (CN^-) released into the bloodstream by the nitroprusside molecule.

Cyanide Intoxication

Nitroprusside infusions carry a considerable risk of cyanide intoxication. In fact, **cyanide accumulation is common during therapeutic infusions of nitroprusside** (15,24,25). The origin of the cyanide is the nitroprusside molecule, which is a ferricyanide complex that contains 5 cyanide atoms bound to an oxidized iron core (see the upper part of Figure 16.3).

When nitroprusside disrupts to release nitric oxide and exert its actions, the cyanide is released into the bloodstream. The fate of this cyanide is shown in Figure 16.3. Two chemical reactions help to remove cyanide from the bloodstream. One involves the binding of cyanide to the oxidized iron in methemoglobin. The other reaction involves the transfer of sulfur from a donor molecule (thiosulfate) to cyanide to form a thiocyanate compound, which is then cleared by the kidneys. The latter (transulfuration) reaction is the principal mechanism for removing cyanide from the human body.

Healthy adults have enough methemoglobin to bind the cyanide in 18 mg of nitroprusside and enough thiosulfate to bind the cyanide in 50 mg of nitroprusside (15). This means that the human body has the capacity to detoxify 68 mg of nitroprusside. At a nitroprusside infusion of 2 μg/kg/minute (therapeutic range) in an 80-kg adult, this 68 mg capacity is reached 500 minutes (8.3 hours) after the onset of infusion. This limited capacity for cyanide removal is reduced further by thiosulfate depletion, which is common in smokers and postoperative patients (15,24). Once the capacity for removal is exceeded, the free cyanide will combine with the oxidized iron in cytochrome oxidase and block the utilization of oxygen in the mitochondria.

Clinical Manifestations

The clinical manifestations of cyanide intoxication are shown in Table 16.5. One of the early signs of cyanide accumulation is nitroprusside tachyphylaxis (15). Signs of impaired oxygen use (i.e., a decrease in oxygen extraction ratio and lactic acidosis) often do not appear until the late stages of cyanide intoxication (26). As a result, the absence of lactic

TABLE 16.5 Diagnosis and Treatment of Cyanide Intoxication

Clinical manifestations	Early stages:	Behavioral changes
		Impaired O_2 extraction
		Nitroprusside tachyphylaxis
	Late stages:	Obtundation and coma
		Generalized seizures
		Lactic acidosis
Laboratory diagnosis	Toxicity	Blood cyanide level
	Mild	0.5–2.5 μg/mL
	Severe	> 2.5 μg/mL
	Fatal	> 3.0 μg/mL
*Management:**	Amyl nitrate inhaler for one min, or	
	Sodium nitrite: 300 mg IV over 15 min plus	
	Sodium thiosulfate: 12.5 g IV over 15 min	

From Hall AH, Rumack BH. Clinical toxicology of cyanide. AnnEmerg Med 1986;15:1067.
*A *Cyanide Antidote Kit* is available from Eli Lilly & Co.

acidosis during nitroprusside infusion does not exclude the possibility of cyanide accumulation (15,24).

Diagnosis

Whole blood cyanide levels can be used to document cyanide intoxication, as shown in Table 16.5. However, the results of cyanide assays are not immediately available (a STAT specimen usually requires 3 to 4 hours to be processed) (24), so immediate decisions regarding cyanide intoxication are often based on the clinical presentation. Nitroprusside tachyphylaxis is an important early marker of cyanide accumulation.

Treatment

Treatment of cyanide intoxication should begin with the inhalation of 100% oxygen. The Cyanide Antidote Kit (Eli Lilly & Co.) can be used as described in Table 16.5 (27). This kit uses nitrates and nitrites (which oxidize the iron in hemoglobin to produce methemoglobin) to promote cyanide binding to methemoglobin and also uses thiosulfate to clear cyanide from the bloodstream.

Because nitrite therapy creates methemoglobinemia, alternative methods of cyanide binding have been explored. The affinity of cyanide for cobalt has led to the use of hydroxocobalamin (100 mL of a 5% solution infused over 15 minutes) (28), which combines with cyanide to form cyanocobalamin (vitamin B_{12}), which is then excreted in the urine. This strategy is popular in Europe, but the lack of a suitable hydroxocobalamin preparation has hampered its use in the United States.

Thiocyanate Intoxication

The most important mechanism for cyanide removal involves the formation of thiocyanate, which is slowly excreted in the urine. When renal function is impaired, thiocyanate can accumulate and produce a toxic syndrome that is distinct from cyanide intoxication (15,24). The clinical features include anxiety, confusion, pupillary constriction, tinnitus, hallucinations, and generalized seizures (15,24). Thiocyanate can also produce hypothyroidism by blocking the thyroid uptake of iodine (24).

The diagnosis of thiocyanate toxicity is established by the serum thiocyanate level. Normal levels are below 10 mg/L, and clinical toxicity is usually accompanied by levels above 100 mg/L (24). Thiocyanate intoxication can be treated by hemodialysis or peritoneal dialysis.

Dosage and Administration

A dose chart for nitroprusside is shown in Table 16.6. Note that thiosulfate is added to the nitroprusside infusate to limit cyanide accumulation. About 500 mg of thiosulfate should be added for every 50 mg of nitroprusside (24).

Nitroprusside should be started at a low dose rate (0.2 μg/kg/min) and then titrated upward every 5 minutes to the desired result.

TABLE 16.6 Nitroprusside Dosage Chart

Infusate: Add 50 mg nitroprusside to 250 mL D_5W for a drug concentration of 200 μg/mL. **Add 500 mg thiosulfate.**

Dosage: Start at 0.2 μg/kg/min and titrate upward to desired effect. Effective dose rates are usually between 0.5 and 5 μg/kg/min. Maximum dose allowed is 10 μg/kg/min for 10 min.

Dose Rate (μg/kg/min)	Body Weight (kg) 50	60	70	80	90	100
	Infusion Rate (mL/hr)					
0.2	4	4	5	6	7	8
0.5	7.5	9	11	12	14	15
1	15	18	21	24	27	30
2	30	36	42	48	54	60
3	45	54	63	72	81	90
5	75	90	105	120	135	150

Satisfactory control of hypertension usually requires dose rates of 2 to 5 μg/kg/min, but the dose rate should be kept below 3 μg/kg/min if possible to limit cyanide accumulation (21). In renal failure, the dose rate should be kept below 1 μg/kg/min to limit thiocyanate accumulation (21). The maximum allowable dose rate is 10 μg/kg/min for only 10 minutes.

NOREPINEPHRINE

Norepinephrine is a popular vasopressor that is often used to correct hypotension when other measures (e.g., volume infusion, dopamine) fail (29). It is the preferred vasopressor agent in septic shock (30).

Actions

Norepinephrine stimulates alpha receptors and produces a dose-dependent increase in systemic vascular resistance. Although the drug can stimulate cardiac β-receptors over a wide range, the effects on cardiac output are variable (29). The vasoconstrictor response to norepinephrine is usually accompanied by a decrease in organ blood flow, particularly in the kidneys (29,30). This is not the case in septic shock, where norepinephrine can increase blood pressure without causing a decrease in renal blood flow or a deterioration in renal function (30,31).

Clinical Uses

Norepinephrine is traditionally used as the last measure for cases of hypotension that are refractory to volume infusion and other hemodynamic drugs (e.g., dobutamine, dopamine). Norepinephrine is the vasopressor of choice in septic shock (30) and should be added when hypotension is not corrected by appropriate volume infusion. Despite the ability to correct hypotension, vasopressor drugs (including norepinephrine) do not improve survival in shock states, including septic shock (30).

Dosage and Administration

Norepinephrine is usually supplied as norepinephrine bitartrate, but the dosage is expressed in terms of norepinephrine (2 mg norepinephrine bitartrate = 1 mg norepinephrine) (29). Dextrose-containing fluids are recommended as the diluent for norepinephrine (29). Two milligrams of norepinephrine can be added to 500 mL of diluent to achieve a drug concentration of 4 μg/mL. The initial dose rate can be as low as 1 μg/min (15 microdrops/min) and titrated upward to the desired effect. The effective dose rate in septic shock is usually between 0.2 and 1.3 μg/kg/min (about 1 to 10 μg/min for a 70 kg patient), but dose rates as high as 5 μg/kg/min may be required (30).

Incompatibilities

Norepinephrine, like all catecholamines, is inactivated at an alkaline pH (29), so alkaline fluids should not be given with norepinephrine.

Adverse Effects

Adverse effects of norepinephrine include local tissue necrosis from drug extravasation and intense systemic vasoconstriction with worsening organ function. As for the latter effect, whenever a vasoconstrictor drug is required to correct hypotension, it is often difficult to distinguish between adverse drug effects and adverse disease effects.

Finally, norepinephrine bitartrate contains sulfites to prevent oxidative decomposition (29), and allergic reactions to sulfites have been reported (particularly in patients with asthma).

REFERENCES

Dobutamine

1. Dobutamine monograph. Mosby's Drug Consult, 2006. Accessed on the MD Consult website (www.MDconsult.com) on Feb 3, 2006.
2. Bayram M, De Luca L, Massie B, et al. Reassessment of dobutamine, dopamine, and milrinone in the management of acute heart failure syndromes. Am J Cardiol 2005;96(suppl):47G–58G.
3. Romson JL, Leung JM, Bellows WH, et al. Effects of dobutamine on hemodynamics and left ventricular performance after cardiopulmonary bypass in cardiac surgical patients. Anesthesiology 1999;91:1318–1327.
4. Hayes MA, Yau EHS, Timmins AC, et al. Response of critically ill patients to treatment aimed at achieving supranormal oxygen delivery and consumption: relationship to outcome. Chest 1993;103:886–895.

5. Klem C, Dasta JF, Reilley TE, et al. Variability in dobutamine pharmacokinetics in unstable critically ill surgical patients. Crit Care Med 1994;22:1926–1932.
6. Rich MW, Imburgia M. Inotropic response to dobutamine in elderly patients with decompensated congestive heart failure. Am J Cardiol 1990;65:519–521.

Dopamine

7. Dopamine monograph. Mosby's Drug Consult, 2006. Accessed on the MD Consult website (www.MDconsult.com) on Feb 3, 2006.
8. Kellum JA, Decker JM. Use of dopamine in acute renal failure: a meta-analysis. Crit Care Med 2001;29:1526–1531.
9. Brath PC, MacGregor DA, Ford JG, Prielipp RC. Dopamine and intraocular pressure in critically ill patients. Anesthesiology 2000;93:1398–1400.
10. Johnsom AG. Source of infection in nosocomial pneumonia [Letter]. Lancet 1993;341:1368.

Nitroglycerin

11. Anderson TJ, Meredith IT, Ganz P, et al. Nitric oxide and nitrovasodilators: similarities, differences and potential interactions. J Am Coll Cardiol 1994;24:555–566.
12. Nitroglycerin. In: McEvoy GK, ed. AHFS Drug Information, 2001. Bethesda, MD: American Society of Health System Pharmacists, 2001:1832–1835.
13. Elkayam U. Nitrates in heart failure. Cardiol Clin 1994;12:73–85.
14. Stamler JS, Loscalzo J. The antiplatelet effects of organic nitrates and related nitroso compounds in vitro and in vivo and their relevance to cardiovascular disorders. J Am Coll Cardiol 1991;18:1529–1536.
15. Curry SC, Arnold-Cappell P. Nitroprusside, nitroglycerin, and angiotensin-converting enzyme inhibitors. In: Toxic effects of drugs used in the ICU. Crit Care Clin 1991;7:555–582.
16. Radermacher P, Santak B, Becker H, et al. Prostaglandin F_I and nitroglycerin reduce pulmonary capillary pressure but worsen ventilation–perfusion distribution in patients with adult respiratory distress syndrome. Anesthesiology 1989;70:601–606.
17. Korn SH, Comer JB. Intravenous nitroglycerin and ethanol intoxication. Ann Intern Med 1985;102:274.
18. Demey HE, Daelemans RA, Verpooten GA, et al. Propylene glycol-induced side effects during intravenous nitroglycerin therapy. Intensive Care Med 1988;14:221–226.
19. Daiber A, Mulsch A, Hink U, et al. The oxidative stress concept of nitrate tolerance and the antioxidant properties of hydralazine. Am J Cardiol 2005; 96(suppl):25i–36i.
20. Gogia A, Mehra A, Parikh S, et al. Prevention of tolerance to the hemodynamic effects of nitrates with concomitant use of hydralazine in patients with chronic heart failure. J Am Coll Cardiol 1995;26:1575–1580.

Nitroprusside

21. Nitroprusside. In: McEvoy GK, ed. AHFS Drug Information, 2001. Bethesda, MD: American Society of Health System Pharmacists, 2001:1816–1820.

22. Guiha NH, Cohn JN, Mikulic E, et al. Treatment of refractory heart failure with infusion of nitroprusside. N Engl J Med 1974;291:587–592.
23. Khot UN, Novaro GM, Popovic ZB, et al. Nitroprusside in critically ill patients with left ventricular dysfunction and aortic stenosis. N Engl J Med 2003;348:1756–1763.
24. Hall VA, Guest JM. Sodium nitroprusside-induced cyanide intoxication and prevention with sodium thiosulfate prophylaxis. Am J Crit Care 1992;2: 19–27.
25. Robin ED, McCauley R. Nitroprusside-related cyanide poisoning: time (long past due) for urgent, effective interventions. Chest 1992;102:1842–1845.
26. Arieff AI. Is measurement of venous oxygen saturation useful in the diagnosis of cyanide poisoning? Am J Med 1992;93:582–583.
27. Kirk MA, Gerace R, Kulig KW. Cyanide and methemoglobin kinetics in smoke inhalation victims treated with the Cyanide Antidote Kit. Ann Emerg Med 1993;22:1413–1418.
28. Curry SC, Connor DA, Raschke RA. Effect of the cyanide antidote hydroxocobalamin on commonly ordered serum chemistry studies. Ann Emerg Med 1994;24:65–67.

Norepinephrine

29. Norepinephrine bitartrate. In: McEvoy GK, ed. AHFS Drug Information, 2001. Bethesda, MD: American Society of Health System Pharmacists, 2001: 1258–1261.
30. Beale RJ, Hollenberg SM, Vincent J-L, et al. Vasopressor and inotropic support in septic shock: an evidence-based review. Crit Care Med 2004;32(suppl): S455–S465.
31. Desairs P, Pinaud M, Bugnon D, et al. Norepinephrine therapy has no deleterious renal effects in human septic shock. Crit Care Med 1989;17:426–429.

Section VI

CRITICAL CARE CARDIOLOGY

We think so because all other people think so, or . . . because we were told to think so, and think we must think so . . .

RUDYARD KIPLING

EARLY MANAGEMENT OF ACUTE CO... S

The ...
tion ...
on a ...
early ...
inter...
tice ...
Am...
the ...

ACI...

Acut...
den ...
one ...
segm...
tion ...
first ...
coro...
are t...
comp...

Figu...
sclero...
leads ...
disru...

Chapter 17

EARLY MANAGEMENT OF ACUTE CORONARY SYNDROMES

The management of patients with acute myocardial ischemia and infarction is one of the few practices in critical care medicine that can save lives on a continued basis, but only when appropriate interventions are used early (often within hours after the initial contact with the patient). Those interventions are described in this chapter using information from practice guidelines published by the American College of Cardiology and American Heart Association (ACC/AHA). These guidelines are listed in the bibliography at the end of the chapter (1–3).

ACUTE CORONARY SYNDROMES

Acute coronary syndromes (ACS) are conditions characterized by the sudden onset of coronary insufficiency as a result of thrombotic occlusion of one or more coronary arteries. Three such conditions are identified: ST-segment elevation myocardial infarction (STEMI), non-ST-segment elevation myocardial infarction (non-STEMI), and unstable angina (UA). The first condition (STEMI) is the result of complete and sustained thrombotic coronary occlusion, while the last two conditions (non-STEMI and UA) are the result of either partial thrombotic coronary occlusion or transient complete occlusion with spontaneous revascularization (1–3).

The seminal event in all these conditions is coronary thrombosis (see Figure 17.1). The nidus for thrombus formation is rupture of an atherosclerotic plaque (4), which exposes the blood to thrombogenic lipids and leads to activation of platelets and clotting factors. The trigger for plaque disruption is not known, but liquefaction caused by local inflammation

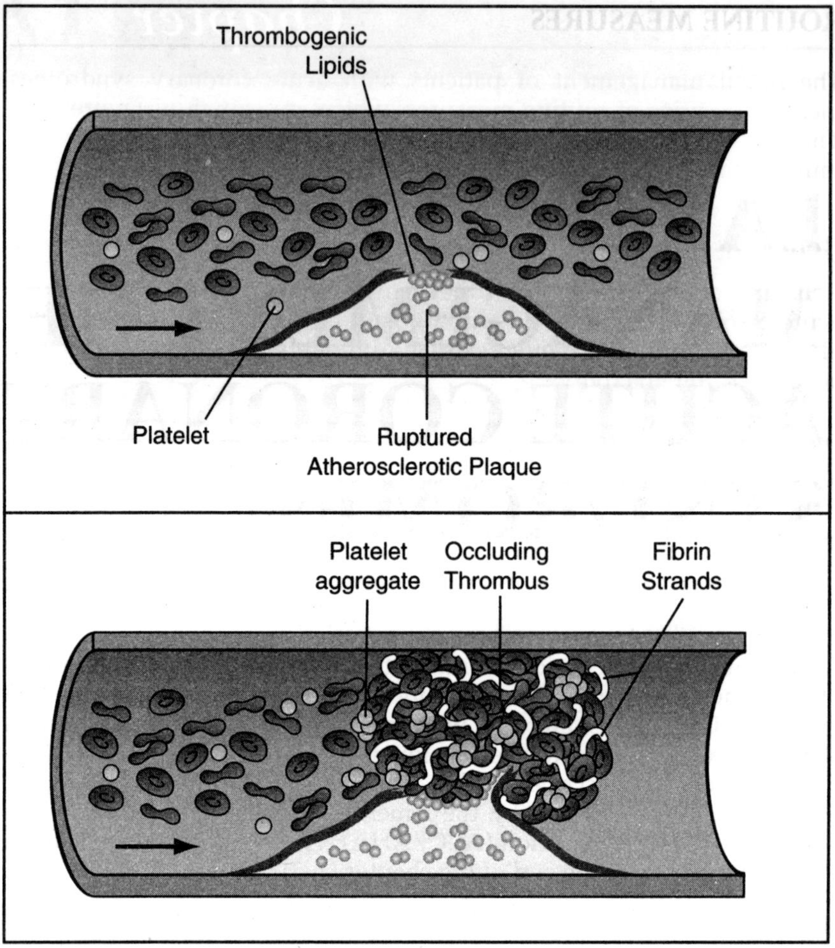

FIGURE 17.1 Illustration showing the pathogenesis of acute coronary syndromes. Rupture of an atherosclerotic plaque leads to activation of platelets and clotting factors (upper panel) and results in the formation of an occlusive thrombus (lower panel).

and inflammatory mediators is believed to be involved (5). Hydraulic stresses may also play a role because plaques that rupture are usually located at branch points or bends in the arterial tree (3,6).

The discovery that coronary thrombosis is responsible for the tissue injury in acute myocardial infarction led to the adoption of several therapeutic measures designed to limit thrombus formation and alleviate thrombotic obstruction. These measures include antiplatelet therapy (aspirin, platelet glycoprotein inhibitors), anticoagulant therapy (heparin), chemical dissolution of clots (fibrinolytic agents), and mechanical disruption of clots (coronary angioplasty). This chapter contains a description of each of these measures and when they should be used.

ROUTINE MEASURES

The initial management of patients with acute coronary syndromes includes a series of routine measures, which are shown in Figure 17.2. These measures are used in all patients and are often initiated during or immediately after the initial patient contact.

Relieving Chest Pain

Relieving chest pain is one of the immediate goals of management in acute coronary syndromes. Pain relief not only promotes well-being, it also helps alleviate unwanted cardiac stimulation from anxiety-induced adrenergic hyperactivity.

Nitroglycerin

Nitroglycerin (0.4 mg sublingual tablets or aerosol spray) is given for up to three doses (each 5 minutes apart) to relieve chest pain. If the pain subsides, intravenous nitroglycerin can be started for continued pain relief (see Chapter 16, Table 16.4, for recommended dose rates for intravenous nitroglycerin). If the chest pain persists after 3 doses of nitroglycerin, immediate administration of morphine is indicated.

Intravenous nitroglycerin is also indicated for persistent or recurrent chest pain due to unstable angina and for acute coronary syndromes associated with hypertension or pulmonary congestion (1–3). In patients with right ventricular infarction, intravenous nitroglycerin should be avoided or used with extreme caution because of the risk of hypotension (aggressive volume loading is needed in this situation to counteract the venodilating effects of nitroglycerin). Finally, nitroglycerin should NOT be used in patients who have taken a phosphodiesterase inhibitor for erectile dysfunction within the past 24 hours (longer for some preparations) because of the high risk for hypotension.

Morphine

Morphine is the drug of choice for chest pain that is refractory to nitroglycerin (1–3). The initial dose is usually 4 mg, given by slow intravenous push (e.g., 1 mg/minute), and this can be repeated every 5 to 10 minutes if necessary. Morphine administration may be followed by a decrease in blood pressure. This is usually the result of a decrease in sympathetic nervous system activity and is not a pathologic process. A drop in blood pressure to hypotensive levels usually indicates hypovolemia and can be corrected by volume infusion (2). Pressor agents should NEVER be used to correct morphine-induced decreases in blood pressure.

Antiplatelet Therapy

Aspirin

Chewable aspirin in a dose of 162 to 325 mg should be given to all patients with ACS who have not taken aspirin prior to presentation (1–3).

Aspirin causes irreversible inhibition of platelet aggregation by inhibiting thromboxane production (7), and aspirin therapy (either alone or in combination with thrombolytic therapy) has been shown to reduce mortality and decrease the rate of re-infarction (8,9). The decrease in short-term (30 day) mortality attributed to aspirin alone is about 2 to 3% (8), which means that for every 100 patients with ACS, there are 2 to 3 fewer deaths attributed to aspirin.

The initial dose of aspirin is usually given as soon as possible after presentation, even though there is no evidence that the beneficial effects of aspirin in ACS are time-dependent (2). Non-enteric-coated aspirin is preferred because of enhanced buccal absorption. The initial aspirin dose (162 to 325 mg) should be followed by a daily dose of 75 to 162 mg, which is continued indefinitely (2). For patients who are unable to receive aspirin because of aspirin allergy or recent GI hemorrhage, alternative therapy with the antiplatelet agents in the next section is advised.

Thienopyridines

The thienopyridines are antiplatelet agents that irreversibly block surface receptors involved in ADP-induced platelet aggregation (7). This mechanism of action differs from that of aspirin, which means that the antiplatelet effects of aspirin and the thienopyridines are additive. The anti-platelet activity of the thienopyridines requires drug activation in the liver, so these drugs are not recommended in patients with liver failure.

There are 2 clinically available drugs in this class: clopidogrel (Plavix) and ticlodipine (Ticlid). Clopidogrel seems to be preferred because of fewer side effects (7). The recommended dose of clopidogrel in ACS is 300 mg initially, followed by 75 mg daily (2). Although clopidogrel is currently recommended as a substitute for aspirin, one large study has shown that combined therapy with clopidogrel and aspirin in ACS is associated with a lower mortality than aspirin therapy alone (10). Combined anti-platelet therapy with clopidogrel and aspirin is already a standard practice following stent placement (2), and more widespread use of combined therapy in ACS is likely to occur.

β-Receptor Blockade

The benefit of β-receptor antagonists in ACS is based on their ability to reduce cardiac work and decrease myocardial energy requirements. Early institution of beta-blocker therapy is recommended for all patients with ACS who do not have a contraindication to β-receptor blockade (1–3). In addition to the usual contraindications (i.e., severe sinus bradycardia with heart rate < 40 bpm, second- or third-degree heart block, decompensated systolic heart failure, hypotension, and reactive airways disease), **β-receptor antagonists are not advised for cocaine-induced myocardial infarction** because of the potential for aggravated coronary vasospasm from unopposed α-receptor activity (11).

Oral beta blocker therapy is suitable for most cases of ACS (1–3). Intravenous therapy is more appropriate for patients with hypertension or troublesome tachyarrhythmias. The agents used most often in clinical trials of ACS are atenolol (Tenormin) and metoprolol (Lopressor). Both are selective β_1-receptor antagonists that can be given orally or intravenously. Lopressor is used in our hospital, and the first dose is usually given within an hour after ACS is first suspected. The oral and intravenous dosing regimens for metoprolol are shown below (12).

Oral regimen: Start with intravenous dose of 2.5 to 5 mg and repeat every 5 minutes if needed to a total dose of 10 mg. Fifteen minutes after the last IV dose, start oral therapy with 50 mg every 6 hours for 48 hours, then 100 mg BID.

IV regimen: Add 5 mg metoprolol to 50 mL D_5W and infuse over 15 to 30 minutes every 6 hours.

Note that the oral regimen begins by giving the drug intravenously. This speeds up the response and reduces the time required to achieve steady-state drug levels in the body.

Angiotensin-Converting-Enzyme Inhibition

Angiotensin-converting-enzyme (ACE) inhibitors are vasodilators that reduce cardiac work and decrease myocardial energy requirements. They may also have an inhibitory effect on the cardiac remodeling that occurs after coronary artery reperfusion and contributes to post-MI heart failure. Oral therapy with ACE inhibitors started in the first 24 hours after onset of acute coronary syndromes has the following effects.

1. Provides a significant survival benefit in patients with anterior MI and acute MI associated with symptomatic heart failure, left ventricular dysfunction (LV ejection fraction <0.40), and tachycardia (2).
2. Provides a modest survival benefit (one life saved for every 200 patients treated) if used in all patients with acute coronary syndromes (13).

Based on these observations, oral therapy with ACE inhibitors is *probably* indicated in all patients with acute coronary syndromes and is *definitely* indicated in the conditions identified in statement #1. Contraindications to ACE inhibitor therapy include hypotension, renal failure (creatinine >2.5 mg/dL), and bilateral renal artery stenosis.

Drug Administration

Any ACE inhibitor can be used, and the first dose should be given within 24 hours after symptom onset (2). To minimize the risk of hypotension (which can be very damaging in the setting of an acute MI), only oral therapy is recommended, and the starting dose is usually reduced and then increased over the next 48 hours. One example of an ACE inhibitor regimen that has proven effective in a large clinical trial (14) is shown in Figure 17.2.

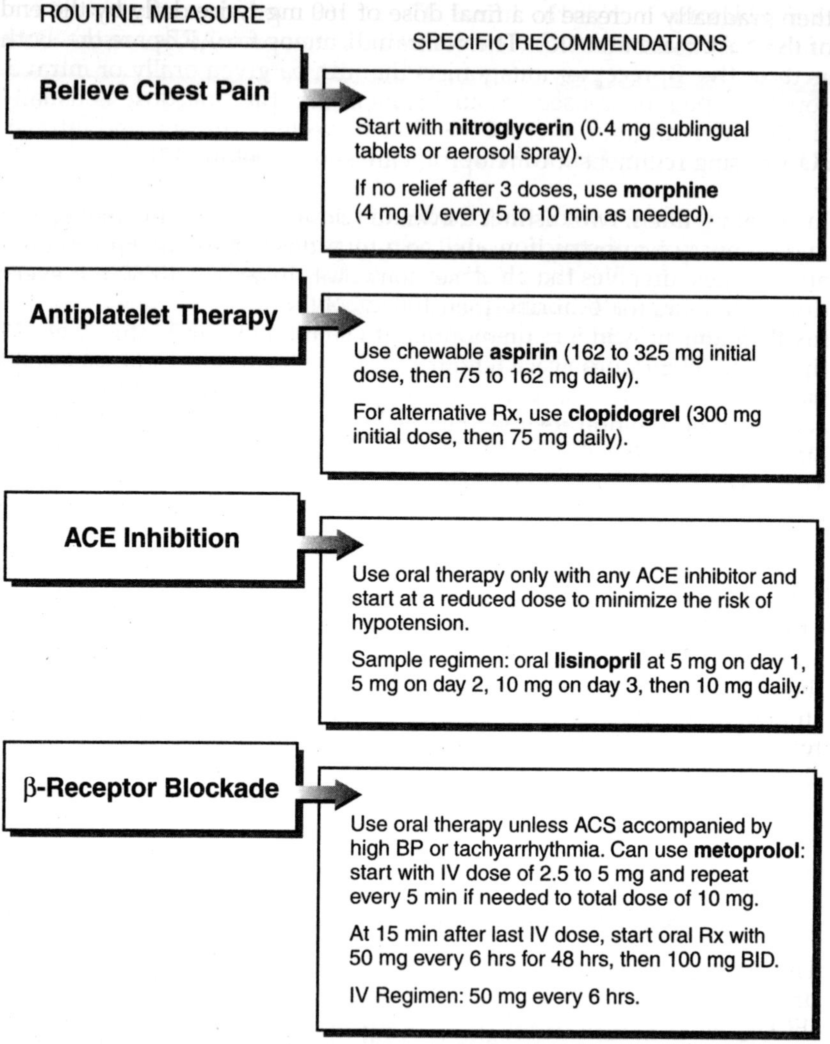

FIGURE 17.2 Routine measures in the early management of acute coronary syndromes. Abbreviations: ACS = acute coronary syndrome, ACE = angiotensin-converting-enzyme.

Angiotensin-Receptor Blockers

Clinical trials have shown that angiotensin-receptor blockers (ARB) produce a survival benefit equivalent to ACE inhibitors in acute MI associated with left ventricular dysfunction (LV ejection fraction <0.40) or symptomatic heart failure (15). As a result, ARBs are considered as a suitable alternative in patients with acute MI complicated by LV dysfunction or heart failure who do not tolerate ACE inhibitors (2). One example of a successful ARB regimen is oral valsartan, 20 mg initially, then gradually increase to a final dose of 160 mg twice daily by the end of the hospitalization (15). The contraindications for ARBs are the same as those mentioned previously for ACE inhibitors.

REPERFUSION THERAPY

In the early 1980s, two distinct modes of therapy were introduced to alleviate thrombotic obstruction and restore patency in occluded coronary arteries. One involves the pharmacologic dissolution of blood clots using drugs that stimulate fibrinolysis (thrombolytic therapy), and the other involves the mechanical disruption of clots using specialized balloon-tipped catheters (coronary angioplasty). These forms of *reperfusion therapy* have had a profound impact on the early management of patients with acute coronary syndromes and are largely responsible for the improved outcomes (reduced morbidity and mortality) reported in recent years. This section describes each type of reperfusion therapy and the relative risks and benefits.

Thrombolytic Therapy

The evaluation of drugs that stimulate fibrinolysis began immediately after the discovery (in 1980) that transmural myocardial infarction was the result of occlusive coronary thrombosis. The first fibrinolytic agent studied was streptokinase, which was shown to produce effective clot lysis when given directly into the affected coronary artery, and later was shown to be equally effective when infused into a peripheral vein (16). In 1986, the first clinical trial of intravenous streptokinase in acute MI was completed, and the results showed fewer deaths in the patients who received thrombolytic therapy (17).

The Initial Electrocardiogram

The survival benefit of thrombolytic therapy in acute coronary syndromes is determined by the findings on the initial electrocardiogram (ECG). This is demonstrated in Figure 17.3, which shows the pooled results of 9 clinical trials comparing thrombolytic therapy (with different fibrinolytic agents) to placebo in patients with acute coronary syndromes (18). **The survival benefit of thrombolytic therapy is greatest in patients who present with new-onset left bundle branch block and ST-segment elevation in the anterior precordial leads, while there is no survival benefit in patients with ST-segment depression** on the initial ECG.

Timing

The effect of thrombolytic therapy on survival is also determined by the time elapsed from the onset of chest pain to initiation of therapy. This is demonstrated in Figure 17.4, which includes data from patients who showed a survival benefit with thrombolytic therapy in the pooled studies depicted in Figure 17.3. This data shows that **the survival benefit of thrombolytic therapy is greatest when therapy is initiated in the first**

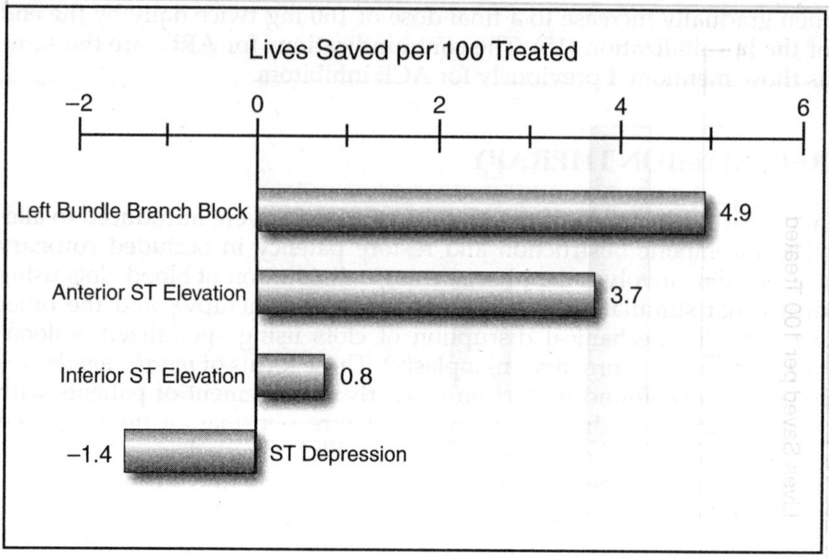

FIGURE 17.3 The survival benefit of thrombolytic therapy in relation to abnormal patterns on the electrocardiogram. (From Reference 18.)

few hours after the onset of chest pain. Thereafter, the survival benefit declines steadily with time and is negligible or lost when the delay to initiation of therapy exceeds 12 hours.

The data in Figure 17.4 highlights the most important feature of thrombolytic therapy: *Time lost is lives lost.* To ensure timely initiation of thrombolytic therapy, emergency rooms in the United States have adopted the following guidelines (2):

1. When a patient with sudden onset of chest pain enters the emergency room, an electrocardiogram should be performed and interpreted within the next 10 minutes (door-to-ECG time $<$10 minutes).
2. Thrombolytic therapy, if indicated, should be started within 30 minutes after the patient enters the emergency room (door-to-needle time $<$30 minutes).

Selection of Candidates

The observations in Figures 17.3 and 17.4 are the basis for the criteria used to select candidates for thrombolytic therapy, which are shown in Table 17.1 (2). Patients are candidates for thrombolytic therapy if coronary angioplasty is not immediately available and all of the following conditions are present: (1) chest pain for at least 30 minutes but less than 12 hours; (2) a 12-lead ECG that shows ST elevation of 0.1 mV (1 mm) or more in two contiguous leads, or a new left bundle branch block; (3) the absence of hypotension or heart failure; and (4) the absence of a

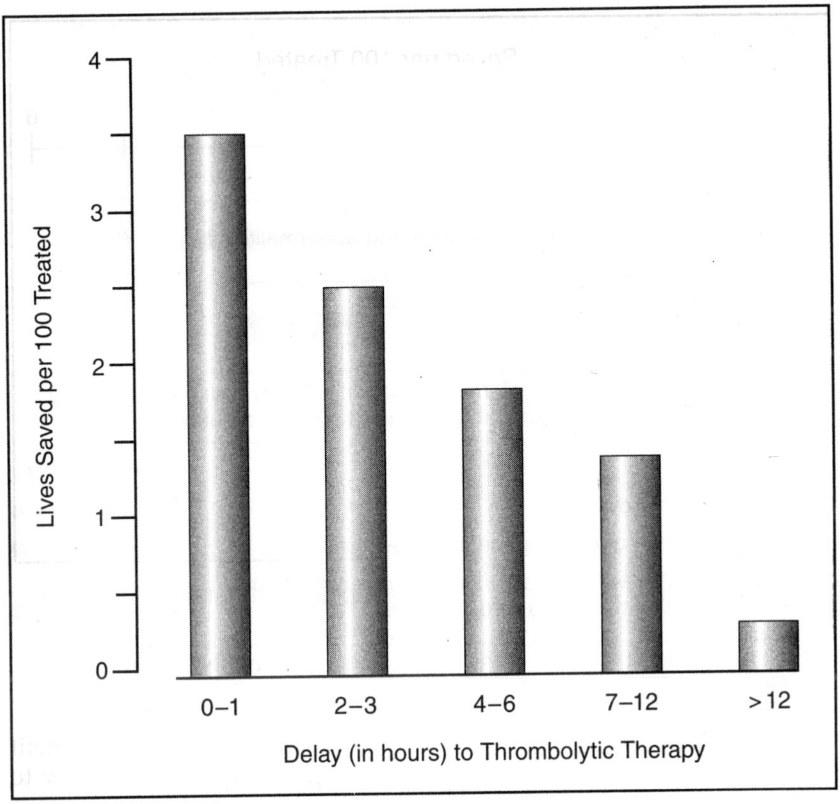

FIGURE 17.4 The survival benefit of thrombolytic therapy as a function of the time elapsed from the onset of chest pain to the initiation of therapy. (From Reference 18.)

contraindication to thrombolytic therapy that would create an unacceptable risk of bleeding (see Table 17.2). The role of coronary angioplasty in these conditions is described later in the chapter.

The most recent ACC/AHA practice guidelines (2) include true posterior MI as a condition that might benefit from thrombolytic therapy if treated within 12 hours of symptom onset. This condition should be suspected when the ECG shows ST-segment depression with upright T waves in precordial leads V_1 through V_4 (19). The discovery of ST-segment elevation in additional precordial leads $V_7 - V_9$ will help confirm the diagnosis of posterior wall MI.

Fibrinolytic Agents

The available fibrinolytic agents and recommended dosing regimens for acute MI are shown in Table 17.3. All of these agents act by converting plasminogen to plasmin, which then breaks fibrin strands into smaller subunits. Some (streptokinase) act on circulating plasminogen and produce a systemic lytic state, while others (alteplase, reteplase,

TABLE 17.1 Reperfusion Strategy for Patients with ST-Elevation Myocardial Infarction (STEMI)

For adults with sudden onset of chest pain, consider the following questions:

	Yes	No
1. Did the chest pain begin more than 30 minutes ago but less than 12 hours ago?	●	○
2. Does the ECG show either of the following abnormalities?	●	○
a) ST elevation ≥ 0.1 mV (1 mm) in at least 2 contiguous precordial leads or 2 adjacent limb leads.		
b) A new, or presumably new, left bundle branch block.		

If the answer is Yes to each of the above, perform **Coronary Angioplasty** if immediately available. Otherwise, proceed to questions below.

	Yes	No
3. Is the patient hypotensive?	○	●
4. Is there evidence of decompensated heart failure?	○	●
5. Is there an unacceptable risk of bleeding as a result of any of the contraindications listed in Table 17.2?	○	●

If the answer is No to each of the above, begin **Thrombolytic Therapy** immediately.

and tenecteplase) act only on plasminogen that is bound to fibrin and produce clot-specific lysis. The site of action (clot-specific versus systemic) has little clinical relevance.

Streptokinase is a bacterial protein that was the first thrombolytic agent evaluated in clinical trials and the first to show improved survival in patients with acute, ST-elevation MI (17). Although it is the least expensive thrombolytic agent, it is also the least favored because it acts as an antigen and produces fever (in 20 to 40% of cases), allergic reactions (in 5% of cases), and accumulation of neutralizing antibodies with repeated use (20).

Alteplase (tissue plasminogen activator or tPA) is a molecular clone of an endogenous plasminogen activator that replaced streptokinase in popularity because it does not produce allergic reactions, and because one large study published in 1993 (the GUSTO trial) showed improved survival with alteplase compared to streptokinase (21). Alteplase has been the favored lytic agent for the past 10 to 15 years, but it may be replaced by the newer lytic agents given as bolus doses, which are easier to administer (22).

Reteplase (rPA) is a molecular variant of tPA that is given in 2 bolus doses 30 minutes apart. It is easier to give than tPA and produces more rapid clot lysis (23). However, clinical trials comparing reteplase and alteplase have shown no difference in mortality rate (24).

Tenecteplase (TNK-tPA) is another variant of tPA that is given as a single bolus. It is the most clot-specific fibrinolytic agent and produces

Table 17.2 Contraindications to Thrombolytic Therapy

Absolute Contraindications:

- Active bleeding other than menses
- Malignant intracranial neoplasm (primary or metastatic)
- Cerebrovascular anomaly (e.g., AV malformation)
- Suspected aortic dissection
- Ischemic stroke within 3 months (but not within 3 hours)
- Prior history of intracranial hemorrhage
- Significant closed-head or facial trauma within 3 months

Relative Contraindications:

- Systolic BP > 180 mm Hg or diastolic BP > 110 mm Hg
- Active bleeding within the past 4 weeks
- Noncompressible vascular punctures
- Major surgery within the past 3 weeks
- Traumatic or prolonged (> 10 min) CPR
- Ischemic stroke over 3 months ago
- Dementia
- Active peptic ulcer disease
- Pregnancy
- Current use of anticoagulants (the higher the INR, the greater the risk of bleeding)

From the practice guidelines in Reference 2.

TABLE 17.3 Thrombolytic Agents

Agent	Dose	Comments
Streptokinase (SK)	1.5 million units IV over 60 min	Allergic reactions and buildup of neutralizing antibodies with repeated use.
Alteplase (tPA)	15 mg IV bolus, + 0.75 mg/kg over 30 min + 0.5 mg/kg over 60 min (90 min total)	Most frequently used lytic agent.
Reteplase (rPA)	10 units as IV bolus and repeat in 30 min	Bolus doses are easier to give and produce more rapid clot lysis than tPA.
Tenecteplase (TNK)	IV bolus of 30 mg for BW < 60 kg, 35 mg for BW = 60–69 kg, 40 mg for BW = 70–79 kg, 45 mg for BW = 80–89 kg, 50 mg for BW ≥ 90 kg	Most clot-specific and rapidly acting lytic agent. Easiest to use because of single bolus dose.

the most rapid clot lysis (22). However, neither of these attributes offers a clinical advantage because clinical trials comparing tenecteplase and alteplase have shown no difference in the incidence of life-threatening bleeding and no difference in mortality rate (25).

In summary, excluding streptokinase because of its unwanted antigen effects, the available fibrinolytic agents are equivalent in terms of survival benefit and risk of bleeding. Bolus fibrinolytic therapy (with reteplase or tenecteplase) is likely to gain in popularity simply because it is easier. Overall, it seems that **the important issue in thrombolytic therapy is not which agent to use, but how quickly to use it.**

Complications

The most feared complication of thrombolytic therapy is intracerebral hemorrhage, which is reported in 0.5 to 1% of cases (22). This may be more common with alteplase when compared to streptokinase (21), but there is no difference between alteplase, reteplase, and tenecteplase in the risk of intracerebral bleeding (22). Extracranial bleeding that requires blood transfusions occurs in 5 to 15% of patients, regardless of the lytic agent used (26). There is no correlation between the risk of hemorrhage and the degree of clot-specificity of the fibrinolytic agents.

The hemorrhagic complications of thrombolytic therapy are the result of systemic fibrinolysis with depletion of circulating fibrinogen levels. If necessary, cryoprecipitate (10 to 15 bags) can be used to achieve a serum fibrinogen level of 1 g/L (26). If bleeding persists, fresh frozen plasma (up to 6 units) can be administered, followed by platelet infusions (10 bags) if needed. The use of antifibrinolytic agents such as epsilon-aminocaproic acid (5 grams given over 15 to 30 minutes) is discouraged for all but the most serious and refractory cases of bleeding because these agents can produce extensive thrombosis (26).

Reocclusion

The benefit of thrombolytic therapy is limited by the risk of reocclusion following clot lysis, which is reported in up to 25% of cases (2,26). This may be a natural consequence of clot dissolution because the exposed thrombin (which had been enmeshed in the thrombus) has prothrombotic effects via platelet activation and an increased rate of thrombin formation (27). To counteract this process, antithrombotic therapy with heparin and antiplatelet agents is given in combination with thrombolytic therapy. This adjunctive therapy is described later in the chapter.

Coronary Angioplasty

The use of balloon-tipped catheters to open occluded arteries (balloon angioplasty) was adapted for use in the coronary arteries in 1977 by a Swiss physician named Andreas Gruntzig. This procedure (*percutaneous coronary angioplasty*) was adopted in the 1980s as an alternative to thrombolytic therapy for patients with acute myocardial infarction. As a result of improved techniques and the introduction of stents to keep arteries open, **coronary angioplasty is now the preferred method of reperfusion therapy for patients with occlusive coronary thrombosis.**

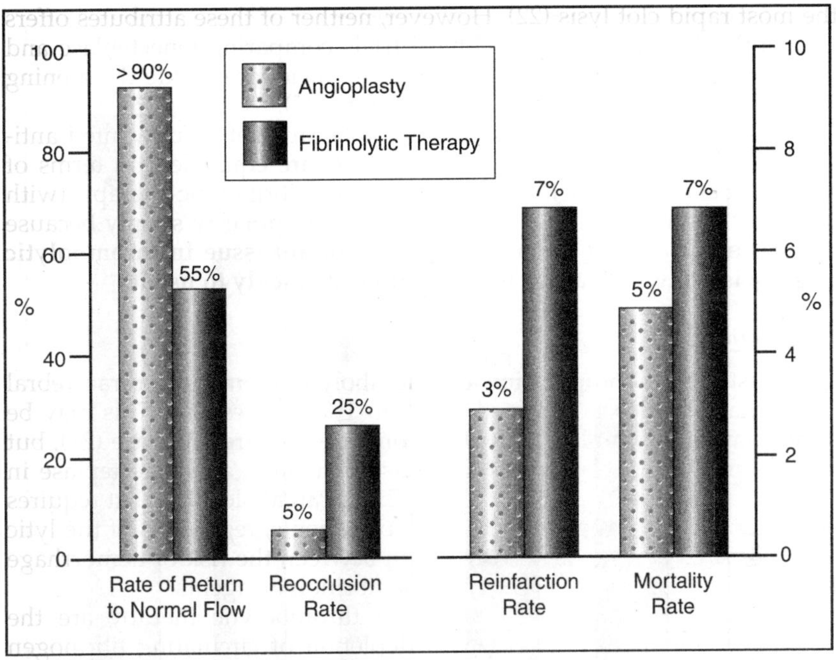

FIGURE 17.5 Comparative effects of primary angioplasty and thrombolytic therapy on vascular events (graph on the left) and clinical outcomes (graph on the right) in patients with ST-elevation myocardial infarction. (Data from References 28–30).

Angioplasty vs. Lytic Therapy

Several clinical trials have compared coronary angioplasty and thrombolytic therapy in patients with ST-elevation MI who present within 12 hours of symptom onset (28–30). The comparative effects on vascular events and clinical outcomes are shown in Figure 17.5. The bar graph on the left (depicting vascular events) shows that angioplasty restores normal flow in infarct-related arteries much more frequently and has a much lower rate of reocclusion than thrombolytic therapy. The bar graph on the right (depicting clinical outcomes), which represents the pooled results of 23 studies (29), shows that angioplasty has a lower reinfarction rate and a lower mortality rate than thrombolytic therapy. These differences in mortality and reinfarction (2% and 4%, respectively) indicate that, **for every 100 patients treated with angioplasty instead of thrombolytic therapy, there are 2 fewer deaths and 4 fewer (non-fatal) recurrent infarctions.**

Timing

The beneficial effects of coronary angioplasty, like those of thrombolytic therapy, are time-dependent. This is demonstrated in Figure 17.6, which shows the mortality rate (at 30 days) for patients with acute MI who underwent angioplasty at different times after arriving at the hospital (31). The time from arrival at the hospital to the angioplasty procedure is

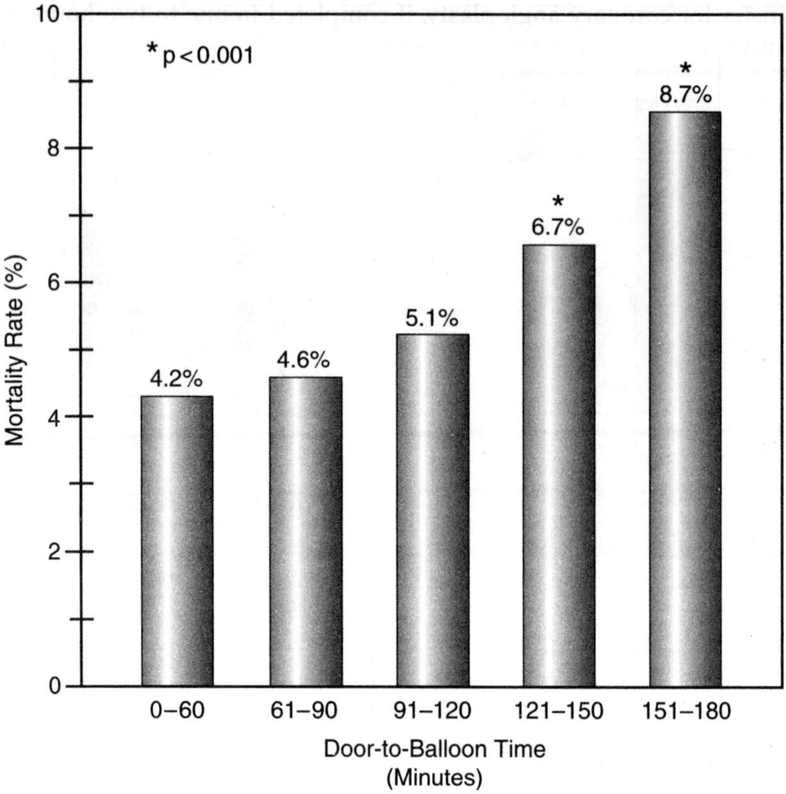

FIGURE 17.6 Mortality rate in patients treated with primary angioplasty as a function of the time period between arrival to the hospital and the angioplasty (door-to-balloon time). Asterisk indicates a significant difference in mortality rate compared to the initial time period (0–60 min). (From Reference 31.)

shown as the "door-to-balloon time" on the horizontal axis of the graph. As demonstrated, mortality rate rises steadily with increasing delays to angioplasty, and the increased mortality becomes significant when the delay to angioplasty exceeds 2 hours. This observation is the basis for the recommendation that **angioplasty should be performed within 90 minutes after the patient arrives in the emergency department** (2). This, of course, only applies to the use of angioplasty for patients with ST-elevation MI who present within 12 hours of symptom onset.

Interhospital Transfer

The major limitation of coronary angioplasty is availability. Less than 25% of hospitals in the United States have facilities for coronary angioplasty, and in Europe, fewer than 10% of hospitals have this capability (32). One solution for the "have-nots" is transfer to a hospital that can perform angioplasty. Clinical studies have shown that interhospital transfer for coronary angioplasty, if completed in one to two hours, can take advantage of the benefits derived from angioplasty and improve clinical outcomes (2,33). The current recommendations for interhospital transfer are stated below (2):

1. If the symptom duration is less than 3 hours, thrombolytic therapy is recommended unless interhospital transfer will not add more than a one-hour delay to treatment.
2. If the symptom duration is longer than 3 hours, interhospital transfer for angioplasty is recommended. The total door-to-balloon time, including the transfer time, should be close to 90 minutes to achieve the optimal benefit of angioplasty.

ADJUNCTS TO REPERFUSION THERAPY

Antithrombotic therapy with antiplatelet agents and heparin has a proven benefit when used with or without reperfusion therapy. When added to reperfusion therapy (particularly thrombolytic therapy), antithrombotic therapy can help to prevent reocclusion and recurrent infarction.

Heparin

Anticoagulation with heparin is beneficial in most patients with acute coronary syndromes, and it may be particularly advantageous in patients who receive fibrinolytic agents to reduce the risk of reocclusion from the prothrombotic effects of thrombin exposed during clot dissolution (described earlier). The effectiveness of heparin in acute coronary syndromes can differ for the two heparin preparations: unfractionated heparin (UFH) and low-molecular-weight heparin (LMWH). (See Chapter 5 for a description of these heparin preparations.) The following is a summary of the ACC/AHA recommendations for the use of UFH and LMWH in acute coronary syndromes.

1. LMWH is preferred to UFH for patients with unstable angina (UA) and non-ST- segment elevation myocardial infarction (non-STEMI) (3,34,35).
2. UFH and LMWH are considered equivalent in patients with ST-segment elevation myocardial infarction (STEMI) who do not undergo reperfusion therapy (2).
3. Despite promising results with LMWH (36), UFH is recommended for patients with STEMI who undergo reperfusion therapy with fibrinolytic agents or angioplasty (2).

Recommended Dose Regimens

The ACC/AHA recommendations for heparin dosing in acute coronary syndromes is shown below (1–3). Enoxaparin is used as the LMWH because this agent has been studied most in acute coronary syndromes.

TABLE 17.4 Enoxaparin Dosage Based on Renal Function

GFR* (mL/min)	SC Dose (mg/kg q 12h)	GFR* (mL/min)	SC Dose (mg/kg q 12h)
≥ 80	1.0	40–49	0.6
70–79	0.9	30–39	0.5
60–69	0.8	20–29	0.4
50–59	0.7	10–19	0.3

*GRF (mL/min) = (140-age) × wt (kg)/72 × serum creatinine (mg/dL). For females, multiply GFR by 0.85.
From Green B, et al. Dosing strategy for enoxaparin in patients with renal impairment presenting with acute coronary syndromes. Br J Clin Pharmacol 2004;59:281.

Enoxaparin: Start with intravenous bolus of 40 mg, and follow with subcutaneous injection of 1 mg/kg twice daily for 5 days (3). Reduced dosing is necessary in renal insufficiency (see Table 17.4)

UFH: Start with intravenous bolus of 60–70 Units/kg, and follow with infusion of 12–15 Units/kg/hr. Adjust infusion to maintain activated partial thromboplastin time (aPTT) at 1.5 to 2 times control (3).

UFH with fibrinolytic agents: Start with intravenous bolus of 60 Units/kg, and follow with infusion of 12 Units/kg/hr. Adjust infusion to maintain aPTT at 1.5 to 2 times control (2).

UFH with angioplasty: Start with intravenous bolus of 70–100 Units/kg, and follow with infusion of 12–15 Units/kg/hr. Adjust infusion to maintain the aPTT at 1.5 to 2 times control (2).

When using UFH, the aPTT should be checked 3 hours after starting the infusion and 6 hours after each dose adjustment. In addition, platelet levels should be checked daily in all patients receiving heparin (because of the risk of heparin-induced thrombocytopenia, described in Chapter 37).

Aspirin

Aspirin is used as an antiplatelet agent in virtually everyone with acute coronary syndromes (except those with aspirin allergy). When used in combination with fibrinolytic agents, aspirin reduces the rate of reinfarction (9). The recommended dosing regimen for aspirin is described earlier in the chapter.

Platelet Glycoprotein Inhibitors

The newest group of drugs added to the war chest for acute coronary syndromes are potent antiplatelet agents that block platelet receptors involved in platelet aggregation. When platelets are activated, specialized glycoproteins on the platelet surface (called IIb/IIIa receptors)

Table 17.5 Platelet Glycoprotein Inhibitors

Agent	Commercial Preparation	Dose
Abciximab	ReoPro	0.25 mg/kg as IV bolus followed by infusion of 0.125 μg/kg/min (maximum 10 μg/min).
Eptifibatide	Integrilin	180 μg/kg as IV bolus followed by infusion of 2 μg/kg/min for up to 96 hrs. For serum creatinine of 2–4 mg/dL, reduce first dose to 130 μg/kg and reduce infusion rate to 0.5 μg/kg/min.*
Tirofiban	Aggrastat	0.4 μg/kg/min for 30 min followed by infusion of 0.1 μg/kg/min. For creatinine clearance < 30 mL/min, reduce both dose rates by 50%.*

*Manufacturer's recommendation.

change configuration and begin to bind fibrinogen. When fibrinogen molecules bind to adjacent platelets, platelet aggregation occurs. The *platelet glycoprotein (IIb/IIIa) inhibitors* bind to the surface receptors on platelets and prevent the binding of fibrinogen. The result is inhibition of platelet aggregation. The IIb/IIIa receptors are the final common pathway for platelet aggregation, so the IIb/IIIa inhibitors are the most powerful antiplatelet agents available (and are sometimes called "superaspirins").

Drug Administration

There are three platelet glycoprotein inhibitors available for clinical use: abciximab (ReoPro), eptifibatide (Integrilin), and tirofiban (Aggrastat). All three are given by intravenous infusion, and the dosing regimen for each agent is shown in Table 17.5.

Abciximab (try to pronounce it!) is a monoclonal antibody that is the most potent, most expensive, and longest-acting drug in the group. After discontinuing abciximab, bleeding times can take 12 hours to normalize (7), and this prolonged action can be a disadvantage when emergency bypass surgery is contemplated.

Eptifibatide (a synthetic peptide) and tirofiban (a tyrosine derivative) are short-acting agents that are cleared by the kidneys. After discontinuing these drugs, bleeding times return to normal in 15 minutes for eptifibatide and 4 hours for tirofiban (7). Dose adjustments in renal insufficiency are recommended for both drugs, and these dose adjustments are included in Table 17.5. Excess dosing in renal insufficiency will result in drug accumulation and increased risk of bleeding. Dose adjustments in renal failure are not necessary for abciximab because it is an antibody and is presumably cleared by the reticuloendothelial system.

Indications

Platelet glycoprotein inhibitors are primarily used in patients with unstable angina (UA) and nonST-elevation myocardial infarction (non-STEMI) when the following conditions are present (3):

1. When coronary angioplasty is planned in the next 24 to 48 hours.
2. When there is evidence of continuing myocardial ischemia (e.g., recurrent angina or angina at rest with transient ST-segment changes).
3. When there are risk factors for recurrent ischemic events, such as age >75 years, heart failure, new or worsening mitral regurgitation, markedly elevated cardiac troponin levels, and cardiogenic shock (3).

The **greatest benefits occur when these agents are used in conjunction with angioplasty** (1–3,38). Abciximab is recommended only when angioplasty is planned and seems a favorite of cardiologists. In the catheterization lab, the initial bolus of abciximab is given after the arterial sheath is placed, and the abciximab infusion is continued for 12 hours after the procedure (39).

Platelet glycoprotein inhibitors are gaining popularity in patients with ST-elevation MI (STEMI), and are usually given in combination with angioplasty or thrombolytic therapy (2,3,37). In the future, expect platelet glycoprotein inhibitors to be combined with low-dose fibrinolytic agents as a prelude to coronary angioplasty (so-called "facilitated angioplasty").

Adverse Effects

The major risk with platelet glycoprotein inhibitors is bleeding. The incidence of bleeding from these agents is difficult to assess because they are often used in combination with aspirin and heparin. Most of the bleeding is mucocutaneous, and intracranial hemorrhage is not a risk with these agents (7,38). Thrombocytopenia is reported in up to 2% of patients who receive abciximab and is more common with repeated use of the drug (38).

Active bleeding is an absolute contraindication to platelet glycoprotein inhibitors. Relative contraindications include major surgery within the past 3 months, stroke in the past 6 months, systolic blood pressure >180 mm Hg or diastolic pressure >110 mm Hg, and severe thrombocytopenia (38).

EARLY COMPLICATIONS

The appearance of decompensated heart failure and cardiogenic shock in the first few days after an acute MI is an ominous sign and usually indicates a mechanical problem like acute mitral regurgitation or cardiac pump failure. Echocardiography is usually needed to uncover the problem, but the mortality in these conditions is high despite timely interventions.

Mechanical Complications

Mechanical complications are usually the result of transmural (ST-elevation) MI. All are serious, and all require prompt action.

Acute mitral regurgitation is the result of papillary muscle rupture and presents with the sudden onset of pulmonary edema and the characteristic holosystolic murmur radiating to the axilla. The pulmonary artery occlusion pressure should show prominent V waves, but this can be a non-specific finding. Diagnosis is by echocardiography, and arterial vasodilators (e.g., hydralazine) are used to relieve pulmonary edema pending surgery. Mortality is 70% without surgery and 40% with surgery (39).

Ventricular septal rupture can occur anytime in the first 5 days after acute MI. The diagnosis can be elusive without cardiac ultrasound. There is a step-up in O_2 saturation from right atrial to pulmonary artery blood, but this is rarely measured. Initial management involves vasodilator (e.g., nitroglycerin) infusions and the intraaortic balloon pump if needed. Mortality is 90% without surgery and 20% to 50% with surgery (2).

Ventricular free wall rupture occurs in up to 6% of cases of STEMI and is more common with anterior MI, fibrinolytic or steroid therapy, and advanced age (2). The first signs of trouble are usually return of chest pains and new ST-segment abnormalities on the ECG. Accumulation of blood in the pericardium often leads to rapid deterioration and cardiovascular collapse from pericardial tamponade. Diagnosis is made by cardiac ultrasound (if time permits), and prompt pericardiocentesis combined with aggressive volume resuscitation is required for hemodynamic support. Immediate surgery is the only course of action, but fewer than half of the patients survive despite surgery (2).

Pump Failure

About 15% of cases of acute MI result in cardiac pump failure and cardiogenic shock (40). Management involves hemodynamic support (usually with intraaortic balloon counterpulsation) followed by reperfusion using coronary angioplasty or coronary bypass surgery. Despite the best intentions, the mortality in this situation is 60 to 80% (40).

Hemodynamic Support

Hemodynamic support should be designed to augment cardiac output without increasing myocardial oxygen consumption. Table 17.6 shows the effects of hemodynamic support on the determinants of myocardial O_2 consumption (preload, contractility, afterload, and heart rate) in decompensated heart failure and cardiogenic shock. As judged by the net effect on myocardial O_2 consumption, vasodilator therapy is superior to dobutamine in heart failure, and the intra-aortic balloon pump (IABP) is superior to dopamine in cardiogenic shock. (See Chapter 14 for more information on the treatment of cardiac pump failure.)

TABLE 17.6 Hemodynamic Support and Myocardial O_2 Consumption

Parameter	Heart Failure		Cardiogenic Shock	
	Vasodilators	Dobutamine	IABP	Dopamine
Preload	↓	↓	↓	↑
Contractility	—	↑↑	—	↑↑
Afterload	↓↓	↓	↓	↑
Heart rate	—	↑	—	↑
Net effect on myocardial VO_2	↓↓↓	↑	↓↓	↑↑↑↑↑

IABP = Intra-aortic balloon pump, VO_2 = oxygen consumption.

Emergency Revascularization

The ACC/AHA guidelines recommend coronary angioplasty when cardiogenic shock appears within 36 hours of acute MI and when the angioplasty can be performed within 18 hours of the onset of shock (2). Coronary artery bypass surgery is considered if the cardiac catheterization reveals multivessel disease that is not amenable to angioplasty or disease involving the left main coronary artery (2).

Arrhythmias

Disturbances of cardiac rhythm are common after acute MI and are not suppressed by prophylactic use of lidocaine (2). The management of serious arrhythmias is described in the next chapter.

Acute Aortic Dissection

Aortic dissection is included in this chapter because the clinical presentation can be mistaken as an acute coronary syndrome, and the condition is often fatal if missed.

Clinical Presentation

The most common complaint is abrupt onset of chest pain. The pain is often sharp and is described as "ripping or tearing" (mimicking the underlying process) in about 50% of cases (41). Radiation to the jaws and arms is uncommon. **The pain can subside spontaneously for hours to days (41,42), and this can be a source of missed diagnoses.** The return of the pain after a pain-free interval is often a sign of impending aortic rupture.

Clinical Findings

Hypertension and aortic insufficiency are each present in about 50% of cases, and hypotension is reported in 25% of cases (41,42). Dissection can cause obstruction of the left subclavian artery, leading to blood pressure differences in the arms, but this finding can be absent in up to 85% of cases (42). Obstruction involving other arteries in the chest can lead to stroke and coronary insufficiency.

Diagnosis

Mediastinal widening on chest x-ray (present in 60% of cases) often raises suspicion for dissection (42). However, the diagnosis requires one of four imaging modalities (43): magnetic resonance imaging (MRI) (sensitivity and specificity, 98%), transesophageal echocardiography (sensitivity, 98%; specificity, 77%), contrast-enhanced computed tomography (sensitivity, 94%; specificity, 87%), and aortography (sensitivity, 88%; specificity, 94%). Thus **MRI is the diagnostic modality of choice for aortic dissection**, but the immediate availability of MRI is limited in some hospitals, and helical CT and transesophageal ultrasound are high-yield alternatives to MRI. Aortography is the least sensitive but provides valuable information for the operating surgeon.

Management

Acute dissection in the ascending aorta is a surgical emergency. Prompt control of hypertension is advantageous prior to surgery to reduce the risk of aortic rupture. Increased flow rates in the aorta create shear forces that promote further dissection, so **blood pressure reduction should not be accompanied by increased cardiac output.** This can be accomplished with the drug regimens shown in Table 17.7 (41,42). One regimen uses a vasodilator (nitroprusside) infusion combined with a β-blocker (esmolol) infusion. The β-blocker is given first to block the vasodilator-induced increase in cardiac output. Esmolol is used as the β-blocker because it has a short duration of action (9 minutes) and is easy to titrate. It can also be stopped just prior to surgery without the risk of residual cardiac suppression during surgery. Single-drug therapy with a combined α and β-receptor antagonist (labetalol) is also effective and is easier to use than the combination drug regimen.

TABLE 17.7 Treating Hypertension in Aortic Dissection

Combined therapy with β-blocker and vasodilator:	
Start with esmolol:	500 μ/kg IV bolus and follow with 50 μg/kg/min. Increase infusion by 25 μg/kg/min every 5 min until heart rate 60–80 bpm. Maximum dose rate is 200 μg/kg/min.
Add nitroprusside:	Start infusion at 0.2 μg/kg/min and titrate upward to desired effect. See the nitroprusside dosage chart in Table 16.6.
Monotherapy with combined α-β receptor antagonist:	
Labetalol:	20 mg IV over 2 min, then infuse 1–2 mg/min to desired effect and stop infusion. Maximum cumulative dose is 300 mg.

A FINAL WORD

The discovery that acute myocardial infarction is the result of blood clots that obstruct coronary arteries has one important implication (besides the improved therapeutic approach to myocardial infarction) that seems overlooked. It disputes the traditional teaching that myocardial infarction is the result of a generalized imbalance between myocardial O_2 delivery and O_2 consumption. This distinction is important because the O_2-imbalance paradigm is the basis for the overzealous use of oxygen breathing and blood transfusions in patients with coronary artery disease. Blood clots (from ruptured atherosclerotic plaques) cause heart attacks, not hypoxia or anemia.

If you have ever wondered why heart attacks are uncommon in patients with progressive shock and multiorgan failure, you now have the answer.

REFERENCES

Clinical Practice Guidelines

1. 2005 American Heart Association Guidelines for Cardiopulmonary Resuscitation and Emergency Cardiovascular Care. Part 8: Stabilization of the patient with acute coronary syndromes. Circulation 2005;112(suppl I):IV89–IV110. (Available online @ http://circ.ahajournals.org/content/vol112/24_suppl/)
2. Antman EM, Anbe DT, Armstrong PW, et al. ACC/AHA guidelines for the management of patients with ST-elevation myocardial infarction: executive summary: a report of the American College of Cardiology/American Heart Association Task Force on Practice Guidelines (Writing Committee to Revise the 1999 Guidelines for the Management of Patients with Acute Myocardial Infarction). Circulation 2004;110:588–636. (Available at www.acc.org/clinical/guidelines/stemi/Guideline1/index.htm)
3. Braunwald E, Antman EM, Beasley JW, et al. ACC/AHA 2002 guideline update for the management of patients with unstable angina and non-ST-segment myocardial infarction: summary article: a report of the American College of Cardiology/American Heart Association Task Force on Practice Guidelines (Committee on the Management of Patients with Unstable Angina). J Am Coll Cardiol 2002;40:1366–1374.

Acute Coronary Syndromes

4. Davies MJ, Thomas AC. Plaque fissuring: the cause of acute myocardial infarction. Br Heart J 1985;53:363–373.
5. Van der Wal AC, Becker AE, van der Loos CM, et al. Site of intimal rupture or erosion of thrombosed coronary atherosclerotic plaques is characterized by an inflammatory process irrespective of the dominant plaque morphology. Circulation 1994;89:36–44.
6. Malek AM, Alper SL, Izumo S. Hemodynamic shear stress and its role in atherosclerosis. JAMA 1999;282:2035–2042.

Routine Measures

7. Patrono C, Coller B, Fitzgerald G, et al. Platelet-active drugs: the relationships among dose, effectiveness, and side effects. Chest 2004;126:234S–264S.
8. ISIS-2 (Second International Study of Infarct Survival) Collaborative group. Randomized trial of intravenous streptokinase, oral aspirin, both, or neither among 17,187 cases os suspected acute myocardial infarction: ISIS-2. Lancet 1988;2:349–360.
9. Roux S, Christellar S, Ludin E. Effects of aspirin on coronary reocclusion and recurrent ischemia after thrombolysis: a meta-analysis. J Am Coll Cardiol 1992;19:671–677.
10. Clopidogrel in Unstable Angina to Prevent Recurrent Events Trial Investigators. Effects of clopidogrel in addition to aspirin in patients with acute coronary syndromes without ST-segment elevation. N Engl J Med 2001;345:494–502.
11. Kloner RA, Hale S. Unraveling the complex effects of cocaine on the heart. Circulation 1993;87:1046–1047.
12. AHFS. Metoprolol succinate and metoprolol tartrate. In McEvoy GK, ed. AHFS drug information, 2001. Bethesda, MD: American Society for Health System Pharmacists, 2001:1622–1629.
13. ACE Inhibitor Myocardial Infarction Collaborative Group. Indications for ACE inhibitors in the early treatment of acute myocardial infarction: systematic overview of individual data from 100,000 patients in randomized trials. Circulation 1998;97:2202–2212.
14. Gruppo Italiano per lo Studio della Sopravvivenza nell'infarto Miocardico (GISSI). GISSI-3. Effects of lisinopril and transdermal glyceryl trinitrate singly and together on 6-week mortality and ventricular function after acute myocardial infarction. Lancet 1994;343:1115–1122.
15. Pfeffer MA, McMurray JJ, Velazquez EJ, et al., for the Valsartan in Acute Myocardial Infarction Trial Investigators. Valsartan, captopril, or both in myocardial infarction complicated by heart failure, left ventricular dysfunction, or both. N Engl J Med 2003;349:1893–1906.

Thrombolytic Therapy

16. Anderson HV, Willerson JT. Thrombolysis in acute myocardial infarction. N Engl J Med 1993;329:703–725.
17. Gruppo Italiano per lo Studio della Streptochinasi nell'Infarto Miocardico (GISSI). Effectiveness of intravenous thrombolytic treatment in acute myocardial infarction. Lancet 1986;1:397–401.
18. Fibrinolytic Therapy Trialists Collaborative Group. Indications for fibrinolytic therapy in suspected acute myocardial infarction: collaborative overview of early mortality and major morbidity results from all randomized trials of more than 1000 patients. Lancet 1994;343:311–322.
19. Boden WE, Kleiger RE, Gibson RS, et al. Electrocardiographic evolution of posterior acute myocardial infarction: importance of early precordial ST-segment depression. Am J Cardiol 1987;59:782–787.
20. Guidry JR, Raschke R, Morkunas AR. Anticoagulants and thrombolytics. In: Blumer JL, Bond GR, eds. Toxic effects of drugs in the ICU: critical care clinics. Vol. 7. Philadelphia: WB Saunders, 1991:533–554.

21. GUSTO Investigators. An international randomized trial comparing four thrombolytic strategies for acute myocardial infarction. N Engl J Med 1993;329:673–682.
22. Llevadot J, Giugliano RP, Antman EM. Bolus fibrinolytic therapy in acute myocardial infarction. JAMA 2001;286:442–449.
23. Smalling RW, Bode C, Kalbfleisch J, et al. More rapid, complete, and stable coronary thrombolysis with bolus administration of reteplase compared with alteplase infusion in acute myocardial infarction. Circulation 1995;91:2725–2732.
24. GUSTO-III Investigators. An international, multicenter, randomized comparison of reteplase with alteplase for acute myocardial infarction. N Engl J Med 1997;337:1118–1123.
25. Assessment of the Safety and Efficacy of a New Thrombolytic (ASSENT-2) Investigators. Single-bolus tenecteplase compared with front-loaded alteplase in acute myocardial infarction. Lancet 1999;354:716–722.
26. Young GP, Hoffman JR. Thrombolytic therapy. Emerg Med Clin 1995;13:735–759.
27. Topol EJ. Acute myocardial infarction: thrombolysis. Heart 2000;83:122–126.

Coronary Angioplasty

28. The GUSTO IIb Angioplasty Substudy Investigators. A clinical trial comparing primary coronary angioplasty with tissue plasminogen activator for acute myocardial infarction. N Engl J Med 1997;336:1621–1628.
29. Keeley EC, Boura JA, Grines CL. Primary angioplasty versus intravenous thrombolytic therapy for acute myocardial infarction: a quantitative review of 23 randomized trials. Lancet 2003;361:13–20.
30. Stone GW, Cox D, Garcia E, et al. Normal flow (TIMI-3) before mechanical reperfusion therapy is an independent determinant of survival in acute myocardial infarction. Circulation 2001;104:636–641.
31. Cannon CP, Gibson CM, Lambrew CT, et al. Relationship of symptom onset to balloon time and door-to-balloon time with mortality in patients undergoing angioplasty for acute myocardial infarction. JAMA 2000;283:2941–2947.
32. Meyer MC. Reperfusion strategies for ST-segment elevation myocardial infarction: an overview of current therapeutic options. Part II: Mechanical reperfusion. Emergency Medicine Reports, Vol 25, April 2004 (Accessed on 1/2/2005 at www.emronline.com/articles/Issues_Abstracts/2004/emr04052004a.html)
33. Andersen HR, Nielsen TT, Rasmussen K, et al. for the DANAMI-2 Investigators. A comparison of coronary angioplasty with fibrinolytic therapy in acute myocardial infarction. N Engl J Med 2003;349:733–742.

Adjuncts to Reperfusion Therapy

34. Wong GC, Gugliano RP, Antman EM. Use of low-molecular-weight heparins in the management of acute coronary syndromes and percutaneous coronary intervention. JAMA 2003;289:331–342.
35. Petersen JL, Mahaffey KW, Hasselblad V, et al. Efficacy and bleeding complications among patients randomized to enoxaparin or unfractionated heparin

for antithrombin therapy in non-ST-segment elevation acute coronary syndromes. JAMA 2004;292:89–96.
36. Theroux P, Welsh RC. Meta-analysis of randomized trials comparing enoxaparin versus unfractionated heparin as adjunctive therapy to fibrinolysis in ST-elevation acute myocardial infarction. Am J Cardiol 2003;91:860–864.
37. Assessment of the Safety and Efficacy of a New Thrombolytic Regimen (ASSENT-3) Investigators. Efficacy and safety of tenectaplase in combination with enoxaparin, abciximab, or unfractionated heparin: the ASSENT-3 randomized trial in acute myocardial infarction. Lancet 2001;358:605–613.
38. Bhatt DL, Topol EJ. Current role of platelet glycoprotein IIb/IIIa inhibitors in acute coronary syndromes. JAMA 2000;284:1549–1558.

Early Complications

39. Thompson CR, Buller CE, Sleeper LA, et al. Cardiogenic shock due to acute severe mitral regurgitation complicating acute myocardial infarction: a report from the SHOCK trial registry. J Am Coll Cardiol 2000;36:1104–1109.
40. Samuels LF, Darze ES. Management of acute cardiogenic shock. Cardiol Clin 2003;21:43–49.

Aortic Dissection

41. Khan IA, Nair CK. Clinical, diagnostic, and management perspectives of aortic dissection. Chest 2002;122:311–328.
42. Knaut AL, Cleveland JC. Aortic emergencies. Emerg Med Clin N Am 2003; 21:817–845.
43. Zegel HG, Chmielewski S, Freiman DB. The imaging evaluation of thoracic aortic dissection. Appl Radiol 1995;(June):15–25.

Chapter 18

TACHYARRHYTHMIAS

Acute arrhythmias are the gremlins of the ICU because they pop up unexpectedly, create some havoc, and are often gone in a flash. The arrhythmias that create the most havoc are the ones that produce rapid heart rates: the *tachyarrhythmias*. This chapter describes the acute management of tachyarrhythmias using clinical practice guidelines developed by consensus groups in the United States and Europe. The published guidelines are listed in the bibliography at the end of chapter (1–3), along with Internet addresses where they can be downloaded at no cost.

CLASSIFICATION

Tachycardias (heart rate above 100 beats/minute) can be the result of *increased automaticity* in pacemaker cells (e.g., sinus tachycardias), *triggered activity* (e.g., ectopic impulses), or a process known as *re-entry*, where a triggered impulse encounters a pathway that blocks propagation in the forward direction but allows the impulse to pass in the return (retrograde) direction. Such retrograde transmission allows a triggered impulse to propagate continually, creating a self-sustaining tachycardia. Re-entry is the most common cause of clinically significant tachycardias.

Tachycardias are classified according to the site of impulse generation in relation to the atrioventricular (AV) conduction system. *Supraventricular tachycardias* (SVT) originate above the AV conduction system and have a normal QRS duration ($\leq$ 0.12 seconds), while *ventricular tachycardias* (VT) originate below the AV conduction system and have a prolonged QRS duration ($>$ 0.12 seconds). Each type of tachycardia can then be subdivided according to regularity of the rhythm (i.e., the regularity of the R–R interval on the ECG). The classification of tachycardias based on the QRS duration and the regularity of the R-R interval is shown in Figure 18.1.

Narrow QRS Complex Tachycardia

The tachycardias associated with a QRS duration of 0.12 seconds or less include sinus tachycardia, atrial tachycardia, AV nodal re-entrant tachycardia (also called paroxysmal supraventricular tachycardia), atrial flutter, and atrial fibrillation.

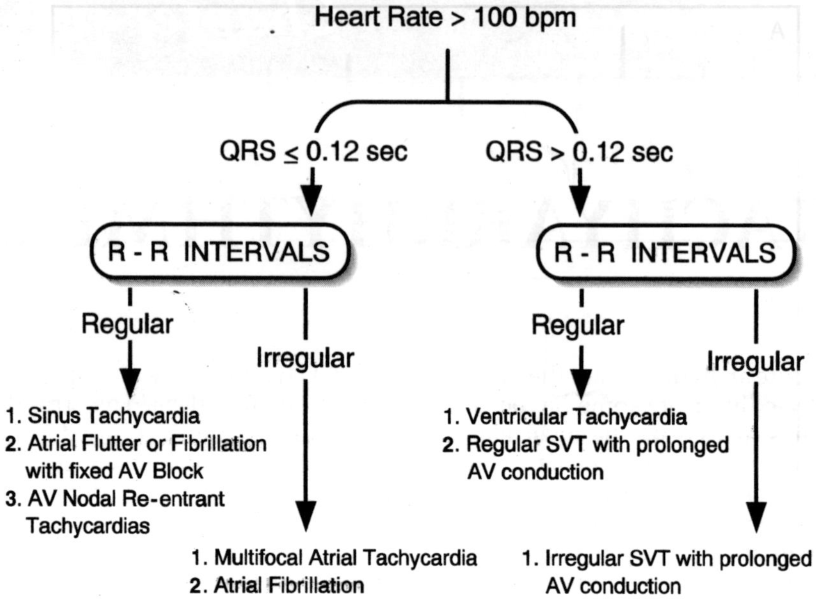

FIGURE 18.1 Classification of the tachycardias based on the QRS duration and the regularity of the R–R interval on the electrocardiogram.

Regular Rhythm

If the R-R intervals are uniform in length (indicating a regular rhythm), the possible arrhythmias include sinus tachycardia, AV nodal re-entrant tachycardia, or atrial flutter with a fixed (2:1, 3:1) AV block. The atrial activity can help to identify each of these rhythms. Uniform P waves with a fixed P–R interval is characteristic of sinus tachycardia; the absence of P waves suggests an AV nodal re-entrant tachycardia (see Figure 18.2), and sawtooth waves are characteristic of atrial flutter.

If the R-R intervals are not uniform in length (indicating an irregular rhythm), the most likely arrhythmias are multifocal atrial tachycardia

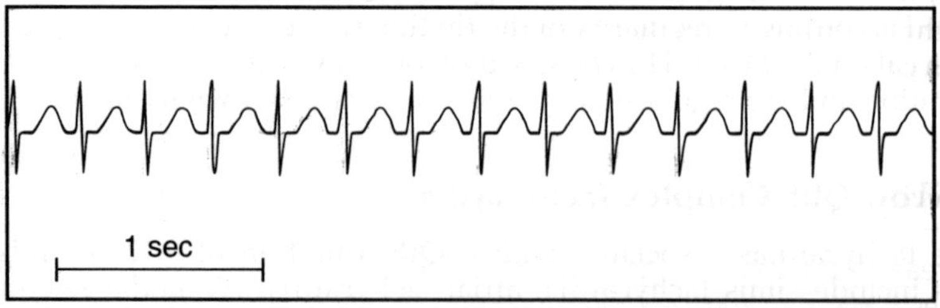

FIGURE 18.2 AV nodal re-entrant tachycardia, which is also called a paroxysmal supraventricular tachycardia. Note the absence of P waves, which are hidden in the QRS complexes.

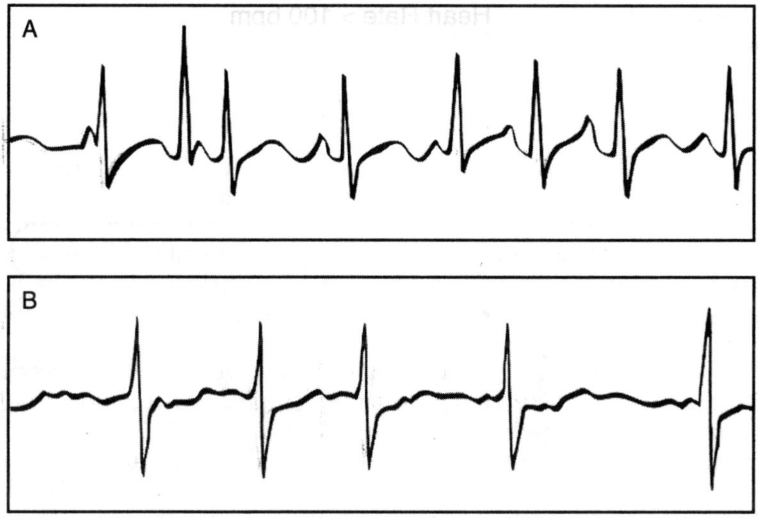

FIGURE 18.3 Multifocal atrial tachycardia (panel A) and atrial fibrillation (panel B). (From the CD ROM that accompanies Critical care nursing: A holistic approach. Philadelphia: Lippincott Williams & Wilkins, 2005.)

and atrial fibrillation. Once again, the atrial activity helps to identify each of these rhythms. Multifocal atrial tachycardia has multiple P wave morphologies and nonuniform PR intervals (Panel A, Figure 18.3), while atrial fibrillation has fibrillatory atrial waves and no identifiable P waves (Panel B, Figure 18.3). The rhythm in atrial fibrillation is highly irregular and is sometimes described as an "irregularly irregular" rhythm (which indicates that no two R-R intervals have the same length).

Wide QRS Complex Tachycardia

A tachycardia with a QRS duration > 0.12 seconds is either ventricular tachycardia (VT) or SVT with aberrant (prolonged) AV conduction. VT is characterized by a regular rhythm and the presence of AV dissociation, while SVT with aberrant conduction can have a regular or irregular rhythm (depending on the rhythm of the inciting SVT). These two arrhythmias can look remarkably similar, as presented later in the chapter.

SINUS TACHYCARDIA

Increased automaticity in the pacemaker cells of the sinoatrial node produces a regular, narrow-complex tachycardia with a gradual onset and rate of 100 to 140 beats/minute. The ECG shows uniform P waves and a fixed P–R interval. Sinus tachycardia can also be the result of re-entry into the sinus node. This variant sinus tachycardia has an abrupt onset, but is otherwise indistinguishable from the increased automaticity type of sinus tachycardia.

Management

Sinus tachycardia is often a response to a systemic illness. It is usually well tolerated (cardiac filling is usually not compromised until the heart rate rises above 180 beats/minute) (4) and does not require primary treatment. **The primary goal of management is to identify and treat the associated illness**. Possible sources of sinus tachycardia in the ICU include systemic infection and inflammation, hypovolemia, and adrenergic drugs.

The major indication for slowing a sinus tachycardia is the presence of myocardial ischemia or infarction. In this situation, β-receptor antagonists can be used to slow the heart rate. (See Chapter 17, Figure 17.2, for an effective β-blocker regimen in acute coronary syndromes.) Because these agents also depress ventricular function, they are not recommended for sinus tachycardia associated with systolic heart failure.

ATRIAL FIBRILLATION

Atrial fibrillation (AF) is the most common cardiac arrhythmia in the general population. (Atrial flutter is considered here as a more organized form of atrial fibrillation rather than a distinct arrhythmia). An estimated 2.2 million adults (or 1% of the adult population) have AF (3). Most are elderly (median age, 75 years) and have either ischemic heart disease, valvular disease, or cardiomyopathy. Contrary to popular perception, few have hyperactive thyroid disease (5). About 15% of patients with AF are relatively young (less than 60 years of age) and have no predisposing conditions (3): this condition is known as *lone atrial fibrillation*.

Postoperative AF

Postoperative AF is reported in 30 to 40% of patients undergoing coronary artery bypass surgery, and 60% of patients undergoing valve surgery, and usually appears in the first 4 postoperative days (6). The etiology is unclear, but risk factors include valvular surgery, advanced age, and failure to resume β-blocker therapy after surgery. β-blockers are preferred for rate control of AF in this setting (7). This arrhythmia is usually self-limited, and more than 90% of patients will convert to sinus rhythm within 6 to 8 weeks (3).

Adverse Consequences

Contraction of the atria is responsible for 25% of the ventricular end-diastolic volume (preload) in the normal heart (4). This atrial contribution to ventricular filling is lost in AF. There is little consequence in the normal heart, but cardiac output can be impaired in patients with diastolic dysfunction due to a noncompliant or stiff ventricle (where ventricular filling volumes are already reduced). This effect is pronounced at rapid heart rates (because of the reduced time for ventricular filling).

The other notable complication of AF is thrombus formation in the left atrium, which can embolize to the cerebral circulation and produce an ischemic stroke. Atrial thrombosis can be demonstrated in 15% of patients who have AF for longer than 3 days (8), and about 6% of patients with chronic AF and certain risk factors (see later) suffer an embolic stroke each year without adequate anticoagulation (3,8). The indications for anticoagulation in AF are presented later.

Management Strategies

The acute management of AF involves 3 strategies: (1) cardioversion to terminate the arrhythmia and restore normal sinus rhythm, (2) drug-induced reduction of the ventricular rate, and (3) anticoagulation to prevent thromboembolism. The following presentation is organized according to these strategies.

Cardioversion

Cardioversion can be accomplished by applying electric shocks (electrical cardioversion) or administering an antiarrhythmic agent (pharmacological cardioversion).

Electrical Cardioversion

Immediate cardioversion using direct-current (DC) electric shocks is indicated for cases of AF associated with severe hemodynamic compromise (hypotension or decompensated heart failure). This procedure is both painful and anxiety-provoking and, if tolerated, pre-medication with a benzodiazepine (e.g., midazolam) and/or an opiate (morphine or fentanyl) is indicated. The individual shocks should be synchronized to the R wave of the QRS complex to prevent electrical stimulation during the vulnerable period of ventricular repolarization, which usually coincides with the peak of the T wave (3). The following protocols are recommended (3).

1. For monophasic shocks, begin with 200 joules (J) for atrial fibrillation and 50 J for atrial flutter. If additional shocks are needed, increase the energy level of each successive shock by 100 J until a maximum shock strength of 400 J is reached. Wait at least one minute between shocks to minimize the risk of cardiac ischemia.
2. For biphasic shocks (which are the waveforms used in many of the newer defibrillator machines), use only half the energy recommended for monophasic shocks.

These regimens should result in successful cardioversion in about 90% of cases (3).

Pharmacologic Cardioversion

Acute pharmacologic cardioversion may be appropriate for first episodes of AF that are less than 48 hours in duration and are not associated with hemodynamic compromise or evidence of cardiac ischemia. In this situation, conversion to sinus rhythm will avoid the need for anticoagulation (see later) and can prevent atrial remodeling that predisposes to recurrent AF (9). However, over 50% of cases of recent-onset AF convert spontaneously to sinus rhythm in the first 72 hours (10), so cardioversion is not necessary in most cases of recent-onset AF unless the symptoms are distressing.

Several antiarrhythmic agents are recommended for the acute termination of AF (flecainide, propafenone, ibutilide, difetilide, and amiodarone), but the only one with a success rate higher than 5 or 10% is **ibutilide**. When patients with recent-onset AF are given ibutilide in the dosing regimen shown in Table 18.1, over 50% will convert to sinus rhythm, and 80% will show a response within 30 minutes of drug administration (11). The only risk associated with ibutilide is torsade de pointes (described later), which is reported in 4% of cases (11). (For information

TABLE 18.1 Intravenous Drug Regimens for Acute Management of Atrial Fibrillation†

Drug	Dose Regimen	Comments
CARDIOVERSION		
Ibutilide	1 mg IV over 10 min and repeat once if needed.	The best agent available for acute cardioversion of AF. Torsade de pointes reported in 4% of cases
ACUTE RATE CONTROL		
Diltiazem	0.25 mg/kg IV over 2 min, then 0.35 mg/kg 15 minutes later if needed. Follow with infusion of 5–15 mg/hr for 24 hrs.	Effective rate control in > 95% of patients. Has negative inotropic actions, but can be used safely in patients with heart failure.
Esmolol	500 μg/kg IV over 1 min, then infuse at 50 μg/kg/min. Increase dose rate by 25 μg/kg/min every 5 min if needed to maximum of 200 μg/kg/min.	Ultra-short-acting β-blocker that permits rapid dose titration to desired effect.
Metoprolol	2.5 to 5 mg IV over 2 min. Repeat every 10–15 min if needed to total of 3 doses.	Easy to use, but bolus dosing is not optimal for exact rate control.
Amiodarone	300 mg IV over 15 min, then 45 mg/hr for 24 hrs.‡	A suitable alternative for patients who do not tolerate more effective rate-reducing drugs.

† From the recommendations in Reference 3.

‡ Data from Reference 17.

on the other antiarrhythmic agents recommended for cardioversion of AF, see Reference #3.)

Intravenous amiodarone is also recommended for acute termination of AF despite evidence of variable and limited efficacy. Bolus administration of amiodarone results in acute cardioversion of AF in less than 5% of cases (12). This agent may be more useful for acute rate control in AF, as described later.

Controlling the Heart Rate

The acute management of AF (particularly chronic or recurrent AF) is most often aimed at reducing the ventricular rate into the range of 60 to 80 bpm (3). If an arterial catheter is in place, monitoring the systolic blood pressure can provide a more physiological end-point for rate control. The systolic blood pressure is a reflection of the stroke volume, and the principal determinant of stroke volume is ventricular end-diastolic volume (this is the Frank-Starling relationship described in Chapter 1). When the heart rate in AF is slow enough to allow for adequate ventricular filling during each period of diastole, the systolic blood pressure (stroke volume) should remain constant with each heart beat. Therefore a constant systolic blood pressure with each heart beat can be used as an end-point of rate control in AF.

The drugs that are used for acute rate control in AF are shown in Table 18.1. These drugs are either calcium-channel blockers (diltiazem) or β-blockers (esmolol and metoprolol), and they act by prolonging conduction through the atrioventricular node, which slows the ventricular response to the rapid atrial rate.

Calcium-Channel Blockers

Verapamil was the original calcium-channel blocker used for acute rate control in AF, but diltiazem (Cardizem) is now preferred because it produces less myocardial depression and is less likely to produce hypotension (3). When given in appropriate doses, **diltiazem will produce satisfactory rate control in 85% of patients with AF** (13). The response to a bolus dose of diltiazem is evident within 5 minutes (see Figure 18.4), and the effect dissipates over the next 1 – 3 hours (14). Because the response is transient, the initial bolus dose of diltiazem should be followed by a continuous infusion. Although diltiazem has mild negative inotropic actions, it has been used safely in patients with heart failure (15).

β-Receptor Antagonists

β-blockers are the preferred agents for rate control when AF is associated with hyperadrenergic states (such as acute MI and post-cardiac surgery) (3,7). Two β-blockers with proven efficacy in AF are **esmolol** (Brevibloc) and **metoprolol** (Lopressor), and their dosing regimens are shown in Table 18.1. Both are cardioselective agents that preferentially block β-1 receptors in the heart. Esmolol is the preferred agent for acute rate control because it is ultra–short-acting (serum half-life of 9 minutes), and the infusion rate can be titrated rapidly to maintain the target heart

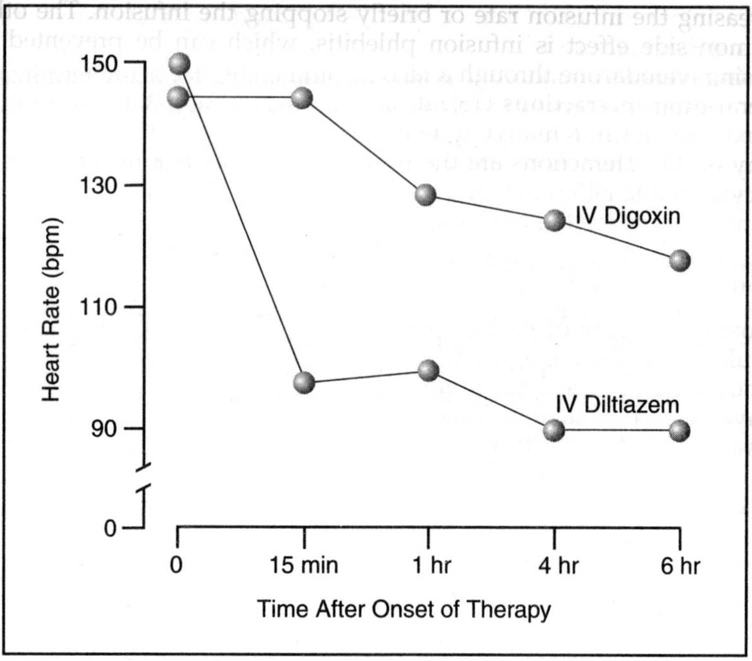

FIGURE 18.4 Comparative effects of IV diltiazem (same dose as in Table 18.1) and IV digoxin (0.5 mg in two divided doses over 6 hours) on acute control of heart rate in patients with recent-onset AF. (Adapted from data in Schreck DM, Rivera AR, Tricarico VJ, et al. Emergency treatment of atrial fibrillation and flutter: comparison of IV digoxin versus IV diltiazem. Ann Emerg Med 1995;25:127.)

rate (16). Because β-blockers and calcium-channel-blockers both have cardiodepressant effects, combined therapy with β-blockers and calcium-channel blockers should be avoided.

Amiodarone

Amiodarone can prolong conduction in the AV node and reduce the ventricular rate in patients with AF. When given in the dosing regimen shown in Table 18.1, intravenous amiodarone can produce an acute reduction in heart rate in 75% of patients with recent-onset AF (17). Although not as effective as diltiazem, amiodarone produces less cardiac depression and is less likely to produce hypotension than diltiazem (17). As a result, amiodarone may be a suitable alternative when other rate-controlling drugs are not tolerated.

The potential **side effects** of short-term intravenous amiodarone include hypotension (15%), infusion phlebitis (15%), bradycardia (5%), and elevated liver enzymes (3%) (11,18). Hypotension is the most common side effect and is related to the vasodilator actions of amiodarone and the solvent (polysorbate 80 surfactant) used to enhance water solubility of the injectable drug (18). Hypotension can usually be managed by decreasing the infusion rate or briefly stopping the infusion. The other common side effect is infusion phlebitis, which can be prevented by infusing amiodarone through a large, central vein. Amiodarone also has several **drug interactions** (18). It increases the serum concentrations of digoxin, warfarin, fentanyl, quinidine, procainamide, and cyclosporine. Many of the interactions are the result of amiodarone's metabolism via the cytochrome P450 enzyme system in the liver. The digoxin and warfarin interactions are the most important in the ICU.

Digoxin

Digoxin, by virtue of its ability to prolong AV conduction, has been a popular and effective agent for long-term rate control in AF. However, it should not be used for immediate rate control in AF because of its delayed onset of action. This is demonstrated in Figure 18.4, which shows the results of a study comparing the effects of IV diltiazem and IV digoxin on acute rate control in patients with recent-onset AF. The heart rate decreased to below 100 bpm (the target rate) promptly in the patients who received diltiazem, while the heart rate remained above 110 bpm after 6 hours in the patients who received digoxin. These results demonstrate that **digoxin is ineffective for acute rate control in AF.**

Anticoagulation

Cerebral embolic stroke (mentioned earlier) is the most devastating complication of AF. Each year about 6% of patients with AF will suffer an embolic stroke if they have certain high-risk conditions for thromboembolism. This can be reduced by 3% with warfarin anticoagulation to achieve an INR between 2.0 to 3.0 (19). In other words, therapeutic anticoagulation with warfarin in high-risk patients is associated with 3 fewer strokes for every 100 patients treated. This benefit requires strict monitoring of warfarin anticoagulation to keep the INR in the therapeutic range (2.0 – 3.0).

Risk Stratification

Table 18.2 shows the different antithrombotic strategies based on the risk factors for thomboembolism in patients with AF (3). The patients with the highest risk for thromboembolism (annual stroke rate > 6%) that will benefit from warfarin anticoagulation include those with rheumatic valvular disease, prosthetic valves, a prior history of thromboembolism, heart failure with comorbid conditions, or advanced age (> 75 years of age). The conditions with a low risk of thromboembolism (annual stroke rate < 2%) can be treated with daily aspirin. The risk of thromboembolism is lowest (the same as the general population) in patients with AF who are younger than 60 years of age and have no evidence of heart disease. This condition is known as *lone atrial fibrillation*, and it does not require any form of antithrombotic therapy.

The benefits of anticoagulation must always be weighed against the risk of hemorrhage, particularly intracerebral bleeding. Warfarin

TABLE 18.2 Risk-Based Antithrombotic Strategies for Patients with Atrial Fibrillation†

I. **Oral Anticoagulation** (INR = 2.0 – 3.0)	
	Age > 75 years
	Age ≥ 60 years plus diabetes or coronary artery disease
	Heart failure with LV ejection fraction < 0.35
	Heart failure with hypertension or thyrotoxicosis
	Prosthetic heart valves (mechanical or tissue)
	Rheumatic mitral valve disease
	Prior thromboembolism
II. **Antiplatelet Therapy** (Aspirin, 325 mg daily)	
	Age < 60 years with heart disease, but no risk factors‡
	Age ≥ 60 years with no risk factors‡
III. **No Therapy Required**	
	Age < 60 years and no heart disease (lone AF)

‡Risk factors include heart failure, LV ejection fraction < 0.35, and history of hyptertension.
†From the ACC/AHA/ECC guidelines for the management of patients with atrial fibrillation (3).

anticoagulation increases the yearly rate of intracerebral hemorrhage by < 1% (19), so the risk:benefit ratio favors anticoagulation in high-risk patients with AF. For patients with a predisposition to bleeding, the decision to anticoagulate is made on a case-by-case basis.

Anticoagulation & Cardioversion

In cases of recent-onset AF that are less than 48 hours in duration, the risk of embolism with cardioversion is low (< 1%), so anticoagulation is not needed prior to elective cardioversion (3). In fact, as mentioned earlier, successful cardioversion of AF that is less than 48 hours in duration will avoid the need for long-term anticoagulation. When the duration of AF is > 48 hours, the risk of embolization with cardioversion is about 6%, and anticoagulation is recommended for 3 weeks before elective cardioversion.

Wolff–Parkinson–White Syndrome

The WPW syndrome (short P–R interval and Δ waves before the QRS) is characterized by recurrent supraventricular tachycardias that originate from an accessory (re-entrant) pathway in the AV conduction system (2). (Re-entrant tachycardias are described later in the chapter.) One of the tachycardias associated with WPW syndrome is atrial fibrillation. Agents that prolong AV conduction and produce effective rate control in conventional AF (such as the calcium-channel blockers) can paradoxically accelerate the ventricular rate (by blocking the wrong pathway) in patients with WPW syndrome. Thus **in cases of AF associated with WPW syndrome, calcium-channel blockers and digoxin are contraindicated**. The treatment of choice is electrical cardioversion or pharmacologic cardioversion with procainamide (20). The dosing regimen for procainamide is presented later.

MULTIFOCAL ATRIAL TACHYCARDIA

Multifocal atrial tachycardia (MAT) is characterized by multiple P wave morphologies and a variable P–R interval (see Figure 18.3). The ventricular rate is highly irregular, and MAT is easily confused with atrial fibrillation when atrial activity is not clearly displayed on the ECG. MAT is a disorder of the elderly (average age = 70), and over half of the cases occur in patients with chronic lung disease (21). The link with lung diseases may be partly due to the bronchodilator theophylline (22). Other associated conditions include magnesium and potassium depletion and coronary artery disease. (21).

Acute Management

MAT can be a difficult arrhythmia to manage, but the steps listed below can be effective.

1. **Discontinue theophylline** (although this is no longer a popular bronchodilator). In one study, this maneuver resulted in conversion to sinus rhythm in half the patients with MAT (22).
2. **Give intravenous magnesium** (unless there is a contraindication) using the following protocol: 2 grams $MgSO_4$ (in 50 mL saline) over 15 minutes, then 6 grams $MgSO_4$ (in 500 mL saline) over 6 hours (23). In one study, this measure was effective in converting MAT to sinus rhythm in 88% of cases, even when serum magnesium levels were normal. The mechanism is unclear, but magnesium's actions as a calcium-channel blocker may be involved.
3. **Correct hypomagnesemia and hypokalemia** if they exist. If both disorders co-exist, the magnesium deficiency must be corrected before potassium replacement is started. (The reason for this is described in Chapter 34.) Use the following replacement protocol: infuse 2 mg $MgSO_4$ (in 50 mL saline) IV over 15 minutes, then infuse 40 mg potassium over 1 hour.
4. If the above measures are ineffective, **give IV metoprolol** if there is no evidence of COPD otherwise, give IV **verapamil** (a calcium-channel blocker). Metoprolol, given according to the regimen in Table 18.2, has been successful in converting MAT to sinus rhythm in 80% of cases (21). The verapamil dose is 75–150 μg/kg IV over 2 minutes (3). Verapamil converts MAT to sinus rhythm in less than 50% of cases, but it can also slow the ventricular rate. Watch for hypotension, which is a common side effect of verapamil.

PAROXYSMAL SUPRAVENTRICULAR TACHYCARDIAS

Paroxysmal supraventricular tachycardias (PSVT) are narrow QRS complex tachycardias that are characterized by an abrupt onset and abrupt termination (unlike sinus tachycardia, which has a gradual onset and gradual resolution). These arrhythmias occur when there is an accessory pathway in the conduction system between atria and ventricles that conducts impulses at a different speed than the normal pathway. This difference in conduction velocities allows an impulse traveling down one pathway (antegrade transmission) to travel up the other pathway (retrograde transmission). This circular transmission of impulses creates a rapid, self-sustaining, *re-entrant tachycardia*. The trigger is an ectopic atrial impulse that travels through either of the two pathways.

There are 5 different types of PSVT, each characterized by the location of the accessory pathway. The most common PSVT is *AV nodal re-entrant tachycardia*, where the accessory pathway is located in the AV node.

AV Nodal Re-entrant Tachycardia

AV nodal re-entrant tachycardia (AVNRT) is one of the most common rhythm disturbances in the general population. It most often occurs in subjects who have no evidence of structural heart disease and is more common in women (2). The onset is abrupt, and there may be distressing palpitations, but there is usually no evidence of heart failure or myocardial ischemia. The ECG shows a narrow QRS complex tachycardia with a regular rhythm and a rate between 140 and 220 bpm. There may be no evidence of atrial activity on the ECG (see Figure 18.2), which is a feature that distinguishes AVNRT from sinus tachycardia.

Acute Management

Maneuvers that increase vagal tone can occasionally terminate AVNRT and can sometimes slow another type of tachycardia to reveal the diagnosis (e.g., sinus tachycardia). The vagal-enhancing maneuvers include the Valsalva maneuver (forced exhalation against a closed glottis), carotid massage, eyeball compression, and facial immersion in cold water (2). The value of these maneuvers is largely unproven, and some of the maneuvers (like eyeball compression or facial immersion in ice water) only add to the patient's distress and delay the termination of the arrhythmia. (Take a patient with AVNRT who is anxious and may be short of breath then stick the patient's face in a sink full of ice water and tell them to hold their breath, and you will know what I mean.)

AVNRT can be terminated quickly by drugs that block the re-entrant pathway in the AV node. The most effective drugs are calcium-channel blockers (verapamil and diltiazem) and adenosine. These agents are equally effective for terminating AVNRT, but adenosine works faster and produces less cardiovascular depression than the calcium-channel blockers.

TABLE 18.3 Intravenous Adenosine for Paroxysmal SVT

Indications: Termination of AV nodal re-entrant tachycardia, particularly in patients with

- Heart failure
- Hypotension
- Ongoing therapy with calcium channel blockers or β-blockers
- WPW syndrome

Contraindications: Asthma, AV block

Dose: For delivery via peripheral veins:

1. Give 6 mg by rapid IV injection and flush with saline.
2. After 2 min, give a second dose of 12 mg if necessary.
3. The 12-mg dose can be repeated once.

Dose adjustments: Decrease dose by 50% for:

- Injection into superior vena cava
- Patients receiving calcium blockers, β-blockers, or dipyridamole

Response: Onset of action < 30 sec. Effects last 1–2 min.

Side effects: Facial flushing (50%)
Sinus bradycardia, AV block (50%)
Dyspnea (35%)
Anginal-type chest pain (20%)
Nausea, headache, dizziness (5–10%)

AV = atrioventricular; VT = ventricular tachycardia; WPW = Wolff–Parkinson–White syndrome.
From References 24–27.

Adenosine (Adenocard)

Adenosine is an endogenous purine nucleotide that briefly depresses activity in the sinus node and AV node (24). When given by rapid intravenous injection in the doses shown in Table 18.3, **adenosine terminates re-entrant tachycardias in over 90% of cases and is effective within 30 seconds of drug injection** (24–26). Each bolus dose of the drug should be followed by a 20 mL saline flush to speed up the drug effect. The effect dissipates in 1 to 2 minutes, so troublesome side effects are gone in a flash. Note in Table 18.3 that the dose of adenosine should be reduced by 50% when the drug is injected through a central venous (CVP) catheter instead of a peripheral vein (27). This recommendation is based on reports of ventricular asystole when standard doses of adenosine are injected through CVP catheters (27).

Adenosine has an important drug interaction with theophylline (the once-popular bronchodilator agent). Theophylline blocks adenosine receptors and antagonizes the actions of adenosine. As a result, therapeutic doses of adenosine may not be effective in patients receiving theophylline, so combined therapy with adenosine and theophylline is not advised. Fortunately, theophylline is disappearing from the medicine cabinets of most asthmatics (because of better bronchodilator effects with (β-agonists), and the significance of the adenosine-theophylline interaction is diminishing.

Side effects are common after adenosine injection, and these are listed in Table 18.3 (26). However, these side effects are fleeting because of adenosine's ultra-short duration of action. Adenosine blocks catecholamine effects on the heart (24), but heart failure is not a problem because of the rapid disappearance of drug effects. One of the significant side effects is bronchoconstriction in asthmatic subjects (28,29), which is why **adenosine should NOT be used in patients with asthma.**

VENTRICULAR TACHYCARDIA

Ventricular tachycardia (VT) is the most feared and life-threatening tachyarrhythmia. Sustained VT (defined as VT that lasts longer than 30 seconds or causes hemodynamic compromise) rarely occurs in the absence of structural heart disease (30), and often indicates a profound disruption of the mechanical and electrical integrity of the heart. The appearance of VT is an ominous sign and requires prompt recognition and management.

Diagnosis

VT is a wide QRS complex tachycardia with a regular rhythm and a rate above 100 bpm. The onset is abrupt, and the hemodynamic consequences vary from no apparent effect to complete loss of pulses and cardiac arrest. VT can be *monomorphic* (QRS complexes are uniform in size and shape) or *polymorphic* (QRS morphology changes continuously). Monomorphic VT is most common and can be difficult to distinguish from an SVT with prolonged AV conduction (see below).

Diagnostic Clues

The single-lead ECG tracings in Figure 18.5 illustrate the difficulty in distinguishing VT from an SVT with aberrant (prolonged) AV conduction. The tracing in the upper panel shows a wide QRS complex tachycardia with a regular rhythm that looks very much like (monomorphic) VT. The tracing in the lower panel shows spontaneous conversion to sinus rhythm. Note that the QRS complex remains unchanged after the arrhythmia is terminated, revealing an underlying bundle branch block. Thus the apparent VT in the upper panel is actually a paroxysmal SVT superimposed on a pre-existing bundle branch block.

VT has two characteristic features on the ECG that can distinguish it from an SVT with aberrant conduction. One of these is *AV dissociation*, where there is no fixed relationship between P waves and QRS complexes. This may not be evident on a single-lead ECG tracing and is more likely to be discovered on a 12-lead ECG (where one of the leads might reveal p waves). The other diagnostic clue for VT is the presence of *fusion*

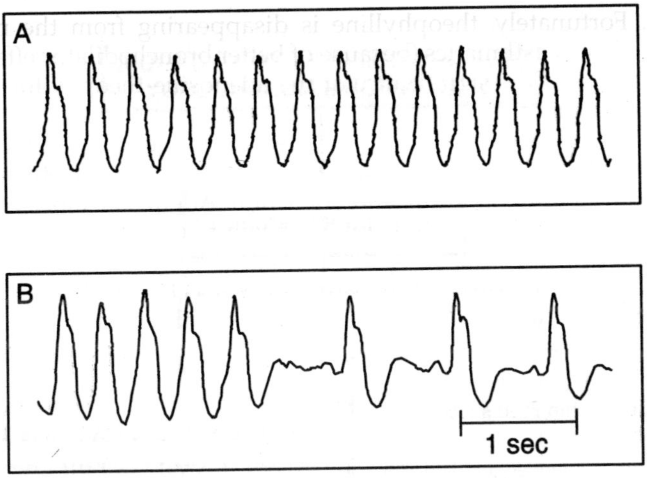

FIGURE 18.5 An SVT with aberrant (prolonged) AV conduction masquerading as VT. Spontaneous conversion to sinus rhythm in the lower panel reveals an underlying bundle branch block. (Tracings courtesy of Dr. Richard M. Greenberg, M.D.)

beats prior to the onset of the arrhythmia. A fusion beat is an irregularly-shaped QRS complex that is caused by retrograde transmission of a ventricular ectopic impulse that merges (fuses) with a normal QRS complex. The presence of a fusion beat (which should be evident on a single-lead ECG tracing) is therefore evidence of ventricular ectopic activity.

If there are no characteristic features of VT on the ECG, the presence or absence of heart disease can be useful, because VT is the cause of 95% of wide complex tachycardias in patients with primary heart disease (31). Therefore **a wide QRS complex tachycardia in any patient with primary heart disease should be treated as probable VT**.

Acute Management

The management of patients with a wide QRS complex tachycardia can proceed as follows. This approach is organized in a flow diagram in Figure 18.6.

1. If there is evidence of hemodynamic compromise, initiate DC cardioversion immediately with an initial shock of 100 J, followed by repetitive shocks of 200, 300, and 360 J, if necessary. This is necessary regardless of whether the rhythm is VT or SVT with aberrant conduction.
2. If there is no evidence of hemodynamic compromise and the diagnosis of VT is certain, intravenous amiodarone should be used to terminate the arrhythmia (see Figure 18.6 for the amiodarone dosing regimen). Lidocaine had been the favored antiarrhythmic agent for terminating VT; however, the most recent guidelines published by the American Heart Association (1) state

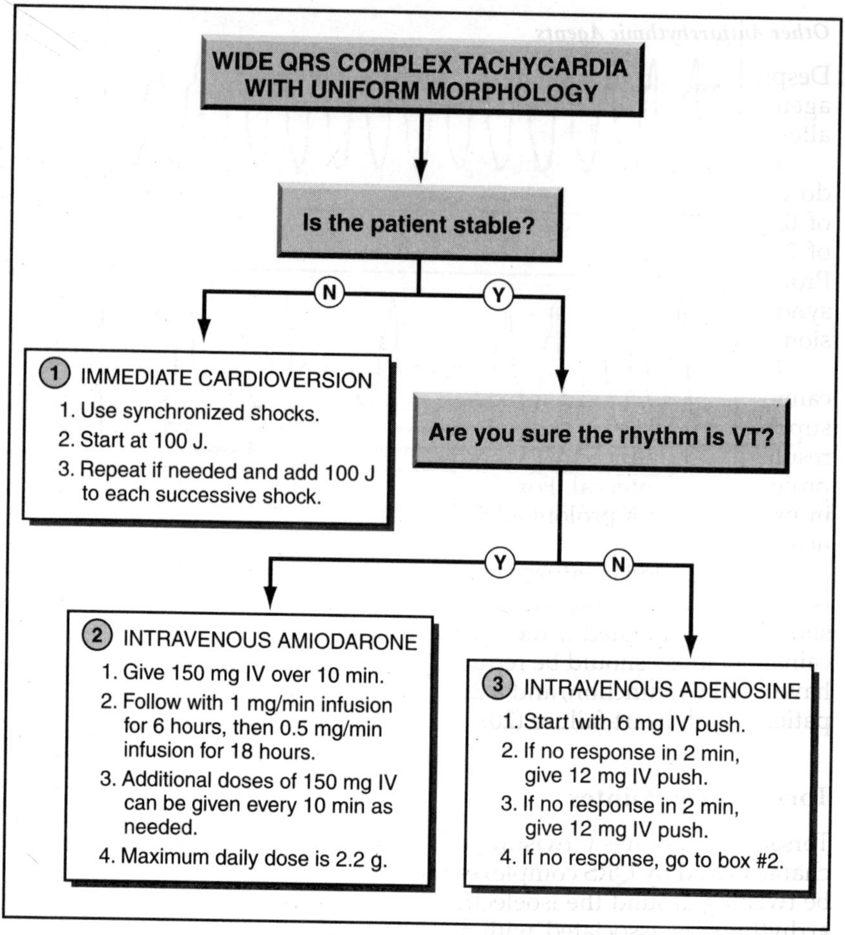

FIGURE 18.6 Flow diagram for the acute management of patients with wide QRS complex tachycardia. (Based on recommendations in the 2005 American Heart Association guidelines for cardiopulmonary resuscitation and emergency cardiovascular care. Circulation 2005;112:IV-67.)

that **amiodarone has replaced lidocaine as the antiarrhythmic agent of choice for terminating VT**. This recommendation may be based on the safety of amiodarone in patients with heart failure because most cases of VT occur in patients with significant cardiac disease.

3. If there is no evidence of hemodynamic compromise and the diagnosis of VT is uncertain, **intravenous adenosine can help to unmask a paroxysmal SVT** (like the rhythm in Figure 18.4). Adenosine will not terminate VT, but it will abruptly terminate most cases of paroxysmal SVT. If the arrhythmia persists after adenosine, VT is the likely diagnosis, and intravenous amiodarone is indicated to terminate the rhythm.

Other Antiarrhythmic Agents

Despite the current preference for amiodarone, other antiarrhythmic agents are effective in suppressing VT, and these drugs can be used as alternatives to amiodarone.

Lidocaine has a long history of success in suppressing VT. The initial dose is 1 to 1.5 mg/kg by bolus injection. After 5 minutes, a second dose of 0.5 to 0.75 mg/kg can be given if needed. A maintenance infusion of 2 to 4 mg/min can be used for continued arrhythmia suppression. Prolonged infusions of lidocaine can produce an excitatory neurotoxic syndrome, particularly in elderly patients. For this reason, lidocaine infusions should not be continued longer than 6 to 12 hours.

Procainamide is considered a second-line drug for VT because it cannot be administered rapidly, which prolongs the time to arrhythmia suppression. Procainamide also prolongs the QT interval, and this can result in drug-induced VT when procainamide is given to patients with a prolonged QT interval. For this reason, procainamide is contraindicated in patients with a prolonged QT interval (>0.44 sec after correction for heart rate).

Procainamide is infused at a rate of 20 mg/min until the arrhythmia is suppressed or a total dose of 17 mg/kg is reached (32). The infusion should be terminated if the QT interval increases by 50% (30). The procainamide dose should be reduced by 50% in patients who are elderly or have renal dysfunction, and a 25% reduction in dose is recommended for patients with heart failure (20).

Torsades De Pointes

Torsades de pointes ("twisting around the points") is a polymorphic VT characterized by QRS complexes that change in amplitude and appear to be twisting around the isoelectric line of the ECG (see Figure 18.7). This arrhythmia is associated with a prolonged QT interval (33), and it can be congenital (idiopathic) or acquired. The acquired form is caused by a variety of drugs and electrolyte disorders that prolong the QT interval. The drugs that can trigger this arrhythmia are listed in Table 18.4 (34,35). The prominent offenders are antiarrhythmic drugs, macrolide and quinolone antibiotics, and psychotropic agents. The electrolyte disorders

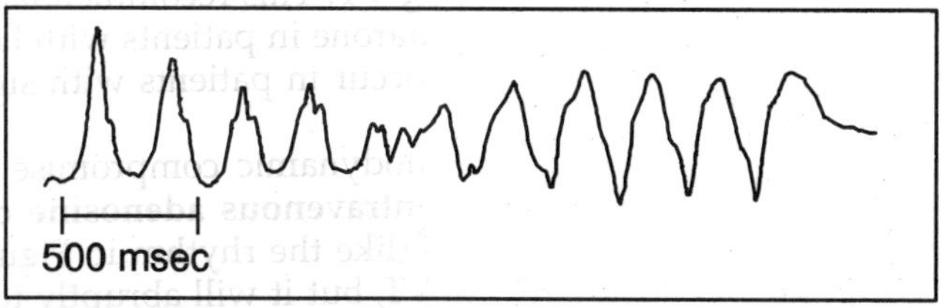

FIGURE 18.7 Torsades de pointes, a polymorphic ventricular tachycardia described as "twisting around (the isoelectric) points." (Tracing courtesy of Dr. Richard M. Greenberg, M.D.)

TABLE 18.4 Drugs That Can Trigger Torsades de Pointes†

Antiarrhythmic Agents		Antimicrobial Agents	Antipsychotic Agents	Other Agents
IA	Quinidine	Clarithromycin	Chlorpromazine	Cisapride
	Procainamide	Erythromycin	Haloperidol	Droperidol
	Flecainide	Gatifoxacin	Thioridazine	Methadone
III	Ibutilide	Levofloxacin		
	Sotalol	Pentamidine		

†From References 34, 35.

that prolong the QT interval and predispose to torsades de pointes are hypokalemia, hypomagnesemia, and hypocalcemia.

Polymorphic VT can also be associated with a normal QT interval. This condition is not torsades de pointes and is simply known as polymorphic VT.

Management

The management of polymorphic VT is guided by the QT interval. This parameter is usually measured in limb lead II and must be corrected for the heart rate. The rate-corrected QT interval (QTc) is equivalent to the measured QT interval divided by the square root of the R-R interval (36). A prolonged QT interval is defined as QTc > 0.44 seconds.

$$QTc = QT/\sqrt{RR}$$

Polymorphic VT with a normal QT interval can be managed with standard antiarrhythmic agents like amiodarone and lidocaine. For cases of torsades de pointes associated with a prolonged QT interval, the management strategy depends on whether the QT prolongation is congenital or acquired.

If the QT prolongation is acquired:

1. Give intravenous magnesium (as magnesium sulfate, $MgSO_4$). Start with 2 grams IV over one minute, and repeat this dose 10 minutes later if needed. Follow with a continuous infusion of 1 gram per hour for the next 6 hours.
2. Correct electrolyte abnormalities if present. Remember that hypokalemia and hypocalcemia may be the result of an underlying magnesium deficiency (even if the serum magnesium levels are normal). In this situation, it is difficult to correct the serum potassium and calcium levels until the magnesium deficit is corrected. Therefore magnesium replacement should be the first order of business in patients with hypokalemia and hypocalcemia. (The importance of magnesium deficiency in hospitalized patients is presented in Chapter 34.)
3. Discontinue any drugs that prolong the QT interval.

If the QT prolongation is a congenital disorder, use ventricular pacing to raise the heart rate above 100 bpm. The rapid rate will shorten the QT interval and reduce the tendency for VT.

A FINAL WORD

Serious or life-threatening tachyarrhythmias are uncommon events in critical care areas other than coronary care units. This is probably because pathologic arrhythmias are triggered by focal areas of myocardial ischemia or focal alterations in myocardial architecture, and most critically ill patients (other than those admitted for coronary insufficiency) do not experience these events during the course of their illness. To gain experience in the diagnosis and management of tachyarrhythmias, spend time in a coronary care unit or an emergency room.

REFERENCES

Clinical Practice Guidelines

1. 2005 American Heart Association Guidelines for Cardiopulmonary Resuscitation and Emergency Cardiovascular Care. Part 7.3: Management of symptomatic bradycardia and tachycardia. Circulation 2005;112(supplI):IV67–IV77. (Available online @ http://circ.ahajournals.org/content/vol112/24_suppl/)
2. Blomstrom-Lunqvist C, Scheinmann MM, Haliot EM, et al. ACC/AHA/ESC guidelines for the management of patients with supraventricular arrhythmias: a report of the American College of Cardiology/American Heart Association Task Force on Practice Guidelines and the European Society of Cardiology Committee on Practice Guidelines, 2003. American College of Cardiology Web Site. Available at http://www.acc.org/clinical/guidelines/arrhythmias/sva_index.pdf
3. Fuster V, Ryden LE, Ansinger RW, et al. ACC/AHA/ESC guidelines for the management of patients with atrial fibrillation: a report of the American College of Cardiology/American Heart Association Task Force on Practice Guidelines and the European Society of Cardiology Committee on Practice Guidelines and Policy Conferences. J Am Coll Cardiol 2001;38:1266i–lxx. (Available @ http://www.acc.org/clinical/guidelines/atrial.fib/as_index.htm)

Atrial Flutter and Fibrillation

4. Guyton AC. The relationship of cardiac output and arterial pressure control. Circulation 1981;64:1079–1088.
5. Siebers MJ, Drinka PJ, Vergauwen C. Hyperthyroidism as a cause of atrial fibrillation in long-term care. Arch Intern Med 1992;152:2063–2064.
6. Hogue CW, Creswell LL, Gutterman DD, et al. American College of Chest Physicians guidelines for the prevention and management of postoperative atrial fibrillation after cardiac surgery: epidemiology, mechanisms, and risks. Chest 2005;128(suppl):9S–16S.

7. Martinez EA, Epstein AE, Bass EB. American College of Chest Physicians guidelines for the prevention and management of postoperative atrial fibrillation after cardiac surgery. Pharmacological control of ventricular rate. Chest 2005;128(suppl):56S–60S.
8. Blackshear JL, Kopecky SL, Litin SC, et al. Management of atrial fibrillation in adults: prevention of thromboembolism and symptomatic treatment. Mayo Clin Proc 1996;71:150–160.
9. Wijffels MC, Kirchhof CJ, Dorland R, Allessie MA. Atrial fibrillation begets atrial fibrillation: a study in awake, chronically instrumented goats. Circulation 1995;92:1954–1968.
10. Danias PG, Caulfield TA, Weigner MJ, et al. Likelihood of spontaneous conversion of atrial fibrillation to sinus rhythm. J Am Coll Cardiol 1998;31:588–592.
11. VerNooy RA, Mounsey P. Antiarrhythmic drug therapy in atrial fibrillation. Cardiol Clin 2004;22:21–34.
12. Trohman RG. Supraventricular tachycardia: implications for the intensivist. Crit Care Med 2000;28(suppl): N129–N135.
13. Ellenbogen KA, Dias VC, Plumb VJ, et al. A placebo-controlled trial of continuous intravenous diltiazem infusion for 24-hour heart rate control during atrial fibrillation and atrial flutter: a multicenter study. J Am Coll Cardiol 1991;18:891–897.
14. Diltiazem injectable monograph. Mosby's Drug Consult, 2006. Accessed from MD Consult Web Site on 3/1/06.
15. Goldenberg IF, Lewis WR, Dias VC, et al. Intravenous diltiazem for the treatment of patients with atrial fibrillation or flutter and moderate to severe congestive heart failure. Am J Cardiol 1994;74:884–889.
16. Gray RJ. Managing critically ill patients with esmolol: an ultra-short-acting β-adrenergic blocker. Chest 1988;93:398–404.
17. Karth GD, Geppert A, Neunteufl T, et al. Amiodarone versus diltiazem for rate control in critically ill patients with atrial tachyarrhythmias. Crit Care Med 2001;29:1149–1153.
18. Chow MSS. Intravenous amiodarone: pharmacology, pharmacokinetics, and clinical use. Ann Pharmacother 1996;30:637–643.
19. Ezekowitz MD, Falk RH. The increasing need for anticoagulant therapy to prevent stroke in patients with atrial fibrillation. Mayo Clin Proc 2004;79: 904–913.
20. Marcus FI, Opie LH. Antiarrhythmic drugs. In: Opie LH, ed. Drugs for the heart. 4th ed. Philadelphia: WB Saunders, 1995:207–246.

Multifocal Atrial Tachycardia

21. Kastor J. Multifocal atrial tachycardia. N Engl J Med 1990;322:1713–1720.
22. Levine J, Michael J, Guanieri T. Multifocal atrial tachycardia: a toxic effect of theophylline. Lancet 1985;1:1–16.
23. Iseri LT, Fairshter RD, Hardeman JL, et al. Magnesium and potassium therapy in multifocal atrial tachycardia. Am Heart J 1985;312:21–26.

Paroxysmal Supraventricular Tachycardias

24. Shen W-K, Kurachi Y. Mechanisms of adenosine-mediated actions on cellular and clinical cardiac electrophysiology. Mayo Clin Proc 1995;70:274–291.

25. Rankin AC, Brooks R, Ruskin JM, et al. Adenosine and the treatment of supraventricular tachycardia. Am J Med 1992;92:655–664.
26. Chronister C. Clinical management of supraventricular tachycardia with adenosine. Am J Crit Care 1993;2:41–47.
27. McCollam PL, Uber W, Van Bakel AB. Adenosine-related ventricular asystole. Ann Intern Med 1993;118:315–316.
28. Cushley MJ, Tattersfield AE, Holgate ST. Adenosine-induced bronchoconstriction in asthma. Am Rev Respir Dis 1984;129:380–384.
29. Bjorck T, Gustafsson LE, Dahlen S-E. Isolated bronchi from asthmatics are hyperresponsive to adenosine, which apparently acts indirectly by liberation of leukotrienes and histamine. Am Rev Respir Dis 1992;145:1087–1091.

Ventricular Tachycardia

30. Gupta AK, Thakur RK. Wide QRS complex tachycardias. Med Clin North Am 2001;85:245–266.
31. Akhtar M, Shenasa M, Jazayeri M, et al. Wide QRS complex tachycardia. Ann Intern Med 1988;109:905–912.
32. Sharma AD, Purves P, Yee R, et al. Hemodynamic effects of intravenous procainamide during ventricular tachycardia. Am Heart J 1990;119:1034–1041.
33. Vukmir RB. Torsades de pointes: a review. Am J Emerg Med 1991;9:250–262.
34. Frothingham R. Rates of torsades de pointes associated with ciprofloxacin, ofloxacin, levofloxacin, gatifloxacin, and moxifloxacin. Pharmacotherapy 2001;21:1468–1472.
35. Roden DM. Drug-induced prolongation of the QT interval. N Engl J Med 2004;350:1013–1022.
36. Garson A Jr. How to measure the QT interval: what is normal? Am J Cardiol 1993;72:14B–16B.

Section VII

ACUTE RESPIRATORY FAILURE

People say life can't exist without air, but it does under water; in fact, it started in the sea.

RICHARD FEYNMAN

Chapter 19

HYPOXEMIA AND HYPERCAPNIA

Over the course of an average ICU stay, about 125 laboratory measurements are performed on each patient, requiring an average of 550 mL of blood per patient (enough to drop the hemoglobin level by 3 g/dL) (1). The most frequently performed laboratory test in the ICU is the arterial blood gas measurement (the simultaneous measurement of PO_2, PCO_2, and pH in arterial blood) (2). This chapter focuses on two abnormalities in the blood gas measurement: a low arterial PO_2 (hypoxemia) and an elevated arterial PCO_2 (hypercapnia). The first part of the chapter describes the relationship between arterial blood gases (PO_2 and PCO_2) and pulmonary gas exchange, and the second part of the chapter presents a physiological approach to identify the sources of hypoxemia and hypercapnia in the individual patient.

PULMONARY GAS EXCHANGE

The adequacy of gas exchange in the lungs is determined by the balance between pulmonary ventilation and capillary blood flow (3–5). This balance is commonly expressed as the ventilation–perfusion (V/Q) ratio. The influence of V/Q ratios on pulmonary gas exchange can be described using a schematic alveolar–capillary unit, as shown in Figure 19.1. The upper panel shows a perfect match between ventilation and perfusion (V/Q = 1). This is the reference point for defining the abnormal patterns of gas exchange.

Dead Space Ventilation

A V/Q ratio above 1.0 (Fig. 19.1, middle panel) describes the condition where ventilation is excessive relative to capillary blood flow. The excess ventilation, known as *dead space ventilation*, does not participate in gas exchange with the blood. There are two types of dead space ventilation.

Anatomic dead space is the gas in the large conducting airways that does not come in contact with capillaries (approximately 50% of the anatomic dead space is in the pharynx). *Physiologic dead space* is the alveolar

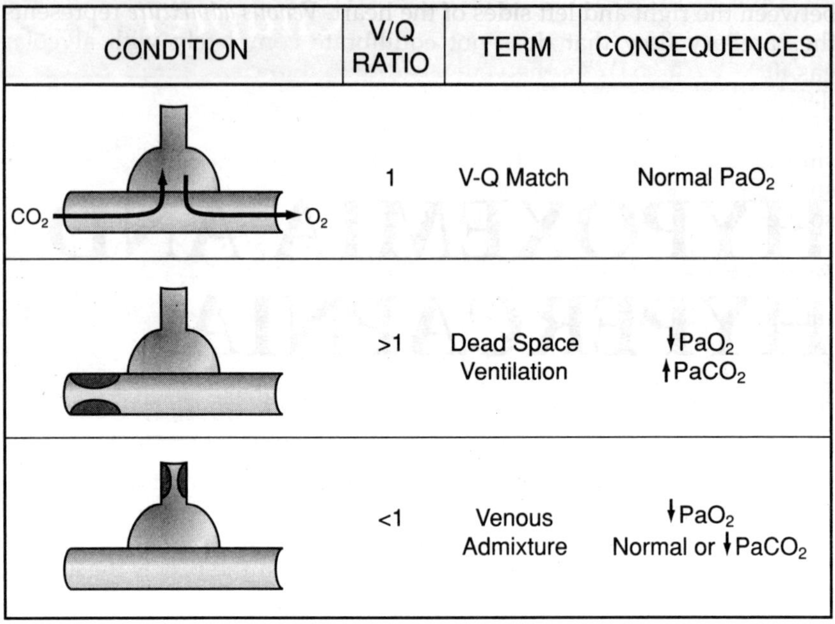

FIGURE 19.1 Ventilation–perfusion (*V/Q*) relationships and associated blood gas abnormalities.

gas that does not equilibrate fully with capillary blood. In normal subjects, dead space ventilation (V_D) accounts for 20 to 30% of the total ventilation (V_T), so $V_D/V_T = 0.2$ to 0.3 (3,5).

Pathophysiology

Dead space ventilation increases when the alveolar–capillary interface is destroyed (e.g., emphysema), when blood flow is reduced (e.g., low cardiac output), or when alveoli are overdistended (e.g., positive-pressure ventilation).

Arterial Blood Gases

An increase in V_D/V_T above 0.3 results in both hypoxemia and hypercapnia (analogous to what would happen if you held your breath). The hypercapnia usually appears when the V_D/V_T rises above 0.5 (5).

Intrapulmonary Shunt

A V/Q ratio below 1.0 (Fig. 19.1, lower panel) describes the condition where capillary blood flow is excessive relative to ventilation. The excess blood flow, known as *intrapulmonary shunt*, does not participate in pulmonary gas exchange. There are two types of intrapulmonary shunt. *True shunt* indicates the total absence of exchange between capillary blood and alveolar gas (V/Q = 0), and is equivalent to an anatomic shunt between the right and left sides of the heart. *Venous admixture* represents the capillary flow that does not equilibrate completely with alveolar gas ($0 < V/Q < 1$). As the venous admixture increases, the V/Q ratio decreases until it reaches true shunt conditions ($V/Q = 0$).

The fraction of the cardiac output that represents intrapulmonary shunt is known as the *shunt fraction*. In normal subjects, intrapulmonary shunt flow (Qs) represents less than 10% of the total cardiac output (Qt), so the shunt fraction (Qs/Qt) is less than 10% (3,4,6).

Pathophysiology

Intrapulmonary shunt fraction increases when small airways are occluded (e.g., asthma), when alveoli are filled with fluid (e.g., pulmonary edema, pneumonia), when alveoli collapse (e.g., atelectasis), or when capillary flow is excessive (e.g., nonembolized regions of lung in pulmonary embolism).

Arterial Blood Gases

The influence of shunt fraction on arterial oxygen and carbon dioxide tensions (PaO_2, $PaCO_2$, respectively) is shown in Figure 19.2. The PaO_2 falls progressively as shunt fraction increases, but the $PaCO_2$ remains constant until the shunt fraction exceeds 50% (6). The $PaCO_2$ is often below normal in patients with increased intrapulmonary shunt as a result of hyperventilation triggered by the disease process (e.g., sepsis) or by the accompanying hypoxemia.

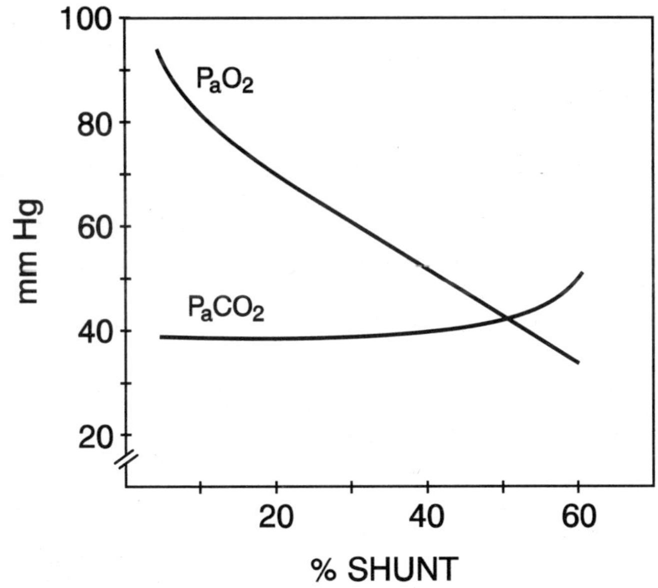

FIGURE 19.2 The influence of shunt fraction on arterial PO_2 (PaO_2) and arterial PCO_2 ($PaCO_2$). (From D'Alonzo GE, Dantzger DR. Mechanisms of abnormal gas exchange. Med Clin North Am 1983;67:557–571.)

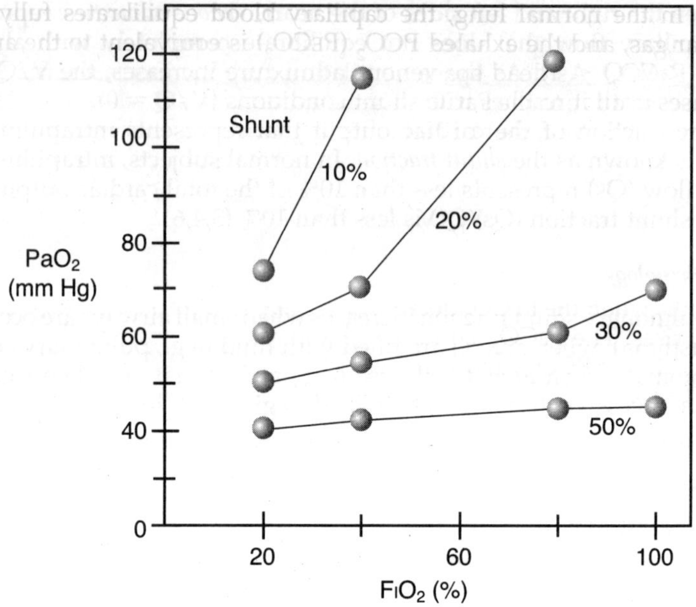

FIGURE 19.3 The influence of shunt fraction on the relationship between the inspired oxygen (FIO_2) and the arterial PO_2 (PaO_2). (From D'Alonzo GE, Dantzger DR. Med Clin North Am 1983;67:557–571.)

Inhaled Oxygen

The shunt fraction also determines the influence of inhaled oxygen on the arterial PO_2. This is shown in Figure 19.3 (6). As intrapulmonary shunt increases from 10 to 50%, an increase in fractional concentration of inspired oxygen (FIO_2) produces less of an increment in the arterial PO_2. When the shunt fraction exceeds 50%, the arterial PO_2 is independent of changes in FIO_2, and the condition behaves like a true (anatomic) shunt. This means that, *in conditions associated with a high shunt fraction* (e.g., acute respiratory distress syndrome), *the FIO_2 can often be lowered to non-toxic levels (FIO_2 below 50%) without further compromising arterial oxygenation*. This can be a valuable maneuver for preventing pulmonary oxygen toxicity.

QUANTITATIVE MEASURES

The following derived variables are used to determine the presence and severity of gas exchange abnormalities in the lungs.

Dead Space Ventilation

The calculation of dead space ventilation (V_D/V_T) is based on the difference between the PCO_2 in exhaled gas and end-capillary (arterial) blood. In the normal lung, the capillary blood equilibrates fully with alveolar gas, and the exhaled PCO_2 (P_ECO_2) is equivalent to the arterial PCO_2 ($PaCO_2$). As dead space ventilation (V_D/V_T) increases, the P_ECO_2 decreases relative to the $PaCO_2$. The Bohr equation shown below (derived by Christian Bohr, father of Neils Bohr) is based on this principle.

$$V_D/V_T = \frac{PaCO_2 - P_ECO_2}{PaCO_2} \qquad (19.1)$$

Thus, when the P_ECO_2 decreases relative to the $PaCO_2$, the calculated V_D/V_T rises. The P_ECO_2 is measured in a random sample of expired gas (mean exhaled PCO_2), and is not measured at the end of expiration (end-tidal PCO_2).

Intrapulmonary Shunt Fraction

The intrapulmonary shunt fraction (Qs/Qt) is derived by the relationship between the O_2 content in arterial blood (CaO_2), mixed venous blood (CvO_2), and pulmonary capillary blood (CcO_2).

$$Qs/Qt = \frac{CcO_2 - CaO_2}{CcO_2 - CvO_2} \qquad (19.2)$$

The problem with this formula is the inability to measure the pulmonary capillary O_2 content (CcO_2) directly. As a result, pure oxygen breathing (to produce 100% oxyhemoglobin saturation in pulmonary capillary blood) is recommended for the shunt calculation. However in this situation, Qs/Qt measures only true shunt.

The A-a PO_2 Gradient

The PO_2 difference between alveolar gas and arterial blood (P_AO_2 − PaO_2) is an indirect measure of ventilation–perfusion abnormalities (7–9). The P_AO_2 − PaO_2 (A-a PO_2) gradient is determined with the alveolar gas equation shown below.

$$P_AO_2 = P_IO_2 - (PaCO_2/RQ) \qquad (19.3)$$

This equation defines the relationship between the PO_2 in alveolar gas (P_AO_2), the PO_2 in inhaled gas (P_IO_2), the PCO_2 in arterial blood ($PaCO_2$), and the respiratory quotient (RQ). The RQ defines the relative rates of exchange of O_2 and CO_2 across the alveolar–capillary interface: $RQ = VCO_2/VO_2$. The P_IO_2 is determined using the fractional concentration of inspired oxygen (F_IO_2), the barometric pressure (P_B), and the partial pressure of water vapor (P_{H_2O}) in humidified gas:

$$P_IO_2 = F_IO_2\,(P_B - P_{H_2O}) \qquad (19.4)$$

TABLE 19.1 Normal Arterial Blood Gases

Age (years)	PaO_2 (mm Hg)	$PaCO_2$ (mm Hg)	A-a PO_2 (mm Hg)
20	84–95	33–47	4–17
30	81–92	34–47	7–21
40	78–90	34–47	10–24
50	75–87	34–47	14–27
60	72–84	34–47	17–31
70	70–81	34–47	21–34
80	67–79	34–47	25–38

All values pertain to room air breathing at sea level.
From the Intermountain Thoracic Society Manual of Uniform Laboratory Procedures. Salt Lake City, 1984:44–45.

If equations 19.3 and 19.4 are combined (for the alveolar PO_2), the A - a PO_2 gradient can be calculated as follows:

$$\text{A-a } PO_2 = [FIO_2\,(P_B - P_{H_2O}) - (PaCO_2/RQ)] - PaO_2 \qquad (19.5)$$

In a healthy subject breathing room air at sea level, $FIO_2 = 0.21$, $P_B = 760$ mm Hg, $P_{H_2O} = 47$ mm Hg, $PaO_2 = 90$ mm Hg, $PaCO_2 = 40$ mm Hg, and RQ = 0.8:

$$\text{A-a } PO_2 = [0.21\,(760 - 47) - (40/0.8)] - 90 = 10 \text{ mm Hg} \qquad (19.6)$$

This represents an idealized rather than normal A-a PO_2 gradient, because the A-a PO_2 gradient varies with age and with the concentration of inspired oxygen.

Influence of Age

As shown in Table 19.1, the normal A-a PO_2 gradient rises steadily with advancing age (8). Assuming that most adult patients in an ICU are 40 years of age or older, the normal A-a PO_2 gradient in an adult ICU patient can be as high as 25 mm Hg when the patient is breathing room air. However, few ICU patients breathe room air and the A-a PO_2 gradient is increased further when oxygen is added to inhaled gas.

Influence of Inspired Oxygen

The influence of inspired oxygen on the A-a PO_2 gradient is shown in Figure 19.4 (9). The A-a PO_2 gradient increases from 15 to 60 mm Hg as the FIO_2 increases from 21% (room air) to 100%. According to this relationship, **the normal A-a PO_2 gradient increases 5 to 7 mm Hg for every 10% increase in FIO_2.** This effect is presumably caused by the loss of regional hypoxic vasoconstriction in the lungs. Hypoxic vasoconstriction in poorly ventilated lung regions diverts blood to more adequately ventilated regions, and this helps to preserve the normal V/Q balance.

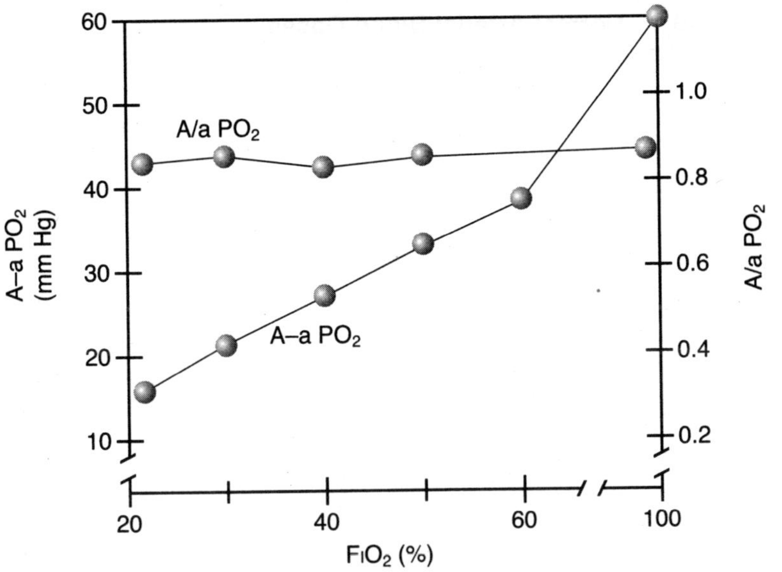

FIGURE 19.4 The influence of F_IO_2 on the alveolar-arterial PO_2 gradient (A-a PO_2) and the arterial–alveolar PO_2 ratio (a/A PO_2) in normal subjects. (From Reference 9.)

Loss of regional hypoxic vasoconstriction during supplemental oxygen breathing maintains blood flow in poorly ventilated lung regions, and this increases intrapulmonary shunt fraction and increases the A-a PO_2 gradient.

Positive-Pressure Ventilation

Positive-pressure mechanical ventilation elevates the pressure in the airways above the ambient barometric pressure. Therefore, when determining the A-a PO_2 gradient in a ventilator-dependent patient, the mean airway pressure should be added to the barometric pressure (10). In the example presented previously, a mean airway pressure of 30 cm H_2O would increase the A-a PO_2 gradient from 10 to 16 mm Hg (a 60% increase). Thus, neglecting the contribution of positive airway pressure during mechanical ventilation will underestimate the degree of abnormal gas exchange.

The a/A PO_2 Ratio

Unlike the A-a PO_2 gradient, the a/A PO_2 ratio is relatively unaffected by the F_IO_2. This is demonstrated in Figure 19.5. The independence of the a/A PO_2 gradient in relation to the F_IO_2 is explained by the equation below.

$$a/A\ PO_2 = 1 - (\text{A-a}\ PO_2)/PaO_2 \qquad (19.7)$$

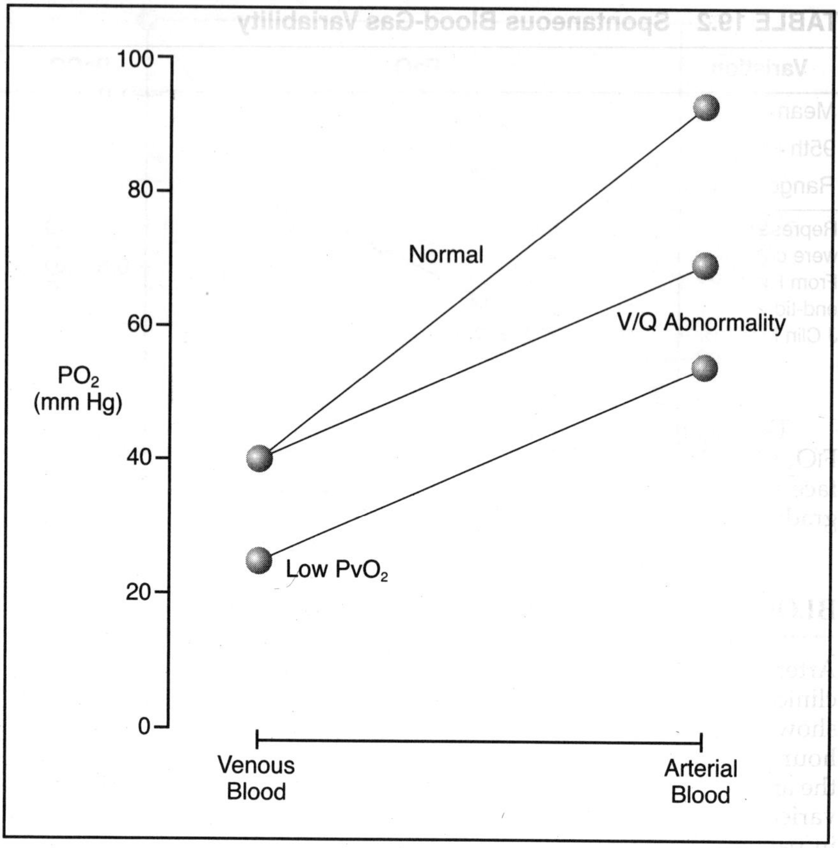

FIGURE 19.5 The influence of a V/Q abnormality on the transition from venous to arterial PO_2 and the added effect of a low mixed venous PO_2 (PvO_2).

Because the alveolar PO_2 is in both the numerator and denominator of the equation, the influence of FiO_2 on the PaO_2 is eliminated. Thus, **the a/A PO_2 ratio is a mathematical manipulation that eliminates the influence of FiO_2 on the A-a PO_2 gradient.** The normal a/A PO_2 ratio is 0.74 to 0.77 when breathing room air, and 0.80 to 0.82 when breathing 100% oxygen (9).

The PaO_2/FiO_2 Ratio

The PaO_2/FiO_2 ratio is used as an indirect estimate of shunt fraction. The following correlations have been reported (11).

PaO_2/FiO_2	Qs/Qt
<200	>20%
>200	<20%

TABLE 19.2 Spontaneous Blood-Gas Variability

Variation	PaO_2	$PaCO_2$
Mean	13 mm Hg	2.5 mm Hg
95th Percentile	±18 mm Hg	±4 mm Hg
Range	2–37 mm Hg	0–12 mm Hg

Represents variation over a 1-hour period in 26 ventilator-dependent trauma victims who were clinically stable.
From Hess D, Agarwal NN. Variability of blood gases, pulse oximeter saturation, and end-tidal carbon dioxide pressure in stable, mechanically ventilated trauma patients. J Clin Monit 1992;8:111.

The major limitation of the PaO_2/FIO_2 ratio is the variability of the FIO_2 when supplemental oxygen is delivered through nasal prongs or a face mask (see Chapter 21). This limitation also applies to the A-a PO_2 gradient.

BLOOD GAS VARIABILITY

Arterial blood gases can vary spontaneously without a change in the clinical condition of the patient. This is demonstrated in Table 19.2, which shows the spontaneous variation in arterial PO_2 and PCO_2 over a one-hour period in a group of clinically stable trauma victims (12). Note that the arterial PO_2 varied by as much as 36 mm Hg, while the arterial PCO_2 varied by as much as 12 mm Hg. This variability has also been observed in patients in a medical ICU (13). Because arterial blood gases can vary spontaneously without a change in the clinical condition of the patient, **routine monitoring of arterial blood gases can be misleading and is not justified.**

HYPOXEMIA

The causes of hypoxemia can be separated into 3 groups based on the physiological process involved (14,15). Each group of disorders can be distinguished by the A-a PO_2 gradient and/or the mixed venous PO_2, as shown in Table 19.3.

TABLE 19.3 Sources of Hypoxemia

Source	A-a PO_2	PvO_2
Hypoventilation	Normal	Normal
V/Q mismatch	Increased	Normal
DO_2/VO_2 imbalance	Increased	Decreased

TABLE 19.4 Alveolar Hypoventilation in the ICU

Brainstem respiratory depression

1. Drugs (e.g., opiates)
2. Obesity-hypoventilation syndrome

Peripheral neuropathy

1. Critical illness polyneuropathy
2. Guillain-Barré syndrome

Muscle weakness

1. Critical illness myopathy
2. Hypophosphatemia
3. Magnesium depletion
4. Myasthenia gravis

Hypoventilation

Alveolar hypoventilation causes both hypoxemia and hypercapnia as a result of a decrease in the total volume of air inhaled (and exhaled) each minute. There is no V/Q imbalance in the lungs, so the A-a PO_2 gradient is not elevated. The common causes of alveolar hypoventilation are listed in Table 19.4. Most cases of hypoventilation in the ICU are the result of drug-induced respiratory depression or neuromuscular weakness. Obesity-related hypoventilation (Pickwickian syndrome) is present in up to one third of morbidly obese patients (body mass index >35 kg/m^2) (16), and this disorder is likely to become much more common as the ranks of the obese continue to grow steadily in number.

Respiratory Muscle Weakness

Most cases of respiratory muscle weakness in the ICU are the result of an idiopathic polyneuropathy and myopathy that is specific to ICU patients, particularly those with sepsis, prolonged mechanical ventilation, and prolonged neuromuscular paralysis (17). (This is described in Chapter 51). The standard method of evaluating respiratory muscle strength is to measure the *maximum inspiratory pressure* (PImax), which is the maximum pressure recorded during a maximum inspiratory effort against a closed valve. The normal PImax varies with age and gender, but most healthy adults can generate a negative PImax of at least 80 cm H_2O (18). A PImax that does not exceed –25 cm H_2O is considered evidence of respiratory muscle failure (19). (See Chapter 51 for more information on neuromuscular weakness syndromes in the ICU.)

V/Q Abnormality

Most cases of hypoxemia are the result of a V/Q mismatch in the lungs. Virtually any lung disease can be included in this category, but the common ones encountered in the ICU are pneumonia, inflammatory lung injury (acute respiratory distress syndrome), obstructive lung disease, hydrostatic pulmonary edema, and pulmonary embolism. The A-a PO_2 gradient is almost always elevated in these conditions, but the elevation can be minimal in patients with severe airways obstruction (which behaves like hypoventilation).

DO_2/VO_2 Imbalance

As explained in Chapter 2, a decrease in systemic O_2 delivery (DO_2) is usually accompanied by an increase in O_2 extraction from capillary blood, and this serves to maintain a constant rate of O_2 uptake (VO_2) into the tissues. The increased O_2 extraction from capillary blood results in a decrease in the PO_2 of venous blood, and this can have a deleterious effect on arterial oxygenation, as explained below.

Mixed Venous PO_2

The oxygen in arterial blood represents the sum of the oxygen in mixed venous (pulmonary artery) blood and the oxygen added from alveolar gas. When gas exchange is normal, the PO_2 in alveolar gas is the major determinant of the arterial PO_2. However when gas exchange is impaired, the contribution of the alveolar PO_2 declines and the contribution of the mixed venous PO_2 rises (20). The greater the impairment in gas exchange, the greater the contribution of the mixed venous PO_2 to the arterial PO_2. (If there is no gas exchange in the lungs, the mixed venous PO_2 would be the sole determinant of the arterial PO_2.)

The diagram in Figure 19.5 demonstrates the influence of mixed venous PO_2 on the arterial PO_2 when gas exchange is impaired. The curves in the graph represent the transition from mixed venous PO_2 to arterial PO_2 in the lungs. The slope of each curve reflects the efficiency of gas exchange in the lungs. Note that the curve representing the V/Q abnormality results in a lower arterial PO_2 because the slope is decreased (indicating impaired oxygen exchange in the lungs) when compared to the normal curve. If this curve begins at a lower mixed venous PO_2, as indicated, the curve shifts downward, resulting in a further decrease in arterial PO_2. This illustrates how a decrease in mixed venous PO_2 can aggravate the hypoxemia caused by a V/Q abnormality. It also indicates that, in the presence of a V/Q abnormality, the mixed venous PO_2 is an important consideration in the evaluation of hypoxemia.

The relationship between O_2 delivery (DO_2), O_2 uptake (VO_2) and the mixed venous PO_2 (PvO_2) is shown below (k is the proportionality constant).

$$PvO_2 = k \times (DO_2/VO_2) \qquad (19.8)$$

Thus, any condition that reduces DO_2 (e.g., low cardiac output, anemia) or increases VO_2 (e.g., hypermetabolism) can decrease the PvO_2 and aggravate the hypoxemia caused by abnormal gas exchange in the lungs.

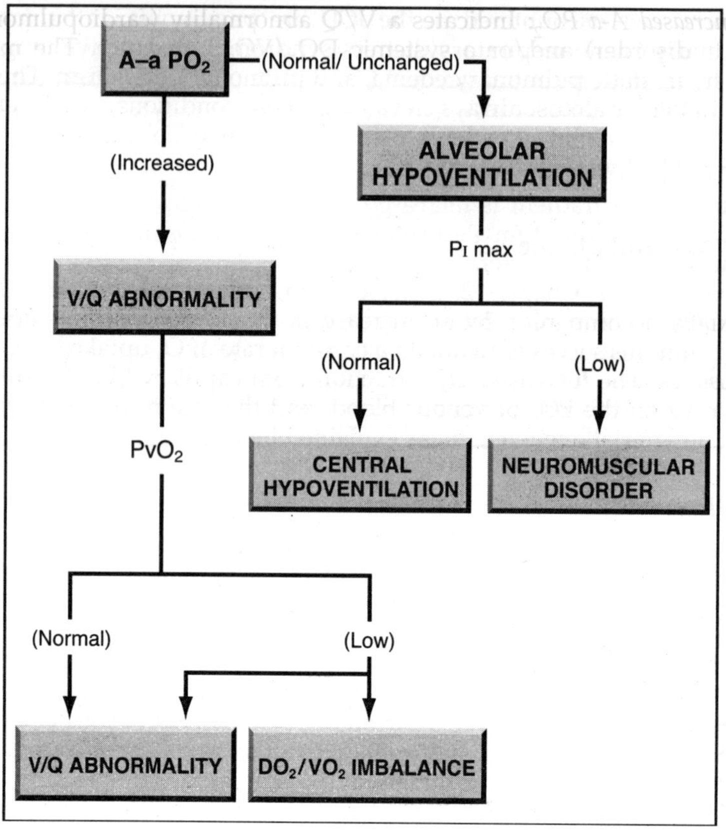

FIGURE 19.6 Flow diagram for the evaluation of hypoxemia.

Diagnostic Evaluation

The evaluation of hypoxemia can proceed according to the flow diagram in Figure 19.6. This approach uses three measures: A-a PO_2 gradient, mixed venous PO_2, and maximum inspiratory pressure. The PO_2 in superior vena cava blood (central venous PO_2) can be used as the mixed venous O_2 when there is no indwelling pulmonary artery catheter.

Step 1: A-a PO_2 Gradient

The first step in the approach involves a determination of the A-a PO_2 gradient. After correcting for age and FIO_2, the A-a PO_2 gradient can be interpreted as follows:

Normal A-a PO_2: Indicates a hypoventilation disorder rather than a cardiopulmonary disorder. In this situation, the most likely problems are drug-induced respiratory depression and neuromuscular weakness. The latter condition can be uncovered by measuring the maximum inspiratory pressure (PImax). This measurement is described in the upcoming section on hypercapnia.

Increased A-a PO_2: Indicates a V/Q abnormality (cardiopulmonary disorder) and/or a systemic DO_2/VO_2 imbalance. The mixed venous (or central venous) PO_2 will help to differentiate between these two disorders.

Step 2: Mixed Venous PO_2

When the A-a gradient is increased, the PO_2 should be measured in a blood sample taken from a central venous catheter or the distal port of a pulmonary artery catheter.

Normal venous PO_2: If the venous PO_2 is 40 mm Hg or higher, the problem is solely a V/Q mismatch in the lungs.

Low venous PO_2: If the venous PO_2 is below 40 mm Hg, there is a DO_2/VO_2 imbalance adding to the hypoxemia created by a V/Q mismatch in the lungs. The source of this imbalance is either a decreased DO_2 (from anemia or a low cardiac output) or an increased VO_2 (from hypermetabolism).

Spurious Hypoxemia

Spurious hypoxemia is a rarely reported phenomenon that is characterized by hypoxemia in an arterial blood sample without corresponding hypoxemia in circulating blood (as measured by pulse oximetry) (21). This phenomenon seems to occur only in patients with hematologic malignancies who have marked leukocytosis (WBC > 100,000) or thrombocytosis (platelet count > 1,000,000). The reduced PO_2 in the blood sample has been attributed to O_2 consumption by activated leukocytes in the sample; a process that has been called *leukocyte larceny* (22). While this is the prevailing explanation, it doesn't explain why marked thrombocytosis can also produce spurious hypoxemia because platelets are not oxygen-guzzlers like activated leukocytes. Regardless of the mechanism, there is no accepted method of preventing spurious hypoxemia (rapid cooling of blood samples has had inconsistent results), so you should be aware of the phenomenon and the value of pulse oximetry for validating in vitro PO_2 measurements (pulse oximetry is described in the next chapter).

HYPERCAPNIA

Hypercapnia is defined as an arterial PCO_2 above 46 mm Hg that does not represent compensation for a metabolic alkalosis (23). The causes of hypercapnia can be identified by considering the determinants of arterial PCO_2 ($PaCO_2$). The $PaCO_2$ is directly related to the rate of CO_2 production (VCO_2) in the body, and is inversely related to the rate of CO_2 elimination by alveolar ventilation (V_A) (3,18). Therefore, $PaCO_2 = k \times (VCO_2/V_A)$, where *k* is a proportionality constant. Alveolar ventilation is the portion of the total ventilation (V_E) that is not dead space ventilation (V_D/V_T); that is, $V_A = V_E\,(1 - V_D/V_T)$. Combining these relationships yields Equation 19.8, which identifies the determinants of $PaCO_2$:

$$PaCO_2 = k \times [VCO_2/V_E(1 - V_D/V_T)] \tag{19.9}$$

This equation identifies three major sources of hypercapnia: (a) increased CO_2 production (VCO_2), (b) hypoventilation ($1/V_E$), and (c) increased dead space ventilation (V_D/V_T).

Hypoventilation

Hypoventilation was discussed briefly in the last section on hypoxemia, and Table 19.4 shows the common causes of hypoventilation. Because hypoxemia is so common in ICU patients, hypercapnia may be the first sign of hypoventilation from neuromuscular weakness or drug-induced respiratory depression in the ICU. This is also the case in obesity-hypoventilation syndrome, where hypercapnia while awake is often the first evidence of daytime hypoventilation. On the other hand, hypercapnia is a relatively late sign in neuromuscular disorders, and does not appear until the maximum inspiratory pressure (described in the hypoxemia section) falls to levels below 50% of normal (19).

V/Q Abnormality

As mentioned earlier, hypercapnia is not a feature of increased intrapulmonary shunt until late in the process (which is why hypercapnia is not a feature of pulmonary edema or other infiltrative lung processes until they are far advanced). Hypercapnia is more a feature of increased dead space ventilation (such as occurs in advanced emphysema, where there is destruction of the alveolar-capillary interface), and the $PaCO_2$ usually begins to rise when dead space ventilation accounts for more than 50% of total ventilation ($V_D/V_T > 0.5$).

Increased CO_2 Production

An increase in CO_2 production is usually related to oxidative metabolism, but non-metabolic CO_2 production is possible when extracellular acids generate hydrogen ions that combine with bicarbonate ions and generate CO_2. Whatever the source, increased CO_2 production is normally accompanied by an increase in minute ventilation, which eliminates the excess CO_2 and maintains a constant arterial PCO_2. Therefore, excess CO_2 production does not normally cause hypercapnia. However when CO_2 excretion is impaired (by neuromuscular weakness or lung disease), an increase in CO_2 production can lead to an increase in $PaCO_2$. Thus, increased CO_2 production is an important factor in promoting hypercapnia only in patients with a reduced ability to eliminate CO_2.

Overfeeding

Overfeeding, or the provision of calories in excess of daily needs, is a recognized cause of hypercapnia in patients with severe lung disease and acute respiratory failure (24). Nutrition-associated hypercapnia occurs predominantly in ventilator-dependent patients, and can delay weaning from mechanical ventilation. Overfeeding with carbohydrates is particularly problematic because oxidative metabolism of carbohydrates

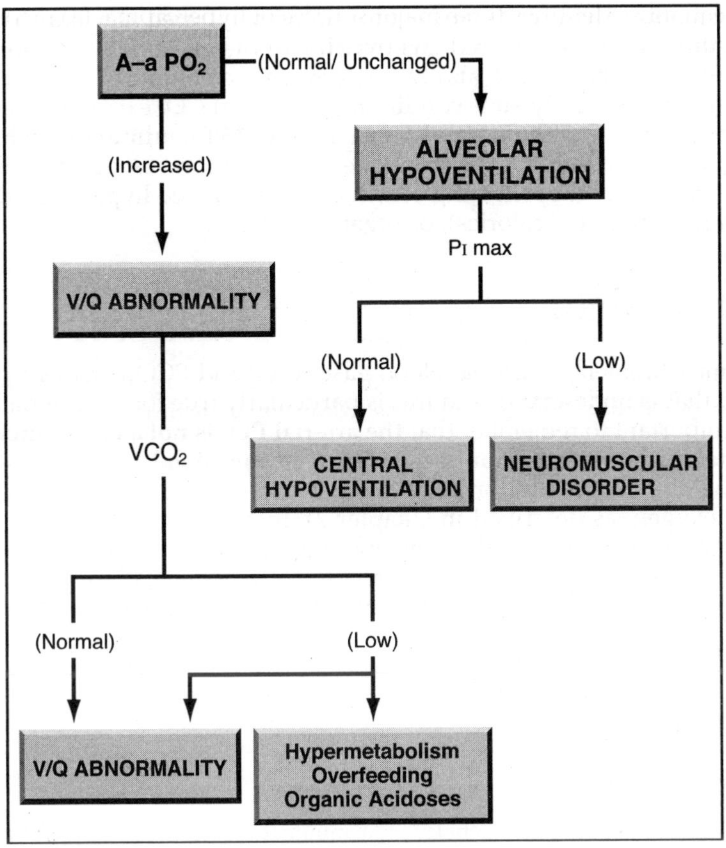

FIGURE 19.7 Flow diagram for the evaluation of hypercapnia.

generates more carbon dioxide than the other nutrient substrates (lipids and proteins).

Diagnostic Evaluation

The bedside evaluation of hypercapnia is shown in Figure 19.7. The evaluation of hypercapnia, like hypoxemia, begins with the A-a PO_2 gradient (25). A normal or unchanged A-a PO_2 gradient indicates that the problem is alveolar hypoventilation (the same as described for the evaluation of hypoxemia). An increased A-a PO_2 gradient indicates a V/Q abnormality (an increase in dead space ventilation) that may or may not be accompanied by an increase in CO_2 production.

Measuring CO_2 Production

The rate of CO_2 production (VCO_2) can be measured at the bedside with specialized metabolic carts that are normally used to perform nutritional assessments. These carts are equipped with infrared devices that can measure the CO_2 in expired gas (much like the end-tidal CO_2 monitors described in Chapter 20), and can determine the volume of CO_2 excreted per minute. In steady-state conditions, the rate of CO_2 excretion is equivalent to the VCO_2. The **normal VCO_2 is 90 to 130 L/minute/m^2**, which is roughly 80% of the VO_2. As mentioned earlier, an increased VCO_2 is evidence for one of the following conditions: generalized hypermetabolism, overfeeding (excess calories), or organic acidoses.

A FINAL WORD

The measurement of arterial blood gases (PO_2 and PCO_2) enjoys a popularity that is undeserved, and this is particularly true for the arterial PO_2. It is important to remember that **the arterial PO_2 is not a useful measure for determining the amount of oxygen in the blood** (this requires the hemoglobin concentration and the percent saturation of hemoglobin with oxygen, as described in Chapter 2). Instead, the PaO_2 (along with the $PaCO_2$) can be useful for evaluating gas exchange in the lungs. A more useful measurement for evaluating the oxygenation of blood is the pulse oximeter measurement of arterial oxyhemoglobin saturation (described in the next chapter).

REFERENCES

Introduction

1. Dale JC, Pruett SK. Phlebotomy: a minimalist approach. Mayo Clin Proc 1993;68:249–255.
2. Raffin TA. Indications for blood gas analysis. Ann Intern Med 1986;105:390–398.

Pulmonary Gas Exchange

3. Dantzger DR. Pulmonary gas exchange. In: Dantzger DR, ed. Cardiopulmonary critical care. 2nd ed. Philadelphia: WB Saunders, 1991:25–43.
4. Lanken PN. Ventilation-perfusion relationships. In: Grippi MA, ed. Pulmonary pathophysiology. Philadelphia: JB Lippincott, 1995:195–210.
5. Buohuys A. Respiratory dead space. In: Fenn WO, Rahn H, eds. Handbook of physiology: respiration. Bethesda: American Physiological Society, 1964:699–714.
6. D'Alonzo GE, Dantzger DR. Mechanisms of abnormal gas exchange. Med Clin North Am 1983;67:557–571.

Quantitative Measures

7. Gammon RB, Jefferson LS. Interpretation of arterial oxygen tension. UpToDate Web Site, 2006. (Accessed 3/11/2006)

8. Harris EA, Kenyon AM, Nisbet HD, et al. The normal alveolar-arterial oxygen tension gradient in man. Clin Sci 1974;46:89–104.
9. Gilbert R, Kreighley JF. The arterial/alveolar oxygen tension ratio: an index of gas exchange applicable to varying inspired oxygen concentrations. Am Rev Respir Dis 1974;109:142–145.
10. Carroll GC. Misapplication of the alveolar gas equation. N Engl J Med 1985;312:586.
11. Covelli HD, Nessan VJ, Tuttle WK. Oxygen derived variables in acute respiratory failure. Crit Care Med 1983;11:646–649.

Blood-Gas Variability

12. Hess D, Agarwal NN. Variability of blood gases, pulse oximeter saturation, and end-tidal carbon dioxide pressure in stable, mechanically ventilated trauma patients. J Clin Monit 1992;8:111–115.
13. Sasse SA, Chen P, Mahutte CK. Variability of arterial blood gas values over time in stable medical ICU patients. Chest 1994;106:187–193.

Hypoxemia

14. Duarte A, Bidani A. Evaluating hypoxemia in the critically ill. J Crit Illness 2005;20:91–93.
15. White AC. The evaluation and management of hypoxemia in the chronic critically ill patient. Clin Chest Med 2001;22:123–134.
16. Nowbar S, Burkhart KM, Gonzalez R, et al. Obesity-associated hypoventilation in hospitalized patients: prevalence, effects, and outcome. Am J Med 2004;116:1–7.
17. Rich MM, Raps EC, Bird SJ. Distinction between acute myopathy syndrome and critical illness polyneuropathy. Mayo Clin Proc 1995;70:198–199.
18. Bruschi C, Cerveri I, Zoia MC, et al. Reference values for maximum respiratory mouth pressures: a population-based study. Am Rev Respir Dis 1992; 146:790–793.
19. Baydur A. Respiratory muscle strength and control of ventilation in patients with neuromuscular disease. Chest 1991;99:330–338.
20. Rossaint R, Hahn S-M, Pappert D, et al. Influence of mixed venous PO_2 and inspired oxygen fraction on intrapulmonary shunt in patients with severe ARDS. J Appl Physiol 1995;78:1531–1536.
21. Lele A, Mirski MA, Stevens RD. Spurious hypoxemia. Crit Care Med 2005;33: 1854–1856.
22. Fox MJ, Brody JS, Weintraub LR. Leukocyte larceny: a cause of spurious hypoxemia. Am J Med 1979;67:742–746.

Hypercapnia

23. Weinberger SE, Schwartzstein RM, Weiss JW. Hypercapnia. N Engl J Med 1989;321:1223–1230.
24. Talpers SS, Romberger DJ, Bunce SB, et al. Nutritionally associated increased carbon dioxide production. Chest 1992;102:551–555.
25. Gray BA, Blalock JM. Interpretation of the alveolar-arterial oxygen difference in patients with hypercapnia. Am Rev Respir Dis 1991;143:4–8.

Chapter 20

OXIMETRY AND CAPNOGRAPHY

The noninvasive detection of blood gases (PO_2, PCO_2) using optical and colorimetric techniques (1,2) is the most significant and useful advance in critical care monitoring in the last quarter century. This chapter describes the monitoring techniques that have become an integral part of daily patient care in the ICU (and in most other areas of the hospital as well). Despite the popularity of these techniques, surveys reveal that 95% of ICU staff members have little or no understanding of how the techniques work (3).

OXIMETRY

All atoms and molecules absorb specific wavelengths of light (this is the source of color in the lighted world). This property is the basis for an optical technique known as *spectrophotometry*, which transmits light of specific wavelengths through a medium to determine the molecular composition of the medium. The absorption of light as it passes through a medium is proportional to the concentration of the substance that absorbs the light and the length of the path that the light travels (this is known as the Lambert-Beer Law). The application of this principle to the detection of hemoglobin in its different forms is known as *oximetry*.

Optical Recognition of Hemoglobin

Hemoglobin (like all proteins) changes its structural configuration when it participates in a chemical reaction, and each of the configurations has a distinct pattern of light absorption. The patterns of light absorption for the different forms of hemoglobin are shown in Figure 20.1. Four different forms of hemoglobin are represented in the figure: oxygenated hemoglobin (HbO_2) deoxygenated hemoglobin (Hb), methemoglobin (met Hb) and carboxyhemoglobin (COHb). Comparing the oxygenated and deoxygenated forms of hemoglobin (HbO_2 and Hb) shows that, in the red region of the light spectrum (660 nm), HbO_2 does not absorb light

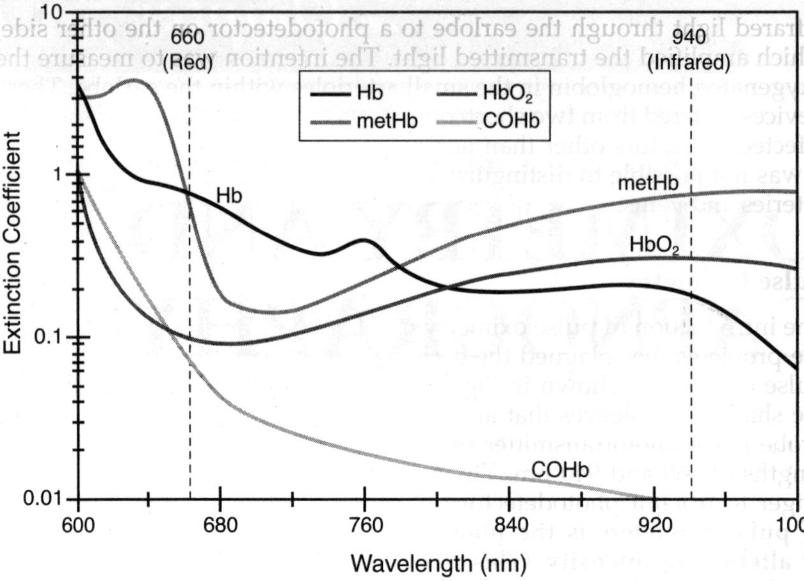

FIGURE 20.1 The absorption spectrum for the different forms of hemoglobin: oxygenated hemoglobin (*HbO*$_2$), deoxygenated hemoglobin (*Hb*), carboxyhemoglobin (*COHb*), and methemoglobin (*metHb*) The vertical lines represent the two wavelengths of light (660 nm and 940 nm) used by pulse oximeters. (Adapted from Barker SJ, Tremper KK. Pulse oximetry: applications and limitations. Internat Anesthesiol Clin 1987;25:155)

as well as Hb (this is why oxygenated blood is more intensely red than deoxygenated blood), while in the infrared region (940 nm), the opposite is true, and HbO_2 absorbs light more effectively than Hb.

Because methemoglobin (metHb) and carboxyhemoglobin (COHb) make up less than 5% of the total hemoglobin pool in most situations (2–4), the transmission of light at 660 nm through a blood sample is determined by the amount of HbO_2 in the sample, while light transmission at 940 nm is determined by amount of Hb in the sample. The amount of HbO_2 can then be compared to the total amount of hemoglobin (HbO_2 + Hb) to express the fraction of the hemoglobin pool that is in the oxygenated form. This is known as *% saturation*, and is derived in Equation 20.1 below.

$$\% \text{ Saturation} = (HbO_2/HbO_2 + Hb) \times 100 \qquad (20.1)$$

This is how most bedside oximeters operate, using two wavelengths of light (660 and 940 nm), and expressing the oxygenated hemoglobin as a percentage of the total hemoglobin.

Early Oximeters

The first bedside oximeters used probes that were clamped onto an earlobe. A light emitting device on one side of the probe sent red and infrared light through the earlobe to a photodetector on the other side, which amplified the transmitted light. The intention was to measure the oxygenated hemoglobin in the small arterioles within the earlobe. These devices suffered from two shortcomings: (*1*) the transmission of light was affected by factors other than hemoglobin (e.g., skin pigments), and (*2*) it was not possible to distinguish between oxyhemoglobin saturation in arteries and veins.

Pulse Oximetry

The introduction of pulse oximetry in the mid-1970s eliminated many of the problems that plagued the early oximeters. The basic operation of a pulse oximeter is shown in Figure 20.2. The probes on pulse oximeters are shaped like sleeves that are placed around a finger. One side of the probe has a phototransmitter that emits monochromatic light at wavelengths of 660 and 940 nm. The light travels through the tissues of the finger to reach a photodetector on the other side. **The unique feature of pulse oximeters is the photodetector, which amplifies only light of alternating intensity.** (This is analogous to an AC amplifier, which amplifies only alternating-current impulses.) Light that strikes a pulsating artery will develop phasic changes in intensity and will be amplified by the photodetector, while light that passes through non-pulsatile tissue will be blocked by the photodetector. This allows pulse oximeters to detect only the hemoglobin in pulsating arteries, and it reduces or eliminates errors created by light absorption in non-pulsatile structures like connective tissue and veins.

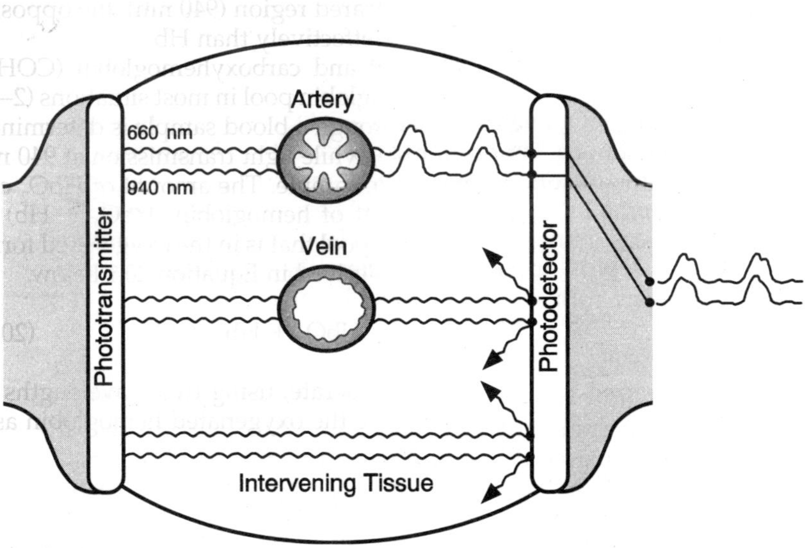

FIGURE 20.2 The principle of pulse oximetry. The photodetector senses only light of alternating intensity (analogous to an AC amplifier).

TABLE 20.1 Variability in Oximetry and Capnometry Recordings

Study Parameters	SpO_2*	SvO_2**	$PETCO_2$*
Time period	60 min	120 min	60 min
Mean variation	1%	6%	2 mm Hg
Range of variation	0–5%	1–19%	0–7 mm Hg

Clinically stable patients. 95% of measurements obtained during mechanical ventilation.
*From Reference 6.
**From Reference 19.

Accuracy

At clinically acceptable levels of arterial oxygenation (SaO_2 above 70%), the O_2 saturation recorded by pulse oximeters (SpO_2) differs by less than 3% from the actual SaO_2 (4,5). SpO_2 also shows a high degree of precision (consistency of repeated measurements). This is demonstrated in Table 20.1 (6), which shows that SpO_2 varies by $\leq$ 2% in most patients who are clinically stable.

Carbon Monoxide Intoxication

Carbon monoxide displaces oxygen from the iron binding sites in hemoglobin, so carbon monoxide intoxication will increase carboxyhemoglobin (COHb) levels and decrease oxyhemoglobin (HbO_2) levels. This should be evident as a decreased arterial O_2 saturation (SaO_2). However, as demonstrated in Figure 20.1, light absorption at 660 nm is similar for carboxyhemoglobin (COHb) and oxygenated hemoglobin (HbO_2). This means that pulse oximeters will mistake COHb for HbO_2, and the SpO_2 will be higher than the actual SaO_2. The difference between the SpO_2 and the SaO_2 ($SpO_2 - SaO_2$), the *pulse oximetry gap*, is equivalent to the COHb level (7).

Because the SpO_2 overestimates the SaO_2 when COHb levels are elevated, **pulse oximetry is unreliable for detecting hypoxemia in carbon monoxide intoxication.** When carbon monoxide intoxication is suspected, an arterial blood sample should be sent to the clinical laboratory for a direct measurement of the COHb level. (Clinical laboratories have multiple-wavelength spectrophotometers that can more precisely measure the different forms of hemoglobin in the blood.)

Methemoglobinemia

The oxidized iron moieties in methemoglobin do not carry oxygen effectively, so accumulation of methemoglobin (metHb) will decrease the SaO_2. Pulse oximetry overestimates the SaO_2 ($SpO_2 > SaO_2$), and the SpO_2 rarely falls below 85% in methemoglobinemia despite much lower levels of SaO_2 (8). Thus, **pulse oximetry should not be used when methemoglobinemia is suspected.** Accurate measurements of metHb, and SaO_2 require the more sophisticated spectrophotometers in clinical laboratories.

Hypotension

Although pulse oximetry is based on the presence of pulsatile blood flow, SpO_2 is an accurate reflection of SaO_2 down to blood pressures as low as 30 mm Hg (9). Damped pulsations also do not affect the accuracy of fingertip SpO_2 recordings taken distal to a cannulated radial artery (10).

For situations where fingertip SpO_2 recordings may be problematic because of severely reduced peripheral blood flow, specialized **oximeter sensors are available that can be placed on the forehead.** These sensors differ from the fingertip sensors because they record light that is reflected back to the skin surface (reflectance spectrophotometry). Forehead sensors respond much more rapidly to changes in SpO_2 than fingertip sensors (11), and they should gain popularity as a suitable alternative to the traditional fingertip sensors.

Anemia

In the absence of hypoxemia, pulse oximetry is accurate down to hemoglobin levels as low as 2 to 3 g/dL (12). With lesser degrees of anemia (Hb between 2.5 and 9 g/dL), SpO_2 underestimates SaO_2 by only 0.5% (12).

Pigments

The effects of dark skin pigmentation on the SpO_2 has varied in different reports. In one study, the SpO_2 was spuriously low in patients with dark skin (13), while in another study, the SpO_2 was spuriously high ($SpO_2 - SaO_2 = 3.5\%$) when the SaO_2 was less than 70% (14). Fingernail polish has a small effect on the SpO_2 when the color is black or brown (SpO_2 2% less than SaO_2), but this effect can be eliminated by placing the probes on the side of the finger (15). The largest pigment effect is produced by methylene blue, which can produce a 65% decrease in SpO_2 when injected intravenously (4). Because methylene blue is used to treat methemoglobinemia, this is another reason to avoid pulse oximetry in patients with methemoglobinemia.

Detecting Hypoventilation

Clinical studies have shown that the SpO_2 can be a sensitive marker of inadequate ventilation (a low PaO_2) when patients are breathing room air, but not when they are breathing supplemental oxygen (16). This is explained by the shape of the oxyhemoglobin dissociation curve. When SpO_2 (or SaO_2) exceeds 90% ($PaO_2 > 60$ mm Hg), the curve begins to flatten, and larger changes in PaO_2 are accompanied by smaller changes in SpO_2. Breathing supplemental oxygen will push the SpO_2 further out onto the flat part of the oxyhemoglobin dissociation curve (the SpO_2 is often >98% during supplemental O_2 breathing), where relatively large changes in PaO_2 are accompanied by minor changes in the SpO_2.

There is a tendency to use supplemental oxygen routinely in the ICU (and the postanesthesia recovery unit) even when the SpO_2 exceeds 90%. Because there is no documented benefit to increasing the SaO_2 far above 90%, **supplemental O_2 can be safely withheld if the SpO_2 is**

92% or higher on room air. This practice will limit unnecessary oxygen administration (to limit the toxic effects of oxygen), and will preserve the sensitivity of pulse oximetry in detecting inadequate ventilation.

When to Use Pulse Oximetry

Considering that the SpO_2 has been called the *fifth vital sign*, it might be more appropriate to consider when *not* to use pulse oximetry. In short, pulse oximetry is indicated in any situation where monitoring arterial oxygenation is considered important. In critically ill patients, at least 15 clinical studies have shown that continuous monitoring of SpO_2 with pulse oximetry is superior to periodic blood gas measurements for detecting episodes of significant hypoxemia (4). The combination of pulse oximetry and end-tidal CO_2 monitoring (described next) should largely replace the more expensive and painful method of arterial blood gas measurements.

Venous Oximetry

The O_2 saturation in the superior vena cava or pulmonary artery can be monitored continuously with specialized catheters that emit red and infrared light from the catheter tip and record the light reflected back from the hemoglobin in circulating erythrocytes (see Figure 20.3) (17). This technique of *reflectance spectrophotometry* is a variant of the *transmission spectrophotometry* used by fingertip probes for pulse oximetry. Most venous oximetry systems process and display the venous O_2 saturation every 5 seconds.

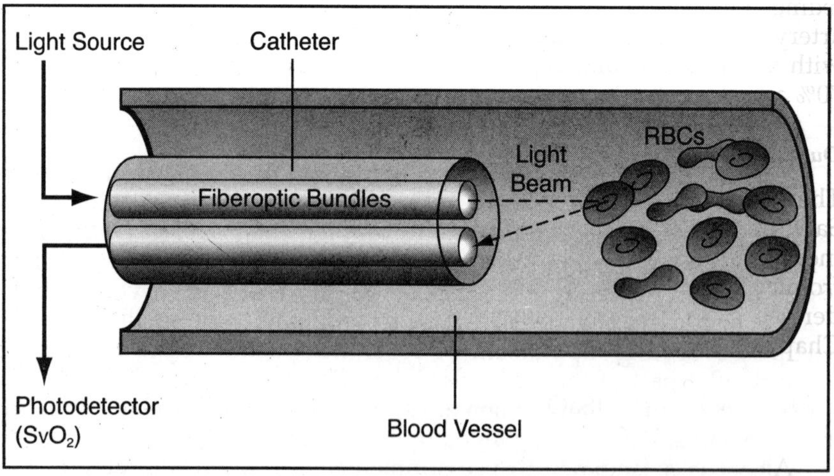

FIGURE 20.3 Continuous measurement of O_2 saturation of hemoglobin in mixed venous blood (SvO_2) using reflectance spectrophotometry.

Mixed Venous O_2 Saturation

The interpretation of mixed venous O_2 saturation (SvO_2) is described in Chapter 11. The SvO_2 is measured in pulmonary artery blood, and is a marker of the balance between whole-body O_2 delivery (DO_2) and O_2 consumption (VO_2): $SvO_2 = DO_2/VO_2$. A decrease in SvO_2 below the normal range of 70 to 75% identifies a state of inadequate O_2 delivery relative to O_2 consumption that could be the result of a decreased DO_2 (from low cardiac output, anemia, or hypoxemia) or an increased VO_2 (from hypermetabolism). (The determinants of DO_2 and VO_2 are described in Chapter 2.)

The continuous measurement of SvO_2 using specialized pulmonary artery catheters is accurate to within 1.5% of the SvO_2 measured in the clinical laboratory (18). Despite this acceptable accuracy, SvO_2 can vary considerably without an apparent change in hemodynamic status. The spontaneous variability of SvO_2 is shown in Table 20.1. The average variation over a 2-hour period is 6%, but can be as high as 19% (19). As a general rule, a greater than 5% variation in SvO_2 that persists for longer than 10 minutes is considered a significant change (20).

Central Venous O_2 Saturation

Continuous monitoring of the central venous O_2 saturation ($ScvO_2$) is achieved with specialized central venous catheters placed in the superior vena cava. The $ScvO_2$ tends to be slightly lower than the SvO_2, and this difference is magnified in the presence of circulatory shock (17). Single measurements of $ScvO_2$ can differ from SvO_2 by as much as 10%, but the difference is reduced (to within 5%) when multiple measurements are obtained (21). The $ScvO_2$ seems most valuable in identifying *trends* in the balance between DO_2 and VO_2.

Central venous oximetry is gaining popularity over mixed venous oximetry because of the cost and morbidity associated with pulmonary artery catheters. Recent guidelines for the early management of patients with severe sepsis and septic shock includes an $ScvO_2$ of greater than 70% as a therapeutic end-point (22).

Dual Oximetry

The predictive value of SvO_2 or $ScvO_2$ can be increased by adding the SaO_2 measured by pulse oximetry (SpO_2). This provides a continuous measure of ($SaO_2 - SvO_2$), which is equivalent to the O_2 extraction from capillary blood (23). The determinants of the ($SaO_2 - SvO_2$) can be derived using the determinants of DO_2 and VO_2 (which are described in Chapter 2):

$$(SaO_2 - SvO_2) = VO_2/Q \times Hb \qquad (20.2)$$

An increase in ($SaO_2 - SvO_2$) above the normal range of 20 to 30% can be the result of increased VO_2 (hypermetabolism), a reduced Q (low cardiac output) or a reduced Hb (anemia). The ($SaO_2 - SvO_2$) may be more valuable as a marker of tissue dysoxia (defined as a state of oxygen-limited metabolism) or impending dysoxia. For example, in the presence of anemia or a low cardiac output, an increase in (SaO_2 – SvO_2) to its maximum level of 50 to 60% indicates that the tissues are no longer able to compensate for further reductions on Hb or cardiac output, which means there is a risk for tissue anaerobiasis. Thus, in a patient with progressive anemia, an (SaO_2 – SvO_2) of 50 to 60% could be used as an indication for transfusion (transfusion trigger).

CAPNOMETRY

Capnometry is the measurement of CO_2 in exhaled gas. This can be achieved with a colorimetric technique, or with infrared spectrophotometry. Both methods are described below.

Colorimetric CO_2 Detection

The colorimetric detection of CO_2 in exhaled gas is a quick and simple method of determining if an endotracheal tube has been placed in the lungs (24,25). This is recommended as a standard practice following attempted intubation because **auscultation for breath sounds is an unreliable method of determining if an endotracheal tube is in the esophagus or lungs** (26).

The most popular colorimetric CO_2 detector in clinical practice is illustrated in Figure 20.4. This device has two ports for attachment: one to the endotracheal tube and the other end to an inflatable resuscitation bag. The central area of the device contains filter paper that is impregnated with a pH-sensitive indicator that changes color as a function of pH. When exhaled gas passes over the filter paper, the CO_2 in the gas is hydrated by a liquid film on the filter paper, and the resulting pH is detected by a color change. The outer perimeter of the chemical reaction area contains color-coded sections indicating the concentrations of exhaled CO_2 associated with each color change. A purple color indicates <0.5% CO_2 in exhaled gas, a tan color indicates 0.5 to <2.0% CO_2 in exhaled gas, and a yellow color indicates 2.0 to 5.0% CO_2 in exhaled gas. (The normal exhaled CO_2 is 5%, which is equivalent to a PCO_2 of 40 mm Hg.)

Predictive Value

The accuracy of this colorimetric device for predicting the success of endotracheal intubation is shown in Table 20.2 (24). For patients who are not in cardiac arrest, the absence of a color change from purple (exhaled CO_2 < 0.5% or exhaled PCO_2 <4 mm Hg) always means the tube is in the esophagus, and the presence of a color change from purple almost always means the tube is in the trachea. However in cardiac arrest victims, the absence of a color change from purple (indicating little or no CO_2 in exhaled gas) is not reliable for predicting if the tube is in the esophagus or trachea. This is explained by the fact that exhaled CO_2

TABLE 20.2 Performance of Colorimetric CO_2 Detector†

	Color on CO_2 Detector	
Patient Group	**Purple ($CO_2 < 0.5\%$)**	**Tan or Yellow ($CO_2 \geqslant 0.5\%$)**
No cardiac arrest (n = 83)	Tube in esophagus in 100% of cases.	Tube in trachea in 99% of cases.
Cardiac arrest (n = 144)	Tube in trachea in 77% of cases and tube in esophagus in 23% of cases.	Tube in trachea in 100% of cases.

† From Ornato JP, et al. Multicenter study of a portable, hand-size, colorimetric end-tidal CO_2 detection device. Ann Emerg Med 1992;21:518.

decreases when cardiac output is reduced, and thus a very low level of exhaled CO_2 in a cardiac arrest victim can be the result of a very low cardiac output rather than esophageal intubation. Therefore, **during cardiac arrest, the lack of a color change from purple on the colorimetric CO_2**

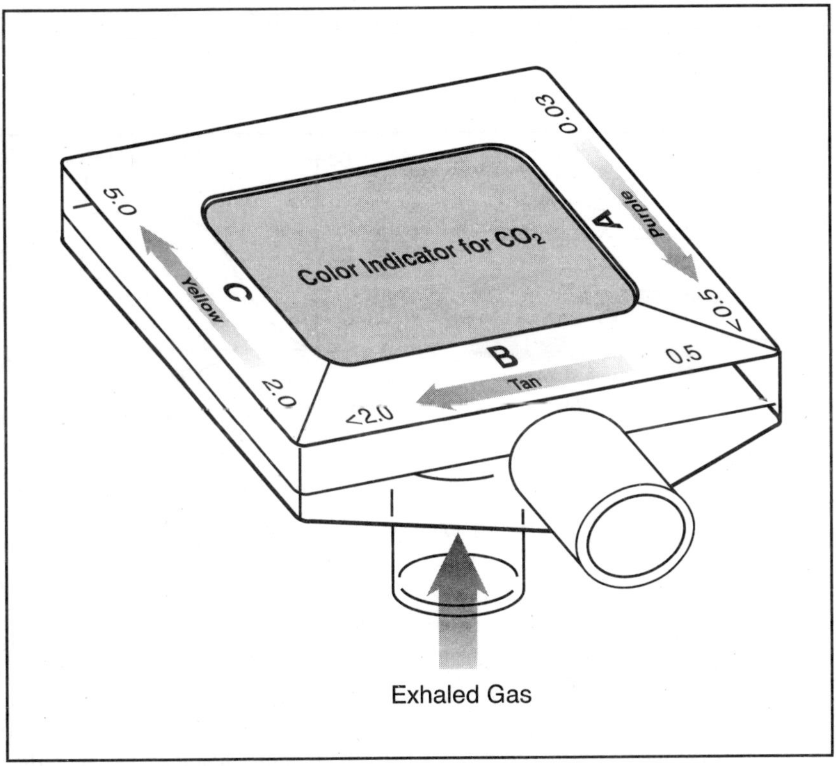

FIGURE 20.4 A disposable device (*Easy Cap II*, Nellcor, Pleasanton, CA) for the colorimetric detection of CO_2 in exhaled gas.

detector (indicating little or no CO_2 in exhaled gas) is not evidence of failure to intubate the lungs.

Feeding Tube Placement

The colorimetric CO_2 detector has been used to detect improper placement of feeding tubes. In one study (27), placement of feeding tubes in the upper airways was always associated with a color change from purple, while placement of feeding tubes in the upper GI tract was never associated with a color change from purple. (See reference 27 for a description of how to attach the CO_2 detector to the feeding tube.) If these results are corroborated, colorimetric CO_2 detection could replace chest films for evaluating the placement of feeding tubes.

Infrared Capnography

Carbon dioxide absorbs light in the infrared spectrum, and this property is the basis for the use of infrared capnography to measure the PCO_2 in exhaled gas (28). This provides a more quantitative measure of exhaled CO_2 than the colorimetric method. Figure 20.5 shows an infrared CO_2 probe that has an airway attachment (which is placed in series with the expiratory tubing during mechanical ventilation) and a fitted transducer. When in place, the probe emits a continuous infrared light beam that travels through the exhaled gas. The photodetector has a rapid response,

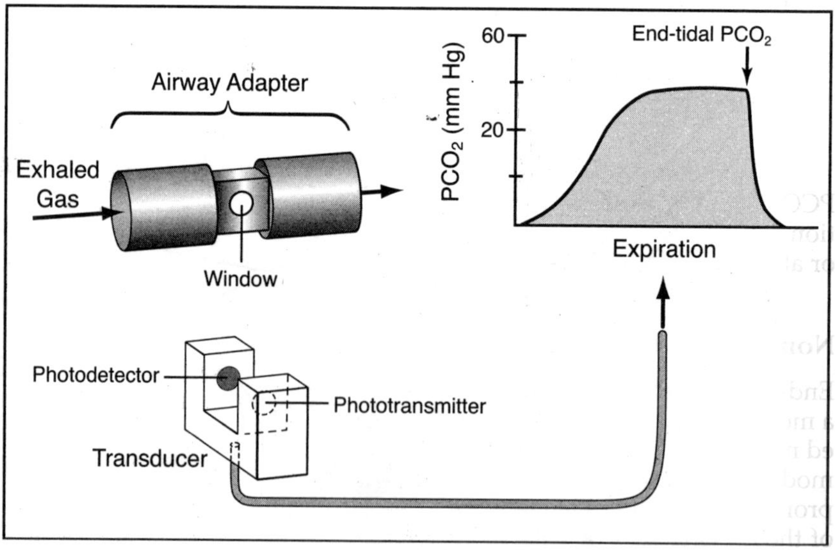

FIGURE 20.5 Infrared capnography. The airway adapter and fitted transducer on the left allow for a steady beam of infrared light to pass through exhaled gas. The photodetector records changes in PCO_2 during each exhalation, as shown in the capnogram on the right.

and can measure changes in PCO_2 during a single exhalation to produce a capnogram like the one shown in Figure 20.5.

Capnography

The shape of the normal capnogram has been described as "the outline of a snake that has swallowed an elephant" (29). The PCO_2 at the onset of expiration is negligible because the gas in the upper airways is first to leave the lungs. As exhalation proceeds, gas from the alveoli begins to contribute to the exhaled gas, and the PCO_2 begins to rise steadily. The rate of rise eventually declines, and the exhaled PCO_2 reaches a plateau near the end of expiration. When gas exchange is normal, the PCO_2 at the very end of expiration (called the *end-tidal PCO_2*) is equivalent to the PCO_2 in end-capillary (arterial) blood.

End-Tidal Versus Arterial PCO_2

When pulmonary gas exchange is normal, the end-tidal PCO_2 ($P_{ET}CO_2$) is only 2 to 3 mm Hg lower than the arterial PCO_2 (2,28). However, **when gas exchange in the lungs is impaired, $P_{ET}CO_2$ decreases relative to $PaCO_2$**, and the ($PaCO_2$ − $P_{ET}CO_2$) difference exceeds 3 mm Hg. This occurs in the following conditions:

- Increased anatomic dead space:
  - Open ventilator circuit
  - Shallow breathing
- Increased physiologic dead space:
  - Obstructive lung disease
- Low cardiac output:
  - Pulmonary embolism
  - Excessive lung inflation (e.g., PEEP)

Although uncommon, the end-tidal PCO_2 can be higher than arterial PCO_2 (30). This is possible in the following situations: when CO_2 production is high and there is a low inspired volume or a high cardiac output, or at high concentrations of inhaled O_2 (the O_2 displaces CO_2 from Hb).

Nonintubated Patients

End-tidal PCO_2 can be monitored in patients who are not intubated using a modified nasal cannula. These are commercially available (Salter divided nasal cannula, DRE Medical, Louisville, KY), or a nasal cannula can be modified as shown in Figure 20.6 (31). The tubing between the two nasal prongs must be occluded (either with a cotton ball inserted through one of the nasal prongs or with a small screw clamp). This allows one nasal prong to be used for oxygen inhalation while the other nasal prong is used to transmit exhaled gas. A 14-gauge intravascular catheter (2 inches long) is inserted into the exhalation side of the nasal cannula to transmit gas to the CO_2 detector. A sidestream CO_2 detector (i.e., one that applies

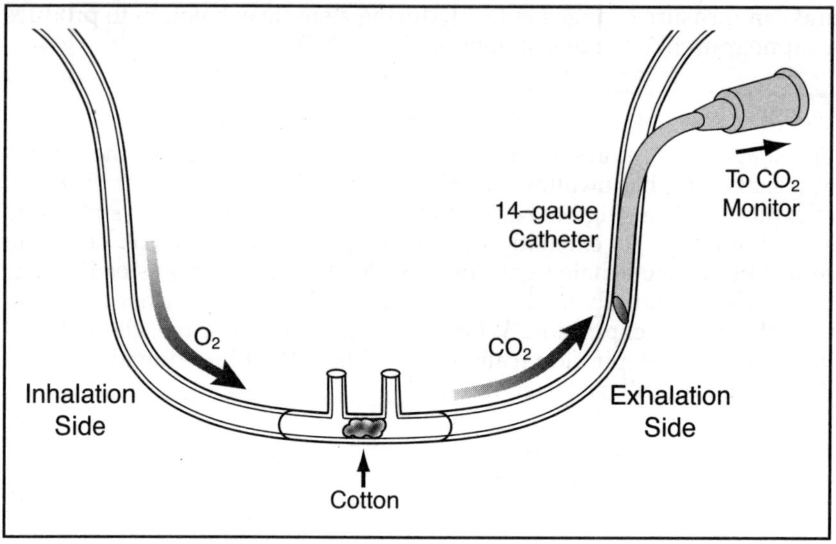

FIGURE 20.6 A modified nasal cannula to measure end-tidal PCO_2 during spontaneous breathing.

suction to draw gas from the tubing) is best suited for this application. If one of these is not available, a mainstream infrared CO_2 detector (such as the one shown in Fig. 20.5) can be used with a suction pump to draw gas samples from the cannula (at 150 mL/minute). The respiratory therapy department should help with this modification.

Clinical Applications

The end-tidal PCO_2 can be used in a number of ways in the ICU. The following are some possible applications.

Monitoring Arterial PCO_2

The end-tidal PCO_2 is most often used as a noninvasive method of monitoring the arterial PCO_2. The continuous (breath-by-breath) measurement of end-tidal PCO_2 provides a real advantage over the traditional method of measuring arterial blood gases periodically. When gas exchange in the lungs is abnormal and the $P_{ET}CO_2$ is lower than the arterial PCO_2, it is still possible to monitor *changes* in end-tidal PCO_2 as a measure of *changes* in arterial PCO_2. The arterial PCO_2 should be measured simultaneously with the end-tidal PCO_2 to establish the $PaCO_2$–$P_{ET}CO_2$ gradient. This gradient should remain the same as long as no other process intervenes to disturb pulmonary gas exchange. Changing ventilator settings will affect the $PaCO_2$–$P_{ET}CO_2$ gradient (32), so the arterial PCO_2 should be measured after each change in ventilator settings to establish the new $PaCO_2$–$P_{ET}CO_2$ gradient.

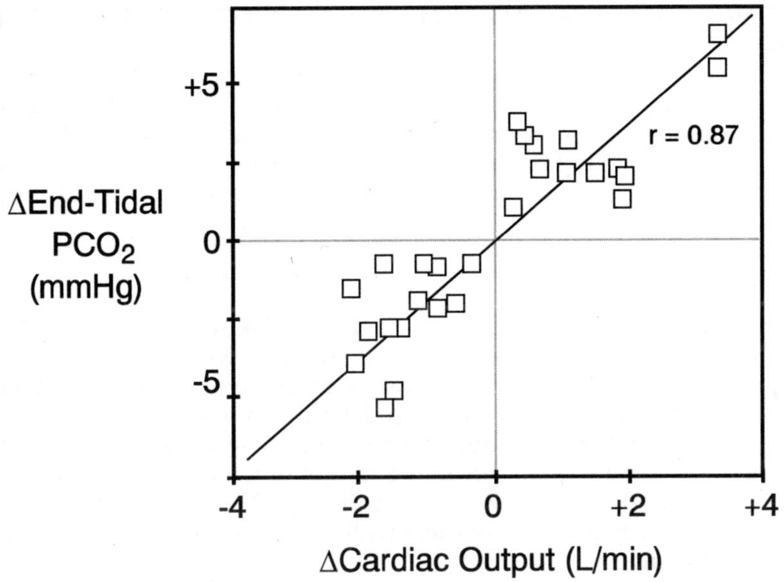

FIGURE 20.7 Relationship between changes in end-tidal PCO_2 and changes in cardiac output in a group of postoperative patients. Correlation coefficient indicated as *r*. (From Reference 33.)

Cardiac Output

There is a close correlation between changes in $P_{ET}CO_2$ and changes in cardiac output, as demonstrated in Figure 20.7 (33). This is the basis for the use of end-tidal PCO_2 to evaluate the effectiveness of chest compressions during CPR, as described in Chapter 15 (see Fig. 15.5). This relationship can also be used to detect changes in cardiac output resulting from aggressive diuresis or short-term volume loading.

Early Detection of Nosocomial Disorders

A decrease in $P_{ET}CO_2$ accompanied by an increase in the $PaCO_2-P_{ET}CO_2$ gradient can be an early manifestation of any of the following conditions:

Overdistention of alveoli from high tidal volumes or PEEP
Migration of an endotracheal tube into a main-stem bronchus (34)
Acute pulmonary embolism (35)
Pneumonia
Pulmonary edema

An increase in the $PaCO_2-P_{ET}CO_2$ gradient can thus serve as an early warning signal for any of these conditions. The use of the $PaCO_2-P_{ET}CO_2$ gradient to detect overdistention of alveoli may be particularly useful in light of the discovery that high tidal volumes, which are common during mechanical ventilation, can be damaging to the lungs (see Chapters 22 and 24 for information on ventilator-induced lung injury).

The end-tidal PCO_2 has become a popular measurement in the evaluation of suspected pulmonary embolism. A normal $PaCO_2-P_{ET}CO_2$ gradient, combined with a normal D-dimer assay, can be used to exclude the diagnosis of acute pulmonary embolism (35). The value of this approach in the ICU (where patients often have an elevated $PaCO_2-P_{ET}CO_2$ gradient) is unclear.

Ventilator Weaning

During weaning from mechanical ventilation, end-tidal CO_2 monitoring can serve several purposes (36). In uneventful weaning (e.g., following surgery), it serves as a noninvasive measure of $PaCO_2$. In difficult or complicated weaning, it can help determine the success or failure of the wean attempt. For example, a progressive rise in $P_{ET}CO_2$ can signal an increase in the work of breathing (a sign of wean failure), whereas a decline in $P_{ET}CO_2$ with a increase in the $PaCO_2-P_{ET}CO_2$ gradient can signal respiratory muscle weakness with shallow breathing (another sign of wean failure).

Controlled Hyperventilation

When induced hyperventilation is used to reduce intracranial pressure (e.g., in patients with closed head injuries), monitoring the end-tidal CO_2 is useful for maintaining the $PaCO_2$ at the desired level (which is usually 25 mm Hg). In this setting, the $PaCO_2-P_{ET}CO_2$ gradient must be checked periodically to maintain the $P_{ET}CO_2$ at a level that corresponds to the target $PaCO_2$.

TRANSCUTANEOUS PCO_2

The latest in noninvasive CO_2 monitoring is a cutaneous CO_2 electrode (TOSCA, Linde Medical Sensors, Basel, Switzerland) that is placed on the earlobe and measures the PCO_2 in the underlying arterioles. The electrode (which is combined with a pulse oximeter sensor) heats the underlying skin to 42°C to dilate surface arterioles and promote the diffusion of CO_2. One study of this device in ICU patients showed a good correlation between transcutaneous PCO_2 and arterial PCO_2 over a wide range of arterial PCO_2 values (from 25 to 100 mm Hg) (37). If proven reliable, the transcutaneous PCO_2 should be more accurate than the end-tidal PCO_2 for monitoring arterial PCO_2 in patients with abnormal pulmonary gas exchange (where end-tidal PCO_2 is lower than arterial PCO_2).

A FINAL WORD

Pulse oximetry is the single most useful monitoring technique that has been introduced in my 25 years of service to critical care medicine. Besides being safe, inexpensive, easy to use, and remarkably reliable, the

SpO_2 measurement is valuable because it provides information about the state of arterial oxygenation (which the PaO_2 does not). In fact, if the SpO_2 is combined with a measurement of the hemoglobin concentration in blood, it is possible to calculate the concentration of oxygen in arterial blood (see Chapter 2, Equation 2.5), which is the parameter that *should* be used (instead of the PaO_2 or SaO_2) to evaluate the state of arterial oxygenation.

REFERENCES

General Reviews

1. Jubran A, Tobin MJ. Monitoring during mechanical ventilation. Clin Chest Med 1996;17:453–473.
2. Soubani AO. Noninvasive monitoring of oxygen and carbon dioxide. Am J Emerg Med 2001;19:141–146.

Pulse Oximetry

3. Stoneham MD, Saville GM, Wilson IH. Knowledge about pulse oximetry among medical and nursing staff. Lancet 1994;344:1339–1342.
4. Wahr JA, Tremper KK. Noninvasive oxygen monitoring techniques. Crit Care Clin 1995;11:199–217.
5. Severinghaus JW, Kelleher JF. Recent developments in pulse oximetry. Anesthesiology 1992;76:1018–1038.
6. Hess D, Agarwal NN. Variability of blood gases, pulse oximeter saturation, and end-tidal carbon dioxide pressure in stable, mechanically ventilated trauma patients. J Clin Monit 1992;8:111–115.
7. Bozeman WP, Myers RAM, Barish RA. Confirmation of the pulse oximetry gap in carbon monoxide poisoning. Ann Emerg Med 1997;30:608–611.
8. Barker SJ, Kemper KK, Hyatt J. Effects of methemoglobinemia on pulse oximetry and mixed venous oximetry. Anesthesiology 1989;70:112–117.
9. Severinghaus JW, Spellman MJ. Pulse oximeter failure thresholds in hypotension and vasoconstriction. Anesthesiology 1990;73:532–537.
10. Morris RW, Nairn M, Beaudoin M. Does the radial arterial line degrade the performance of a pulse oximeter? Anesth Intensive Care 1990;18:107–109.
11. Bebout DE, Mannheimer PD, Wun CC. Site-dependent differences in the time to detect changes in saturation during low perfusion. Crit Care Med 2001;29:A115.
12. Jay GD, Hughes L, Renzi FP. Pulse oximetry is accurate in acute anemia from hemorrhage. Ann Emerg Med 1994;24:32–35.
13. Ries AL, Prewitt LM, Johnson JJ. Skin color and ear oximetry. Chest 1989;96: 287–290.
14. Bickler PE, Feiner JR, Severinghaus JW. Effects of skin pigmentation on pulse oximeter accuracy at low saturations. Anesthesiology 2005;102:715–719.
15. Chan ED. What is the effect of fingernail polish on pulse oximetry? Chest 2003;123:2163–2164.
16. Fu ES, Downs JB, Schweiger JW, et al. Supplemental oxygen impairs detection of hypoventilation by pulse oximetry. Chest 2004;126:1552–1558.

Venous Oximetry

17. Rivers EP, Ander DS, Powell D. Central venous oxygen saturation monitoring in the critically ill patient. Curr Opin Crit Care 2001;7:204–211.
18. Armaganidis A, Dhinaut JF, Billard JL, et al. Accuracy assessment for three fiberoptic pulmonary artery catheters for SvO_2 monitoring. Intensive Care Med 1994;20:484–488.
19. Noll ML, Fountain RL, Duncan CA, et al. Fluctuation in mixed venous oxygen saturation in critically ill medical patients: a pilot study. Am J Crit Care 1992;3:102–106.
20. Krafft P, Steltzer H, Heismay M, et al. Mixed venous oxygen saturation in critically ill septic shock patients. Chest 1993;103:900–906.
21. Dueck MH, Kilmek M, Appenrodt S, et al. Trends but not individual values of central venous oxygen saturation agree with mixed venous oxygen saturation during varying hemodynamic conditions. Anesthesiology 2005;103: 249–257.
22. Dellinger RP, Carlet JM, Masur H, et al. Surviving Sepsis Campaign guidelines for management of severe sepsis and septic shock. Crit Care Med 2004;32:858–873.
23. Bongard FS, Leighton TA. Continuous dual oximetry in surgical critical care. Ann Surg 1992;216:60–68.

Colorimetric CO_2 Detection

24. Ornato JP, Shipley JB, Racht EM, et al. Multicenter study of a portable, hand-size, colorimetric end-tidal carbon dioxide detection device. Ann Emerg Med 1992;21:518–523.
25. Deem S, Bishop MJ. Evaluation and management of the difficult airway. Crit Care Clin 1995;11:1–27.
26. Mizutani AR, Ozake G, Benumoff JL, et al. Auscultation cannot distinguish esophageal from tracheal passage of tube. J Clin Monit 1991;7:232–236.
27. Preza-Araujo CE, Melhado ME, Guitierrez FJ, et al. Use of capnometry to verify feeding tube placement. Crit Care Med 2002;30:2255–2259.

Infrared Capnography

28. Stock MC. Capnography for adults. Crit Care Clin 1995;11:219–232.
29. Gravenstein JS, Paulus DA, Hayes TJ. Capnography in clinical practice. Boston: Butterworth-Heinemann, 1989:11.
30. Moorthy SS, Losasso AM, Wilcox J. End-tidal PCO_2 greater than $PaCO_2$. Crit Care Med 1984;12:534–535.
31. Roy J, McNulty SE, Torjman MC. An improved nasal prong apparatus for end-tidal carbon dioxide monitoring in awake, sedated patients. J Clin Monit 1991;7:249–252.
32. Hoffman RA, Kreiger PB, Kramer MR, et al. End-tidal carbon dioxide in critically ill patients during changes in mechanical ventilation. Am Rev Respir Dis 1989;140:1265–1268.
33. Shibutani K, Shirasaki S, Braatz T, et al. Changes in cardiac output affect $PETCO_2$, CO_2 transport, and O_2 uptake during unsteady state in humans. J Clin Monit 1992;8:175–176.

34. Gandhi SK, Munshi CA, Bardeen-Henschel A. Capnography for detection of endobronchial migration of an endotracheal tube. J Clin Monit 1991;7: 35–38.
35. Rodger MA, Gwynne J, Rasuli P. Steady-state end-tidal alveolar dead space fraction and D-dimer: Bedside tests to exclude pulmonary embolism. Chest 2001;120:115–119.
36. Healey CJ, Fedullo AJ, Swinburne AJ, et al. Comparison of noninvasive measurements of carbon dioxide tension during weaning from mechanical ventilation. Crit Care Med 1987;15:764–767.

Transcutaneous PCO_2

37. Bendjelid K, Schutz N, Stotz M, et al. Transcutaneous PCO_2 monitoring in critically ill adults: clinical evaluation of a new sensor. Crit Care Med 2005; 33:2203–2206.

Chapter 21

OXYGEN INHALATION THERAPY

For as a candle burns out much faster in dephlogisticated than in common air, so we might, as may be said, live out too fast . . . in this pure kind of air.

Joseph Priestley

One of the rare sights in any ICU is a patient who is *not* receiving supplemental oxygen to breathe. The overzealous use of oxygen is often without justification (without evidence of impaired tissue oxygenation) and is even more often without consideration of the toxic effects of oxygen. This chapter begins by highlighting the shortcomings in the indications and end-points of supplemental oxygen administration. This is followed by a brief description of the methods used to provide supplemental oxygen. The final section of the chapter focuses on the dark side of oxygen; i.e., the tendency for oxygen to produce widespread and lethal cell injury.

THE NEED FOR SUPPLEMENTAL OXYGEN

Oxygen inhalation should be used to prevent or correct tissue hypoxia, but in most cases it seems to be a knee-jerk response to the mere presence of a serious illness. This is supported by a survey showing that over 50% of hospitalized patients were receiving supplemental oxygen without a written order (1). This section will briefly examine the need for supplemental oxygen.

Tissues are Normally Hypoxic

The care of critically ill patients is dominated by the fear of tissue hypoxia. However, the tissues of the human body normally operate in a low-oxygen environment. As described in Chapter 2, oxygen does not dissolve readily in water, which is why we need hemoglobin to transport

TABLE 21.1 Total Volume of Oxygen in Tissues

	Interstitial Fluid	Intracellular Fluid
PO_2	15 mm Hg	5 mm Hg
O_2 Content‡	0.45 mL/L	0.15 mL/L
Total Volume†	16 L	23 L
Volume of O_2	9.6 mL	3.5 mL

‡Based on solubility coefficient for O_2 in water at 37°C = 0.03 mL/L/mm Hg.
†Volume estimates based on total body water (TBW) = 42 liters, intracellular volume = 55% of TBW, and interstitial volume = 0.38% of TBW.

oxygen to the tissues. The concentration of (dissolved) oxygen in tissues is determined by the PO_2 in the tissues and the solubility coefficient of oxygen in water. This is shown in the equation below (which is similar to Equation 2.2 in Chapter 2).

$$\text{Dissolved } O_2 \text{ (mL/dL)} = 0.003 \times PO_2 \qquad 21.1$$

where 0.003 is the solubility coefficient of O_2 in water (expressed as mL O_2 per 100 mL blood per mm Hg PO_2) at a body temperature of 37°C. Experimental observations show that the intracellular PO_2 is about 5 mm Hg (1) and the tissue (interstitial) PO_2 is about 15 mm Hg (2). This corresponds to an O_2 concentration of 0.15 mL/L inside cells and 0.45 mL/L in the interstitial fluid. Using the estimated volume of the body fluid compartments shown in Table 21.1, the total volume of oxygen in the tissues of the human body is only about 13 mL. This demonstrates that the tissues of the human body normally operate in an oxygen deficient environment.

Tolerance to Arterial Hypoxemia

The standard indications for supplemental oxygen are an arterial PO_2 (PaO_2) less than 60 mm Hg or an arterial O_2 saturation (SaO_2) less than 90% (4). However, clinical observations show that severe degrees of hypoxemia are tolerated without evidence of inadequate tissue oxygenation (5–7). This is demonstrated in Table 21.2, which shows the arterial PO_2 and corresponding blood lactate level in seven patients with severe hypoxemia ($PaO_2 < 40$ mm Hg) due to acute exacerbation of chronic obstructive lung disease (5). The normal blood lactate levels (<4 mmol/L) show no evidence of a switch to anaerobic metabolism in any of the patients with severe hypoxemia, even at arterial PO_2 levels as low as 22 mm Hg. This observation has been corroborated in patients with acute respiratory distress syndrome (6).

The available evidence is stated best in the study shown in Table 21.2: *In the resting patient, even the most severe clinical hypoxemia due to pulmonary insufficiency does not itself lead to generalized tissue anaerobiasis* (5).

TABLE 21.2 Severe Hypoxemia without Evidence of Anaerobic Metabolism

Patient	Arterial PO_2 (mm Hg)	Blood Lactate (mmol/L)
1	22	0.90
2	30	0.25
3	32	0.86
4	33	1.57
5	34	2.03
6	37	2.08
7	39	1.12

Data from Reference 5.

Remember this statement when considering the use of supplemental oxygen based on measures of arterial oxygenation.

THE END-POINT OF OXYGEN INHALATION

The standard end-point of supplemental oxygen inhalation is a satisfactory increase in the PaO_2 or SaO_2 (what is satisfactory seems to differ with individual physicians). The problem with this approach is demonstrated in Figure 21.1. The graphs in this figure show the discrepancy between changes in arterial PO_2 and changes in systemic oxygen transport during supplemental oxygen administration (8). Note that arterial PO_2 increases from 61 to 83 mm Hg (36% change, $P < 0.01$) while the rate of oxygen transport decreases from 12.8 to 12.1 mL/minute/kg (5% change, not significant). Thus, **an increase in arterial PO_2 during oxygen inhalation should not be used as evidence for an increase in tissue oxygen availability (8,9).** This is consistent with the observation that oxygen inhalation does not protect against myocardial ischemia (10).

Oxygen and Systemic Blood Flow

The lack of improvement in systemic oxygen transport during oxygen inhalation is explained by the **tendency for oxygen to reduce systemic blood flow.** There are two mechanisms for this effect. First, oxygen acts as a vasoconstrictor in all vascular beds except the pulmonary circulation (where it acts as a vasodilator) (11,12). Second, oxygen inhalation is often associated with a decrease in cardiac output (8,9,13). Although this is caused partly by reversal of the cardiac stimulatory effects of hypoxemia, oxygen also has negative inotropic effects on the heart, and oxygen inhalation can reduce cardiac output in the absence of hypoxemia (13). The ability of oxygen to reduce systemic blood flow emphasizes the need to adopt measures other than the PaO_2 and SaO_2 to evaluate the success of oxygen inhalation.

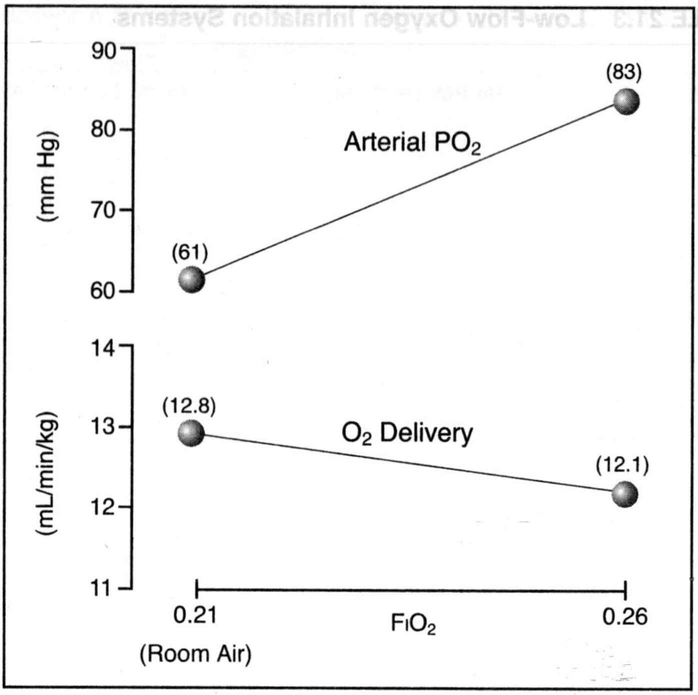

FIGURE 21.1 Effects of oxygen inhalation (F_IO_2 = 0.26) on arterial oxygenation and systemic oxygen transport. Points on the graph represent mean values for the group of patients studied. (Data from DeGaute JP et al. Oxygen delivery in acute exacerbation of chronic obstructive pulmonary disease. Effects of controlled oxygen therapy. Am Rev Respir Dis 1981;124:26.)

METHODS OF OXYGEN INHALATION

Oxygen delivery systems are classified as low-flow or high-flow systems (14). Low-flow delivery systems, which include nasal prongs, face masks, and masks with reservoir bags, provide a reservoir of oxygen for the patient to inhale. When the patient's minute ventilation exceeds the flow rates of these devices, the oxygen reservoir is drained, and room air is inhaled to meet the patient's additional needs. The final concentration of inhaled oxygen (F_IO_2) is determined by the size of the oxygen reservoir, the rate at which the reservoir is filled, and the ventilatory demands of the patient. In contrast to the variable F_IO_2 with low-flow systems, high-flow oxygen delivery systems provide a constant F_IO_2. This is achieved by delivering oxygen at flow rates that exceed the patient's peak inspiratory flow rate, or by using devices that entrain a fixed proportion of room air.

Nasal Prongs

Nasal prongs deliver a constant flow of oxygen to the nasopharynx and oropharynx, which acts as an oxygen reservoir (average capacity = 50 mL,

TABLE 21.3 Low-Flow Oxygen Inhalation Systems

Device	Reservoir Capacity	Oxygen Flow (L/min)	Approximate (FIO_2)*
Nasal cannula	50 mL	1	0.21–0.24
		2	0.24–0.28
		3	0.28–0.34
		4	0.34–0.38
		5	0.38–0.42
		6	0.42–0.46
Oxygen face mask	150–250 mL	5–10	0.40–0.60
Mask–reservoir bag:	750–1250 mL		
Partial rebreather		5–7	0.35–0.75
Nonrebreather		5–10	0.40–1.0

*Estimated value based on a tidal volume of 500 mL, a respiratory rate of 20 breaths/min, and an inspiratory: expiratory time ratio of 1:2.
From Reference 14.

or about one-third of the anatomic dead space) (15). The relationship between the oxygen flow rate and the FIO_2 in normal subjects is shown in Table 21.3 (15). As the oxygen flow rate increases from 1 to 6 L/min, the FIO_2 increases from 0.24 to 0.46. This relationship varies with changes in the patients' minute ventilation: when minute ventilation increases and exceeds the flow rate of O_2, the excess ventilation is drawn from room air, and the FIO_2 begins to decline. This is demonstrated below, which shows the relationship between minute ventilation (V_E) and the FIO_2 at a constant flow rate through the nasal cannula (16).

O_2 Flow	V_E	FIO_2
6 L/min	5 L/min	0.60
6 L/min	10 L/min	0.44
6 L/min	20 L/min	0.32

In this case, a fourfold increase in minute ventilation above the O_2 flow rate provided by the nasal cannula resulted in a 48% reduction in FIO_2. This demonstrates the limitations of O_2 delivery through nasal prongs in patients who have high ventilatory demands.

Advantages and Disadvantages

Nasal prongs are easy to use and well tolerated by most patients. The major disadvantage of nasal prongs is the inability to achieve high concentrations of inhaled O_2 in patients who have a high minute ventilation.

Low-Flow Oxygen Masks

Face masks add 100 to 200 mL to the capacity of the oxygen reservoir. These devices fit loosely on the face, which allows room air to be inhaled, if needed. Standard face masks deliver oxygen at flow rates between 5 and 10 L/min. The minimum flow rate of 5 L/min is needed to clear exhaled gas from the mask. Low-flow oxygen masks can achieve a maximum FIO_2 of approximately 0.60.

Advantages and Disadvantages

Standard face masks can provide a slightly higher maximum FIO_2 than nasal prongs. However, this difference can be small and insignificant. In general, face masks are considered to have the same drawbacks as nasal prongs.

Masks with Reservoir Bags

The addition of a reservoir bag to a standard face mask increases the capacity of the oxygen reservoir by 600 to 1000 mL (depending on the size of the bag). If the reservoir bag is kept inflated, the patient will inhale only the gas contained in the bag. There are two types of mask–reservoir bag devices. The one shown in Figure 21.2 is a partial rebreathing system. This device allows the gas exhaled in the initial phase of expiration to return to the reservoir bag. As exhalation proceeds, the expiratory flow rate declines, and when the expiratory flow rate falls below the oxygen flow rate, exhaled gas can no longer return to the reservoir bag. The initial part of expiration contains gas from the upper airways (anatomic dead space), so the gas that is rebreathed is rich in oxygen and largely devoid of CO_2. Partial rebreather devices can achieve a maximum FIO_2 of 70 to 80%.

The modified device in Figure 21.3 is a nonrebreathing system. This device has a one-way valve that prevents any exhaled gas from returning to the reservoir bag. Nonrebreather devices permit inhalation of pure oxygen (FIO_2 = 1.0).

Advantages and Disadvantages

The principal advantage of the reservoir bags is the greater ability to control the composition of inhaled gas. However, because the masks must create a tight seal on the face, it is not possible to feed patients by mouth or nasoenteral tube when these devices are in use. Aerosolized bronchodilator therapy is also not possible with reservoir bag devices.

High-Flow Oxygen Masks

High-flow oxygen inhalation devices provide complete control of the inhaled gas mixture and deliver a constant FIO_2 regardless of changes in ventilatory pattern. The operation of a high-flow oxygen mask is shown in Figure 21.4 (17). Oxygen is delivered to the mask at low flow rates, but at the inlet of the mask, the oxygen is passed through a narrowed

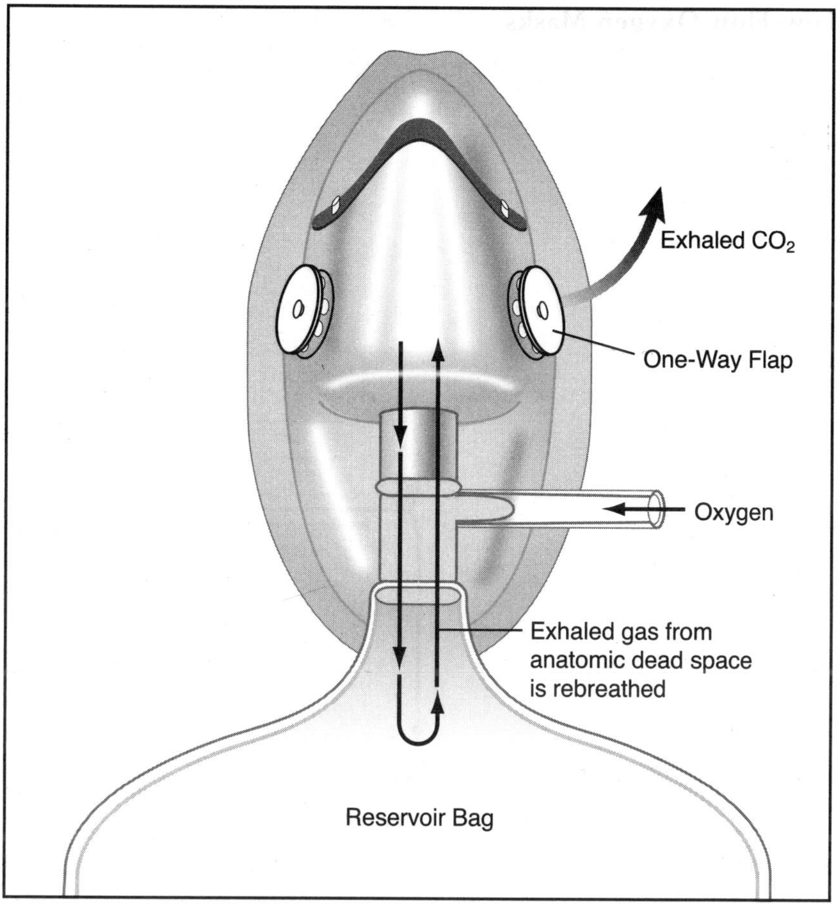

FIGURE 21.2 Partial rebreathing system. The initial 100 to 150 mL of exhaled gas (anatomic dead space) is returned to the reservoir bag for rebreathing.

orifice, and this creates a high-velocity stream of gas (analogous to the effect created by a nozzle on a garden hose). This high-velocity jet stream generates a shearing force known as viscous drag that pulls room air into the mask. The volume of room air that moves into the mask (which determines the FIO_2) can be varied by varying the size of the openings (called entrainment ports) on the mask. These masks can increase the FIO_2 to a maximum of 0.50. At any given FIO_2, the proportion of inhaled gas provided by entrained room air remains constant; that is, FIO_2 remains fixed regardless of changes in oxygen flow rate or changes in inspiratory flow rate.

Advantages and Disadvantages

The major advantage of high-flow oxygen masks is the ability to deliver a constant FIO_2. This feature is desirable in patients with chronic

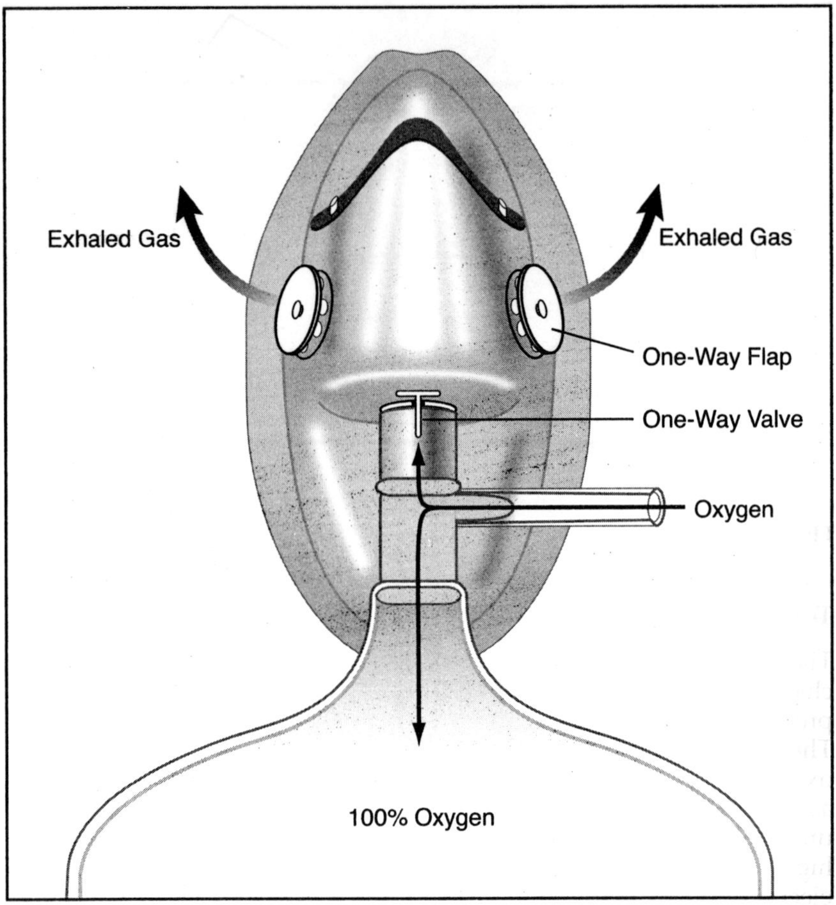

FIGURE 21.3 Nonrebreathing system. A one-way valve prevents exhaled gas from returning to the reservoir bag.

hypercapnia because an inadvertent increase in FIO_2 in these patients can lead to further CO_2 retention. The major drawback with these masks is the inability to deliver high concentrations of inhaled O_2.

THE DARK SIDE OF OXYGEN

The overzealous and unregulated use of supplemental oxygen must be tempered by the potential for oxygen to act as a powerful and even lethal toxin (18). In fact, contrary to the notion that oxygen protects cells from injury, the accumulated evidence suggests that oxygen (via the production of toxic metabolites) is *responsible* for much of the cell injury in critically ill patients. The following is a brief description of the dark (toxic) side of oxygen.

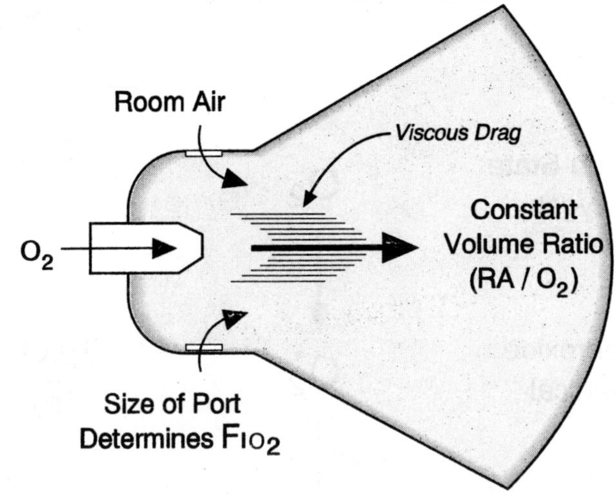

FIGURE 21.4 High-flow oxygen inhalation device. *RA* = room air.

Toxic Metabolites of Oxygen

The metabolism of oxygen takes place at the end of the electron transport chain in mitochondria, where electrons that accumulate as a result of ATP production are removed by using the electrons to reduce oxygen to water. The reaction sequence for this process is shown in Figure 21.5. Molecular oxygen has two unpaired electrons in its outer orbitals, which qualifies it as a *free radical.* (A free radical is an atom or molecule with one or more unpaired electrons in its outer orbitals.) Although most free radicals are highly-reactive, oxygen is only sluggishly reactive because the unpaired electrons in its outer orbitals have the same directional spin.

According to Pauli's Exclusion Principle (proposed by the Austrian physicist Wolfgang Pauli), no two electrons can occupy the same orbital if they have the same directional spin. This means it is not possible to add an electron pair to oxygen and reduce it to water in a one-step reaction because one orbital would have two electrons with the same directional spin, which is a quantum impossibility. This *spin restriction* limits oxygen metabolism to a series of single-electron reduction reactions, and this process produces a series of highly reactive intermediates.

The intermediates in oxygen metabolism, which are shown in Figure 21.5, include the superoxide radical, hydrogen peroxide, and the hydroxyl radical. All are powerful *oxidants* capable of damaging cell membranes, denaturing proteins, and breaking DNA into strands. The hydroxyl radical is the most reactive molecule known to biochemistry, and usually enters a reaction within three molecular diameters of its point of origin (18).

Granulocyte Activation

The activation of granulocytes (as part of the inflammatory response) involves a marked (up to 20-fold) increase in oxygen consumption (19).

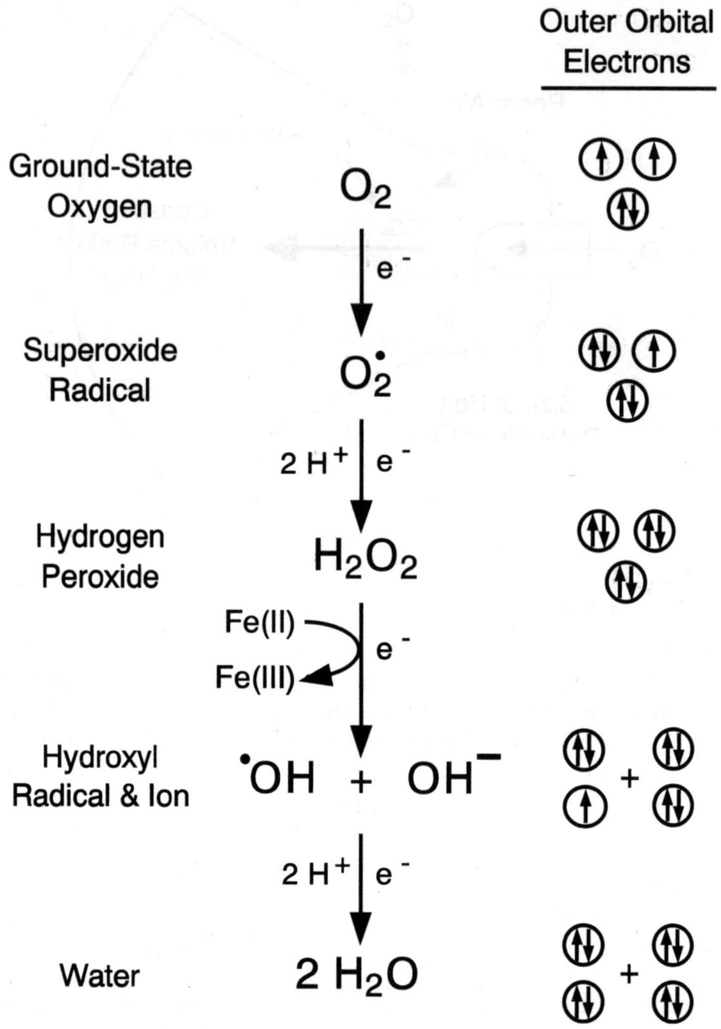

FIGURE 21.5 The metabolism of molecular oxygen to water, which occurs as a series of four single-electron reduction reactions. Orbital diagrams on the right side of the figure show the electron configuration *(arrows)* in the outer orbitals of each reactant.

This is known as the *respiratory burst,* and its purpose is to produce toxic oxygen metabolites, which are stored in cytoplasmic granules. These metabolites are released as part of the inflammatory response, and they can damage and destroy invading microorganisms. They can also damage and destroy the tissues of the host if adequate *antioxidant* protection is not available (see next). **Toxic oxygen metabolites have been implicated in the inflammatory-mediated cell injury that occurs in the acute respiratory distress syndrome (ARDS) and the systemic inflammatory response syndrome** (see Chapter 40) (20,21).

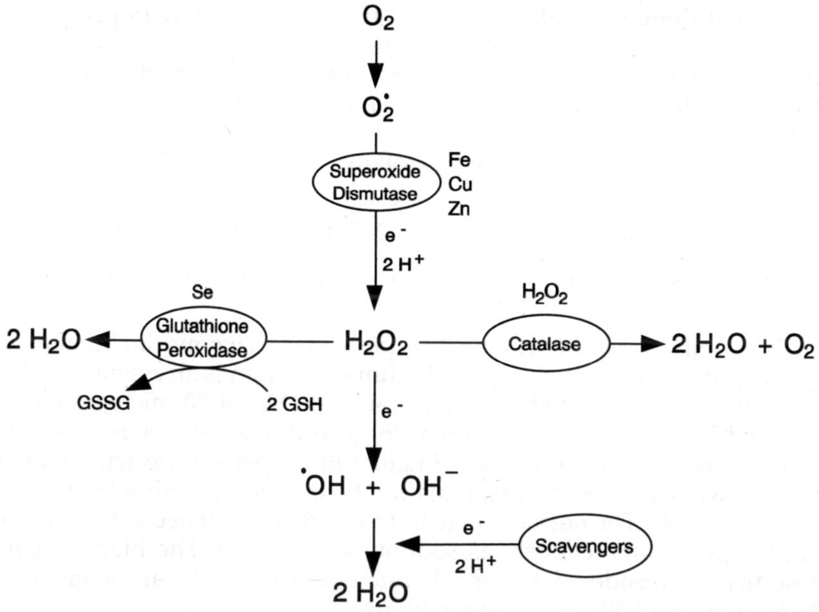

FIGURE 21.6 Actions of antioxidant enzymes and free radical scavengers. Cofactors for superoxide dismutase can be iron (*Fe*), zinc (*Zn*) or copper (*Cu*). The cofactor for glutathione peroxidase is selenium (*Se*). *GSH* = reduced glutathione, *GSSG* = oxidized glutathione, which is a dipeptide connected by a disulfide bridge.

Antioxidant Protection

Oxidative (oxygen-related) injury is kept in check by a vast array of endogenous antioxidants (22). (An antioxidant is a substance that delays or reduces the oxidation of a suitable substrate.) Some of the more important ones are described next.

Enzyme Antioxidants

Normally, about 98% of the oxygen in mitochondria is reduced completely to water, and less than 2% of the toxic metabolites escape into the cytoplasm (23). This is a tribute to the actions of some enzymes that are highlighted in Figure 21.6.

Superoxide dismutase promotes the conversion of the superoxide radical to hydrogen peroxide. Although considered an antioxidant, superoxide dismutase promotes the production of another toxic oxygen metabolite (hydrogen peroxide) and, if clearance mechanisms for hydrogen peroxide are defective, superoxide dismutase can act as a prooxidant (24).

Catalase is an iron-containing heme protein that reduces hydrogen peroxide to water. It is present in most cells, and the lowest concentrations are in cardiac cells and neurons. Inhibition of the catalase enzyme does not enhance the toxicity of hydrogen peroxide for endothelial cells (25), so this enzyme may have a limited role in preventing oxidative cell injury.

Glutathione peroxidase enhances the reduction of hydrogen peroxide to water by first removing electrons from glutathione in its reduced form and then donating the electrons to hydrogen peroxide. The oxidized glutathione (GSSG) is then returned to its reduced state (GSH) by a reductase enzyme that transfers the reducing equivalents from NADPH. The total reaction can be written as follows:

$$\text{Peroxidase reaction: } H_2O_2 + 2\,GSH \rightarrow 2\,H_2O + GSSG$$

$$\text{Reductase reaction: } NADPH + H^+ + GSSG \rightarrow 2\,GSH + NADP$$

The activity of the glutathione peroxidase enzyme in humans is dependent on the trace element **selenium**. Selenium is an essential nutrient with a recommended daily allowance (RDA) of 70 micrograms for men and 55 micrograms for women (26). The absence of dietary selenium produces measurable differences in glutathione peroxidase activity after just one week (27). Selenium status can be monitored with whole blood selenium levels. The normal range is 0.5 to 2.5 mg/L. If needed, selenium can be given intravenously as sodium selenite (28). The highest daily dose that is considered safe is 200 micrograms, which can be given in divided doses of 50 μg IV every 6 hours.

Glutathione is a sulfur-containing tripeptide that is one of the major antioxidants in the human body, and is present in *molar* concentrations (0.5-10 mM/L) in most cells (29,30). It is found in all organs, but is particularly prevalent in the lung, liver, endothelium and intestinal mucosa. It is synthesized de novo within cells, and it remains sequestered in cells. Plasma levels of glutathione are three orders of magnitude lower than intracellular levels, and exogenous glutathione administration has little effect on intracellular levels (31). The popular mucolytic agent **N-acetylcysteine** is a glutathione analogue capable of crossing cell membranes and enhancing intracellular glutathione activity. This is the mechanism for the beneficial effects of N-acetylcysteine in acetaminophen toxicity (see Chapter 53).

Other Antioxidants

Vitamin E (alpha-tocopherol) is a lipid-soluble vitamin that is found within most cell membranes and helps to block oxidative injury to cell membranes. It is considered the major lipid-soluble antioxidant in the human body. The normal concentration of vitamin E in plasma is 1 mg/dL, and a level below 0.5 mg/dL is evidence of deficiency (32). Vitamin E deficiency may be common in critically ill patients (33), so it seems wise to check the vitamin E status in patients who are at risk for oxygen-related injury (see later).

Vitamin C (ascorbic acid) is a water-soluble antioxidant that operates primarily in the extracellular space. Vitamin C is found in abundance in the lung, where it may play a protective role in inactivating pollutants that enter the airways.

Caeruloplasmin and transferrin account for most of the antioxidant activity in plasma (34). The antioxidant activity of both proteins is related to their actions in limiting free iron in plasma. Caeruloplasmin oxidizes iron from the Fe (II) to the Fe (III) state, and transferrin binds iron in the oxidized or Fe(III) state. Free iron can promote oxidant cell injury by enhancing the formation of hydroxyl radicals (see Fig. 21.5) (35). The tendency for free iron to promote oxidant injury may be the reason that most of the iron in the body is sequestered and very little is allowed to roam free in plasma.

Oxidant Stress

The risk of oxidant-induced (oxygen-induced) tissue injury is determined by the balance between oxidant and antioxidant activities. When oxidant activity exceeds the neutralizing capacity of the antioxidants, the excess or unopposed oxidant activity can promote tissue injury. This condition of unopposed biological oxidation is known as *oxidant stress.*

Pulmonary Oxygen Toxicity

Inhaled O_2 can damage the lungs in any concentration, but the lungs are normally well-endowed with antioxidant activity (particularly glutathione and vitamin C) that protects the lungs from O_2 toxicity at the usual concentrations of inhaled O_2. When the inhaled O_2 exceeds the protective capacity of the endogenous antioxidants in the lungs, the result is a progressive and potentially lethal form of inflammatory lung injury that is clinically indistinguishable from the acute respiratory distress syndrome (ARDS), which is described in the next chapter.

Species Differences

The tendency to develop pulmonary oxygen toxicity varies in different species. For example, laboratory rats will die of respiratory failure after 5 to 7 days of breathing pure O_2, while sea turtles can breathe pure O_2 indefinitely without harm (36). This species-specific effect is important because experimental studies of pulmonary oxygen toxicity have been conducted almost solely in laboratory rats. As a result, little is known about the tendency of humans to develop pulmonary oxygen toxicity. In healthy volunteers, inhalation of 100% oxygen for brief periods of time (6 to 12 hours) results in a tracheobronchitis and a decrease in vital capacity believed to be a result of absorption atelectasis (37). The longest exposure to 100% oxygen in humans includes 5 patients with irreversible coma (3 to 4 days) and one healthy volunteer (4.5 days) (38,39). In all these cases, prolonged exposure to oxygen resulted in a pulmonary syndrome very much like ARDS.

What FIO_2 is Toxic?

Based on the observation that oxygen inhalation reduces the vital capacity when the FIO_2 is 0.60 or higher (37), the toxic level of FIO_2 was set at 0.60. The consensus seems to be that exposure to an FIO_2 above 0.60 for longer than 48 hours constitutes a toxic exposure to oxygen. The problem with adopting one FIO_2 that applies to all patients is that it neglects the contribution of endogenous antioxidants to the risk of oxygen toxicity. If the antioxidant stores in the lungs are depleted, oxygen toxicity will develop at an FIO_2 that is much lower than 0.60. Antioxidant depletion may be common in ICU patients (40,41), which means that an FIO_2 below 0.60 may not be safe in ICU patients. Thus, it seems more reasonable to assume that **any FIO_2 above 0.21 (room air) can represent a toxic exposure to oxygen in ICU patients**. Therefore, the best practice is to reduce the FIO_2 to the lowest tolerable level in all ICU patients. (Remember that, even though an FIO_2 of 0.4 may seem safe, it is about twice the normal dose of a potentially toxic gas.)

Promoting Antioxidant Protection

Little attention has been given to supporting antioxidant protection to limit the risk of pulmonary oxygen toxicity. While it is not yet possible to evaluate the adequacy of antioxidant protection in individual patients, two measures may be helpful. The first is to maintain the recommended daily intake of selenium (70 μg/day for men and 55 μg/day in women), and the second is to monitor and correct deficiencies in vitamin E stores. A reliable measure of oxidant stress in exhaled breath is sorely needed to evaluate the risk of pulmonary oxygen toxicity in individual patients.

A FINAL WORD

There is little doubt that the use of oxygen in the ICU is excessive and dangerous. The routine use of oxygen should be abandoned, and the PaO_2 and SaO_2 should be replaced as markers of the need for inhaled oxygen because they bear no relationship to the integrity of tissue oxygenation. Possible replacements would be the SvO_2 and the (SaO_2 – SvO_2): When cardiac output and serum hemoglobin are adequate, inhaled oxygen should be indicated for an $SvO_2 \leq 50\%$, or an (SaO_2 – SvO_2) $\geq 50\%$ (see Chapter 11 for a description of these measurements). Finally, more attention must be given to the antioxidant status of individual patients to assess the risk of pulmonary oxygen toxicity.

REFERENCES

The Need for Supplemental Oxygen

1. Small D, Duha A, Wieskopf B, et al. Uses and misuses of oxygen in hospitalized patients. Am J Med 1992;92:591–595.
2. Whalen WJ, Riley J. A microelectrode for measurement of intracellular PO_2. J Appl Physiol 1967;23:798–801.
3. Sair M, Etherington PJ, Winlove CP, Evans TW. Tissue oxygenation and perfusion in patients with systemic sepsis. Crit Care Med 2001;29:1343–1349.
4. Kallstrom TJ. AARC Clinical Practice Guideline: oxygen therapy for adults in the acute care facility: 2002 revision & update. Respir Care 2002;47:717–720.
5. Eldridge FE. Blood lactate and pyruvate in pulmonary insufficiency. N Engl J Med 1966;274:878–883.

6. Lundt T, Koller M, Kofstad J. Severe hypoxemia without evidence of tissue hypoxia in the adult respiratory distress syndrome. Crit Care Med 1984;12: 75–76.
7. Abdelsalam M. Permissive hypoxemia: Is it time to change our approach? Chest 2006;129:210–211.

The End-Point of Oxygen Inhalation

8. Corriveau ML, Rosen BJ, Dolan GF. Oxygen transport and oxygen consumption during supplemental oxygen administration in patients with chronic obstructive pulmonary disease. Am J Med 1989;87:633–636.
9. Lejeune P, Mols P, Naeije R, et al. Acute hemodynamic effects of controlled oxygen therapy in decompensated chronic obstructive pulmonary disease. Crit Care Med 1984;12:1032–1035.
10. Kavanaugh PB, Cheng DCH, Sandler AN, et al. Supplemental oxygen does not reduce myocardial ischemia in premedicated patients with critical coronary artery disease. Anesth Analg 1993;76:950–956.
11. Packer M, Lee WH, Medina N, Yushak M. Systemic vasoconstrictor effects of oxygen administration in obliterative pulmonary vascular disorders. Am J Cardiol 1986;57:853–858.
12. Bongard O, Bounameaux H, Fagrell B. Effects of oxygen on skin microcirculation in patients with peripheral arterial occlusive disease. Circulation 1992; 86:878–886.
13. Daly WJ, Bondurant S. Effects of oxygen breathing on the heart rate, blood pressure and cardiac index of normal men—resting, with reactive hyperemia, and after atropine. J Clin Invest 1962;41:126–132.

Methods of Oxygen Inhalation

14. Vines DL, Shelledy DC, Peters J. Current respiratory care: Oxygen therapy, oximetry, bronchial hygiene. J Crit Illness 2000;15:507–515.
15. Shapiro BA, Kacmarek RM, Cane RD, et al. Clinical application of respiratory care. 4th ed. St. Louis: CV Mosby, 1991:123–134.
16. O'Connor BS, Vender JS. Oxygen therapy. Crit Care Clin 1995;11:67–78.
17. Scacci R. Air entrainment masks: jet mixing is how they work. The Bernoulli and Venturi principles is how they don't. Respir Care 1979;24:928–931.

The Dark Side of Oxygen

18. Halliwell B, Gutteridge JMC. Oxygen is a toxic gas: an introduction to oxygen toxicity and reactive oxygen species. In: Free radicals in biology and medicine. 3rd ed. Oxford: Oxford University Press, 1999:1–104.
19. Anderson BO, Brown JM, Harken A. Mechanisms of neutrophil-mediated tissue injury. J Surg Res 1991;51:170–179.
20. Fink M. Role of reactive oxygen and nitrogen species in acute respiratory distress syndrome. Curr Opin Crit Care 2002;8:6–11.
21. Alonso de Vega JM, Diaz J, Serrano E, Carbonell LF. Oxidative stress in critically ill patients with systemic inflammatory response syndrome. Crit Care Med 2002;30:1782–1788.

22. Halliwell B, Gutteridge JMC. Antioxidant defenses. In: Free radicals in biology and medicine. 3rd ed. Oxford: Oxford University Press, 1999:105–245.
23. Liochev SI, Fridovich I. The role of $O_2^{\bullet}$ in the production of $HO^{\bullet}$ in vitro and in vivo. Free Radic Biol Med 1994;16:29–33.
24. Michiels C, Raes M, Toussant O, et al. Importance of Se-glutathione, peroxidase, catalase, and CU/ZN-SOD for cell survival against oxidative stress. Free Rad Biol Med 1994;17:235–248.
25. Suttorp N, Toepfer W, Roka L. Antioxidant defense mechanisms of endothelial cells: glutathione redox cycle versus catalase. Am J Physiol 1986;251:C671–C680.
26. National Research Council. Subcommittee. On the tenth edition of the RDAs. 10th ed. Washington, DC: Academic Press, 1989:220.
27. Sando K, Hoki M, Nezu R, et al. Platelet glutathione peroxidase activity in long-term total parenteral nutrition with and without selenium supplementation. J Parent Enteral Nutr 1992;16:54–58.
28. World Health Organization. Selenium. Environmental Health Criteria 58. Geneva, Switzerland, 1987.
29. Meister A. On the antioxidant effects of ascorbic acid and glutathione. Biochem Pharmacol 1992;44:1905–1915.
30. Cantin AM, Begin R. Glutathione and inflammatory disorders of the lung. Lung 1991;169:123–138.
31. Robinson M, Ahn MS, Rounds JD, et al. Parenteral glutathione monoester enhances tissue antioxidant stores. J Parent Enteral Nutr 1992;16:413–418.
32. Meydani M. Vitamin E. Lancet 1995;345:170–176.
33. Pincemail J, Bertrand Y, Hanique G, et al. Evaluation of vitamin E deficiency in patients with adult respiratory distress syndrome. Ann N Y Acad Sci 1989; 570:498–500.
34. Halliwell B, Gutteridge JMC. Role of free radicals and catalytic metal ions in human disease. Methods Enzymol 1990;186:1–85.
35. Herbert V, Shaw S, Jayatilleke E, et al. Most free-radical injury is iron-related: it is promoted by iron, hemin, haloferritin and vitamin C, and inhibited by desferrioxamine and apoferritin. Stem Cells 1994;12:289–303.
36. Fanburg BL. Oxygen toxicity: why can't a human be more like a turtle? Intensive Care Med 1988;3:134–136.
37. Lodato RF. Oxygen toxicity. Crit Care Clin 1990;6:749–765.
38. Barber RE, Hamilton WK. Oxygen toxicity in man. N Engl J Med 1970;283: 1478–1483.
39. Winter PM, Smith G. The toxicity of oxygen. Anesthesiology 1972;37:210–212.
40. Hawker FH, Stewart PM, Switch PJ. Effects of acute illness on selenium homeostasis. Crit Care Med 1990;18:442–446.
41. Pincemail J, Bertrand Y, Hanique G, et al. Evaluation of vitamin E deficiency in patients with adult respiratory distress syndrome. Ann N Y Acad Sci 1989; 570:498–500.

Chapter 22

ACUTE RESPIRATORY DISTRESS SYNDROME

Physicians think they do a lot for a patient when they give his disease a name.

Immanuel Kant

The condition described in this chapter has had several names over the years, including *shock lung, non-cardiogenic pulmonary edema, adult respiratory distress syndrome, acute lung injury,* and most recently, *acute respiratory distress syndrome,* or *ARDS*. None of these names provides any useful information about the condition, which is a type of inflammatory lung injury that is neither a primary disease or a single entity. Rather, it is an expression of myriad other diseases that produce diffuse inflammation in the lungs, often accompanied by inflammatory injury in other organs (1–3). It is also the leading cause of acute respiratory failure in the United States.

PATHOGENESIS

The first clinical report of ARDS included 12 patients with diffuse infiltrates on chest roentgenogram and hypoxemia that was resistant to supplemental oxygen (4). Seven patients died (mortality = 60%), and autopsy findings revealed dense infiltration of the lungs with leukocytes and proteinaceous material, similar to the photomicrograph in Figure 22.1. There was no evidence of infection, which indicated that ARDS is principally an inflammatory condition.

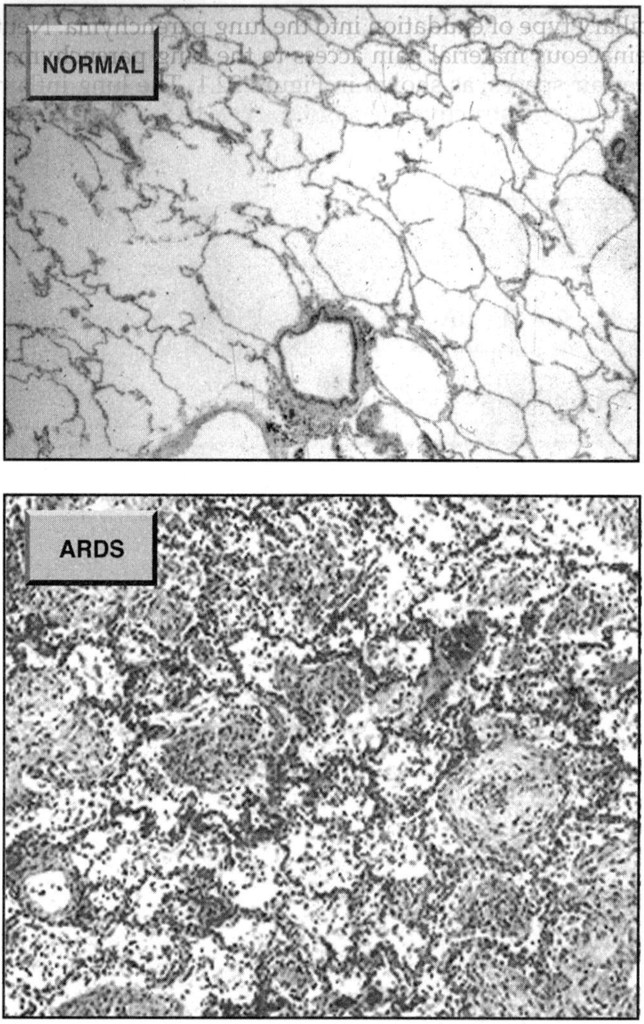

FIGURE 22.1 Microscopic images of a normal lung and a lung in the advanced stages of ARDS. Note the dense infiltration of inflammatory cells in ARDS and the obliteration of the distal airspaces. (Photomicrograph of ARDS courtesy of Martha L Warnock, MD, University of California at San Francisco, San Francisco, CA. Image digitally retouched.)

Inflammatory Injury

The basic pathology of ARDS is a diffuse inflammatory process that involves both lungs. The lung consolidation in ARDS is believed to originate from a systemic activation of circulating neutrophils (5). The activated neutrophils become sticky and adhere to the vascular endothelium in the pulmonary capillaries. The neutrophils then release the contents of their cytoplasmic granules (i.e., proteolytic enzymes and toxic oxygen metabolites), and this damages the endothelium and leads to a leaky-capillary type of exudation into the lung parenchyma. Neutrophils and proteinaceous material gain access to the lung parenchyma and fill the alveolar air spaces, as shown in Figure 22.1. The lung inflammation in ARDS is often destructive, and the resulting lung damage promotes further inflammation, creating a vicious cycle that leads to progressive respiratory insufficiency.

Fibrin deposition in the lungs is another characteristic feature of ARDS, and this fibrin can undergo remodeling and produce pulmonary fibrosis (similar to the process that occurs in wound healing) (6). The source of fibrin is a procoagulant state triggered by release of tissue factor from the lungs (6). The involvement of the coagulation system in ARDS has important implications for the possible role of anticoagulation and fibrinolytic therapy in ARDS (see later).

Thus, **ARDS is the result of inflammatory lung injury**. Although it is often referred to as a type of pulmonary edema (e.g., leaky capillary or noncardiogenic pulmonary edema), this is misleading because the lungs are filled with an inflammatory exudate rather than watery edema fluid. This has important implications for the role of diuretic therapy in ARDS (see later).

Predisposing Conditions

A variety of clinical disorders can predispose to ARDS, and the common ones are indicated on the body map in Figure 22.2. The one feature

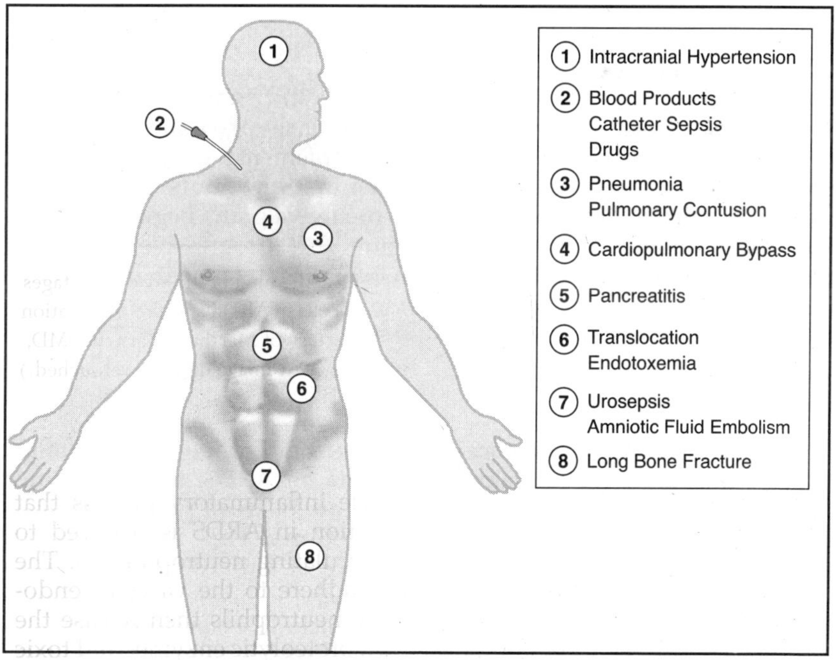

FIGURE 22.2 Clinical conditions that predispose to ARDS.

TABLE 22.1 Predisposing Factors and Mortality in ARDS

	Incidence of ARDS (%)		
Predisposing Factor	ARDS	No ARDS	Mortality (%)
Sepsis syndrome	41	69	50
Multiple transfusions	36	70	35
Pulmonary contusion	22	49	12
Aspiration of gastric contents	22	48	21
Multiple fractures	11	49	9
Drug overdose	9	35	4
All high-risk conditions	26	62	19

Data from Hudson LD et al. (7).

shared by all of these conditions is the ability to trigger a systemic inflammatory response. The incidence of ARDS in some high-risk conditions is shown in Table 22.1 (7). Overall, one of every four patients with a predisposing condition develops ARDS (see bottom of the table), and ARDS is most prevalent in patients with sepsis syndrome (defined as an infection associated with fever and leukocytosis). Note the negative impact of ARDS on survival.

CLINICAL FEATURES

The earliest clinical signs of ARDS include tachypnea and progressive hypoxemia, which is often refractory to supplemental oxygen. The chest roentgenogram can be unrevealing in the first few hours of the illness. However, within 24 hours, the chest roentgenogram begins to reveal bilateral pulmonary infiltrates (see Figure 22.3). Progressive hypoxemia requiring mechanical ventilation often occurs in the first 48 hours of the illness.

Diagnostic Criteria

In 1994, a consensus conference of experts from Europe and the United States published a set of diagnostic criteria for ARDS, which is shown in Table 22.2 (1). The hallmarks of ARDS are bilateral pulmonary infiltrates, severe hypoxemia (PaO_2/FIO_2 <200 mm Hg), the presence of a predisposing condition, and no evidence of left-heart failure (either clinically or by measuring a pulmonary artery occlusion pressure that is ≤18 mm Hg). Note that these criteria also include a condition known as *acute lung injury*. This is a less severe form of ARDS, and is distinguished from ARDS by the PaO_2/FIO_2 ratio.

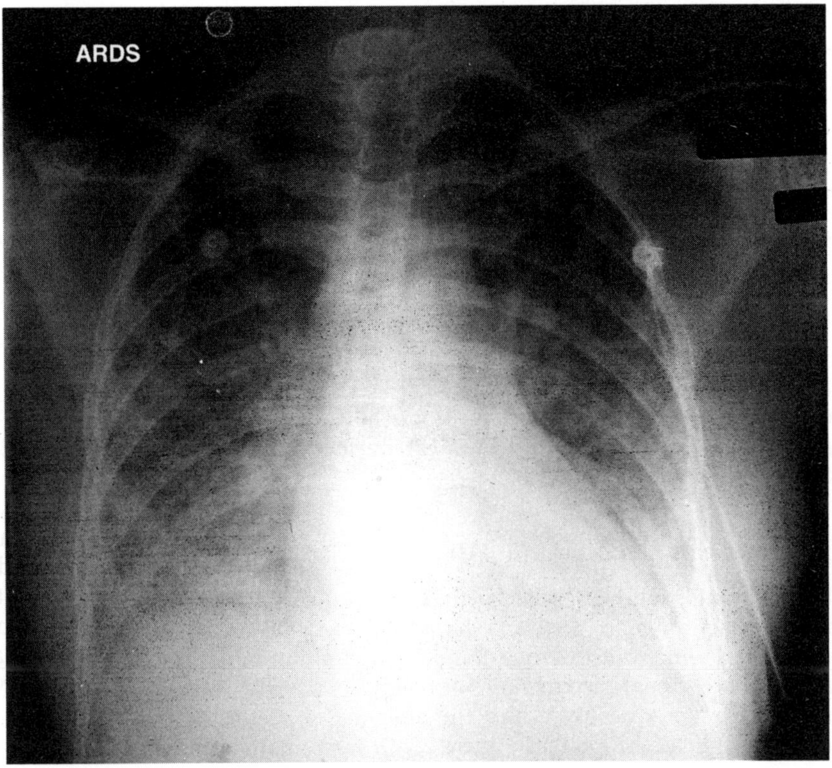

FIGURE 22.3 Upright portable chest x-ray from a patient with ARDS. The infiltrate appears to be homogeneous or equally distributed throughout both lower lung fields. The actual location of the infiltrates in ARDS is shown in Figure 22.4.

Lack of Specificity

The diagnosis of ARDS based on clinical criteria in Table 22.2 can be problematic because many of the clinical features of ARDS are shared by other causes of acute respiratory failure (8). This is demonstrated in Table 22.3, which compares the diagnostic features of ARDS with the clinical features of severe pneumonia, acute pulmonary embolism, and

TABLE 22.2 Diagnostic Criteria for ALI and ARDS†

1. Acute Onset
2. Presence of a predisposing condition.
3. Bilateral infiltrates on frontal chest x-ray.
4. PaO_2 / FiO_2 < 200 mm Hg for ARDS, < 300 mm Hg for ALI
5. Pulmonary artery occlusion pressure ≤18 mm Hg or no clinical evidence of left atrial hypertension.

†From the consensus conference report in Reference 8.
ALI = acute lung injury, *ARDS* = acute respiratory distress syndrome.

TABLE 22.3 Features Shared by ARDS & Other Causes of Acute Respiratory Failure

Feature	ARDS	Severe Pneumonia	Pulmonary Embolism	Cardiogenic Lung Edema
Acute Onset	√	√	√	√
Fever, Leukocytosis.	√	√	√	If Acute MI
Bilateral infiltrates	√	√		√
$PaO_2 / FiO_2 < 200$ mm Hg	√	√	√	
PAOP $\leq$18 mm Hg	√	√	√	

cardiogenic pulmonary edema. Note the perfect match between ARDS and severe pneumonia, and the near-perfect match between ARDS and acute pulmonary embolism.

ARDS Versus Cardiogenic Edema

For patients who present with bilateral pulmonary infiltrates, the usual concern is to distinguish between ARDS and cardiogenic pulmonary edema (although a bilateral pneumonia is also a consideration). The appearance of the chest x-ray is usually of little or no value. A homogeneous infiltrate and the absence of pleural effusions is more characteristic of ARDS (see Figure 22.3), while patchy infiltrates emanating from the hilum and prominent pleural effusions is more characteristic of cardiogenic pulmonary edema. However, there is considerable overlap in these characteristics (e.g., pleural effusions can appear in ARDS), and the consensus view is that **chest roentgenograms are not reliable for distinguishing ARDS from cardiogenic pulmonary edema** (1,9,10).

Severity of Hypoxemia

The severity of the hypoxemia can sometimes help distinguish ARDS from cardiogenic pulmonary edema. In the early stages of ARDS, the hypoxemia is often more pronounced than the chest roentgenogram abnormalities, whereas in the early stages of cardiogenic pulmonary edema, the roentgenogram abnormalities are often more pronounced than the hypoxemia. However, there are exceptions, and severe hypoxemia can occur in cardiogenic pulmonary edema if the mixed venous oxygen pressure (PO_2) is reduced from a low cardiac output (see Figure 19.4).

Pitfalls of the Wedge Pressure

As indicated in Table 22.2, the pulmonary capillary wedge pressure (PCWP) is considered to be a valuable measurement for differentiating ARDS from cardiogenic pulmonary edema. The problem here is that **the wedge pressure is not a measure of capillary hydrostatic pressure**, as explained in Chapter 10. The PCWP is a measure of left-atrial pressure (and is obtained in the absence of flow), and left-atrial pressure cannot be the same as the pulmonary capillary pressure in the presence of blood flow. That is, **if the wedge (left-atrial) pressure were equivalent to the pressure in the pulmonary capillaries, there would be no pressure gradient for flow in the pulmonary veins**. Thus, the capillary hydrostatic pressure must be higher than the wedge pressure.

The wedge pressure will therefore underestimate the actual capillary hydrostatic pressure. This difference is small in the normal lung, but in severe ARDS, the capillary hydrostatic pressure can be double the wedge pressure, as explained in Chapter 10. If this is the case, then a PCWP of 15 mm Hg could represent cardiogenic pulmonary edema because the capillary hydrostatic pressure may be twice this or 30 mm Hg. Because of this discrepancy, **the wedge pressure should be abandoned as a diagnostic criterion for ARDS**.

Bronchoalveolar Lavage

The most reliable method for confirming or excluding the diagnosis of ARDS is *bronchoalveolar lavage*. This procedure can be performed at the bedside using a flexible fiberoptic bronchoscope that is advanced into one of the involved lung segments. Once in place, the lung segment is lavaged with isotonic saline. The lavage fluid is then analyzed for neutrophil density and protein concentration, as described below (11).

Neutrophils

In normal subjects, neutrophils make up less than 5% of the cells recovered in lung lavage fluid, whereas in patients with ARDS, as many as 80% of the recovered cells are neutrophils (11). A low neutrophil count in lung lavage fluid can be used to exclude the diagnosis of ARDS, while a high neutrophil count is considered evidence of ARDS (even though pneumonia can produce similar results).

Total Protein

Because inflammatory exudates are rich in proteinaceous material, lung lavage fluid that is similarly rich in protein can be used as evidence of lung inflammation. When the protein concentration in lung lavage fluid is expressed as a fraction of the total protein concentration, the following criteria can be applied (12):

$$\text{Protein (lavage/serum)} < 0.5 = \text{Hydrostatic edema}$$
$$\text{Protein (lavage/serum)} > 0.7 = \text{Lung inflammation}$$

Thus, lung inflammation is expected to produce a protein concentration that is greater than 70% of the protein concentration in serum. Although a positive test result is not specific for ARDS, it can be used as evidence of ARDS if other causes of lung inflammation (e.g., pneumonia) can be excluded on clinical grounds.

Bronchoalveolar lavage has not gained widespread acceptance as a diagnostic tool for ARDS, probably because most ICU physicians use the diagnostic criteria in Table 22.2 to evaluate possible ARDS. Considering the nonspecific nature of these diagnostic criteria (as shown in Table 22.3), more reliable diagnostic methods like bronchoalveolar lavage are probably underutilized.

MANAGEMENT OF ARDS

In the 40 years since ARDS was first described, only one therapeutic manipulation has proven effective in improving survival in ARDS: the use of low tidal volume mechanical ventilation. This is not really a specific therapy for ARDS, but is a lessening of the harmful effects of mechanical ventilation on the lungs. The realization that conventional mechanical ventilation is injurious to the lungs is one of the most important discoveries in critical care medicine in the last quarter-century.

Lung-Protective Ventilation

Since the introduction of positive-pressure mechanical ventilation, large inflation volumes (tidal volumes) have been used to reduce the presumed tendency for atelectasis during mechanical ventilation. The standard tidal volumes are 10 to 15 mL/kg, which are twice the size of tidal volumes used during quiet breathing (6 to 7 mL/kg). In patients with ARDS, these large inflation volumes are delivered into lungs that have a marked reduction in functional volume. The decreased functional volume in ARDS is evident in the CT images in Figure 22.4. Note the dense lung consolidation in the posterior or dependent lung regions, and the small region of uninvolved lung in the anterior one third of the thorax.

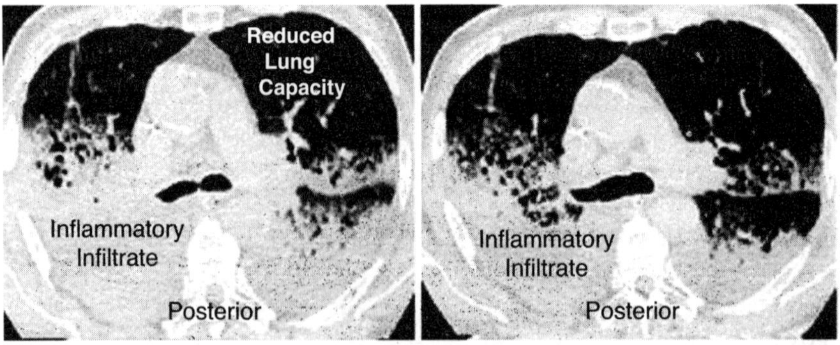

FIGURE 22.4 Computed tomographic images of lung slices in the region of the hilum in a patient with ARDS. The lung consolidation is not homogeneous, but is confined to the posterior or dependent lung regions. The uninvolved lung in the anterior one-third of the thorax represents the functional portion of the lung in ARDS. (CT images digitally retouched from Rouby J-J, et al. Crit Care Med 2003;31[suppl]:S285–S295.)

Conventional chest radiographs in ARDS show what appears to be a homogeneous pattern of lung infiltration; however, CT images reveal that the lung infiltration in ARDS is not spread evenly throughout the lungs, but rather is confined to dependent lung regions (13). The remaining area of uninvolved lung is the functional portion of the lungs in ARDS. Because the functional lung volume in ARDS is markedly reduced, the large inflation volumes delivered by mechanical ventilation cause overdistention and rupture of the distal airspaces. This condition is called *ventilator-induced lung injury.*

Ventilator-Induced Lung Injury

Overdistention and rupture of the distal airspaces during mechanical ventilation is a volume-related rather than pressure-related injury (14), and is called *volutrauma.* (Pressure-related lung injury is called *barotrauma.*) Excessive inflation volumes produce stress fractures in the alveolar capillary interface, and this leads to infiltration of the distal airspaces with inflammatory cells and proteinaceous material. The resulting clinical condition, known as ventilator-induced lung injury (VILI), is strikingly similar to ARDS (14).

The organ injury from mechanical ventilation may not be confined to the lungs. Bronchoalveolar lavage studies have shown that volutrauma is accompanied by release of inflammatory cytokines from neutrophils that infiltrate the lungs (15). This effect is not explained by mechanical forces (volume and pressure), and is called *biotrauma.* Some have suggested that the cytokines released in the lungs could enter the systemic circulation and travel to distant organs to produce widespread inflammatory injury and multiorgan failure (16). This would mean that mechanical ventilation is as lethal as severe sepsis and other causes of multiorgan failure.

Low-Volume Ventilation

A total of 5 clinical trials have compared mechanical ventilation with low tidal volumes (usually 6 mL/kg) and conventional tidal volumes (usually 12 mL/kg) in patients with ARDS. In two trials, low tidal volumes were associated with fewer deaths, and in 3 trials, there was no survival benefit associated with low tidal volumes (17). The pooled results of all five trials suggests a benefit with low tidal volumes, particularly when the end-inspiratory plateau pressure (which correlates with the risk of volutrauma) is above 30 cm H_2O. (See Chapter 24 for an explanation of this pressure.)

The most successful trial of low tidal volume ventilation in ARDS was conducted by the ARDS Clinical Network (a network created by governmental health agencies to perform multicenter trials of ARDS treatments). This study enrolled over 800 patients with ARDS, and compared ventilation with tidal volumes of 6 mL/kg and 12 mL/kg using *predicted body weight* (which is the weight at which lung volumes are normal). Ventilation with low tidal volumes was associated with a 9% (absolute) reduction in mortality when the end-inspiratory plateau pressure was <30 cm H_2O (18).

TABLE 22.4 Protocol for Low Volume Ventilation in ARDS[†]

GOALS: TV = 6 mL/kg, Ppl < 30 cm H_2O, pH = 7.30 − 7.45

I. FIRST STAGE:

1. Calculate patient's **predicted** body weight (PBW)[‡]

   Males: PBW = 50 + [2.3 × (height in inches − 60)]

   Females: PBW = 45.5 + [2.3 × (height in inches − 60)]
2. Set initial tidal volume (TV) to 8 mL/kg PBW.
3. Add positive end-expiratory pressure (PEEP) at 5 − 7 cm H_2O,
4. Reduce TV by 1 mL/kg every 2 hours until TV = 6 mL/kg PBW.

II. SECOND STAGE

1. When TV down to 6 mL/kg, measure plateau pressure (Ppl).
   A. Target Ppl < 30 cm H_2O.
   B. If Ppl > 30 cm H_2O, decrease TV in 1 mL/kg steps until Ppl drops below 30 cm H_2O or TV down to 4 mL/kg.

III. THIRD STAGE

1. Monitor arterial blood gases for respiratory acidosis.
   A. Target pH = 7.30 − 7.45
   B. If pH 7.15 − 7.30, increase respiratory rate (RR) until pH > 7.30 or RR = 35 bpm.
   C. If pH < 7.15, increase RR to 35 bpm. If pH still < 7.15, increase TV at 1 mL/kg increments until pH > 7.15.

[‡]The predicted body weight is the weight at which lung volumes are normal.
[†]Protocol from the ARDS Clinical Network web site (www.ardsnet.org).

A protocol for low volume ventilation recommended by the ARDS Clinical Network is shown in Table 22.4. This protocol is designed to achieve three goals: (1) maintain a tidal volume of 6 mL/kg using predicted body weight, (2) keep the end-inspiratory plateau pressure below 30 cm H_2O, and (3) avoid severe respiratory acidosis.

Permissive Hypercapnia

One of the consequences of low volume ventilation is a reduction in CO_2 elimination via the lungs leading to hypercapnia and respiratory acidosis. Allowing hypercapnia to persist in favor of maintaining lung-protective low-volume ventilation is known as *permissive hypercapnia* (19). The limits of tolerance to hypercapnia and respiratory acidosis are unclear, but individual reports show that $PaCO_2$ levels as high as 375 mm Hg and pH levels as low as 6.6 are remarkably free of serious side effects as long as tissue oxygenation is adequate (20). One of the more troublesome side effects of hypercapnia is brainstem respiratory stimulation with subsequent hyperventilation, which often requires neuromuscular blockade to prevent ventilator asynchrony.

There are few guidelines that identify a safe and appropriate level of hypercapnic acidosis. However, data from clinical trials of permissive hypercapnia show that arterial PCO_2 levels of 60 to 70 mm Hg and arterial pH levels of 7.2 to 7.25 are safe for most patients (21). Often, the perceived risk of hypercapnic acidosis in individual patients is determined by the perceived benefit of maintaining low-volume ventilation to protect the lungs from volutrauma.

Positive End-Expiratory Pressure

(For a full description of this pressure, see Chapter 25.) Low-volume ventilation can be accompanied by collapse of terminal airways at the end of expiration and re-opening of the airways during lung inflation. This repetitive opening and closing of terminal airways can itself be a source of lung injury (possibly by creating shear forces that damage the airway epithelium) (22). Positive end-expiratory pressure (PEEP) can mitigate this problem by acting as a stent to keep small airways open at the end of expiration. For this reason, the addition of low-level PEEP (5–7 cm H_2O) has become a standard practice during low-volume ventilation. There is no added benefit to the use of higher levels of PEEP in this condition (23).

PEEP is also used as an aid to arterial oxygenation in ARDS. The hypoxemia in ARDS can be refractory to increased (and potentially toxic) concentrations of inhaled oxygen, and the addition of PEEP often allows a reduction in the fractional concentration of inhaled oxygen (FIO_2) to safer levels. The recommended combinations of PEEP and FIO_2 for promoting arterial oxygenation in ARDS is shown in Table 22.5. These combinations represent the consensus views of members of the ARDS Clinical Network.

It is important to emphasize that the use of PEEP to promote arterial oxygenation is a flawed practice because PEEP can decrease cardiac output and this effect can counteract a PEEP-induced increase in arterial oxygenation. The effects of PEEP are described in more detail in Chapter 25.

Fluid Management

Fluid management in ARDS is usually aimed at reducing extravascular lung water with diuretics. While this approach has shown modest benefits in clinical measures like lung compliance, gas exchange, and length

TABLE 22.5 FIO_2: PEEP Combinations for Promoting Arterial Oxygenation in ARDS†

GOAL: PaO_2 = 55–80 mm Hg or SpO_2 = 88–95%								
FIO_2	0.3	0.4	0.4	0.5	0.5	0.6	0.7	0.7
PEEP	5	5	8	8	10	10	10	12
FIO_2	0.7	0.8	0.9	0.9	0.9	1.0	1.0	1.0
PEEP	14	14	14	16	18	20	22	24

†From the ARDS Clinical Network web site (www.ardsnet.org).

of time on the ventilator, there is little evidence of a consistent survival benefit (24,25). The following are some problems with diuretic therapy in ARDS that deserve mention.

The Pitfalls of Diuretic Therapy in ARDS

The first problem with the use of diuretic therapy in ARDS is the nature of the lung infiltration. While diuretics can remove the watery edema fluid that forms as a consequence of heart failure, **the lung infiltration in ARDS is an inflammatory process, and diuretics don't reduce inflammation**. The photomicrograph of ARDS in Figure 22.1, which shows dense infiltration of the lungs with inflammatory cells, illustrates why diuretic therapy has had limited success in the treatment of ARDS (26).

The second problem with diuretic therapy in ARDS is the risk for hemodynamic compromise. Most patients with ARDS are receiving positive-pressure mechanical ventilation, and venous pressures must be high enough to exceed the positive intrathoracic pressure and maintain venous return to the heart. Aggressive diuretic therapy can reduce venous pressures and compromise venous return to the heart. This will ultimately compromise systemic oxygen transport (via a reduction in cardiac output), which is the single most important parameter to support in acute respiratory failure.

The hemodynamic risks of diuretic therapy in ARDS can be minimized by monitoring cardiac filling pressures and cardiac output using a pulmonary artery catheter. Diuretic therapy can then be tailored to achieve the lowest cardiac filling pressures that do not compromise cardiac output and systemic oxygen transport. Although the popularity of pulmonary artery catheters is rapidly declining, this is a situation where the information provided by the catheter would play an important role in patient management.

Promoting Oxygen Transport

The ultimate goal of management in hypoxemic respiratory failure is to maintain oxygen delivery to the vital organs. The oxygen transport parameters are described in detail in Chapter 2, and the determinants of systemic oxygen delivery (DO_2) are shown in the equation below.

$$DO_2 = Q \times 13.6 \times Hb \times SaO_2 \qquad (22.1)$$

Q is cardiac output, Hb is blood hemoglobin concentration, and SaO_2 is the arterial oxyhemoglobin saturation. **Systemic oxygen delivery should be maintained at a normal rate of 900 to 1100 mL/min or 520 to 600 mL/min/m^2 when adjusted for body size** (see Table 2.3 in Chapter 2 for the normal ranges of the oxygen transport parameters). Promoting systemic oxygen delivery is achieved by providing support for each of the variables identified in Equation 22.1. Support for the SaO_2 has already been described in the section on ventilator management. Support for the other two components of O_2 delivery (cardiac output and hemoglobin) is described briefly in the sections that follow.

Cardiac Output

The cardiac output should be maintained at 5–6 L/min or 3–4 L/min/m^2 when adjusted for body size. If the cardiac output is below these normal ranges, check the central venous pressure or wedge pressure. If these pressures are not elevated, volume infusion is indicated. Despite the fear that infused fluids will move out into the lungs, the tendency for fluids to move into the lungs should be the same for ARDS and pneumonia (and there is no fear of volume infusion in pneumonia).

If volume infusion is not indicated, dobutamine is preferred over vasodilators for augmenting the cardiac output (26) because vasodilators will increase intrapulmonary shunt and will add to the gas exchange abnormality in ARDS. (See Table 16.2 for a dobutamine dose chart.) **Dopamine should be avoided in ARDS because it constricts pulmonary veins**, and this will cause an exaggerated rise in the pulmonary capillary hydrostatic pressure.

Hemoglobin

Transfusion is often recommended to keep the Hb above 10 g/dL, but this practice has no scientific basis or documented benefit, even in ventilator-dependent patients (27). Considering that blood transfusions can *cause* ARDS, and that this complication may be much more common than is currently recognized (28), it is wise to avoid transfusing blood products in patients with ARDS. **If there is no evidence of tissue dysoxia or impending dysoxia (e.g., an oxygen extraction ratio ≥50%), there is no need to correct anemia with blood transfusions.**

Pharmacotherapy

Despite nearly forty years of active research in search of a cure, ARDS remains an untreatable condition. The lack of effective therapy for ARDS may be reflection of the fact that ARDS is not an independent entity, but exists only as an expression of another disease entity.

Steroids

High-dose steroid therapy has no effect on ARDS when given within 24 hours of the onset of illness (29,30). However when steroids are given later in the course of illness, during the fibrinoproliferative phase that begins 7–14 days after the onset of illness, there is a definite survival benefit (31). One of the successful regimens involved methylprednisolone in a dose of 2 to 3 mg/kg/day. The benefit of steroids in late ARDS may be explained by the ability of steroids to promote collagen breakdown and inhibit fibrosis (25).

The Casualties

The medical literature is littered with failed therapies in ARDS. Some of the more notable failures are surfactant (in adults), nitric oxide, pentoxyphylline, lisophylline, ibuprofen, prostaglandin E_1, ketoconazole (inhibits thromboxane) and *N*-acetylcysteine (an antioxidant) (24,25).

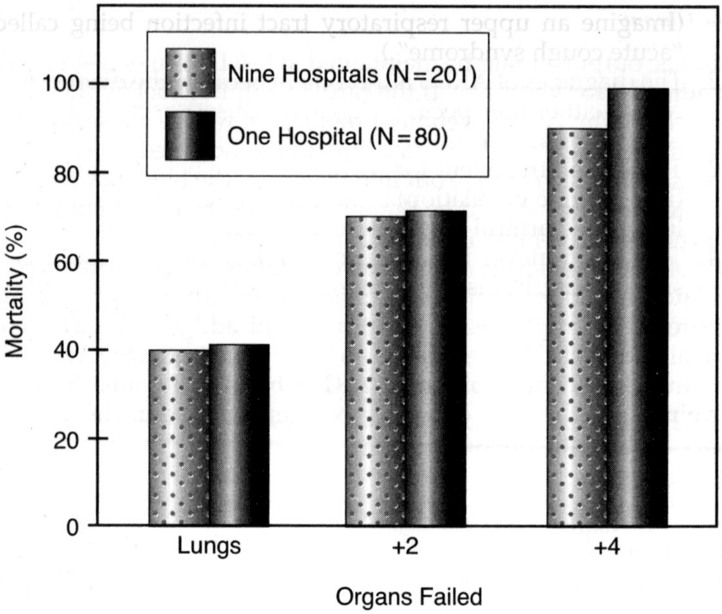

FIGURE 22.5 Multiorgan failure and survival in ARDS. (Results of the multicenter study from Reference 33. Results of the single center study from Reference 34.)

A Case of Misdirection?

Although the treatment of ARDS has been directed at the lungs, **most of the deaths from ARDS are not due to respiratory failure**. Fewer than 40% of deaths in ARDS are the result of respiratory failure (32–36). The majority of deaths are attributed to multiple organ failure. Age is also an important factor, with mortality being as much as five times higher in patients over 60 years of age (37).

The influence of multiorgan failure on survival in ARDS is shown in Figure 22.5. Included in this graph are the results of a multicenter study (33) and the results of a study conducted at a single hospital (34). Both show a steady rise in mortality as more organs fail in addition to the respiratory failure. This demonstrates that ARDS is often just one part of a multiorgan illness, and it emphasizes the limitations of management strategies that focus primarily on the lungs.

A FINAL WORD

ARDS has been a major problem since it was first described in 1967. Some of the notable problems are listed below.

1. The name "acute respiratory distress syndrome" is a problem because it uses symptomatology to describe a disease entity.

(Imagine an upper respiratory tract infection being called the "acute cough syndrome".)

2. The diagnosis of ARDS is a problem because the diagnostic criteria are either nonspecific (e.g., acute onset) or flawed (using the wedge pressure as the hydrostatic pressure).
3. There is no treatment for ARDS. The one beneficial intervention (low-volume ventilation) is not really a treatment, but is a lessening of the harmful effects of mechanical ventilation.
4. There may never be a treatment for ARDS because it is not a single entity, but is an expression of several diverse conditions.

REFERENCES

Reviews

1. Ware LB, Matthay MA. The acute respiratory distress syndrome. N Engl J Med 2000;342:1334–1349.
2. Abraham E, Matthay MA, Dinarello C, et al. Consensus conference definitions for sepsis, septic shock, acute lung injury and acute respiratory distress syndrome: time for a reevaluation. Crit Care Med 2000;28:232–235.
3. The Fourth Margaux Conference on Critical Illness. Acute lung injury: understanding mechanisms of injury and repair. Crit Care Med 2003;31(suppl):S183–S337.

Pathogenesis

4. Petty TL. The acute respiratory distress syndrome: historical perspective. Chest 1994;105(suppl):44S–46S.
5. Abraham E. Neutrophils and acute lung injury. Crit Care Med 2003;31(suppl): S195–S199.
6. Idell S. Coagulation, fibrinolysis, and fibrin deposition in acute lung injury. Crit Care Med 2003;31(suppl):S213–S220.
7. Hudson LD, Milberg JA, Anardi D, et al. Clinical risks for development of the acute respiratory distress syndrome. Am Rev Respir Crit Care Med 1995; 151:293–301.

Clinical Features

8. Bernard GR, Artigas A, Brigham KL, et al. The American–European Consensus Conference on ARDS: definitions, mechanisms, relevant outcomes, and clinical trial coordination. Am Rev Respir Crit Care Med 1994;149:818–824.
9. Aberle DR, Brown K. Radiologic considerations in the adult respiratory distress syndrome. Clin Chest Med 1990;11:737–754.
10. Weiner-Kronish JP, Matthay MA. Pleural effusions associated with hydrostatic and increased permeability pulmonary edema. Chest 1988;93:852–858.
11. Idell S, Cohen AB. Bronchoalveolar lavage in patients with the adult respiratory distress syndrome. Clin Chest Med 1985;6:459–471.

12. Sprung CL, Long WM, Marcial EH, et al. Distribution of proteins in pulmonary edema: the value of fractional concentrations. Am Rev Respir Dis 1987;136:957–963.

Lung-Protective Ventilation

13. Rouby J-J, Puybasset L, Nieszkowska A, Lu Q. Acute respiratory distress syndrome: lessons from computed tomography of the whole lung. Crit Care Med 2003;31(suppl):S285–S295.
14. Dreyfuss D, Saumon G. Ventilator-induced lung injury. Am J Respir Crit Care Med 1998;157:294–323.
15. Ranieri VM, Suter PM, Tortorella C, et al. Effect of mechanical ventilation on inflammatory mediators in patients with acute respiratory distress syndrome: a randomized controlled trial. JAMA 1999;282:54–61.
16. Ranieri VM, Giunta F, Suter P, et al. Mechanical ventilation as a mediator of multisystem organ failure in acute respiratory distress syndrome. JAMA 2000;284:43–44.
17. Fan E, Needham DM, Stewart TE. Ventilator management of acute lung injury and acute respiratory distress syndrome. JAMA 2005;294:2889–2896.
18. The Acute Respiratory Distress Syndrome Network. Ventilation with lower tidal volumes as compared with traditional tidal volumes for acute lung injury and the acute respiratory distress syndrome. N Engl J Med 2000;342: 1301–1308.
19. Bidani A, Tzouanakis AE, Cardenas VJ, et al. Permissive hypercapnia in acute respiratory failure. JAMA 1994;272:957–962.
20. Potkin RT, Swenson ER. Resuscitation from severe acute hypercapnia: determinants of tolerance and survival. Chest 1992;102:1742–1745.
21. Hickling KG, Walsh J, Henderson S, et al. Low mortality rate in adult respiratory distress syndrome using low-volume, pressure-limited ventilation with permissive hypercapnia: a prospective study. Crit Care Med 1994;22:1568–1578.
22. Muscedere JG, Mullen JBM, Gan K, et al. Tidal ventilation at low airway pressures can augment lung injury. Am J Respir Crit Care Med 1994;149: 1327–1334.
23. The National Heart, Lung, and Blood Institute ARDS Clinical Network. Higher versus lower positive end-expiratory pressures in patients with acute respiratory distress syndrome. N Engl J Med 2004;351:327–336.

Fluid Management

24. Brower RG, Ware LB, Berthiaume Y, et al. Treatment of ARDS. Chest 2001; 120:1347–1367.
25. McIntyre RC Jr, Pulido EJ, Bensard DD, et al. Thirty years of clinical trials in acute respiratory distress syndrome. Crit Care Med 2000;28:3314–3331.

Promoting Oxygen Transport

26. Broaddus VC, Berthiaume Y, Biondi JW, et al. Hemodynamic management of the adult respiratory distress syndrome. J Intensive Care Med 1987;2:190–213.

27. Hebert PC, Blajchman MA, Cook DJ, et al. Do blood transfusions improve outcomes related to mechanical ventilation? Chest 2001;119:1850–1857.
28. Goodnough LT. Risks of blood transfusion. Crit Care Med 2003;31(suppl): S678–S686.

Pharmacotherapy

29. Bernard GR, Luce JM, Sprung CL, et al. High-dose corticosteroids in patients with adult respiratory distress syndrome. N Engl J Med 1987;317: 1565–1570.
30. Bone RC, Fischer CJ Jr, Clemmer TP, et al. Early methylprednisolone treatment for septic syndrome and the adult respiratory distress syndrome. Chest 1987;92:1032–1036.
31. Meduri GU, Chinn A. Fibrinoproliferation in late adult respiratory distress syndrome. Chest 1994;105(suppl):127S–129S.

A Case of Misdirection?

32. Montgomery AB, Stager MA, Carrico J, et al. Causes of mortality in patients with the adult respiratory distress syndrome. Am Rev Respir Dis 1985;132: 485–489.
33. Bartlett RH, Morris AH, Fairley B, et al. A prospective study of acute hypoxic respiratory failure. Chest 1986;89:684–689.
34. Gillespie DJ, Marsh HMM, Divertie MB, et al. Clinical outcome of respiratory failure in patients requiring prolonged (>24 hours) mechanical ventilation. Chest 1986;90:364–369.
35. Suchyta MR, Clemmer TP, Elliott CG, et al. The adult respiratory distress syndrome: a report of survival and modifying factors. Chest 1992;101: 1074–1079.
36. Rubenfeld GD, Caldwell E, Peabody E, et al. Incidence and outcomes of acute lung injury. N Engl J Med 2005;353:1685–1693.

Chapter 23

SEVERE AIRFLOW OBSTRUCTION

This chapter describes the acute management of patients with severe airflow obstruction as a result of asthma and chronic obstructive lung disease. The focus here is on the use of pharmacologic agents (bronchodilator drugs and corticosteroids) to relieve airways obstruction (1,2). The use of mechanical ventilation in these disorders is described in the next section of the book.

BEDSIDE MONITORING

The clinical examination is notoriously inaccurate in assessing the presence and severity of airflow obstruction (3). As a result, objective measures of airflow obstruction are needed to aid in the evaluation and treatment of diseases that involve the airways. The standard index of airflow obstruction requires measurement of the forced expiratory volume in one second (FEV_1) and the forced vital capacity (FVC): the ratio FEV_1/FVC is used as the measure of airflow obstruction (e.g., an FEV_1/FVC ratio less than 0.7 indicates the presence of airflow obstruction). Unfortunately, these measurements are not easily obtained at the bedside. The following are some measurements that are easily performed at the bedside and can be used as alternative measures of airflow obstruction.

Peak Expiratory Flow Rate

The *peak expiratory flow rate* (PEFR) is the greatest flow velocity that can be obtained during a forced exhalation starting with the lungs fully inflated. The PEFR can be measured with a hand held device like the one in Figure 23.1. This device (the Mini-Wright™ peak flowmeter) is about 6 inches in length, and weighs only 3 ounces. The patient holds the device in a horizontal position close to the mouth and inhales as much air as possible (to total lung capacity). The patient then exhales as forcefully as possible into the mouthpiece of the device. The flow of exhaled gas follows a contour like the one illustrated in Figure 23.1, with the peak flow occurring very early in exhalation, when the elastic recoil of the lungs

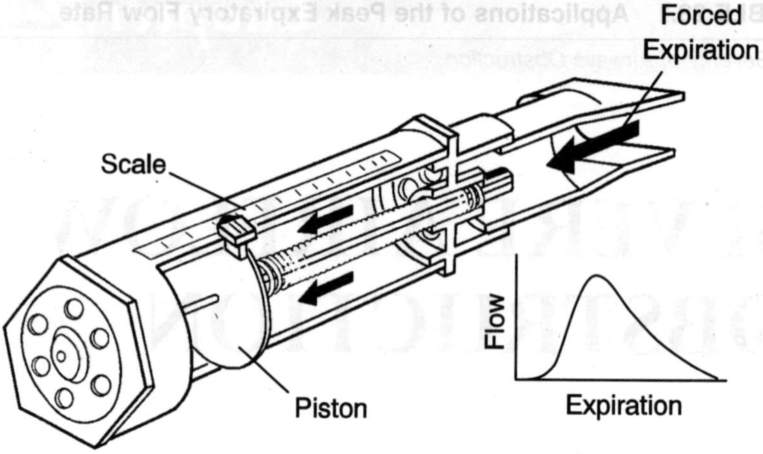

FIGURE 23.1 A hand-held device for measuring peak expiratory flow rate (the highest point on the expiratory flow contour).

is the highest and the caliber of the airways is the greatest. The flow of exhaled gas displaces a spring-loaded piston in the peak flowmeter, and a pointer attached to the piston records the displacement on a calibrated scale etched on the outer surface of the device. The pointer remains at the point of maximal displacement, which is the PEFR in liters per minute (L/min). This maneuver is repeated twice, and the highest of the three measurements is recorded as the PEFR at that time (1).

The PEFR is an effort-dependent measurement, and is reliable only when the expiratory effort is maximal (4). Therefore, it is important to observe the patient during the peak flow maneuver to determine if a maximum effort is being expended. If not, the measurement is unreliable and should be discarded.

The Normal PEFR

The PEFR varies with age, gender, race, and height (5,6), and thus reference tables are needed to interpret the PEFR in individual patients (these tables are included in the Appendix at the end of the text). Predictive formulae are also available (6), but are tedious to use. The following are some general statements regarding the normal or expected PEFR.

1. The normal range of PEFR is 500 to 700 L/min for men and 380 to 500 L/min for women (5,6). At any given age, the PEFR in an average-sized male is at least 50% higher than the PEFR in an average-sized female.
2. In both sexes, the PEFR is 15 to 20% lower at age 70 than at age 20 (5).
3. The PEFR has a diurnal variation of 10 to 20%, with the nadir in the early morning (7,8). The relevance of this in hospitalized patients (where diurnal rhythms may be lost) is not known.

TABLE 23.1 Applications of the Peak Expiratory Flow Rate

I. *Severity of Airways Obstruction*	
PEFR (% Predicted)	Interpretation
>70	Mild obstruction
50–70	Moderate obstruction
<50	Severe obstruction
<30	Respiratory failure
II. *Bronchodilator Responsiveness*	
PEFR (% Increase)	Interpretation
>15	Favorable response
10–15	Equivocal response
<10	Poor response

An alternative to the normal PEFR is the *personal best* PEFR, which is obtained when the patient is free of symptoms. This eliminates the multiple variables that must be considered when identifying the normal PEFR.

Clinical Applications

The PEFR can be used to evaluate the severity of airways obstruction and the response to bronchodilator therapy using the criteria shown in Table 23.1 (1). An example of how these criteria can be used is shown in the flow diagram in Figure 23.2.

Bronchodilator Need

Inhaled bronchodilators are often ordered routinely for hospitalized patients with a history of chronic obstructive lung disease (COPD) without determining if an individual patient responds favorably to bronchodilators. This practice does not seem justified because patients with COPD are poorly responsive to inhaled bronchodilators (which is one of the features that distinguishes COPD from asthma). The PEFR can help by providing a bedside test of bronchodilator responsiveness (see Table 23.1). The PEFR can be recorded just before, and again 20 minutes after, a bronchodilator aerosol treatment (the respiratory therapy department will perform the peak flow measurements on request). If the PEFR increases by 15% or more after the treatment (indicating a favorable response), then therapy with bronchodilator aerosols can be continued. If the post-bronchodilator PEFR does not change or increases by less than 10% (indicating a poor response), inhaled bronchodilators are not justified. This test can be performed more than once to add validity to the results.

Peak Inspiratory Pressure

Aerosol bronchodilator treatments are given routinely to ventilator dependent patients, often without documented need or benefit. One method

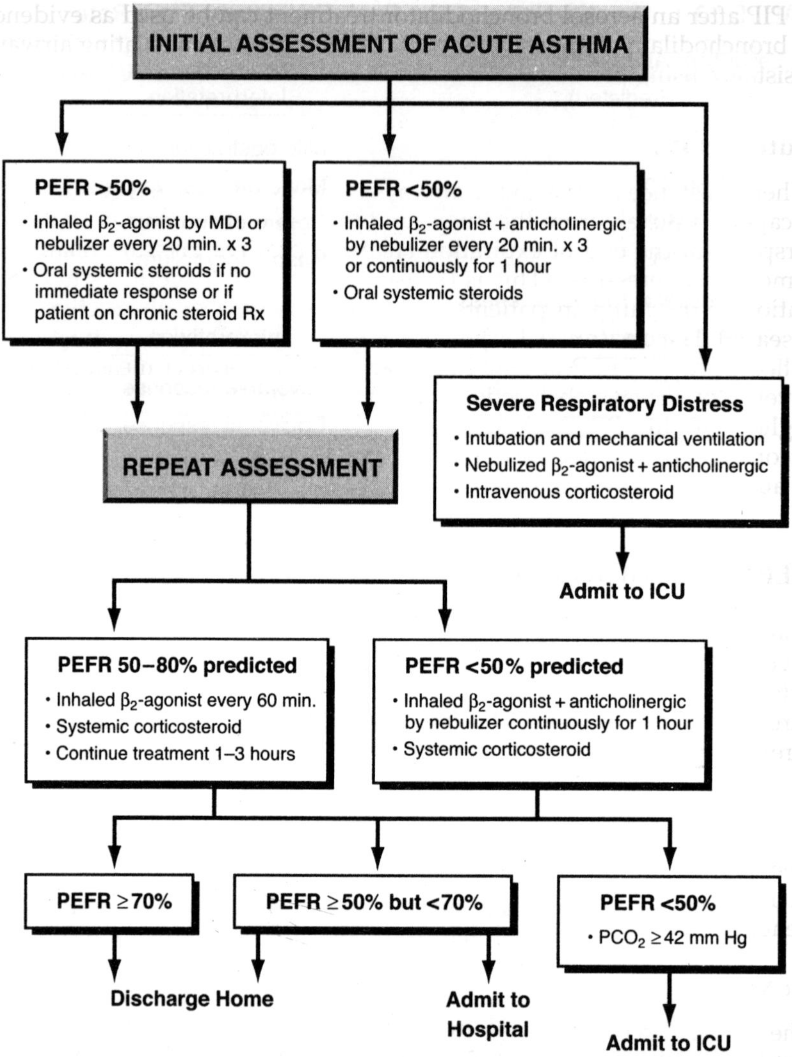

FIGURE 23.2 Protocol for the early management of acute asthma in the emergency department. *PEFR* = peak expiratory flow rate. (Adapted from the National Asthma Education Program, Expert Panel Report 2 [1].)

of assessing bronchodilator responsiveness during positive-pressure mechanical ventilation is to monitor changes in the peak inspiratory pressure (PIP), which is the pressure in the proximal airways at the end of each lung inflation. This pressure varies in the same direction as changes in the tidal volume and changes in the resistance to flow in the endotracheal tube and airways, and it varies in the opposite direction with changes in the distensibility (compliance) of the lungs. If a bronchodilator treatment has effectively decreased airways resistance, the PIP will also decrease. Therefore, assuming all other variables are constant, a decrease in PIP after an aerosol bronchodilator treatment can be used as evidence of bronchodilator responsiveness (9). A technique for calculating airways resistance using proximal airways pressures is described in Chapter 24.

Auto-PEEP

When resistance to flow in the airways is increased, exhaled gas does not escape completely from the lungs, and the gas that remains in the distal airspaces at the end of expiration creates a positive pressure relative to atmospheric pressure. (This is the same process that produces hyperinflation of the lungs in patients with severe asthma or obstructive lung disease.) The *positive end-expiratory pressure* (PEEP) in this situation is called intrinsic PEEP or *auto-PEEP*, and it is an indirect measure of the severity of airways obstruction. (The greater the airflow obstruction, the higher the auto-PEEP.) A favorable bronchodilator response should be accompanied by a decrease in the level of auto-PEEP. The measurement of auto-PEEP is described in Chapter 26.

AEROSOL DRUG THERAPY

The management of patients with severe airflow obstruction usually involves the administration of drugs directly into the airways. This is achieved by creating aerosols of drug solutions that can be inhaled directly into the airways. The following is a brief description of the different methods of aerosol therapy.

Aerosol Generators

The two devices used to generate bronchodilator aerosols are depicted in Figure 23.3 (see reference 10 for a detailed description of aerosol generators).

Jet Nebulizer

The jet nebulizer operates on the same principle as the high flow oxygen mask shown in Figure 21.4. One end of a narrow capillary tube is submerged in the drug solution, and a rapidly flowing stream of gas is passed over the other end of the tube. This gas jet creates a viscous drag that draws the drug solution up the capillary tube, and when the solution reaches the gas jet, it is pulverized to form the aerosol spray, which is then carried to the patient with the inspiratory gas flow. Small volume jet nebulizers use a reservoir volume of 3 to 6 mL (drug solution plus saline diluent) and can completely aerosolize the reservoir volume in less than 10 minutes.

Metered-Dose Inhaler

The metered dose inhaler (MDI) operates in much the same way as a canister of hair spray. The device has a pressurized canister that contains a drug solution with a boiling point below room temperature. When the canister is squeezed between the thumb and fingers, a valve opens that

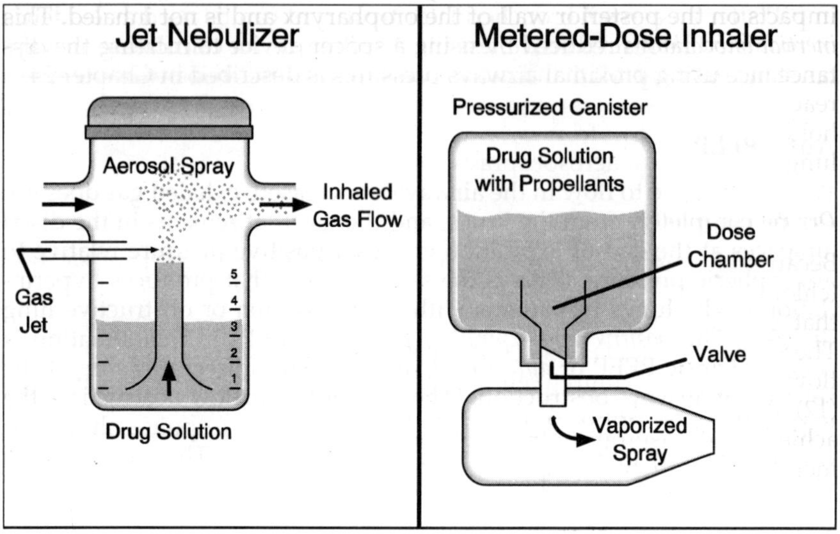

FIGURE 23.3 Small-volume aerosol generators.

releases a fixed volume of the drug solution. The liquid immediately vaporizes when it emerges from the canister, and a liquid propellant in the solution creates a high-velocity spray. The spray emerging from the canister can have a velocity in excess of 30 meters per second (over 60 miles per hour) (11). Because of the high velocity of the emerging spray, when an MDI is placed in the mouth, most of the aerosol spray

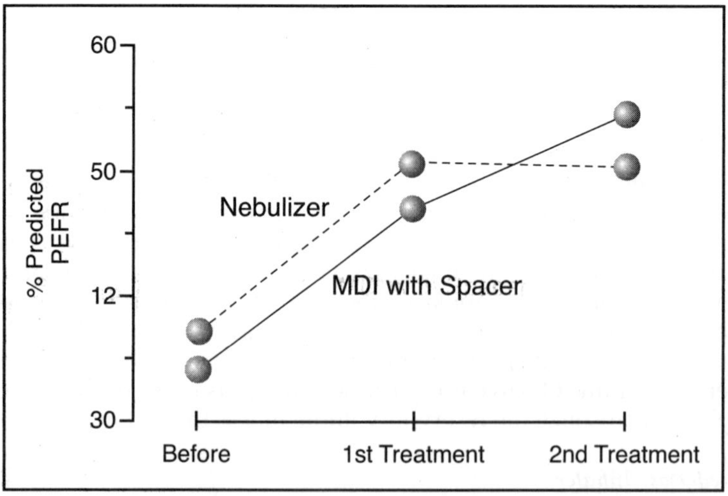

FIGURE 23.4 Bronchodilator responses to albuterol delivered by a nebulizer (2.5 mg per treatment) and a metered-dose inhaler (*MDI*) (0.4 mg per treatment) in patients with acute exacerbation of asthma. *PEFR* = peak expiratory flow rate. (Data from Idris AH, et al. Emergency department treatment of severe asthma. Chest 1993;103:665–672.)

impacts on the posterior wall of the oropharynx and is not inhaled. This *inertial impaction* is reduced by using a spacer device to increase the distance between the MDI and mouth (this reduces the velocity of the spray reaching the mouth). Spacer devices (which are usually chambers that hold several sprays from an MDI) are now used routinely to improve lung deposition of aerosol sprays from MDIs.

Dry Powder Inhalers

Because of concern for the environmental hazards of liquid propellants (chlorofluorocarbons) used in MDIs, alternative inhalers were developed that produce micronized particles from powdered drug preparations. These *dry powder inhalers* require patients to generate high inspiratory flow rates (≥60 L/min) to ensure proper drug deposition in the airways (12). Because patients with severe airflow obstruction may not be able to achieve high inspiratory flow rates, dry powder inhalers are not recommended for patients with severe airflow obstruction.

Nebulizer versus Metered-Dose Inhaler

The dose of bronchodilators delivered by nebulizers is much greater than the dose delivered by MDIs (see Table 23.2), but the bronchodilator

TABLE 23.2 Drug Therapy for Acute Exacerbation of Asthma

Drug Preparation	Dose	Comment
Short-Acting β_2-Receptor Agonist		
Albuterol nebulizer solution (5 mg/mL)	2.5–5 mg every 20 min × 3 doses, or 10–15 mg/hr continuously, then 2.5–10 mg every 1–4 hrs as needed.	Dilute nebulizer solution to 5 mL and deliver at gas flows of 6–8 L/min.
Albuterol by MDI (90 μg/puff)	4–8 puffs every 20 min up to 4 hrs, then every 1–4 hrs. as needed.	As effective as nebulizer Rx if patients able to cooperate.
Anticholinergic Agent		
Ipatropium bromide nebulizer solution (0.25 mg/mL)	0.5 mg every 20 min for 3 doses, then every 2–4 hours as needed.	Can mix in same nebulizer with albuterol. Should not be used as first-line therapy.
Ipatropium bromide by MDI (18 μg/puff)	4–8 puffs as needed.	MDI delivery has not been studied in acute asthma.
Corticosteroids		
Methylprednisolone (IV) prednisolone (oral) or prednisone (oral)	120–180 mg/day in 3 or 4 divided doses for 48 hrs, then 60–80 mg/day until PEFR reaches 70% of predicted.	No difference in efficacy between IV and oral drug administration. Takes hours for drug effect to become evident.

From Reference 1. Drug doses are for adults only.

response is often the same with both devices. This is demonstrated in Figure 23.4, which compares the response to a commonly used bronchodilator (albuterol) administered with a hand-held nebulizer (2.5 mg albuterol per treatment) or MDI with a spacer device (4 puffs or 0.36 mg albuterol per treatment) in a group of patients with severe asthma (13). After two treatments with each type of aerosol device, the increase in PEFR is equivalent. Thus, despite an almost tenfold difference in total drug dose (5 mg via nebulizer versus 0.7 mg via MDI), the bronchodilator response is the same. This discrepancy in drug doses is partly explained by the extensive drug loss (via condensation) in jet nebulizers.

Mechanical Ventilation

Both nebulizers and MDIs can be used to deliver effective bronchodilator treatments in ventilator-dependent patients (14,15). Aerosol deposition in the lungs with either device is reduced in intubated, mechanically ventilated patients compared with non-intubated, spontaneously breathing subjects (15), so the dose of aerosol bronchodilator may need to be increased in ventilator-dependent patients. The response to MDIs is best when a spacer is used (15): the spacer is connected to the inspiratory limb of the ventilator tubing (via a Y-connector), and five puffs from the MDI are actuated into the spacer and are inhaled during the ensuing lung inflations. Regardless of the aerosol device used, drug delivery into the airways can be enhanced by (16): (*a*) turning the humidifier off, (*b*) decreasing the inspiratory flow rate, and (*c*) increasing the inspiratory time.

Summary

Equivalent bronchodilator responses to nebulizer and metered-dose aerosols have been documented in both spontaneously breathing and ventilator-dependent patients (14–17). The lower doses used by MDIs provides a less costly method of aerosol bronchodilator therapy than nebulizer drug treatments. Because of the benefits in cost and labor, **metered-dose inhalers should be the favored method of aerosol bronchodilator therapy in the hospital setting.**

ACUTE MANAGEMENT OF ASTHMA

The management of adult patients with an acute exacerbation of asthma is summarized in Table 23.2 and Figure 23.2.

β_2-Receptor Agonists

The favored bronchodilators in asthma are drugs that stimulate β-adrenergic receptors in bronchial smooth muscle (β-2 subtype) to promote smooth muscle relaxation (12). Aerosol delivery of these β_2-*agonists* is the preferred mode of treatment because it is more effective than oral (18) or intravenous (19) drug therapy, and has fewer side effects. Short-acting β_2-agonists are preferred for the acute management of asthma because these drugs can be given in rapid succession with less risk of drug accumulation in the body. The most extensively used short-acting β_2-agonist is **albuterol**, which has a rapid onset of action (less than 5 minutes) when inhaled, and a bronchodilator effect that lasts 2–5 hours (12). Other short-acting β_2-agonists available for use in acute asthma include metaproterenol, bitolterol, pibuterol, and levalbuterol, but none of these agents has been studied as extensively as albuterol in acute asthma. For this reason, the description of β_2-agonist therapy in acute asthma will focus only on albuterol.

Intermittent versus Continuous Aerosol Therapy

For acute exacerbation of asthma, there are two recommended regimens for aerosol therapy with albuterol (1,2). The first regimen involves a series of repetitive 20-minute treatments using a nebulizer (with an albuterol dose of 2.5–5 mg per treatment) or an MDI (4–8 puffs per treatment with a dose of 90 µg albuterol per puff). The second regimen involves more continuous one-hour nebulizer treatments using 10–15 mg albuterol per treatment. Studies of these two regimens have revealed the following:

1. When using repetitive aerosol treatments every 20 minutes, there is no advantage to using an albuterol dose greater than 2.5 mg per treatment (20,21).
2. Most studies show no difference in efficacy between the continuous and repetitive aerosol regimens in acute asthma (20,22).

Continuous aerosol therapy is favored by many because it is easier to administer than the repetitive aerosol treatments.

Parenteral Therapy

For the rare asthmatic patient who does not tolerate bronchodilator aerosols (usually because of excessive coughing) parenteral therapy can be given using subcutaneous epinephrine (0.3 to 0.5 mg every 20 minutes for 3 doses) or subcutaneous terbutaline (0.25 mg every 20 minutes for 3 doses) (1). It is important to remember that parenteral β-agonist therapy (including intravenous therapy) offers no advantage over inhaled therapy, and is more likely to produce unwanted side effects (19,23)

Side Effects

High-dose aerosol therapy with β_2-agonists can produce a number of side effects, including tachycardia, tremors (from stimulation of skeletal muscle β_2-receptors), hyperglycemia, and a decrease in serum potassium, magnesium, and phosphate levels (12,24,25). Cardiac ischemia has been reported, but is rare (24). The **decrease in serum potassium** is the result of a β-receptor mediated shift of potassium into cells. This effect is particularly notable because large doses of inhaled β_2-agonists (e.g., 20 mg albuterol) can be used for the acute management of hyperkalemia (26).

Anticholinergic Agents

Despite conflicting results from clinical trials, aerosolized anticholinergic agents are recommended in combination with β_2-agonists for the treatment of acute asthma (1,27). The only anticholinergic agent approved for clinical use in the United States is **ipatropium bromide**, a derivative of atropine that blocks muscarinic receptors in the airways. The recommended aerosol dose in acute asthma is 0.5 mg (which can be mixed with albuterol in the nebulizer) every 20 minutes for 3 doses, then every 2 to 4 hours as needed, or 4–8 puffs (18 μg per puff) by MDI (1). Systemic absorption is minimal, so anticholinergic side effects (tachycardia, dry mouth, blurred vision, urinary retention) are minimal. Ipatropium is not a first-line bronchodilator drug in asthma, and is recommended in combination with β_2-agonist bronchodilator therapy.

Corticosteroids

Corticosteroids have enjoyed a 50-year reign of popularity in the management of asthma. The reason for this popularity is the anti-inflammatory effects of corticosteroids. In acute asthma, bronchospasm is an early manifestation, but lasts only 30 to 60 minutes. A second episode of airway obstruction occurs 3 to 8 hours later, and is caused by inflammation and edema in the walls of the small airways (28). Thus, bronchodilators should be effective in the early stages of acute asthma, whereas anti-inflammatory agents like corticosteroids should be effective in the later stages. This may explain why steroid effects may not be apparent for 12 hours after therapy is started (29).

The relative potencies of the different therapeutic corticosteroids is shown in Table 23.3. Note that dexamethasone is the most potent anti-inflammatory corticosteroid. If the efficacy of steroids in asthma is due to their anti-inflammatory actions, then why is dexamethasone almost never used to treat asthma? I will leave you to consider the answer to this question.

Steroids in Acute Asthma

According to the National Asthma Education Program (1,2), steroids are recommended for virtually *all* patients with acute asthma (see Fig. 23.2), even those who respond favorably to bronchodilators (where steroids are

TABLE 23.3 Comparison of Therapeutic Corticosteroids

Corticosteroid	Equivalent Dose (mg)	RAIA*	RSR†
Hydrocortisone	20	1	20
Prednisone	5	3.5	1
Methylprednisolone	4	5	0.5
Dexamethasone	0.75	30–40	0

*RAIA = relative anti-inflammatory activity.
†RSR = relative sodium retention.
From Zeiss CR. Intense pharmacotherapy. Chest 1992;101(Suppl):407S.

used to prevent relapse). The steroid preparations used most often in acute asthma are **methylprednisolone** (for intravenous therapy) and **prednisone** (for oral therapy), and the recommended dose of either is 30 to 40 mg every 6 hours (120 to 160 mg daily) for the first 48 hours, then 60 to 80 mg daily until the PEFR normalizes or reaches baseline levels. The following statements regarding steroid therapy in acute asthma deserve mention:

1. There is no difference in efficacy between oral and intravenous steroids (29).
2. The beneficial effects of steroids may not be apparent until 12 hours after therapy is started (29). Therefore, steroid therapy should not be expected to influence the clinical course of asthma in the emergency department.
3. There is no clearly defined dose-response curve for steroids, which means that higher doses of steroids are not superior to lower doses (29).
4. A 10-day course of steroids can be stopped abruptly without a tapering dose (30).
5. Some clinical studies show *no* benefit from steroid therapy in acute asthma (31–33).

Despite the overwhelming popularity of steroids in acute asthma, clinical studies often show meager (if any) responses to these agents in the acute care setting. This is consistent with the continued but unjustified popularity of steroids in other inflammatory conditions like septic shock and acute respiratory distress syndrome.

Steroid Myopathy

A myopathy has been reported in ventilator-dependent asthmatic patients treated with high dose steroids and neuromuscular blocking agents (34). Unlike the traditional steroid myopathy, which is characterized by proximal muscle weakness, the myopathy in ventilator dependent asthmatics involves both proximal and distal muscles, and is often associated with rhabdomyolysis. The etiology of this destructive myopathy is unknown, but the combination of steroids and paralyzing drugs is somehow involved. The muscle weakness can be prolonged and can hamper weaning from mechanical ventilation. Once the disorder is suspected, rapid taper of the paralyzing agents and steroids is advised. This disorder is usually reversible. (For more information on muscle weakness syndromes in ventilator-dependent patients, see Chapter 51.)

Other Measures

The following are some additional recommendations for the management of acute asthma:

1. The presence of wheezing does not always mean the presence of asthma. Other causes of wheezing include acute left heart failure (cardiac asthma), upper airway obstruction (wheezing may be

inspiratory), bronchopneumonia (wheezing may be localized), and anaphylaxis.

2. Supplemental oxygen is not justified if the arterial O_2 saturation measured by pulse oximetry is 92% or higher.
3. Chest x-rays are not necessary unless there is suspicion of pneumonia (e.g., fever and purulent sputum), acute pulmonary edema, or some other intrathoracic problem.
4. Arterial blood gases are not necessary unless the patient is *in extremis*, is cyanotic, or is refractory to initial bronchodilator therapy.
5. Antibiotics are not necessary unless there is specific evidence of a *treatable* infection.

Asthma is not a single disease entity, which means that the evaluation and management of acute asthma should be tailored to the individual patient, not the condition. The heterogeneity of asthma may explain why some patients respond promptly to therapy (with bronchodilators and steroids), while others do not.

CHRONIC OBSTRUCTIVE PULMONARY DISEASE

Chronic obstructive pulmonary disease (COPD) is the term used to describe patients with constant airflow obstruction (FEV_1/FVC <70%) as a result of chronic bronchitis or emphysema. This condition is distinguished from asthma by limited responsiveness to bronchodilator therapy and the steady or chronic nature of the symptomatology (which usually involves dyspnea). Patients with COPD experience 1 or 2 episodes a year where there is a worsening of their dyspnea over a few days, often accompanied by an increase in the quantity or quality of sputum production. These *exacerbations* of COPD are responsible for about half a million hospital admissions yearly in the United States, and half of these admissions require care in an ICU (35).

Bronchodilator Therapy

Despite the limited responsiveness to bronchodilators that characterizes COPD, bronchodilators are used routinely in patients with COPD (often without objective evidence of benefit). For acute exacerbations of COPD, the same aerosol bronchodilators used in the acute management of asthma (albuterol and ipatropium) are recommended, but the aggressive use of bronchodilators in acute asthma (see Fig. 23.2) is not advocated for exacerbations of COPD. Also unlike asthma, the bronchodilating effects of ipatropium are equal to those of the β_2-agonists like albuterol, and ipatropium can be used alone as a bronchodilator in acute exacerbations of COPD (36,37). The common practice is to combine β_2-agonists and ipatropium, although at least three clinical studies do not support this practice (37).

Corticosteroids

A short course (2 weeks) of corticosteroid therapy is recommended for all patients with acute exacerbation of COPD (35–37). One example of an effective two-week steroid regimen is shown below (38).

Methylprednisolone: 125 mg IV every 6 hrs on days 1–3, then

Prednisone: 60 mg once daily on days 4–7,
40 mg once daily on days 8–11,
20 mg once daily on days 12–15.

This regimen was used in the largest clinical trial of steroid therapy in acute exacerbations of COPD (38), and the results are shown in Figure 23.5 (the shaded area highlights the difference between patients who received steroids and patients who received placebo). The steroid-treated patients show a greater increase in FEV_1 in the first day of treatment (although the difference in FEV_1 is only about 120 mL, which may not be clinically significant), and this effect lasts for at least three days. It is lost by two weeks (the time when steroids are usually discontinued). The only significant side effect of this steroid treatment protocol is hyperglycemia, which occurs mostly in diabetic patients (38).

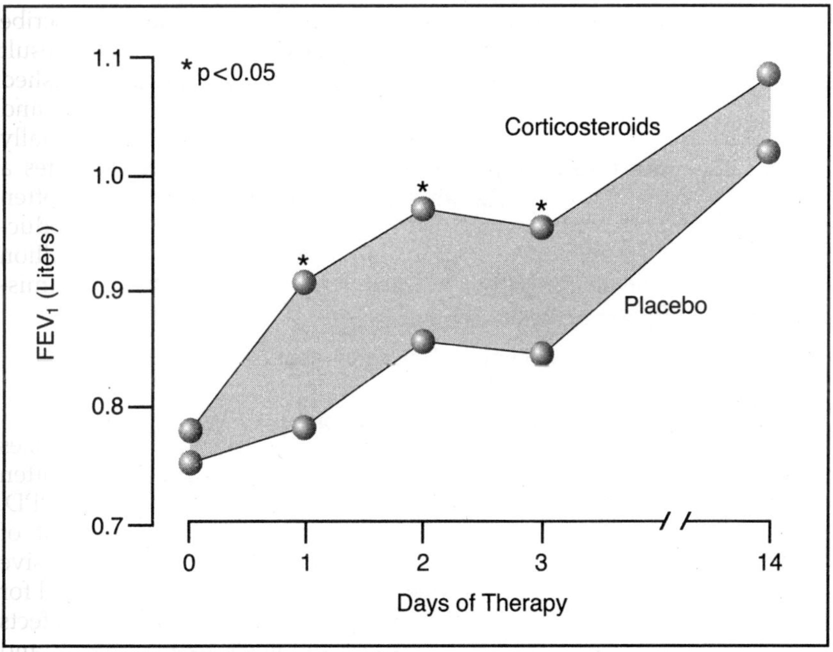

FIGURE 23.5 Effects of a two-week course of steroid therapy on airway function in patients with acute exacerbation of COPD. FEV_1, is the forced expired volume in one second. Asterisks mark a significant difference between steroid-treated and placebo-treated patients (From Reference 38).

Antibiotics

Infection in the upper airways is believed to be the culprit in 80% of cases of acute exacerbation of COPD, and bacteria are isolated in about 50 to 60% of cases (39). The infections are usually polymicrobial, and the most frequent isolates that can be treated with antimicrobial agents are *Chlamydia pneumoniae, Haemophilus influenzae,* and *Streptococcus pneumoniae* (39).

Despite the prevalence of airway infection, the benefit of antimicrobial therapy in acute exacerbation of COPD has been debated for years. The major concern is that repeated use of antibiotics in this patient population had led to the emergence of antimicrobial resistance in many of the isolates (37,39). The most recent evidence using pooled data from 11 clinical trials indicates that antimicrobial therapy is justified (because of greater increments in airflow and more rapid resolution of symptoms) in patients with severe exacerbations who are at risk for a poor outcome (37). Sputum cultures are not necessary, and **antibiotic selection is based on the likelihood of a poor outcome**. A protocol for antibiotic selection based on risk assessment is shown in Table 23.4. The optimal duration of antimicrobial therapy is not known: the common practice is to continue therapy for at least 7 days.

Oxygen Inhalation

In patients with severe COPD and chronic hypercapnia, the unregulated use of inhaled oxygen can result in further increases in arterial PCO_2. This phenomenon was first described in 1967 (40), and the rise in PCO_2 was attributed to relative hypoventilation from loss of hypoxic

TABLE 23.4 Antibiotic Selection for Acute Exacerbation of COPD Based on Risk Assessment

I. *Risk Assessment:*		
Answer the following questions:	YES	NO
1. Is the FEV_1 less than 50% of predicted?	☐	☐
2. Does the patient have cardiac disease or other significant comorbid conditions?	☐	☐
3. Has the patient had 3 or more exacerbations in the previous 12 months?	☐	☐
If the answer is YES to at least one of these questions, the patient is considered to be high-risk for an unfavorable outcome.		
II. *Antibiotic Selection*		
High Risk Patients: Amoxicillin-clavulanate or a newer fluoroquinolone (gatifloxacin, levofloxacin, or moxifloxacin),		
Low Risk Patients: Doxycycline, a second-generation cephalosporin (e.g., cefuroxime) or a newer macrolide (azithromycin or clarithromycin).		

From Sethi S. Acute exacerbation of COPD: A "multipronged" approach. J Respir Dis 2002; 23:217–225.

ventilatory drive. This is no longer considered to be the explanation for this phenomenon because the oxygen-induced rise in arterial PCO_2 is not accompanied by a decrease in ventilatory drive (41). (An increase in dead space ventilation may play a role in this phenomenon.) Regardless of the mechanism, it is important to avoid unregulated use of inhaled oxygen in patients with hypercapnic COPD to prevent unwanted increases in arterial PCO_2. The best practice in this regard is to monitor the arterial oxyhemoglobin saturation (SaO_2) with pulse oximetry and maintain the SaO_2 at about 90% and *no higher*. There is no evidence that raising the SaO_2 above 90% will increase tissue oxygenation, so the common practice of maintaining the SaO_2 at 95% or higher has no scientific basis.

A FINAL WORD

The acute management of asthma and COPD can be reduced to the following simple scheme: *Give bronchodilators and steroids and wait to see what happens* (add antibiotics to the scheme for COPD). This is the same scheme that has been used for the past 30 to 40 years—only the drugs change with time.

REFERENCES

Clinical Practice Guidelines

1. National Asthma Education and Prevention Program Expert Panel Report 2. Guidelines for the diagnosis and management of asthma. NIH Publication No. 97-4051, July, 1997. (Available at www.nhlbi.nih.gov/guidelines/asthma)
2. National Asthma Education and Prevention Program Expert Panel Report. Guidelines for the diagnosis and management of asthma. Update on selected topics, 2002. NIH Publication No. 02-5074, June, 2003. (Available at www.nhlbi.nih.gov/guidelines/asthma)

Bedside Monitoring

3. Shim CS, Williams MH. Evaluation of the severity of asthma: patients versus physicians. Am J Med 1980;68:11–13.
4. Tantucci C. The best peak expiratory flow is flow-limited and effort-independent in normal subjects. Am J Respir Crit Care Med 2002;165:1304–1308.
5. Leiner GC. Expiratory peak flow rate: Standard values from normal subjects. Am Rev Respir Dis 1963;88:644.
6. Hankinson J, Odencrantz J, Ferdan K. Spirometric reference values from a sample of the general U.S. population. Am Rev Respir Crit Care Med 1999;159:179–187.
7. Quackenboss JJ, Lebowitz MD, Kryzyzanowski M. The normal range of diurnal changes in peak expiratory flow rate. Am Rev Respir Dis 1991;143:323–330.
8. Jain P, Kavuru MS, Emerman CL, et al. Utility of peak expiratory flow monitoring. Chest 1998;114:861–876.

9. Gay PC, Rodarte JR, Tayyab M, et al. Evaluation of bronchodilator responsiveness in mechanically ventilated patients. Am Rev Respir Dis 1987;136:880–885.

Aerosol Drug Therapy

10. Kacmarek RM. Humidity and aerosol therapy. In: Pierson DJ, Kacmarek RM, eds. Foundations of respiratory care. New York: Churchill Livingstone, 1992: 793–824.
11. Clarke SW, Newman SP. Differences between pressurized aerosol and stable dust particles. Chest 1981;80(suppl):907–908.
12. Dutta EJ, Li JTC. β-agonists. Med Clin North Am 2002;86:991–1008.
13. Idris AH, McDermott MF, Raucci JC, et al. Emergency department treatment of severe asthma: metered-dose inhaler plus holding chamber is equivalent in effectiveness to nebulizer. Chest 1993;103:665–672.
14. Dhand R, Tobin MJ. Pulmonary perspective: inhaled bronchodilator therapy in mechanically ventilated patients. Am J Respir Crit Care Med 1997;156: 3–10.
15. AARC Clinical Practice Guideline. Selection of device, administration of bronchodilator, and evaluation of response to therapy in mechanically ventilated patients. Respir Care 1999;44:105–113.
16. Mantous CA, Hall JB. Update on using therapeutic aerosols in mechanically ventilated patients. J Crit Illness 1996;11:457–468.
17. Smalldone GC. Aerosolized bronchodilators in the intensive care unit. Am Rev Respir Crit Care Med 1999;159:1029–1030.

Management of Acute Asthma

18. Shim C, Williams MH. Bronchial response to oral versus aerosol metaproterenol in asthma. Ann Intern Med 1980;93:428–431.
19. Salmeron S, Brochard L. Mal H, et al. Nebulized versus intravenous albuterol in hypercapnic acute asthma. Am J Respir Crit Care Med 1994;149:1466–1470.
20. Rubenfeld JMF, Georgas SN. The treatment of acute severe asthma in the adult: an overview. Formulary 2003;38:538–544.
21. Emerman CL, Cydulka RK, McFadden ER. Comparison of 2.5 vs 7.5 mg of inhaled albuterol in the treatment of acute asthma. Chest 1999;115:92–96.
22. Rodrigo GJ, Rodrigo C. Continuous vs. intermittent beta-agonists in the treatment of acute adult asthma: a systematic review with meta-analyses. Chest 2002;122:1982–1987.
23. Travers AH, Rowe BH, Barker S, et al. The effectiveness of IV beta-agonists in treating patients with acute asthma in the emergency department: a meta-analysis. Chest 2002;122:1200–1207.
24. Truwit JD. Toxic effect of bronchodilators. Crit Care Clin 1991;7:639–657.
25. Bodenhamer J, Bergstrom R, Brown D, et al. Frequently nebulized beta agonists for asthma: effects on serum electrolytes. Ann Emerg Med 1992;21:1337–1342.
26. Allon M, Dunlay R, Copkney C. Nebulized albuterol for acute hyperkalemia in patients on hemodialysis. Ann Intern Med 1989;110:426–429.

27. Rodrigo G, Rodrigo C. The role of anticholinergics in acute asthma treatment: an evidence-based evaluation. Chest 2002;121:1977–1987.
28. Kay AB. Asthma and inflammation. J Allergy Clin Immunol 1991;87:893–945.
29. Rodrigo G, Rodrigo C. Corticosteroids in the emergency department therapy of acute adult asthma: an evidence-based evaluation. Chest 1999;116:285–295.
30. Cydulka RK, Emerman CL. A pilot study of steroid therapy after emergency department treatment of acute asthma: is a taper needed? J Emerg Med 1998; 16:15–19.
31. Stein LM, Cole RP. Early administration of corticosteroids in emergency room treatment of asthma. Ann Intern Med 1990;112:822–827.
32. Bowler SD, Mitchell CA, Armstrong JG. Corticosteroids in acute severe asthma: effectiveness of low doses. Thorax 1992;47:584–587.
33. Morrell F, Orriols R, de Gracia J, et al. Controlled trial of intravenous corticosteroids in severe acute asthma. Thorax 1992;47:588–591.
34. Griffin D, Fairman N, Coursin D, et al. Acute myopathy during treatment of status asthmaticus with corticosteroids and steroidal muscle relaxants. Chest 1992;102:510–514.

Chronic Obstructive Pulmonary Disease

35. Stoller JK. Acute exacerbations of chronic obstructive pulmonary disease. N Engl J Med 2002;346:988–994.
36. Snow V, Lascher S, Mottur-Pilson C, for the Joint Expert Panel on COPD of the American College of Chest Physicians and the American College of Physicians-American Society of Internal Medicine. The evidence base for management of acute exacerbations of COPD. Chest 2001;119:1185–1189.
37. McCrory DC, Brown C, Gelfand SE, et al. Management of acute exacerbations of COPD: a summary and appraisal of published evidence. Chest 2001; 119:1190–1209.
38. Niewoehner DE, Erbland ML, Deupree RH, et al. Effect of systemic glucocorticoids on exacerbations of chronic obstructive pulmonary disease. N Engl J Med 1999;340:1941–1947.
39. Sethi S. Acute exacerbations of COPD: a "multipronged" approach. J Respir Dis 2002;23:217–225.
40. Campbell EJM. The J. Burns Amberson Lecture: The management of acute respiratory failure in chronic bronchitis and emphysema. Am Rev Respir Dis 1967; 96:626–639.
41. Aubier M, Murciano D, Fournier M, et al. Central respiratory drive in acute respiratory failure or patients with chronic obstructive pulmonary disease. Am Rev Respir Dis 1980;122:191–199.

Section VIII

MECHANICAL VENTILATION

All who drink of this remedy will recover . . . except those in whom it does not help, who will die. Therefore, it is obvious that it fails only in incurable diseases.

GALEN

Chapter 24

PRINCIPLES OF MECHANICAL VENTILATION

". . . an opening must be attempted in the trunk of the trachea, into which a tube of reed or cane should be put; you will then blow into this, so that the lung may rise again . . . and the heart becomes strong . . ."

Andreas Vesalius (1555)

Vesalius is credited with the first description of positive-pressure ventilation, but it took 400 years to apply his concept to patient care. The occasion was the polio epidemic of 1955, when the demand for assisted ventilation outgrew the supply of negative-pressure tank ventilators (known as *iron lungs*). In Sweden, all medical schools shut down and medical students worked in 8-hour shifts as human ventilators, manually inflating the lungs of afflicted patients. In Boston, the nearby Emerson Company made available a prototype positive-pressure lung inflation device, which was put to use at the Massachusetts General Hospital, and became an instant success. Thus began the era of positive-pressure mechanical ventilation (and the era of intensive care medicine).

CONVENTIONAL MECHANICAL VENTILATION

The first positive-pressure ventilators were designed to inflate the lungs until a preset pressure was reached. This type of *pressure-cycled* ventilation fell out of favor because the inflation volume varied with changes in the mechanical properties of the lungs. In contrast, *volume-cycled* ventilation, which inflates the lungs to a predetermined volume, delivers a constant alveolar volume despite changes in the mechanical properties of the lungs. For this reason, volume-cycled ventilation has become the standard method of positive-pressure mechanical ventilation (1–3).

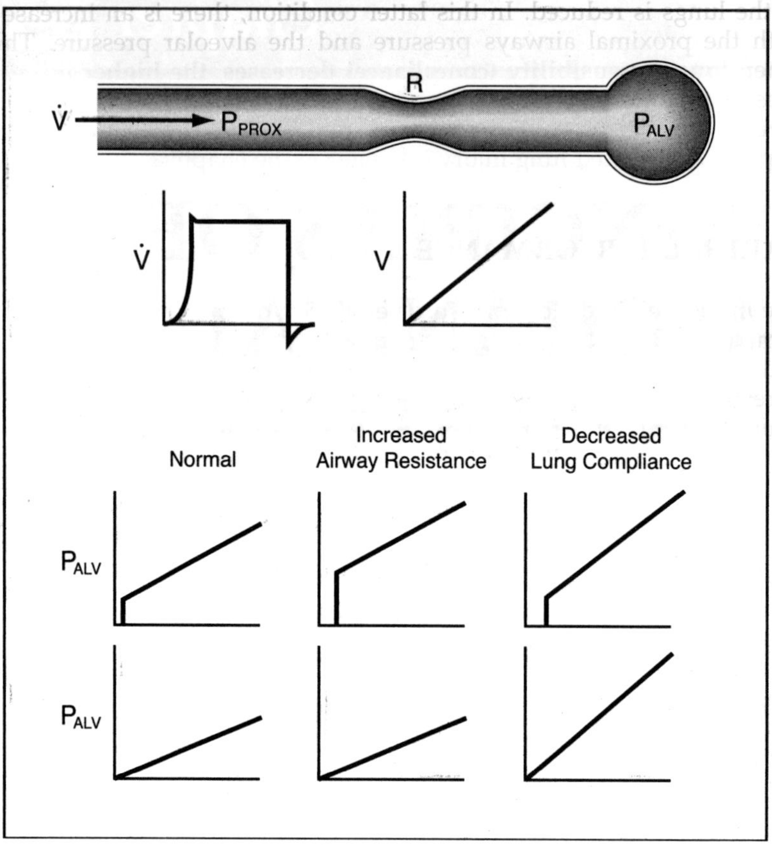

FIGURE 24.1 Waveforms produced by constant-flow, volume-cycled ventilation. $\dot{V}$ = inspiratory flow rate, V = inspiratory volume, R = flow resistance in the airways, P_{prox} = proximal airway pressure, P_{ALV} = alveolar pressure.

Inflation Pressures

The waveforms produced by volume-cycled ventilation are shown in Figure 24.1. The lungs are inflated at a constant flow rate, and this produces a steady increase in lung volume. The pressure in the proximal airways (P_{prox}) shows an abrupt initial rise, followed by a more gradual rise through the remainder of lung inflation. However, the pressure in the alveoli (P_{ALV}) shows only a gradual rise during lung inflation.

The early, abrupt rise in proximal airway pressure is a reflection of flow resistance in the airways. An increase in airways resistance magnifies the initial rise in proximal airway pressure, while the alveolar pressure at the end of lung inflation remains unchanged. Thus, **when resistance in the airways increases,** higher inflation pressures are needed to deliver the inflation volume, but **the alveoli are not exposed to the higher inflation pressures.** This is not the case when the distensibility (compliance) of the lungs is reduced. In this latter condition, there is an increase in both the proximal airways pressure and the alveolar pressure. Thus, **when lung distensibility (compliance) decreases, the higher inflation pressures** needed to deliver the inflation volume **are transmitted to the alveoli.** The increase in alveolar pressure in noncompliant lungs can lead to pressure-induced lung injury (see later in the chapter).

CARDIAC PERFORMANCE

The influence of positive-pressure ventilation on cardiac performance is complex, and involves changes in preload and afterload for both the right and left sides of the heart (4). To describe these changes, it is important to review the influence of intrathoracic pressure on transmural pressure, which is the pressure that determines ventricular filling (preload) and the resistance to ventricular emptying (afterload).

Transmural Pressure

The transmission of intrathoracic pressure into the lumen of intrathoracic blood vessels is described briefly in Chapter 10 (see Fig. 10.1). The influence of lung mechanics on this pressure transmission is illustrated in Figure 24.2. The panel on the left shows what happens when a normal lung is inflated with 700 mL from a positive-pressure source. In this situation, the increase in alveolar pressure is completely transmitted into the pulmonary capillaries, and there is no change in transmural pressure (P_{tm}) across the capillaries. However, when the same lung inflation

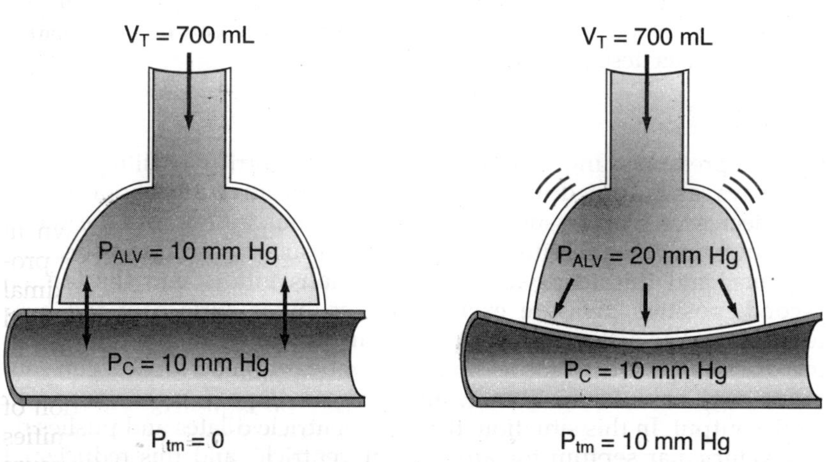

FIGURE 24.2 Alveolar–capillary units showing the transmission of alveolar pressure (P_{ALV}) to the pulmonary capillaries in normal and noncompliant (stiff) lungs. P_c = capillary hydrostatic pressure, P_{tm} = transmural pressure across the capillary wall, V_T = tidal volume delivered by the ventilator.

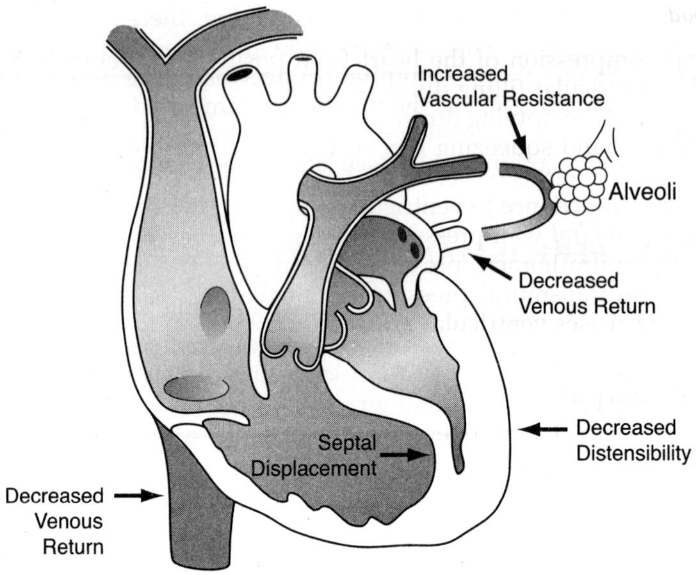

FIGURE 24.3 The mechanisms whereby positive-pressure ventilation can decrease ventricular filling (preload).

occurs in lungs that are not easily distended (panel on the right), the increase in alveolar pressure is not completely transmitted into the capillaries and the transmural pressure increases. This increase in transmural pressure acts to compress the capillaries. Therefore, in conditions associated with a decrease in lung compliance (e.g., pulmonary edema, pneumonia), positive-pressure lung inflation tends to compress the heart and intrathoracic blood vessels (5–7). This compression can be beneficial or detrimental, as described below.

Preload

Positive-pressure lung inflation can reduce ventricular filling in several ways, as indicated in Figure 24.3. First, positive intrathoracic pressure decreases the pressure gradient for venous inflow into the thorax (although positive-pressure lung inflations also increase intra-abdominal pressure, and this tends to maintain venous inflow into the thorax). Second, positive pressure exerted on the outer surface of the heart reduces cardiac distensibility, and this can reduce ventricular filling during diastole. Finally, compression of pulmonary blood vessels can raise pulmonary vascular resistance, and this can impede right ventricular stroke output. In this situation, the right ventricle dilates and pushes the interventricular septum toward the left ventricle, and this reduces left ventricular chamber size and left ventricular filling. This phenomenon, known as *ventricular interdependence*, is one of the mechanisms whereby right heart failure can impair the performance of the left side of the heart (see Fig. 14.4).

Afterload

Whereas compression of the heart from positive intrathoracic pressure impedes ventricular filling during diastole, this same compression *facilitates* ventricular emptying during systole. This latter effect is easy to visualize (like a hand squeezing the ventricles during systole) and can also be explained in terms of ventricular afterload. That is, ventricular afterload, or the impedance to ventricular emptying, is a function of the peak systolic *transmural* wall pressure (see Fig. 1.4). Incomplete transmission of positive intrathoracic pressure into the ventricular chambers will decrease the transmural pressure across the ventricles during systole, and this decreases ventricular afterload.

Cardiac Output

Positive-pressure lung inflation tends to reduce ventricular filling during diastole but enhances ventricular emptying during systole. The overall effect of positive-pressure ventilation on cardiac output depends on whether the effect on preload or afterload predominates. **When intravascular volume is normal** and intrathoracic pressures are not excessive, the effect on afterload reduction predominates, and **positive-pressure ventilation increases cardiac stroke output.** The increase in stroke volume causes an increase in systolic blood pressure during lung inflation; a phenomenon known as *reverse pulsus paradoxus*. This is demonstrated in Figure 1.5. The favorable influence of positive intrathoracic pressure on cardiac output is one mechanism that could explain the ability of chest compressions to increase cardiac output during cardiac arrest (see Chapter 15).

The beneficial actions of positive-pressure ventilation on cardiac output are reversed by hypovolemia. **When intravascular volume is reduced,** the predominant effect of positive intrathoracic pressure is to reduce ventricular preload and, in this setting, **positive-pressure ventilation decreases cardiac stroke output.** This emphasizes the importance of avoiding hypovolemia in the management of ventilator-dependent patients.

INDICATIONS FOR MECHANICAL VENTILATION

The decision to intubate and initiate mechanical ventilation has always seemed more complicated than it should be. Instead of presenting the usual list of clinical and physiologic indications for mechanical ventilation, the following simple rules should suffice.

RULE 1. The indication for intubation and mechanical ventilation is thinking of it. There is a tendency to delay intubation and mechanical ventilation as long as possible in the hopes that it will be unnecessary. However, elective intubation carries far fewer dangers than emergency intubation, and thus delays in intubation create unnecessary dangers for the patient. If the patient's condition is severe enough for intubation and mechanical ventilation to be considered, then proceed without delay.

RULE 2. Intubation is not an act of personal weakness. Housestaff tend to apologize on morning rounds when they have intubated a patient during the evening, almost as though the intubation was an act of weakness on their part. Quite the contrary, intubation carries the strength of conviction, and no one will be faulted for gaining control of the airways in an unstable patient.

RULE 3. Initiating mechanical ventilation is not the "kiss of death." The perception that "once on a ventilator, always on a ventilator" is a fallacy that should never influence the decision to initiate mechanical ventilation. Being on a ventilator does not create ventilator dependence; having a severe cardiopulmonary or neuromuscular diseases does.

A NEW STRATEGY FOR MECHANICAL VENTILATION

In the early days of positive-pressure mechanical ventilation, large inflation volumes were recommended to prevent alveolar collapse (8). Thus, **whereas the tidal volume during spontaneous breathing is normally 5 to 7 mL/kg (ideal body weight), the standard inflation volumes during volume-cycled ventilation have been twice as large, or 10 to 15 mL/kg.** This volume discrepancy is even greater with the addition of mechanical *sighs,* which are 1.5 to two times greater than standard inflation volumes (or 15 to 30 mL/kg) and are delivered 6 to 12 times per hour.

The large inflation volumes used in conventional mechanical ventilation can damage the lungs (3), and can even promote injury in distant organs through the release of inflammatory cytokines (9). The discovery of *ventilator-induced lung injury* is drastically changing the way that mechanical ventilation is delivered. This topic has been described in Chapter 22, and will be briefly reviewed here.

Ventilator-Induced Lung Injury

In lung diseases that most often require mechanical ventilation (e.g., acute respiratory distress syndrome [ARDS], pneumonia), the pathologic changes are not uniformly distributed throughout the lungs. This is even the case for pulmonary conditions like ARDS that appear to be distributed homogeneously throughout the lungs on the chest x-ray (see Fig. 22.4) (10). Because inflation volumes are distributed preferentially to regions of normal lung function, inflation volumes tend to overdistend the normal regions of diseased lungs. This tendency to overdistend normal lung regions is exaggerated when large inflation volumes are used.

The **hyperinflation of normal lung regions during mechanical ventilation can produce stress fractures at the alveolar-capillary interface** (11,12). An example of such a fracture is shown in Figure 24.3 (12). The electron micrographs in this figure are from the lungs of a patient with ARDS who required excessively high ventilatory pressures to maintain adequate arterial oxygenation. These fractures may be the result of excessive alveolar pressures (*barotrauma*) or excessive alveolar volumes (*volutrauma*) (13). Alveolar rupture like that in Figure 24.4 can have three adverse consequences. The first is accumulation of alveolar gas in

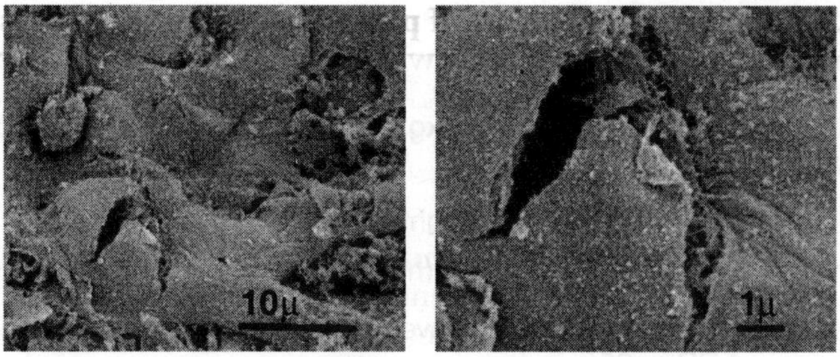

FIGURE 24.4 Electron micrograph showing a tear at the alveolar-capillary interface in a post-mortem specimen from a patient with ARDS. Scales shown in lower right corner of each image. (From Hotchkiss JR, Simonson DA, Marek DJ, et al. Pulmonary microvascular fracture in a patient with acute respiratory distress syndrome. Crit Care Med 2002; 30:2368–2370.) Image digitally retouched.

the pulmonary parenchyma (pulmonary interstitial emphysema), mediastinum (pneumomediastinum), or pleural cavity (pneumothorax). The second adverse consequence is a condition of inflammatory lung injury that is indistinguishable from ARDS (14). The third and possibly worst consequence is multiorgan injury from release of inflammatory mediators into the bloodstream (9). This latter process is known as *biotrauma*.

Lung-Protective Ventilation

The risk of lung injury with large inflation volumes has prompted clinical studies evaluating lower tidal volumes for positive-pressure ventilation. The largest study to date included over 800 patients with ARDS (15), and compared ventilation with tidal volumes of 6 mL/kg and 12 mL/kg using *predicted body weight* (which is the weight at which lung volumes are normal). Ventilation with low tidal volumes was associated with a 9% (absolute) reduction in mortality when the end-inspiratory "plateau pressure" was <30 cm H_2O (this pressure is described later in the chapter).

Low volume or *lung protective ventilation* is now recommended for all patients with ARDS, but there is evidence that ventilator-induced lung injury also occurs in conditions other than ARDS (16). Therefore, lung protective ventilation with low tidal volumes is considered a beneficial strategy for all patients with acute respiratory failure. A protocol for low volume ventilation is shown in Table 24.1. This protocol is adapted from the protocol for lung protective ventilation in ARDS, which is shown in Table 22.4. This strategy is designed to achieve and maintain a tidal volume of 6 mL/kg (using the patient's predicted body weight).

Positive End-Expiratory Pressure

Low tidal volumes can result in airway collapse, particularly at the end of expiration. Repeated opening and closing of airways at the end of expiration can become a source of lung injury (possibly by generating excessive shear forces that can damage the airways epithelium) (17).

TABLE 24.1 Protocol for Lung Protective Ventilation

1. Select assist-control mode and $FIO_2 = 100\%$.
2. Set initial tidal volume (V_T) at 8 mL/kg using the patient's *predicted body weight* (PBW).

   Males: PBW = 50 + [2.3 × (height in inches − 60)]

   Females: PBW = 45.5 + [2.3 × (height in inches − 60)]
3. Select respiratory rate (RR) to achieve pre-ventilator minute ventilation, but do not exceed RR = 35/min.
4. Add positive end-expiratory pressure (PEEP) at 5 − 7 cm H_2O.
5. Reduce V_T by 1 mL/kg every 2 hours until V_T = 6 mL/kg.
6. Adjust FIO_2 and PEEP to keep $PaO_2 > 55$ mm Hg or $SaO_2 > 88\%$.
7. When V_T is down to 6 mL/kg, measure:

   a) Plateau pressure (Ppl)

   b) Arterial PCO_2 and pH

   If Ppl > 30 cm H_2O or pH < 7.30, follow recommendations in Table 22.4.

Protocol from the ARDS Clinical Network website (www.ardsnet.org).

Airways collapse can be mitigated by adding positive end-expiratory pressure (PEEP). This pressure (which is described in the next chapter) acts as a stent to keep small airways open at the end of expiration.

Permissive Hypercapnia

Another consequence of low volume ventilation is a reduction in CO_2 elimination via the lungs, which can lead to hypercapnia and respiratory acidosis. Allowing hypercapnia to persist in favor of maintaining low volume ventilation is known as *permissive hypercapnia* (18). This is described in Chapter 22.

MONITORING LUNG MECHANICS

During spontaneous breathing, the mechanical properties of the lungs (i.e., elastic recoil of the lungs and resistance to flow in the airways) can be monitored with pulmonary function tests. However, these tests are not easily performed during mechanical ventilation. In this setting, the proximal airways pressures can be used to assess pulmonary function (1,19,20).

Proximal Airway Pressures

Positive-pressure mechanical ventilators have a pressure gauge that monitors the proximal airway pressure during each respiratory cycle. The components of this pressure are illustrated in Figure 24.5.

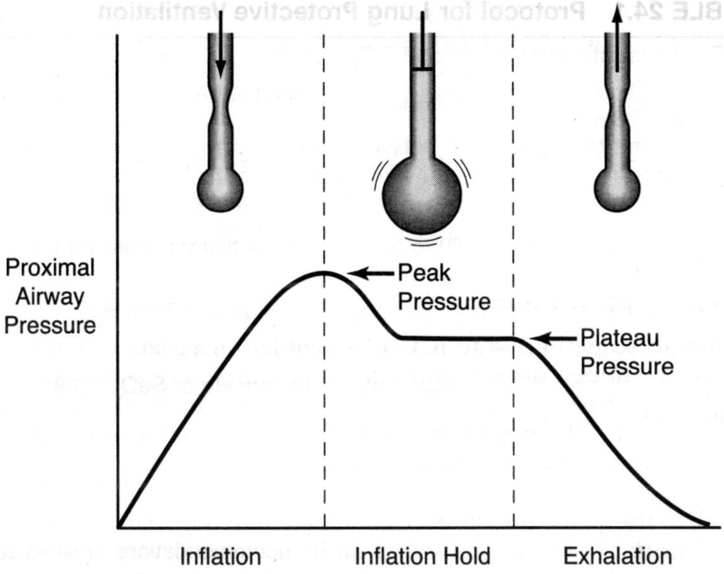

FIGURE 24.5 Proximal airway pressure at the end of a positive-pressure lung inflation (peak pressure) and during an inflation-hold maneuver (plateau pressure), which is performed by occluding the expiratory limb of the ventilator circuit to prevent lung deflation. These pressures can be used to evaluate the mechanical properties of the lungs (see Fig. 24.6).

End-Inspiratory Peak Pressure

The peak pressure at the end of inspiration (P_{peak}) is a function of the inflation volume, the flow resistance in the airways, and the elastic recoil force of the lungs and chest wall. At a constant inflation volume, the peak pressure varies directly with changes in airflow resistance and elastic recoil force (elastance) of the lungs and chest wall

$$P_{peak} \approx (\text{Resistance} + \text{Elastance}) \tag{24.1}$$

Therefore, when the inflation volume is constant, an increase in peak inspiratory pressure indicates an increase in airway resistance or an increase in the elastic recoil force of the lungs (or both).

End-Inspiratory Plateau Pressure

The contribution of resistance and elastance to the peak inspiratory pressure can be distinguished by occluding the expiratory tubing at the end of inspiration, as shown in Figure 24.5. When the inflation volume is held in the lungs, the proximal airway pressure decreases initially and then reaches a steady level, which is called the end-inspiratory *plateau pressure*. Because no airflow is present when the plateau pressure is created, the pressure is not a function of flow resistance in the airways. Instead, the plateau pressure ($P_{plateau}$) is directly related to the elastic recoil force (elastance) of the lungs and chest wall.

$$P_{plateau} \approx \text{Elastance} \tag{24.2}$$

Therefore, the difference between end-inspiratory peak and plateau pressures is proportional to the flow resistance in the airways.

$$(P_{peak} - P_{plateau}) \approx \text{Airways Resistance} \tag{24.3}$$

Practical Applications

A common scenario in any ICU is a ventilator-dependent patient who develops a sudden deterioration in cardiopulmonary status (this could include hypotension, hypoxemia, or respiratory distress). The flow diagram in Figure 24.6 demonstrates how the proximal airways pressures can be used to quickly evaluate these patients.

1. If the peak pressure is increased but the plateau pressure is unchanged, the problem is an increase in airways resistance. In this situation, the major concerns are obstruction of the tracheal tube, airway obstruction from secretions, and acute bronchospasm. Therefore, airways suctioning is indicated to clear secretions, followed by an aerosolized bronchodilator treatment if necessary.
2. If the peak and plateau pressures are both increased, the problem is a decrease in distensibility of the lungs and chest wall. In this situation, the major concerns are pneumothorax, lobar atelectasis, acute pulmonary edema, and worsening pneumonia or ARDS. Active contraction of the chest wall and increased abdominal pressure can also decrease the distensibility of the thorax. Finally, a patient with obstructive lung disease who becomes tachypneic can develop auto-PEEP, and this increases the peak and plateau pressures as well (see Chapter 26).
3. If the peak pressure is decreased, the problem may be an air leak in the system (e.g., tubing disconnection, cuff leak). In this situation, the lungs should be manually inflated while listening for a cuff leak. A decrease in peak pressure can also be due to hyperventilation, when the patient is generating enough of a negative intrathoracic pressure to "pull" air into the lungs.
4. If no change in peak pressure occurs, it does not necessarily mean that there has been no change in lung mechanics. The sensitivity of the proximal airways pressures in detecting changes in lung mechanics is unknown. When the pressures do not change, the evaluation should proceed as it would without the aid of proximal airway pressures.

Bronchodilator Responsiveness

Ventilator-dependent patients often receive aerosolized bronchodilator treatments routinely, without documented need or benefit. The proximal

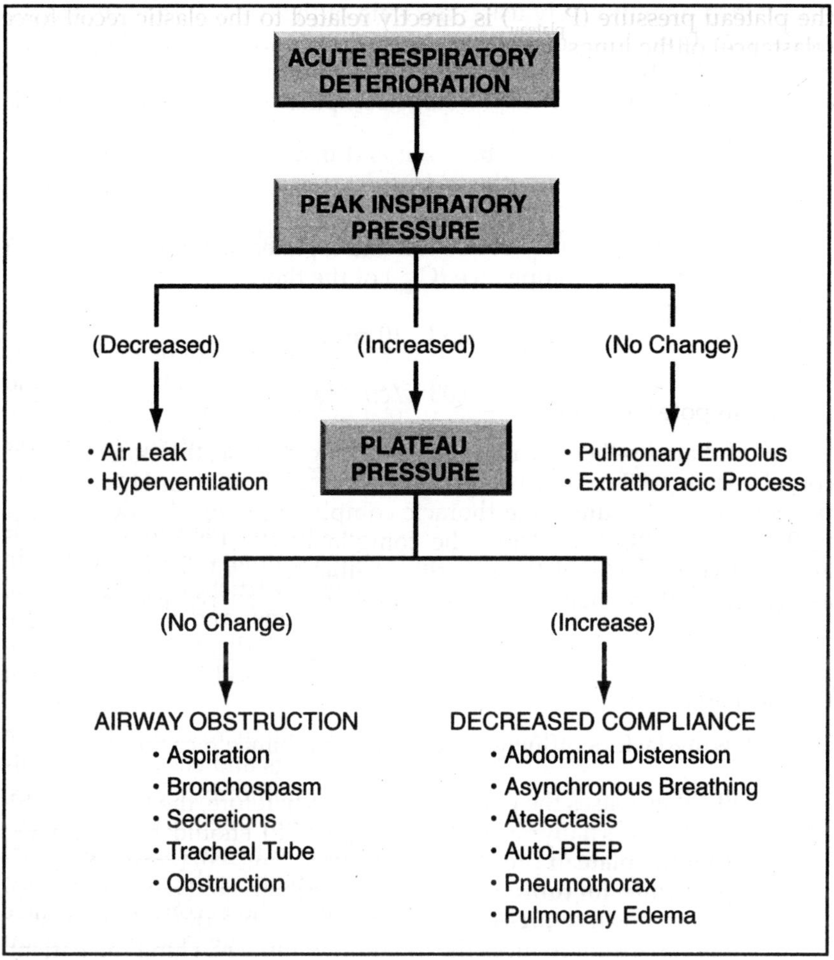

FIGURE 24.6 The use of proximal airway pressures to evaluate a patient with acute respiratory decompensation.

airway pressures can be used to evaluate bronchodilator responsiveness during mechanical ventilation. Bronchodilation represents a decrease in airways resistance, so a positive bronchodilator response should be accompanied by a decrease in the peak inspiratory pressure (assuming lung elastance stays the same). If an aerosol bronchodilator treatment is not accompanied by a decrease in peak inspiratory pressure, then there is little justification for continuing the aerosol treatments.

Thoracic Compliance

Compliance (distensibility) is the reciprocal of elastance. The compliance of the lungs and chest wall (called thoracic compliance) can be determined quantitatively using the ratio of the tidal volume (V_T) to the elastic recoil pressure (i.e., plateau pressure). Since the plateau pressure is measured in the absence of airflow, the resulting compliance is called a "static" compliance. Thus, the static compliance (C_{stat}) of the thorax is derived as:

$$C_{stat} = V_T/P_{plateau} \tag{24.4}$$

For a tidal volume (V_T) of 500 mL and a plateau pressure ($P_{plateau}$) of 10 cm H_2O, the static compliance (C_{stat}) of the thorax is:

$$\begin{aligned} C_{stat} &= 0.5\ L/10\ cm\ H_2O \\ &= 0.05\ L/cm\ H_2O \end{aligned} \tag{24.5}$$

In intubated patients with no known lung disease, the static thoracic compliance is 0.05 to 0.08 L/cm H_2O (or 50 to 80 mL/cm H_2O) (19). In patients with stiff lungs, the thoracic compliance is much lower at 0.01 to 0.02 L/cm H_2O (21). Thus, the compliance determination provides an objective measure of the severity of illness in pulmonary disorders associated with a change in lung compliance (e.g., pulmonary edema and ARDS).

Considerations

The following factors influence the static compliance measurement.

1. **PEEP** increases the plateau pressure. Therefore, the level of PEEP (either externally applied or auto-PEEP) should be subtracted from the plateau pressure for the compliance determination.
2. The **connector tubing** between the ventilator and patient expands during positive-pressure lung inflations, and the volume lost in this expansion reduces the inflation volume reaching the patient. The volume lost is a function of the peak inflation pressure and the inherent compliance of the tubing. The usual compliance of connector tubing is 3 mL/cm H_2O, which means that 3 mL of volume is lost for every 1 cm H_2O increase in inflation pressure. Thus, if the inflation volume from the ventilator is 700 mL and the peak inspiratory pressure is 40 cm H_2O, then (3 × 40) 120 mL will be lost to expansion of the ventilator tubing and the inflation volume reaching the patient will be (700 − 120) 580 mL. Because of this discrepancy, the predetermined volume setting on the ventilator should not be used as the inflation volume for the compliance calculation. Instead, the exhaled volume, which is usually displayed digitally on the ventilator panel, should be used.
3. Because the proximal airways pressures are transthoracic pressures (i.e., measured relative to atmospheric pressure) and not transpulmonary pressures (i.e., measured relative to intrapleural pressure), the compliance measurement includes the chest

wall as well as the lungs. Because contraction of the chest wall muscles can reduce the compliance (distensibility) of the chest wall, the compliance determination should be performed only during passive ventilation. However during passive ventilation, the chest wall can account for 35% of the total thoracic compliance (20,21).

Airway Resistance

The resistance to airflow during inspiration (R_{insp}) can be determined as the ratio of the pressure gradient needed to overcome airways resistance ($P_{peak} - P_{plateau}$) and the inspiratory flow rate (V_{insp}):

$$R_{insp} = (P_{peak} - P_{plateau})/V_{insp} \tag{24.6}$$

This resistance represents the summed resistances of the connector tubing, the tracheal tube, and the airways. Because the resistance of the connector tubing and tracheal tube should remain constant (assuming the tracheal tube is clear of secretions), changes in R_{insp} should represent changes in airways resistance.

A sample calculation of inspiratory resistance is shown below using an inspiratory flow rate of 60 L/min (1.0 L/sec), a peak pressure of 20 cm H_2O, and a plateau pressure of 10 cm H_2O.

$$\begin{aligned} R_{insp} &= (20 - 10) \text{ cm } H_2O/1 \text{ L/sec} \\ &= 10 \text{ cm } H_2O/\text{L/sec} \end{aligned} \tag{24.7}$$

The minimal flow resistance in large-bore endotracheal tubes is 3 to 7 cm H_2O/L/sec (22), so nonpulmonary resistive elements can contribute a considerable fraction of the total inspiratory resistance.

Limitations

The major limitations of the inspiratory resistance measurement are the contributions of resistive elements not in the lung and the relative insensitivity of the resistance measured during inspiration. Airflow obstruction is usually measured during expiration, when the airways have the greatest tendency to collapse. The distending pressures delivered by the ventilator during lung inflation keep the airways open, and thus the resistance to flow during inspiration does not measure the tendency for the airways to collapse during expiration (20).

A FINAL WORD

After mechanical ventilation was introduced into clinical practice, there was a flurry of interest in developing newer modes of ventilation that would benefit patients with respiratory failure. This type of "more is better" approach was based on a perception that mechanical ventilation is a type of therapy for patients with respiratory failure (one example of this perception are the claims that positive end-expiratory pressure can drive water out of the lungs in patients with pulmonary edema). However, there is nothing therapeutic about mechanical ventilation. In fact, the most significant discovery about mechanical ventilation since it was first introduced is the fact that it damages the lungs (and indirectly damages other organs as well).

Mechanical ventilation is a technique that opposes the normal physiology of ventilation (by creating positive pressure instead of negative pressure to ventilate the lungs) and, in this sense, it is not surprising that it is problematic. The current trend of using lower tidal volumes during mechanical ventilation is a step in the right direction because a "lesser is better" strategy is the only one that makes sense with a technique that is so unphysiological.

REFERENCES

Reviews

1. Tobin MJ. Advances in mechanical ventilation. N Engl J Med 2001;344:1986–1996.
2. Fan E, Needham DM, Stewart TE. Ventilatory management of acute lung injury and acute respiratory distress syndrome. JAMA 2005;294:2889–2896.
3. Dreyfuss D, Saumon G. Ventilator-induced lung injury. Am Rev Respir Crit Care Med 1998;157:294–323.

Cardiac Performance

4. Pinsky MR. Cardiovascular issues in respiratory care. Chest 2005;128:592S–597S.
5. Versprille A. The pulmonary circulation during mechanical ventilation. Acta Anesthesiol Scand 1990;34(suppl):51–62.
6. Venus B, Cohen LE, Smith RA. Hemodynamics and intrathoracic pressure transmission during controlled mechanical ventilation and positive end-expiratory pressure in normal and low compliant lungs. Crit Care Med 1988; 16:686–690.
7. Kiiski R, Takala J, Kari A, et al. Effect of tidal volume on gas exchange and oxygen transport in the adult respiratory distress syndrome. Am Rev Respir Dis 1992;146:1131–1135.

Strategies for Mechanical Ventilation

8. Bendixen HH, Egbert LD, Hedley-White J, et al. Respiratory care. St. Louis: Mosby, 1965:137–153.
9. Ranieri VM, Giunta F, Suter P, et al. Mechanical ventilation as a mediator of multisystem organ failure in acute respiratory distress syndrome. JAMA 2000;284:43–44.

10. Gattinoni L, Caironi P, Pelosi P, et al. What has computed tomography taught us about the acute respiratory distress syndrome? Am J Respir Crit Care Med 2001;164:1701–1711.
11. Costello ML, Mathieu-Costello OA, West JB. Stress failure of alveolar epithelial cells studied by scanning electron microscopy. Am Rev Respir Dis 1992;145:1446–1455.
12. Hotchkiss JR, Simonson DA, Marek DJ, et al. Pulmonary microvascular fracture in a patient with acute respiratory distress syndrome. Crit Care Med 2002;30:2368–2370.
13. Bray JC, Cane RD. Mechanical ventilatory support and pulmonary parenchymal injury: positive airway pressure or alveolar hyperinflation? Intensive Crit Care Digest 1993;12:33–36.
14. Timby J, Reed C, Zeilander S, et al. "Mechanical" causes of pulmonary edema. Chest 1990;98:973–979.
15. The Acute Respiratory Distress Syndrome Network. Ventilation with lower tidal volumes as compared with traditional tidal volumes for acute lung injury and the acute respiratory distress syndrome. N Engl J Med 2000;342:1301–1308.
16. Gajic O, Dara S, Mendez JL, et al. Ventilator-associated lung injury in patients without acute lung injury at the onset of mechanical ventilation. Crit Care Med 2004;32:1817–1824.
17. Muscedere JG, Mullen JBM, Gan K, et al. Tidal ventilation at low airway pressures can augment lung injury. Am J Respir Crit Care Med 1994;149:1327–1334.
18. O'Croinin D, Ni Chonghaile M, Higgins B, et al. Bench-to-bedside review: permissive hypercapnia. Crit Care 2005;9:51–59.

Monitoring Lung Mechanics

19. Tobin MJ. Respiratory monitoring. JAMA 1990;264:244–251.
20. Marini JJ. Lung mechanics determinations at the bedside: instrumentation and clinical application. Respir Care 1990;35:669–696.
21. Katz JA, Zinn SE, Ozanne GM, et al. Pulmonary, chest wall, and lung–thorax elastances in acute respiratory failure. Chest 1981;80:304–311.
22. Marini JJ. Strategies to minimize breathing effort during mechanical ventilation. Crit Care Clin 1990;6:635–662.

Chapter 25

MODES OF ASSISTED VENTILATION

In the half century since positive ... least 15 ... duced, ... claims that ... plication ... the work of ... (1–3). Most of these ventilatory ... ventilation more effective, safe, ... have done instead is make positive ... cated than it needs to be.

ASSIST-CONTROL VENTILATION

As des... pressu... instead ... *volume-*... mechan... of minu... trolled ... This continuous ...

Ventilatory Pattern

The upper panel in Figure 25.1 ... produced by assist-control ventilation ...

Chapter 25

MODES OF ASSISTED VENTILATION

Development in most fields of medicine appears to occur according to sound scientific principles. However, exceptions can be found, and the development of mechanical ventilatory support is one of them.

J. Rasanen

In the half century since positive-pressure ventilation first appeared, at least 15 different modes of positive-pressure ventilation have been introduced, each with claims that it will improve gas exchange, prevent complications, or reduce the work of breathing during mechanical ventilation (1–3). Most of these ventilatory modes have failed to make mechanical ventilation more effective, safer, or more tolerable for patients. What they have done instead is make positive-pressure ventilation more complicated than it needs to be.

ASSIST-CONTROL VENTILATION

As described in the last chapter, the most popular method of positive-pressure lung inflation involves the use of a constant inflation volume instead of a constant inflation pressure. This method, which is called *volume-cycled ventilation*, allows the patient to initiate or "trigger" each mechanical breath (assisted ventilation) but can also deliver a preset level of minute ventilation if the patient is unable to trigger the ventilator (controlled ventilation). This combination is called *assist-control ventilation*.

Ventilatory Pattern

The upper panel in Figure 25.1 shows the changes in airway pressure produced by assist-control ventilation (ACV). The tracing begins with a

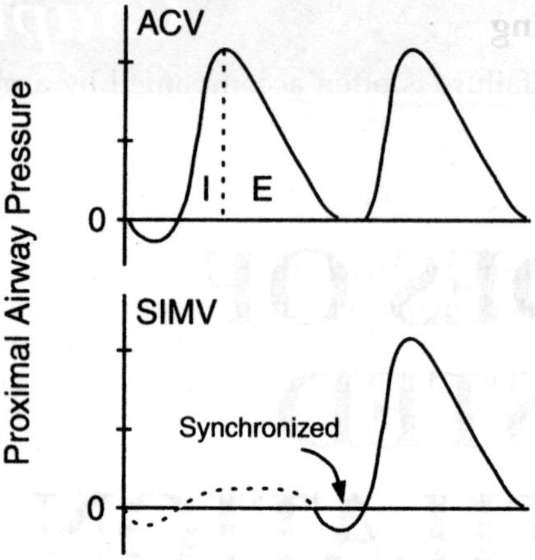

FIGURE 25.1 Airway pressure patterns in assist-control ventilation (*ACV*) and synchronized intermittent mandatory ventilation (*SIMV*). Spontaneous breaths are indicated by dashed lines, and machine breaths are indicated by solid lines. The mechanical breath in the upper panel indicates the period of lung inflation (*I*) and deflation (*E*).

negative-pressure deflection, which is the result of a spontaneous inspiratory effort by the patient. When the negative pressure reaches a certain level (which is usually set at −2 to −3 cm H_2O), a pressure-activated valve in the ventilator opens, and a positive-pressure breath is delivered to the patient. The second machine breath in the tracing is identical to the first, but it is not preceded by a spontaneous ventilatory effort. The first breath is an example of *assisted ventilation,* and the second breath is an example of *controlled ventilation.*

Respiratory Cycle Timing

As mentioned in Chapter 24, volume-cycled ventilation has traditionally employed large inflation volumes (10 to 15 mL/kg or about twice the normal tidal volume during spontaneous breathing). To allow patients sufficient time to passively exhale these large volumes, the time allowed for exhalation should be at least twice the time allowed for lung inflation (see Fig. 25.1) The ratio of inspiratory time to expiratory time, which is called the I:E ratio, should then be maintained at 1:2 or higher (1). This is accomplished by using an inspiratory flow rate that is at least twice the expiratory flow rate. At a normal respiratory rate, an inspiratory flow rate of 60 L/min will inflate the lungs quickly enough to allow the time needed to exhale the inflation volume. However, when a patient has obstructive lung disease and can't exhale quickly, the I:E ratio can fall below 1:2, and an increase in inspiratory flow rate may be needed to achieve the appropriate I:E ratio.

Work of Breathing

Acute respiratory failure is often accompanied by a marked increase in the work of breathing, and patients who are working hard to breathe are often placed on mechanical ventilation to rest the respiratory muscles and reduce the work of breathing. However, the assumption that the diaphragm rests during mechanical ventilation is incorrect because **the diaphragm is an involuntary muscle that never rests.** The contraction of the diaphragm is dictated by the activity of respiratory neurons in the lower brainstem, and these cells fire automatically and are not silenced by mechanical ventilation. Only death can silence the brainstem respiratory centers, and the diaphragm follows suit. This means that the diaphragm does not relax when the ventilator is triggered and delivers the mechanical breath, but it continues to contract throughout inspiration. Because of the continued contraction of the diaphragm, mechanical ventilation may have little impact on the work of breathing (4).

Ventilatory Drive

The activity of the diaphragm is largely dictated by the output from the brainstem respiratory neurons, and this output, which is often referred to as the *ventilatory drive*, is increased as much as three to four times above normal in acute respiratory failure (mechanism unknown) (1,5). **Reducing ventilatory drive is the appropriate measure for decreasing the workload of the respiratory muscles**. Promoting patient comfort with sedation might help in this regard (6). Altering the mechanism for triggering the ventilator can also help, as described next.

The Trigger Mechanism

The traditional method of assisted ventilation uses a decrease in airways pressure generated by the patient to open a pressure-sensitive valve and initiate the ventilator breath. The threshold pressure is usually set at a low level of −1 to −3 cm H_2O. Although this does not seem excessive, many ventilator-dependent patients have positive end-expiratory pressure (PEEP), and this adds to the pressure that must be generated to trigger the ventilator. For example, if a patient has +5 cm H_2O of PEEP and the trigger pressure is −2 cm H_2O, a pressure of 7 cm H_2O must be generated to trigger a ventilator breath. This may not seem like much, but the diaphragm generates only 2 to 3 cm H_2O during quiet breathing in healthy adults, so generating a pressure of 7 cm H_2O will require more than twice the normal effort of the diaphragm. The increased effort needed to reach the trigger pressure would explain the observation that about one-third of inspiratory efforts in ventilator-dependent patients fail to trigger the ventilator (7).

Inspiratory flow offers advantages over inspiratory pressure as a trigger mechanism because flow triggering (usually at 2 L/min) does not require a decrease in airway pressure, and therefore should require less effort. Studies comparing flow and pressure triggering have been inconsistent except for patients with chronic obstructive pulmonary disease (COPD), where the work of breathing is less with flow triggering (8). Some ventilators provide flow-triggering as an option (e.g., Bird 8400 ST) but don't expect much.

Disadvantages

Based on an unfounded fear that mechanical ventilation will be accompanied by progressive atelectasis, large tidal volumes have been employed for volume-cycled ventilation. These volumes are about twice the normal tidal volumes in adults (12 to 15 mL/kg vs. 6 to 8 mL/kg, respectively). This practice has changed in recent years, and the preferred tidal volumes for mechanical ventilation have been cut in half to the range of 6 to 8 mL/kg. The conditions that prompted this change are described next.

Ventilator-Induced Lung Injury

The topic of ventilator-induced lung injury (VILI) is described in Chapters 22 and 24, and is only briefly mentioned here. High inflation volumes overdistend alveoli and promote alveolar rupture (see Figure 24.4). This process is known as *volutrauma,* and it incites an inflammatory response in the lungs that can produce a condition of inflammatory lung injury similar to the acute respiratory distress syndrome (ARDS) (9). Inflammatory mediators in the lungs can be released into the systemic circulation and this can lead to inflammatory injury in distant organs (10). This condition of multiorgan injury from local injury in the lungs is known as *biotrauma.*

The discovery of volutrauma led to studies comparing ventilation with conventional tidal volumes (12 to 15 mL/kg) and reduced tidal volumes (6 mL/kg). Some of these studies showed improved outcomes associated with the low-volume *lung-protective ventilation* (11). As a result, the recommended inflation volumes for volume-cycled ventilation have been cut in half to 6 to 8 mL/kg (see Tables 22.4 and 24.1).

VILI has been described almost exclusively in patients with ARDS, but there is evidence that this condition can occur in any patient with underlying pulmonary disease (12). The recommendation for low-volume ventilation is thus being applied to all ventilator-dependent patients.

Auto-PEEP

Assist-control ventilation can be problematic for patients who are breathing rapidly or have reduced expiratory airflow because there may not be enough time to exhale the large tidal volumes. The air that remains in the alveoli at the end-of expiration creates a positive end-expiratory pressure (PEEP) that is known as *auto-PEEP.* This pressure can impair cardiac output and can also increase this risk of pulmonary barotrauma (pressure-induced injury). The lower tidal volumes that are now being adopted for volume-cycled ventilation will reduce the risk of auto-PEEP, but will not eliminate this problem. (The deleterious effects of PEEP are described later in the chapter, and the condition of auto-PEEP is described in Chapter 26.)

INTERMITTENT MANDATORY VENTILATION

The problem of incomplete emptying of the lungs with rapid breathing during assist-control ventilation led to the introduction of *intermittent mandatory ventilation* (IMV). This mode of ventilation was introduced in 1971 to ventilate neonates with respiratory distress syndrome, who typically have respiratory rates in excess of 40 breaths/minute. IMV is designed to provide only partial ventilatory support: it combines periods of assist-control ventilation with periods where patients are allowed to breathe spontaneously. The periods of spontaneous breathing help to prevent progressive lung hyperinflation and auto-PEEP in patients who breathe rapidly, and was also intended to prevent respiratory muscle atrophy from prolonged periods of mechanical ventilation.

Ventilatory Pattern

The lower portion of Figure 25.1 shows the pattern of ventilation associated with IMV. The initial negative and positive deflection in the tracing represents a spontaneous breath (dashed line). The second spontaneous breath triggers an assisted ventilator breath (solid line). Thus, IMV combines assisted ventilation with spontaneous breathing. The ventilatory pattern in Figure 25.1 is called *synchronized* IMV because the assisted breaths are synchronized to coincide with spontaneous inspiratory efforts.

When IMV is first set up for a patient, the rate of assisted lung inflations is usually set at 10 breaths/minute. This rate can then be adjusted upward or downward as needed until the patient is breathing comfortably and gas exchange is adequate. The period of spontaneous breathing is poorly tolerated by patients, and it is now a common practice to use pressure-support ventilation (described later in the chapter) at 10 cm H_2O during the spontaneous breathing periods. The addition of pressure-supported breathing has been shown to decrease the work of breathing during IMV (7), and this has improved patient tolerance. However, when IMV is employing both volume-cycled ventilation and pressure-supported ventilation, it is no longer providing partial ventilatory support, and is functioning more like assist-control ventilation than IMV.

Disadvantages

The principal disadvantages of IMV are an increased work of breathing and a decreased cardiac output.

Work of Breathing

The spontaneous breathing during IMV takes place through a high-resistance circuit (the tracheal tube and ventilator tubing) and this can increase the inspiratory work of breathing. The addition of pressure-supported spontaneous breathing has been effective in minimizing this problem, as described above (13). The increased work of breathing attributed to pressure-based triggering, which was described previously for assist-control ventilation, can also be a problem with IMV, and the use of inspiratory airflow to trigger the ventilator breaths has been shown to reduce the work of breathing during IMV (7).

Cardiac Output

As described in Chapter 24, positive-pressure ventilation can reduce cardiac output by reducing ventricular preload, or can increase cardiac output by reducing ventricular afterload. In patients with a normal intravascular volume, the afterload effect predominates, and positive-pressure ventilation usually augments cardiac output (14). This effect is particularly evident in patients with left ventricular dysfunction, where positive-pressure ventilation can serve as a ventricular-assist device (15). IMV has the opposite effect, and decreases cardiac output in patients with left-ventricular dysfunction (15).

Summary

In summary, IMV provides few benefits over assist-control ventilation. The principal benefit of IMV is for the patient who is breathing rapidly because volume-cycled (assist-control) ventilation for these patients creates a risk for hyperinflation, auto-PEEP, and volutrauma. The risk of ventilator-induced lung injury may be lower with IMV than assist-control because less time is devoted to volume-cycled ventilation with IMV. This, however, is unproven. Finally, IMV should be avoided in patients with respiratory muscle weakness or left-ventricular dysfunction.

PRESSURE-CONTROLLED VENTILATION

Pressure-controlled ventilation (PCV) uses a constant pressure to inflate the lungs. This mode of ventilation was frowned upon because the inflation volumes can be variable (this is explained later). However, there has been a resurgence of interest in PCV because the risk for ventilator-induced lung injury may be lower with PCV, as explained in the next section.

The pattern of ventilation associated with PCV is shown in Figure 25.2. Ventilation with PCV is completely controlled by the ventilator, with no participation by the patient (similar to the control mode in assist-control ventilation).

Benefits and Risks

The perception that ventilator-induced lung injury may be less of a risk with PCV is based on the tendency for lower inflation volumes and lower airways pressures during PCV. However, there is no evidence to support

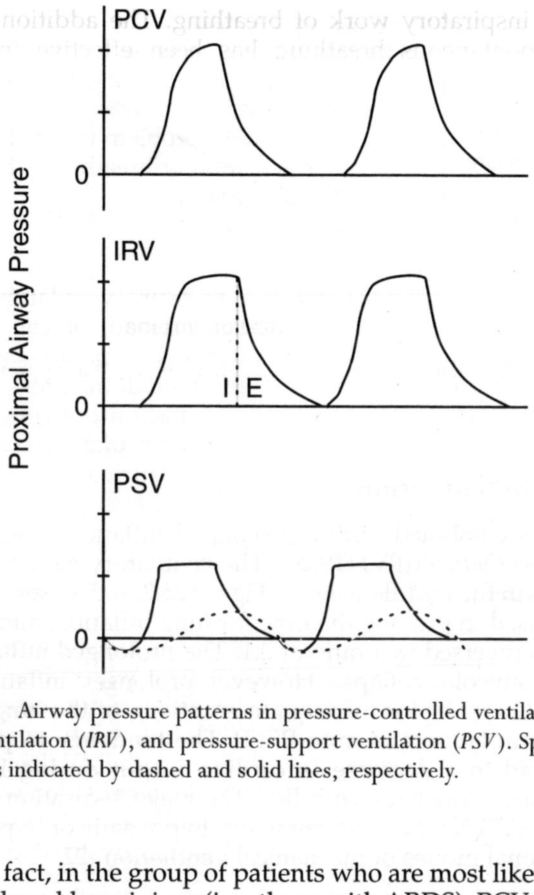

FIGURE 25.2 Airway pressure patterns in pressure-controlled ventilation (*PCV*), inverse ratio ventilation (*IRV*), and pressure-support ventilation (*PSV*). Spontaneous and machine breaths indicated by dashed and solid lines, respectively.

this claim. In fact, in the group of patients who are most likely to develop ventilator-induced lung injury (i.e., those with ARDS), PCV may not provide adequate ventilation.

The major advantage of PCV is the decelerating inspiratory flow pattern. In volume-cycled ventilation, the inspiratory flow rate is constant throughout lung inflation, whereas in pressure-controlled ventilation the inspiratory flow decreases exponentially during lung inflation (to keep the airway pressure at the pre-selected value). This decelerating flow pattern reduces peak airway pressures and can improve gas exchange (16–18).

The major disadvantage of PCV is the tendency for inflation volumes to vary with changes in the mechanical properties of the lungs. This is illustrated in Figure 25.3. The inflation volume increases as the peak inflation pressure increases (dashed lines). However, at a constant peak inflation pressure, the inflation volume decreases as the airway resistance increases or the lung compliance decreases. Therefore, any change in lung mechanics during PCV can lead to a change in inflation volumes. Because of the influence of lung mechanics on inflation volumes during PCV, this method of mechanical ventilation seems best suited for patients with neuromuscular disease (and normal lung mechanics).

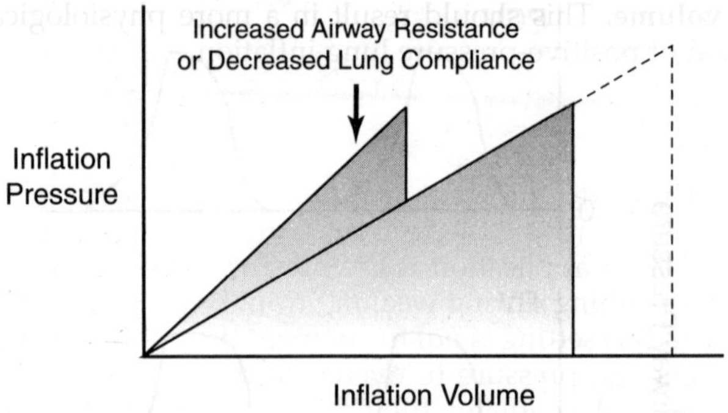

FIGURE 25.3 The determinants of lung inflation volume during pressure-cycled ventilation.

Inverse Ratio Ventilation

When PCV is combined with a prolonged inflation time, the result is *inverse ratio ventilation* (IRV) (19,20). The ventilatory pattern produced by IRV is shown in the middle panel of Figure 25.2. A decrease in inspiratory flow rate is used to prolong the time for lung inflation, and the usual I:E ratio of 1:2 is reversed to a ratio of 2:1. The prolonged inflation time can help prevent alveolar collapse. However, prolonged inflation times also increase the tendency for inadequate emptying of the lungs, which can lead to hyperinflation and auto-PEEP. **The tendency to produce auto-PEEP can lead to a decrease in cardiac output during IRV** (21), and this is the major drawback with IRV. The major indication for IRV is for patients with ARDS who have refractory hypoxemia or hypercapnia during conventional modes of mechanical ventilation (22).

PRESSURE-SUPPORT VENTILATION

Pressure-augmented breathing that allows the patient to determine the inflation volume and respiratory cycle duration is called *pressure-support ventilation* (PSV) (23). This method of ventilation is used to augment spontaneous breathing, not to provide full ventilatory support.

Ventilatory Pattern

The ventilatory pattern produced by PSV is shown in the lower panel of Figure 25.2. At the onset of each spontaneous breath, the negative pressure generated by the patient opens a valve that delivers the inspired gas at a pre-selected pressure (usually 5 to 10 cm H_2O). The patient's inspiratory flow rate is adjusted by the ventilator as needed to keep the inflation pressure constant, and when the patient's inspiratory flow rate falls below 25% of the peak inspiratory flow, the augmented breath is terminated. By recognizing the patient's inherent inspiratory flow rate, **PSV allows the patient to dictate the duration of lung inflation and the**

inflation volume. This should result in a more physiologically acceptable method of positive-pressure lung inflation.

Clinical Uses

PSV can be used to augment inflation volumes during spontaneous breathing or to overcome the resistance of breathing through ventilator circuits. The latter application is the most popular and is used to limit the work of breathing during weaning from mechanical ventilation. The goal of PSV in this setting is not to augment the tidal volume, but merely to provide enough pressure to overcome the resistance created by the tracheal tubes and ventilator tubing. Inflation pressures of 5 to 10 cm H_2O are appropriate for this purpose. PSV has also become popular as a noninvasive method of mechanical ventilation (24,25). In this situation, PSV is delivered through specialized face masks or nasal masks, using inflation pressures of 20 cm H_2O.

POSITIVE END-EXPIRATORY PRESSURE

Collapse of distal airspaces at the end of expiration is a common occurrence in ventilator-dependent patients, and the resulting atelectasis impairs gas exchange and adds to the severity of the respiratory failure. The driving force for this atelectasis is a decreased lung compliance, which is a consequence of the pulmonary disorders that are common in ventilator-dependent patients (i.e., ARDS and pneumonia). To counterbalance the tendency for alveolar collapse at the end of expiration, a positive pressure is created in the airways at end-expiration. This *positive end-expiratory pressure (PEEP)* has become a standard measure in the management of ventilator-dependent patients.

PEEP is created by placing a pressure-relief valve in the expiratory limb of the ventilator circuit, and setting the threshold pressure on the valve to correspond to the desired PEEP. The valve allows exhalation to proceed until the expiratory pressure decreases to the pre-selected pressure on the valve. At this point, airflow will cease (because there is no longer a pressure gradient across the valve) and, in the absence of airflow, the pressure at the valve is equivalent to alveolar pressure, which is the PEEP.

Airway Pressure Profile

The pressure profile with PEEP is shown in Figure 25.4. Note that the entire pressure waveform is displaced upward, resulting in an increase in peak airway pressure and mean airway pressure. The relationship between PEEP, peak intrathoracic pressure, and mean intrathoracic pressure is summarized below.

1. The complications of PEEP are not directly related to the PEEP level, but are determined by the peak and mean airway pressures during ventilation with PEEP.

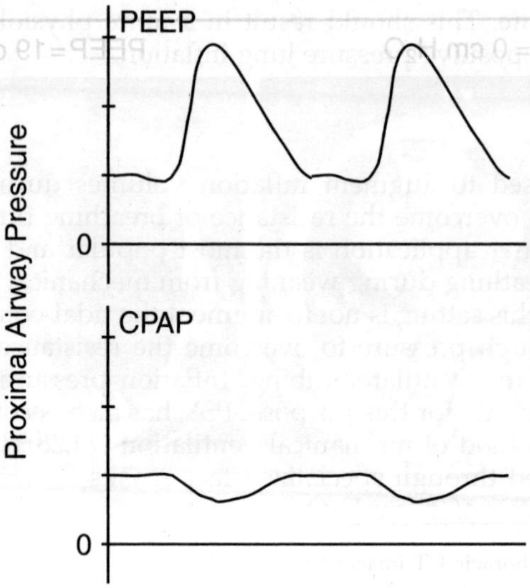

FIGURE 25.4 Airway pressure patterns in volume-cycled ventilation with positive end-expiratory pressure (*PEEP*), and in spontaneous breathing with continuous positive airway pressure (*CPAP*).

2. The peak airway pressure determines the risk of barotrauma (e.g., pneumothorax).
3. The mean airway pressure determines the cardiac output response to PEEP.
4. When airway pressures are used to evaluate lung mechanics (see Figs. 24.5 and 24.6), the PEEP level should be subtracted from the pressures.

Lung Recruitment

PEEP acts like a stent for the distal airspaces and counterbalances the compressive force generated by the elastic recoil of the lungs. In addition to preventing atelectasis, PEEP can also open collapsed alveoli and reverse atelectasis. This effect is demonstrated in Figure 25.5 (26). The thoracic CT image on the left shows consolidation in the posterior (dependent) regions of the both lungs, and this disappears after the application of PEEP. The PEEP has restored aeration in the area of atelectasis. This effect is known as *lung recruitment*, and it increases the available surface area in the lungs for gas exchange (26,27).

Recruitable Lung

The effect of PEEP shown in Figure 25.5 will result in improved gas exchange in the lungs. However, PEEP does not always have such a beneficial effect, and it can be harmful. In fact, PEEP can result in overdistention of normal lung regions, and this can injure the lungs in a manner similar to ventilator-induced lung injury. The important variable

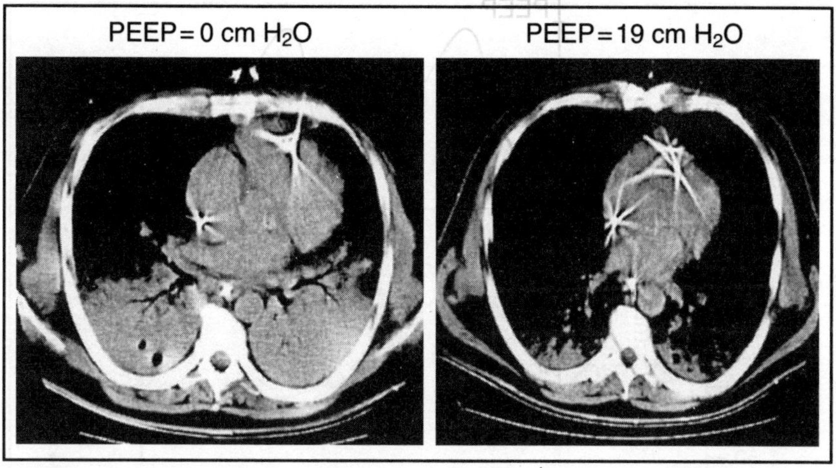

FIGURE 25.5 Thoracic CT images from a patient with ARDS showing resolution of atelectasis (recruitment) in response to PEEP. Images from Barbas CSV. Lung recruitment maneuvers in acute respiratory distress syndrome and facilitating resolution. Crit Care Med 2003;31(suppl):S265–S271.

for determining whether PEEP will have a favorable or unfavorable response is the relative volume of "recruitable lung" (i.e., areas of atelectasis that can be aerated). If there is recruitable lung, then PEEP will have a favorable effect and will improve gas exchange in the lungs. However if there is no recruitable lung, PEEP can overdistend the lungs (because the lung volume is lower if areas of atelectasis cannot be aerated) and produce an injury similar to ventilator-induced lung injury.

Preliminary studies in ARDS show that the volume of recruitable lung varies widely (from 2% to 25% of total lung volume) in individual patients (27). Although it is not possible to measure recruitable lung volume reliably, the appearance of atelectasis on CT images can sometimes help. Areas of atelectasis that contain pockets of aeration are most likely to represent recruitable lung, whereas areas of atelectasis that are airless are unlikely to be recruitable (27).

The PaO_2/FIO_2 Ratio

The effects of PEEP on lung recruitment can be monitored with the PaO_2/FIO_2 ratio, which is a measure of the efficiency of oxygen exchange across the lungs. The PaO_2/FIO_2 ratio is usually below 300 in acute respiratory failure, and below 200 in cases of ARDS. If PEEP has a favorable effect and converts areas of atelectasis to functional alveolar-capillary units, there will be an increase in the PaO_2/FIO_2 ratio. However, if PEEP is harmful by overdistending the lungs, the PaO_2/FIO_2 ratio will decrease. An example of a beneficial response in the PaO_2/FIO_2 ratio is shown in Figure 25.6.

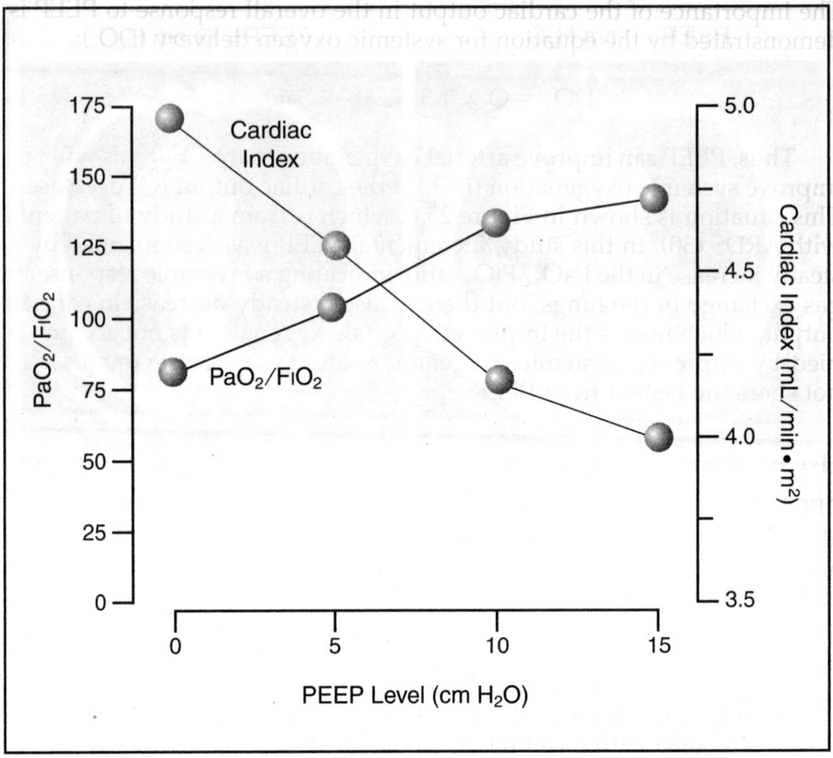

FIGURE 25.6 Effects of positive end-expiratory pressure (*PEEP*) on arterial oxygenation (PaO_2/FIO_2) and cardiac output in patients with ARDS. From Gainnier M, Michelet P, Thirion X, et al. Prone position and positive end-expiratory pressure in acute respiratory distress syndrome. Crit Care Med 2003;31:2719–2726.

Cardiac Performance

PEEP has the same influence on the determinants of cardiac performance as positive-pressure ventilation (described in Chapter 24), but the ability to decrease ventricular preload is more prominent with PEEP. PEEP can decrease cardiac output by several mechanisms, including reduced venous return, reduced ventricular compliance, increased right ventricular outflow impedance, and ventricular external constraint by hyperinflated lungs (28,29). The decrease in cardiac output from PEEP is particularly prominent in hypovolemic patients. PEEP can also increase cardiac output by reducing left ventricular afterload, but the significance of this response is unclear.

Oxygen Transport

The tendency for PEEP to reduce cardiac output is an important consideration because the beneficial effects of PEEP on lung recruitment and gas exchange in the lungs can be erased by the cardiodepressant effects.

The importance of the cardiac output in the overall response to PEEP is demonstrated by the equation for systemic oxygen delivery (DO_2):

$$DO_2 = Q \times 1.3 \times Hb \times SaO_2 \qquad (25.1)$$

Thus, PEEP can improve arterial oxygenation (SaO_2), but this will not improve systemic oxygenation (DO_2) if the cardiac output (Q) decreases. This situation is shown in Figure 25.6, which is from a study of patients with ARDS (30). In this study, incremental PEEP was accompanied by a steady increase in the PaO_2/FiO_2 ratio, indicating a favorable response in gas exchange in the lungs, but there is also a steady decrease in cardiac output, which means the improved arterial oxygenation is not accompanied by improved systemic oxygenation, and the systemic organs will not share the benefit from PEEP.

Use of PEEP

PEEP is used almost universally in ventilator-dependent patients, presumably as a preventive measure for atelectasis. This practice is unproven, and it creates unnecessary work to trigger a ventilator breath (as described earlier). The few situations where PEEP is indicated are included below:

1. When the chest x-ray shows diffuse infiltrates (e.g., ARDS) and the patient requires toxic levels of inhaled oxygen to maintain adequate arterial oxygenation. In this situation, PEEP can increase the PaO_2/FiO_2 ratio, and this would permit reduction of the FiO_2.
2. When low-volume, lung-protective ventilation is used. In this situation, PEEP is needed to prevent repeated opening and closing of distal airspaces because this can damage the lungs and add to the severity of the clinical condition(s).

PEEP is not recommended for localized lung disease like pneumonia because the applied pressure will preferentially distribute to normal regions of the lung and this could lead to overdistention and rupture of alveoli (ventilator-induced lung injury) (31). In lung-protective ventilation, a PEEP level of 5 to 10 cm H_2O is adequate because higher levels of PEEP are not associated with a better outcome (32).

Misuse of PEEP

Considering that PEEP is used almost universally in ventilator-dependent patients, misuse of PEEP must be common. The following statements are based on personal observations on the misuses of PEEP:

1. PEEP should not be used routinely in intubated patients because **there is no "physiologic PEEP"** that is generated by glottic closure. The alveolar pressure at end-expiration is zero in healthy adults. Neonates can generate PEEP by grunting, but this gift is lost by adulthood.

2. PEEP should not be used to reduce lung water in patients with pulmonary edema. In fact, **PEEP increases the water content of the lungs** (33,34), possibly by impeding lymphatic drainage from the lungs.

CONTINUOUS POSITIVE AIRWAYS PRESSURE

Spontaneous breathing in which a positive pressure is maintained throughout the respiratory cycle is called *continuous positive airway pressure* (CPAP). The airway pressure pattern with CPAP is shown in Figure 25.4. Note that the patient does not have to generate a negative airway pressure to receive the inhaled gas. This is made possible by a specialized inhalation valve that opens at a pressure above atmospheric pressure. This eliminates the extra work involved in generating a negative airway pressure to inhale. CPAP should be distinguished from *spontaneous PEEP*. In spontaneous PEEP, a negative airway pressure is required for inhalation. Spontaneous PEEP has been replaced by CPAP because of the reduced work of breathing with CPAP.

Clinical Uses

The major uses of CPAP are in nonintubated patients. CPAP can be delivered through specialized face masks equipped with adjustable, pressurized valves. CPAP masks have been used successfully to postpone intubation in patients with acute respiratory failure (35,36). However, these masks must be tight-fitting, and they cannot be removed for the patient to eat. Therefore, they are used only as a temporary measure. Specialized nasal masks may be better tolerated. CPAP delivered through nasal masks (nasal CPAP) has become popular in patients with obstructive sleep-apnea (37). In this situation, the CPAP is used as a stent to prevent upper airway collapse during negative pressure breathing. Nasal CPAP has also been used successfully in patients with acute exacerbation of chronic obstructive lung disease (38,39).

A FINAL WORD

Since mechanical ventilation is a support measure and not a treatment modality, nothing that is done with a ventilator will have a favorable impact on the outcome of the primary illness. On the other hand, mechanical ventilation can have a negative impact on outcomes by creating adverse effects. This means that the best mode of mechanical ventilation is the one with the fewest adverse effects. It also means that, if we really want to improve outcomes in ventilator-dependent patients, less attention should be directed to the knobs on ventilators, and more attention should be directed at the diseases that create ventilator dependency.

REFERENCES

Reviews

1. Tobin MJ. Advances in mechanical ventilation. N Engl J Med 2001;344:1986–1996.
2. Tobin MJ. Patient-ventilator interaction. Am J Respir Crit Care Med 2001; 163:1059–1063.
3. Branson RD. Functional principles of positive pressure ventilators: implications for patient-ventilator interaction. Respir Care Clin North Am 2005; 11:119–145.

Assist-Control Ventilation

4. Marini JJ, Capps JS, Culver BH. The inspiratory work of breathing during assisted mechanical ventilation. Chest 1985;87:612–618.
5. Fernandez R, Blanch L, Antigas A. Respiratory center activity during mechanical ventilation. J Crit Care 1991;6:102–111.
6. Izurieta R, Rabatin J. Sedation during mechanical ventilation: a systematic review. Crit Care Med 2002;30:2644–2648.
7. Leung P, Jubran A, Tobin MJ. Comparison of assisted ventilator modes on triggering, patients' effort, and dyspnea. Am J Respir Crit Care Med 1997;155: 1940–1948.
8. Laureen H, Pearl R. Flow triggering, pressure triggering, and autotriggering during mechanical ventilation. Crit Care Med 2000;28:579–581.

Ventilator-Induced Lung Injury

9. Dreyfuss D, Saumon G. Ventilator-induced lung injury. Am Rev Respir Crit Care Med 1998;157:294–323.
10. Ranieri VM, Giunta F, Suter P, Slutsky AS. Mechanical ventilation as a mediator of multisystem organ failure in acute respiratory distress syndrome. JAMA 2000;284:43–44.
11. The Acute Respiratory Distress Syndrome Network. Ventilation with lower tidal volumes as compared with traditional tidal volumes for acute lung injury and the acute respiratory distress syndrome. N Engl J Med 2000;342: 1301–1308.
12. Gajic O, Dara S, Mendez JL, et al. Ventilator-associated lung injury in patients without acute lung injury at the onset of mechanical ventilation. Crit Care Med 2004;32:1817–1824.

Intermittent Mandatory Ventilation

13. Sassoon CSH, Del Rosario N, Fei R, et al. Influence of pressure- and flow-triggered synchronous intermittent mandatory ventilation on inspiratory muscle work. Crit Care Med 1994;22:1933–1941.
14. Pinsky MR. Cardiovascular issues in respiratory care. Chest 2005;128(suppl): 592S–597S.

15. Mathru M, et al. Hemodynamic responses to changes in ventilatory patterns in patients with normal and poor left ventricular reserve. Crit Care Med 1982; 10:423–426.

Pressure-Controlled Ventilation

16. Shelledy DC, Rau JL, Thomas-Goodfellow L. A comparison of the effects of assist-control, SIMV, and SIMV with pressure-support on ventilation, oxygen consumption, and ventilatory equivalent. Heart Lung 1995;24:67–75.
17. Rappaport SH, Shipner R, Yoshihara G, et al. Randomized, prospective trial of pressure-limited versus volume controlled ventilation in severe respiratory failure. Crit Care Med 1994;22:22–32.
18. Yang SC, Yang SP. Effects of inspiratory waveform on lung mechanics, gas exchange, and respiratory metabolism in COPD patients during mechanical ventilation. Chest 2002;122:2096–2104.

Inverse Ratio Ventilation

19. Marcy TW, Marini JJ. Inverse ratio ventilation in ARDS: rationale and implementation. Chest 1991;100:494–504.
20. Malarkkan N, Snook NJ, Lumb AB. New aspects of ventilation in acute lung injury. Anesthesia 2003;58:647–667.
21. Yanos J, Watling SM, Verhey J. The physiologic effects of inverse ratio ventilation. Chest 1998;114:834–838.
22. Wang SH, Wei TS. The outcome of early pressure-controlled inverse ratio ventilation on patients with severe acute respiratory distress syndrome in surgical intensive care unit. Am J Surg 2002;183:151–155.

Pressure-Support Ventilation

23. Hess DR. Ventilator waveforms and the physiology of pressure support ventilation. Respir Care 2005;50:166–186.
24. Hess DR. The evidence for noninvasive positive-pressure ventilation in the care of patients in acute respiratory failure: a systematic review of the literature. Respir Care 2004;49:810–829.
25. Caples SM, Gay PC. Noninvasive positive pressure ventilation in the intensive care unit: a concise review. Crit Care Med 2005;33:2651–2658.

Positive End-Expiratory Pressure

26. Barbas CSV, Lung recruitment maneuvers in acute respiratory distress syndrome and facilitating resolution. Crit Care Med 2003;31(suppl):S265–S271.
27. Gattinoni L, Cairon M, Cressoni M, et al. Lung recruitment in patients with the acute respiratory distress syndrome. N Engl J Med 2006;354:1775–1786.
28. Schmitt J-M, Viellard-Baron A, Augarde R, et al. Positive end-expiratory pressure titration in acute respiratory distress syndrome patients: impact on right ventricular outflow impedance evaluated by pulmonary artery Doppler flow velocity measurements. Crit Care Med 2001;29:1154–1158.

29. Takata M, Robotham JL. Ventricular external constraint by the lung and pericardium during positive end-expiratory pressure. Am Rev Respir Dis 1991; 43:872–875.
30. Gainnier M, Michelet P, Thirion X, et al. Prone position and positive end-expiratory pressure in acute respiratory distress syndrome. Crit Care Med 2003; 31:2719–2726.
31. Hawker FH, Torzillo PJ, Southee AE. PEEP and "reverse mismatch": a case where less PEEP is best. Chest 1991;99:1034–1036.
32. Brower RG, Lanken PN, MacIntyre N, et al. Higher versus lower positive end-expiratory pressures in patients with the acute respiratory distress syndrome. N Engl J Med 2004;351:327–336.
33. Petty TL. The use, abuse, and mystique of positive end-expiratory pressure. Am Rev Respir Dis 1988;138:475–478.
34. Saul GM, Freeley TW, Mihm FG. Effect of graded PEEP on lung water in noncardiogenic pulmonary edema. Crit Care Med 1982;10:667–669.

Continuous Positive Airway Pressure

35. Hess DR. Noninvasive positive-pressure ventilation and ventilator-associated pneumonia. Respir Care 2005;50:924–931.
36. Brochard L, Mancebo J, Elliott MW. Noninvasive ventilation for acute respiratory failure. Eur Respir J 2002;19:712–721.
37. Pack AI. Advances in sleep-disordered breathing. Am J Respir Crit Care Med 2006;173:7–15.
38. de Lucas P, Tarancon C, Puente L, et al. Nasal continuous positive airway pressure in patients with COPD in acute respiratory failure. Chest 1993;104: 1694–1697.
39. Majid A, Hill NS. Noninvasive ventilation for acute respiratory failure. Curr Opin Crit Care 2005;11:77–81.

Chapter 26

THE VENTILATOR-DEPENDENT PATIENT

This chapter describes the practices and common concerns involved in the care of ventilator-dependent patients. The focus in this chapter is on issues that are directly related to artificial airways (endotracheal and tracheostomy tubes) and positive-pressure ventilation. The complicating illnesses that can develop in ventilator-dependent patients, such as nosocomial infections, are described elsewhere.

ARTIFICIAL AIRWAYS

Positive-pressure ventilation is delivered through a variety of plastic tubes that are passed into the trachea through the vocal cords (endotracheal tubes) or are inserted directly into the trachea (tracheostomy tubes) (1–3). These tubes are equipped with an inflatable balloon at the distal end (called a cuff) that is used to seal the trachea and prevent positive-pressure inflation volumes from escaping out through the larynx. The complications created by these tubes are related to their path of entry into the trachea, and to pressure-induced injury of the tracheal mucosa from the inflated cuffs. The major complications are indicated in Figure 26.1 (2–4).

Endotracheal Intubation

The patient who has been recently intubated will have an endotracheal tube inserted through the nose or mouth. These tubes vary in length from 25 to 35 cm, and are sized according to their internal diameter, which varies from 5 to 10 mm (e.g., a "size 7" endotracheal tube will have an internal diameter of 7 mm). The volume capacity of endotracheal tubes is 35 to 45 mL (5), which is about half the volume of the anatomic dead space in adults (1 mg/kg). The decrease in anatomic dead space associated with endotracheal intubation has no apparent significance.

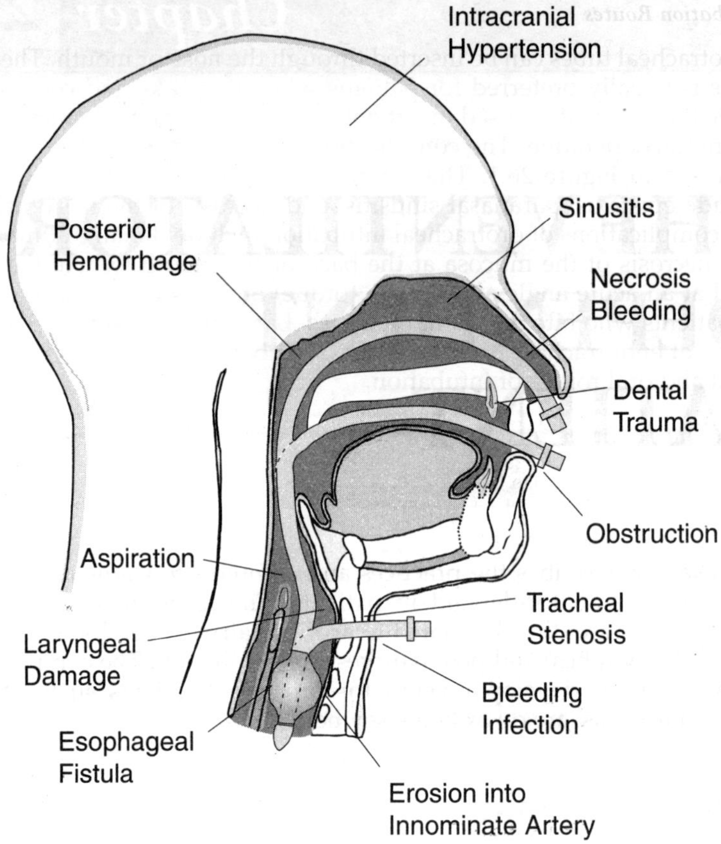

FIGURE 26.1 Complications of endotracheal intubation (nasal and oral routes) and tracheostomy.

The Work of Breathing

Endotracheal tubes increase the resistance to airflow. This resistance is directly related to the length of the tube, and inversely related to the diameter of the tube (e.g., tubes that are longer and narrower will create a greater resistance to airflow). An increased resistance to airflow will require a higher pressure gradient to ensure the same rate of airflow. During spontaneous breathing, a greater negative intrathoracic pressure will be needed to maintain a constant inspiratory flow rate when a subject is breathing through a long and narrow tube. This increases the work of breathing. High flow rates create turbulent flow, and this increases resistance further, so the work of breathing through endotracheal tubes is particularly high when patients are in respiratory distress.

The work of breathing created by endotracheal tubes is important when weaning patients from the ventilator. In general, **the diameter of endotracheal tubes should be at least 7 mm, and preferably 8 mm, to limit the influence of the tube on the work of breathing**. (The process of weaning patients from the ventilator is described in the next chapter.)

Intubation Routes

Endotracheal tubes can be inserted through the nose or mouth. The nasal route is usually preferred for patients who are awake and cooperative, while the oral route is used in patients who have an altered mental status or are uncooperative. The complications associated with each route are indicated in Figure 26.1. The complications of nasotracheal intubation include epistaxis, paranasal sinusitis, and necrosis of the nasal mucosa. The complications of orotracheal intubation include dental trauma, pressure necrosis of the mucosa at the back of the mouth (where the tubes bend at an acute angle and exert a torque) and obstruction of the tubes by patients who bite down on the tubes. Laryngeal damage is a complication of endotracheal (translaryngeal) intubation, and occurs with both nasal and oral routes of intubation.

Proper Tube Position

Evaluation of endotracheal tube position is mandatory after intubation, and should be repeated on a regular basis until the patient is extubated or receives a tracheostomy. Some useful radiographic landmarks for evaluating endotracheal tube position are shown in Table 26.1 (6). The vocal cords are usually situated at the interspace between the fifth and sixth cervical vertebrae (C5–C6). If not visible, the main carina is usually over the interspace between the fourth and fifth thoracic vertebrae (T4–T5) on a portable chest x-ray film. **When the head is in a neutral position, the tip of the endotracheal tube should be 3 to 5 cm above the carina**, or midway between the carina and vocal cords. The head is in the neutral position when the inferior border of the mandible projects over the lower cervical spine (C5–C6). Note that flexion or extension of the head and

TABLE 26.1 Radiographic Evaluation of Tracheal Intubation

	Radiographic Location
Anatomic Structures	
Vocal Cords	Usually over the C4–C5 interspace
Carina	Usually over the T4–T5 interspace
Head and Neck Position	
Neutral Position	Inferior border of mandible is over C5–C6
Flexion	Mandible is over T1–T2
Extension	Mandible is above C4
Tracheal Tube Position	
Head in Neutral Position	Tip of the tube should be midway between the vocal cords and carina, or 3–5 cm above the carina
Head Flexed	Tip of tube will descend 2 cm
Head Extended	Tip of tube will ascend 2 cm

From Goodman LR, Putman CE, eds. Critical care imaging. 3rd ed, Philadelphia: WB Saunders, 1992:35–56.

neck causes a 2 cm displacement of the tip of the endotracheal tube (6). The total displacement of 4 cm with changes in head position represents about one-third of the length of the trachea.

Migration of Tubes

Endotracheal tubes can migrate in either direction along the trachea (from manipulation of the tube during suctioning, turning, etc.), and when tubes move distally into the lungs, they often end up in the right mainstem bronchus (which runs a straight course down from the trachea). What can happen next is shown in Figure 26.2; i.e., selective ventilation of one lung results in progressive atelectasis in the non-ventilated lung. Delivering the entire tidal volume to one lung can also result in alveolar rupture and pneumothorax in the ventilated lung (which is not the case in Figure 26.2).

There are two measures that can reduce the incidence of endotracheal tube migration into one of the mainstem bronchi. First, for orotracheal intubations, don't allow the tip of the endotracheal tube to advance further than 21 cm from the teeth in women and 23 cm from the teeth in men (7). Second, monitor the position of the endotracheal tube on

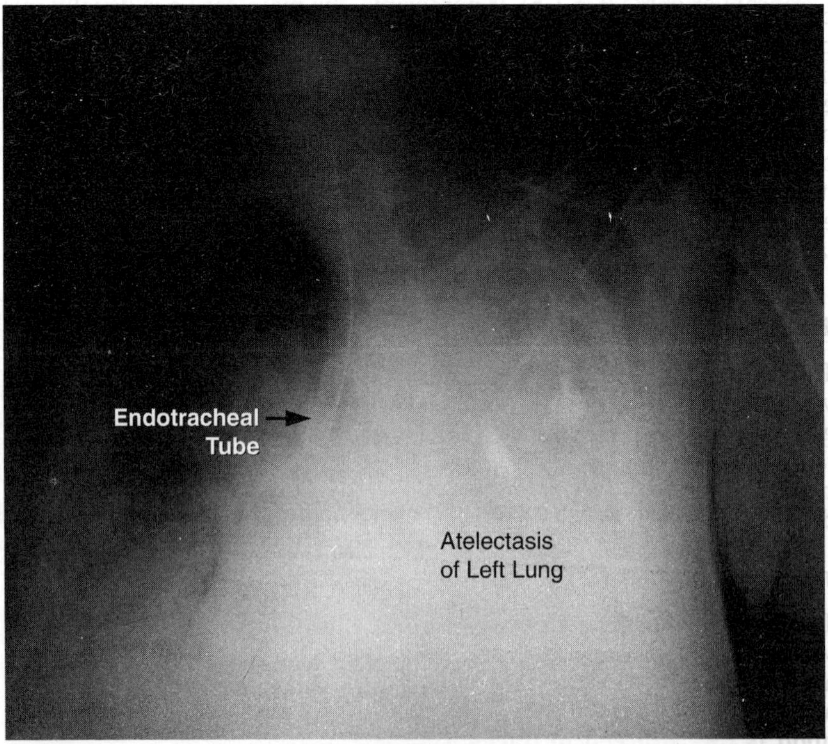

FIGURE 26.2 Portable chest x-ray showing the tip of an endotracheal tube in the right lung. The opacification of the left hemothorax represents atelectasis of the left lung. Image is digitally enhanced.

regularly-scheduled chest x-rays (which is a common practice in ventilator-dependent patients), and keep the tip of the tube at least 3 cm above the main carina (where the trachea bifurcates to form the right and left mainstem bronchi.

Paranasal Sinusitis

Nasotracheal (and nasogastric) tubes can obstruct the ostia that drain the paranasal sinuses, and this predisposes to a purulent sinusitis (8,9). The maxillary sinus is almost always involved (see Fig. 39.3). The presence of an air-fluid level by sinus radiography suggests the diagnosis, but confirmation requires aspiration of infected material from the involved sinus. The significance of paranasal sinusitis is unclear. It may be an important consideration when all other causes of fever have been eliminated (9), but in the routine evaluation of fever in the ICU, sinusitis is often not evaluated and there are no apparent adverse consequences. This complication has also been reported with orotracheal tubes (9). See Chapter 39 for more information on sinusitis in the ICU.

Laryngeal Damage

The risk for laryngeal injury with endotracheal tubes is a major concern, and is the principal reason for performing tracheostomies when prolonged intubation is anticipated. The spectrum of laryngeal damage includes ulceration, granulomas, vocal cord paresis, and laryngeal edema. Some type of laryngeal damage is usually evident after 72 hours of translaryngeal intubation (10), and laryngeal edema is reported in 5% of cases. Fortunately, most cases of laryngeal injury do not result in significant airways obstruction, and the injury resolves within weeks after extubation (11). The problem of laryngeal edema after tracheal decannulation is described in Chapter 27.

Tracheostomy

Tracheostomy is preferred in patients who require prolonged mechanical ventilation. There are several advantages with tracheostomy, including greater patient comfort, more effective clearing of secretions, reduced resistance for breathing, and reduced risk of laryngeal injury (12). Tracheostomy patients can ingest food orally and can even vocalize using specially designed tracheostomy tubes.

Tracheostomy Timing

The optimal time for performing a tracheostomy can vary widely in individual patients. However, the following recommendation can be used as a general guideline (12): **After 5 to 7 days of endotracheal intubation, assess the likelihood of extubation in the following week: if the likelihood is low, proceed to tracheostomy**. This recommendation is based on the observation that the clinical course in the first week is predictive of the final outcome in patients with ventilator-dependent respiratory failure (13).

Techniques

Tracheostomy can be performed as an open surgical procedure, or by percutaneous placement of the tracheostomy tube at the bedside. There are three percutaneous techniques; each involves puncturing the anterior wall of the trachea with a needle and then passing a guidewire through the needle into the trachea. The guidewire is then used to advance the tracheostomy tube into the trachea. The original technique, *percutaneous dilatational tracheostomy*, uses dilator catheters advanced over the guidewire to create a tract for the tracheostomy tube (14), similar to the Seldinger technique used to insert vascular catheters (see Fig. 6.3). In experienced hands, each of the percutaneous techniques can be performed successfully and safely (12).

The technique known as *cricothyroidotomy* is used only for emergency access to the airway. The trachea is entered through the cricothyroid membrane, just below the larynx, and there is high incidence of laryngeal injury and subglottic stenosis. Patients who survive following a cricothyroidotomy should have a regular tracheostomy (surgical or percutaneous) as soon as they are stable (12).

Complications

The morbidity and mortality associated with tracheostomy has declined in recent years. Combining surgical and percutaneous tracheostomy, the mortality rate is less than 1%, and major adverse events occur in 5 to 10% of cases (12). The acute complications of most concern are bleeding and infection. A comparison of surgical and percutaneous tracheostomy from pooled studies showed less bleeding and fewer infections with the percutaneous technique (15). However, the results of individual studies are conflicting, and the local expertise with each procedure will probably determine the technique with the fewest complications at each hospital.

One acute complication that deserves mention is accidental decannulation. If the tracheostomy tube is dislodged before the stoma tract is mature (which takes about one week) the tract closes quickly, and blind reinsertion of the tube can create false tracts. To minimize the risk of a bad outcome in this situation, the patient should be reintubated orally before attempting to reinsert the tracheostomy tube.

The most feared complication of tracheostomy is **tracheal stenosis**, which is a late complication that appears in the first 6 months after the tracheostomy tube is removed. Most cases of tracheal stenosis occur at the tracheotomy site, and are caused by tracheal narrowing after the stoma closes. The incidence of tracheal stenosis ranges from zero to 15% in individual reports (12), but most cases are asymptomatic.

Cuff Management

Positive-pressure ventilation requires a seal in the trachea that prevents gas from escaping out through the larynx during lung inflation, and this seal is created by inflatable balloons (called cuffs) that surround the distal portions of endotracheal tubes and tracheostomy tubes. An illustration

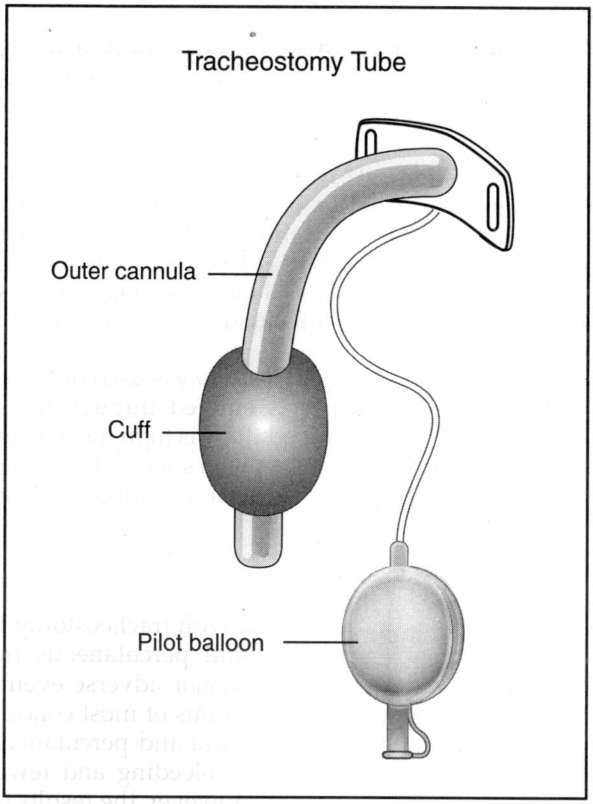

FIGURE 26.3 Illustration of a tracheostomy tube with an inflated cuff.

of a tracheostomy tube with an inflated cuff is shown in Figure 26.3. The cuff is attached to a pilot balloon that has a one-way valve. Cuff inflation is accomplished by attaching a syringe to the pilot balloon and injecting air. When the cuff is inflated, the pilot balloon will also inflate. Air is injected until there is no evidence of a leak around the cuff (i.e., there is no difference between inspiratory and expiratory volumes). **The pressure in the cuff** (measured with a pressure gauge attached to the pilot balloon) **should not exceed 25 mm Hg (35 cm H_2O)** (4). This pressure limit is based on the assumption that the capillary hydrostatic pressure in the wall of the trachea is 25 mm Hg, and thus external (cuff) pressures above 25 mm Hg can compress the underlying capillaries and produce ischemic injury and tracheal necrosis. The cuffs are elongated, which allows for greater dispersion of pressure, and this high-volume, low-pressure design allows for a tracheal seal at relatively low pressures.

The risk of pressure-induced tracheal injury can be virtually eliminated by using tracheal tubes that have a **foam rubber cuff that is normally inflated at atmospheric pressure** (an example is the Bivona Fome-Cuf tracheostomy tube). When the tube is inserted, the cuff must be manually deflated by applying suction from a syringe. Once in place, the cuff is allowed to inflate and create a tracheal seal. This cuff design allows the trachea to be sealed at atmospheric (zero) pressure, which eliminates the risk of pressure-induced injury in the wall of the trachea.

Aspiration

Contrary to popular belief, **cuff inflation to create a tracheal seal does not prevent aspiration of mouth secretions and tube feedings into the lower airways.** Aspiration of saliva and liquid tube feedings has been documented in over 50% of ventilator-dependent patients with tracheostomies and, in over three-fourths of the cases, the aspiration is clinically silent (16). Considering that approximately 1 L of saliva is normally produced each day (the normal rate of saliva production is 0.6 mL/min) and that each *micro*liter of saliva contains approximately 1 billion microorganisms, the danger associated with aspiration of mouth secretions is considerable (17). This emphasizes the value of oral decontamination described in Chapter 4.

Cuff Leaks

Cuff leaks are usually detected by sounds generated during lung inflation (created by gas flowing through the vocal cords). When a cuff leak becomes audible, the volume of the leak can be estimated as the difference between the desired inflation volume and the exhaled volume recorded by the ventilator. Cuff leaks are rarely caused by disruption of the cuff (18), and are usually the result of nonuniform contact between the cuff and the wall of the trachea.

If a cuff leak is apparent, the patient should be separated from the ventilator and the lungs should be manually inflated with an anesthesia bag. If the cuff leak involves an endotracheal tube, the tube should be replaced (or a fiberoptic instrument can be advanced through the tube to make sure it is still in the lungs). Air should never be added to the cuff blindly because the tube may be coming out of the trachea, and cuff inflation will damage the vocal cords. If the cuff leak involves a tracheostomy tube, air can be added to the cuff in an attempt to produce a seal. If this eliminates the leak, the cuff pressure should be measured. If the cuff pressure is above 35 cm H_2O, or the leak persists despite adding volume, the tracheostomy tube should be replaced.

CLEARING SECRETIONS

Routine suctioning to clear secretions is a standard practice in the care of intubated patients. This section will focus on measures that are used to liquify respiratory secretions to aid in their removal.

Physicochemical Properties

The respiratory secretions create a blanket that covers the mucosal surface of the airways. This blanket has a hydrophilic (water soluble) layer, and a hydrophobic (water insoluble) layer. The hydrophilic layer faces inward, and keeps the mucosal surface moist. The hydrophobic layer faces outward, towards the lumen of the airways. This outer layer is composed of a meshwork of mucoprotein strands (called mucus threads) held together by disulfide bridges. This meshwork traps particles and debris in the airways, and the combination of the mucoprotein meshwork and the trapped debris is what determines the viscoelastic behavior of the respiratory secretions.

Saline Instillation

Saline is often instilled into the trachea to facilitate the clearing of secretions, but this practice is ill-advised for two reasons. First, according to the physicochemical properties of respiratory secretions just described, the layer that contributes to the viscoelastic properties of respiratory secretions is not water soluble, which means that **saline cannot liquify or reduce the viscosity of respiratory secretions**. Adding saline to thick, respiratory secretions is like pouring water over grease.

The second problem with saline instillation is the risk for infection. As mentioned in Chapter 7, bacteria form biofilms on prosthetic devices (see Fig. 7.2), and bacterial biofilms have been demonstrated on the inner surface of endotracheal tubes and tracheostomy tubes (19). Saline injections into tracheal tubes can dislodge these bacterial biofilms. In a study using endotracheal tubes from extubated patients, the results showed that injection of 5 mL of saline can dislodge up to 300,000 colonies of viable bacteria from the inner surface of the tubes (20). Therefore, **saline injection provides a vehicle for transporting bacteria into the lower airways.** This observation deserves much more attention than it receives.

Mucolytic Therapy

The accumulation of tenacious secretions can result in a condition like the one shown in Figure 26.4, where a waterless "plug" is completely obstructing a major airway. In this situation, a mucolytic agent like *N*-acetylcysteine (Mucomyst) can help to disrupt the plug and relieve the obstruction. *N*-acetylcysteine (NAC) is a sulfhydryl-containing tripeptide that is better known as the antidote for acetaminophen overdose, but is primarily a mucolytic agent that acts by disrupting the disulfide bridges between mucoprotein strands in sputum (21). The drug is available in a liquid preparation (10 or 20% solution) that can be given as an aerosol spray, or injected directly into the airways (Table 26.2). Aerosolized NAC should be avoided when possible because it is irritating to the airways and can provoke coughing and bronchospasm (particularly in asthmatics). Direct instillation of NAC into the tracheal tube is preferred, especially when there is an obstruction.

If intratracheal injection of NAC does not relieve an obstruction, bronchoscopy should be performed (the NAC is then applied directly to the mucous plug). Following relief of the obstruction, NAC can be instilled two or three times a day for the next day or two. Daily use of NAC is not advised because the drug solution is hypertonic (even with the saline additive) and can provoke bronchorrhea.

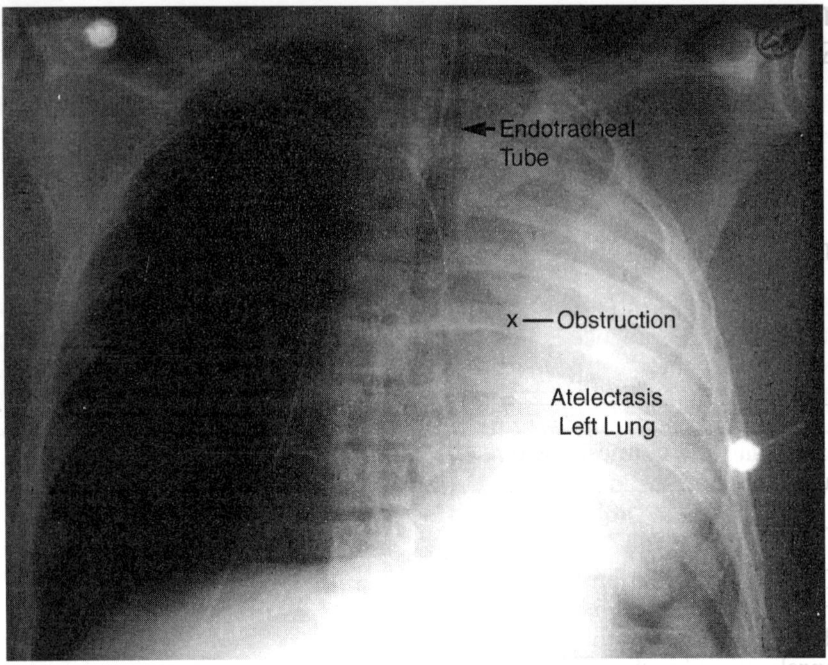

FIGURE 26.4 Portable chest x-ray of an intubated patient showing atelectasis of the left lung, which is usually caused by a mucous plug in the left mainstem bronchus.

ALVEOLAR RUPTURE

The problem of ventilator-induced lung injury described in Chapters 22 and 24 has its ultimate expression in clinically apparent alveolar rupture, which occurs in up to one-fourth of patients receiving positive-pressure ventilation (22).

Clinical Presentation

Escape of gas from the alveoli can produce a variety of clinical manifestations. The alveolar gas can dissect along tissue planes and produce *pulmonary interstitial emphysema,* and can move into the mediastinum and produce *pneumomediastinum.* Mediastinal gas can move into the neck to produce *subcutaneous emphysema,* or can pass below the diaphragm to produce *pneumoperitoneum.* Finally, if the rupture involves the visceral pleura, gas will collect in the pleural space and produce a *pneumothorax*. Each of these entities can occur alone or in combination with the others (22,23).

Pneumothorax

Radiographic evidence of pneumothorax occurs in 5 to 15% of ventilator-dependent patients (22,23). Risk factors include high inflation pressures

TABLE 26.2 Mucolytic Therapy with N-acetylcysteine (NAC)

Aerosol therapy:	• Use 10% NAC solution. • Mix 2.5 mL NAC with 2.5 mL saline and place mixture (5 mL) in a small volume nebulizer for aerosol delivery. • *Warning*: this can provoke bronchospasm, and is not recommended in asthmatics.
Tracheal injection:	• Use 20% NAC solution. • Mix 2 mL NAC with 2 mL saline and inject 2 mL aliquots into the trachea. • *Warning*: Excessive volumes can produce bronchorrhea.

and inflation volumes, positive end-expiratory pressure (PEEP), and diffuse lung injury.

Clinical Presentation

Clinical manifestations are either absent, minimal, or nonspecific. The **most valuable clinical sign is subcutaneous emphysema** in the neck and upper thorax, which is pathognomonic of alveolar rupture. Breath sounds are unreliable in ventilator-dependent patients because sounds transmitted from the ventilator tubing can be mistaken for airway sounds.

Radiographic Detection

The radiographic detection of pleural air can be difficult **in the supine position,** because **pleural air does not collect at the lung apex** when patients are supine (23,24). Figure 26.5 illustrates this difficulty. In this case of a traumatic pneumothorax, the chest x-ray is unrevealing, but the CT scan reveals an anterior pneumothorax on the left. Pleural air will collect in the most superior region of the hemithorax and, in the supine position, this region is just anterior to both lung bases. Therefore, **basilar and subpulmonic collections of air are characteristic of pneumothorax in the supine position** (24).

Redundant Skin Folds

When the film cartridge used for portable chest x-ray examinations is placed under the patient, the skin on the back can fold over on itself, and the edge of this redundant skin fold creates a radiographic shadow that can be mistaken for a pneumothorax. The radiographic appearance of a redundant skin fold is shown in Figure 26.6. Note that there is a gradual increase in radiodensity that suddenly ends as a wavy line. The increase in density is produced by the skin that is folded back on itself. A pneumothorax would appear as a sharp white line with dark shadows (air) on either side.

When a redundant skin fold is suspected, a repeat chest film should be obtained (it may be wise to alert the x-ray technician to make sure the film cartridge is flush on the patient's back). The shadow should disappear if it is due to a redundant skin fold.

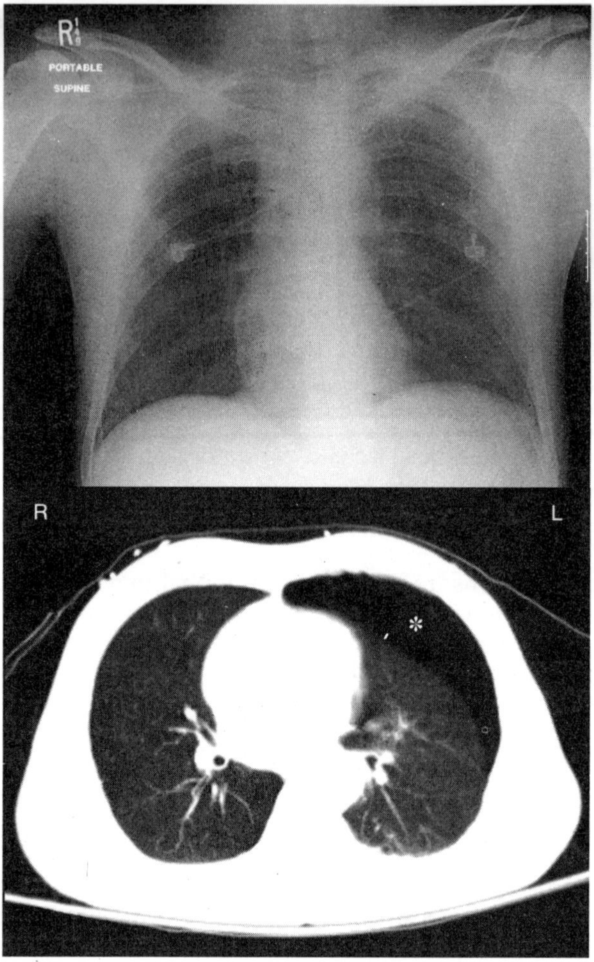

FIGURE 26.5 A portable chest x-ray and CT image of the thorax in a young male with blunt trauma to the chest. An anterior pneumothorax is evident on the CT image (indicated by the asterisk) but is not apparent on the chest x-ray.

Pleural Evacuation

Evacuation of pleural air is accomplished by inserting a chest tube through the fourth or fifth intercostal space along the mid-axillary line. The tube should be advanced in an anterior and superior direction (because this is where pleural air collects in the supine position). The pleural space is drained of fluid and air using a three-chamber system like the one shown in Figure 26.7 (25).

Collection Chamber

The first bottle in the system collects fluid from the pleural space and allows air to pass through to the next bottle in the series. Because the inlet

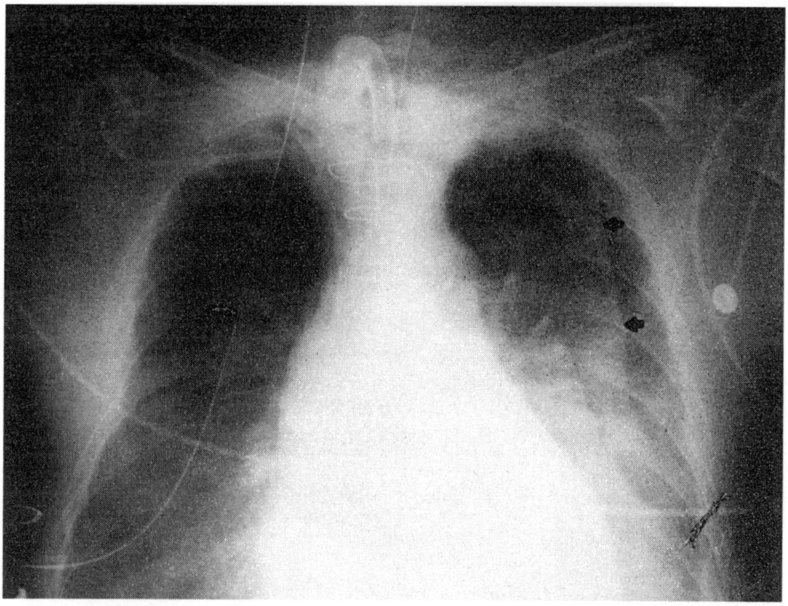

FIGURE 26.6 Portable chest x-ray showing a wavy line in the left hemithorax. This line is the edge of a redundant skin fold, and not the edge of the lung.

of this chamber is not in direct contact with the fluid, the pleural fluid that is collected does not impose a back pressure on the pleural space.

Water-Seal Chamber

The second bottle acts as a one-way valve that allows air to escape from the pleural space but prevents air from entering the pleural space. This one-way valve is created by submerging the inlet tube under water. This imposes a back-pressure on the pleural space that is equal to the depth that the tube is submerged. The positive pressure in the pleural space then prevents atmospheric air (at zero pressure) from entering the pleural space. The water thus "seals" the pleural space from the surrounding atmosphere. This water-seal pressure is usually 2 cm H_2O.

Air that is evacuated from the pleural space passes through the water in the second bottle and creates bubbles. Thus, the presence of bubbles in the water-seal chamber (called bubbling) is used as evidence for a continuing bronchopleural air leak.

Suction-Control Chamber

The third bottle in the system is used to set a maximum limit on the negative suction pressure that is imposed on the pleural space. This maximum pressure is determined by the height of the water column in the air inlet tube. Negative pressure (from wall suction) draws the water down the air inlet tube, and when the negative pressure exceeds the height of the water column, air is entrained from the atmosphere. Therefore, the pressure in the bottle can never become more negative than the height of the water column in the air inlet tube.

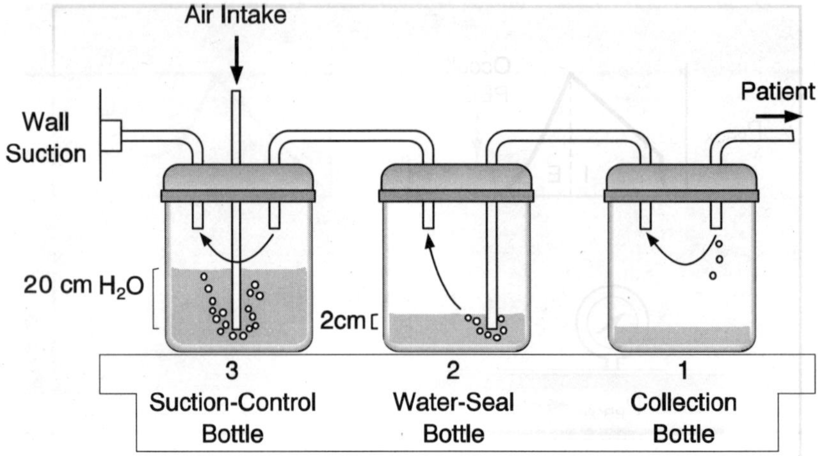

FIGURE 26.7 A standard pleural drainage system for evacuating air and fluid from the pleural space.

Water is added to the suction-control chamber to achieve a water level of 20 cm. The wall suction is then activated and slowly increased until bubbles appear in the water. This bubbling indicates that atmospheric air is being entrained, and thus the maximum negative pressure has been achieved. The continuous bubbling causes water evaporation, so it is imperative that the height of the water in this chamber is checked periodically, and more water is added when necessary.

Why Suction?

The practice of using suction to evacuate pleural air is unnecessary and potentially harmful. Although there is a perception that suction will help the lungs reinflate, the lungs will reinflate without the use of suction. Furthermore, creating a negative pressure in the pleural space also creates a higher transpulmonary pressure (the pressure difference between alveoli and the pleural space), and this increases the rate of the air flowing through the bronchopleural fistula. Thus, **applying suction to the pleural space increases bronchopleural air leaks,** and this can keep bronchopleural fistulas patent. If a persistent air leak is present when suction is applied to the pleural space, the suction should be discontinued. Any air that collects in the pleural space will continue to be evacuated when the pleural pressure becomes more positive than the water-seal pressure.

INTRINSIC PEEP

As mentioned in Chapter 25, mechanical ventilation with high inflation volumes and rapid rates can (and probably often does) produce PEEP as a result of incomplete alveolar emptying during expiration (26–28). The illustration in Figure 26.8 helps explain this phenomenon.

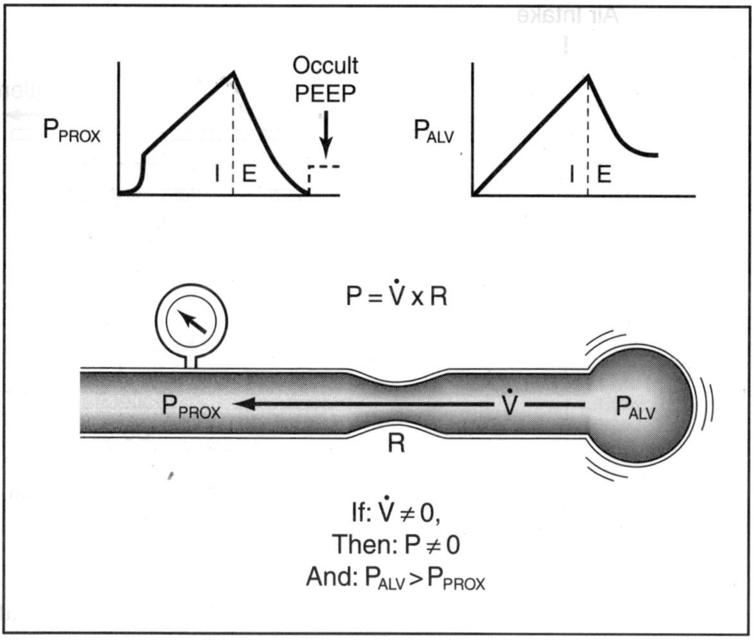

FIGURE 26.8 The features of intrinsic PEEP resulting from inadequate alveolar emptying. The presence of airflow ($\dot{V}$) at end-expiration indicates a pressure drop from the alveolus (P_{ALV}) to the proximal airways (P_{prox}). As shown at the top of the figure, the proximal airway pressure returns to zero at end-expiration while the alveolar pressure remains positive; hence the term *occult* PEEP. The upper left panel illustrates the end-expiratory occlusion method for detecting occult PEEP.

Pathogenesis

Under normal circumstances, there is no airflow at the end of expiration, and thus end-expiratory pressure is the same in the alveoli and proximal airways. On the other hand, when alveolar emptying is incomplete during expiration, airflow is present at the end of expiration, and this creates a pressure drop from the alveoli to the proximal airways at end-expiration. Thus in this situation, alveolar pressure will be positive relative to atmospheric (zero) pressure at end-expiration (i.e., PEEP). As shown in the upper portion of Figure 26.8, the positive alveolar pressure is not evident on the proximal airways pressure tracing, and hence this is an *occult* PEEP (26). More popular terms for this pressure are *intrinsic PEEP, auto-PEEP,* and *dynamic hyperinflation* (27). The latter term is usually reserved for PEEP produced by obstructive airways disease (see below).

Predisposing Factors

The factors that predispose to hyperinflation and intrinsic PEEP can be separated into ventilation-associated and disease-associated factors. The ventilatory factors that promote hyperinflation include high inflation volumes, rapid breathing, and a relative decrease in exhalation time relative to inhalation time. The disease-related factor that promotes hyperinflation is airways obstruction (as occurs in asthma and chronic obstructive pulmonary disease [COPD]). All three factors are operative in ventilator-dependent patients with obstructive airways disease.

In patients with asthma and COPD, intrinsic PEEP is probably universal during conventional volume-cycled mechanical ventilation (27–29). Intrinsic PEEP is also common in ventilator-dependent patients with ARDS (30), but the absolute level is low (<3 cm H_2O).

Consequences

Cardiac Performance

Intrinsic PEEP has the same effects on cardiac performance as extrinsic PEEP, which are described in Chapter 25. However, because intrinsic PEEP is often overlooked, the cardiac suppression from intrinsic PEEP can be life-threatening. Intrinsic PEEP from overly aggressive ventilation has been implicated as an occult cause of cardiac arrest (31), and failed cardiopulmonary resuscitation (32).

Alveolar Rupture

Intrinsic PEEP increases peak inspiratory airway pressures, and this will predispose to pressure-induced alveolar rupture (barotrauma). Hyperinflation-induced alveolar rupture and pneumothorax are particular concerns in ventilator-dependent asthmatic patients (29).

Work of Breathing

Intrinsic PEEP increases the work of breathing in several ways. To begin with, PEEP increases the pressure that must be generated to trigger the ventilator (e.g., if the ventilator breath is triggered at a pressure of −2 cm H_2O and there is an end-expiratory pressure of 5 cm H_2O, then the total pressure that must be generated to trigger the ventilator is 7 cm H_2O). In addition, hyperinflation places the lungs on a flatter portion of the pressure-volume curve, so higher pressures are needed to inhale the tidal volume. (To appreciate this effect, take a deep breath, and then try to breathe in further.) Finally, hyperinflation flattens the diaphragm and this (according to the Law of LaPlace; $T = Pr$) will increase the muscle tension needed to generate a given change in thoracic pressure. The sum of all of these factors can lead to a considerable increase in the work of breathing, and this could impede efforts to wean from mechanical ventilation (see Chapter 27).

Thoracic Compliance

Intrinsic PEEP increases the end-inspiratory pressures in the proximal airways (both peak and plateau pressures). When intrinsic PEEP goes undetected, the increase in plateau pressure is misinterpreted as a decrease in the compliance of the lungs and chest wall. Therefore, **failure to consider intrinsic PEEP can result in an underestimation of thoracic**

compliance. When thoracic compliance is calculated (see Chapter 24), the level of intrinsic PEEP should be subtracted from the measured plateau pressure and the resulting pressure should be used to calculate thoracic compliance.

Cardiac Filling Pressures

As mentioned in Chapter 10, the presence of PEEP can cause a spurious increase in cardiac filling pressures: central venous pressure (CVP) and pulmonary artery occlusion pressure (PAOP). This effect is due to transmission of PEEP into the lumen of intrathoracic vessels, resulting in an increase in intravascular pressure with little or no increase in transmural pressure (the physiologically important pressure).

A simple method for correcting the CVP and PAOP in the presence of intrinsic PEEP is to measure the level of intrinsic PEEP with the end-expiratory occlusion method and then subtract this pressure from the CVP or PAOP measured at end-expiration. Although PEEP is not always fully transmitted into vessels (33), the degree of transmission of intrinsic PEEP into vessels is difficult to determine because of the dynamic nature of this pressure.

Monitoring Intrinsic PEEP

Intrinsic PEEP is easy to detect but difficult to quantify. The easiest method of detection is listening for the presence of airflow at the end of expiration, which has been shown to be a sensitive but not specific method of detection (34). Expiratory flow tracings can also be used to detect intrinsic PEEP. The most accurate method of measuring intrinsic PEEP is to measure intraesophageal (pleural) pressure at end-expiration. The most popular method of monitoring intrinsic PEEP is the end-expiratory occlusion method.

End-Expiratory Occlusion

During controlled ventilation (i.e., when the patient is completely passive), intrinsic PEEP can be uncovered by occluding the expiratory tubing at the end of expiration (27). This maneuver blocks airflow and allows the pressure in the proximal airways to equilibrate with alveolar pressure. Thus, **a sudden rise in proximal airways pressure with end-expiratory occlusion is evidence of intrinsic PEEP** (see the upper left panel in Fig. 26.8). Unfortunately, accuracy requires that the occlusion occur at the very end of expiration, just before the next breath (because expiratory flow can persist until the end of expiration), and this is not possible on a consistent basis when the occlusion is performed manually.

Response to Extrinsic PEEP

The application of extrinsic PEEP normally increases the peak inspiratory airway pressure by an equivalent amount. However, in the presence of intrinsic PEEP, the peak inspiratory pressure may not change when extrinsic PEEP is applied (this is explained below). Therefore, **failure**

of extrinsic PEEP to produce an increase in peak inspiratory airway pressure is evidence of intrinsic PEEP (35–37). Furthermore, the level of extrinsic PEEP that first produces a rise in peak inspiratory pressures can be taken as the quantitative level of occult PEEP (35).

Management

The methods used to prevent or reduce hyperinflation and occult PEEP are all directed at promoting alveolar emptying during expiration. Ventilator-induced hyperinflation can be minimized by avoiding excessive inflation volumes, and by optimizing the time allowed for exhalation. These measures are described in Chapters 24 and 25.

Extrinsic PEEP

When hyperinflation is due to small airway collapse at end-expiration, as occurs in patients with asthma and COPD, the application of extrinsic PEEP can help keep the small airways open at end-expiration. The level of extrinsic PEEP must be enough to counterbalance the pressure causing small airways collapse (the *critical closing pressure*) but should not exceed the level of intrinsic PEEP (so that it does not impair expiratory flow) (36). To accomplish this, the level of extrinsic PEEP should match the level of intrinsic PEEP. The appropriate level of extrinsic PEEP is difficult to determine because of inaccuracies in measuring intrinsic PEEP. An alternative method is to apply external PEEP and measure the changes in end-expiratory plateau pressure. If this pressure decreases with external PEEP, this indicates that external PEEP has effectively decreased internal PEEP (37). The clinical significance of all of this, however, is unclear.

A FINAL WORD

The patient's clinical course in the first few days of mechanical ventilation will give you a fairly accurate indication of what is coming. If the patient is not improving, proceed to tracheostomy as soon as it can be done safely. (Tracheostomies are more comfortable for patients, and they allow more effective airway care.) Most of the day-to-day management in the ICU is aimed at preventing other adverse events (such as pneumothorax), and remaining vigilant for adverse events so they can be treated or corrected quickly. You will learn that, in many cases, you are (unfortunately) not the one controlling the course of the patient's illness.

REFERENCES

Reviews

1. 2005 American Heart Association Guidelines for Cardiopulmonary Resuscitation and Emergency Cardiovascular Care. Part 7.1: Adjuncts for airway control and ventilation. Circulation 2005; 112 (Suppl I):IV51–IV57. (Available online @ http://circ. ahajournals.org/content/vol112/24_ suppl/)

2. Gray AW. Endotracheal tubes. Crit Care Clin 2003;24:379–387.
3. Sue RD, Susanto I. Long-term complications of artificial airways. Clin Chest Med 2003;24:457–471.
4. Heffner JE, Hess D. Tracheostomy management in the chronically ventilated patient. Clin Chest Med 2001;22:561–568.

Endotracheal Intubation

5. Habib MP. Physiologic implications of artificial airways. Chest 1989;96:180–184.
6. Goodman LR. Pulmonary support and monitoring apparatus. In: Goodman LR, Putman CE, eds. Critical care imaging. 3rd ed. Philadelphia: WB Saunders, 1992:35–59.
7. Owen RL, Cheney FW. Endotracheal intubation: a preventable complication. Anesthesiology 1987;67:255–257.
8. Rouby J-J, Laurent P, Gosnach M, et al. Risk factors and clinical relevance of nosocomial maxillary sinusitis in the critically ill. Am J Respir Crit Care Med 1994;150:776–783.
9. van Zanten AR, Dixon JM, Nipshagen MD, et al. Hospital-acquired sinusitis is a common cause of fever of unknown origin in orotracheally intubated critically ill patients. Crit Care 2005;9:R583–R590.
10. Gallagher TJ. Endotracheal intubation. Crit Care Clin 1992;8:665–676.
11. Colice GL. Resolution of laryngeal injury following translaryngeal intubation. Am Rev Respir Dis 1992;145:361–364.

Tracheostomy

12. Tracheotomy: application and timing. Clin Chest Med 2003;24:389–398.
13. Estenssoro E, Dubin A, Laffaire E, et al. Incidence, clinical course, and outcome in 217 patients with acute respiratory distress syndrome. Crit Care Med 2002;30:2450–2456.
14. Ciagla P. Technique, complications, and improvements in percutaneous dilatational tracheostomy. Chest 1999;115:1229–1230.
15. Freeman BD, Isabella K, Lin N, et al. A meta-analysis of prospective trials comparing percutaneous and surgical tracheostomy in critically ill patients. Chest 2000;118:1412–1418.
16. Elpern EH, Scott MG, Petro L, et al. Pulmonary aspiration in mechanically ventilated patients with tracheostomies. Chest 1994;105:563–566.
17. Estes RJ, Meduri GU. The pathogenesis of ventilator-associated pneumonia: mechanisms of bacterial transcolonization and airway inoculation. Intensive Care Med 1995;21:365–383.
18. Kearl RA, Hooper RG. Massive airway leaks: an analysis of the role of endotracheal tubes. Crit Care Med 1993;21:518–521.

Clearing Secretions

19. Adair CG, Gorman SP, Feron BM, et al. Implications of endotracheal tube biofilm for ventilator-associated pneumonia. Intensive Care Med 1999;25:1072–1076.

20. Hagler DA, Traver GA. Endotracheal saline and suction catheters: sources of lower airways contamination. Am J Crit Care 1994;3:444–447.
21. Holdiness MR. Clinical pharmacokinetics of *N*-acetylcysteine. Clin Pharmacokinet 1991;20:123–134.

Alveolar Rupture

22. Gammon RB, Shin MS, Buchalter SE. Pulmonary barotrauma in mechanical ventilation. Chest 1992;102:568–572.
23. Marcy TW. Barotrauma: detection, recognition, and management. Chest 1993; 104:578–584.
24. Tocino IM, Miller MH, Fairfax WR. Distribution of pneumothorax in the supine and semirecumbent critically ill adult. Am J Radiol 1985;144:901–905.
25. Kam AC, O'Brien M, Kam PCA. Pleural drainage systems. Anesthesia 1993; 48:154–161.

Intrinsic PEEP

26. Pepe P, Marini JJ. Occult positive end-expiratory pressure in mechanically ventilated patients with airflow obstruction. Am Rev Respir Dis 1982;126: 166–170.
27. Blanch L, Bernabe F, Lucangelo U. Measurement of air trapping, intrinsic positive end-expiratory pressure, and dynamic hyperinflation in mechanically ventilated patients. Respir Care 2005;50:110–123.
28. Mughal MM, Culver DA, Minai OA, et al. Auto-positive end-expiratory pressure: mechanisms and treatment. Cleve Clin J Med 2005;72:801–809.
29. Shapiro JM. Management of respiratory failure in status asthmaticus. Am J Respir Med 2002;1:409–416.
30. Hough CL, Kallet RH, Ranieri M, et al. Intrinsic positive end-expiratory pressure in Acute Respiratory Distress Syndrome (ARDS) Network subjects. Crit Care Med 2005;33:527–532.
31. Rosengarten PL, Tuxen DV, Scheinkestel C, et al. Circulatory arrest induced by intermittent positive pressure ventilation in a patient with severe asthma. Anesth Intensive Care 1991;19:118–121.
32. Rogers PL, Schlichtig R, Miro A, et al. Auto-PEEP during CPR: an "occult" cause of electromechanical dissociation. Chest 1991;99:492–493.
33. Teboul J-L, Pinsky MR, Mercat A, et al. Estimating cardiac filling pressure in mechanically ventilated patients with hyperinflation. Crit Care Med 2000;28: 3631–3636.
34. Kress JP, O'Connor MF, Schmidt GA. Clinical examination reliably detects intrinsic positive end-expiratory pressure in critically ill, mechanically ventilated patients. Am J Respir Crit Care Med 1999;159:290–294.
35. Slutsky AS. Mechanical ventilation. Chest 1993;104:1833–1859.
36. Tobin MJ, Lodato RF. PEEP, auto-PEEP, and waterfalls. Chest 1989;96:449–451.
37. Caramez MP, Borges JB, Tucci MR, et al. Paradoxical responses to positive end-expiratory pressure in patients with airway obstruction during controlled ventilation. Crit Care Med 2005;33:1519–1528.

Chapter 27

DISCONTINUING MECHANICAL VENTILATION

Discontinuing mechanical ventilation is a rapid and uneventful process for most patients, but for one of every four or five patients, the transition to spontaneous breathing is a prolonged process that can consume almost half of the total time on a ventilator. This chapter describes the process of discontinuing mechanical ventilation, and the principal causes of difficulty in the transition to spontaneous breathing (1–4).

READINESS CRITERIA

The management of patients who require mechanical ventilation requires constant vigilance for signs indicating that ventilatory support may no longer be necessary. When patients begin to show evidence of clinical improvement, the criteria listed in Table 27.1 can be used to identify possible candidates for removal of ventilatory support. In general, oxygenation should be adequate while breathing non-toxic levels of inhaled oxygen, and patients should be hemodynamically stable with minimal or no vasopressor support. Patients should be aware of their surroundings when not sedated, and should be free of any reversible conditions (e.g., sepsis or electrolyte abnormalities) that can add to the difficulty of removing ventilatory support.

When the criteria in Table 27.1 have been satisfied, the patient should be removed from the ventilator briefly to obtain the measurements listed in Table 27.2. These measurements have been used to predict the likelihood that the patient will tolerate a trial of spontaneous breathing. Unfortunately, none of these measurements, when used in isolation, can predict with certainty which patients are ready to resume spontaneous breathing (1,5,6). However, when taken together, these measurements provide an impression of how difficult it will be for the patient to resume

Table 27.1 Checklist for Identifying Patients who Can be Considered for a Trial of Spontaneous Breathing

Respiratory Criteria:

- ☑ $PaO_2 \geq 60$ mm Hg on $FIO_2 \leq 40$–50% and PEEP ≤ 5–8 cm H_2O
- ☑ $PaCO_2$ normal or baseline (except for permissive hypercapnia).
- ☑ Patient is able to initiate an inspiratory effort.

Cardiovascular Criteria:

- ☑ No evidence of myocardial ischemia.
- ☑ Heart rate ≤ 140 beats/minute.
- ☑ Blood pressure normal without vasopressors or with minimum vasopressor support (e.g., dopamine < 5 μg/kg/min).

Adequate Mental Status:

- ☑ Patient is arousable, or Glasgow Coma Score ≥ 13.

Absence of Correctible Comorbid Conditions:

- ☑ Patient is afebrile.
- ☑ There are no significant electrolyte abnormalities.

From Reference 1.

spontaneous breathing. Two of the more predictive measurements are described next.

Rapid-Shallow Breathing Index

Rapid and shallow breathing is common in patients who do not tolerate spontaneous breathing (6). An index of rapid and shallow breathing is provided by the ratio of respiratory rate to tidal volume (RR/V_T), which is also called the *rapid-shallow breathing index*. This ratio is normally 40 to

Table 27.2 Measurements Used to Identify Patients Who Will Tolerate a Spontaneous Breathing Trial (SBT)

Measurement*	Reference Range in Adults	Threshold for Successful SBT†
Tidal Volume (V_T)	5–7 mL/kg	4–6 mL/kg
Respiratory Rate (RR)	10–18 bpm	30–38 bpm
Total Ventilation (V_E)	5–6 L/min	10–15 L/min
RR/V_T Ratio	40–50/L	60–105/L
Maximum Inspiratory Pressure (PImax)	−90 to −120 cm H_2O	−15 to −30 cm H_2O

*All measurements should be obtained during spontaneous breathing.
†From Reference 1.

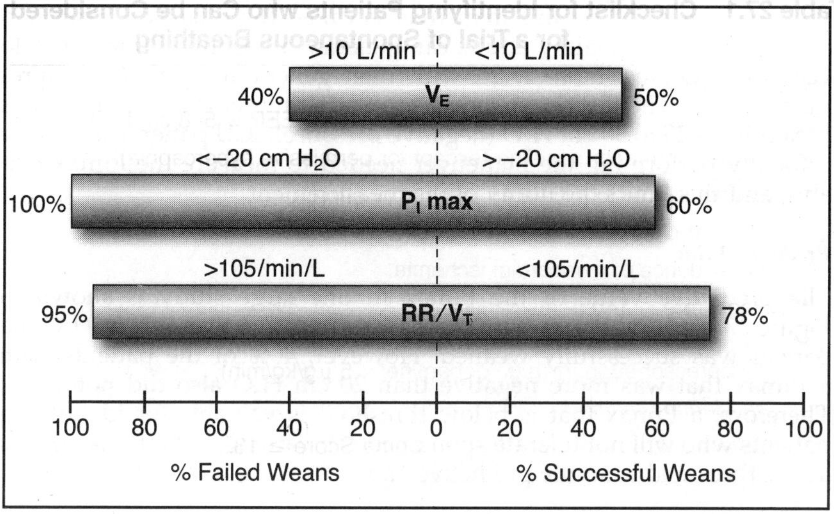

FIGURE 27.1 The predictive value of selected measurements obtained during spontaneous breathing. V_E = minute ventilation, *Pimax* = maximum inspiratory pressure, RR/V_T = ratio of respiratory rate to tidal volume. (Data from Yang K, Tobin MJ. A prospective study of indexes predicting the outcome of weaning from mechanical ventilation. N Engl J Med 1991;324:1445 – 1450.)

50/L, and is often above 100/L in patients who do not tolerate spontaneous breathing.

Predictive Value

The original study of the predictive value of the RR/V_T ratio is shown in Figure 27.1 (6). When the RR/V_T ratio was above 105 /L, 95% of the attempts to discontinue (wean) mechanical ventilation failed. However when the RR/V_T ratio was below 105, 80% of the wean attempts were successful. Therefore, the results of this study establish a **threshold RR/V_T ratio of approximately 100/L for predicting success or failure** to resume spontaneous breathing.

Other studies have shown that that the threshold RR/V_T ratio may differ in specific groups of patients (2), and that serial measurements of the RR/V_T ratio during a spontaneous breathing trial may be more predictive than measurements obtained at the onset of the trial (7). Nevertheless, the threshold RR/V_T ratio of 100/L remains useful because it can identify which patients might have difficulty during the spontaneous breathing trial.

Maximum Inspiratory Pressure

The strength of the diaphragm and other muscles of inspiration can be evaluated by having a patient exhale to residual lung volume and then inhale as forcefully as possible against a closed valve (8). The airway pressure generated by this maneuver is called the *maximum inspiratory pressure* (PImax). Healthy adults can generate a negative PImax of 90 to 120 cm H_2O (see Table 27.2), with men generating higher pressures than women. The threshold PImax for predicting return to spontaneous breathing is 20 to 30 cm H_2O (negative pressure). ICU patients may have difficulty performing the maneuver needed to measure the PImax reliably, and this limits the utility of the measurement.

Predictive Value

The predictive value of the PImax in one large study is shown in Figure 27.1 (6). When the PImax was less negative than 20 cm H_2O, no patient was successfully weaned. However, 40% of the patients with a PImax that was more negative than 20 cm H_2O also did not wean. Therefore, a PImax that is below threshold is valuable for identifying patients who will not tolerate spontaneous breathing, but a PImax that is above threshold has little predictive value.

THE SPONTANEOUS BREATHING TRIAL

The spontaneous breathing trial (SBT) can be conducted while the patient is still connected to the ventilator circuit, or the patient can be removed completely from the ventilator and allowed to breathe from an independent source of oxygen. The latter technique is often referred to as a *T-piece trial* because the breathing circuit is shaped like the letter *T* (see Figure 27.3). The advantages and disadvantages of each method are described next. There is no evidence that either method is superior to the other for allowing patients to be removed from the ventilator permanently (1).

Breathing Through the Ventilator

Spontaneous breathing trials are usually conducted while the patient is attached to the ventilator. The advantage of this method is the ability to monitor the tidal volume and respiratory rate during spontaneous breathing to detect the rapid and shallow breathing that often signals failure to sustain spontaneous breathing. The drawback with this method is an increased work of breathing, which is due to: 1) the negative pressure that must be generated to open an actuator valve in the ventilator and receive the inhaled oxygen mixture, and 2) the resistance created by the ventilator tubing between the patient and the ventilator. To counteract this increased work of breathing, *pressure-support ventilation* (described in Chapter 25) is used routinely during spontaneous breathing trials.

Pressure-Support Ventilation

The goal of pressure-support ventilation (PSV) during a spontaneous breathing trial is to add enough inspiratory pressure to reduce the work of breathing through the endotracheal tube and ventilator circuit without augmenting the spontaneous tidal volume. A positive pressure of

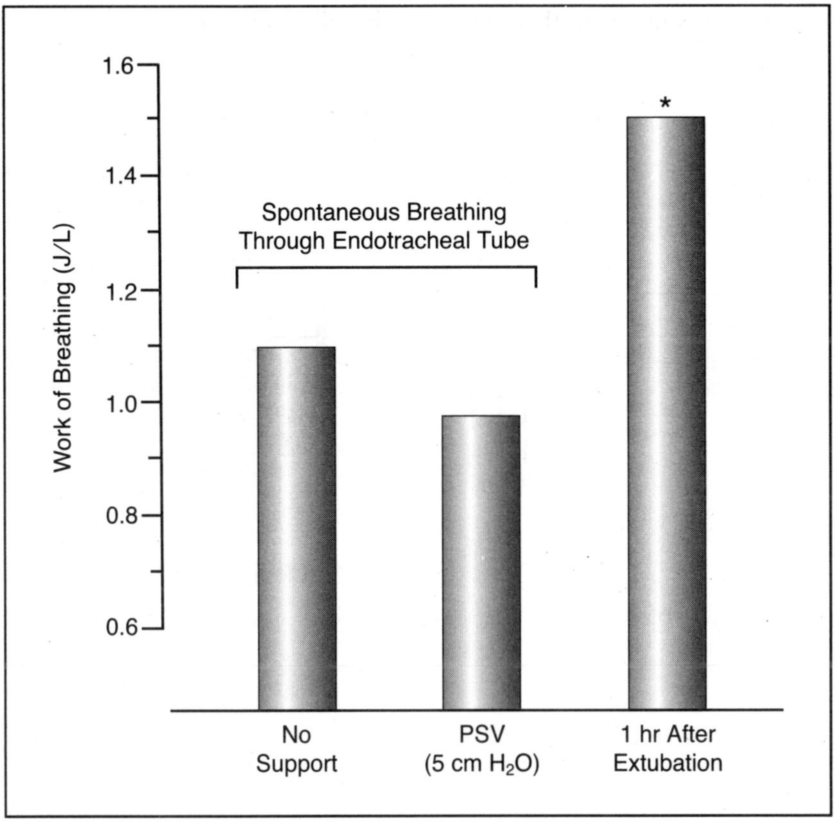

FIGURE 27.2 The work of breathing during spontaneous breathing trials conducted with and without the aid of pressure-support ventilation (PSV) at 5 cm H_2O, and one hour after extubation. Work is expressed in joules per liter (J/L). The asterisk indicates a significant difference from the other conditions ($p < 0.05$). All patients in this study were removed from ventilatory support without incident. (Adapted from Mehta S, Nelson DL, Klinger JR, et al. Prediction of post-extubation work of breathing. Crit Care Med 2000; 28:1341–1346, with permission.)

5–7 cm H_2O is routinely used for this purpose. The effect of this practice is shown in Figure 27.2. In this group of patients (who tolerated spontaneous breathing), the use of pressure support ventilation (PSV) at 5 cm H_2O is associated with a small but insignificant decrease in the work of breathing. Note also that the work of breathing is much higher after the endotracheal tubes are removed! (This observation is discussed again at the end of the chapter.)

The graph in Figure 27.2 indicates that: 1) **inspiratory pressure support is not necessary during spontaneous breathing trials,** and 2) breathing through endotracheal tubes and ventilator circuits is not associated with an increased work of breathing, at least in comparison to the early time period following extubation. These conclusions may only apply to

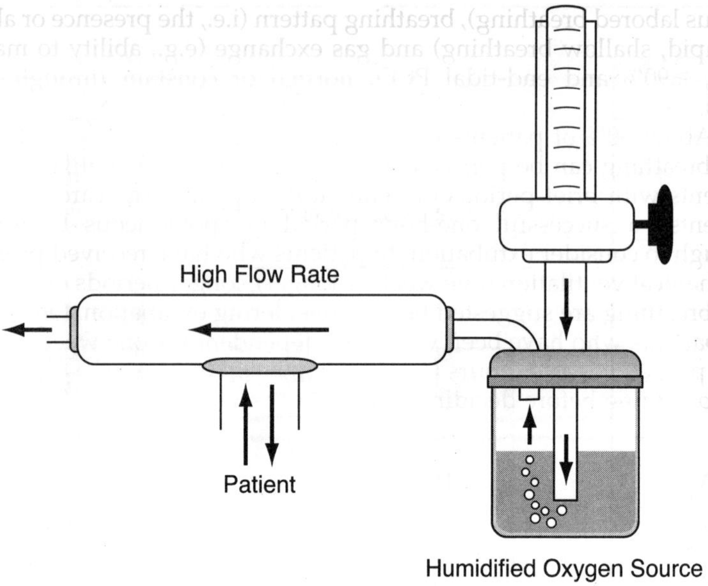

FIGURE 27.3 Diagram of the T-shaped circuit used for spontaneous breathing trials when the patient is disconnected from the ventilator.

patients who can sustain spontaneous breathing (like the patients used in the study in Figure 27.2), but they may apply to all patients as well.

Breathing Through the T-Piece

Spontaneous breathing trials can be conducted with the patient disconnected from the ventilator using the T-shaped circuit design shown in Figure 27.3. The inhaled gas is delivered at a high flow rate (greater than the patient's inspiratory flow rate) through the upper arm of the apparatus. The high flow rate serves two purposes. First, it creates a "suction effect" that carries the exhaled gas out of the apparatus and prevents rebreathing of exhaled gas. Second, it prevents the patient from inhaling room air from the exhalation side of the apparatus.

The disadvantage of T-piece trials is the inability to monitor the patient's spontaneous tidal volume and respiratory rate. The assumed advantage is less work of breathing when compared to spontaneous breathing while connected to the ventilator. T-piece trials are often preferred in patients who are breathing rapidly or have a high minute ventilation.

Protocol

The recommended protocol is to allow 30 to 120 minutes for the initial trial of spontaneous breathing (1). Although not mentioned, it is wise to increase the F_{IO_2} by 10% for the period of spontaneous breathing. Success or failure is judged by a combination of patient appearance (comfortable versus labored breathing), breathing pattern (i.e., the presence or absence of rapid, shallow breathing) and gas exchange (e.g., ability to maintain SaO_2 ≥90% and end-tidal PCO_2 normal or constant throughout the trial).

About 80% of patients who tolerate 30 to 120 minutes of spontaneous breathing can be permanently removed from the ventilator (1). For patients with brief periods of ventilatory support (e.g., cardiac surgery patients), a successful one-hour period of spontaneous breathing is enough to consider extubation. In patients who have received prolonged mechanical ventilation (one week or longer), longer periods of spontaneous breathing are suggested before considering extubation. Our practice for patients who have been ventilator-dependent for one week or longer is to permit at least 8 hours (and sometimes up to 24 hours) of spontaneous breathing before deciding to remove the ventilator from the room.

An Approach to Rapid Breathing

Patients who are being removed from ventilatory support often experience anxiety and a sense of dyspnea, and these patients often breathe rapidly even though they are ventilating adequately (9,10). Therefore, for patients who begin to breathe rapidly during the spontaneous breathing trials, it is important to distinguish anxiety from ventilatory failure requiring continued mechanical ventilation. The flow diagram in Figure 27.4 shows a simple approach to this problem using the patient's spontaneous tidal volume. Anxiety is accompanied by hyperventilation, where the tidal volume is usually increased, whereas ventilatory failure is usually accompanied by a decrease in tidal volume (rapid shallow breathing). Therefore, **an increase in tidal volume suggests anxiety, whereas a decrease in tidal volume suggests continued need for ventilatory support.** When the tidal volume is unchanged or increased, the arterial PCO_2 can also be helpful i.e., a decrease in arterial PCO_2 indicates that ventilation is adequate and suggests that anxiety is the problem. In this case, judicious use of sedation should be considered. On the other hand, if the arterial PCO_2 is normal or increasing, the patient should be returned immediately to ventilatory support. (Remember that a normal arterial PCO_2 in the face of a high minute ventilation is a sign of ventilatory failure.)

Abdominal Paradox

The respiratory movements of the abdomen can be a useful sign of success or failure to tolerate spontaneous breathing. Normally, abdominal movements during breathing provide information about the functional integrity of the diaphragm (11). When the diaphragm contracts, it descends into the abdomen and increases intraabdominal pressure. This pushes the anterior wall of the abdomen outward. However, when the diaphragm is weak, the negative intrathoracic pressure created by the accessory muscles of respiration pulls the diaphragm upward into the thorax. This decreases the intraabdominal pressure and causes a paradoxical inward displacement of the abdomen during inspiration. This

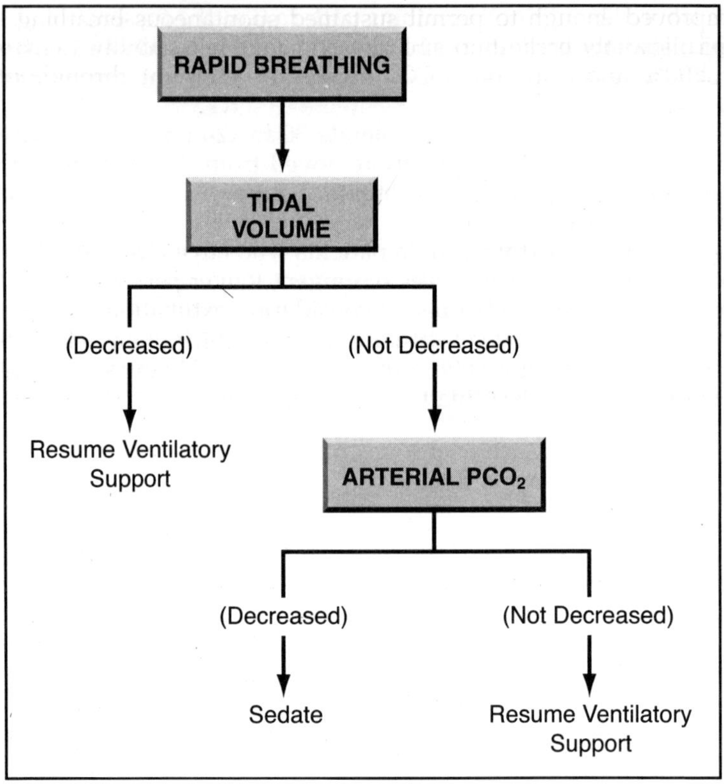

FIGURE 27.4 An approach to the patient who is breathing rapidly during a spontaneous breathing trial.

phenomenon is called *abdominal paradox*, and it is sign of a diaphragmatic weakness if it occurs during quiet breathing.

During labored breathing, contraction of the accessory muscles of inspiration can overcome the contractile force of the diaphragm and pull the diaphragm up into the thorax during inspiration. This results in abdominal paradox in the face of an actively contracting diaphragm. Because quiet breathing may be uncommon during a spontaneous breathing trial, **the appearance of abdominal paradox during weaning** is not necessarily a sign of diaphragm weakness. However, it is a sign of labored breathing, and **should prompt immediate return to full ventilatory support.**

FAILURE OF SPONTANEOUS BREATHING

Failure to sustain spontaneous breathing is usually a sign that the pathologic condition requiring ventilatory support needs more time to improve. Therefore, patients who require continued ventilatory support should have **a daily trial of spontaneous breathing** to identify when the condition has improved enough to permit sustained spontaneous breathing. This method allows the earliest possible detection of when spontaneous breathing will be tolerated (12–14). The following conditions can add to the difficulty of discontinuing mechanical ventilation, and each of these conditions should be considered in patients who fail spontaneous breathing trials.

Low Cardiac Output

The transition from positive-pressure ventilation to negative-pressure spontaneous breathing can result in a decrease in cardiac output (caused by an increase in left-ventricular afterload) (15). This can add to the difficulty of spontaneous breathing by promoting pulmonary congestion (which reduces lung compliance) and also by impairing diaphragm function. The diaphragm depends heavily on cardiac output (like the heart, the diaphragm maximally extracts oxygen), and **a drop in cardiac output can decrease the strength of diaphragmatic contractions** (16). Low cardiac output can also promote hypoxemia through a decrease in mixed venous O_2 saturation (see Figure 19.5 in Chapter 19). These deleterious effects of a low cardiac output should be considered in patients with cardiac dysfunction who do not tolerate spontaneous breathing. Some simple methods of detecting a low cardiac output are described next.

Detecting a Low Cardiac Output

The following are two measurements can be used to detect a low cardiac output in patients who are not tolerating spontaneous breathing. Neither method requires a pulmonary artery catheter. Each measurement should be performed at the beginning of a spontaneous breathing trial, and repeated when the patient is experiencing difficulty.

O_2 EXTRACTION: (SaO_2 - SvO_2). A decrease in cardiac output will increase O_2 extraction in the systemic capillaries, and this will be reflected in an increase in the (SaO_2 - SvO_2) difference (see Chapter 2). The SaO_2 is easily monitored with a pulse oximeter, and the SvO_2 can be measured with a central venous catheter in the superior vena cava. (See Chapter 20 for a description of the difference between "mixed venous" and "central venous" O_2 saturation.) The (SaO_2 - SvO_2) is normally about 25%, and it will increase to 50% in low output states.

ARTERIAL-END TIDAL PCO_2 GRADIENT: ($PaCO_2$ – $P_{ET}CO_2$). The arterial and end-tidal PCO_2 are equivalent in healthy subjects. A decrease in cardiac output will decrease end-tidal PCO_2 relative to arterial PCO_2, and this will be reflected in an increase in the ($PaCO_2$ – $P_{ET}CO_2$) difference. An increase in dead-space ventilation from lung disease will also increase the ($PaCO_2$ – $P_{ET}CO_2$) gradient, so it is important to monitor changes in the gradient during the spontaneous breathing trial. (See Chapter 20 for a description of the end-tidal PCO_2 measurement.)

Myocardial Ischemia

In patients with coronary artery disease, failure to tolerate spontaneous breathing is occasionally associated with acute myocardial ischemia (17).

The ischemia is often silent, and will not be detected without an electrocardiogram. Therefore, an ECG should be obtained in patients with coronary artery disease who do not tolerate spontaneous breathing.

Continuous Positive Airway Pressure

For patients who show evidence of a reduced cardiac output during spontaneous breathing, continuous positive airway pressure (CPAP) can help by eliminating the increased afterload caused by negative intrathoracic pressures. (See Chapter 25 for a description of CPAP.) Noninvasive ventilation with **CPAP has been used effectively in patients with acute cardiogenic pulmonary edema,** and can reduce the need for intubation and mechanical ventilation in these patients (18). The same benefits can be gained by adding CPAP to facilitate removal from mechanical ventilation. In patients who show a favorable response, CPAP can be continued after extubation (by face mask) if necessary.

Overfeeding

An increase in the daily intake of calories is associated with an increase in metabolic CO_2 production, as demonstrated in Figure 27.5 (19). If the daily intake of calories exceeds the daily caloric requirements (the resting

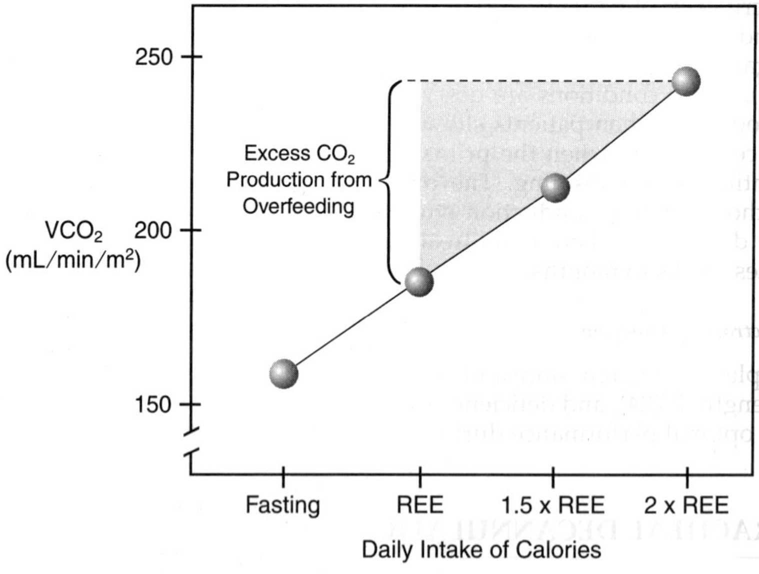

FIGURE 27.5 The influence of daily caloric intake on metabolic CO_2 production (VCO_2) in mechanically ventilated patients. REE is the resting energy expenditure (in kcal/24 hours). Each data point represents a mean value. (Data from Talpers S, Romberger DJ, Bunce SB, et al. Nutritionally associated increased carbon dioxide production. Chest 1992;102:551.)

energy expenditure in Figure 27.5), the excess CO_2 that is produced must be removed by the lungs. This requires an increase in minute ventilation, and this can add to the difficulty of sustaining spontaneous breathing in patients who are ventilator-dependent (19). To avoid this problem, ventilator-dependent patients should have their daily energy needs measured with indirect calorimetry (not estimated with conventional formulas) and their daily caloric intake should be matched to daily needs (see Chapter 45 for a description of how to measure daily energy needs).

Respiratory Muscle Weakness

The role of respiratory muscle weakness in failure to discontinue mechanical ventilation is unclear. The general belief is that the diaphragm becomes weak during mechanical ventilation (20), like muscles that are immobilized. However, **the diaphragm is not a voluntary muscle** that will stop contracting during mechanical ventilation. The diaphragm is controlled by the respiratory neurons in the lower brainstem, and these cells fire automatically throughout life. In fact, the output of these respiratory neurons to the diaphragm (called *ventilatory drive*) is increased in respiratory failure (21), and the activity of the diaphragm will likewise be increased.

Critical Illness Polyneuropathy and Myopathy

There are two conditions that can produce respiratory muscle weakness in critically ill patients: *critical illness polyneuropathy and myopathy*. These conditions often accompany cases of severe systemic sepsis with multiorgan failure, and they can prolong the need for mechanical ventilation (22). These conditions are described in Chapter 51. They are often first recognized when patients show a continued need for ventilatory assistance at a time when the primary condition that prompted mechanical ventilation is subsiding. The diagnosis is usually made by exclusion (although nerve conduction studies and electromyography can secure the diagnosis). There is no treatment for these disorders, and recovery takes weeks to months.

Electrolyte Depletion

Depletion of magnesium and phosphorous can impair respiratory muscle strength (23,24), and deficiencies in these electrolytes should be corrected for optimal performance during the spontaneous breathing trials.

TRACHEAL DECANNULATION

For patients who have proven that they no longer require ventilatory support, the next step is to remove the tracheal tube. There are 2 concerns prior to removing these tubes. First, is the patient able to protect the airway and clear secretions? Second, is there any evidence of laryngeal injury that would compromise breathing after the tube is removed?

Protecting the Airway

Patients should be alert and able to follow commands prior to removing tracheal tubes. The ability to protect the airway is determined with the gag and cough reflexes, and also by the volume of respiratory secretions. Cough strength can be assessed by placing a file card or piece of paper 1-2 cm from the end of the tracheal tube and asking the patient to cough. If wetness appears on the card, the cough strength is considered adequate (25). The absence of a cough or gag reflex will not prevent removal of tracheal tubes, but it will identify the patients who need to be watched closely after the tubes are removed.

Laryngeal Edema

Severe laryngeal edema is reported in as many as 40% of cases of prolonged translaryngeal intubation (26), and about 5% of patients can develop significant upper airway obstruction following extubation (27). Laryngeal edema is a particular concern in cases where the intubation was traumatic or required multiple attempts, or when multiple reintubations were necessary because of self-extubation. However, virtually any patient subjected to translaryngeal intubation can develop significant laryngeal edema.

The Cuff-Leak Test

The cuff-leak test is designed to identify patients with severe laryngeal edema prior to removal of the endotracheal tube. The test is performed while the patient is receiving volume-cycled ventilation, and it involves measuring the volume of gas exhaled through the endotracheal tube before and after deflating the cuff. If there is no obstruction at the level of the larynx, cuff deflation will cause exhaled gas to flow around the endotracheal tube, and the volume exhaled through the tube will decrease. Therefore, **a decrease in exhaled volume after cuff deflation is used as evidence against the presence of a significant obstruction at the level of the larynx**. However, there is no agreement about the magnitude of the volume change that is significant. Different studies have used volumes of 110 mL, 140 mL, and a 25% change in volume as the threshold that separates the presence and absence of significant upper airways obstruction (26–28).

One problem with the cuff-leak test is the lack of agreement on the volume change after cuff deflation that signifies a patent upper airway. This may not be possible because factors other than upper airway patency can influence the volume change after cuff deflation. One source of variability in exhaled volumes after cuff deflation is an inspiratory volume leak (29). Air that escapes out of the lungs during positive-pressure lung inflation will result in a decrease in exhaled volume through the endotracheal tube, and this volume will vary according to lung compliance and airways resistance. Therefore, the mechanical properties of the lungs are a source of individual variation in results of the cuff-leak test. Another source of variability is the diameter of the endotracheal tube relative to the diameter of the trachea. Tubes that fit snugly in the trachea can create an obstruction to expiratory flow after cuff deflation that will be misinterpreted as indicating a significant upper airway obstruction.

Thus, there are multiple factors that can influence the results of the cuff-leak test, and this creates doubt about the predictive value of the test.

Fenestrated Tracheostomy Tubes

Laryngeal obstruction is also possible after removal of tracheostomy tubes (30). In this case, the laryngeal damage can be the result of the endotracheal tube that was present prior to tracheostomy, or can be caused by ischemic injury to the larynx during the tracheostomy procedure. Detection of laryngeal obstruction is sometimes possible using a fenestrated (windowed) tracheostomy tube like the one shown in Figure 27.6. When the inner cannula is removed, the fenestration allows airflow through the larynx. When the opening of the tube is capped and the cuff is deflated, the patient must breathe entirely through the mouth, and any difficulty in breathing in this situation could be the result of obstruction at the level of the larynx. When this occurs, direct laryngoscopy can be used to identify a source of laryngeal obstruction. Fenestrated tracheostomy tubes are also available without a cuff: these tubes can be used to test the patency of the upper airways, but they must be replaced by cuffed tubes if the patient is placed back on the ventilator.

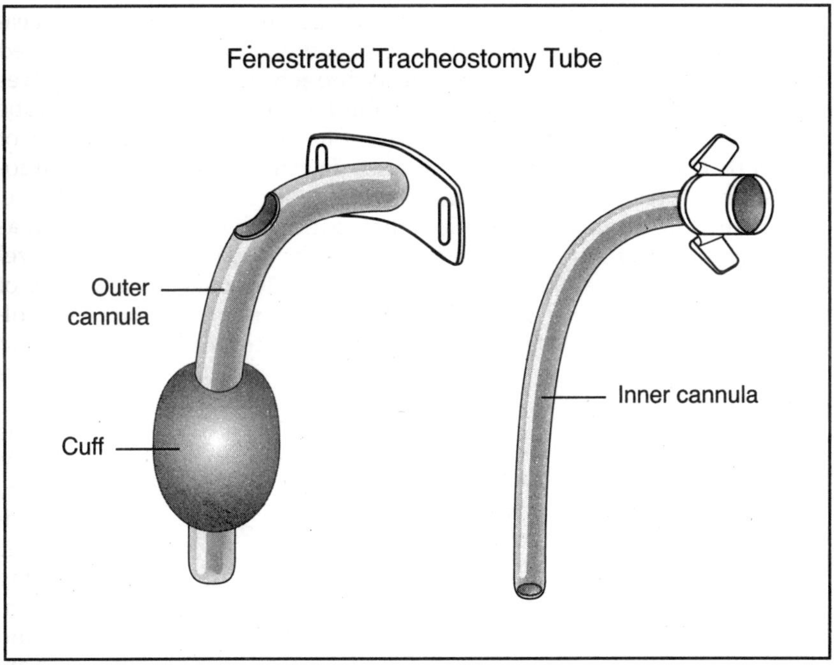

FIGURE 27.6 A fenestrated tracheostomy tube. When the inner cannula is removed, the fenestration (window) allows air to flow through the larynx, and this can be used to test the patency of the larynx before tracheal decannulation.

Steroids for Anything That Swells?

The antiinflammatory actions of steroids (see Table 23.3) is somehow used to justify the use of steroids for cases of traumatic edema. One example of this *steroids for anything that swells* philosophy (31) is the use of steroids for traumatic cerebral edema, and another example is the use of steroids to treat intubation-induced laryngeal edema. Few studies have evaluated the effects of steroids on post-extubation laryngeal edema in adults, and the results of the available studies are inconclusive. One study shows no effect when intravenous methylprednisolone (40 mg) is given one hour before extubation (32), while another study shows a beneficial effect when intravenous methylprednisolone is given 24 hours before extubation (either as a single dose of 40 mg or in repeated doses of 40 mg every 6 hrs) (28). Further study is required, but it seems unlikely that one dose of steroids (or one day of therapy) will reverse the cumulative effects of days of trauma to the larynx.

The Postextubation Period

The Work of Breathing

The cross-sectional area of the glottis (the narrowest portion of the upper airway) is 66 mm^3 in the average-sized adult, whereas the cross-sectional area of an average-sized adult tracheal tube (8 mm internal diameter) is 50 mm^3 (33). The narrower cross-sectional area of the tracheal tube creates an increased resistance to airflow, so the work of breathing should be greater when breathing through endotracheal tubes. However, as shown in Figure 27.2, removal of endotracheal tubes is accompanied by an *increased* work of breathing (at least in the early period following removal). This is a consistent observation in patients who otherwise do well after extubation, and it is unexplained.

There is a popular perception that patients who do not tolerate spontaneous breathing while intubated might breathe easier after the tube is removed. The observation in Figure 27.2 proves otherwise, and shows that **endotracheal tubes should never be removed based on the assumption that it will be easier for the patient to breathe**.

Posrtextubation Stridor

Laryngeal obstruction following extubation is signaled by the onset of **stridor**. Because the obstruction is extrathoracic, the stridor occurs during inspiration (i.e., the negative intrathoracic pressure is transmitted to the larynx and causes inspiratory narrowing). Postextubation stridor is not always an indication for immediate reintubation. If the patient is not *in extremis*, **aerosolized epinephrine** (2.5 mL of 1% epinephrine) is a popular intervention. This is effective in treating post-extubation stridor in children (34), but similar efficacy in adults is unproven. A racemic mixture of epinephrine (which has equal amounts of the l-isomer and d-isomer) has been popular in this situation, but the standard (l-isomer) epinephrine preparation is equally effective (33).

Breathing a helium-oxygen (heliox) gas mixture has also been used in patients with postextubation stridor (27). Helium is less dense than air, and it flows more readily through regions of reduced cross-sectional area, where flow is turbulent. Although heliox has theoretical advantages in patients with postextubation laryngeal edema, the influence of heliox breathing in preventing reintubation has not been studied.

A FINAL WORD

The most important issue in discontinuing mechanical ventilation is not how to do it, but when to do it; i.e., recognizing when a patient is ready to try spontaneous breathing. A trial of spontaneous breathing is usually indicated when the patient is afebrile, alert, hemodynamically OK, and able to oxygenate while breathing 50% oxygen or less with a minimum of applied PEEP. Once these criteria are satisfied, start the spontaneous breathing trial and continue it as long as tolerated. If the patient does well, then consider extubation, but make sure the extubation can be done safely before proceeding. For patients who do not tolerate periods of spontaneous breathing, be patient and repeat the spontaneous breathing trial every day.

For patients who require prolonged ventilatory support, there is nothing you can do to make the patient less ventilator-dependent (other than treating the primary disease process). Your principal task is to provide general support while the primary disease process improves, and to use whatever measures are available to reduce the risk of complications that can keep the patient on a ventilator (e.g., acute pulmonary embolism).

REFERENCES

Clinical Practice Guidelines

1. MacIntyre NR, Cook DJ, Ely EW Jr, et al. Evidence-based guidelines for weaning and discontinuing ventilatory support: a collective task force facilitated by the American College of Chest Physicians, the American Association for Respiratory Care, and the American College of Critical Care Medicine. Chest 2001;120(suppl):375S–395S. Accessed in June, 2006 at www.chestjournal.org/cgi/content/full/120/6_suppl/375S.

Reviews

2. Epstein SK. Controversies in weaning from mechanical ventilation. J Intensive Care Med 2001;16:270–286.
3. Nevins ML, Epstein SK. Weaning from prolonged mechanical ventilation. Clin Chest Med 2001;22:13–33.
4. Scheinhorn DJ, Chao DC, Stearn-Hassenpflug M. Liberation from prolonged mechanical ventilation. Crit Care Clin 2002;18:569–595.

Readiness Criteria

5. MacIntyre NR. Respiratory mechanics in the patient who is weaning from the ventilator. Respir Care 2005;50:275–286.
6. Yang K, Tobin MJ. A prospective study of indexes predicting the outcome of trials of weaning from mechanical ventilation. N Engl J Med 1991;324:1445–1450.
7. Kreiger BP, Isber J, Breitenbucher A, et al. Serial measurements of the rapid-shallow breathing index as a predictor of weaning outcome in elderly medical patients. Chest 1997;112:1029–1034.
8. Marini JJ, Smith TC, Lamb V. Estimation of inspiratory muscle strength in mechanically ventilated patients: the measurement of maximal inspiratory pressure. J Crit Care 1986;1:32–38.

Spontaneous Breathing Trial

9. Mehta S, Nelson DL, Klinger JR, et al. Prediction of post-extubation work of breathing. Crit Care Med 2000;28:1341–1346.
10. Bouley GH, Froman R, Shah H. The experience of dyspnea during weaning. Heart Lung 1992;21:471–476.
11. Mier-Jedrzejowicz A, Brophy C, Moxham J, et al. Assessment of diaphragm weakness. Am Rev Respir Dis 1988;137:877–883.

Failure of Spontaneous Breathing

12. Esteban A, Frutos F, Tobin MJ, et al. A comparison of four methods of weaning patients from mechanical ventilation. N Engl J Med 1995;332:345–350.
13. Ely W, Baker AM, Dunagen DP, et al. Effect of duration of mechanical ventilation of identifying patients capable of breathing spontaneously. N Engl J Med 1996;335:1864–1869.
14. Frutos-Vivar F, Esteban A. When to wean from a ventilator: an evidence-based strategy. Cleve Clin J Med 2003;70:389–397.
15. Pinsky MR. Cardiovascular issues in respiratory care. Chest 2005;128:592S–597S.
16. Nishimura Y, Maeda H, Tanaka K, et al. Respiratory muscle strength and hemodynamics in heart failure. Chest 1994;105:355–359.
17. Srivastava S, Chatila W, Amoateng-Adjepong Y, et al. Myocardial ischemia and weaning failure in patients with coronary artery disease: an update. Crit Care Med 1999;27:2109–2112.
18. Park M, Sangean MC, Volpe M, et al. Randomized, prospective trial of oxygen, continuous positive airway pressure, and bilevel airway pressure by face mask in acute cardiogenic pulmonary edema. Crit Care Med 2004;32:2407–2415.
19. Talpers SS, Romberger DJ, Bunce SB, et al. Nutritionally associated increased carbon dioxide production. Chest 1992;102:551–555.
20. Vassilakopoulos T, Petrof BJ. Ventilator-induced diaphragmatic dysfunction. Am Rev Respir Crit Care Med 2004;169:336–341.
21. Fernandez R, Blanch L, Antigas A. Respiratory center activity during mechanical ventilation. J Crit Care 1991;6:102–111.

22. Hudson LD, Lee CM. Neuromuscular sequelae of critical illness. N Engl J Med 2003;348:745–747.
23. Benotti PN, Bistrian B. Metabolic and nutritional aspects of weaning from mechanical ventilation. Crit Care Med 1989;17:181–185.
24. Malloy DW, Dhingra S, Solren F, et al. Hypomagnesemia and respiratory muscle power. Am Rev Respir Dis 1984;129:427–431.

Tracheal Decannulation

25. Khamiees M, Raju P, DeGirolamo A, et al. Predictors of extubation outcome in patients who have successfully completed a spontaneous breathing trial. Chest 2001;120:1262–1270.
26. Chung Y-H, Chao T-Y, Chiu C-T, et al. The cuff-leak test is a simple tool to verify severe laryngeal edema in patients undergoing long-term mechanical ventilation. Crit Care Med 2006;34:409–414.
27. Kriner EJ, Shafazand S, Colice GL. The endotracheal tube cuff leak test as a predictor for postextubation stridor. Respir Care 2005;50:1632–1638.
28. Cheng K-C, Hou C-C, Huang H-C, et al. Intravenous injection of methylprednisolone reduces the incidence of post-extubation stridor in intensive care unit patients. Crit Care Med 2006;34:1345–1350.
29. Prinianakis G, Alexopoulou C, Mamidakis E, et al. Determinants of the cuff-leak test: a physiological study. Crit Care 2005;9:R24–R31.
30. Colice C, Stukel T, Dain B. Laryngeal complications of prolonged intubation. Chest 1989;96:877–884.
31. Shemie S. Steroids for anything that swells: dexamethasone and postextubation airway obstruction. Crit Care Med 1996;24:1613–1614.
32. Gaussorgues P, Boyer F, Piperno D, et al. Do corticosteroids prevent postintubation laryngeal edema? A prospective study of 276 adults. Crit Care Med 1988;16:649–652.
33. Kaplan JD, Schuster DP. Physiologic consequences of tracheal intubation. Clin Chest Med 1991;12:425–432.
34. Nutman J, Brooks LJ, Deakins K, et al. Racemic versus l-epinephrine aerosol in the treatment of postextubation laryngeal edema: results from a prospective, randomized, double-blind study. Crit Care Med 1994;22:1591–1594.

Section IX

ACID-BASE DISORDERS

Life is a struggle, not against sin, not against Money Power . . but against hydrogen ions.

H.L. Mencken

Chapter 28

ACID-BASE INTERPRETATIONS

Seek simplicity, and distrust it.

Alfred North Whitehead

Disorders of acid-base balance can be found in as many as nine of every 10 patients in the ICU (1), which means that acid-base disorders may be the most common clinical problems you will encounter in the ICU. This chapter presents a structured approach to the identification of acid-base disorders based on a set of well-defined rules that can be applied to arterial blood gas (ABG) and serum electrolyte measurements (2–6).

BASIC CONCEPTS

The hydrogen ion concentration $[H^+]$ in extracellular fluid is determined by the balance between the partial pressure of carbon dioxide (PCO_2) and the concentration of bicarbonate (HCO_3) in the fluid. This relationship is expressed as follows (1):

$$[H^+]\ (\text{nEq/L}) = 24 \times (PCO_2/HCO_3) \tag{28.1}$$

Using a normal arterial PCO_2 of 40 mm Hg and a normal serum HCO_3 concentration of 24 mEq/L, the normal $[H^+]$ in arterial blood is $24 \times (40/24) = 40$ nEq/L.

Hydrogen Ion Concentration and pH

Note that the $[H^+]$ in extracellular fluid is expressed in *nano*equivalents (nEq) per liter. A nanoequivalent is *one-millionth* of a milliequivalent, so there are millions more sodium, chloride, and other ions measured in mEq than there are hydrogen ions. Because nanoequivalents represent such a small amount, the $[H^+]$ is routinely expressed in pH units, which

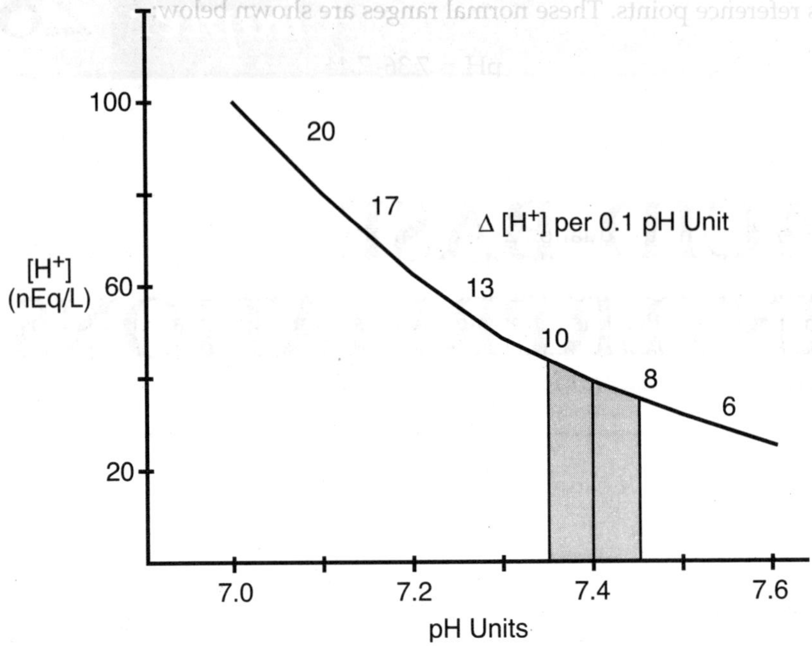

FIGURE 28.1 The relationship between hydrogen ion concentration [H^+] and pH. The numbers above the curve indicate the change in [H^+] associated with a change of 0.1 pH unit. The *shaded area* shows the normal pH range in extracellular fluid.

are derived by taking the negative logarithm (base 10) of the [H^+] in nEq/L. The relationship between pH and [H^+] is shown in Figure 28.1. A normal [H^+] of 40 nEq/L corresponds to a pH of 7.40. Because the pH is a negative logarithm of the [H^+], changes in pH are inversely related to changes in [H^+] (e.g., a decrease in pH is associated with an increase in [H^+]).

Inspection of the curve in Figure 28.1 reveals that, as the pH decreases from 7.60, the slope of the curve progressively increases, which means there is a progressively larger change in [H^+] for a given change in pH. The numbers above the curve indicate the change in [H^+] associated with each change of 0.1 pH units. At the acidotic end of the curve, the change in [H^+] for a given change in pH is more than threefold greater than at the alkalotic end of the curve (20 nEq/L versus 6 nEq/L per 0.1 pH unit, respectively). Therefore, the acid-base consequences of a given change in pH depend on the baseline acid-base status of the patient.

Types of Acid-Base Disorders

The different types of acid-base disorders can be defined using the normal ranges for pH, PCO_2, and HCO_3 concentration in extracellular fluid as reference points. These normal ranges are shown below:

$$pH = 7.36\text{–}7.44$$

$$PCO_2 = 36\text{–}44 \text{ mm Hg} \quad (28.2)$$

$$HCO_3 = 22\text{–}26 \text{ mEq/L}$$

According to Equation 28.1, a change in either the PCO_2 or the HCO_3 will cause a change in the pH of extracellular fluid. When the change involves the PCO_2, the condition is called a *respiratory* acid-base disorder: an increase in PCO_2 is a *respiratory acidosis,* and a decrease in PCO_2 is a *respiratory alkalosis.* When the change involves the HCO_3, the condition is called a *metabolic* acid-base disorder: a decrease in HCO_3 is a *metabolic acidosis,* and an increase in HCO_3 is a *metabolic alkalosis.* If any of these changes causes the pH to change to a value outside the normal range, the suffix *emia* is used to describe the acid-base derangement: acid*emia* is the condition where the pH falls below 7.36, and alkal*emia* is the condition where the pH rises above 7.44.

Acid-Base Control

The $[H^+]$ in extracellular fluid normally varies less than 10 nEq/L (see the shaded area in Fig. 28.1). The determinants of extracellular fluid pH in Equation 28.1 indicate that tight control of the pH requires a fairly constant PCO_2/HCO_3 ratio. Thus, a change in one of the determinants (PCO_2 or HCO_3) must be accompanied by a proportional change in the other determinant to keep the PCO_2/HCO_3 ratio (and the pH) constant. Thus, an increase in PCO_2 (respiratory acidosis) must be accompanied by an increase in HCO_3 (metabolic alkalosis) to keep the pH constant. This is how the control system for acid-base balance operates. A respiratory disorder (change in PCO_2) always initiates a complementary metabolic response (that alters the HCO_3), and vice-versa. These complementary changes in $PaCO_2$ and HCO_3 are shown in Table 28.1. The initial change in PCO_2 or HCO_3 is called the *primary* acid-base disorder, and the subsequent response is called the *compensatory* or *secondary* acid-base disorder.

TABLE 28.1 Primary Acid-Base Disorders and Associated Compensatory Changes

$$[H^+] = 24 \times PCO_2/HCO_3$$

Primary Disorder	Primary Change	Compensatory Change*
Respiratory acidosis	Increased PCO_2	Increased HCO_3
Respiratory alkalosis	Decreased PCO_2	Decreased HCO_3
Metabolic acidosis	Decreased HCO_3	Decreased PCO_2
Metabolic alkalosis	Increased HCO_3	Increased PCO_2

*Compensatory changes are designed to keep the PCO_2/HCO_3 ratio constant.

Compensatory responses are not strong enough to keep the pH constant (they do not correct the acid-base derangement); they only to limit the change in pH that results from a primary change in PCO_2 or HCO_3.

Respiratory Compensation

Metabolic acid-base disorders elicit prompt ventilatory responses that are mediated by peripheral chemoreceptors located in the carotid body at the carotid bifurcation in the neck. A metabolic acidosis stimulates these chemoreceptors and initiates an increase in ventilation and a subsequent decrease in arterial PCO_2 ($PaCO_2$). A metabolic alkalosis silences the chemoreceptors and produces a prompt decrease in ventilation and increase in arterial $PaCO_2$. The respiratory compensation for primary metabolic acid-base disturbances can be described quantitatively using the top two equations shown in Figure 28.2.

COMPENSATION FOR METABOLIC ACIDOSIS. The ventilatory response to a metabolic acidosis will reduce the $PaCO_2$ to a level that is defined by Equation 28.3 (7). (The HCO_3 in this equation is the measured bicarbonate concentration in plasma, expressed in mEq/L.)

$$\text{Expected } PaCO_2 = (1.5 \times HCO_3) + (8 \pm 2) \tag{28.3}$$

For example, if a metabolic acidosis results in a serum HCO_3 of 15 mEq/L, the expected $PaCO_2$ is $(1.5 \times 15) + (8 \pm 2) = 30.5 \pm 2$ mm Hg. If the measured $PaCO_2$ is equivalent to the expected $PaCO_2$, then the respiratory compensation is adequate, and the condition is called a *compensated metabolic acidosis*. If the measured $PaCO_2$ is higher than the expected $PaCO_2$ (>32.5 mm Hg in this example), the respiratory compensation is not adequate, and there is a respiratory acidosis in addition to the metabolic acidosis. This acid-base disturbance is called a *primary metabolic acidosis with a superimposed respiratory acidosis*. If the PCO_2 is lower than expected (lower than 28.5 mm Hg in the example), there is a respiratory alkalosis in addition to the compensated metabolic acidosis. This acid-base disturbance is called a *primary metabolic acidosis with a superimposed respiratory alkalosis*.

COMPENSATION FOR METABOLIC ALKALOSIS. The compensatory response to metabolic alkalosis has varied in different reports, but the equation shown below has proven reliable, at least up to a HCO_3 level of 40 mEq/L (8).

$$\text{Expected } PaCO_2 = (0.7 \times HCO_3) + (21 \pm 2) \tag{28.4}$$

For example, if a metabolic alkalosis is associated with a plasma HCO_3 of 40 mEq/L, the expected PCO_2 is $(0.7 \times 40) + (21 \pm 2) = 49 \pm 2$ mm Hg. If the measured $PaCO_2$ is equivalent to the expected $PaCO_2$, then the respiratory compensation is adequate, and the condition is called a *compensated metabolic alkalosis*. If the measured $PaCO_2$ is higher than the expected $PaCO_2$ (>51 mm Hg in this example), the respiratory compensation is not adequate, and there is a respiratory acidosis in addition to the metabolic alkalosis. This condition is called a *primary metabolic*

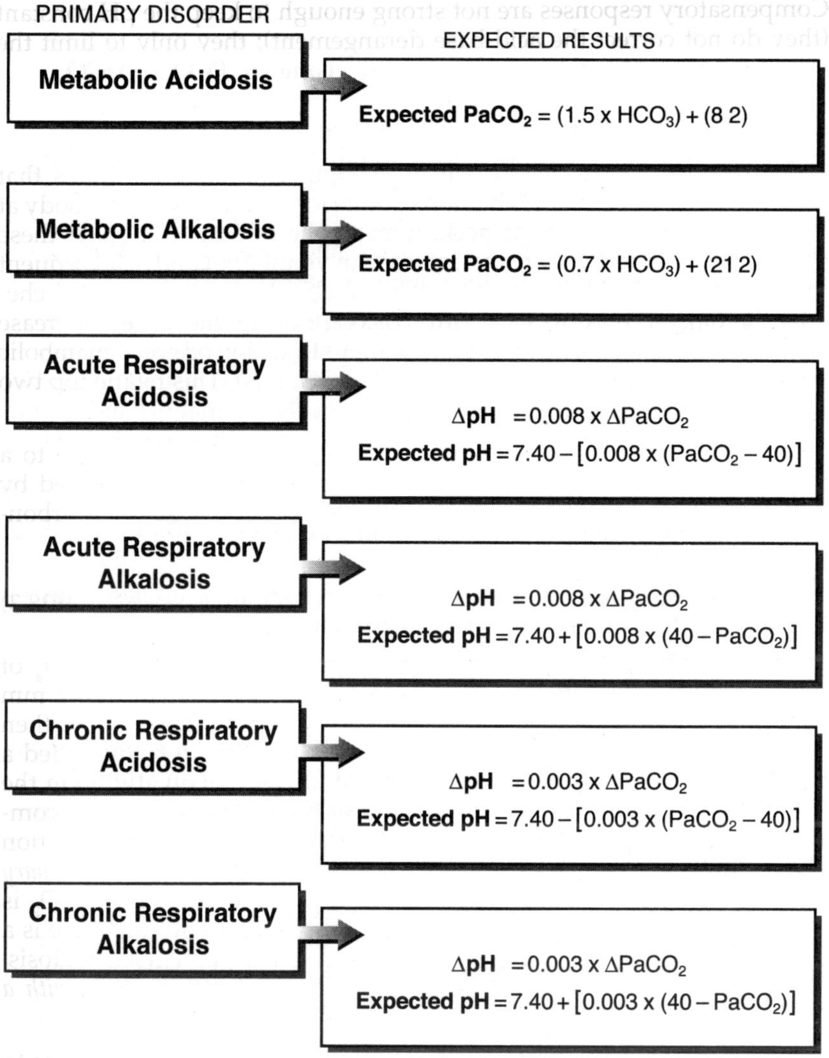

FIGURE 28.2 Useful formulas for acid-base interpretations.

alkalosis with a superimposed respiratory acidosis. If the $PaCO_2$ is lower than expected (lower than 47 mm Hg in the example), there is an additional respiratory alkalosis, and this condition is called a *primary metabolic alkalosis with a superimposed respiratory alkalosis.*

Metabolic Compensation

The compensatory response to primary changes in $PaCO_2$ takes place in the kidneys, and involves an adjustment in HCO_3 reabsorption in the proximal tubules. An increase in $PaCO_2$ (respiratory acidosis) results in an increased HCO_3 reabsorption and a subsequent increase in serum

HCO_3 levels, while a decrease in $PaCO_2$ (respiratory alkalosis) results in a decreased HCO_3 reabsorption and a subsequent decrease in plasma HCO_3 levels. These compensatory responses are slow to develop (unlike the ventilatory response to metabolic acid-base disorders, which is prompt). Compensation begins to appear in 6 to 12 hours and is fully developed after a few days. Because of this delay in renal compensation, respiratory acid-base disorders are classified as acute (before renal compensation begins) and chronic (after renal compensation is fully developed). The changes in pH that are expected in acute and chronic respiratory acid-base disorders are defined by the equations shown in Figure 28.2.

ACUTE RESPIRATORY ACID-BASE DISORDERS. Prior to the onset of renal compensation, a change in $PaCO_2$ of 1 mm Hg will produce a change in xpH of 0.008 pH units: $\Delta pH = 0.008 \times \Delta PaCO_2$ (2,3). This relationship is incorporated into Equation 28.5 using 7.40 for the normal pH and 40 mm Hg for the normal $PaCO_2$. This equation then defines the expected pH for an *acute respiratory acidosis*.

$$\text{Expected pH} = 7.40 - [0.008 \times (PaCO_2 - 40)] \qquad (28.5)$$

The expected arterial pH for an *acute respiratory alkalosis* can be described in the same manner using Equation 28.6.

$$\text{Expected pH} = 7.40 + [0.008 \times (40 - PaCO_2)] \qquad (28.6)$$

For example, starting with a normal pH of 7.40, an acute increase in $PaCO_2$ from 40 to 60 mm Hg is expected to result in an arterial pH of $[7.40 - (0.008 \times 20)]$ 7.24 pH units, and a sudden drop in $PaCO_2$ from 40 to 25 mm Hg is expected to result in an arterial pH of $[7.40 + (0.008 \times 15)]$ 7.56 pH units.

CHRONIC RESPIRATORY ACID-BASE DISORDERS. When the compensatory response in the kidneys is fully developed, the arterial pH changes only 0.003 pH units for every 1 mm Hg change in $PaCO_2$: $\Delta pH = 0.003 \times \Delta PaCO_2$ (3). This relationship is incorporated into Equation 28.7 using 7.40 as a normal arterial pH and 40 mm Hg as a normal $PaCO_2$. This equation describes the expected change in pH for a *chronic (compensated) respiratory acidosis*.

$$\text{Expected pH} = 7.40 - [0.003 \times (PaCO_2 - 40)] \qquad (28.7)$$

The expected arterial pH for a *chronic (compensated) respiratory alkalosis* is described in a similar fashion in Equation 28.8.

$$\text{Expected pH} = 7.40 + [0.003 \times (40 - PaCO_2)] \qquad (28.8)$$

For example, a patient with emphysema and chronic CO_2 retention who usually has a $PaCO_2$ of 60 mm Hg is expected to have the following arterial pH (from Equation 28.7): $7.40 - (0.003 \times 20) = 7.34$ pH units. The expected pH for an acute rise in $PaCO_2$ to 60 mm Hg (from Equation 28.5) is: $7.40 - (0.008 \times 20) = 7.24$ pH units. Therefore, the renal compensation for an acute rise in $PaCO_2$ to 60 mm Hg is expected to increase the arterial pH by 0.1 pH units.

A STEPWISE APPROACH TO ACID-BASE INTERPRETATION

The following is a structured approach to the diagnosis of acid-base disorders using rules of acid-base interpretation based on the material just presented. This approach has three distinct stages. The first two stages will allow you to identify major acid-base abnormalities using only three variables: pH, $PaCO_2$, and serum HCO_3 concentration. The last stage allows you to further investigate cases of metabolic acidosis using commonly measured serum electrolytes. Several examples are provided along the way as instructional aids.

Stage I: Identify the Primary Acid-Base Disorder

In the first stage of the approach, the measured $PaCO_2$ and pH are used to determine if an acid-base disturbance is present and, if so, to identify the primary acid-base disorder.

RULE 1: An acid-base abnormality is present if either the $PaCO_2$ or the pH is outside the normal range. (A normal pH or $PaCO_2$ does not exclude the presence of an acid-base abnormality, as explained in Rule 3.)

RULE 2: If the pH and $PaCO_2$ are both abnormal, compare the directional change. If both change in the same direction (both increase or decrease), the primary acid-base disorder is metabolic, and if both change in opposite directions, the primary acid-base disorder is respiratory.

EXAMPLE: Consider a patient with an arterial pH of 7.23 and a $PaCO_2$ of 23 mm Hg. The pH and $PaCO_2$ are both reduced (indicating a primary metabolic problem) and the pH is low (indicating acidemia), so the problem is a *primary metabolic acidosis*.

RULE 3: If either the pH or $PaCO_2$ is normal, there is a mixed metabolic and respiratory acid-base disorder (one is an acidosis and the other is an alkalosis). If the pH is normal, the direction of change in $PaCO_2$ identifies the respiratory disorder, and if the $PaCO_2$ is normal, the direction of change in the pH identifies the metabolic disorder.

EXAMPLE: Consider a patient with an arterial pH of 7.37 and a $PaCO_2$ of 55 mm Hg. The pH is normal, so there is a mixed metabolic and respiratory acid-base disorder. The $PaCO_2$ is elevated, so the respiratory disorder is an acidosis, and thus the metabolic disorder must be an alkalosis. Therefore, this is a *combined respiratory acidosis and metabolic alkalosis*. There is no primary acid-base disorder in this situation; both disorders are equivalent in severity (which is why the pH is normal).

Remember that the compensatory responses to a primary acid-base disturbance are never strong enough to correct the pH, but act to reduce the severity of the change in pH. Therefore, a normal pH in the presence of an acid-base disorder always signifies a mixed respiratory and metabolic acid-base disorder. (It is sometimes easier to think of this situation as a condition of overcompensation for one of the acid-base disorders.)

Stage II: Evaluate Compensatory Responses

The second stage of the approach is for cases where a primary acid-base disorder has been identified in Stage I. (If a mixed acid-base disorder was identified in Stage I, go directly to Stage III.) The goal in Stage II is to determine if the compensatory responses are adequate and if there are additional acid-base derangements.

RULE 4: If there is a primary metabolic acidosis or alkalosis, use the measured serum bicarbonate concentration in Equation 28.3 or 28.4 to identify the expected $PaCO_2$. If the measured and expected $PaCO_2$ are equivalent, the condition is fully compensated. If the measured $PaCO_2$ is higher than the expected $PaCO_2$, there is a superimposed respiratory acidosis. If the measured PCO_2 is less than the expected PCO_2, there is a superimposed respiratory alkalosis.

EXAMPLE: Consider a patient with a $PaCO_2$ of 23 mm Hg, an arterial pH of 7.32, and a serum HCO_3 of 15 mEq/L. The pH is acidemic and the pH and PCO_2 change in the same direction, so there is a primary metabolic acidosis. Equation 28.3 should be used to calculate the expected PCO_2: $(1.5 \times 15) + (8 \pm 2) = 30.5 \pm 2$ mm Hg. The measured $PaCO_2$ (23 mm Hg) is lower than the expected $PaCO_2$, so there is an additional respiratory alkalosis. Therefore, this condition can be described as a *primary metabolic acidosis with a superimposed respiratory alkalosis.*

RULE 5: If there is a respiratory acidosis or alkalosis, use the $PaCO_2$ to calculate the expected pH using Equations 28.5 and 28.7 (for respiratory acidosis) or Equations 28.6 and 28.8 (for respiratory alkalosis). Compare the measured pH to the expected pH to determine if the condition is acute, partially compensated, or fully compensated. For respiratory acidosis, if the measured pH is lower than the expected pH for the acute, uncompensated condition, there is a superimposed metabolic acidosis, and if the measured pH is higher than the expected pH for the chronic, compensated condition, there is a superimposed metabolic alkalosis. For respiratory alkalosis, if the measured pH is higher than the expected pH for the acute, uncompensated condition, there is a superimposed metabolic alkalosis, and if the measured pH is below the expected pH for the chronic, compensated condition, there is a superimposed metabolic acidosis.

EXAMPLE: Consider a patient with a $PaCO_2$ of 23 mm Hg and a pH of 7.54. The $PaCO_2$ and pH change in opposite directions so the primary problem is respiratory and, since the pH is alkalemic, this is a primary respiratory alkalosis. The expected pH for an acute respiratory alkalosis is described in Equation 28.6, and is $7.40 + [0.008 \times (40 - 23)] = 7.54$. This is the same as the measured pH, so this is an *acute, uncompensated respiratory alkalosis*. If the measured pH was higher than 7.55, this would be evidence of a superimposed metabolic alkalosis.

Stage III: Use The "Gaps" to Evaluate Metabolic Acidosis

The final stage of this approach is for patients with a metabolic acidosis, and it involves two determinations known as *gaps*. The first is the *anion gap*, which is an estimate of unmeasured anions that helps to identify the cause of a metabolic acidosis. The second gap is a comparison of the change in the anion gap and the change in the serum HCO_3 concentration: the gap between the two (known as the *gap-gap*) can uncover mixed metabolic disorders (e.g., a metabolic acidosis and alkalosis) that would otherwise go undetected. These two measurements are described in the next section.

THE ANION GAP

The anion gap is an estimate of the relative abundance of unmeasured anions, and is used to determine if a metabolic acidosis is due to an accumulation of non-volatile acids (e.g., lactic acid) or a net loss of bicarbonate (e.g., diarrhea) (5,9,10).

Measuring the Anion Gap

To achieve electrochemical balance, the concentration of negatively-charged anions must equal the concentration of positively-charged cations. All ions participate in this balance, including those that are routinely measured, such as sodium (Na), chloride (CL), and bicarbonate (HCO_3), and those that are not measured. The unmeasured cations (UC) and unmeasured anions (UA) are included in the electrochemical balance equation shown below:

$$Na + UC = (CL + HCO_3) + UA \tag{28.9}$$

Rearranging the terms in this equation yields Equation 28.10.

$$Na - (CL + HCO_3) = UA - UC \tag{28.10}$$

The difference (UA − UC) is a measure of the relative abundance of unmeasured anions and is called the *anion gap* (AG). The difference between the two groups reveals an anion excess (anion gap) of 12 mEq/L, and much of this difference is due to the albumin concentration.

Reference Range

The normal value of the AG was originally set at 12 ± 4 mEq/L (range = 8 to 16 mEq/L) (9). With the adoption of newer automated systems that more accurately measure serum electrolytes, **the normal value of the AG has decreased to 7 ± 4 mEq/L** (range = 3 to 11 mEq/L) (11). This newer reference range has not been universally adopted, and this is a source of error in the interpretation of the AG.

Influence of Albumin

Another source of error in the interpretation of the AG occurs when the contribution of albumin is overlooked. As indicated in Table 28.2, albumin is major source of unmeasured anions, and **a 50% reduction in**

TABLE 28.2 Determinants of the Anion Gap

Unmeasured Anions	Unmeasured Cations
Albumin (15 mEq/L)*	Calcium (5 mEq/L)
Organic Acids (5 mEq/L)	Potassium (4.5 mEq/L)
Phosphate (2 mEq/L)	Magnesium (1.5 mEq/L)
Sulfate (1 mEq/L)	
Total UA: (23 mEq/L)	Total UC: (11 mEq/L)
Anion Gap = UA − UC = 12 mEq/L	

*If albumin is reduced by 50%, anion gap = 4 mEq/L

the albumin concentration will result in a 75% reduction in the anion gap. Since hypoalbuminemia is common in ICU patients, the influence of albumin on the AG must be considered in all ICU patients.

Two methods have been proposed to correct the AG for the influence of albumin in patients with a low serum albumin. One method is to calculate the expected AG using just the albumin and phosphate concentrations (6,12), since these variables are responsible for a majority of the normal anion gap.

$$\text{Expected AG (mEq/L)} = [2 \times \text{albumin (g/dL)}] + [0.5 \times PO_4 \text{ (mg/dL)}] \quad (28.11)$$

The calculated AG using the traditional method [Na − (CL + HCO_3)] is then compared to the expected AG. If the calculated AG is greater than the expected AG, the difference is attributed to unmeasured anions from non-volatile acids. The second method of adjusting the AG in hypoalbuminemic patients involves the following equation (where the factor 4.5 is the normal albumin concentration in g/dL) (13):

$$\text{Adjusted AG} = \text{Observed AG} + 2.5 \times [4.5 - \text{measured albumin (g/dL)}] \quad (28.12)$$

Thus, a patient with a calculated AG of 10 mEq/L and a serum albumin of 2 g/dL would have an adjusted AG that is [10 + (2.5 × 2.5)] = 16 mEq/L. This represents a 60% increase in the AG, and this difference could transform a seemingly normal AG into an elevated AG.

The choice of method is up to you. The important issue is to use some method of adjusting the AG in patients with a low serum albumin.

Interpreting the Anion Gap

Metabolic acidoses are characterized as having an elevated AG or a normal AG (5,10). Those with an elevated AG are caused by the addition of a fixed (non-volatile) acid to the extracellular fluid, and those with

TABLE 28.3 Interpretation of the Anion Gap (AG)

High AG Acidoses	Normal AG Acidoses
Lactic acidosis	Diarrhea
Ketoacidosis	Isotonic saline infusion
End-stage renal failure	Early renal insufficiency
Methanol ingestion	Renal tubular acidosis
Ethylene glycol ingestion	Acetazolamide
Salicylate toxicity	Ureteroenterostomy

a normal AG are the result of a net increase in chloride concentration in the extracellular fluid. The conditions in each category are shown in Table 28.3.

High Anion Gap

When a fixed acid is added to the extracellular space, the acid dissociates to produce hydrogen ions and anions. The hydrogen ions combine with bicarbonate (HCO_3) to form carbonic acid and, according to the relationship AG = Na − (CL + HCO_3), the decreased HCO_3 results in an increased AG. The **usual causes of an elevated AG** metabolic acidosis are **lactic acidosis, ketoacidosis,** and **end-stage renal failure** (where hydrogen ion secretion in the distal tubules is impaired) (9). Elevated AG acidosis can also be seen in certain toxic ingestions, including **methanol** (which forms formic acid), **ethylene glycol** (which forms oxalic acid), **propylene glycol** (which accelerates the formation of lactic acid and pyruvic acid), and **salicylates** (which form salicylic acid) (10).

Normal Anion Gap

When a metabolic acidosis is caused by the loss of bicarbonate ions from the extracellular fluid, the bicarbonate loss is counterbalanced by a gain of chloride ions to maintain electrical charge neutrality. Some believe the increase in chloride comes first, and the loss of HCO_3 is a secondary phenomenon to maintain electrical neutrality (6). Because the increase in chloride concentration is proportional to the decrease in bicarbonate concentration, the relationship AG = Na − (CL + HCO_3) remains unchanged. (In the high AG metabolic acidoses, the loss of HCO_3 is not accompanied by increased CL because the anions from the dissociated acids balance the loss of HCO_3.) Because normal AG metabolic acidoses are accompanied by increased chloride concentrations, they are often referred to as **hyperchloremic metabolic acidoses.**

The common **causes of a normal AG metabolic acidosis** include **diarrhea** (where there is loss of HCO_3 in the stool), **early renal insufficiency** (which is accompanied by increased HCO_3 losses in the urine), and **infusion of isotonic saline.** The chloride concentration in isotonic saline is much higher than in extracellular fluid (154 mEq/L vs.

100 mEq/L, respectively), so infusion of isotonic saline raises the chloride concentration in extracellular fluid, and this is accompanied by increased HCO_3 losses in urine to maintain electrical neutrality (14). This condition has been called "dilutional acidosis," but this is a misnomer because the decreased HCO_3 in this condition is not a dilutional effect but is a specific response to the increased chloride concentration in the extracellular space. Other less common causes of a normal AG metabolic acidosis are **renal tubular acidosis, acetazolamide** (a carbonic anhydrase inhibitor that increases HCO_3 losses in urine), and **fistulas between the ureters and GI tract** (which promote HCO_3 losses in stool).

Reliability

The reliability of the AG in detecting lactic acidosis has been questioned because there are numerous reports of lactic acidosis with a normal anion gap (15,16). However in most of the reported cases, the influence of hypoalbuminemia in reducing the AG was not considered. The general consensus at this time is that the AG is a reliable marker of conditions associated with fixed acid accumulation (e.g., lactic acidosis) as long as the confounding influence of hypoalbuminemia is considered (12,13).

The "Gap-Gap"

In the presence of a high AG metabolic acidosis, it is possible to detect another metabolic acid-base disorder (a normal AG metabolic acidosis or a metabolic alkalosis) by comparing the AG excess (the difference between the measured and normal AG) to the HCO_3 deficit (the difference between the measured and normal HCO_3 concentration in plasma). The ratio (AG excess/HCO_3 deficit) is shown below using 12 mEq/L as the normal AG and 24 mEq/L as the normal plasma HCO_3 concentration.

$$\text{AG Excess}/HCO_3\ \text{deficit} = (\text{Measured AG} - 12)/(24 - \text{Measured } HCO_3) \qquad (28.13)$$

This ratio is sometimes called the *gap-gap* because it is a measure of the difference (gap) between the increase in AG and the decrease in HCO_3 concentration in extracellular fluid. This ratio can be used as follows.

Mixed Metabolic Acidoses

When a fixed acid accumulates in extracellular fluid (i.e., high AG metabolic acidosis), the decrease in serum HCO_3 is equivalent to the increase in AG, and the gap-gap (AG Excess/HCO_3 deficit) ratio is unity (= 1). However, when a hyperchloremic acidosis appears, the decrease in HCO_3 is greater than the increase in the AG, and the ratio (AG excess/HCO_3 deficit) falls below unity (< 1). Therefore, **in the presence of a high AG metabolic acidosis, a "gap-gap" (AG excess/HCO_3 deficit) ratio of less than 1 indicates the co-existence of a normal AG metabolic acidosis** (2,17).

Diabetic ketoacidosis (DKA) is an example of a condition that can be associated with a high AG and a normal AG metabolic acidosis (18). DKA first presents with a high AG metabolic acidosis, but after therapy with isotonic saline begins, the high AG acidosis begins to resolve (as the keto-acids are cleared) and a normal AG acidosis begins to appear (due to the saline infusion). In this situation, the serum bicarbonate remains low, but the gap-gap (AG excess/HCO_3 deficit) ratio begins to fall progressively below 1. Monitoring the serum HCO_3 alone will therefore create a false impression that the ketoacids are not being cleared. This is one example of the clinical utility of the gap-gap ratio.

Metabolic Acidosis and Alkalosis

When alkali is added in the presence of a high AG acidosis, the decrease in serum bicarbonate is less than the increase in AG, and the gap-gap (AG excess/HCO_3 deficit) ratio is greater than unity (>1). Therefore, **in the presence of a high AG metabolic acidosis, a gap-gap (AG excess/HCO_3 deficit) ratio of greater than 1 indicates the co-existence of a metabolic alkalosis.** This is an important consideration because metabolic alkalosis is common in the ICU due to the frequent use of nasogastric suction and diuretics.

ARTERIAL vs. VENOUS BLOOD

The evaluation of acid-base disorders relies heavily on arterial blood gas (ABG) measurements, however the acid-base status in arterial blood is unlikely to reflect the acid-base status in peripheral tissues, particularly in hemodynamically unstable patients. Venous blood should be a more accurate representation of what is occurring in the tissues. The discrepancy between the acid-base status in arterial and venous blood during cardiopulmonary resuscitation is shown in Figure 28.3 (19). Note that the arterial blood has a normal pH, while the venous blood shows severe acidemia (pH = 7.15). Although these are extreme conditions, this serves to demonstrate that, in critically ill patients, the acid-base status of arterial blood may not be an accurate reflection of the acid-base conditions in peripheral tissues. At least remember this when you are performing CPR.

A FINAL WORD

The reliance on the PCO_2-HCO_3 relationship to evaluate acid-base status has been criticized because the $PaCO_2$ and HCO_3 are both dependent variables (each depends on the other) and thus it is not possible to detect acid-base conditions that operate independently of these variables (6). There are alternate methods of acid-base analysis (see reference 6), but these involve complex equations and are not easily implemented

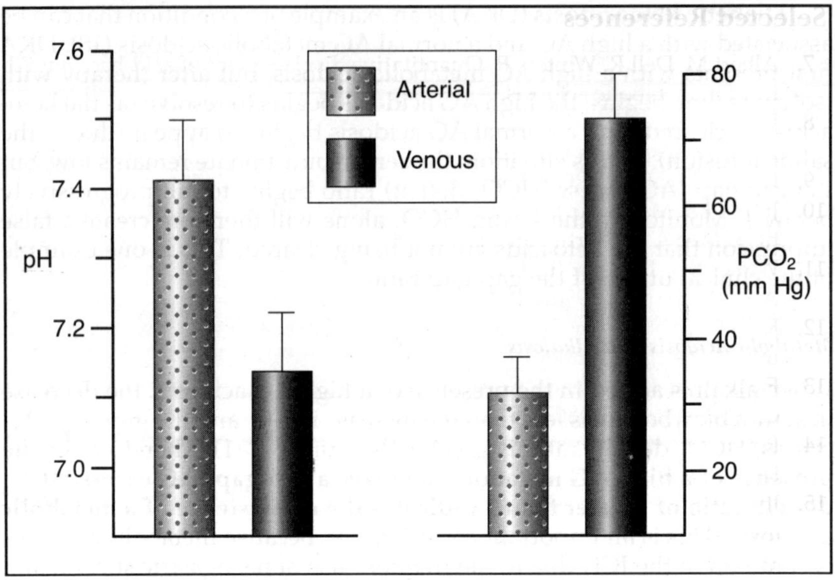

FIGURE 28.3 Acid-base parameters in arterial and venous blood during cardiopulmonary resuscitation. *Height of the vertical columns* indicates the mean; *cross-bars* indicate standard deviation. Study group: 16 adult patients. (From Weil MH, Rackow EC, Trevino R, et al. Difference in acid-base state between venous and arterial blood during cardiopulmonary resuscitation. N Engl J Med 1986;315:153–156.)

at the bedside. Furthermore, there is no convincing evidence that other systems of acid-base analysis provide any real clinical benefit over the traditional method presented in this chapter.

REFERENCES

Introduction

1. Gilfix BM, Bique M, Magder S. A physical chemical approach to the analysis of acid-base balance in the clinical setting. J Crit Care 1993;8:187–197.

Reviews

2. Narins RG, Emmett M. Simple and mixed acid-base disorders: a practical approach. Medicine 1980;59:161–187.
3. Morganroth ML. An analytical approach to diagnosing acid-base disorders. J Crit Illness 1990;5:138–150.
4. Whittier WL, Rutecki GW. Primer on clinical acid-base problem solving. Dis Mon 2004;50:117–162.
5. Casaletto JJ. Differential diagnosis of metabolic acidosis. Emerg Med Clin North Am 2005;23:771–787.
6. Kellum JA. Determinants of plasma acid-base balance. Crit Care Clin 2005; 21:329–346.

Selected References

7. Albert M, Dell R, Winters R. Quantitative displacement of acid-base equilibrium in metabolic acidosis. Ann Intern Med 1967;66:312–315.
8. Javaheri S, Kazemi H. Metabolic alkalosis and hypoventilation in humans. Am Rev Respir Dis 1987;136:1011–1016.
9. Emmet M, Narins RG. Clinical use of the anion gap. Medicine 1977;56:38–54.
10. Judge BS. Metabolic acidosis: differentiating the causes in the poisoned patient. Med Clin North Am 2005;89:1107–1124.
11. Winter SD, Pearson JR, Gabow PA, et al. The fall of the serum anion gap. Arch Intern Med 1990;150:311–313.
12. Kellum JA, Kramer DJ, Pinsky MJ. Closing the gap: a simple method of improving the accuracy of the anion gap. Chest 1996;110:185.
13. Figge J, Jabor A, Kazda A, Fencl V. Anion gap and hypoalbuminemia. Crit Care Med 1998;26:1807–1810.
14. Powner DJ, Kellum JA, Darby JM. Concepts of the strong ion difference applied to large volume resuscitation. J Intensive Care Med 2001;16:169–176.
15. Iberti TS, Liebowitz AB, Papadakos PJ, et al. Low sensitivity of the anion gap as a screen to detect hyperlactatemia in critically ill patients. Crit Care Med 1990;18:275–277.
16. Schwartz-Goldstein B, Malik AR, Sarwar A, Brandtsetter RD. Lactic acidosis associated with a normal anion gap. Heart Lung 1996;25:79–80.
17. Haber RJ. A practical approach to acid-base disorders. West J Med 1991;155: 146–151.
18. Paulson WD. Anion gap-bicarbonate relationship in diabetic ketoacidosis. Am J Med 1986;81:995–1000.
19. Weil MH, Rackow EC, Trevino R. Difference in acid-base state between venous and arterial blood during cardiopulmonary resuscitation. N Engl J Med 1986;315:153–156.

Chapter 29

ORGANIC ACIDOSES

It is incident to physicians, beyond all other men, to mistake subsequence for consequence.
Samuel Johnson

This chapter describes the clinical disorders associated with the production of organic (carbon-based) acids. The characteristic feature of these disorders is a metabolic acidosis with a high anion gap (see Chapter 28 for a description of the anion gap) (1–3). The main focus of the chapter is lactic acidosis and ketoacidosis. The final section contains a brief description of the metabolic acidoses associated with toxic ingestions of ethylene glycol and methanol.

LACTIC ACIDOSIS

Lactate Metabolism

Lactate is the end product of anaerobic glycolysis, as shown below:

$$\text{Glucose} + 2\text{ATP} + 2\text{H}_2\text{PO}_4 \rightarrow 2\text{Lactate} + 2\text{ADP} + 2\text{H}_2\text{O} \qquad (29.1)$$

Note that this reaction produces lactate, a negatively charged ion, *not* lactic acid. The hydrogen ions needed to convert lactate to lactic acid must be generated by the hydrolysis of ATP (4–6). Therefore, lactate is not synonymous with lactic acid, and **hyperlactatemia is not synonymous with lactic acidosis.** Most of the lactate production occurs in skeletal muscle, bowel, brain, and erythrocytes. The lactate generated in these tissues can be taken up by the liver and converted to glucose (via gluconeogenesis) or can be used as a primary oxidative fuel.

The Lactate Shuttle

As described in Chapter 11, lactate can serve as an alternate fuel source (see Table 11.3). This is demonstrated in Figure 29.1 The anaerobic metabolism

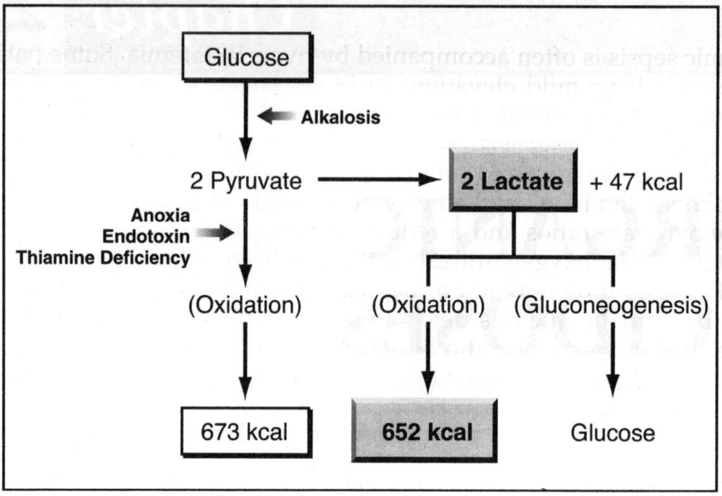

FIGURE 29.1 The salient features of glucose and lactate metabolism.

of one mole of glucose generates 47 kilocalories (kcal), which is only 7% of the energy yield from complete oxidation of glucose (673 kcal) (7). This energy difference can be erased by the oxidation of lactate, which generates 652 kcal per mole of glucose (326 kcal per mole of lactate) (7). The use of lactate as an oxidative fuel (called the *lactate shuttle*) has been described in exercise (8).

The lactate shuttle could also operate in critically ill patients. For example, there is evidence that the hyperlactatemia in sepsis is due to inhibition of glucose utilization by endotoxin (see Fig. 29.1). If the effects of endotoxin predominated in one organ (e.g., skeletal muscle), lactate that is generated could be used as a source of energy by other vital organs, such as the heart and central nervous system. In fact, both of these organs can use lactate as an energy source. This view of lactate is very different than the traditional view of lactate as a source of acidosis that can damage tissues.

Causes of Hyperlactatemia

Circulatory Shock

An increase in blood lactate levels in patients who are hemodynamically unstable is taken as evidence of impaired oxygen utilization by cells (cell dysoxia). This condition is generally known as *circulatory shock.* The degree of elevation in blood lactate levels is directly correlated with the mortality rate in circulatory shock, as shown in Figure 11.5 (9). It is important to emphasize that a decrease in systemic oxygen delivery, as occurs with anemia and hypoxemia, is not a cause of hyperlactatemia.

Sepsis

Systemic sepsis is often accompanied by hyperlactatemia. Some patients with sepsis have mild elevations of blood lactate (2 to 5 mEq/L) with a normal lactate:pyruvate ratio and a normal blood pH. These patients have *stress hyperlactatemia*, which is considered a result of hypermetabolism without impaired cellular oxygen utilization (10). Patients with septic shock can have marked elevations in blood lactate with increased lactate:pyruvate ratios and a reduced blood pH. These patients have a defect in cellular oxygen utilization that has been called *cytopathic hypoxia* (11). This condition may not be associated with impaired tissue oxygenation, but may be due to a defect in oxygen utilization in mitochondria. One contributing factor could be endotoxin-mediated inhibition of pyruvate dehydrogenase, the enzyme that initiates pyruvate oxidation in the mitochondria (see Fig. 11.6) (11,12).

Thiamine Deficiency

Thiamine serves as a co-factor for the pyruvate dehydrogenase enzyme that initiates pyruvate oxidation in the mitochondria (see Fig. 29.1). Therefore, it is no surprise that thiamine deficiency can be accompanied by hyperlactatemia (13). Because thiamine deficiency may be common in critically ill patients, this diagnosis should be considered in all cases of unexplained hyperlactatemia in the ICU. (See Chapter 45 for information on the diagnosis of thiamine deficiency.)

Drugs

A variety of drugs can produce hyperlactatemia, including nucleoside reverse transcriptase inhibitors, acetaminophen, epinephrine, metformin, propofol, and nitroprusside (3,14). In most of these cases (except epinephrine), the lactic acidosis indicates a defect in oxygen utilization, and carries a poor prognosis.

Propylene Glycol

Propylene glycol is an alcohol used to enhance the water solubility of many hydrophobic intravenous medications, including lorazepam, diazepam, esmolol, nitroglycerin, and phenytoin. About 55–75% of propylene glycol is metabolized by the liver and the primary metabolites are lactate and pyruvate (15). Propylene glycol toxicity from solvent accumulation has been reported in 19% to 66% of ICU **patients receiving high dose lorazepam or diazepam** for more than 2 days (15,16). Signs of toxicity include agitation, coma, seizures, tachycardia, hypotension, and hyperlactatemia (which can exceed 10 mEq/L). The clinical presentation can mimic that of systemic sepsis.

Propylene glycol toxicity is probably much more common than suspected in patients receiving infusions of lorazepam and diazepam. (15). This condition should be suspected in any patient with unexplained hyperlactatemia who is on a continuous infusion of one of these drugs. If suspected, the drug infusion should be stopped and another sedative agent selected. Midazolam does not have propylene glycol as a solvent, and could be used for short-term sedation. An assay for propylene glycol in blood is available, but the acceptable range has not been determined.

Lactic Alkalosis

Severe alkalosis (respiratory or metabolic) can raise blood lactate levels as a result of increased activity of pH dependent enzymes in the glycolytic pathway (17). When liver function is normal, the liver clears the extra lactate generated during alkalosis, and *lactic alkalosis* becomes evident only when the blood pH is 7.6 or higher. However, in patients with impaired liver function, hyperlactatemia can be seen with less severe degrees of alkalemia.

Other Causes

Other possible causes of hyperlactatemia in patients in the ICU are **seizures** (from increased lactate production), **hepatic insufficiency** (from reduced lactate clearance), and **acute asthma** (possibly from enhanced lactate production by the respiratory muscles) (18–20). Hyperlactatemia associated with hepatic insufficiency is often mild and not accompanied by lactic acidosis (18). Hyperlactatemia that accompanies generalized seizures can be severe but is transient (19). Hyperlactatemia during nitroprusside infusions is a manifestation of cyanide intoxication and is an ominous sign (see Chapter 16).

Diagnosis

The Anion Gap

As described in Chapter 28, the anion gap should be elevated in lactic acidosis, but there are numerous reports of a normal anion gap in patients with lactic acidosis (19,21). As a result, **the anion gap should not be used as a screening test for lactic acidosis.** For more information on the anion gap, see Chapter 28.

Blood Lactate

Lactate concentrations can be measured in plasma or whole blood. If immediate measurements are unavailable, the blood sample should be placed on ice to retard lactate production by red blood cells in the sample. A lactate level above 2 mEq/L is abnormal, but in patients with sepsis, a blood lactate level above 4 mEq/L may have more prognostic value (as explained earlier).

D-Lactic Acidosis

The lactate produced by mammalian tissues is a levo-isomer (bends light to the left), whereas a dextro-isomer of lactate (bends light to the right) is produced by certain strains of bacteria that can populate the bowel (22). D-lactate generated by bacterial fermentation in the bowel can gain access to the systemic circulation and produce a metabolic acidosis, often combined with a metabolic encephalopathy (23). Most cases of D-lactic acidosis have been reported after extensive small bowel resection or after jejunoileal bypass for morbid obesity (22–24).

Diagnosis

D-lactic acidosis can produce an elevated anion gap, but the standard laboratory assay for blood lactate measures only L-lactate. If D-lactic acidosis is suspected, you must request the laboratory to perform D-lactate assay.

ALKALI THERAPY FOR LACTIC ACIDOSIS

The primary goal of therapy in lactic acidosis is to correct the underlying metabolic abnormality. Alkali therapy aimed at correcting the pH is of questionable value (25). The following is a brief summary of the pertinent issues regarding alkali therapy for lactic acidosis.

Acidosis Is Not Harmful

The principal fear from acidosis is the risk of impaired myocardial contractility (26). However, in the intact organism, acidemia is often accompanied by an increase in cardiac output (27). This is explained by the ability of acidosis to stimulate catecholamine release from the adrenals and to produce vasodilation. Therefore, impaired contractility from acidosis is less of a concern in the intact organism. Furthermore, acidosis may have a protective role in the setting of clinical shock. For example, extracellular acidosis has been shown to protect energy-depleted cells from cell death (27a).

Bicarbonate Is Not an Effective Buffer

Sodium bicarbonate is the standard buffer used for lactic acidosis, but has limited success in raising the serum pH (27b). This can be explained by the titration curve for the carbonic acid-bicarbonate buffer system, which is shown in Figure 29.2. The HCO_3 buffer pool is generated by the dissociation of carbonic acid (H_2CO_3):

$$CO_2 + H_2O \leftrightarrow H_2CO_3 \leftrightarrow H^+ + HCO_3^- \qquad (29.2)$$

The dissociation constant (pK) for carbonic acid (i.e., the pH at which the acid is 50% dissociated) is 6.1, as indicated on the titration curve. Buffers are most effective within 1 pH unit on either side of the pK, so the effective range of the bicarbonate buffer system should be an extracellular pH between 5.1 and 7.1 pH units (indicated by the shaded area on the titration curve). Therefore, **bicarbonate is not expected to be an effective buffer in the usual pH range of extracellular fluid.** Bicarbonate is not

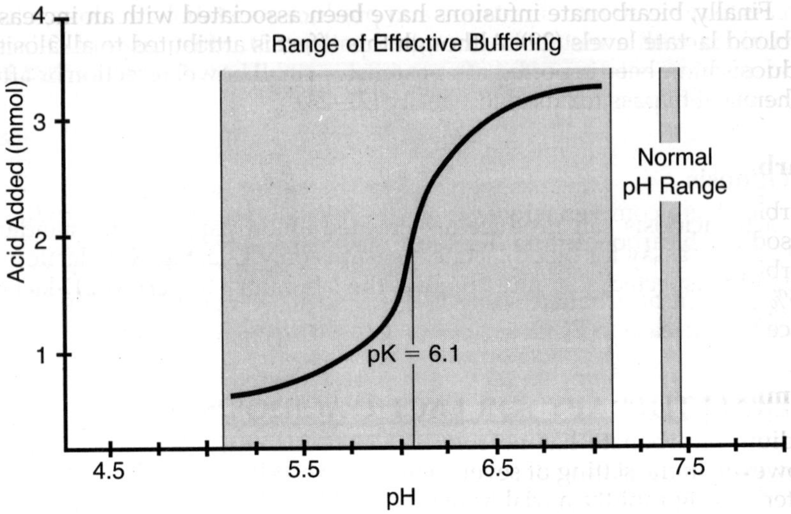

FIGURE 29.2 The titration curve for the carbonic acid-bicarbonate buffer system. The large, shaded area indicates the effective pH range for the bicarbonate buffer system, which does not coincide with the normal pH range for extracellular fluid. (Adapted from Comroe JH. Physiology of respiration. Chicago: Yearbook Medical Publishers, 1974;203.)

really a buffer (at least in the pH range we live in); rather, it is a transport form for carbon dioxide in blood (see Fig. 2.5).

Bicarbonate Can Be Harmful

A number of undesirable effects are associated with sodium bicarbonate therapy. One of these is the ability to generate CO_2 and actually lower the intracellular pH and cerebrospinal fluid pH (28,29). In fact, considering that **the PCO_2 is 200 mm Hg in standard bicarbonate solutions** (see Table 29.1), bicarbonate is really a CO_2 burden (an acid load!) that must be removed by the lungs.

TABLE 29.1 Bicarbonate-Containing Buffer Solutions

	7.5% $NaHCO_3$	Carbicarb
Sodium	0.9 mEq/mL	0.9 mEq/mL
Bicarbonate	0.9 mEq/mL	0.3 mEq/mL
Dicarbonate	—	0.3 mEq/mL
PCO_2	>200 mm Hg	3 mm Hg
Osmolality	1461 mOsm/kg	1667 mOsm/kg
pH (25°C)	8.0	9.6

Finally, bicarbonate infusions have been associated with an increase in blood lactate levels (29). Although this effect is attributed to alkalosis-induced augmentation of lactate production, it is not a desirable effect for a therapy of lactic acidosis.

Carbicarb

Carbicarb is a commercially available buffer solution that is a 1:1 mixture of sodium bicarbonate and disodium carbonate. As shown in Table 29.1, Carbicarb has less bicarbonate and a much lower PCO_2 than the standard 7.5% sodium bicarbonate solution. As a result, Carbicarb does not produce the increase in PCO_2 seen with sodium bicarbonate infusions (28).

Summary

Sodium bicarbonate has no role in the management of lactic acidosis. However, in the setting of severe acidosis (pH < 7.1) where the patient is deteriorating rapidly, a trial infusion of bicarbonate can be attempted by administering one-half of the estimated bicarbonate deficit (29).

$$HCO_3 \text{ deficit (mEq)} = 0.6 \times \text{wt (kg)} \times (15 - \text{measured } HCO_3) \quad (29.3)$$

(where 15 mEq/L is the end-point for the plasma HCO_3). If cardiovascular improvement occurs, bicarbonate therapy can be continued to maintain the plasma HCO_3 at 15 mEq/L. If no improvement or further deterioration occurs, further bicarbonate administration is not warranted.

KETOSIS

In conditions of reduced nutrient intake, adipose tissue releases free fatty acids, which are then taken up in the liver and metabolized to form the ketones acetoacetate and β-hydroxybutyrate. These ketones are released from the liver and can be used as oxidative fuels by vital organs such as the heart and central nervous system. The oxidative metabolism of ketones yields 4 kcal/g, which is a greater energy yield than the 3.4 kcal/g produced by carbohydrate metabolism (see Chapter 45).

The normal concentration of ketones in the blood is negligible (less than 0.1 mmol/L), but blood ketone levels increase tenfold after just 3 days of starvation. Ketones are strong acids, and progressive ketosis eventually produces a metabolic acidosis. The prevalence of acetoacetate (AcAc) and β-hydroxybutyrate (β-OHB) in blood is determined by the following redox reaction:

$$\text{AcAc} + \text{NADH} \leftrightarrow \beta\text{-OHB} + \text{NAD} \quad (29.4)$$

The balance of this reaction favors the formation of β-OHB. In conditions of enhanced ketone production, the β-OHB:AcAc ratio ranges from 3:1 in diabetic ketoacidosis, to as high as 8:1 in alcoholic ketoacidosis. The concentration of ketones in the blood in diabetic and alcoholic ketoacidosis is shown in Figure 29.3. Note the preponderance of β-hydroxybutyrate

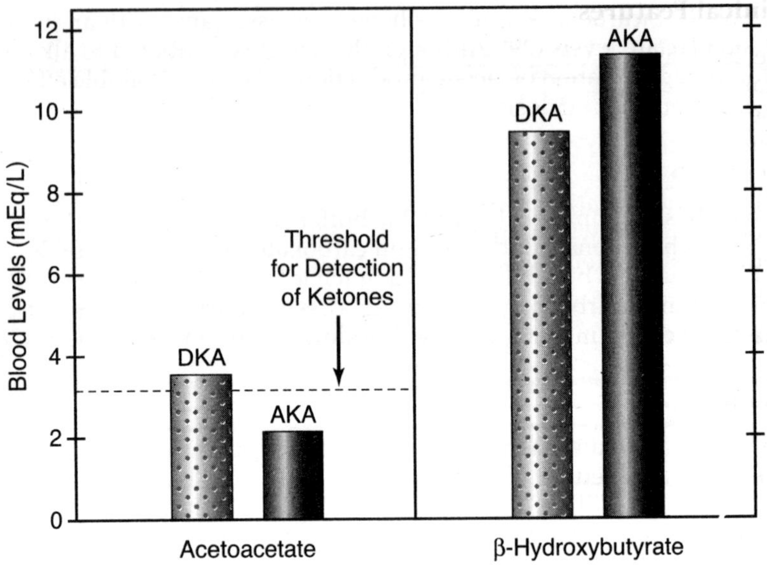

FIGURE 29.3 The concentrations of acetoacetate and β-hydroxybutyrate in the blood in diabetic ketoacidosis (DKA) and alcoholic ketoacidosis (AKA). The horizontal dashed line represents the minimum concentration of acetoacetate required to produce a positive nitroprusside reaction.

in both conditions. Because of this preponderance, ketoacidosis is more accurately called β-*hydroxybutyric acidosis.*

The Nitroprusside Reaction

The nitroprusside reaction is a colorimetric method for detecting acetoacetate and acetone in blood and urine. The test can be performed with tablets (Acetest) or reagent strips (Ketostix, Labstix, Multistix). A detectable reaction requires a minimum acetoacetate concentration of 3 mEq/L. Because this reaction **does not detect the predominant ketoacid β-hydroxybutyrate** (30), it is an insensitive method for monitoring the severity of ketoacidosis. This is illustrated in Figure 29.3. In alcoholic ketoacidosis, the total concentration of ketoacids in blood is 13 mEq/L, which represents more than a hundredfold increase over the normal concentration of blood ketones, yet the nitroprusside reaction will be negative because the acetoacetate concentration is below 3 mEq/L.

DIABETIC KETOACIDOSIS

Diabetic ketoacidosis (DKA) is usually seen in insulin-dependent diabetic patients, but in 20% of cases, there is no previous history of diabetes mellitus. DKA is most often the result of inappropriate insulin dosing, but some patients have a concurrent illness, most commonly an infection (30).

Clinical Features

The hallmark of DKA is the combination of hyperglycemia, a serum bicarbonate below 20 mEq/L, and an elevated anion gap. The blood glucose is usually above 250 mg/dL, but it may only be mildly elevated or even normal in about 20% of cases (30). There is no correlation between the severity of the hyperglycemia and the severity of the ketoacidosis (31). Semiquantitative methods for detecting ketones (acetoacetate) in blood and urine will be positive. However, as mentioned earlier, these methods will underestimate the severity of the ketonemia.

The Anion Gap

The increase in ketoacids should produce an elevated anion gap; however, this is variable, and the anion gap can be normal in DKA (32). The renal excretion of ketones is accompanied by an increase in chloride reabsorption in the renal tubules, and the resulting hyperchloremia limits the increase in the anion gap.

Management

The management of DKA is summarized in Table 29.2. The following are some of the details.

Insulin

Insulin therapy is given intravenously, starting with a bolus dose of 0.1 units per kilogram body weight (some do not feel this is necessary) and followed with a continuous infusion at 0.1 U/kg per hour. Because insulin adsorbs to intravenous tubing, the initial 50 mL of infusate should be run through the IV setup before the insulin drip is started. The blood glucose levels should be measured every 1 to 2 hours during intravenous

TABLE 29.2 Management of Diabetic Ketoacidosis

Insulin:	0.1 U/kg IV push, then 0.1 U/kg/hr by continuous infusion. Decrease dose rate 50% when serum HCO_3 rises above 16 mEq/L.	
Fluids:	Start with 0.9% saline, 1 L/hr for the first 2 hours. Follow with 0.45% saline at 250–500 mL/hr. Total fluid deficit is usually 50–100 mL/kg.	
Potassium:	If serum K = ____ mEq/L, give ____ mEq over next hour.	
	<3	40
	3–4	30
	4–5	20
	5–6	10
	>6	0
Phosphate:	If serum PO_4 is below 1.0 mg/dL, give 7.7 mg/kg over 4 hours.	

insulin therapy. The goal is to decrease the blood glucose by 50 to 75 mg/dL per hour (33). If this goal is not achieved, the insulin infusion rate should be doubled (33). Fingerstick glucose determinations can be performed if the blood glucose is below 500 mg/dL.

Fluids

Volume deficits average 50 to 100 mL/kg (or 4 to 8 L for a 175 lb adult). If no evidence of hypovolemic shock exists, crystalloid fluids are appropriate for volume replacement. Fluid therapy begins with 0.9% (isotonic) saline infused at a rate of approximately 1 L/hour for the first 2 hours. This is followed by infusion of 0.45% (half normal) saline at 250 to 500 mL/hour. When the blood glucose falls to 250 mg/dL, dextrose can be used in the intravenous fluids and the infusion rate is dropped to 100 to 250 mL/hour.

If evidence of hypovolemic shock (e.g., hypotension, reduced urine output) does exist, fluid replacement should begin with colloid fluids until the blood pressure normalizes. The preferred colloid in this situation is 5% albumin because 6% hetastarch increases the serum amylase levels, and elevated amylase is a common finding in DKA (in up to 80% of cases) and may represent subclinical pancreatitis (30).

Potassium

Potassium depletion is almost universal in DKA, and the average deficit is 3 to 5 mEq/kg. However, the serum potassium is often normal (74% of patients) or elevated (22% of patients) at presentation. The serum potassium falls during insulin therapy (transcellular shift), and this fall can be dramatic. Therefore, potassium replacement should be started as soon as possible (Table 29.2), and the serum potassium should be monitored hourly for the first 4 to 6 hours of therapy.

Phosphate

Phosphorous depletion is also common in DKA and averages 1 to 1.5 mmol/kg. However, phosphorous replacement seems to have little impact on the outcome in DKA, and therefore phosphate replacement is not recommended routinely (30). The serum phosphate level should be measured 4 hours after the start of therapy. If the level is severely depressed (less than 1 mg/dL), phosphate replacement is advised (see Table 29.2 for the recommended replacement dose).

Bicarbonate

Bicarbonate therapy does not improve the outcome in DKA, and is not recommended, regardless of the severity of the acidemia (30).

Monitoring Acid-Base Status

The serum bicarbonate may not be a reliable parameter for following the acid-base changes in DKA. Fluid replacement therapy often produces a hyperchloremic acidosis by promoting ketoacid excretion in the urine, which increases chloride reabsorption in the renal tubules. This can keep the bicarbonate from rising despite a resolving ketoacidosis. In this situation, the *pattern* of the acidosis is changing (i.e., changing from a high anion gap to a low anion gap acidosis). Therefore, monitoring the pattern of the acidosis as therapy proceeds can be more informative. This is accomplished by monitoring the gap gap: i.e., the **anion gap excess : bicarbonate deficit ratio,** as described in Chapter 28. This ratio is 1.0 in pure ketoacidosis, and decreases toward zero as the ketoacidosis resolves and is replaced by the hyperchloremic acidosis. When the ketones have been cleared from the bloodstream, the ratio approaches zero.

ALCOHOLIC KETOACIDOSIS

Alcoholic ketoacidosis (AKA) is a complex acid-base disorder that occurs in chronic alcoholics and usually appears 1 to 3 days after a period of heavy binge drinking (34). Several mechanisms seem to be involved in the ketosis, including reduced nutrient intake (which initiates enhanced ketone production), hepatic oxidation of ethanol (which generates NADH and enhances β-hydroxybutyrate formation), and dehydration (which impairs ketone excretion in the urine).

Clinical Features

Patients with AKA tend to be chronically ill and have several comorbid conditions. The presentation usually includes nausea, vomiting, and abdominal pain (34). Electrolyte abnormalities are common, particularly the *hypos* (e.g., hyponatremia, hypokalemia, hypophosphatemia, hypomagnesemia, hypoglycemia). Mixed acid-base disorders are also common in AKA. More than half the patients can have lactic acidosis (caused by other conditions), and metabolic alkalosis occurs in patients with protracted vomiting.

Diagnosis

The diagnosis of AKA is suggested by the clinical setting (i.e., after a period of binge drinking), an elevated anion gap, and the presence of ketones in the blood or urine. However, **the nitroprusside reaction for detecting ketones can be negative in AKA.** This is shown in Figure 29.3. The oxidation of ethanol in the liver generates NADH, and this favors the conversion of acetoacetate to β-hydroxybutyrate and results in a low concentration of acetoacetate in blood and urine. Even though most cases of AKA have a positive nitroprusside reaction for ketones (34), the severity of the ketoacidosis is significantly underestimated.

Management

The management of AKA is notable for its simplicity. Infusion of dextrose-containing saline solutions is all that is required. The glucose helps retard hepatic ketone production, while the infused volume promotes the renal clearance of ketones. The ketoacidosis usually resolves within 24 hours. Other electrolyte deficiencies are corrected as needed. Bicarbonate therapy is unnecessary (34).

TOXIC ALCOHOLS

Two alcohols are noted for their ability to generate organic acids: ethylene glycol and methanol. These are called toxic alcohols, but this is not meant to imply that ethanol is nontoxic.

Ethylene Glycol

Ethylene glycol is an alcohol solvent used primarily in antifreeze and deicing solutions. Toxic exposure to ethylene glycol is the leading cause of death from chemical agents in the United States (35). About 70% of toxic exposures are unintentional, but only 15% of life-threatening exposures are unintentional (36).

Pathophysiology

Ethylene glycol can be ingested, inhaled, or absorbed through the skin. Most life-threatening exposures involve ingestion. Absorption from the GI tract is rapid, and 80% of the ingested dose is metabolized in the liver. Metabolism by alcohol dehyrogenase in the liver produces glycolic acid, as shown in Figure 29.4. This is the major metabolite of ethylene glycol,

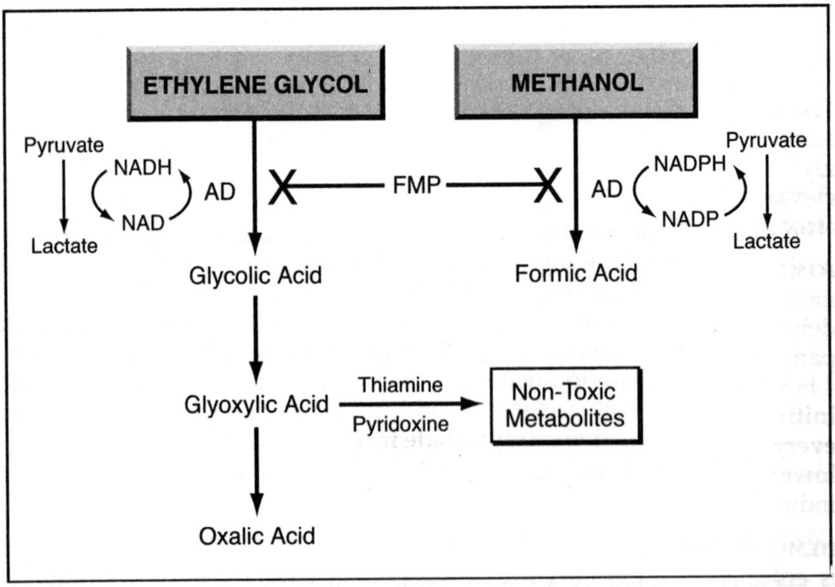

FIGURE 29.4 The metabolism of ethylene glycol and methanol. AD = alcohol dehydrogenase. FMP = fomepizole

and it produces a metabolic acidosis with an elevated anion gap (37). The formation of glycolic acid also involves the conversion of NAD to NADH, and this promotes the conversion of pyruvate to lactate. As a result, serum lactate levels are also elevated in ethylene glycol poisoning (37,38).

The final metabolite of ethylene glycol is oxalic acid, which can combine with calcium to form a calcium oxalate complex that precipitates in the renal tubules. The calcium oxalate crystals (which are recognizable on microscopic examination of the urine) can damage the renal tubules and produce acute renal failure.

Clinical Presentation

Early signs of ethylene glycol intoxication include nausea, vomiting, and apparent inebriation (altered mental status, slurred speech, and ataxia). Because ethylene glycol is odorless, there is no odor of alcohol on the breath. Severe cases are accompanied by depressed consciousness, coma, generalized seizures, renal failure, pulmonary edema, and cardiovascular collapse (37). Renal failure can be a late finding (i.e., 24 hours after ingestion).

Laboratory studies show a metabolic acidosis with an elevated anion gap and an elevated osmolal gap (see Chapter 32 for a description of the osmolal gap). Serum lactate levels can be elevated (usually 5 to 6 mEq/L) (37,38). Hypocalcemia can be present, and calcium oxalate crystals are visualized in the urine in about 50% of cases (39). A plasma assay for ethylene glycol is available, and a level > 25 mg/dL is considered toxic, and deserving of immediate therapy (36,37). Plasma levels can be misleading because metabolism of the parent compound can result in negligible plasma levels in patients who present late after ingestion.

Treatment

The results of the ethylene glycol assay are often not available immediately, and therapy is started based on a high clinical suspicion of ethylene glycol intoxication (e.g., metabolic acidosis with elevated anion gap, elevated osmolal gap, and oxaluria). Treatment involves inhibition of alcohol dehydrogenase, and hemodialysis if necessary.

FOMEPIZOLE. The traditional use of ethanol to inhibit alcohol dehydrogenase has been replaced by the drug fomepizole, which inhibits alcohol dehydrogenase (see Figure 29.4) without the side effects that accompany ethanol. The best results are obtained when therapy begins within 4 hours of ingestion. The recommended dosage is: **15 mg/kg IV as an initial dose, then 10 mg/kg every 12 hours for 48 hours, then 15 mg/kg every 12 hours until the plasma ethylene glycol level is 25 mEq/L or lower** (37,40). The increased dose at 48 hours compensates for a self-induced increase in fomepizole metabolism.

HEMODIALYSIS. The clearance of ethylene glycol and all its metabolites is enhanced by hemodialysis. The indications for immediate hemodialysis include severe acidemia (pH < 7.1), and evidence of significant end-organ damage (e.g., coma, seizures, and renal insufficiency) (37,40).

Multiple courses of hemodialysis may be necessary. Fomepizole should be dosed every 4 hours if hemodialysis is continued (37).

ADJUNCTS. Thiamine (100 mg IV daily) and pyridoxine (100 mg IV daily) can divert glyoxylic acid to non-toxic metabolites (see Figure 29.4). Despite evidence that these measures improve outcome, they are recommended based on theoretical benefit (37).

Methanol

Methanol (which is popularly known as *wood alcohol* because it was first distilled from wood) is a simple alcohol that is a common ingredient in shellac, varnish, windshield washer fluid, and solid cooking fuel (Sterno) (37,41).

Pathophysiology

Like ethylene glycol, methanol is rapidly absorbed from the GI tract and is metabolized by alcohol dehydrogenase in the liver (see Figure 29.4). The metabolite, formic acid, is a mitochondrial toxin that acts by inhibiting cytochrome oxidase. Tissues that are particularly susceptible to damage are the retina, optic nerve, and basal ganglia (41). Serum lactate levels can be elevated for the same reason as explained for ethylene glycol, but the added mitochondrial toxicity of formic acid can result in higher serum lactate levels.

Clinical Presentation

Early signs (within 6 hours of ingestion) include signs of apparent inebriation without the odor of ethanol (as in ethylene glycol intoxication). Later signs (6 to 24 hours after ingestion) include visual disturbances (e.g., scotoma, blurred vision, complete blindness), depressed consciousness, coma, and generalized seizures. Pancreatitis has also been described (37). Examination of the retina can reveal papilledema and generalized retinal edema.

Laboratory studies show the same acid-base abnormalities and elevated osmolal gap as described for ethylene glycol intoxication (although lactate levels may be higher). Pancreatic enzymes can be also be elevated, and elevated CPK from rhabdomyolysis has been reported (37). A plasma assay for methanol is available, and a level above 25 mg/dL is considered toxic (and deserving of treatment). As explained with ethylene glycol, plasma levels can be misleading in patients who present late after ingestion because the parent compound can be completely degraded by this time.

Treatment

Treatment is the same as described for ethylene glycol, except: visual impairment is an indication for dialysis, and adjunctive therapy with thiamine and pyridoxine is not indicated.

A FINAL WORD

The most important take-home message in this chapter is the fact that acidosis *per se* is not harmful, and does not require treatment. The problem with lactic acidosis and ketoacidosis is not the acidosis, but the underlying condition causing the acidosis. Lactic acidosis has a high mortality when it is caused by circulatory shock, but it is the shock that causes the high mortality, not the acidosis. The other point that deserves emphasis is the fact that bicarbonate is not much of a buffer in the pH range that we live with (see Figure 29.2), so even if alkali therapy was desirable, bicarbonate is not a good choice.

REFERENCES

General Reviews

1. Gauthier PM, Szerlip HM. Metabolic acidosis in the intensive care unit. Crit Care Clin 2002;18:289–308.
2. Casaletto JJ. Differential diagnosis of metabolic acidosis. Emerg Med Clin North Am 2005;23:771–787.
3. Judge BS. Metabolic acidosis: differentiating the causes in the poisoned patient. Med Clin North Am 2005;89:1107–1124.

Lactic Acidosis

4. Mizock BA, Falk JL. Lactic acidosis in critical illness. Crit Care Med 1992;20: 80–93.
5. Stacpoole PW. Lactic acidosis. Endocrinol Metab Clin North Am 1993;22:221–245.
6. Aberti KGMM, Cuthbert C. The hydrogen ion in normal metabolism: a review. CIBA Foundation Symposium 87. Metabolic acidosis. London: Pitman Books, 1982;1–15.
7. Lehninger AL. Bioenergetics. New York: WA Benjamin, 1965:16.
8. Brooks GA. Lactate production under fully aerobic conditions: the lactate shuttle during rest and exercise. Fed Proc 1986;45:2924–2929.
9. Weil MH, Afifi AA. Experimental and clinical studies on lactate and pyruvate as indicators of the severity of acute circulatory failure (shock). Circulation 1970;16:989–1001.
10. Mizock BA. Metabolic derangements in sepsis and septic shock. Crit Care Clin 2000;16:319–336.
11. Fink MP. Cytopathic hypoxia. Crit Care Clin 2001;17:219–238.
12. Curtis SE, Cain SM. Regional and systemic oxygen delivery/uptake relations and lactate flux in hyperdynamic, endotoxin-treated dogs. Am Rev Respir Dis 1992;145:348–354.
13. Campbell CH. The severe lactic acidosis of thiamine deficiency: acute, pernicious or fulminating beriberi. Lancet 1984;1:446–449.
14. Yann-Erick C, Cariou A, Monchi M, et al. Detecting life-threatening lactic acidosis related to nucleoside-analog treatment of human immunodeficiency virus-infected patients and treatment with L-carnitine. Crit Care Med 2003;31:1042–1047.

15. Wilson KC, Reardon C, Theodore AC, et al. Propylene glycol toxicity: a severe iatrogenic illness in ICU patients receiving IV benzodiazepines. Chest 2005;128:1674–1681.
16. Arroglia A, Shehab N, McCarthy K, et al. Relationship of continuous infusion lorazepam to serum propylene glycol concentration in critically ill adults. Crit Care Med 2004;32:1709–1714.
17. Bersin RM, Arieff AI. Primary lactic alkalosis. Am J Med 1988;85:867–871.
18. Kruse JA, Zaidi SAJ, Carlson RW. Significance of blood lactate levels in critically ill patients with liver disease. Am J Med 1987;83:77–82.
19. Brivet F, Bernadin M, Cherin P, et al. Hyperchloremic acidosis during grand mal seizure acidosis. Intensive Care Med 1994;20:27–31.
20. Mountain RD, Heffner JE, Brackett NC, et al. Acid-base disturbances in acute asthma. Chest 1990;98:651–655.
21. Iberti TS, Liebowitz AB, Papadakos PJ, et al. Low sensitivity of the anion gap as a screen to detect hyperlactatemia in critically ill patients. Crit Care Med 1990;18:275–277.
22. Anonymous. The colon, the rumen, and d-lactic acidosis. Lancet 1990;336:599–600 (editorial).
23. Thurn JR, Pierpoint GL, Ludvigsen CW, et al. D-lactate encephalopathy. Am J Med 1985;79:717–720.
24. Bustos D, Ponse S, Pernas JC, et al. Fecal lactate and the short bowel syndrome. Dig Dis Sci 1994;39:2315–2319.

Alkali Therapy

25. Forsythe SM, Schmidt GA. Sodium bicarbonate for the treatment of lactic acidosis. Chest 2000;117:260–267.
26. Sonnett J, Pagani FD, Baker LS, et al. Correction of intramyocardial hypercarbic acidosis with sodium bicarbonate. Circ Shock 1994;42:163–173.
27. Mehta PM, Kloner RA. Effects of acid-base disturbance, septic shock, and calcium and phosphorous abnormalities on cardiovascular function. Crit Care Clin 1987;3:747–758.
27a. Gores GJ, Nieminen AL, Fleischman KE, et al. Extracellular acidosis delays onset of cell death in ATP-depleted hepatocytes. Am J Physiol 1988; 255:C315–C322.
27b. Graf H, Arieff AI. The use of sodium bicarbonate in the therapy of organic acidoses. Intensive Care Med 1986;12:286–288.
28. Rhee KY, Toro LO, McDonald GG, et al. Carbicarb, sodium bicarbonate, and sodium chloride in hypoxic lactic acidosis. Chest 1993;104:913–918.
29. Rose BD. Clinical physiology of acid-base and electrolyte disorders. 4th ed. New York: McGraw-Hill, 1994;590.

Diabetic Ketoacidosis

30. Charfen MA, Fernandez-Frackelton M. Diabetic ketoacidosis. Emerg Med Clin North Am 2005;23:609–628.
31. Brandt KR, Miles JM. Relationship between severity of hyperglycemia and metabolic acidosis in diabetic ketoacidosis. Mayo Clin Proc 1988;63:1071–1074.
32. Gamblin GT, Ashburn RW, Kemp DG, et al. Diabetic ketoacidosis presenting with a normal anion gap. Am J Med 1986;80:758–760.

33. Kitabachi AE, Umpierrez GE, Murphy MB, et al. American Diabetes Association. hyperglycemic crisis in diabetes. Diabetes Care 2004;27(Suppl):S94–S102.

Alcoholic Ketoacidosis

34. Wrenn KD, Slovis CM, Minion GE, et al. The syndrome of alcoholic ketoacidosis. Am J Med 1991;91:119–128.

Toxic Alcohols

35. Watson WA, Litovitz TL, Klein-Schwartz W, et al. Annual report of the American Association of Poison Control Centers Toxic Exposure Surveillance System. Am J Emerg Med 2004;22:335–404.
36. Caravati EM, Erdman AR, Christianson G, et al. Ethylene glycol exposure: an evidence-based consensus guideline for out-of-hospital management. Clin Toxicol 2005;43:327–345.
37. Weiner SW. Toxic alcohols. In Goldfrank LR, Flomenbaum NE, Hoffman RS, et al., eds. Goldfrank's toxicologic emergencies. 7th ed. New York: McGraw-Hill, 2002: 1447–1459.
38. Gabow PA, Clay K, Sullivan JB, et al. Organic acids in ethylene glycol intoxication. Ann Intern Med 1986;105:16–20.
39. Borkan SC. Extracorporeal therapies for acute intoxications. Crit Care Clin 2002;18:393–420.
40. Brent J, McMartin K, Phillips S, et al. Fomepizole for the treatment of ethylene glycol poisoning. N Engl J Med 1999;340:832–838.
41. Barceloux DG, Bond GR, Krenzelok EP, et al. American Academy of Clinical Toxicology practice guidelines on the treatment of methanol poisoning. J Toxicol Clin Toxicol 2002;40:415–446.

Chapter 30

METABOLIC ALKALOSIS

Although the spotlight usually falls on metabolic acidosis, one of every three acid-base disorders in hospitalized patients is a metabolic *alkalosis* (1). In the ICU, the prevalence of metabolic alkalosis is determined by the popularity of diuretics and nasogastric decompression. However, the real culprit in ICU-related metabolic alkalosis is chloride depletion, aided by the inherent tendency of body fluids to remain electrically neutral (1–3).

ORIGINS OF METABOLIC ALKALOSIS

Metabolic alkalosis is characterized by an increase in extracellular bicarbonate (HCO_3) concentration without an associated decrease in arterial PCO_2 (see Table 28.1 in Chapter 28). The inciting event can be loss of fixed (nonvolatile) acid or gain in bicarbonate in the extracellular fluid. The kidneys have a prominent role in the development and maintenance of metabolic alkalosis, and the mechanisms involved are described next.

Renal Mechanisms of Acid-Base Control

The participation of the kidneys in acid-base control is illustrated in Figure 30.1. There are two principal mechanisms: bicarbonate reabsorption in the proximal tubules, and hydrogen ion secretion in the distal tubules.

Bicarbonate Reabsorption

Bicarbonate is readily filtered at the glomerulus, and most (80%) of the filtered HCO_3 is returned to the bloodstream in the proximal tubules. The mechanism of HCO_3 reabsorption in the proximal tubules is shown in the left panel of Figure 30.1. Hydrogen ions (H^+) are released into the lumen of the proximal tubules by a sodium-hydrogen (Na^+-H^+) transporter protein on the luminal surface of the tubular epithelial cells. The H^+ reacts with HCO_3 to form carbonic acid, which dissociates immediately to form CO_2 and H_2O. The CO_2 moves across the wall of the renal

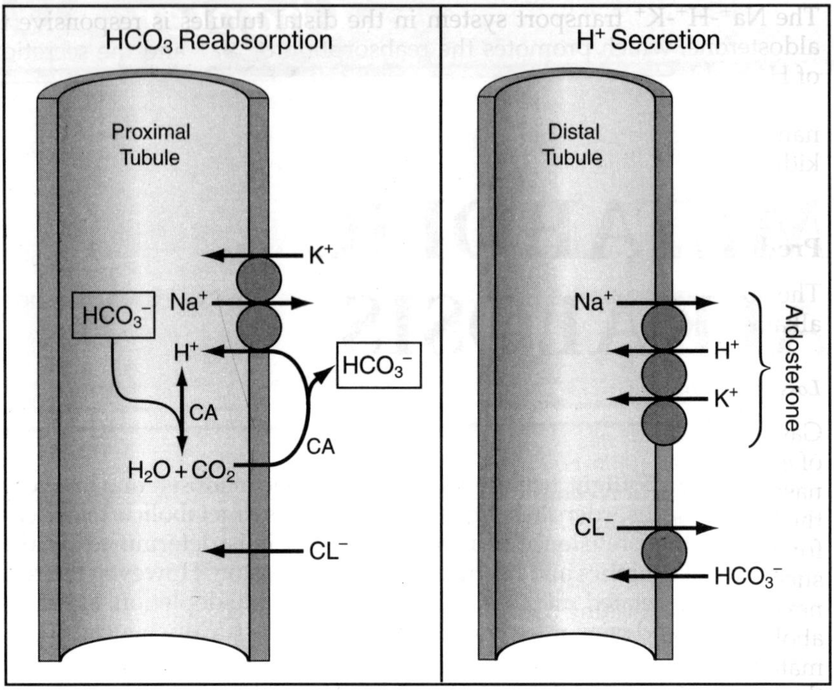

FIGURE 30.1 Mechanisms of acid-base control in the kidneys. CA = carbonic anhydrase.

tubule and is hydrated in the process to regenerate the HCO_3 and H^+. The HCO_3 moves into the bloodstream and the H^+ is transported back into the lumen of the renal tubule for another go-round. The reactions in this sequence are facilitated by the enzyme carbonic anhydrase (the importance of this will surface later in the chapter).

For every molecule of HCO_3 that is reabsorbed and added back to the extracellular fluid, one molecule of chloride moves in the opposite direction (from extracellular fluid to the lumen of the renal tubules). This maintains electrical neutrality in the extracellular fluid. **The reciprocating relationship between chloride and bicarbonate plays a pivotal role in the development of metabolic alkalosis,** as will be explained.

Hydrogen Ion Secretion

The kidneys are responsible for removing fixed (nonvolatile) acids from the body, and this occurs in the distal tubules, where H^+ is secreted into the lumen of the tubules and excreted in the urine (see the panel on the right in Figure 30.1). The secretion of H^+ is accomplished by a Na^+-H^+ transport protein (like the one in the proximal tubule) and a membrane pump that can move potassium as well as H^+ into the renal tubules.

The Na^+-H^+-K^+ transport system in the distal tubules is responsive to aldosterone, which promotes the reabsorption of Na^+ and the secretion of H^+ and K^+.

The renal mechanisms of acid-base control are the major determinants of bicarbonate concentration in extracellular fluid. As such, the kidneys are involved in most cases of metabolic alkalosis in the ICU.

Predisposing Conditions

The following conditions are responsible for most cases of metabolic alkalosis in ICUs.

Loss of Gastric Secretions

Gastric secretions are rich in hydrogen and chloride ions (concentration of each is 50 to 100 mEq/L), and loss of these secretions from vomiting or nasogastric suction can produce a profound metabolic alkalosis. Despite the loss of gastric acid, chloride depletion is the major factor responsible for the metabolic alkalosis that accompanies vomiting and nasogastric suctioning. Chloride depletion stimulates HCO_3 reabsorption in the kidneys, and the resulting increase in extracellular fluid HCO_3 creates a metabolic alkalosis. The HCO_3 that is added to the extracellular fluid must match the chloride that is lost to maintain electrical neutrality. Therefore, the severity of the alkalosis is determined (at least partly) by the magnitude of the chloride loss. Other factors that contribute to the alkalosis from loss of gastric secretions are hypovolemia and hypokalemia.

Diuretics

Thiazide diuretics and "loop" diuretics like furosemide promote metabolic alkalosis by increasing the urinary loss of electrolytes and free water. The following electrolytes are involved:

1. The principal action of these diuretics is to increase **sodium** loss in urine (natriuresis). However, an equivalent amount of **chloride** is also lost in urine because chloride excretion in the urine usually follows the sodium excretion. The increased urinary chloride excretion is known as *chloruresis,* and diuretics that promote chloride loss in the urine are known as *chloriuretic* diuretics (2).
2. **Potassium** loss in the urine is also increased by these diuretics because sodium delivery to the distal tubules is increased, and this promotes potassium secretion via the sodium–potassium exchange pump in the distal tubule (see Fig. 30.1).
3. Magnesium reabsorption in the kidneys usually mirrors sodium reabsorption, so these diuretics also promote **magnesium** loss in the urine. Magnesium depletion plays an important role in diuretic induced potassium depletion, as described in Chapter 34.

An additional mechanism for diuretic-induced metabolic alkalosis is volume depletion, as described next.

Volume Depletion

Volume depletion promotes metabolic alkalosis in two ways. Sodium and bicarbonate reabsorption are directly linked (by the Na^+-H^+ transporter) so the increased sodium reabsorption in response to volume depletion is accompanied by an increase in bicarbonate reabsorption. Volume depletion also stimulates renin release and thereby promotes the formation of aldosterone, which will promote H^+ secretion in the distal tubules.

Volume depletion has a longstanding relationship with metabolic alkalosis, as shown by the term *contraction alkalosis*. However, the importance of volume depletion as an independent source of metabolic alkalosis is being questioned because volume resuscitation does not correct metabolic alkalosis without chloride repletion (2). Because volume depletion is often associated with chloride depletion, the distinction may not be important, as long as isotonic saline is used to correct the volume deficits.

Hypokalemia

Hypokalemia is associated with a transcellular shift of H^+ into cells, and an increase in H^+ secretion in the distal tubules: both of these effects favor the development of a metabolic alkalosis. The enhanced secretion of H^+ in the distal tubules involves a Na^+-H^+ transporter (see Figure 30.1) that requires adequate delivery of sodium to the distal tubules. In the setting of hypovolemia, most of the filtered sodium is reabsorbed in the proximal tubules, and the effects of hypokalemia on H^+ secretion are minimal. The transcellular shift of H^+ is considered the most important mechanism favoring metabolic alkalosis from hypokalemia in ICU patients.

Organic Anions

The administration of organic anions such as lactate (in lactated Ringer's solution), acetate (in parenteral nutrition solutions), and citrate (in banked blood) could produce a metabolic alkalosis. However, only citrate administration in blood transfusions is capable of causing a metabolic alkalosis (4), and a minimum of 8 units of blood must be transfused before the plasma HCO_3 begins to rise (5).

Chronic CO_2 Retention

The compensatory response to CO_2 retention is a metabolic alkalosis that results from an increased bicarbonate reabsorption in the kidneys. According to the scheme shown in Figure 30.1 (left panel), CO_2 can directly stimulate HCO_3 reabsorption. If chronic hypercapnia is corrected suddenly (e.g., by overventilation during brief periods of mechanical ventilation), the compensatory metabolic alkalosis will become a primary acid-base disorder. The metabolic alkalosis in this case should not be a concern because it is an adaptive response to prevent severe acidosis from CO_2 retention.

CLINICAL CONSEQUENCES

Despite the potential for harm, metabolic alkalosis has no apparent deleterious effects in most patients. The following adverse effects are the ones most often mentioned.

Neurologic Manifestations

The neurologic manifestations attributed to alkalosis include depressed consciousness, generalized seizures, and carpopedal spasms. However, these manifestations are almost always associated with respiratory alkalosis, not metabolic alkalosis. This is explained by the greater tendency for respiratory alkalosis to influence the acid-base status of the central nervous system.

Hypoventilation

Unlike the ability of metabolic acidosis to stimulate ventilation, **metabolic alkalosis does not cause significant respiratory depression or CO_2 retention** in most patients. The magnitude of increase in serum bicarbonate that is needed to cause significant respiratory depression can be determined using the equation shown below.

$$\text{Expected } PaCO_2 = (0.7 \times HCO_3) + (21 \pm 2) \tag{30.1}$$

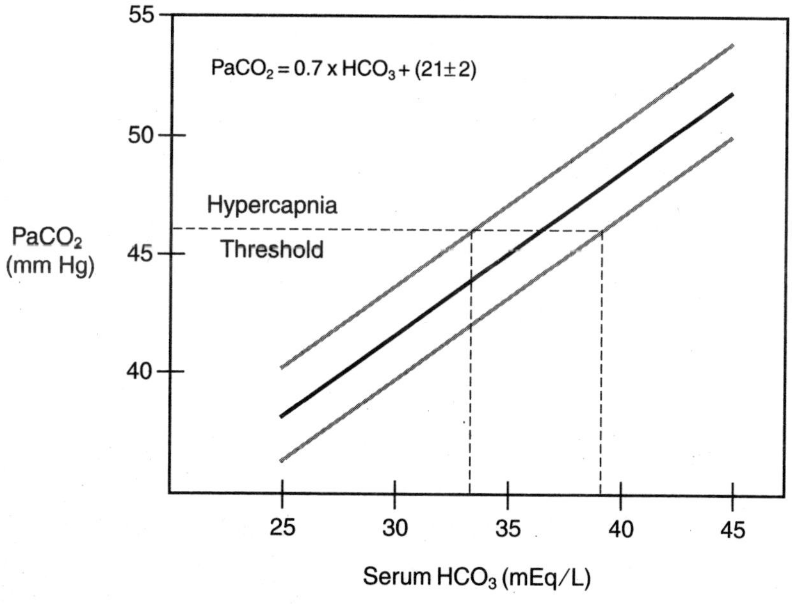

FIGURE 30.2 The relationship between serum bicarbonate (HCO_3) and arterial PCO_2 ($PaCO_2$) from the equation shown at the top of the graph. Note that the serum HCO_3 must rise above 30 to 35 mEq/L to produce hypercapnia (i.e., $PaCO_2$ above 46 mm Hg).

This equation was presented in Chapter 28 (Equation 28.4) as a means of identifying if the respiratory response to metabolic alkalosis is appropriate (6). This equation is used to plot the relationship between serum HCO_3 and arterial PCO_2 shown in Figure 30.2. The threshold for hypercapnia (which is an arterial PCO_2 of 46 mm Hg in this graph) corresponds to a serum HCO_3 of 34 to 39 mEq/L. Therefore, significant hypoventilation is not expected in metabolic alkalosis until the serum HCO_3 reaches the mid-thirties range.

Systemic Oxygenation

Alkalosis has a number of effects that, in combination, can threaten tissue oxygen availability. These effects are indicated in Figure 30.3, and each is summarized below. Once again, these effects are more prominent with respiratory alkalosis.

1. Severe alkalemia (pH > 7.6) can produce widespread vasoconstriction. Alkalosis increases the fraction of serum calcium that is bound to albumin, and the resultant decrease in ionized (free) calcium can promote widespread vasoconstriction that compromises tissue perfusion. Myocardial contractility is often reduced, and cardiac output decreases.
2. Alkalosis shifts the oxyhemoglobin dissociation curve to the left (Bohr effect), so that hemoglobin is less willing to release oxygen into the tissues.

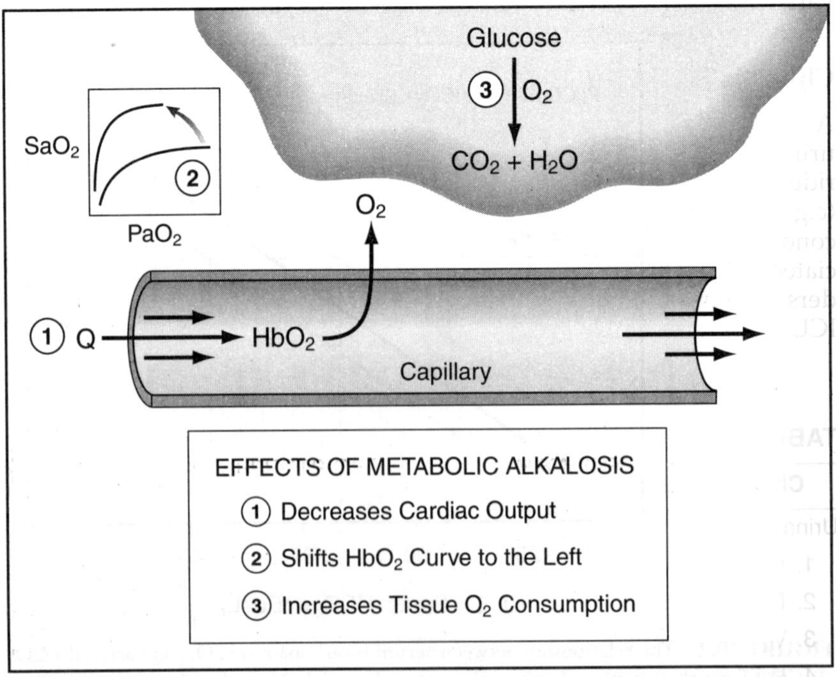

FIGURE 30.3 Effects of metabolic alkalosis on the determinants of tissue oxygenation.

3. Intracellular alkalosis increases the activity of enzymes in the glycolytic pathway, and the rate of glycolysis subsequently increases (7).

Therefore, metabolic alkalosis can decrease tissue oxygen availability while increasing tissue oxygen demands. The clinical significance of these effects is unclear, but they certainly deserve attention in patients with circulatory failure or circulatory shock.

THE EVALUATION

Metabolic alkaloses are traditionally classified as chloride-responsive or chloride-resistant, based on the urinary chloride concentration (see Table 30.1).

Chloride-Responsive Alkalosis

A *chloride-responsive* metabolic alkalosis is characterized by a low urinary chloride concentration (i.e., less than 15 mEq/L), indicating chloride depletion. This type of metabolic alkalosis is the result of gastric acid loss, diuretic therapy, volume depletion, or renal compensation for hypercapnia. As indicated by the inciting conditions, volume depletion is common in chloride responsive metabolic alkalosis. The majority of cases of metabolic alkalosis in hospitalized patients are the chloride-responsive variety.

Chloride-Resistant Alkalosis

A *chloride-resistant* metabolic alkalosis is characterized by an elevated urinary chloride concentration (i.e., above 25 mEq/L). Most cases of chloride resistant alkalosis are caused by primary mineralocorticoid excess (e.g., hyperadrenal conditions) or severe potassium depletion (these two conditions often co-exist). This type of metabolic alkalosis is usually associated with volume expansion rather than volume depletion. The disorders associated with chloride-resistant alkalosis are uncommon in the ICU, with the possible exception of aggressive corticosteroid therapy.

TABLE 30.1 Classification of Metabolic Alkalosis

Chloride-Responsive	Chloride-Resistant
Urinary chloride <15 mEq/L:	Urinary chloride >25 mEq/L:
1. Loss of gastric acid	1. Mineralocorticoid excess
2. Diuretics	2. Potassium depletion
3. Volume depletion	
4. Posthypercapnia	

Spot Urine Chloride

When the cause of a metabolic alkalosis is unclear, the concentration of chloride in a random (spot) urine sample can help identify the possible sources of the problem. One source of error occurs in the early stages of diuretic therapy, when the urinary chloride concentration is elevated in a chloride-responsive metabolic alkalosis. Another benefit of measuring the spot urinary chloride concentration is in selecting the appropriate therapy to correct the alkalosis. These are described next.

MANAGEMENT

Because most metabolic alkaloses in hospitalized patients are chloride-responsive, chloride replacement is the mainstay of therapy for metabolic alkalosis. The chloride can be replaced as sodium chloride, potassium chloride, or hydrochloric acid (HCl).

Saline Infusion

Because volume depletion is common in chloride-responsive metabolic alkalosis, infusion of isotonic saline (0.9% sodium chloride) is the most common method of chloride replacement in this condition. The volume of isotonic saline needed can be determined by estimating the chloride (Cl) deficit, as shown below:

$$\text{Cl deficit (mEq)} = 0.2 \times \text{wt (kg)} \times (\text{normal Cl} - \text{actual Cl}) \qquad (30.2)$$

The factor 0.2 represents the extracellular volume as a fraction of body weight. Once the chloride deficit is determined, the volume of isotonic saline needed to correct the deficit is the ratio: Cl deficit/154, where 154 is the chloride concentration in isotonic saline. This method is summarized in Table 30.2.

EXAMPLE. A patient who weighs 70 kg and has a metabolic alkalosis from repeated vomiting with a serum chloride of 80 mEq/L. Using a

TABLE 30.2 Saline Infusions for Metabolic Alkalosis

Step 1: *Calculate the chloride (Cl) deficit.*

$$\text{Cl deficit (mEq)} = 0.3 \times \text{wt (kg)} \times (100 - \text{plasma [Cl]})$$

Step 2: *Determine the volume of isotonic saline to correct the Cl deficit.*

$$\text{Volume of saline (L)} = \text{Chloride Deficit}/154$$

From References 2 and 3.

normal serum chloride of 100 mEq/L, the chloride deficit is $0.2 \times 70 \times (100 - 80) = 280$ mEq. The volume of isotonic saline needed to correct this deficit is $280/154 = 1.8$ liters.

Potassium Chloride

The administration of potassium chloride is not an effective method of chloride repletion because the maximum rate of potassium infusion that is safe is 40 mEq/hour (see Chapter 33). Therefore, potassium chloride administration is indicated only for patients who are hypokalemic. However, because hypokalemia can promote metabolic alkalosis, correcting hypokalemia is an important measure for correcting a metabolic alkalosis.

It is important to emphasize that the administration of **potassium chloride will not replenish potassium stores if there is concurrent magnesium depletion** (8). Therefore, it is important to identify and correct magnesium depletion before attempting to replace potassium deficits (see Chapter 34 for information on identifying and correcting magnesium deficiency).

Hydrochloric Acid Infusions

Infusions of dilute solutions of hydrochloric acid (HCl) produces the most rapid correction of metabolic alkalosis (1). However, because of the risks involved (see later), HCl infusions are reserved for patients with severe alkalemia (pH greater than 7.5) who are not candidates for saline infusions or potassium replacement, or have failed these therapies.

Method

The "dose" of HCl is determined by estimating the hydrogen ion (H^+) deficit with the equation below (see Table 30.3).

$$H^+ \text{ deficit (mEq)} = 0.5 \times \text{wt (kg)} \times (\text{actual } HCO_3 - \text{desired } HCO_3) \quad (30.3)$$

TABLE 30.3 Infusions of Hydrochloric Acid for Severe or Refractory Metabolic Alkalosis

Step 1: *Calculate the hydrogen ion (H^+) deficit.*

$$H^+ \text{ deficit (mEq)} = 0.5 \times \text{wt (kg)} \times (\text{actual } HCO_3 - \text{desired } HCO_3)$$

Step 2: *Determine the volume of 0.1 N HCl needed to correct the H^+ deficit.*

$$\text{Volume of 0.1N HCl (L)} = H^+ \text{ deficit}/100$$

From References 2 and 3.

The factor 0.5 represents the volume of distribution for H^+ (relative to body weight) and is larger than the chloride space because some of the H^+ will end up inside cells. The desired HCO_3 should be above the normal range (the goal is not to correct the alkalosis, but to reduce the severity), and can be set halfway between the actual and normal HCO_3.

The preferred HCl solution for intravenous use is 0.1N HCl, which contains 100 mEq H^+ per liter (similar to the H^+ concentration of 50 to 100 mEq/L in gastric secretions). The volume of 0.1N HCl needed to correct the H^+ deficit is determined as the ratio (H^+ deficit/100), as shown in Table 30.3. Because HCl solutions are sclerosing, they must be infused through a large, central vein (9), and **the infusion rate should not exceed 0.2 mEq/kg/hr** (3).

EXAMPLE. Consider a patient who weighs 70 kg and has a plasma HCO_3 of 45 mEq/L and an arterial pH of 7.59. Using a desired plasma HCO_3 of 35 mEq/L, the H^+ deficit is $0.5 \times 70 \times 10 = 350$ mEq. The corresponding volume of 0.1N HCl is $350/100 = 3.5$ L, and the maximum infusion rate is $(0.2 \times 70)/100 = 0.14$ L/hour (2.3 ml/minute).

Adverse Effects

The major concern with HCl infusions is the corrosive effects of the HCl solutions. Extravasation of HCl solutions can produce severe tissue necrosis, even when the solution is infused through a central vein (10). Solutions more concentrated than 0.1N HCl can also corrode the intravascular catheters (11)!

Gastric Acid Suppression

Inhibition of gastric acid secretion (with histamine H_2 receptor antagonists or proton pump inhibitors) has been recommended for patients who require continued nasogastric suction. However, it is important to point out **gastric acid suppression will substitute sodium chloride losses for hydrochloric acid losses, so chloride will continue to be lost.** Considering that chloride depletion plays a major role in the metabolic alkalosis from upper GI losses, the rationale for gastric acid suppression in this setting needs to be reevaluated.

Chloride-Resistant Alkalosis

The management of chloride-resistant metabolic alkalosis is aimed at treating the underlying cause of the mineralocorticoid excess (e.g., hyperadrenalism, heart failure) and correcting potassium deficits. The carbonic anhydrase inhibitor, acetazolamide, can also be used to relieve the alkalosis in this condition (see below).

Acetazolamide

Acetazolamide (Diamox) blocks HCO_3 reabsorption in the kidneys by inhibiting the carbonic anhydrase enzyme involved in the $CO_2 \leftrightarrow HCO_3$

reaction sequence (see Figure 30.1). The increase in HCO_3 loss in urine is accompanied by an increase in sodium loss in urine, and this produces a diuretic effect. Therefore, acetazolamide has a dual benefit in patients with chloride-resistant metabolic alkalosis because most of these patients have an increased extracellular volume. The recommended dose is 5 to 10 mg/kg IV (or PO), and the maximum effect occurs after an average of 15 hours (12).

Acetazolamide promotes potassium depletion as well as volume depletion, and it should not be used in cases of chloride resistant metabolic alkalosis that are associated with hypokalemia or volume depletion.

A FINAL WORD

The final word for this chapter is *chloride*: i.e., most cases of metabolic alkalosis in the ICU are associated with (and probably caused by) chloride depletion, and most cases are corrected by giving chloride as NaCl, KCl, or HCl. Metabolic alkalosis seems to have very few deleterious effects that are apparent clinically, so treating the alkalosis is probably not as important as correcting the condition that produces the alkalosis.

REFERENCES

Reviews

1. Khanna A, Kurtzman NA. Metabolic alkalosis. Respir Care 2001;46:354–365.
2. Galla JH. Metabolic alkalosis. J Am Soc Nephrol 2000;11:360–375. (Available at http://jasn.asnjournals.org/cgi/reprint/11/2/369, Accessed June, 2006)
3. Androgue HJ, Madias N. Management of life-threatening acid-base disorders. Part 2. N Engl J Med 1998;338:107–111

Selected References

4. Driscoll DF, Bistrian BR, Jenkins RL. Development of metabolic alkalosis after massive transfusion during orthotopic liver transplantation. Crit Care Med 1987;15:905–908.
5. Rose BD, Post TW. Metabolic alkalosis. In: Clinical physiology of acid-base and electrolyte disorders. 5th ed. New York: McGraw-Hill, 2001, pp 551–577.
6. Javaheri S, Kazemi H. Metabolic alkalosis and hypoventilation in humans. Am Rev Respir Dis 1987;136:1011–1016.
7. Rastegar HR, Woods M, Harken AH. Respiratory alkalosis increases tissue oxygen demand. J Surg Res 1979;26:687–692.
8. Whang R, Flink EB, Dyckner T, et al. Mg depletion as a cause of refractory potassium depletion. Arch Intern Med 1985;145:1686–1689.
9. Brimioulle S, Vincent JL, Dufaye P, et al. Hydrochloric acid infusion for treatment of metabolic alkalosis: effects on acid-base balance and oxygenation. Crit Care Med 1985;13:738–742.

10. Jankauskas SJ, Gursel E, Antonenko DR. Chest wall necrosis secondary to hydrochloric acid use in the treatment of metabolic alkalosis. Crit Care Med 1989;17:963–964.
11. Kopel R, Durbin CG. Pulmonary artery catheter deterioration during hydrochloric infusion for the treatment of metabolic alkalosis. Crit Care Med 1989; 17:688–689.
12. Marik PE, Kussman BD, Lipman J, Kraus P. Acetazolamide in the treatment of metabolic alkalosis in critically ill patients. Heart Lung 1991;20:455–458.

Section X

RENAL AND ELECTROLYTE DISORDERS

It is the internal environment (not the external world) that provides the physical needs for life.

CLAUDE BERNARD

Chapter 31

OLIGURIA AND ACUTE RENAL FAILURE

Lack of urine output in the acutely hypovolemic patient is renal success, not renal failure.

Ronald V. Maier, MD

An acute decrease in urine output can represent a functional adaptation, as Dr. Maier points out, but more often it represents trouble. The trouble is acute renal failure, which develops in about 5% of patients admitted to the ICU, and has a mortality rate of 60% (1). Acute renal failure is similar to the acute respiratory distress syndrome (ARDS) in that it is not a primary disease, but is a complication of other disease processes, most notably severe sepsis and septic shock (2,3). As a result, the mortality rate in acute renal failure mirrors the mortality rate of the primary diseases. Since these primary diseases have a high mortality, it is not surprising that the mortality rate in acute renal failure has not changed in the last 50 years (4), and that acute hemodialysis has had little or no impact on mortality. This latter observation seems to have escaped the notice of the "evidence-based medicine" crowd, who preach that an intervention should be discarded if it does not improve mortality.

GENERAL CONSIDERATIONS

Oliguria

Oliguria is traditionally defined as a urine output of less than 400 mL/day (5), but no one waits 24 hours to make the diagnosis, so this translates to a urine output of less than 16.6 mL/hr. Another definition of oliguria, based on body weight, is a urine output less that 0.5 mL/kg/hr (2).

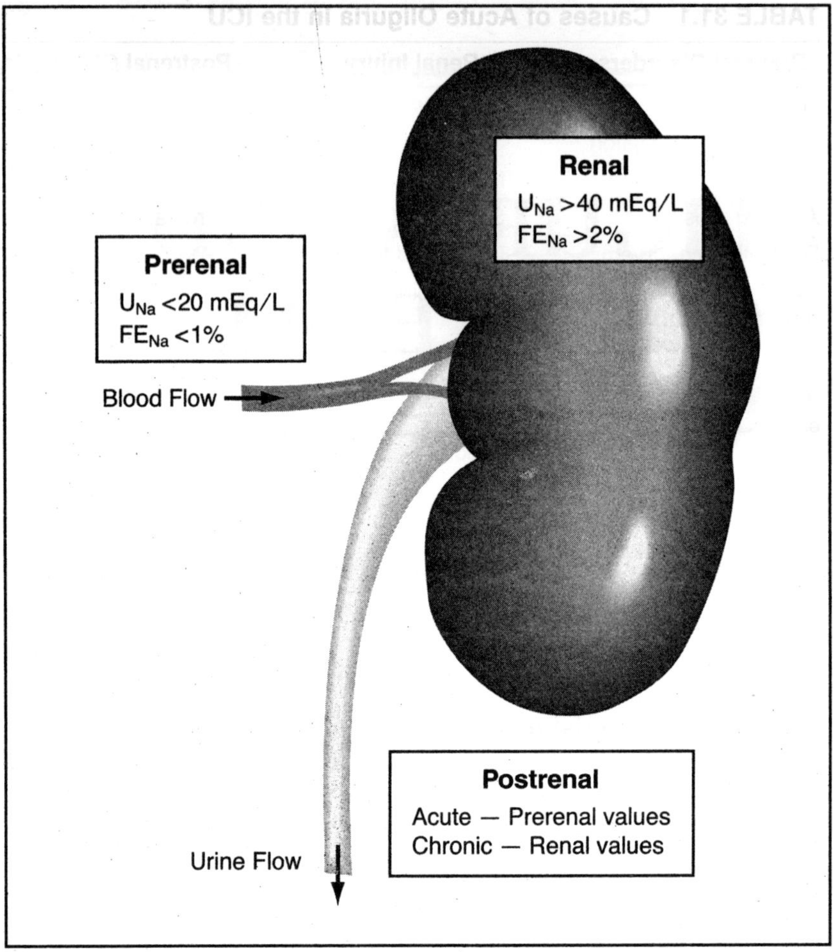

FIGURE 31.1 Classification of oliguria and acute renal failure based on the anatomic location of the problem.

The weight-based definition corresponds to a urine output of 35 to 40 mL/hr for a 70 to 80 kg adult, which is more than twice the urine output in the traditional definition of oliguria. The difference between these definitions is probably not significant (although this has never been addressed), but you should at least be aware that there is more than one definition of oliguria.

The causes of oliguria are traditionally separated into three categories, as illustrated in Figure 31.1. Each category is named according to the anatomic location of the problem responsible for the oliguria. The conditions in each category that are encountered in ICU patients are listed in Table 31.1.

TABLE 31.1 Causes of Acute Oliguria in the ICU

Prerenal Disorders	Renal Injury	Postrenal Obstruction
Hypovolemia	Circulatory shock	Papillary necrosis
Mechanical ventilation	Severe sepsis	Retroperitoneal mass
Cardiomyopathy	Multiorgan failure	Urethral stricture
Aortic stenosis	Surgery†	Prostatic hypertrophy
Dissecting aneurysm	Drugs and toxins‡	
Drugs that impair renal autoregulation*	Myoglobinuria	
	Radiocontrast dye	

*Includes nonsteroidal antiinflammatory agents (ketorolac), angiotensin-converting enzyme inhibitors, and angiotensin receptor blockers.
† Cardiac surgery and abdominal aortic aneurysm repair.
‡ Includes nephrotoxic drugs (aminoglycosides, amphotericin, cisplatin), drugs that cause acute interstitial nephritis (see Table 31.4), and nephrotoxins (e.g., ethylene glycol).

Prerenal Conditions

The prerenal sources of oliguria are located proximal to the kidneys and are characterized by a decrease in renovascular flow. The disorders in this category include **low cardiac output** from hypovolemia, mechanical ventilation, aortic stenosis, and end-stage cardiomyopathy, as well as drugs that impair renal autoregulation (e.g., angiotensin-converting enzyme inhibitors). Prerenal disorders are responsible for about 30 to 40% of cases of oliguria in the ICU (3). The oliguria in these conditions can usually be corrected by correcting the underlying disorder, but prolonged or severe prerenal conditions can lead to renal injury and oliguric renal failure.

Renal Injury

The intrinsic renal disorders encountered in the ICU usually fall into two categories: acute tubular necrosis (ATN), or acute interstitial nephritis (AIN). ATN is responsible for over 50% of cases of acute oliguria in the ICU (3), and is most often caused by inflammatory injury (including sepsis), circulatory shock, and toxic injury from drugs (e.g., aminoglycosides), radiocontrast dye, and myoglobinuria. ATN is described briefly below, while AIN is described later in the chapter.

ATN and GFR

ATN is characterized by (oxidative) injury to the renal tubular epithelial cells with sloughing of the cells into the lumen of the renal tubules (see Fig. 31.2). The sloughed cells create an obstruction that increases the pressure in the proximal tubules. This decreases the net filtration pressure across the glomerular capillaries and reduces the glomerular filtration rate (GFR). This process is called *tubulo-glomerular feedback.*

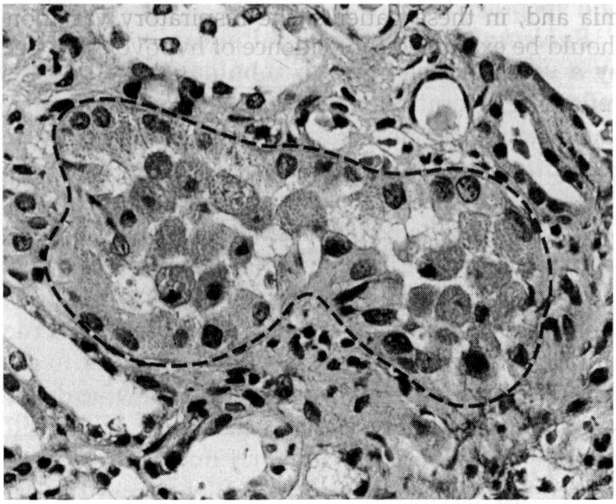

FIGURE 31.2 Photomicrograph of acute tubular necrosis (ATN) showing a proximal tubule (outlined by the dotted line) filled with exfoliated epithelial cells. (From Racusen LC. Histopathology of acute renal failure. New Horiz 1995;3:662–668.)

Postrenal Obstruction

Obstruction distal to the renal parenchyma is responsible for only about 10% of cases of oliguria in the ICU (3). The obstruction can involve the most distal portion of the renal collecting ducts (papillary necrosis), the ureters (extraluminal obstruction from a retroperitoneal mass), or the ureters (strictures or extraluminal obstruction from prostatic enlargement). Ureteral obstruction from stones does not cause oliguria unless there is a solitary functional kidney.

EVALUATION OF OLIGURIA

The initial evaluation of the oliguric patient should be aimed at identifying prerenal or reversible causes of oliguria. Prompt evaluation is necessary because prolonged or severe prerenal conditions can lead to oliguric renal failure, which is not immediately reversible. The following measurements can help to distinguish between prerenal and renal causes of oliguria.

Central Venous Catheters

Most patients in the ICU will have a central venous catheter, and these catheters permit 2 measurements that are useful in the evaluation of oliguria. The first measurement is the central venous pressure (CVP). The CVP will overestimate cardiac filling volumes in critically ill patients (as described in Chapter 12), but a central venous pressure that is very low (1–2 mm Hg) can be used as evidence of hypovolemia. In ventilator-dependent patients, a CVP as high as 10 to 12 mm Hg could represent hypovolemia and, in these patients, the respiratory variation in blood pressure should be examined for evidence of hypovolemia (see below).

The other measurement available with CVP catheters is the *central venous oxyhemoglobin saturation* ($ScvO_2$), which is described in Chapter 11. An $ScvO_2$ that is below 50% can indicate a low cardiac output (when the arterial O_2 saturation and hemoglobin levels are normal), and an $ScvO_2$ that is close to 25 or 30% is probable evidence of a low cardiac output (unless the patient is severely anemic). In patients with systemic sepsis, an $ScvO_2$ below 70% is considered abnormal (6).

Respiratory Variation in Blood Pressure

As explained in Chapters 1 and 24, positive-pressure lungs inflations during mechanical ventilation will augment cardiac stroke output and increase the systolic blood pressure (see Fig. 1.5), but only when cardiac filling volumes are adequate. When cardiac filling volumes are inadequate, positive-pressure lung inflations will reduce the cardiac stroke output and decrease the systolic blood pressure. Therefore **in ventilator-dependent patients, a decrease in blood pressure shortly after each lung inflation can be used as evidence of inadequate cardiac filling.**

Evaluation of the Urine

Urine Microscopy

Microscopic examination of the urine sediment is the easiest and least expensive diagnostic procedure. The presence of abundant tubular epithelial cells with epithelial cell casts is virtually pathognomonic of ATN. In addition, the presence of white cell casts identifies an interstitial nephritis, and the presence of pigmented casts identifies myoglobinuria. If urine microscopy is unrevealing, measuring the sodium concentration in a spot urine sample can be useful.

Spot Urine Sodium

When renal perfusion is diminished, sodium reabsorption increases and urinary sodium excretion decreases. On the other hand, intrinsic renal disease is usually accompanied by a decrease in sodium reabsorption and an increase in sodium excretion in the urine. Therefore, in the setting of oliguria, **a urine sodium below 20 mEq/L usually indicates a prerenal condition** (5). However, a urine sodium above 40 mEq/L does not rule out a prerenal condition when it is superimposed on an underlying case of chronic renal insufficiency (where there is obligatory sodium loss in the urine), or when there is ongoing diuretic therapy. Elderly patients can also have an obligatory loss of sodium in the urine. Therefore, a urine sodium above 40 mEq/L must be interpreted according to the clinical setting.

Fractional Excretion of Sodium

The fractional excretion of sodium (FE_{Na}) is the fraction of sodium filtered at the glomerulus that is excreted in the urine. This is equivalent to the sodium clearance divided by the creatinine clearance, as shown in

TABLE 31.2 Quantitative Assessment of Renal Function

Creatinine Clearance (Men):

$$CL_{Cr}(\text{mL/min}) = \frac{(140 - \text{age}) \times \text{weight (kg)}}{72 \times \text{Serum creatinine (mg/dL)}}$$

Creatinine Clearance (Women):

$$CL_{Cr}\ (\text{mL/min}) = 0.85 \times CL_{Cr} \text{ for men}$$

Fractional Excretion of Sodium:

$$FE_{Na} = \frac{\text{Urine [Na] / Plasma [Na]}}{\text{Urine [Cr] / Plasma [Cr]}} \times 100$$

Table 31.2 (7). The FE_{Na} is normally less than 1%; i.e., less than 1% of the filtered sodium is excreted in the urine. In the setting of oliguria, the FE_{Na} provides the following information:

$$\begin{aligned} FE_{Na} < 1\% &= \text{probable prerenal condition} \\ FE_{Na} > 2\% &= \text{probable renal injury} \end{aligned} \qquad (31.1)$$

There are some exceptions to these criteria: e.g., the FE_{Na} can be less than 1% in ATN due to myoglobinuria (5). Despite the occasional exception, **the FE_{Na} is one of the most reliable urinary parameters for distinguishing prerenal from renal causes of oliguria.** However, it is a cumbersome determination to perform, and this limits its popularity.

Serum Creatinine Concentration

A *change* in the serum creatinine concentration can be used to identify patients with renal injury and renal failure (2) as shown in Table 31.3. The serum creatinine can also be used to calculate the creatinine clearance, as shown in Table 31.2 (8). The creatinine clearance overestimates the GFR because creatinine is secreted by the renal tubules. However, changes in creatinine clearance can be used to track changes in GFR. The changes in creatinine clearance expected in acute renal failure are shown in Table 31.3.

TABLE 31.3 Criteria for the Diagnosis of Acute Renal Injury and Acute Renal Failure

Condition	Serum Creatinine	Creatinine Clearance
Renal Injury	2 × baseline	>50% decrease
Renal Failure	3 × baseline or acute rise ≥0.5 mg/dL to ≥4 mg/dL	≥75% decrease

From Reference 2.

INITIAL MANAGEMENT

The principal task in the early management of the oliguric patient is to identify and correct volume deficits and discontinue any drugs that could be a source of oliguric renal failure.

Fluid Challenge

If there is evidence or suspicion of inadequate ventricular filling based on the evaluation described in the last section, then immediate volume infusion is warranted. Fluid challenges of 500 mL to 1,000 mL for crystalloid fluids and 300 mL to 500 mL for colloid fluids, infused over 30 minutes, have been proposed for patients with severe sepsis and septic shock (9), and these recommendations can be applied to all patients who require volume infusion. The fluid challenges are continued until there is a response or until you are concerned about volume overload.

There is no evidence to favor crystalloid or colloid fluids for volume infusions. Colloid fluids are more likely to expand the plasma volume and less likely to expand the extracellular fluid volume than crystalloid fluids (see Chapter 13). In patients with hypoalbuminemia, 5% albumin should be seriously considered for volume resuscitation.

Don't Use Low-Dose Dopamine

Despite more than thirty years of use as a renal vasodilator, low-dose dopamine (2 μg/kg/min) has shown no evidence of benefit in patients with acute oliguric renal failure (10,11). In fact, low-dose dopamine can have deleterious effects on hemodynamics (decreased splanchnic blood flow) immune function (inhibition of T-cell lymphocyte function) and endocrine function (inhibition of thyroid-stimulating hormone release from the pituitary) (11). For these reasons, the use of low-dose dopamine in patients with acute oliguria is (borrowing the title from reference 11) *bad medicine.*

Furosemide

In patients with acute oliguric renal failure, there is little or no chance of increasing urine output with furosemide because less than 10% of the injected drug will reach the site of action in the renal tubules (12). If furosemide is used in an attempt to promote urine flow, it should be given by continuous infusion as described in Chapter 14.

SPECIFIC RENAL DISORDERS

Inflammatory Renal Injury

Acute, oliguric renal failure is reported in about 25% of patients with severe sepsis and 50% of patients with septic shock (13). It also occurs in patients with systemic inflammation without evidence of infection (see Chapter 40). In these clinical settings, acute renal failure appears to be just one part of a more widespread systemic illness associated with dysfunction and failure in multiple organs (14). The culprit in these conditions is the inflammatory response, which has been called *malignant intravascular inflammation* (15). The management of this condition is supportive, and is described in Chapter 40.

Contrast-Induced Renal Failure

Iodinated radiocontrast agents can produce acute renal injury and renal failure, and contrast-induced nephropathy is now considered the third leading cause of acute renal failure in hospitalized patients (16). The renal injury usually becomes apparent as a rising serum creatinine within 72 hours after the procedure. Predisposing conditions include diabetes, hypertension, pre-existing renal disease, congestive heart failure, and the osmolality and volume of iodinated contrast agent used during the procedure. Oliguria is uncommon, but can occur in patients with pre-existing renal disease. Most cases resolve within 2 weeks, and few require hemodialysis (16). The mechanism of renal injury is multifactorial, and includes hyperosmolar injury to the endothelium of small vessels in the kidney, and oxidative injury to the renal tubular epithelial cells.

Prevention

The most effective strategy for prevention of contrast-induced nephropathy in high-risk patients is intravenous hydration (if permitted) combined with the antioxidant *N*-acetylcysteine. The following regimen is recommended (16,17):

Volume infusion: Isotonic saline at 100 to 150 mL/hr started at 3 to 12 hours before the procedure. For emergent procedures, at least 300 to 500 mL isotonic saline should be infused just prior to the procedure. Urine output should be maintained at 150 mL/hr for at least 6 hours after the procedure (16).

N-acetylcysteine: 600 mg by mouth twice daily from 24 hours before, to 24 hours after, the procedure (16), or for emergent procedures such as primary angioplasty, 600 mg IV just before the procedure and 600 mg orally twice daily for 48 hours after the procedure (18).

N-acetylcysteine is an intracellular glutathione surrogate that is used as the antidote for acetaminophen hepatotoxicity (see Chapter 53). Oral administration of *N*-acetylcysteine is poorly tolerated because the sulfur content has a pungent taste (like rotten eggs). Intravenous *N*-acetylcysteine was recently approved for use in acetaminophen overdose, and is considered safe except for rare cases of anaphylaxis.

The physician performing the contrast procedure should be informed when patients are at risk for contrast-induced nephropathy. Although contrast agents with reduced osmolality are now used routinely to limit the risk of contrast-induced nephropathy, limiting the volume of the contrast agent to 100 mL is also beneficial (16).

TABLE 31.4 Drugs That Can Cause Interstitial Nephritis

Antibiotics	CNS Drugs	Diuretics
Aminoglycosides	Carbamazepine	Acetazolamide
Amphotericin B	Phenobarbital	Furosemide
Cephalosporins	Phenytoin	Thiazides
Fluoroquinolones	***NSAIDs***	***Others***
Penicillins	Aspirin	Acetaminophen
Sulfonamides	Ibuprofen	ACE Inhibitors
Vancomycin	Ketorolac	Iodinated dyes
	Naproxen	Ranitidine

NSAIDs = nonsteroidal antiinflammatory drugs, *ACE* = angiotensin-converting enzyme.
From Reference 19.

Acute Interstitial Nephritis (AIN)

AIN is an inflammatory condition that involves the renal interstitium and presents as acute renal failure, usually without oliguria (19). Most cases are the result of a hypersensitivity drug reaction, but infections (usually viral or atypical pathogens) can also be involved. The drugs most often implicated in AIN are listed in Table 31.4. Antibiotics are the most common offenders, particularly the penicillins.

AIN can be difficult to distinguish from ATN. In cases of drug-induced AIN, the characteristic signs of a hypersensitivity reaction (e.g., fever, rash, eosinophilia) may not be present. The onset of renal injury usually occurs within 2 weeks after starting the drug, but delayed reactions occurring months after the onset of drug therapy have been reported (17). The presence of eosinophils and leukocyte casts on urine microscopy are the most characteristic diagnostic findings. A renal biopsy can secure the diagnosis, but is rarely obtained.

In suspected cases of AIN, any possible offending agents should be discontinued. Oral prednisone at a dose of 0.5 to 1 mg/kg daily for one to four weeks may help to speed recovery (19,20). Complete resolution can take months.

Myoglobinuric Renal Failure

Acute renal failure develops in about one-third of patients with diffuse muscle injury (rhabdomyolysis) (21,22). The culprit is myoglobin, which is released by the injured muscle and is capable of damaging the renal tubular epithelial cells after it is filtered through the glomerulus. The source of cell injury may be the iron moiety in heme (23), which is capable of oxidative cell injury via the production of hydroxyl radicals (see Chapter 21, Fig. 21.5). This would also explain why hemoglobin can produce a similar type of renal tubular injury.

The common causes of rhabdomyolysis are trauma, infection, immobility (in alcoholics), drugs (e.g., lipid lowering agents) and electrolyte abnormalities (e.g., hypophosphatemia). The risk of renal failure is not related to any single abnormality, but is more likely when there is a combination of abnormalities. For example, one study of trauma victims with rhabdomyolysis revealed that the best predictor of acute renal failure was the combination of a serum creatinine >1.5, a creatine kinase (CPK) >5,000 IU/L, a base deficit ≤4, and myoglobin in the urine (23). The serum creatinine is not an accurate index of renal function in rhabdomyolysis because the enhanced creatine release from skeletal muscle adds to the serum creatinine. The principal conditions that predispose to renal injury are hypovolemia and acidosis.

Myoglobin in Urine

Myoglobin can be detected in urine with the orthotoluidine dipstick reaction (Hemastix) that is used to detect occult blood in urine. If the test is positive, the urine should be centrifuged (to separate erythrocytes) and the supernatant should be passed through a micropore filter (to remove hemoglobin). A persistently positive test after these measures is evidence of myoglobin in urine.

The presence of myoglobin in urine does not identify patients with a high risk of renal injury, but **the absence of myoglobin in urine identifies patients with a low risk of renal injury** (22).

Management

The plasma levels of potassium and phosphate must be monitored carefully in rhabdomyolysis because these electrolytes are released by injured skeletal muscle and the concentration in plasma can increase dramatically, especially when renal function is impaired. Aggressive **volume resuscitation** to prevent hypovolemia and maintain renal blood flow is one of the most effective measures for preventing or limiting the renal injury in rhabdomyolysis. Alkalinizing the urine can also help to limit the renal injury, but this is difficult to accomplish and is often not necessary. About 30% of patients who develop myoglobinuric renal failure will require dialysis (22).

RENAL REPLACEMENT THERAPY

About 70% of patients with acute renal failure will require some form of renal replacement therapy (RRT). The usually indications for RRT are volume overload, uremic encephalopathy, and difficult-to-control hyperkalemia and metabolic acidosis. There is a growing body of RRT techniques, including hemodialysis, hemofiltration, hemodiafiltration, high flux dialysis, and plasmafiltration. Each employs a different method of water and solute transport. The presentation that follows is limited to the techniques of hemodialysis and hemofiltration.

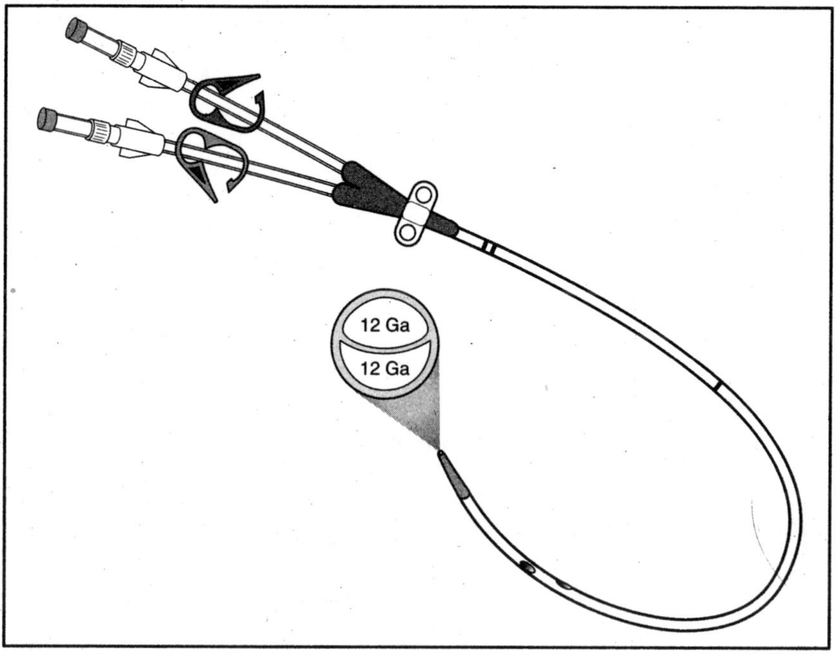

FIGURE 31.3 A double lumen venous catheter used for hemodialysis. The internal diameter of each lumen is about twice the diameter of each lumen in a triple-lumen central venous catheter (see Figure 6.4).

Hemodialysis

Hemodialysis removes solutes by diffusion, which is driven by the concentration gradient of the solutes across a semipermeable membrane. To maintain this concentration gradient, blood and dialysis fluid are driven in opposite directions across the diffusional barrier (dialysis membrane): this technique is known as *countercurrent exchange* (24). A blood pump is used to move blood in one direction across the dialysis membrane at a rate of 200 to 300 mL/min. The dialysis fluid on the other side of the membrane moves twice as fast, or at 500 to 800 mL/min (24).

Vascular Access

A large-bore, double-lumen vascular catheter like the one shown in Figure 31.3 is required to perform intermittent hemodialysis. Each lumen of the catheter in this figure has a diameter that is roughly twice the diameter of each lumen in a standard central venous catheter (see the triple-lumen catheter in Figure 6.4 and compare lumen sizes using Table 6.1). Because flow through rigid tubes varies directly with the fourth power of the radius (see the Hagen-Poiseuille equation in Figure 1.6), a catheter lumen that is doubled in size will allow ($2^4 = 16$) a 16-fold greater flow

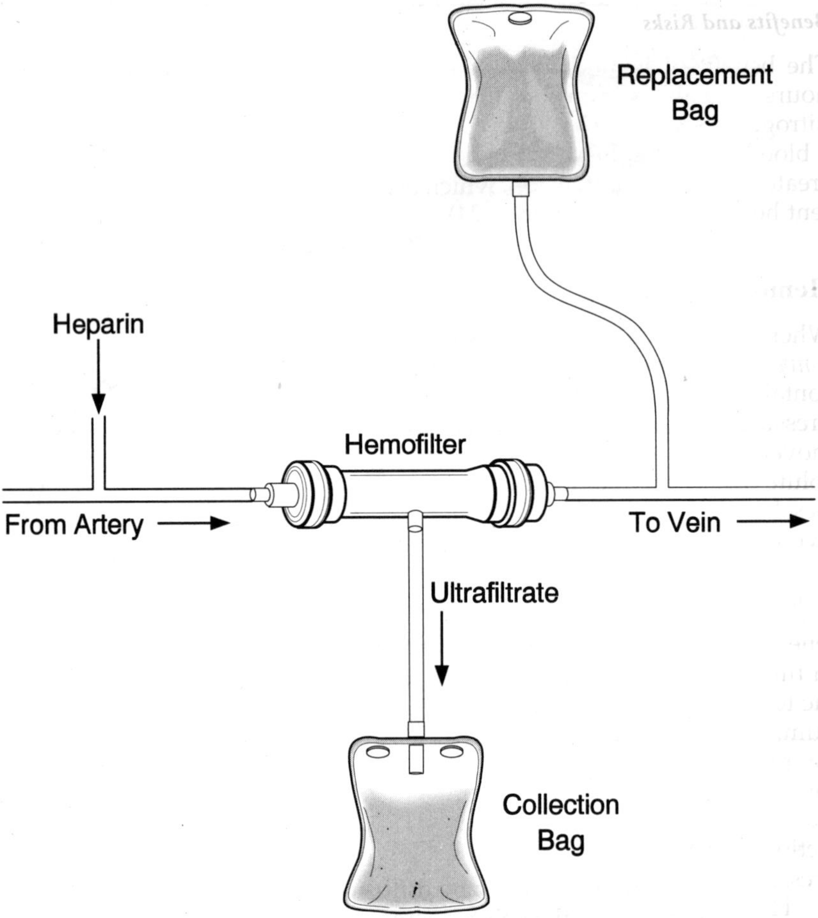

FIGURE 31.4 The technique of continuous arteriovenous hemofiltration (CAVH).

rate. The large-bore catheter in Figure 31.3 is thus well-suited for the high flow needed to perform intermittent hemodialysis. Blood is withdrawn from one lumen of the catheter, pumped through the dialysis chamber, and then returned to the patient through the other lumen.

The large-bore dialysis catheters are placed in either the internal jugular vein or the femoral vein. The subclavian vein is not recommended because there is a high incidence of vascular stenosis and this makes the ipsilateral arm veins unsuitable for chronic dialysis access if renal function does not recover (25). The internal jugular vein is preferred because of the risk for venous thrombosis with femoral vein cannulation (see Table 6.3), but awake patients are intolerant of the limited neck mobility associated with cannulation of the internal jugular vein with these large-bore catheters.

Benefits and Risks

The benefit of hemodialysis is rapid clearance of solutes. Only a few hours of dialysis is needed to remove a day's worth of accumulated nitrogenous waste. The disadvantage of dialysis is the need to maintain a blood flow of at least 300 mL/min through the dialysis chamber. This creates a risk of hypotension, which occurs in about one-third of intermittent hemodialysis treatments (24).

Hemofiltration

Whereas hemodialysis removes solutes by diffusion, hemofiltration uses *convection* for solute transport. Convection is a method where a solute-containing fluid is driven across a permeable membrane by exerting a pressure difference across the membrane. The solutes are cleared by the movement of the fluid across the membrane. Since the fluid "drags" the solute across the membrane, this method of solute transport is known as *solvent drag* (24). Because the removal of solutes by convection is relatively slow, hemofiltration is performed continuously.

Continuous Hemofiltration

One technique of continuous hemofiltration is illustrated in Figure 31.4. In this case, the hemofilter is placed between an artery and a vein, and the technique is called *continuous arteriovenous hemofiltration* (CAVH). No pumps are required for CAVH. The arteriovenous pressure difference is the pressure gradient for flow through the filter. The pressure gradient for water movement across the filter is the mean blood pressure on one side, and the vertical distance between the filter and the ultrafiltrate collection bag on the other side. If the collection bag is lowered, the filtration pressure will increase.

Hemofiltration can remove large volumes of fluid (up to 3 liters per hour) so a replacement fluid is needed to prevent hypovolemia. This is shown in the CAVH circuit in Figure 31.4. The replacement fluid also decreases the plasma concentration of waste products that are removed in the ultrafiltrate. That is, the concentration of solutes in the ultrafiltrate is the same as in the blood, so the plasma concentration of waste products will not decrease unless a waste-free fluid is used to replace the fluid that is removed.

Benefits

Since hemofiltration is driven by pressure and not flow, high flow rates are not needed, and **there is a much less risk of hypotension** with CAVH. The removal of solutes is also more gradual and more physiological with continuous hemofiltration. One shortcoming of CAVH is that it is not suitable for use in patients with hypotension. The technique of *continuous venovenous hemofiltration* (CVVH) uses a pump to generate a pressure, and can be used in hypotensive patients.

In general, the benefits of continuous renal replacement therapy are leading to a gradual disappearance of intermittent hemodialysis in the ICU.

A FINAL WORD

A sudden and precipitous drop in urine output is rarely a sign of simple dehydration that will be corrected with fluids. Instead, it is usually an ominous sign of failure involving of one of the major organ systems in the body. In the setting of sepsis, the appearance of oliguria usually heralds the beginning of multiple organ failure, which often has a fatal outcome. This condition of multiorgan failure, which can be viewed as the gradual process of dying (the more organs that fail, the closer the patient is to death), is described in Chapter 40.

REFERENCES

Introduction

1. Uchino S, Kellum JA, Bellomo R, et al. Acute renal failure in critically ill patients: a multinational, multicenter study. JAMA 2005;294:813–818.

Reviews

2. Bellomo R. Defining, quantifying, and classifying acute renal failure. Crit Care Clin 2005;21:223–237.
3. Abernathy VE, Lieberthal W. Acute renal failure in the critically ill patient. Crit Care Clin 2002;18:203–222.
4. Singri N, Ahya SN, Levin ML. Acute renal failure. JAMA 2003;289:747–751.
5. Klahr S, Miller SB. Acute oliguria. N Engl J Med 1998;338:671–675.

Evaluation of Oliguria

6. Dellinger RP, Carlet JM, Masur H, et al. Surviving sepsis campaign guidelines for management of severe sepsis and septic shock. Crit Care Med 2004; 32:858–873.
7. Steiner RW. Interpreting the fractional excretion of sodium. Am J Med 1984; 77:699–702.
8. Cockroft DW, Gault MN. Prediction of creatinine clearance from serum creatinine. Nephron 1976;16:31–41.

Initial Management

9. Vincent J-L, Gerlach H. Fluid resuscitation in severe sepsis and septic shock: an evidence-based review. Crit Care Med 2004;32(suppl):S451–S454.
10. Kellum JA, Decker JM. Use of dopamine in acute renal failure: a meta-analysis. Crit Care Med 2001;29:1526–1531.
11. Holmes CL, Walley KR. Bad medicine: low-dose dopamine in the ICU. Chest 2003;123:1266–1275.
12. Brater DC, Anderson SA, Brown-Cartwright D. Response to furosemide in chronic renal insufficiency: rationale for limited doses. Clin Pharmacol Ther 1986;40:134–139.

Specific Renal Disorders

13. Schrier RW, Wang W. Acute renal failure and sepsis. N Engl J Med 2004;351: 159–169.
14. Balk RA. Pathogenesis and management of multiple organ dysfunction or failure in severe sepsis and septic shock. Crit Care Clin 2000;16:337–352.
15. Pinsky MR, Vincent J-L, Deviere J, et al. Serum cytokine levels in human septic shock: relation to multiple-system organ failure and mortality. Chest 1993;103:565–575.
16. McCullough PA, Soman S. Contrast-induced nephropathy. Crit Care Clin 2005;21:261–280.
17. Liu R, Nair D, Ix J, et al. *N*-acetylcysteine for the prevention of contrast-induced nephropathy. A systematic review and meta-analysis. J Gen Intern Med 2005;20:193–200.
18. Marenzi G, Assanelli E, Marana I, et al. *N*-acetylcysteine and contrast-induced nephropathy in primary angioplasty. N Engl J Med 2006;354:2772–2782.
19. Taber SS, Mueller BA. Drug-associated renal dysfunction. Crit Care Clin 2006;22:357–374.
20. Ten RM, Torres VE, Millner DS, et al. Acute interstitial nephritis. Mayo Clin Proc 1988;3:921–930.
21. Beetham R. Biochemical investigation of suspected rhabdomyolysis. Ann Clin Biochem 2000; 2000:37:581–587.
22. Sharp LS, Rozycki GS, Feliciano DV. Rhabdomyolysis and secondary renal failure in critically ill surgical patients. Am J Surg 2004;188:801–806.
23. Visweswaran P, Guntupalli J. Rhabdomyolysis. Crit Care Clin 1999;15:415–428.

Renal Replacement Therapy

24. O'Reilly P, Tolwani A. Renal replacement therapy III. IHD, CRRT, SLED. Crit Care Clin 2005;21:367–378.
25. Hernandez D, Diaz F, Rufino M, et al. Subclavian vascular access stenosis in dialysis patients: natural history and risk factors. J Am Soc Nephrol 1998;9: 1507–1511.

Chapter 32

HYPERTONIC AND HYPOTONIC CONDITIONS

This chapter describes the diagnosis and management of conditions associated with abnormalities in total body water. These conditions typically present with abnormalities in the plasma sodium concentration (hypernatremia and hyponatremia) that are sometimes mistaken as problems in sodium balance (1,2). This chapter presents a very simple approach to hypernatremia and hyponatremia based on a clinical assessment of the extracellular volume. The very first part of the chapter contains a quick review of the determinants of water movement between fluid compartments.

BASIC CONCEPTS

The following is a description of the forces that determine the movement of water between the intracellular and extracellular fluid compartments.

Osmotic Activity

The activity (concentration) of solute particles in a solution is inversely related to the activity (concentration) of water molecules in the solution. The solute activity in a solution is also called the *osmotic activity* and is expressed in osmoles (osm). The total osmotic activity in a solution is the sum of the individual osmotic activities of all the solute particles in the solution. For monovalent ions, the osmotic activity in milliosmoles (mOsm) per unit volume is equivalent to the concentration of the ions in milliequivalents (mEq) per unit volume. Thus, the osmotic activity in isotonic saline (0.9% sodium chloride) is as follows:

$$\begin{aligned} 0.9\%\ \text{NaCl} &= 154\ \text{mEq Na/L} + 154\ \text{mEq Cl/L} \\ &= 154\ \text{mOsm Na/L} + 154\ \text{mOsm Cl/L} \qquad (32.1) \\ &= 308\ \text{mOsm/L} \end{aligned}$$

Osmolarity is the osmotic activity per volume of solution (solutes plus water) and is expressed as mOsm/L (3,4). **Osmolality** is the osmotic activity per volume of water and is expressed as mOsm/kg H_2O. The osmotic activity of body fluids usually is expressed in relation to the volume of water (i.e., osmolality). However, the volume of water in body fluids is far greater than the volume of solutes, so there is little difference between the osmolality and osmolarity of body fluids. Thus, the terms osmolality and osmolarity can be used interchangeably to describe the osmotic activity in body fluids.

Tonicity

When two solutions are separated by a membrane that allows the passage of water but not solutes, the water passes from the solution with the lower osmotic activity to the solution with the higher osmotic activity. The *relative* osmotic activity in the two solutions is called the **effective osmolality**, or **tonicity.** The solution with the higher osmolality is described as hypertonic, and the solution with the lower osmolality is described as hypotonic. Thus, the tendency for water to move into and out of cells is determined by the relative osmolality (tonicity) of the intracellular and extracellular fluids.

When the membrane separating two fluids is permeable to both solutes and water, and a solute is added to one of the fluids, the solute equilibrates fully across the membrane. In this situation, the solute increases the osmolality of both fluids, but there will be no movement of water between compartments (because there is no difference in osmolality between the two compartments). A solute that behaves in this manner is urea, which is freely permeable across cell membranes. Therefore, an increase in the urea concentration in extracellular fluid (i.e., an increase in the blood urea nitrogen or BUN) will increase the osmolality of the extracellular fluid, but this does not draw water out of cells because urea does not create a difference in osmolality between extracellular and intracellular fluid. Thus, **azotemia (increased BUN) is a hyperosmotic condition, but not a hypertonic condition.**

Plasma Osmolality

The osmolality of the extracellular fluids can be measured in the clinical laboratory using the freezing point of plasma (a solution containing 1 osm/L will freeze at −1.86°C). This is the *freezing point depression* method for measuring osmolality.

The osmolality of the extracellular fluids can also be calculated using the concentrations of sodium, chloride, glucose, and urea in plasma (these are the major solutes in extracellular fluid). The calculation below uses a plasma sodium (Na^+) of 140 mEq/L, a plasma glucose of 90 mg/dL, and a BUN of 14 mg/dL (3,5).

$$\begin{aligned} \text{Plasma osmolality} &= (2 \times \text{Plasma Na}^+) + \frac{\text{Glucose}}{18} + \frac{\text{BUN}}{2.8} \\ &= (2 \times 140) + \frac{90}{18} + \frac{14}{2.8} \qquad (32.2) \\ &= 290 \text{ mOsm/kg H}_2\text{O} \end{aligned}$$

The sodium concentration is doubled to include the osmotic contribution of chloride. The serum glucose and urea are measured in milligrams per deciliter, and the factors 18 and 2.8 (the atomic weights divided by 10) are used to convert mg/dL to mOsm/kg H_2O.

Osmolal Gap

Because solutes other than sodium, chloride, glucose, and urea are present in the extracellular fluid, the measured plasma osmolality will be greater than the calculated plasma osmolality. This osmolar gap (i.e., the difference between the measured and calculated plasma osmolality) is normally as much as 10 mOsm/kg H_2O (3,5). An increase in the osmolar gap occurs when certain toxins (e.g., ethanol, methanol, ethylene glycol, or the unidentified toxins that accumulate in renal failure) are in the extracellular fluid (6). Therefore, the osmolar gap has been proposed as a screening test for identifying the presence of toxins in the extracellular fluid. In the case of renal failure, the osmolar gap has been recommended as a reliable test for distinguishing acute from chronic renal failure: the osmolar gap is expected to be normal in acute renal failure and elevated in chronic renal failure (7). In reality, the osmolar gap is used infrequently.

Plasma Tonicity

Because urea passes freely across cell membranes, the effective osmolality or tonicity of the extracellular fluid can be calculated by eliminating urea (BUN) from the plasma osmolality equation.

$$\begin{aligned}\text{Plasma tonicity} &= (2 \times \text{Plasma Na}^+) + \frac{\text{Glucose}}{18}\\ &= (2 \times 140) + \frac{90}{18} \\ &= 285\ \text{mOsm/kg H}_2\text{O}\end{aligned} \tag{32.3}$$

Because the concentration of urea contributes little to the total solute concentration in extracellular fluids, there is little difference between the osmolality and tonicity of the extracellular fluid. This equation establishes the plasma sodium concentration as the principal determinant of the effective osmolality of extracellular fluid. Because the effective osmolality determines the tendency for water to move into and out of cells, **the plasma sodium concentration is the principal determinant of the relative volumes of the intracellular and extracellular fluids.**

HYPERNATREMIA

The normal plasma (serum) sodium concentration is 135 to 145 mEq/L. Therefore, hypernatremia (i.e., a serum sodium concentration above 145 mEq/L) can be the result of loss of fluid that has a sodium

TABLE 32.1 Change in Total Body Sodium and Water in Hypernatremia and Hyponatremia

Condition	Extracellular Volume	Total Body Sodium	Total Body Free Water
Hypernatremia	Decreased	↓	↓↓
	Normal	—	↓
	Increased	↑↑	↑
Hyponatremia	Decreased	↓↓	↓
	Normal	—	↑
	Increased	↑	↑↑

concentration below 135 mEq/L (hypotonic fluid loss) or gain of fluid that has a sodium concentration above 145 mEq/L (hypertonic fluid gain). Each of these conditions can be identified by assessing the state of the extracellular volume as shown in Table 32.1 (1,8,9).

Extracellular Volume

If invasive hemodynamic monitoring is available, the state of the intravascular volume can be evaluated by the relationship between the cardiac filling pressures and the cardiac output. For example, the combination of reduced cardiac filling pressures and a low cardiac output is evidence of hypovolemia (see the section on *Hemodynamic Subsets* in Chapter 9). In the absence of hypoproteinemia (which shifts fluids from the intravascular to extravascular space), the state of the intravascular volume can be used as a reflection of the state of the extracellular volume (ECV).

If invasive hemodynamic monitoring is not available, the evaluation of hypovolemia described in Chapter 12 can be used to detect a decreased ECV. The clinical detection of an increased ECV can be difficult because the absence of edema does not exclude the presence of a high ECV (edema may not be apparent until the ECV has increased 4 to 5 liters) and the presence of edema can be misleading because edema in ICU patients can be the result of immobility, hypoalbuminemia, or venous congestion from high intrathoracic pressures (in ventilator-dependent patients).

Once the state of the ECV is determined, the strategies shown in Figure 32.1 can be applied.

Low ECV indicates loss of hypotonic fluids. Common causes are excessive diuresis, vomiting, and diarrhea. The management strategy is to replace the sodium deficit quickly (to maintain plasma volume) and to replace the free water deficit slowly (to prevent intracellular overhydration).

Normal ECV indicates a net loss of free water. This can be seen in diabetes insipidus, or when loss of hypotonic fluids (e.g., diuresis) is

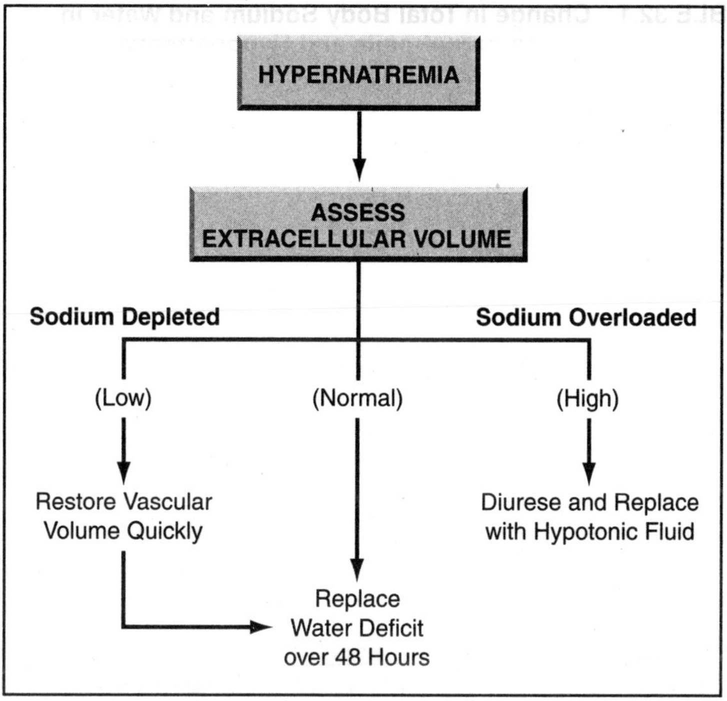

FIGURE 32.1 Management of hypernatremia based on the extracellular volume.

treated by replacement with isotonic saline in a 1:1 volume-to-volume ratio. The management strategy is to replace the free water deficit slowly (to prevent intracellular overhydration).

High ECV indicates a gain of hypertonic fluids. This is seen with aggressive use of hypertonic saline or sodium bicarbonate solutions. The management strategy is to induce sodium loss in the urine with diuresis and to replace the urine volume loss with fluids that are hypotonic to the urine.

Each of these conditions is described in more detail in the following sections.

HYPOVOLEMIC HYPERNATREMIA

The most common cause of hypernatremia is loss of hypotonic body fluids. The concentration of sodium in body fluids that are commonly lost is shown in Table 32.2. With the exception of small bowel and pancreatic secretions, loss of any of these body fluids will result in hypernatremia.

Consequences

All of the body fluids listed in Table 32.2 contain sodium, so the loss of these fluids will be accompanied by deficits in total body sodium as well

TABLE 32.2 Sodium Concentration in Body Fluids

Fluids Commonly Lost	Sodium Concentration (mEq/L)
Urine*	<10
Diarrhea	40
Gastric secretions	55
Sweat	80
Furosemide diuresis	75
Pancreatic secretions	145
Small bowel secretions	145

*Urinary sodium concentration varies according to daily sodium intake.

as total body water (TBW). The sodium deficits predispose to hypovolemia, whereas the free water deficits predispose to hypertonicity in the extracellular fluids. Therefore, the two consequences of hypotonic fluid loss are hypovolemia and hypertonicity.

Hypovolemia

The most immediate threat with hypotonic fluid loss is hypovolemia, which predisposes to hypoperfusion of the vital organs (8,9). Fortunately, hypovolemia is not as prominent when hypotonic fluids are lost as when whole blood is lost. This is because the resultant hypertonicity draws water out of cells, and this helps maintain the volume of the extracellular (intravascular) fluid compartment.

Hypertonicity

The hypertonicity of the extracellular fluids predisposes to cellular dehydration. The most serious consequence of hypertonic hypernatremia is a metabolic encephalopathy (10). Clinical findings include depressed consciousness that can progress to frank coma, generalized seizures, and focal neurological deficits (10). Hypernatremic encephalopathy has an associated mortality of up to 50% (10), but management should proceed slowly.

Volume Replacement

The most immediate concern in hypovolemic hypernatremia is to replace volume deficits and maintain the cardiac output. Volume replacement can be guided by the cardiac filling pressures, cardiac output, urine output, etc. When solute losses are severe and hemodynamic compromise is present, infusions of colloid fluids (5% albumin or 6% hetastarch) will restore the intravascular volume much more effectively than infusion of crystalloid fluids, as described in Chapter 13. When crystalloid fluids are used for volume resuscitation in hypertonic dehydration, isotonic fluids (e.g., 0.9% sodium chloride) are preferred to hypotonic fluids (e.g., half-normal saline) to reduce the risk of cellular edema.

Free Water Replacement

When hypovolemia has been corrected, the next step is to calculate and replace the free water deficit. The calculation of free water deficit is based on the assumption that the product of TBW and plasma sodium concentration (P_{Na}) is always constant.

$$\text{Current TBW} \times \text{Current } P_{Na} = \text{Normal TBW} \times \text{Normal } P_{Na} \qquad (32.4)$$

Substituting 140 mEq/L for a normal P_{Na} and rearranging terms yields the following relationship:

$$\text{Current TBW} = \text{Normal TBW} \times (140/\text{Current } P_{Na}) \qquad (32.5)$$

The normal TBW (in liters) is usually 60% of lean body weight (in kg) in men and 50% of lean body weight in women (11). However, in hypernatremia associated with free water deficits, the normal TBW should be approximately 10% less than usual (11). Thus in men, the normal TBW is 0.5 × body weight (kg), and in women, the normal TBW is 0.4 × body weight (in kg). Once the current TBW is calculated, the water deficit is taken as the difference between the normal and current TBW.

$$\text{TBW deficit (L)} = \text{Normal TBW} - \text{Current TBW} \qquad (32.6)$$

Sample Calculation

Assume that an adult man with a lean body weight of 70 kg has a plasma sodium of 160 mEq/L. The normal TBW will be 0.5 × 70 = 35 L. The current TBW will be 35 × 140/160 = 30.5 L. The TBW deficit will be 35 − 30.5 = 4.5 L.

The volume needed to correct the water deficit is determined by the concentration of sodium in the replacement fluid. This volume can be determined as follows (12):

$$\text{Replacement volume (L)} = \text{TBW deficit} \times (1/1 - X) \qquad (32.7)$$

where X is the ratio of the sodium concentration in the resuscitation fluid to the sodium concentration in isotonic saline (154 mEq/L). If the water deficit is 4.5 L and the resuscitation fluid is half-normal saline (Na = 75 mEq/L), the replacement volume will be 4.5 × (1/0.5) = 9 liters (or twice the free water deficit)

Cerebral Edema

The brain cells initially shrink in response to a hypertonic extracellular fluid, but cell volume is restored within hours. This restoration of cell volume is attributed to the generation of osmotically active substances called idiogenic osmoles (8). Once the brain cell volume is restored to normal, the aggressive replacement of free water can predispose to cerebral edema and seizures. To limit the risk of cerebral edema, **free water**

deficits should be replaced slowly so that serum sodium decreases no faster than 0.5 mEq/L per hour (typically requires 48 to 72 hours) (8,10).

HYPERTONIC SYNDROMES

Diabetes Insipidus

The most noted cause for hypernatremia without apparent volume deficits is diabetes insipidus (DI), which is a condition of impaired renal water conservation (1,13,14). This condition results in excessive loss of urine that is almost pure water (devoid of solute). The underlying problem in DI is related to antidiuretic hormone (ADH), a hormone secreted by the posterior pituitary gland that promotes water reabsorption in the distal tubule. Two defects related to ADH can occur in DI:

Central DI is caused by failure of ADH release from the posterior pituitary (15). Common causes of central DI in critically ill patients include traumatic brain injury, anoxic encephalopathy, meningitis, and brain death (16). The onset is heralded by polyuria that usually is evident within 24 hours of the inciting event.

Nephrogenic DI is caused by defective end-organ responsiveness to ADH. Possible causes of nephrogenic DI in critically ill patients include amphotericin, dopamine, lithium, radiocontrast dyes, hypokalemia, aminoglycosides, and the polyuric phase of ATN (14,17). The defect in urine concentrating ability in nephrogenic DI is not as severe as it is in central DI.

Diagnosis

The hallmark of DI is a dilute urine in the face of hypertonic plasma. In central DI, the urine osmolarity is often below 200 mOsm/L, whereas in nephrogenic DI, the urine osmolarity is usually between 200 and 500 mOsm/L (16). The diagnosis of DI is confirmed by noting the urinary response to fluid restriction. Failure of the urine osmolarity to increase more than 30 mOsm/L in the first few hours of complete fluid restriction is diagnostic of DI. The fluid losses can be excessive during fluid restriction in DI (particularly central DI), and thus fluid restriction must be monitored carefully. Once the diagnosis of DI is confirmed, the response to vasopressin (5 units intravenously) will differentiate central from nephrogenic DI. In central DI, the urine osmolarity increases by at least 50% almost immediately after vasopressin administration, whereas in nephrogenic DI, the urine osmolarity is unchanged after vasopressin.

Management

The fluid loss in DI is almost pure water, so the replacement strategy is aimed at replacing free water deficits only. The water deficit is calculated as described previously, and the free water deficit is corrected slowly (over 2 to 3 days) to limit the risk of cerebral edema. In central DI, vasopressin administration is also required to prevent ongoing free water losses. The usual dose is 2 to 5 units of aqueous vasopressin subcutaneously every

4 to 6 hours (14). The serum sodium must be monitored carefully during vasopressin therapy because water intoxication and hyponatremia can occur if the central DI begins to resolve.

Non-Ketotic Hyperglycemia

The formula for plasma tonicity presented earlier predicts that hyperglycemia will be accompanied by a hypertonic extracellular fluid. When progressive hyperglycemia does not result in ketosis, the major clinical consequence is a hypertonic encephalopathy similar to the one described for hypernatremia (10). The syndrome of **nonketotic hyperglycemia** (NKH) usually is seen in patients who have enough endogenous insulin to prevent ketosis. The condition usually is precipitated by a physiological stress (e.g., infection, trauma), and the patients may or may not have a prior history of diabetes mellitus (11). The plasma glucose is often 1000 mg/dL or higher (11) (whereas in ketoacidosis, the plasma glucose is usually below 800 mg/dL). The persistent loss of glucose in the urine produces an osmotic diuresis that can lead to profound volume losses.

Clinical Manifestations

Patients with NKH usually have an altered mental status and may show signs of hypovolemia. The altered mental status can progress to frank coma when the plasma tonicity rises above 330 mOsm/kg H_2O (11). Advanced cases of encephalopathy can be accompanied by generalized seizures and focal neurological deficits, as described for hypernatremic encephalopathy.

Fluid Management

The fluid management of NKH is similar to that described for hypovolemic hypernatremia. Volume deficits tend to be more profound in NKH than in simple hypovolemic hypernatremia because of the osmotic diuresis that accompanies the glycosuria. Therefore, rapid correction of the plasma volume (i.e., with 5% albumin or isotonic saline) may be necessary.

Free Water Deficit

Once the plasma volume is restored, free water deficits are estimated and replaced slowly. However when calculating the free water deficit that accompanies hyperglycemia, it is necessary to correct the plasma sodium for the increase in plasma glucose. This is because the hyperglycemia draws water from the intracellular space, and this creates a dilutional effect on the plasma sodium concentration. The decrease in plasma sodium in hypernatremia can vary according to the state of the ECV. In general, **for every 100 mg/dL increment in the plasma glucose, the plasma sodium should fall by 1.6 to 2 mEq/L** (11,18). Therefore, for a patient with a plasma glucose of 1000 mg/dL and a measured plasma sodium of 145 mEq/L, the actual or corrected plasma sodium will average $145 + (900/100 \times 1.8) = 161$ mEq/L (the factor 1.8 is taken as the average value between 1.6 and 2 mEq/L).

The restoration of brain cell volume can occur rapidly in hypertonic states due to hyperglycemia (11). Therefore, the free water replacement should be particularly judicious in NKH.

Insulin Therapy

Because insulin drives both glucose and water into cells, insulin therapy can aggravate hypovolemia. Therefore, in patients who are hypovolemic, insulin should be withheld until the vascular volume is restored. Once this is accomplished, insulin therapy can be given as advised for diabetic ketoacidosis (see Chapter 29). The insulin requirement will diminish as the hypertonic condition is corrected, so plasma glucose concentrations should be monitored hourly during intravenous insulin therapy in NKH.

HYPERVOLEMIC HYPERNATREMIA

Hypernatremia from hypertonic fluid gain is uncommon. Possible causes are hypertonic saline resuscitation, sodium bicarbonate infusions for metabolic acidosis (see Table 37.1), and ingestion of excessive amounts of table salt (19).

Management

In patients with normal renal function, excess sodium and water are excreted rapidly. When renal sodium excretion is impaired, it might be necessary to increase renal sodium excretion with a diuretic (e.g., furosemide). Because the sodium concentration in urine during furosemide diuresis is approximately 75 mEq/L, excessive urine output will aggravate the hypernatremia (because the urine is hypotonic to plasma). Therefore, urine volume losses must be partially replaced with a fluid that is hypotonic to the urine.

HYPONATREMIA

Hyponatremia (serum sodium less than 135 mEq/L) (20) has been reported in 50% of hospitalized patients with neurologic disorders (21), 40% of hospitalized patients with acquired immunodeficiency syndrome (22), 5% of hospitalized elderly patients (23) and 1% of postoperative patients (24). Hyponatremic patients can have twice the mortality rate of patients with a normal plasma sodium (22,23), but a causal link is unproven.

Pseudohyponatremia

Plasma is 93% water by volume, and sodium is restricted to this aqueous phase of plasma. The traditional method of measuring the sodium concentration in plasma (flame photometry) uses the entire volume of the sample, which includes both the aqueous and nonaqueous phases of plasma. Sodium is present only in the aqueous phase of plasma, so the measured sodium concentration in plasma will be lower than the actual sodium concentration. Plasma is normally 93% water by volume, so the difference in measured and actual plasma sodium is negligible in normal subjects.

Extreme elevations in plasma lipids or proteins will increase the volume of the nonaqueous phase of plasma. In this situation, the measured plasma sodium concentration can be significantly lower than the actual (aqueous phase) sodium concentration. This condition is called *pseudohyponatremia*(1,25).

Ion-Specific Electrodes

Many clinical laboratories now have ion-specific electrodes that measure sodium activity in water only. Therefore, for patients with marked elevations in plasma lipids or plasma proteins, ask the hospital laboratory to use an ion-specific electrode to measure the plasma sodium concentration.

HYPOTONIC HYPONATREMIA

True or hypotonic hyponatremia represents an increase in free water relative to sodium in the extracellular fluids. It does *not* necessarily represent an increase in the volume of extracellular fluids. As shown in Table 32.1, the ECV can be low, normal, or high in patients with hyponatremia. The diagnostic approach to hyponatremia can begin with an assessment of the ECV, as shown in Figure 32.2 (1,8,21). (The assessment of ECV is described earlier, for the assessment of hypernatremia.)

Hypovolemic Hyponatremia

This condition is characterized by fluid losses combined with volume replacement using a fluid that is hypotonic to the lost fluid (e.g., diuresis replaced by drinking tap water). The result is a net loss of sodium relative to free water, which decreases both the ECV and the extracellular sodium concentration. The concentration of sodium in a random (spot) urine sample can sometimes help determine if the sodium loss is renal or extrarenal in origin.

Site of Sodium Loss	Urine Sodium
Renal	>20 mEq/L
Extrarenal	<10 mEq/L

Renal sodium losses would be seen in diuretic overuse, adrenal insufficiency and in cerebral salt-wasting syndrome; whereas extrarenal sodium losses can occur with diarrhea and persistent vomiting (1,26).

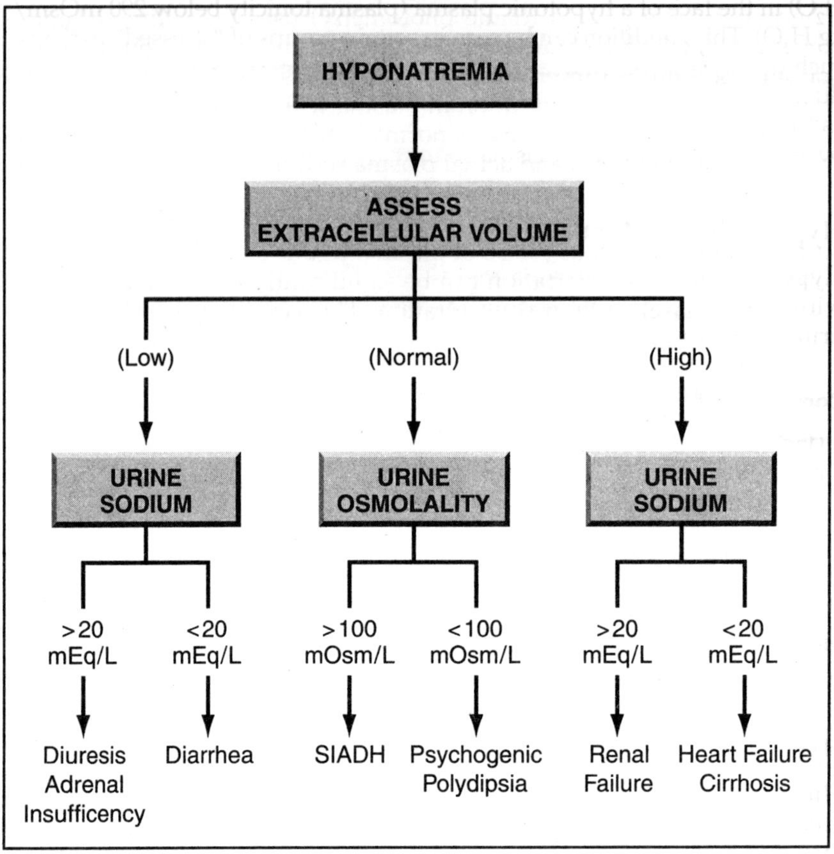

FIGURE 32.2 Diagnostic approach to hyponatremia. *SIADH* = syndrome of inappropriate antidiuretic hormone.

Isovolemic Hyponatremia

Isovolemic hyponatremia is characterized by a small gain in free water, but not enough to be clinically detected (approximately 5 L of excess water is necessary to produce detectable peripheral edema in the average-size adult). In this situation, the major disorders to consider are inappropriate (nonosmotic) release of ADH and acute water intoxication (psychogenic polydipsia). The urine sodium and urine osmolality will help distinguish between these two disorders.

Clinical Disorder	Urine Sodium	Urine Osmolality
Inappropriate ADH	>20 mEq/L	>100 mOsm/kg H_2O
Water intoxication	<10 mEq/L	<100 mOsm/kg H_2O

The inappropriate (nonosmotic) release of ADH is characterized by an inappropriately concentrated urine (urine osmolality above 100 mOsm/kg

H_2O) in the face of a hypotonic plasma (plasma tonicity below 290 mOsm/kg H_2O). This condition can be seen in certain groups of "stressed" patients, such as patients who have undergone recent surgery. It can also be produced by a variety of tumors and infections. This latter condition is known as the *syndrome of inappropriate ADH* (SIADH), and it can be accompanied by severe hyponatremia (plasma sodium below 120 mEq/L).

Hypervolemic Hyponatremia

Hypervolemic hyponatremia represents an excess of sodium and water, with the water gain exceeding the sodium gain. In this situation, the urine sodium can sometimes help identify the source of the problem.

Common Causes	Urine Sodium
Heart failure	$<$20 mEq/L
Renal failure	$>$20 mEq/L
Hepatic failure	$<$20 mEq/L

The urine sodium can be misleading if the patient is also receiving diuretics (which are commonly used in these conditions). The clinical picture is usually helpful, although these conditions can co-exist in critically ill patients.

Hyponatremic Encephalopathy

The most feared complication of hyponatremia is a life-threatening metabolic encephalopathy that is often associated with cerebral edema, increased intracranial pressure, and seizures, and can be accompanied by the adult respiratory distress syndrome (27–29). Severe cases can progress to respiratory arrest.

Correction of the hyponatremia can also be associated with an encephalopathy that is characterized by demyelinating lesions, pituitary damage, and oculomotor nerve palsies (28). This is usually seen when the sodium concentration is corrected too rapidly. A specific demyelinating disorder known as *central pontine myelinolysis* has also been attributed to rapid correction of hyponatremia (30). These conditions can be irreversible and even fatal, and the next section contains some recommendations to limit the risk of central nervous system injury.

MANAGEMENT STRATEGIES

The management of hyponatremia is determined by the state of the ECV (i.e., low, normal, or high) and by the presence or absence of neurological symptoms. Symptomatic hyponatremia requires more aggressive corrective therapy than asymptomatic hyponatremia. However, to limit the risk of a demyelinating encephalopathy, **the rate of rise in plasma sodium should not exceed 0.5 mEq/L per hour and the final plasma sodium**

concentration should not exceed 130 mEq/L (27). The general management strategies based on the ECV are as follows:

Low ECV: Infuse hypertonic saline (3% NaCl) in symptomatic patients, and isotonic saline in asymptomatic patients.

Normal ECV: Combine furosemide diuresis with infusion of hypertonic saline in symptomatic patients, or isotonic saline in asymptomatic patients.

High ECV: Use furosemide-induced diuresis in asymptomatic patients. In symptomatic patients, combine furosemide diuresis with judicious use of hypertonic saline.

Sodium Replacement

When corrective therapy requires the infusion of isotonic saline or hypertonic saline, the replacement therapy can be guided by the calculated sodium deficit. This is determined as follows (using a plasma sodium of 130 mEq/L as the desired end-point of replacement therapy):

$$\text{Sodium deficit (mEq)} = \text{Normal TBW} \times (130 - \text{Current } P_{Na}) \quad (32.8)$$

The normal TBW (in liters) is 60% of the lean body weight (in kg) in men, and 50% of the lean body weight in women. Thus, for a 60 kg woman with a plasma sodium of 120 mEq/L, the sodium deficit will be $0.5 \times 60 \times (130 - 120) = 300$ mEq.

Because 3% sodium chloride contains 513 mEq of sodium per liter, the volume of hypertonic saline needed to correct a sodium deficit of 300 mEq will be 300/513 = 585 mL. Using a maximum rate of rise of 0.5 mEq/L per hour for the plasma sodium (to limit the risk of a demyelinating encephalopathy), the sodium concentration deficit of 10 mEq/L in the previous example should be corrected over at least 20 hours. Thus, the maximum rate of hypertonic fluid administration will be 585/20 = 29 mL/hour. If isotonic saline is used for sodium replacement, the replacement volume will be 3.3 times the replacement volume of the hypertonic 3% saline solution.

A FINAL WORD

To design an effective approach to hypernatremia and hyponatremia, it is essential to understand that these conditions are the result of a problem with water balance more than sodium balance. The approach in this chapter shows you how to identify the problem with water and sodium balance in any patient using one determination: i.e., an assessment of the extracellular volume.

REFERENCES

Reviews

1. Verbalis JG. Disorders of body water homeostasis. Best Pract Res Clin Endocrinol Metab 2003;17:471–503.

2. Rose BD, Post TW. The total body water and the plasma sodium concentration. In: Clinical physiology of acid-base and electrolyte disorders. 5th ed. New York: McGraw-Hill, 2001: 241–257.

Basic Concepts

3. Gennari FJ. Current concepts: serum osmolality: uses and limitations. N Engl J Med 1984;310:102–105.
4. Erstad BL. Osmolality and osmolarity: narrowing the terminology gap. Pharmacotherapy 2003;23:1085–1086.
5. Turchin A, Seifter JL, Seely EW. Clinical problem-solving: mind the gap. N Engl J Med 2003;349:1465–1469.
6. Purssell RA, Lynd LD, Koga Y. The use of the osmole gap as a screening test for the presence of exogenous substances. Toxicol Rev 2004;23:189–202.
7. Sklar AH, Linas SL. The osmolal gap in renal failure. Ann Intern Med 1983;98:481–482.

Hypernatremia

8. Adrogue HJ, Madias NE. Hypernatremia. N Engl J Med 2000;342:1493–1499.
9. McGee S, Abernethy WB 3rd, Simel DL. The rational clinical examination: Is this patient hypovolemic? JAMA 1999;281:1022–1029.
10. Arieff AI, Ayus JC. Strategies for diagnosing and managing hypernatremic encephalopathy. J Crit Illness 1996;11:720–727.
11. Rose BD, Post TW. Hyperosmolal states: hyperglycemia. In: Clinical physiology of acid-base and electrolyte disorders. 5th ed. New York: McGraw-Hill, 2001: 794–821.
12. Marino PL, Krasner J, O'Moore P. Fluid and electrolyte expert. Philadelphia: WB Saunders, 1987.
13. Makaryus AN, McFarlane SI. Diabetes insipidus: diagnosis and treatment of a complex disease. Cleve Clin J Med 2006;73:65–71.
14. Blevins LS Jr, Wand GS. Diabetes insipidus. Crit Care Med 1992;20:69–79.
15. Ghirardello S, Malattia C, Scagnelli P, et al. Current perspective on the pathogenesis of central diabetes insipidus. J Pediatr Endocrinol Metab 2005;18:631–645.
16. Geheb MA. Clinical approach to the hyperosmolar patient. Crit Care Clin 1987;3:797–815.
17. Garofeanu CG, Weir M, Rosas-Arellano MP, et al. Causes of reversible nephrogenic diabetes insipidus: a systematic review. Am J Kidney Dis 2005;45:626–637.
18. Moran SM, Jamison RL. The variable hyponatremic response to hyperglycemia. West J Med 1985;142:49–53.
19. Ofran Y, Lavi D, Opher D, et al. Fatal voluntary salt intake resulting in the highest ever documented sodium plasma level in adults (255 mmol L-1): a disorder linked to female gender and psychiatric disorders. J Intern Med 2004;256:525–528.

Hyponatremia

20. Adrogue HJ, Madias NE. Hyponatremia. N Engl J Med 2000;342:1581–1589.
21. Diringer MN, Zazulia AR. Hyponatremia in neurologic patients: consequences and approaches to treatment. Neurologist 2006;12:117–126.

22. Tang WW, Kaptein EM, Feinstein EI, et al. Hyponatremia in hospitalized patients with the acquired immunodeficiency syndrome (AIDS) and the AIDS-related complex. Am J Med 1993;94:169–174.
23. Terzian C, Frye EB, Piotrowski ZH. Admission hyponatremia in the elderly: factors influencing prognosis. J Gen Intern Med 1994;9:89–91.
24. Ayus JC, Wheeler JM, Arieff AI. Postoperative hyponatremic encephalopathy in menstruant women. Ann Intern Med 1992;117:891–897.
25. Weisberg LS. Pseudohyponatremia: a reappraisal. Am J Med 1989; 86:315–318.
26. Maesaka JK, Gupta S, Fishbane S. Cerebral salt-wasting syndrome: does it exist? Nephron 1999;82:100–109.
27. Ayus JC, Arieff AI. Pathogenesis and prevention of hyponatremic encephalopathy. Endocrinol Metab Clin North Am 1993;22:425–446.
28. Arieff AI, Ayus JC. Pathogenesis of hyponatremic encephalopathy: current concepts. Chest 1993;103:607–610.
29. Ayus JC, Arieff AI. Pulmonary complications of hyponatremic encephalopathy: noncardiogenic pulmonary edema and hypercapnic respiratory failure. Chest 1995;107:517–521.
30. Brunner JE, Redmond JM, Haggar AM, et al. Central pontine myelinolysis and pontine lesions after rapid correction of hyponatremia: a prospective magnetic resonance imaging study. Ann Neurol 1990;27:61–66.

Chapter 33

POTASSIUM

Early sea-living organisms exhibited a preference for intracellular potassium and a disdain for intracellular sodium, which eventually changed the composition of the oceans from a potassium salt solution to a sodium salt solution. This behavior is also found in mammalian organisms, in whom potassium is the major intracellular cation and sodium is the major extracellular cation. This pattern is the result of the sodium–potassium exchange pump on cell membranes, which sequesters potassium and extrudes sodium. In humans, only 2% of the total body potassium stores are found outside cells. This lack of extracellular representation limits the value of the plasma (extracellular) potassium concentration as an index of total body potassium stores.

POTASSIUM DISTRIBUTION

The marked discrepancy between the intracellular and extracellular content of potassium is illustrated in Figure 33.1. The total body potassium content in healthy adults is approximately 50 mEq/kg (1–3), so a 70-kg adult will have 3500 mEq of total body potassium. However, only 70 mEq (2% of the total amount) is found in the extracellular fluids. Because the plasma accounts for approximately 20% of the extracellular fluid volume, the potassium content of plasma will be about 15 mEq, which is about 0.4% of the total amount of potassium in the body. This suggests that the plasma potassium will be an insensitive marker of changes in total body potassium stores.

Serum Potassium

The relationship between changes in total body potassium and changes in serum potassium is curvilinear, as shown in Figure 33.2 (4,5). The slope of the curve decreases on the "deficit" side of the graph, indicating that the change in serum potassium is much smaller when potassium is depleted than when potassium accumulates. In an averaged-size adult with a normal serum potassium concentration (i.e., 3.5 to 5.5 mEq/L), a total body potassium deficit of 200 to 400 mEq is required to produce a 1 mEq/L decrease in serum potassium, whereas a total body potassium

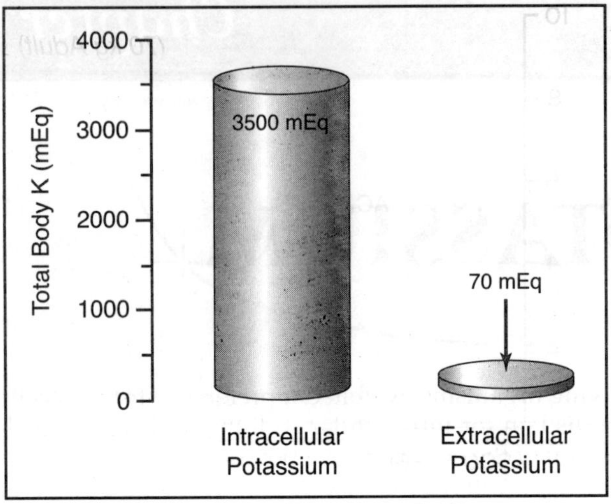

FIGURE 33.1 The intracellular and extracellular potassium content in a 70-kg adult with a total body potassium of 50 mEq/L.

excess of 100 to 200 mEq is required to produce a 1 mEq/L rise in serum potassium (5). In other words, potassium depletion must be twice as great as potassium accumulation to produce a significant (1 mEq/L) change in the serum potassium concentration. This difference is due to the large pool of intracellular potassium, which can replenish extracellular stores when potassium is lost.

HYPOKALEMIA

Hypokalemia is a serum potassium concentration below 3.5 mEq/L. The causes of hypokalemia can be classified according to whether an intracellular shift of potassium (transcellular shift) occurred or whether a decrease in total body potassium content (potassium depletion) occurred (3,6). The following are some of the possible causes of hypokalemia that are likely to be encountered in the ICU.

Transcellular Shift

Potassium movement into cells is facilitated by stimulation of β_2-adrenergic receptors on muscle cell membranes. Inhaled **β-agonist bronchodilators** (e.g., albuterol) are well known for their ability to reduce the serum potassium concentration, but this effect is mild (0.5 mEq/L or less) in the usual therapeutic doses (7). A more significant effect is seen when inhaled β-agonists are given in combination with glucose and insulin (7) or diuretics (8). Other factors that promote the transcellular shift of potassium into cells include **alkalosis** (respiratory or metabolic), **hypothermia** (accidental or induced), and **insulin.** Alkalosis has a variable and unpredictable effect on the serum potassium (9). Hypothermia causes a transient drop in serum potassium that usually resolves during

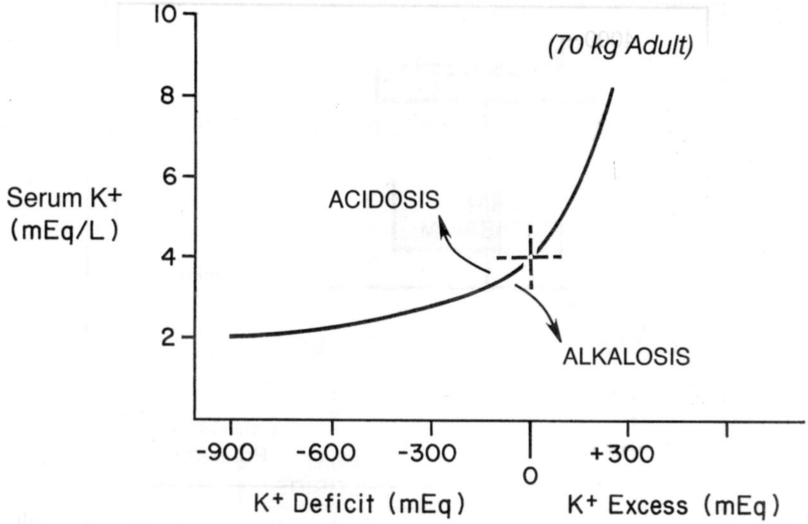

FIGURE 33.2 The relationship between the serum potassium concentration and changes in total body potassium content. (Redrawn from Brown RS. Extrarenal potassium homeostasis Kidney Int 1986;30:116–127.)

rewarming (10). Lethal cases of hypothermia can be accompanied by *hyper*kalemia because of widespread cell death (11).

Potassium Depletion

Potassium depletion can be the result of either renal or extrarenal potassium losses. The site of potassium loss can often be identified by using a combination of urinary potassium and chloride concentrations, as shown in Figure 33.3.

Renal Potassium Loss

The leading cause of renal potassium wasting is **diuretic therapy.** Other causes likely to be seen in the ICU include nasogastric drainage, alkalosis, and magnesium depletion. The urinary chloride is low (less than 15 mEq/L) when nasogastric drainage or alkalosis is involved, and it is high (greater than 25 mEq/L) when magnesium depletion or diuretics are responsible. **Magnesium depletion** impairs potassium reabsorption across the renal tubules and may play a very important role in promoting and sustaining potassium depletion in critically ill patients, particularly those receiving diuretics (12).

Extrarenal Potassium Loss

The major cause of extrarenal potassium loss is **diarrhea.** The potassium concentration in stool is 75 mEq/L, but because the stool volume is normally 200 mL or less each day, little potassium is lost. In diarrheal states, the daily volume of stool can be as high as 10 L, and thus severe or prolonged diarrhea can result in significant potassium depletion.

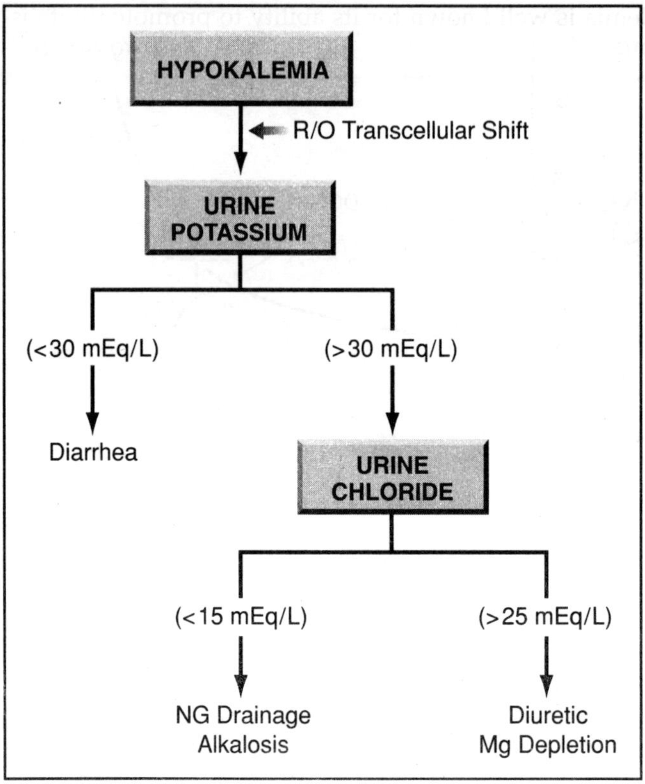

FIGURE 33.3 Diagnostic approach to hypokalemia.

Clinical Manifestations

Severe hypokalemia (serum K^+ below 2.5 mEq/L) can be accompanied by diffuse muscle weakness (3). Milder degrees of hypokalemia (serum K^+ 2.5 to 3.5 mEq/L) are often asymptomatic. Abnormalities in the ECG, including prominent U waves (more than 1 mm in height), flattening and inversion of T waves, and prolongation of the QT interval, can be present in more than half of the cases (13). None of these changes are specific for hypokalemia. The T wave changes and U waves can be seen with digitalis or left ventricular hypertrophy, and QT prolongation can be seen with hypocalcemia and hypomagnesemia.

Arrhythmias

There is a misconception about the ability of hypokalemia to promote cardiac arrhythmias. **Hypokalemia alone does not produce serious ventricular cardiac arrhythmias** (3,13). Hypokalemia is often combined with other conditions that can promote arrhythmias (e.g., magnesium depletion, digitalis, myocardial ischemia), and the hypokalemia may enhance the proarrhythmic effects of these other conditions (3).

Hypokalemia is well known for its ability to promote digitalis-induced arrhythmias.

MANAGEMENT OF HYPOKALEMIA

The first concern in hypokalemia is to eliminate or treat any condition that promotes transcellular potassium shifts (e.g., alkalosis) (3). If the hypokalemia is due to potassium depletion, proceed as described in the following section.

Potassium Deficit

If the hypokalemia is due to potassium depletion, a potassium deficit of 10% of the total body potassium stores is expected for every 1 mEq/L decrease in the serum potassium (14). The correlation between potassium deficits and the severity of hypokalemia is shown in Table 33.1. These estimates do not consider any contribution from transcellular potassium shifts, and thus they are meant only as rough guidelines for gauging the severity of potassium depletion.

Potassium Replacement

Solutions

The usual replacement fluid is potassium chloride, which is available as a concentrated solution (from 1 and 2 mEq/mL) in ampules containing 10, 20, 30, and 40 mEq of potassium. These solutions are extremely hyperosmotic (the 2 mEq/L solution has an osmolality of 4000 mOsm/L H_2O) and must be diluted (15). A potassium phosphate solution is also available (contains 4.5 mEq potassium and 3 mM phosphate per mL) and is preferred by some for potassium replacement in diabetic ketoacidosis (because of the phosphate depletion that accompanies ketoacidosis).

TABLE 33.1 Potassium Deficits in Hypokalemia*

	Potassium Deficit	
Serum Potassium (mEq/L)	mEq	% Total Body K
3.0	175	5
2.5	350	10
2.0	470	15
1.5	700	20
1.0	875	25

*Estimated deficits for a 70 kg adult with a total body potassium content of 50 mEq/kg.

Infusion Rate

The standard method of intravenous potassium replacement is to add 20 mEq of potassium to 100 mL of isotonic saline and infuse this mixture over 1 hour (16). The **maximum rate** of intravenous potassium replacement is usually set at **20 mEq/hour** (16), but dose rates up to 40 mEq/hour occasionally may be necessary (e.g., with serum K^+ below 1.5 mEq/L or serious arrhythmias), and dose rates as high as 100 mEq/hour have been used safely (17). A large central vein should be used for infusion because of the irritating properties of the hyperosmotic potassium solutions. However, if the desired replacement rate is greater than 20 mEq/hour, the infusion should not be given through a central venous catheter because of the theoretical risk of transient hyperkalemia in the right heart chambers, which can predispose to cardiac standstill. In this situation, the potassium dose can be split and administered via two peripheral veins.

Response

The serum potassium may be slow to rise at first, because of the position on the flat part of the curve in Figure 33.2. Full replacement usually takes a few days, particularly if potassium losses are ongoing. If the hypokalemia seems refractory to replacement therapy, the serum magnesium level should be checked. **Magnesium depletion** promotes urinary potassium losses and **can cause refractory hypokalemia** (18). The management of hypomagnesemia is presented in Chapter 34.

HYPERKALEMIA

While hypokalemia is often well tolerated, hyperkalemia (serum K^+ greater than 5.5 mEq/L) can be a serious and life-threatening condition (3,19,20).

Pseudohyperkalemia

Potassium release from traumatic hemolysis during the venipuncture can produce a spurious elevation in serum potassium. This is more common than suspected, and has been reported in 20% of blood samples with an elevated serum potassium (21). Potassium release from muscles distal to a tourniquet can also be a source of spuriously high serum potassium levels (22). Because of the risk of spurious hyperkalemia, an unexpected finding of hyperkalemia in an asymptomatic patient should always prompt a repeat measurement before any diagnostic or therapeutic measures are initiated.

Potassium release from cells during clot formation in the specimen tube can also produce pseudohyperkalemia when severe leukocytosis (white blood cell count greater than 50,000/mm^3) or thrombocytosis (platelet count greater than 1 million/mm^3) is present. When this condition is suspected, the serum potassium should be measured in an unclotted blood sample.

Urine Potassium

Hyperkalemia can be caused by potassium release from cells (transcellular shift) or by impaired renal potassium excretion. If the source of the hyperkalemia is unclear, the urinary potassium concentration can be helpful. A high urine potassium (greater than 30 mEq/L) suggests a transcellular shift, and a low urine potassium (less than 30 mEq/L) indicates impaired renal excretion.

Transcellular Shift

Acidosis traditionally has been listed as a cause of hyperkalemia because of the tendency for acidosis to both enhance potassium release from cells and reduce renal potassium excretion. However, hyperkalemia does not always accompany respiratory acidosis (9), and **no clear evidence exists that organic acidoses** (i.e., lactic acidosis and ketoacidosis) **can produce hyperkalemia** (9). Although hyperkalemia can accompany acidoses associated with renal failure and renal tubular acidosis, hyperkalemia in these instances may be caused by impaired renal potassium excretion.

Rhabdomyolysis can release large amounts of potassium into the extracellular fluid, but if renal function is normal, the extra potassium is promptly cleared by the kidneys. For example, severe exercise can raise the serum potassium to 8 mEq/L, but the hyperkalemia resolves with a half-time of 25 seconds (23).

Drugs that can promote hyperkalemia via transcellular potassium shifts include β-receptor antagonists and digitalis (Table 33.2). Serious hyperkalemia (i.e., serum potassium above 7 mEq/L) is possible only with digitalis toxicity.

Impaired Renal Excretion

Renal insufficiency can produce hyperkalemia when the glomerular filtration rate falls below 10 mL/minute or the urine output falls below 1 L/day (24). Exceptions are interstitial nephritis and hyporeninemic

TABLE 33.2 Drugs That Can Cause Hyperkalemia

ACE Inhibitors*	NSAIDs
Angiotensin Recepter Blockers*	Pentamidine
β-Blockers	Potassium penicillin
Cyclosporine	Tacrolimus
Digitalis	TMP–SMX
Diuretics (K-sparing)	Succinylcholine
Heparin	

ACE = angiotensin converting enzyme, *NSAIDs* = nonsteroidal antiinflammatory drugs, *TMP–SMX* = trimethoprim–sulfamethoxazole.

*Especially when combined with K-sparing diuretics.

hypoaldosteronism (24). The latter condition is seen in elderly diabetic patients who have defective renin release in response to reduced renal blood flow.

Adrenal insufficiency is a well known cause of hyperkalemia from impaired renal potassium excretion, but is not a common cause of hyperkalemia in the ICU.

Drugs that impair renal potassium excretion are considered one of the leading causes of hyperkalemia (3,25). A list of common offenders is shown in Table 33.2. The drugs most commonly implicated are angiotensin-converting enzyme inhibitors, angiotensin receptor blockers, potassium sparing diuretics, and nonsteroidal antiinflammatory drugs (25,26). Other potential offenders in the ICU are heparin, trimethoprim–sulfamethoxazole, and pentamidine (27–29). All of these agents promote hyperkalemia by inhibiting or blocking the renin–angiotensin–aldosterone system, and all promote hyperkalemia particularly when given with potassium supplements.

Blood Transfusions

Massive blood transfusions (i.e., when the transfusion volume exceeds the estimated blood volume) can promote hyperkalemia when given to patients with circulatory shock (30). Potassium leakage from erythrocytes results in a steady rise in plasma potassium levels in stored blood. In whole blood, the plasma potassium rises an average of 1 mEq/L/day. However, because one unit of whole blood contains 250 mL of plasma, this represents an increase of only 0.25 mEq/day in the plasma potassium content per unit of whole blood. After 14 days of storage, the plasma potassium load is 4.4 mEq per unit of whole blood and 3.1 mEq per unit of packed red cells (31).

The potassium load in blood transfusions normally is cleared by the kidneys, and thus no sustained rise in plasma potassium occurs. However, in patients with circulatory shock, the extra potassium from blood transfusions can accumulate and produce hyperkalemia. Furthermore, when the volume of distribution for potassium is curtailed by widespread hypoperfusion, the potassium accumulation can be rapid and life-threatening.

Clinical Manifestations

The most serious consequence of hyperkalemia is the slowing of electrical conduction in the heart. The ECG can begin to change when the serum potassium reaches 6.0 mEq/L, and it is always abnormal when the serum potassium reaches 8.0 mEq/L (24). Figure 33.4 illustrates the ECG changes associated with progressive hyperkalemia.

The earliest change in the ECG is a tall, tapering (tented) T wave that is most evident in precordial leads V_2 and V_3. Similar "peaked T" waves have been observed in metabolic acidosis (32). As the hyperkalemia progresses, the P wave amplitude decreases and the PR interval lengthens. The P waves eventually disappear and the QRS duration becomes prolonged. The final event is ventricular asystole.

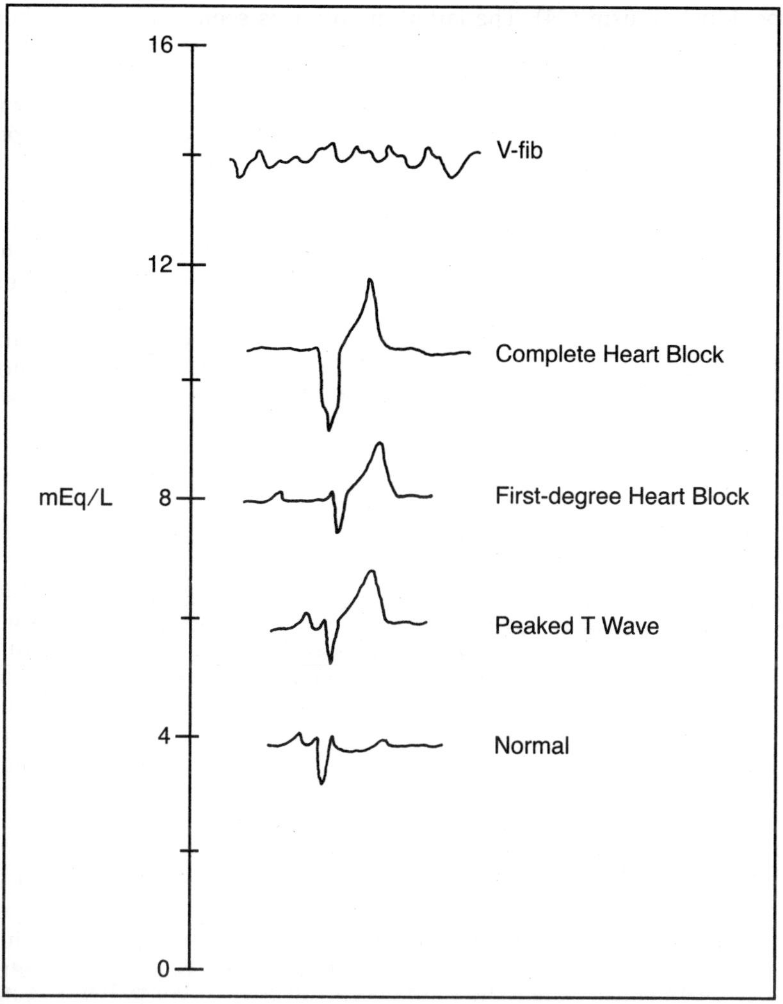

FIGURE 33.4 The ECG manifestations of progressive hyperkalemia. (Adapted from Burch GE, Winsor T. A primer of electrocardiography. Philadelphia: Lea & Febiger, 1966:143.)

MANAGEMENT OF HYPERKALEMIA

The acute management of hyperkalemia is guided by the serum potassium level and the ECG (3,20). The therapeutic maneuvers are outlined in Table 33.3.

Membrane Antagonism

Calcium directly antagonizes the membrane actions of potassium (33). When hyperkalemia is severe (i.e., above 7 mEq/L) or accompanied by advanced ECG changes (i.e., loss of P waves and prolonged QRS duration), **calcium gluconate** is administered in the dose shown in Table 33.3. If there

TABLE 33.3 Acute Management of Hyperkalemia

Condition	Treatment	Comment
ECG changes or serum K >7 mEq/L	Calcium gluconate (10%): 10 mL IV over 3 minutes; can repeat in 5 minutes	Response lasts only 20 to 30 minutes. *Do not* give bicarbonate after calcium.
ECG changes and circulatory compromise	Calcium chloride (10%): 10 mL IV over 3 minutes	Calcium chloride contains 3 times more calcium than calcium gluconate.
AV block refractory to calcium treatment	1. 10 U regular insulin in 500 mL of 20% dextrose: infuse over 1 hour 2. Transvenous pacemaker	Insulin–dextrose treatment should drop the serum K by 1 mEq/L for 1 to 2 hours.
Digitalis cardiotoxicity	1. Magnesium sulfate: 2 g as IV bolus 2. Digitalis specific antibodies if necessary	*Do not* use calcium for the hyperkalemia of digitalis toxicity.
After acute phase or when no ECG changes	Kayexalate: oral dose of 30 g in 50 mL of 20% sorbitol, or rectal dose of 50 g in 200 mL 20% sorbitol as a retention enema	Oral dosing is preferred. Enemas poorly tolerated by patients and nurses.

is no response to calcium within a few minutes, a second dose can be given. A third dose will not be effective if there was no response to the second dose of calcium. The response to calcium lasts only 20 or 30 minutes, so other therapies should be initiated to enhance potassium clearance.

Calcium must be given cautiously to patients on digitalis because hypercalcemia can potentiate digitalis cardiotoxicity. For patients receiving digitalis, the calcium gluconate should be added to 100 mL of isotonic saline and infused over 20 to 30 minutes. If the hyperkalemia is a manifestation of digitalis toxicity, calcium is contraindicated.

When hyperkalemia is accompanied by evidence of circulatory compromise, **calcium chloride** is preferred to calcium gluconate. One ampule (10 mL) of 10% calcium chloride contains three times more elemental calcium than one ampule of 10% calcium gluconate (see Table 35.3), and the extra calcium in calcium chloride may prove beneficial in promoting cardiac contraction and maintaining peripheral vascular tone.

Transcellular Shift

Insulin–Dextrose

Combined therapy with insulin and dextrose will drive potassium into muscle cells and decrease the serum potassium by an average of 1 mEq/L.

However, this is a temporary effect, and other maneuvers aimed at enhancing potassium clearance are also required.

Sodium Bicarbonate

The administration of sodium bicarbonate (44 to 88 mEq) can also shift potassium into cells. However, the most common acidotic condition associated with hyperkalemia is renal failure, and in this condition, insulin–dextrose is much more effective in lowering the serum potassium than bicarbonate (34). Furthermore, bicarbonate binds calcium and should not be given after calcium is administered. For these reasons, there is little value in using bicarbonate to treat hyperkalemia.

Enhanced Clearance

Measures aimed at enhancing the removal of potassium from the body can be used alone in mild cases of hyperkalemia (i.e., serum K less than 7 mEq/L) without advanced ECG changes or can serve as a follow-up to calcium and insulin–dextrose therapy.

Exchange Resin

Sodium polystyrene sulfonate (Kayexalate) is a cation exchange resin that can enhance potassium clearance across the gastrointestinal mucosa (gastrointestinal dialysis). This resin can be given orally or by retention enema, and it is mixed with 20% sorbitol to prevent concretion. For each mEq of potassium removed, 2 to 3 mEq of sodium are added. If there is concern about the added sodium, one or two doses of furosemide can be used to enhance natriuresis.

Loop Diuretics

The loop diuretics furosemide and ethacrynic acid enhance urinary potassium excretion. These agents can be used as a follow-up measure to calcium and insulin–dextrose. This approach is ineffective in renal failure.

Hemodialysis

Hemodialysis is the most effective method of lowering the serum potassium in patients with renal failure (3,20).

A FINAL WORD

The following points about potassium deserve emphasis:

1. Since only 2% of the potassium is outside cells, it is unlikely that the serum potassium concentration is an accurate reflection of total body potassium stores. However, we use the serum potassium as a reflection of total body potassium, so there's

a fundamental problem in the way we interpret and manage changes in serum potassium.

2. There is often a rush to correct even mild cases of hypokalemia (serum K^+ between 3 and 3.5 mEq/L). This is usually not necessary, because hypokalemia is well-tolerated, and does not create a risk of arrhythmias unless there are other arrhythmogenic conditions (such as digitalis toxicity).
3. If hypokalemia is really due to potassium depletion, don't expect an extra 40 mEq of potassium to correct the problem because for each 0.5 mEq/L decrease in serum K^+, you will have to replace about 175 mEq of potassium to replenish total body K^+ stores.
4. Don't forget that hypokalemia associated with diuretic therapy is often the result of magnesium depletion, and that potassium replacement will not correct the problem unless magnesium is also replaced.

REFERENCES

Potassium Distribution

1. Rose BD, Post TW. Potassium homeostasis. In: Clinical physiology of acid-base and electrolyte disorders. 5th ed. New York: McGraw-Hill, 2001:372–402.
2. Halperin ML, Kamel KS. Potassium. Lancet 1998;352:135–140.
3. Schaefer TJ, Wolford RW. Disorders of potassium. Emerg Med Clin North Am 2005;23:723–747, viii–ix.
4. Brown RS. Extrarenal potassium homeostasis. Kidney Int 1986;30:116–127.
5. Sterns RH, Cox M, Feig PU, et al. Internal potassium balance and the control of the plasma potassium concentration. Medicine 1981;60:339–354.

Hypokalemia

6. Glover P. Hypokalaemia. Crit Care Resusc 1999;1:239–251.
7. Allon M, Copkney C. Albuterol and insulin for treatment of hyperkalemia in hemodialysis patients. Kidney Int 1990;38:869–872.
8. Lipworth BJ, McDevitt DG, Struthers AD. Prior treatment with diuretic augments the hypokalemic and electrocardiographic effects of inhaled albuterol. Am J Med 1989;86:653–657.
9. Adrogue HJ, Madias NE. Changes in plasma potassium concentration during acute acid-base disturbances. Am J Med 1981;71:456–467.
10. Bernard SA, Buist M. Induced hypothermia in critical care medicine: a review. Crit Care Med 2003;31:2041–2051.
11. Schaller MD, Fischer AP, Perret CH. Hyperkalemia: a prognostic factor during acute severe hypothermia. JAMA 1990;264:1842–1845.
12. Salem M, Munoz R, Chernow B. Hypomagnesemia in critical illness: a common and clinically important problem. Crit Care Clin 1991;7:225–252.
13. Flakeb G, Villarread D, Chapman D. Is hypokalemia a cause of ventricular arrhythmias? J Crit Illness 1986;1:66–74.

14. Stanaszek WF, Romankiewicz JA. Current approaches to management of potassium deficiency. Drug Intell Clin Pharm 1985;19:176–184.
15. Trissel LA. Handbook on injectable drugs. 13th ed. Bethesda, MD: American Society of Health System Pharmacists, 2005:1230.
16. Kruse JA, Carlson RW. Rapid correction of hypokalemia using concentrated intravenous potassium chloride infusions. Arch Intern Med 1990;150:613–617.
17. Kim GH, Han JS. Therapeutic approach to hypokalemia. Nephron 2002;92 (suppl 1):28–32.
18. Whang R, Flink EB, Dyckner T, et al. Magnesium depletion as a cause of refractory potassium repletion. Arch Intern Med 1985;145:1686–1689.

Hyperkalemia

19. Williams ME. Endocrine crises: hyperkalemia. Crit Care Clin 1991;7:155–174.
20. Evans KJ, Greenberg A. Hyperkalemia: a review. J Intensive Care Med 2005; 20:272–290.
21. Rimmer JM, Horn JF, Gennari FJ. Hyperkalemia as a complication of drug therapy. Arch Intern Med 1987;147:867–869.
22. Don BR, Sebastian A, Cheitlin M, et al. Pseudohyperkalemia caused by fist clenching during phlebotomy. N Engl J Med 1990;322:1290–1292.
23. Medbo JI, Sejersted OM. Plasma potassium changes with high intensity exercise. J Physiol 1990;421:105–122.
24. Williams ME, Rosa RM. Hyperkalemia: disorders of internal and external potassium balance. J Intensive Care Med 1988;3:52–64.
25. Perazella MA. Drug-induced hyperkalemia: old culprits and new offenders. Am J Med 2000;109:307–314.
26. Palmer BF. Managing hyperkalemia caused by inhibitors of the renin-angiotensin-aldosterone system. N Engl J Med 2004;351:585–592.
27. Oster JR, Singer I, Fishman LM. Heparin-induced aldosterone suppression and hyperkalemia. Am J Med 1995;98:575–586.
28. Greenberg S, Reiser IW, Chou SY, et al. Trimethoprim-sulfamethoxazole induces reversible hyperkalemia. Ann Intern Med 1993;119:291–295.
29. Peltz S, Hashmi S. Pentamidine-induced severe hyperkalemia. Am J Med 1989;87:698–699.
30. Leveen HH, Pasternack HS, Lustrin I, et al. Hemorrhage and transfusion as the major cause of cardiac arrest. JAMA 1960;173:770–777.
31. Michael JM, Dorner I, Bruns D, et al. Potassium load in CPD-preserved whole blood and two types of packed red blood cells. Transfusion 1975;15:144–149.
32. Dreyfuss D, Jondeau G, Couturier R, et al. Tall T waves during metabolic acidosis without hyperkalemia: a prospective study. Crit Care Med 1989;17: 404–408.
33. Bosnjak ZJ, Lynch C, III. Cardiac electrophysiology. In: Yaksh T, Lynch C, III, Zapol WM, et al, eds. Anesthesia: biologic foundations. New York: Lippincott-Raven, 1998:1001–1040.
34. Blumberg A, Weidmann P, Shaw S, et al. Effect of various therapeutic approaches on plasma potassium and major regulating factors in terminal renal failure. Am J Med 1988;85:507–512.

Chapter 34

MAGNESIUM

Magnesium is the second most abundant intracellular cation in the human body (potassium being the first), where it serves as a cofactor for more than 300 enzyme reactions that involve adenosine triphosphate (1–4). One of the magnesium-dependent enzyme systems is the membrane pump that generates the electrical gradient across cell membranes. As a result, magnesium plays an important role in the activity of electrically excitable tissues (1,2,5–7). Magnesium also regulates the movement of calcium into smooth muscle cells, which gives it a pivotal role in the maintenance of cardiac contractile strength and peripheral vascular tone (5).

MAGNESIUM BALANCE

The content and distribution of magnesium in the human body is shown in Table 34.1 (8). The average-size adult contains approximately 24 g (1 mole, or 2000 mEq) of magnesium; a little over half is located in bone, whereas less than 1% is located in plasma. This lack of representation in the plasma limits the value of the plasma magnesium concentration as an index of total body magnesium stores. This is particularly true in patients with magnesium deficiency, in whom **serum magnesium levels can be normal in the face of total body magnesium depletion** (8,9).

Serum Magnesium

Serum is favored over plasma for magnesium assays because the anticoagulant used for plasma samples can be contaminated with citrate or other anions that bind magnesium (8). The normal range for serum magnesium depends on the daily magnesium intake, which varies according to geographic region. The normal range for healthy adults residing in the United States is shown in Table 34.2 (10).

Ionized Magnesium

Only 67% of the magnesium in plasma is in the ionized (active) form, and the remaining 33% is either bound to plasma proteins (19% of the total) or chelated with divalent anions such as phosphate and sulfate (14% of the total) (11). The standard assay for magnesium (i.e., spectrophotometry)

TABLE 34.1 Magnesium Distribution in Adults

Tissue	Weight (kg)	Magnesium Content (mEq)	Total Body Magnesium (%)
Bone	12	1060	53
Muscle	30	540	27
Soft Tissue	23	384	19
RBC	2	10	0.7
Plasma	3	6	0.3
Total	70 kg	2000 mEq	100%

From: Elin RJ. Assessment of magnesium status. Clin Chem 1987;33:1965–1970.

measures all three fractions of magnesium. Therefore, when the serum magnesium is abnormally low, it is impossible to determine whether the problem is a decrease in the ionized (active) fraction or a decrease in the bound fractions (e.g., hypoproteinemia) (12). The level of ionized magnesium can be measured with an ion-specific electrode (13) or by ultrafiltration of plasma (14), but these techniques are not routinely available for clinical use. However, because the total amount of magnesium in plasma is small, the difference between the ionized and bound magnesium *content* may not be large enough to be clinically relevant.

Urinary Magnesium

The normal range for urinary magnesium excretion is shown in Table 34.2. Under normal circumstances, only small quantities of magnesium are excreted in the urine. When magnesium intake is deficient, the kidneys conserve magnesium and urinary magnesium excretion falls to negligible levels. This is shown in Figure 34.1. After the start of a magnesium deficient diet, the urinary magnesium excretion promptly falls to negligible levels and the serum magnesium remains in the normal range. This illustrates the relative value of urinary magnesium over serum magnesium levels in the detection of magnesium deficiency. This is discussed again later in this chapter.

TABLE 34.2 Reference Ranges for Magnesium*

Fluid	Traditional Units	SI Units
Serum magnesium:		
Total	1.4–2.0 mEq/L	0.7–1.0 mmol/L
Ionized	0.8–1.1 mEq/L	0.4–0.6 mmol/L
Urinary magnesium	5–15 mEq/24 hr	2.5–7.5 mmol/24 hr

*Pertains to healthy adults residing in the United States. From: Lowenstein FW, Stanton MF. Serum magnesium levels in the United States, 1971–1974. J Am Coll Nutr 1986;5:399–414.

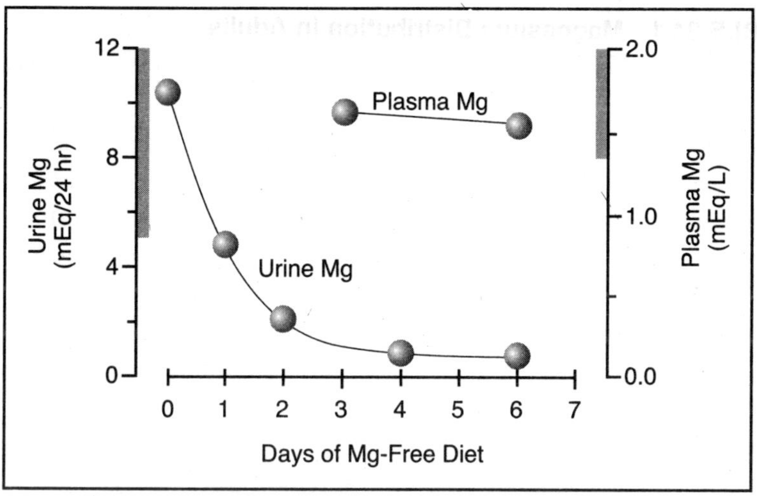

FIGURE 34.1 Urinary and plasma magnesium levels in a healthy volunteer placed on a magnesium-free diet. Solid bars on the vertical axes indicate the normal range for urine and plasma magnesium. (Adapted from Shils ME. Experimental human magnesium deficiency. Medicine 1969;48:61–82.)

MAGNESIUM DEFICIENCY

Magnesium deficiency is common in hospitalized patients (1–3). Hypomagnesemia is reported in up to 20% of patients on medical wards and in as many as 65% of patients in ICUs (1–3). Because magnesium depletion may not be accompanied by hypomagnesemia, the incidence of magnesium depletion is even higher than indicated by the surveys of hypomagnesemia. In fact, magnesium depletion has been described as "the most underdiagnosed electrolyte abnormality in current medical practice" (15).

Predisposing Conditions

Because serum magnesium levels have a limited ability to detect magnesium depletion, recognizing the conditions that predispose to magnesium depletion may be the only clue of an underlying electrolyte imbalance. The common predisposing conditions for magnesium depletion are listed in Table 34.3.

Diuretic Therapy

Diuretics are the leading cause of magnesium deficiency. Drug-induced inhibition of sodium reabsorption also interferes with magnesium reabsorption, and the resultant urinary magnesium losses can parallel urinary sodium losses. Urinary magnesium excretion is most pronounced with the loop diuretics (furosemide and ethacrynic acid). Magnesium deficiency has been reported in 50% of patients receiving chronic therapy

TABLE 34.3 Markers of Possible Magnesium Depletion

Predisposing Conditions	Clinical Findings
Drug therapy:*	Electrolyte abnormalities:*
Furosemide (50%)	Hypokalemia (40%)
Aminoglycosides (30%)	Hypophosphatemia (30%)
Amphotericin, pentamidine	Hyponatremia (27%)
Digitalis (20%)	Hypocalcemia (22%)
Cisplatin, cyclosporine	Cardiac manifestations:
Diarrhea (secretory)	Ischemia
Alcohol abuse (chronic)	Arrhythmias (refractory)
Diabetes mellitus	Digitalis toxicity
Acute MI	Hyperactive CNS Syndrome

*Numbers in parentheses indicate incidence of associated hypomagnesemia.

with furosemide (16). The thiazide diuretics show a similar tendency for magnesium depletion, but only in elderly patients (17). Magnesium depletion is not a complication of therapy with "potassium-sparing" diuretics such as triamterene (18).

Antibiotic Therapy

The antibiotics that promote magnesium depletion are the aminoglycosides, amphotericin and pentamidine (19,20). The aminoglycosides block magnesium reabsorption in the ascending loop of Henle, and hypomagnesemia has been reported in 30% of patients receiving aminoglycoside therapy (20). The other risk associated with antibiotic use occurs with antibiotic-associated diarrhea, which can be accompanied by significant magnesium losses in the stool.

Other Drugs

A variety of other drugs have been associated with magnesium depletion, including digitalis, epinephrine, and the chemotherapeutic agents cisplatin and cyclosporine (19,21). The first two agents shift magnesium into cells, whereas the latter two promote renal magnesium excretion.

Alcohol-Related Illness

Hypomagnesemia is reported in 30% of hospital admissions for alcohol abuse, and in 85% of admissions for delirium tremens (22,23). The magnesium depletion in these conditions is due to a number of factors, including generalized malnutrition and chronic diarrhea. In addition, there is an association between magnesium deficiency and thiamine deficiency (24). Magnesium is required for the transformation of thiamine into thiamine pyrophosphate, so magnesium deficiency can promote thiamine deficiency in the face of adequate thiamine intake. For this reason, the magnesium status should be monitored periodically in patients receiving daily thiamine supplements.

Secretory Diarrhea

A high concentration of magnesium (10 to 14 mEq/L) is present in secretions from the lower gastrointestinal tract (25), and thus secretory diarrhea can be accompanied by profound magnesium depletion (23). Upper tract secretions are not rich in magnesium (1 to 2 mEq/L), so vomiting does not pose a risk for magnesium depletion.

Diabetes Mellitus

Magnesium depletion is common in insulin-dependent diabetic patients, probably as a result of urinary magnesium losses that accompany glycosuria (26). Hypomagnesemia is reported in only 7% of admissions for diabetic ketoacidosis, but the incidence increases to 50% over the first 12 hours after admission (27), probably as a result of insulin-induced movement of magnesium into cells.

Acute Myocardial Infarction

As many as 80% of patients with acute myocardial infarction (MI) can have hypomagnesemia in the first 48 hours after the event (28). The mechanism is unclear but may be due to an intracellular shift of magnesium caused by endogenous catecholamine excess.

Clinical Manifestations

Although no clinical manifestations are specific for magnesium deficiency, the following clinical findings are suggestive of an underlying magnesium deficiency (Table 34.3).

Associated Electrolyte Abnormalities

Magnesium depletion is often accompanied by depletion of other electrolytes, such as potassium, phosphate, and calcium (See Table 34.3) (29). As mentioned in Chapter 33, the **hypokalemia** that accompanies magnesium depletion can be refractory to potassium replacement therapy, and magnesium repletion is often necessary before potassium repletion is possible (30).

The **hypocalcemia** that accompanies magnesium depletion is due to impaired parathormone release (31) combined with an impaired end-organ response to parathormone (32). In addition, magnesium deficiency may act on bone directly to reduce calcium release, independent of parathyroid hormone (33). As with the hypokalemia, the hypocalcemia from magnesium depletion is difficult to correct unless magnesium deficits are corrected.

Hypophosphatemia is a cause rather than effect of magnesium depletion. The mechanism is enhanced renal magnesium excretion (34). Therefore, when hypophosphatemia accompanies hypomagnesemia, the phosphate stores should be replenished to ensure adequate repletion of magnesium stores.

Arrhythmias

Because magnesium is required for proper function of the membrane pump on cardiac cell membranes, magnesium depletion will depolarize cardiac cells and promote tachyarrhythmias. Because both digitalis and magnesium deficiency act to inhibit the membrane pump, magnesium deficiency will magnify the digitalis effect and **promote digitalis cardiotoxicity.** Intravenous magnesium can suppress digitalis-toxic arrhythmias, even when serum magnesium levels are normal (35,36). Intravenous magnesium can also **abolish refractory arrhythmias** (i.e., unresponsive to traditional antiarrhythmic agents) in the absence of hypomagnesemia (37). This effect may be due to a membrane-stabilizing effect of magnesium that is unrelated to magnesium repletion.

One of the most serious arrhythmias associated with magnesium depletion is **torsades de pointes** (polymorphous ventricular tachycardia). The role of magnesium in this arrhythmia is discussed in Chapter 18.

Neurologic Findings

The neurologic manifestations of magnesium deficiency include altered mentation, generalized seizures, tremors, and hyperreflexia. All are uncommon, nonspecific, and have little diagnostic value.

A neurologic syndrome described recently that can abate with magnesium therapy deserves mention. The clinical presentation is characterized by ataxia, slurred speech, metabolic acidosis, excessive salivation, diffuse muscle spasms, generalized seizures, and progressive obtundation (38). The clinical features are often brought out by loud noises or bodily contact, and thus the term **reactive central nervous system magnesium deficiency** has been used to describe this disorder. This syndrome is associated with reduced magnesium levels in cerebrospinal fluid, and it resolves with magnesium infusion. The prevalence of this disorder is unknown at present.

Diagnosis

As mentioned several times, the serum magnesium level is an insensitive marker of magnesium depletion. When magnesium depletion is due to nonrenal factors (e.g., diarrhea), the urinary magnesium excretion is a more sensitive test for magnesium depletion (39). However, because most cases of magnesium depletion are due to enhanced renal magnesium excretion, the diagnostic value of urinary magnesium excretion may be limited.

Magnesium Retention Test

In the absence of renal magnesium wasting, the urinary excretion of magnesium in response to a magnesium load may be the most sensitive index of total body magnesium stores (40,41). This method is outlined

TABLE 34.4 Renal Magnesium Retention Test

Indications:

1. For suspected magnesium deficiency when the serum magnesium concentration is normal.
2. Can be useful for determining the end-point of magnesium replacement therapy.
3. Is *not* reliable in the setting of renal magnesium wasting or when renal function is impaired.

Contraindications:

1. Cardiovascular instability or renal failure.

Methodology*:

1. Add 24 mmol of magnesium (6 g of $MgSO_4$) to 250 mL of isotonic saline and infuse over 1 hour.
2. Collect urine for 24 hours, beginning at the onset of the magnesium infusion.
3. A urinary magnesium excretion of less than 12 mmol (24 mEq) in 24 hours (i.e., less than 50% of the infused magnesium) is evidence of total body magnesium depletion.

*Magnesium infusion protocol. From: Clague JE, Edwards RH, Jackson MJ. Intravenous magnesium loading in chronic fatigue syndrome. Lancet 1992;340:124–125.

in Table 34.4. The normal rate of magnesium reabsorption is close to the maximum tubular reabsorption rate (T_{max}), so most of the infused magnesium will be excreted in the urine when magnesium stores are normal. However, when magnesium stores are deficient, the magnesium reabsorption rate is much lower than the T_{max}, so more of the infused magnesium will be reabsorbed and less will be excreted in the urine. When less than 50% of the infused magnesium is recovered in the urine, magnesium deficiency is *likely*, and when more than 80% of the infused magnesium is excreted in the urine, magnesium deficiency is *unlikely*. This test can be particularly valuable in determining the end-point of magnesium replacement therapy (i.e., magnesium replacement is continued until urinary magnesium excretion is at least 80% of the infused magnesium load). It is important to emphasize that this test will be unreliable in patients with impaired renal function or when there is ongoing renal magnesium wasting.

MAGNESIUM REPLACEMENT THERAPY

Preparations

The magnesium preparations available for oral and parenteral use are listed in Table 34.5 (42,43). The oral preparations can be used for daily maintenance therapy (5 mg/kg in normal subjects) and for correcting

TABLE 34.5 Oral and Parenteral Magnesium Preparations

Preparation	Elemental Magnesium
Oral preparations:	
Magnesium chloride enteric coated tablets	64 mg (5.3 mEq)
Magnesium oxide tablets (400 mg)	241 mg (19.8 mEq)
Magnesium oxide tablets (140 mg)	85 mg (6.9 mEq)
Magnesium gluconate tablets (500 mg)	27 mg (2.3 mEq)
Parenteral solutions:	
Magnesium sulfate (50%)*	500 mg/mL (4 mEq/mL)
Magnesium sulfate (12.5%)	120 mg/mL (1 mEq/mL)

*Should be diluted to a 20% solution for intravenous injection.

mild, asymptomatic magnesium deficiency. However, because intestinal absorption of oral magnesium is erratic, parenteral magnesium is preferred for treating symptomatic or severe magnesium deficiency.

Magnesium Sulfate

The standard intravenous preparation is magnesium sulfate ($MgSO_4$). **Each gram of magnesium sulfate has 8 mEq (4 mmol) of elemental magnesium** (6). A 50% magnesium sulfate solution (500 mg/mL) has an osmolarity of 4000 mOsm/L (43), so it must be diluted to a 10% (100 mg/mL) or 20% (200 mg/mL) solution for intravenous use. Saline solutions should be used as the diluent for magnesium sulfate. Ringer's solutions should not be used because the calcium in Ringer's solutions will counteract the actions of the infused magnesium.

Replacement Protocols

The following magnesium replacement protocols are recommended for patients with normal renal function (44).

Mild, Asymptomatic Hypomagnesemia

The following guidelines can be used for patients with mild hypomagnesemia and no apparent complications (44):

1. Assume a total magnesium deficit of 1 to 2 mEq/kg.
2. Because 50% of the infused magnesium can be lost in the urine, assume that the total magnesium requirement is twice the magnesium deficit.
3. Replace 1 mEq/kg for the first 24 hours, and 0.5 mEq/kg daily for the next 3 to 5 days.
4. If the serum magnesium is greater than 1 mEq/L, oral magnesium can be used for replacement therapy.

Moderate Hypomagnesemia

The following therapy is intended for patients with a serum magnesium level less than 1 mEq/L or when hypomagnesemia is accompanied by other electrolyte abnormalities:

1. Add 6 g $MgSO_4$ (48 mEq Mg) to 250 or 500 mL isotonic saline and infuse over 3 hours.
2. Follow with 5 g $MgSO_4$ (40 mEq Mg) in 250 or 500 mL isotonic saline infused over the next 6 hours.
3. Continue with 5 g $MgSO_4$ every 12 hours (by continuous infusion) for the next 5 days.

Life-Threatening Hypomagnesemia

When hypomagnesemia is associated with serious cardiac arrhythmias (e.g., torsades de pointes) or generalized seizures, do the following:

1. Infuse 2 g $MgSO_4$ (16 mEq Mg) intravenously over 2–5 minutes.
2. Follow with 5 g $MgSO_4$ (40 mEq Mg) in 250 or 500 mL isotonic saline infused over the next 6 hours.
3. Continue with 5 g $MgSO_4$ every 12 hours (by continuous infusion) for the next 5 days.

Serum magnesium levels will rise after the initial magnesium bolus but will begin to fall after 15 minutes. Therefore, it is important to follow the bolus dose with a continuous magnesium infusion. Serum magnesium levels may normalize after 1 to 2 days, but it will take several days to replenish the total body magnesium stores.

Hypomagnesemia and Renal Insufficiency

Hypomagnesemia is not common in renal insufficiency but can occur when severe or chronic diarrhea is present and the creatinine clearance is greater than 30 mL/minute. When magnesium is replaced in the setting of renal insufficiency, no more than 50% of the magnesium in the standard replacement protocols should be administered (44), and the serum magnesium should be monitored carefully.

MAGNESIUM ACCUMULATION

Magnesium accumulation occurs almost exclusively in patients with impaired renal function. In one survey of hospitalized patients, hypermagnesemia (i.e., a serum magnesium greater than 2 mEq/L) was reported in 5% of patients (45).

Predisposing Conditions

Hemolysis

The magnesium concentration in erythrocytes is approximately three times greater than that in serum (46), so hemolysis can increase the plasma magnesium. This can occur either in vivo from a hemolytic anemia or in vitro from traumatic disruption of erythrocytes during phlebotomy. In hemolytic anemia, the serum magnesium is expected to rise by 0.1 mEq/L for every 250 mL of erythrocytes that lyse completely (46), so hypermagnesemia is expected only with massive hemolysis.

Renal Insufficiency

The renal excretion of magnesium becomes impaired when the creatinine clearance falls below 30 mL/minute (47). However, hypermagnesemia is not a prominent feature of renal insufficiency unless magnesium intake is increased.

Others

Other conditions that can predispose to mild hypermagnesemia are diabetic ketoacidosis (transient), adrenal insufficiency, hyperparathyroidism, and lithium intoxication (47).

Clinical Features

The clinical consequences of progressive hypermagnesemia are listed below (47).

Manifestation	Serum Magnesium
Hyporeflexia	>4 mEq/L
1st° AV Block	>5 mEq/L
Complete Heart Block	>10 mEq/L
Cardiac Arrest	>13 mEq/L

Magnesium has been described as nature's physiologic calcium blocker (48), and most of the serious consequences of hypermagnesemia are due to calcium antagonism in the cardiovascular system. Most of the cardiovascular depression is the result of cardiac conduction delays. Depressed contractility and vasodilation are not prominent.

Management

Hemodialysis is the treatment of choice for severe hypermagnesemia. Intravenous calcium gluconate (1 g IV over 2 to 3 minutes) can be used to antagonize the cardiovascular effects of hypermagnesemia *temporarily*, until dialysis is started (49). If fluids are permissible and some renal function is preserved, aggressive volume infusion combined with furosemide may be effective in reducing the serum magnesium levels in less advanced cases of hypermagnesemia.

A FINAL WORD

The following points about magnesium deserve emphasis:

1. Because 99% of the magnesium in the body is inside cells, the serum magnesium is not a sensitive marker of total body magnesium stores, and serum magnesium levels can be normal in patients who are magnesium depleted. The urine magnesium is a better marker of magnesium depletion (except in patients receiving furosemide, which increases urinary magnesium losses).
2. Magnesium depletion is probably very common in ICU patients, particularly in patients with secretory diarrhea and patients receiving furosemide and aminoglycosides.
3. Magnesium is a cofactor for all ATPase reactions, so magnesium depletion could lead to defects in cellular energy utilization.
4. Magnesium should be given daily to all ICU patients except those with renal insufficiency. Magnesium supplements are particularly important in patients receiving furosemide.
5. Magnesium depletion may be the cause of diuretic-associated hypokalemia, and magnesium repletion is often necessary in these cases before the serum potassium will return to normal.
6. In patients with hypomagnesemia, magnesium replacement will correct the serum magnesium before total body stores of magnesium are repleted. The best indicator of magnesium repletion is the urinary excretion of magnesium (see Table 34.4)

REFERENCES

General Reviews

1. Noronha JL, Matuschak GM. Magnesium in critical illness: metabolism, assessment, and treatment. Intensive Care Med 2002;28:667–679.
2. Tong GM, Rude RK. Magnesium deficiency in critical illness. J Intensive Care Med 2005;20:3–17.
3. Weisinger JR, Bellorin-Font E. Magnesium and phosphorus. Lancet 1998;352: 391–396.
4. Rude RK, Shils ME. Magnesium. In: Shils ME, Shike M, Ross AC, et al. eds. Modern nutrition in health and disease. 10th ed. Philadelphia: Lippincott Williams & Wilkins, 2006:223–247.
5. White RE, Hartzell HC. Magnesium ions in cardiac function: regulator of ion channels and second messengers. Biochem Pharmacol 1989;38:859–867.
6. McLean RM. Magnesium and its therapeutic uses: a review. Am J Med 1994; 96:63–76.
7. Marino PL. Calcium and magnesium in critical illness: a practical approach. In: Sivak ED, Higgins TL, Seiver A, eds. The high risk patient: management of the critically ill. Baltimore: Williams & Wilkins, 1995:1183–1195.

Magnesium Balance

8. Elin RJ. Assessment of magnesium status. Clin Chem 1987;33:1965–1970.
9. Reinhart RA. Magnesium metabolism: a review with special reference to the relationship between intracellular content and serum levels. Arch Intern Med 1988;148:2415–2420.
10. Lowenstein FW, Stanton MF. Serum magnesium levels in the United States, 1971–1974. J Am Coll Nutr 1986;5:399–414.
11. Altura BT, Altura BM. A method for distinguishing ionized, complexed and protein-bound Mg in normal and diseased subjects. Scand J Clin Lab Invest 1994;217:83–87.
12. Kroll MH, Elin RJ. Relationships between magnesium and protein concentrations in serum. Clin Chem 1985;31:244–246.
13. Alvarez-Leefmans FJ, Giraldez F, Gamino SM. Intracellular free magnesium in excitable cells: its measurement and its biologic significance. Can J Physiol Pharmacol 1987;65:915–925.
14. Munoz R, Khilnani P, Salem M. Ionized hypomagnesemia: a frequent problem in critically ill neonates. Crit Care Med 1991;19:S48.

Magnesium Depletion

15. Whang R. Magnesium deficiency: pathogenesis, prevalence, and clinical implications. Am J Med 1987;82:24–29.
16. Dyckner T, Wester PO. Potassium/magnesium depletion in patients with cardiovascular disease. Am J Med 1987;82:11–17.
17. Hollifield JW. Thiazide treatment of systemic hypertension: effects on serum magnesium and ventricular ectopic activity. Am J Cardiol 1989;63:22G–25G.
18. Ryan MP. Diuretics and potassium/magnesium depletion: directions for treatment. Am J Med 1987;82:38–47.
19. Atsmon J, Dolev E. Drug-induced hypomagnesaemia: scope and management. Drug Safety 2005;28:763–788.
20. Zaloga GP, Chernow B, Pock A, et al. Hypomagnesemia is a common complication of aminoglycoside therapy. Surg Gynecol Obstet 1984;158:561–565.
21. Whang R, Oei TO, Watanabe A. Frequency of hypomagnesemia in hospitalized patients receiving digitalis. Arch Intern Med 1985;145:655–656.
22. Balesteri FJ. Magnesium metabolism in the critically ill. Crit Care Clin 1985;5:217–226.
23. Martin HE. Clinical magnesium deficiency. Ann N Y Acad Sci 1969;162:891–900.
24. Dyckner T, Ek B, Nyhlin H, et al. Aggravation of thiamine deficiency by magnesium depletion: a case report. Acta Med Scand 1985;218:129–131.
25. Kassirer J, Hricik D, Cohen J. Repairing body fluids: principles and practice. 1st ed. Philadelphia: WB Saunders, 1989:118–129.
26. Sjogren A, Floren CH, Nilsson A. Magnesium deficiency in IDDM related to level of glycosylated hemoglobin. Diabetes 1986;35:459–463.
27. Lau K. Magnesium metabolism: normal and abnormal. In: Arieff AI, DeFronzo RA, eds. Fluids, electrolytes, and acid base disorders. New York: Churchill Livingstone, 1985:575–623.

28. Abraham AS, Rosenmann D, Kramer M, et al. Magnesium in the prevention of lethal arrhythmias in acute myocardial infarction. Arch Intern Med 1987; 147:753–755.

Clinical Manifestations

29. Whang R, Oei TO, Aikawa JK, et al. Predictors of clinical hypomagnesemia: hypokalemia, hypophosphatemia, hyponatremia, and hypocalcemia. Arch Intern Med 1984;144:1794–1796.
30. Whang R, Flink EB, Dyckner T, et al. Magnesium depletion as a cause of refractory potassium repletion. Arch Intern Med 1985;145:1686–1689.
31. Anast CS, Winnacker JL, Forte LR, et al. Impaired release of parathyroid hormone in magnesium deficiency. J Clin Endocrinol Metab 1976;42:707–717.
32. Rude RK, Oldham SB, Singer FR. Functional hypoparathyroidism and parathyroid hormone end-organ resistance in human magnesium deficiency. Clin Endocrinol 1976;5:209–224.
33. Graber ML, Schulman G. Hypomagnesemic hypocalcemia independent of parathyroid hormone. Ann Intern Med 1986;104:804–805.
34. Dominguez JH, Gray RW, Lemann J Jr. Dietary phosphate deprivation in women and men: effects on mineral and acid balances, parathyroid hormone and the metabolism of 25-OH-vitamin D. J Clin Endocrinol Metab 1976;43: 1056–1068.
35. Cohen L, Kitzes R. Magnesium sulfate and digitalis-toxic arrhythmias. JAMA 1983;249:2808–2810.
36. French JH, Thomas RG, Siskind AP, et al. Magnesium therapy in massive digoxin intoxication. Ann Emerg Med 1984;13:562–566.
37. Tzivoni D, Keren A. Suppression of ventricular arrhythmias by magnesium. Am J Cardiol 1990;65:1397–1399.
38. Langley WF, Mann D. Central nervous system magnesium deficiency. Arch Intern Med 1991;151:593–596.

Diagnosis

39. Fleming CR, George L, Stoner GL, et al. The importance of urinary magnesium values in patients with gut failure. Mayo Clin Proc 1996;71:21–24.
40. Clague JE, Edwards RH, Jackson MJ. Intravenous magnesium loading in chronic fatigue syndrome. Lancet 1992;340:124–125.
41. Hebert P, Mehta N, Wang J, et al. Functional magnesium deficiency in critically ill patients identified using a magnesium-loading test. Crit Care Med 1997;25:749–755.

Magnesium Replacement Therapy

42. DiPalma JR. Magnesium replacement therapy. Am Fam Physician 1990;42: 173–176.
43. Trissel LA. Handbook on injectable drugs. 13th ed. Bethesda, MD: American Social Health System Pharmacists, 2005.
44. Oster JR, Epstein M. Management of magnesium depletion. Am J Nephrol 1988;8:349–354.

Magnesium Accumulation

45. Whang R, Ryder KW. Frequency of hypomagnesemia and hypermagnesemia: requested vs routine. JAMA 1990;263:3063–3064.
46. Elin RJ. Magnesium metabolism in health and disease. Dis Mon 1988;34:161–218.
47. Van Hook JW. Hypermagnesemia. Crit Care Clin 1991;7:215–223.
48. Iseri LT, French JH. Magnesium: nature's physiologic calcium blocker. Am Heart J 1984;108:188–193.
49. Mordes JP, Wacker WE. Excess magnesium. Pharmacol Rev 1977;29:273–300

Chapter 35

CALCIUM AND PHOSPHORUS

Calcium and phosphorus are responsible for much of the structural integrity of the bony skeleton. Although neither is found in abundance in the soft tissues, both play an important role in vital cell functions. Phosphorus participates in aerobic energy production, whereas calcium participates in several diverse processes, such as blood coagulation, neuromuscular transmission, and smooth muscle contraction. Considering the important functions of these electrolytes, it is surprising that abnormalities in calcium and phosphorus balance are so well tolerated.

CALCIUM

Calcium is the most abundant electrolyte in the human body (the average adult has more than half a kilogram of calcium), but 99% is in bone (1,2). In the soft tissues, calcium is 10,000 times more concentrated than in the extracellular fluids (2,3).

Plasma Calcium

The calcium in plasma is present in three forms, as depicted in Figure 35.1. Approximately half of the calcium is ionized (biologically active) and the remainder is complexed (biologically inactive) (1). In the inactive form, 80% of calcium is bound to albumin, while 20% is complexed to plasma anions such as proteins and sulfates. The concentration of total and ionized calcium in plasma is shown in Table 35.1. These values may vary slightly in different clinical laboratories.

Total versus Ionized Calcium

The calcium assay used by most clinical laboratories measures all three fractions of calcium, which can be misleading. The column on the right in Figure 35.1 demonstrates the effects of a decrease in the concentration of albumin in plasma. Because albumin is responsible for 80% of the protein-bound calcium in plasma, a decrease in albumin decreases the

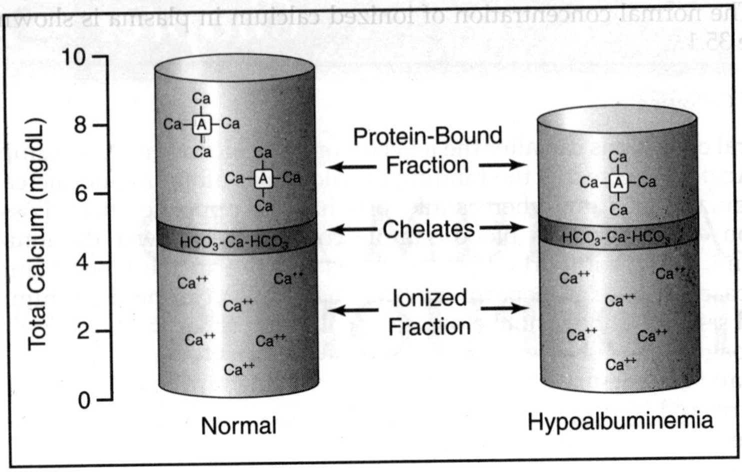

FIGURE 35.1 The three fractions of calcium in plasma and the contribution of each to the total calcium concentration. The column on the right shows how a decrease in plasma albumin can reduce the total plasma calcium without affecting the ionized calcium.

amount of calcium in the protein-bound fraction. The total calcium in plasma decreases by the same amount, but the ionized calcium remains unchanged. Because the ionized calcium is the physiologically active fraction, the hypocalcemia caused by hypoalbuminemia is not physiologically significant. The hypocalcemia that is physiologically significant is *ionized* hypocalcemia (4,5).

A variety of correction factors have been proposed for adjusting the plasma calcium concentration in patients with hypoalbuminemia. However, none of these correction factors are reliable (4,6), and the **only method of identifying true (ionized) hypocalcemia in the face of hypoalbuminemia is to measure the ionized fraction of calcium in plasma**.

Ionized Calcium Measurement

Ionized calcium can be measured in whole blood, plasma, or serum with ion-specific electrodes that are now available in most clinical laboratories

TABLE 35.1 Normal Ranges for Calcium and Phosphorus in Blood

Serum Electrolyte	Traditional Units (mg/dL)	Conversion Factor*	SI Units (mmol/L)
Total calcium	9.0–10.0	0.25	2.2–2.5
Ionized calcium	4.5–5.0	0.25	1.1–1.3
Phosphorus	2.5–5.0	0.32	0.8–1.6

*Multiply traditional units by conversion factor to derive SI Units or divide SI units by conversion factor to derive tranditional units.

(7). The normal concentration of ionized calcium in plasma is shown in Table 35.1.

Blood Collection

Several conditions can alter the level of ionized calcium in blood samples (7). Acidosis decreases the binding of calcium to albumin and increases the ionized calcium, whereas alkalosis has the opposite effect. Loss of carbon dioxide from a blood sample could falsely lower the ionized calcium, so it is important to avoid gas bubbles in the blood sample. Anticoagulants (e.g., heparin, citrate, and EDTA) can bind calcium, so blood samples should not be placed in collection tubes that contain these anticoagulants. Tubes with red stoppers ("red top" tubes) contain silicone and are adequate for measuring ionized calcium in serum samples. Heparinized syringes can be used for measuring ionized calcium in whole blood. Although heparin also binds calcium, the effect is minimal if the heparin level is less than 15 U/mL of blood (7).

Ionized Hypocalcemia

Ionized hypocalcemia has been reported in 15 to 50% of admissions to the ICU (8). The common disorders associated with ionized hypocalcemia in ICU patients are listed in Table 35.2. Hypoparathyroidism is a leading cause of hypocalcemia in outpatients, but is not a consideration in the ICU unless neck surgery has been performed recently.

Predisposing Conditions

Magnesium Depletion

Magnesium depletion promotes hypocalcemia by inhibiting parathormone secretion and reducing end-organ responsiveness to parathormone (see Chapter 34). Hypocalcemia from magnesium depletion is refractory to calcium replacement therapy, and magnesium repletion often corrects the hypocalcemia without calcium replacement.

TABLE 35.2 Causes of Ionized Hypocalcemia in the ICU

Alkalosis	Fat embolism
Blood transfusions (15%)	Magnesium depletion (70%)
Cardiopulmonary bypass	Pancreatitis
Drugs:	Renal insufficiency (50%)
Aminoglycosides (40%)	Sepsis (30%)
Cimetidine (30%)	
Heparin (10%)	
Theophylline (30%)	

Numbers in parentheses show the frequency of ionized hypocalcemia reported in each condition.

Sepsis

Sepsis is a common cause of hypocalcemia in the ICU (8,9). The mechanism is unclear, but it may involve an increase in calcium binding to albumin caused by elevated levels of circulating free fatty acids. Hypocalcemia is independent of the vasodilation that accompanies sepsis (9), and thus the clinical significance of the hypocalcemia in sepsis is unclear.

Alkalosis

As mentioned earlier, alkalosis promotes the binding of calcium to albumin and can reduce the fraction of ionized calcium in blood. Symptomatic hypocalcemia is more common with respiratory alkalosis than with metabolic alkalosis. Infusions of sodium bicarbonate can also be accompanied by ionized hypocalcemia because calcium directly binds to the infused bicarbonate.

Blood Transfusions

Ionized hypocalcemia has been reported in 20% of patients receiving blood transfusions (8). The mechanism is calcium binding by the citrate anticoagulant in banked blood. Hypocalcemia from blood transfusions usually is transient, and resolves when the infused citrate is metabolized by the liver and kidneys (8). In patients with renal or hepatic failure, a more prolonged hypocalcemia can result. Although hypocalcemia from blood transfusions could impede blood coagulation, this is not considered to be a significant effect and calcium infusions are no longer recommended in massive blood transfusions.

Drugs

A number of drugs can bind calcium and promote ionized hypocalcemia (8). The ones most often used in the ICU are aminoglycosides, cimetidine, heparin, and theophylline.

Renal Failure

Ionized hypocalcemia can accompany renal failure as a result of phosphate retention and impaired conversion of vitamin D to its active form in the kidneys. The treatment is aimed at lowering the phosphate levels in blood with antacids that block phosphorus absorption in the small bowel. However, the value of this practice is unproven. The acidosis in renal failure can decrease the binding of calcium to albumin, so hypocalcemia in renal failure does not imply ionized hypocalcemia.

Pancreatitis

Severe pancreatitis can produce ionized hypocalcemia through several mechanisms. The prognosis is adversely affected by the appearance of hypocalcemia (10), although a causal relationship has not been proven.

Clinical Manifestations

The clinical manifestations of hypocalcemia are related to enhanced cardiac and neuromuscular excitability and reduced contractile force in cardiac muscle and vascular smooth muscle.

Neuromuscular Excitability

Hypocalcemia can be accompanied by tetany (of peripheral or laryngeal muscles), hyperreflexia, paresthesias, and seizures (11). Chvōstek's and Trousseau's signs are often listed as manifestations of hypocalcemia. However, **Chvostek's sign is nonspecific** (it is present in 25% of normal adults), and **Trousseau's sign is insensitive** (it can be absent in 30% of patients with hypocalcemia) (12).

Cardiovascular Effects

The cardiovascular complications of hypocalcemia include hypotension, decreased cardiac output, and ventricular ectopic activity. These complications are rarely seen in mild cases of ionized hypocalcemia (i.e., ionized calcium 0.8 to 1.0 mmol/L). However, advanced stages of ionized hypocalcemia (i.e., ionized calcium less than 0.65 mmol/L) can be associated with heart block, ventricular tachycardia and refractory hypotension (8).

Calcium Replacement Therapy

The treatment of ionized hypocalcemia should be directed at the underlying cause of the problem. However, symptomatic hypocalcemia is considered a medical emergency (8), and the treatment of choice is intravenous calcium. The calcium solutions and dosage recommendations for intravenous calcium replacement are shown in Table 35.3.

TABLE 35.3 Intravenous Calcium Replacement Therapy

Solution	Elemental Calcium	Unit Volume	Osmolarity
10% Calcium chloride	27 mg (1.36 mEq)/mL	10-mL ampules	2000 mOsm/L
10% Calcium gluconate	9 mg (0.46 mEq)/mL	10-mL ampules	680 mOsm/L

For symptomatic hypocalcemia:

1. Infuse calcium into a large central vein if possible. If a peripheral vein is used, calcium gluconate should be used.
2. Give a bolus dose of 200 mg elemental calcium (8 mL of 10% calcium chloride or 22 mL of 10% calcium gluconate) in 100 mL isotonic saline over 10 minutes.
3. Follow with a continuous infusion of 1–2 mg elemental calcium per kg per hour for 6–12 hours.

Calcium Salt Solutions

The two most popular calcium solutions for intravenous use are 10% calcium chloride and 10% calcium gluconate. Both solutions have the same concentration of calcium salt (i.e., 100 mg/mL), but **calcium chloride contains three times more elemental calcium than calcium gluconate.** One 10-mL ampule of 10% calcium chloride contains 272 mg (13.6 mEq) of elemental calcium, whereas one 10-mL ampule of 10% calcium gluconate contains only 90 mg (4.6 mEq) of elemental calcium (8).

Dosage Recommendations

The intravenous calcium solutions are hyperosmolar and should be given through a large central vein if possible. If a peripheral vein is used, calcium gluconate is the preferred solution because of its lower osmolarity (Table 35.3). A bolus dose of 100 mg elemental calcium (diluted in 100 mL isotonic saline and given over 5–10 minutes) should raise the total serum calcium by 0.5 mg/dL, but levels will begin to fall after 30 minutes (8). Therefore, the bolus dose of calcium should be followed by a continuous infusion at a dose rate of 0.5 to 2 mg/kg/hr (elemental calcium) for at least 6 hours. Individual responses will vary, so calcium dosing should be guided by the level of ionized calcium in blood (8).

Caution

Intravenous calcium replacement can be risky in select patient populations. Calcium infusions can promote vasoconstriction and ischemia in any of the vital organs (13). The risk of calcium-induced ischemia should be particularly high in patients with low cardiac output who are already vasoconstricted. In addition, aggressive calcium replacement can promote intracellular calcium overload, which can produce a lethal cell injury (14), particularly in patients with circulatory shock. Because of these risks, calcium infusions should be used judiciously. **Intravenous calcium is indicated only for patients with symptomatic hypocalcemia or an ionized calcium level below 0.65 mmol/L** (8).

Maintenance Therapy

The daily maintenance dose of calcium is 2–4 g in adults. This can be administered orally using calcium carbonate (e.g., Oscal) or calcium gluconate tablets (500 mg calcium per tablet).

HYPERCALCEMIA

Hypercalcemia is not nearly as common as hypocalcemia: it is reported in less than 1% of hospitalized patients (15). In 90% of cases, the underlying cause is hyperparathyroidism or malignancy (16,17). Less common causes include prolonged immobilization, thyrotoxicosis, and drugs (lithium, thiazide diuretics). Malignancy is the most common cause of severe hypercalcemia (i.e., total serum calcium above 14 mg/dL or ionized calcium above 3.5 mmol/L) (17).

Clinical Manifestations

The manifestations of hypercalcemia usually are nonspecific and can be categorized as follows (16):

1. **Gastrointestinal (GI):** nausea, vomiting, constipation, ileus, and pancreatitis
2. **Cardiovascular:** hypovolemia, hypotension, and shortened QT interval
3. **Renal:** polyuria and nephrocalcinosis
4. **Neurologic:** confusion and depressed consciousness, including coma

These manifestations can become evident when the total serum calcium rises above 12 mg/dL (or the ionized calcium rises above 3.0 mmol/L), and they are almost always present when the serum calcium is greater than 14 mg/dL (or the ionized calcium is above 3.5 mmol/L) (17).

Management

Treatment is indicated when the hypercalcemia is associated with adverse effects, or when the serum calcium is greater than 14 mg/dL (ionized calcium above 3.5 mmol/L). The management of hypercalcemia is summarized in Table 35.4 (1,16,17).

Saline Infusion

Hypercalcemia usually is accompanied by hypercalciuria, which produces an osmotic diuresis. This eventually leads to hypovolemia, which reduces calcium excretion in the urine and precipitates a rapid rise in the serum calcium. Therefore, volume infusion to correct hypovolemia and promote renal calcium excretion is the first goal of management for hypercalcemia. Isotonic saline is recommended for the volume infusion because natriuresis promotes renal calcium excretion.

Furosemide

Saline infusion will not return the calcium to normal levels. This requires the addition of furosemide (40 to 80 mg IV every 2 hours) to further promote urinary calcium excretion. The goal is an hourly urine output of 100 to 200 mL/minute. The hourly urine output **must** be replaced with isotonic saline. Failure to replace urinary volume losses is counterproductive, and favors a return to hypovolemia.

Calcitonin

Although saline and furosemide will correct the hypercalcemia acutely, this approach does not treat the underlying cause of the problem, which (in malignancy) is enhanced bone resorption. Calcitonin is a naturally occurring hormone that inhibits bone resorption. It is available as salmon calcitonin, which is given subcutaneously or intramuscularly in a dose

TABLE 35.4 Management of Severe Hypercalcemia

Agent	Dose	Comment
Isotonic saline	Variable	Initial treatment of choice. Goal is rapid correction of hypovolemia.
Furosemide	40–80 mg IV every 2 hours	Add to isotonic saline to maintain a urine output of 100–200 mL/hr.
Calcitonin	4 Units/kg IM or SC every 12 hours	Response is evident within a few hours. Maximum drop in serum calcium is only 0.5 mmol/L.
Hydrocortisone	200 mg IV daily in 2–3 divided doses	Used as an adjunct to calcitonin.
Bisphosphonates		More potent than calcitonin, but complete response requires 4–10 days.
Pamidronate	90 mg IV over 2 hours	Reduce dose to 60 mg in renal impairment.
Zoledronate	4 mg IV over 15 minutes	Equivalent to pamidronate in efficacy.
Plicamycin	25 μg/kg IV over 4 hours; can repeat every 2 hours	More rapid effect than pamidronate, but potential for toxic side effects limits the use of this agent.

of 4 U/kg every 12 hours. The response is rapid (onset within a few hours), but the effect is mild (the maximum drop in serum calcium is 0.5 mmol/L).

Hydrocortisone

Corticosteroids can reduce the serum calcium by impeding the growth of lymphoid neoplastic tissue and enhancing the actions of vitamin D. Steroids are usually combined with calcitonin and can be particularly useful in the hypercalcemia associated with multiple myeloma or renal failure (1,16,17). The standard regimen uses hydrocortisone, 200 mg IV daily in 2 or 3 divided doses.

Intravenous Bisphosphonates

Calcitonin can be used for rapid reduction of serum calcium, but the mild response will not keep the calcium in the normal range. A group of compounds known as *bisphosphonates* (pyrophosphate derivatives) are more potent inhibitors of bone resorption and maintain a normal serum calcium. However, their onset of action is delayed, and thus they are not useful when rapid control of serum calcium is desired.

Zoledronate (4 mg over 15 minutes) or **Pamidronate** (90 mg over 2 hours) are the bisphosphonates of choice for the management of severe hypercalcemia (17). The peak effect is seen in 2 to 4 days, and serum calcium normalizes within 4–7 days in 60–90% of cases. The dose may be repeated in 4–10 days, if necessary.

Plicamycin

Plicamycin (formerly mithramycin) is an antineoplastic agent that inhibits bone resorption. It is similar to the bisphosphonates in that it is more potent than calcitonin but has a delayed onset of action. The dose is 25 μg/kg (intravenously over 4–6 hours), which can be repeated in 24–48 hours if necessary (17). Because of the potential for serious side effects (e.g., bone marrow suppression), plicamycin has largely been replaced by pamidronate.

Dialysis

Dialysis (hemodialysis or peritoneal dialysis) is effective in removing calcium in patients with renal failure (17).

PHOSPHORUS

The average adult has 500–800 g of phosphorus (18,19). Most is contained in organic molecules such as phospholipids and phosphoproteins, and 85% is located in the bony skeleton. The remaining 15% in soft tissues is present as free, inorganic phosphorus. Unlike calcium, inorganic phosphorus is predominantly intracellular in location, where it participates in glycolysis and high energy phosphate production. The normal concentration of inorganic phosphorus in plasma is shown in Table 35.1.

Hypophosphatemia

Hypophosphatemia (serum PO_4 less than 2.5 mg/dL or 0.8 mmol/L) is reported in 17 to 28% of critically ill patients (20,21) and can be the result of an intracellular shift of phosphorus, an increase in the renal excretion of phosphorus, or a decrease in phosphorus absorption from the GI tract. Most cases of hypophosphatemia are due to movement of PO_4 into cells.

Predisposing Conditions

Glucose Loading

The movement of glucose into cells is accompanied by a similar movement of PO_4 into cells, and if the extracellular content of PO_4 is marginal, this intracellular PO_4 shift can result in hypophosphatemia. Glucose loading is the most common cause of hypophosphatemia in hospitalized patients (20,22), usually seen during refeeding in alcoholic, malnourished, or debilitated patients. It can occur with oral feedings, enteral tube feedings, or with total parenteral nutrition. The influence of parenteral

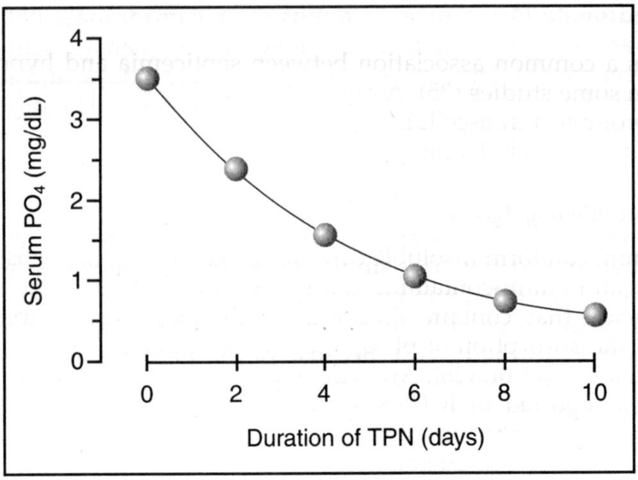

FIGURE 35.2 The cumulative effect of total parenteral nutrition (*TPN*) on the serum phosphate level. (Data from Knochel JP. The pathophysiology and clinical characteristics of severe hypophosphatemia. Arch Intern Med 1977;137:203–220.)

nutrition on serum PO_4 levels is shown in Figure 35.2. Note the gradual decline in the serum PO_4 and the severe degree of hypophosphatemia (serum PO_4 <1 mg/dL) after 7 days of intravenous nutrition. The risk of hypophosphatemia is one of the reasons why parenteral nutrition regimens are advanced gradually for the first few days.

As mentioned, oral and enteral feedings create a similar risk of hypophosphatemia, particularly in debilitated or malnourished patients. In fact, hypophosphatemia may be responsible for the progressive weakness and inanition that characterizes the refeeding syndrome in malnourished patients (22).

Respiratory Alkalosis

Respiratory alkalosis can increase intracellular pH, and this accelerates glycolysis. The increase in glucose utilization is accompanied by an increase in glucose and phosphorus movement into cells (23). This may be an important source of hypophosphatemia in ventilator-dependent patients because overventilation and respiratory alkalosis is common in these patients.

β-Receptor Agonists

Stimulation of β-adrenergic receptors can move PO_4 into cells and promote hypophosphatemia. This effect is evident in patients treated with β-agonist bronchodilators. In one study of patients with acute asthma who were treated aggressively with nebulized albuterol (2.5 mg every 30 minutes), the serum PO_4 decreased by 1.25 mg/dL (0.4 mmol/L) 3 hours after the onset of therapy (24). However, the significance of this effect is unclear.

Sepsis

There is a common association between septicemia and hypophosphatemia in some studies (25). A causal relationship is unproven, but sepsis could promote a transcellular shift of PO_4 as a result of elevated levels of endogenous catecholamines.

Phosphate-Binding Agents

Aluminum can form insoluble complexes with inorganic phosphates. As a result, aluminum-containing compounds such as sucralfate (Carafate), or antacids that contain aluminum hydroxide (e.g., Amphogel) can impede the absorption of phosphate in the upper GI tract and promote phosphate depletion (26). An increased incidence of hypophosphatemia has been reported in ICU patients receiving the cytoprotective agent sucralfate for prophylaxis of stress ulcer bleeding (24). However, a causal relationship between sucralfate and phosphate depletion has not been established.

Diabetic Ketoacidosis

The osmotic diuresis from glycosuria promotes the urinary loss of PO_4, and patients with prolonged or severe hyperglycemia are often phosphate depleted. As mentioned in Chapter 29, phosphate depletion is almost universal in diabetic ketoacidosis, but it does not become evident until insulin therapy drives PO_4 into cells. Because phosphate supplementation does not alter the outcome in diabetic ketoacidosis (see Chapter 29), the significance of the phosphate depletion in this disorder is unclear.

Clinical Manifestations

Hypophosphatemia is often clinically silent, even when the serum PO_4 falls to extremely low levels. In addition, serum PO_4 levels do not necessarily reflect the severity of tissue phosphorous deficit (21). In one study of patients with severe hypophosphatemia (i.e., serum PO_4 less than 1.0 mg/dL), none of the patients showed evidence of harmful effects (27). Despite the apparent lack of harm, phosphate depletion creates a risk for impaired energy production in all aerobic cells.

Aerobic Energy Production

Phosphate depletion has several effects that could impair cellular energy production; these are summarized in Figure 35.3. To begin with, each of the following determinants of systemic oxygen delivery can be adversely affected by phosphate depletion.

1. **Cardiac output:** Phosphate depletion can impair myocardial contractility and reduce cardiac output. Hypophosphatemic patients with heart failure have shown improved cardiac performance after phosphate supplementation (28).

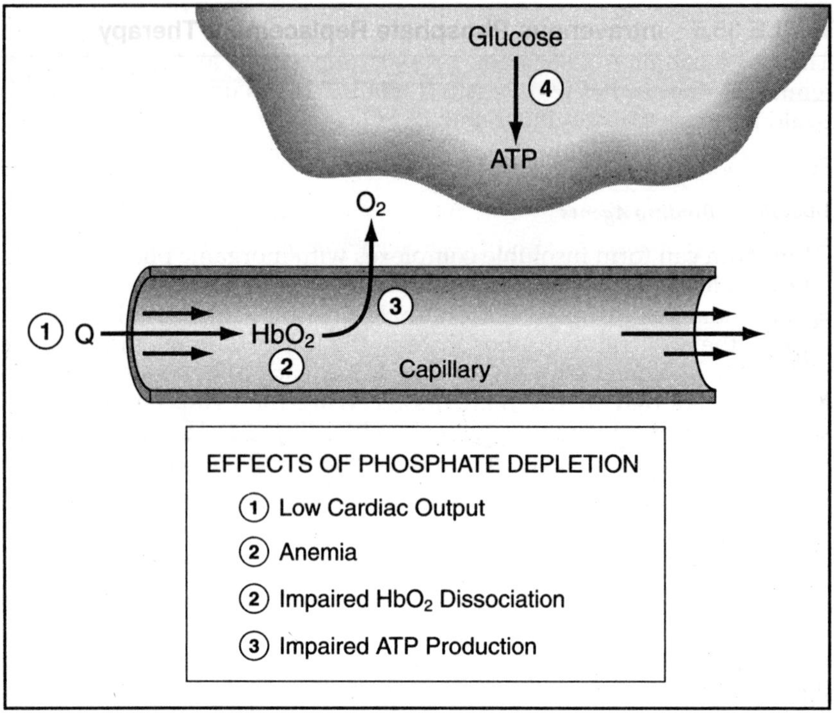

FIGURE 35.3 The effects of phosphate depletion that can impair cellular energy production.

2. **Hemoglobin:** Reduction of high energy phosphate production from glycolysis in erythrocytes can reduce the deformability of red cells. This may explain why severe hypophosphatemia can be accompanied by a hemolytic anemia (26).
3. **Oxyhemoglobin dissociation:** Phosphate depletion is accompanied by depletion of 2,3-diphosphoglycerate, and this shifts the oxyhemoglobin dissociation curve to the left. When this occurs, hemoglobin is less likely to release oxygen to the tissues.

In addition to the adverse effects on tissue oxygen availability, phosphate depletion can directly impede cellular energy production by reducing the availability of inorganic phosphorus for high-energy phosphate production and decreasing the activity of the glycolytic pathway.

Muscle Weakness

One of the possible consequences of impaired energy production from phosphate depletion is skeletal muscle weakness. Biochemical evidence of skeletal muscle disruption (e.g., elevated creatine kinase levels in blood) is common in patients with hypophosphatemia, but overt muscle weakness is usually absent (29). There is one report of respiratory muscle weakness

TABLE 35.5 Intravenous Phosphate Replacement Therapy

Solution	Phosphorus Content	Other Content
Sodium phosphate	93 mg (3 mmol)/mL	Na^+: 4.0 mEq/mL
Potassium phosphate	93 mg (3 mmol)/mL	K^+: 4.3 mEq/mL

*Dosage Recommendations**

For severe hypophosphatemia (PO_4 <1 mg/dL) without adverse effects:
IV dose is 0.6 mg (0.02 mmol) per kg body weight per hour
For hypophosphatemia (PO_4 <2 mg/dL) with adverse effects:
IV dose is 0.9 mg (0.03 mmol) per kg body weight per hour
Monitor serum PO_4 level every 6 hours.

*In patients with renal dysfunction, slower dose rates are advised.
*From Zaloga G. Divalent cations: calcium, magnesium, and phosphorus. In Chernow B, ed. The pharmacologic approach to the critically ill patient., 3rd ed. Baltimore: Williams & Williams, 1994, pp 777–804.

and failure to wean from mechanical ventilation in patients with severe hypophosphatemia (30). However, other studies show that respiratory muscle weakness is common in hypophosphatemia but is not clinically significant in most patients (31). At present, the evidence linking phosphate depletion with clinically significant skeletal muscle weakness is scant.

Phosphorus Replacement Therapy

Intravenous phosphorus replacement is recommended for all patients with severe hypophosphatemia (i.e., serum PO_4 below 1.0 mg/dL or 0.3 mmol/L) and for patients with hypophosphatemia of any degree who also have cardiac dysfunction, respiratory failure, muscle weakness, or impaired tissue oxygenation. The phosphate solutions and dosage recommendations are shown in Table 35.5 (32,33).

Once the serum PO_4 rises above 2 mg/dL, phosphate replacement can be continued using oral phosphate preparations like Neutra-Phos or K-Phos. The oral replacement dosage is 1200–1500 mg phosphorus daily. Remember that sucralfate and phosphate-binding antacids need to be discontinued when oral phosphate preparations are used. The tendency for oral phosphate preparations to promote diarrhea limits the use of high-dosage oral PO_4 replacement therapy.

Maintenance Therapy

The normal daily maintenance dose of phosphate is 1,200 mg if given orally (18). As shown in Table 35.6, the content of enteral feeding formulas varies widely, and thus enteral nutrition may not provide the daily phosphorus requirements without additional supplementation.

In patients who cannot tolerate enteral nutrition, daily phosphate requirements are provided intravenously. The IV maintenance dose of PO_4 is approximately 800 mg/day (this dose is lower than the oral

TABLE 35.6 The Phosphorus Content of Enteral Tube Feedings

Formula	Phosphorus (mg/L)	Formula	Phosphorus (mg/L)
AlitraQ	733	Nutrivent	1200
Compleat Regular	760	Osmolite/1 Cal/1.2 Cal	535/760/1200
Criticare HN	530	Peptamen/1.5	700/1000
Ensure/HN	1268/758	Perative	870
Ensure Plus/HN	845/1000	Pulmocare	1060
Glucerna	705	Nutren Replete	1000
Impact	800	Resource Arginaid Extra	850
Isocal/HN	530/850	TraumaCal	750
Isosource/HN	1100/1200	TwoCal HN	1057
Jevity	760	Ultracal	1000
Nutren 1.0/2.0	668/1341	Vivonex Plus/RTF/TEN	560/670/500

maintenance dose because only 70% of orally administered phosphate is absorbed from the GI tract).

Hyperphosphatemia

Most cases of hyperphosphatemia in the ICU are the result of impaired PO_4 excretion from **renal insufficiency** or PO_4 release from cells because of **widespread cell necrosis** (e.g., rhabdomyolysis or tumor lysis). Hyperphosphatemia can also be seen in diabetic ketoacidosis but, as described earlier, this disorder is almost always accompanied by phosphate depletion, which becomes evident after the onset of insulin therapy.

Clinical Manifestations

The clinical manifestations of hyperphosphatemia include formation of insoluble calcium–phosphate complexes (with deposition into soft tissues) and acute hypocalcemia (with tetany) (11). However, information is lacking about the prevalence or significance of these manifestations.

Management

There are two approaches to hyperphosphatemia. The first is to promote PO_4 binding in the upper GI tract, which can lower the serum PO_4 even in the absence of any oral intake of phosphate (i.e., GI dialysis). Sucralfate or aluminum-containing antacids can be used for this purpose. In patients with significant hypocalcemia, calcium acetate tablets (PhosLo, Braintree Labs) can help raise the serum calcium while lowering the serum PO_4. Each calcium acetate tablet (667 mg) contains 8.45 mEq elemental calcium. The recommended dose is 2 tablets three times a day (34,35).

The other approach to hyperphosphatemia is to enhance PO_4 clearance with hemodialysis. This is reserved for patients with renal failure, and is rarely necessary.

A FINAL WORD

A few points about calcium deserve emphasis:

1. For patients with hypoalbuminemia, do not use any of the correction factors proposed for adjusting the plasma calcium concentration (because they are unreliable). You must measure the ionized calcium in these patients.
2. Magnesium depletion, which is common in ICU patients, should always be considered as a possible cause of hypocalcemia.
3. Because calcium infusions can be damaging, intravenous calcium should be reserved only for cases of symptomatic hypocalcemia, or when ionized calcium levels fall below 0.65 mmol/L.

And for phosphorus:

1. Watch the plasma PO_4 levels carefully when starting parenteral nutrition because of the risk for hypophosphatemia. This also applies to the practice of using continuous insulin infusions for tight glycemic control.
2. Watch for hypophosphatemia in patients receiving sucralfate for prophylaxis of stress ulcer bleeding.

REFERENCES

Calcium Reviews

1. Bushinsky DA, Monk RD. Electrolyte quintet: calcium. Lancet 1998;352:306–311.
2. Baker SB, Worthley LI. The essentials of calcium, magnesium and phosphate metabolism, part I: physiology. Crit Care Resusc 2002;4:301–306.
3. Weaver CM, Heaney RP. Calcium. In: Shils ME, Shike M, Ross AC, et al., eds. Modern nutrition in health and disease. 10th ed. Philadelphia: Lippincott Williams & Wilkins, 2006:194–210.

Plasma Calcium

4. Slomp J, van der Voort PH, Gerritsen RT, et al. Albumin-adjusted calcium is not suitable for diagnosis of hyper- and hypocalcemia in the critically ill. Crit Care Med 2003;31:1389–1393.
5. Koch SM, Warters RD, Mehlhorn U. The simultaneous measurement of ionized and total calcium and ionized and total magnesium in intensive care unit patients. J Crit Care 2002;17:203–205.

6. Byrnes MC, Huynh K, Helmer SD, et al. A comparison of corrected serum calcium levels to ionized calcium levels among critically ill surgical patients. Am J Surg 2005;189:310–314.
7. Forman DT, Lorenzo L. Ionized calcium: its significance and clinical usefulness. Ann Clin Lab Sci 1991;21:297–304.

Hypocalcemia

8. Zaloga GP. Hypocalcemia in critically ill patients. Crit Care Med 1992;20:251–262.
9. Burchard KW, Simms HH, Robinson A, et al. Hypocalcemia during sepsis: relationship to resuscitation and hemodynamics. Arch Surg 1992;127:265–272.
10. Steinberg W, Tenner S. Acute pancreatitis. N Engl J Med 1994;330:1198–1210.
11. Baker SB, Worthley LI. The essentials of calcium, magnesium and phosphate metabolism, part II: disorders. Crit Care Resusc 2002;4:307–315.
12. Zaloga G. Divalent cations: calcium, magnesium, and phosphorus. In: Chernow B, ed. The pharmacologic approach to the critically ill patient. 3rd ed. Baltimore: Williams & Williams, 1994:777–804.
13. Shapiro MJ, Mistry B. Calcium regulation and nonprotective properties of calcium in surgical ischemia. New Horiz 1996;4:134–138.
14. Trump BF, Berezesky IK. Calcium-mediated cell injury and cell death. FASEB J 1995;9:219–228.

Hypercalcemia

15. Shek CC, Natkunam A, Tsang V, et al. Incidence, causes and mechanism of hypercalcaemia in a hospital population in Hong Kong. Q J Med 1990;77: 1277–1285.
16. Ziegler R. Hypercalcemic crisis. J Am Soc Nephrol 2001;12(suppl 17):S3–S9.
17. Stewart AF. Clinical practice: hypercalcemia associated with cancer. N Engl J Med 2005;352:373–379.
18. Knochel JP. Phosphorous. In: Shils ME, Shike M, Ross AC, et al., eds. Modern nutrition in health and disease. 10th ed Philadelphia: Williams &Williams, 2006:211–222.

Hypophosphatemia

19. Bugg NC, Jones JA. Hypophosphataemia: pathophysiology, effects and management on the intensive care unit. Anaesthesia 1998;53:895–902.
20. French C, Bellomo R. A rapid intravenous phosphate replacement protocol for critically ill patients. Crit Care Resusc 2004;6:175–179.
21. Fiaccadori E, Coffrini E, Fracchia C, et al. Hypophosphatemia and phosphorus depletion in respiratory and peripheral muscles of patients with respiratory failure due to COPD. Chest 1994;105:1392–1398.
22. Marinella MA. Refeeding syndrome and hypophosphatemia. J Intensive Care Med 2005;20:155–159.
23. Paleologos M, Stone E, Braude S. Persistent, progressive hypophosphataemia after voluntary hyperventilation. Clin Sci 2000;98:619–625.
24. Bodenhamer J, Bergstrom R, Brown D, et al. Frequently nebulized beta-agonists for asthma: effects on serum electrolytes. Ann Emerg Med 1992;21:1337–1342.

25. Halevy J, Bulvik S. Severe hypophosphatemia in hospitalized patients. Arch Intern Med 1988;148:153–155.
26. Brown GR, Greenwood JK. Drug- and nutrition-induced hypophosphatemia: mechanisms and relevance in the critically ill. Ann Pharmacother 1994; 28:626–632.
27. King AL, Sica DA, Miller G, et al. Severe hypophosphatemia in a general hospital population. South Med J 1987;80:831–835.
28. Davis SV, Olichwier KK, Chakko SC. Reversible depression of myocardial performance in hypophosphatemia. Am J Med Sci 1988;295:183–187.
29. Singhal PC, Kumar A, Desroches L, et al. Prevalence and predictors of rhabdomyolysis in patients with hypophosphatemia. Am J Med 1992;92:458–464.
30. Agusti AG, Torres A, Estopa R, et al. Hypophosphatemia as a cause of failed weaning: the importance of metabolic factors. Crit Care Med 1984;12:142–143.
31. Gravelyn TR, Brophy N, Siegert C, et al. Hypophosphatemia-associated respiratory muscle weakness in a general inpatient population. Am J Med 1988;84:870–876.
32. Clark CL, Sacks GS, Dickerson RN, et al. Treatment of hypophosphatemia in patients receiving specialized nutrition support using a graduated dosing scheme: results from a prospective clinical trial. Crit Care Med 1995;23:1504–1511.
33. Miller SJ, Simpson J. Medication-nutrient interactions: hypophosphatemia associated with sucralfate in the intensive care unit. Nutr Clin Pract 1991; 6:199–201.
34. Kraft MD, Btaiche IF, Sacks GS, et al. Treatment of electrolyte disorders in adult patients in the intensive care unit. Am J Health Syst Pharm 2005;62: 1663–1682.
35. Lorenzo Sellares V, Torres Ramirez A. Management of hyperphosphataemia in dialysis patients: role of phosphate binders in the elderly. Drugs Aging 2004;21:153–165.

Section XI

TRANSFUSION PRACTICES IN CRITICAL CARE

Nothing is so firmly believed as that which is least known.

FRANCIS JEFFREY (1773–1850)

Chapter 36

ANEMIA AND RED BLOOD CELL TRANSFUSIONS IN THE ICU

One of the important discoveries, I believe . . . is the realization that anemia is well tolerated . . . providing blood volume is maintained.

Daniel J. Ullyot, M.D. (1992)

Anemia is almost universal in patients who spend more than a few days in the ICU (1), and about half of ICU patients with anemia are given one or more transfusions of concentrated erythrocytes (packed red blood cells) to correct the problem (2). This practice of **transfusing red blood cells to correct anemia is one of the most fickle and arbitrary interventions in critical care medicine**. Few ICUs employ practice guidelines to standardize transfusion therapy (2), and in most cases blood transfusions are given without documented evidence of need or benefit. The fear of anemia is pervasive but unfounded, because (as indicated in the introductory quote) anemia does not compromise tissue oxygenation as long as the intravascular volume (and hence cardiac output) is maintained. The relative importance of blood volume over blood cells is demonstrated by the fact that hypovolemia is a recognized cause of circulatory shock (impaired tissue oxygenation), whereas anemia is not. The important role of blood volume in supporting tissue oxygenation is often overlooked, even by the American Red Cross, whose popular slogan, *blood saves lives*, deserves a more accurate update like the one shown in Figure 36.1.

This chapter presents the current knowledge on the indications, methods, and complications of erythrocyte transfusions (3–6). Transfusion practices that are physiologically unsound or unproven are highlighted to emphasize the shortcomings that continue to plague this area of clinical practice.

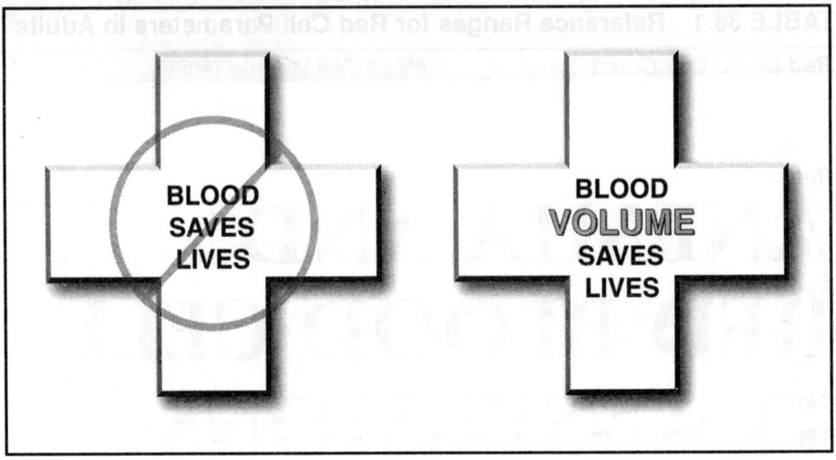

FIGURE 36.1 The slogan of the American Red Cross, shown on the left, is less accurate than the amended statement on the right, which recognizes the contribution of volume to the life-saving effects of blood transfusions.

ANEMIA IN THE ICU

Surveys have consistently shown that anemia is common on admission to the ICU (60% of patients in one study) and is almost universal by the end of the first week after admission (1,2). However, these results can be misleading because they are based on the hemoglobin concentration in blood as a marker of anemia. This is explained in the next section.

The Definition of Anemia

Anemia is defined as a *decrease in the oxygen carrying capacity of blood*. The oxygen carrying capacity of blood is a function of the total volume of circulating red blood cells, so anemia can be defined as a *decrease in the total red cell volume*. This parameter can be measured using chromium-tagged erythrocytes (see Table 36.1 for the normal values), but the methodology is not readily available in the clinical setting. Therefore, clinicians use an alternative definition of anemia that is based on the hematocrit and hemoglobin concentration in blood (see Table 36.1 for the reference ranges of these measurements). However, this practice is problematic, as described next.

The Problem

The problem with the clinical definition of anemia is the influence of the plasma volume on the hematocrit and hemoglobin concentration. This is demonstrated in Figure 36.2, which shows the postural changes in hematocrit and plasma volume in a group of healthy adults (7). When changing from the standing to supine positions, interstitial fluid in the lower extremities moves into the bloodstream and increases the plasma volume. The hematocrit then decreases by dilution. The absolute changes

TABLE 36.1 Reference Ranges for Red Cell Parameters in Adults

Red Blood Cell Count	***Mean Cell Volume (MCV)***
Males: $4.6 - 6.2 \times 10^{12}$ /L	Males: $80 - 100 \times 10^{-15}$L
Females: $4.2 - 5.4 \times 10^{12}$ /L	Females: same
Reticulocyte Count	***Hematocrit***
Males: $25 - 75 \times 10^{9}$ /L	Males: 40 – 54%
Females: same	Females: 38 – 47%
Red Blood Cell Volume*	***Hemoglobin***†
Males: 26 mL/kg	Males: 14 – 18 g/dL
Females: 24mL/kg	Females: 12 – 16 g/dL

*Normal values are 10% lower in the elderly (≥ 65 yrs of age).

†Normal values are 0.5 g/dL lower in blacks.

Sources: (*1*) Walker RH (ed). Technical Manual of the American Association of Blood Banks. 10th ed. Arlington, VA: American Association of Blood Banks, 1990:649–650; (*2*) Hillman RS, Finch CA. Red cell manual. 6th ed. Philadelphia: FA Davis, 1994:46.

in hematocrit (4.1%) and plasma volume (420 mL) in Figure 36.2 are equivalent to one unit of whole blood. The dilutional decrease in hematocrit could therefore be misinterpreted as indicating a red blood cell deficit, and this could lead to the inappropriate transfusion of one unit of blood (packed red blood cells).

Changes in plasma volume are expected in critically ill patients for the following reasons: (1) These patients are often hemodynamically unstable, and this is often associated with fluid shifts between the extravascular and intravascular compartments, (2) hypoalbuminemia is common in critically ill patients, and this will shift fluid out of the vascular compartment, and (3) intravenous fluids (which will increase plasma volume) and diuretics (which will decrease plasma volume) are used frequently in critically ill patients. Because of the risk that plasma volume is changing, **the hematocrit and hemoglobin are unreliable markers of anemia in critically ill patients**. This has been confirmed in clinical studies (8,9).

Common Causes of Anemia in the ICU

There are two conditions that are recognized for favoring the development of anemia in ICU patients: (1) systemic inflammation, and (2) repeated phlebotomy for laboratory studies. Failure of erythropoiesis could also occur without these two predisposing conditions if the energy needs of erythropoiesis are not satisfied.

The Burden of Erythropoiesis

The average adult has as many as 6 *trillion* (6×10^{12}) RBCs per liter of blood (see Table 36.1) (10). Using a blood volume of 5 liters, this corresponds to a total of about 30 trillion RBCs in circulating blood. The average turnover of circulating RBCs is 1% per day (11), which means

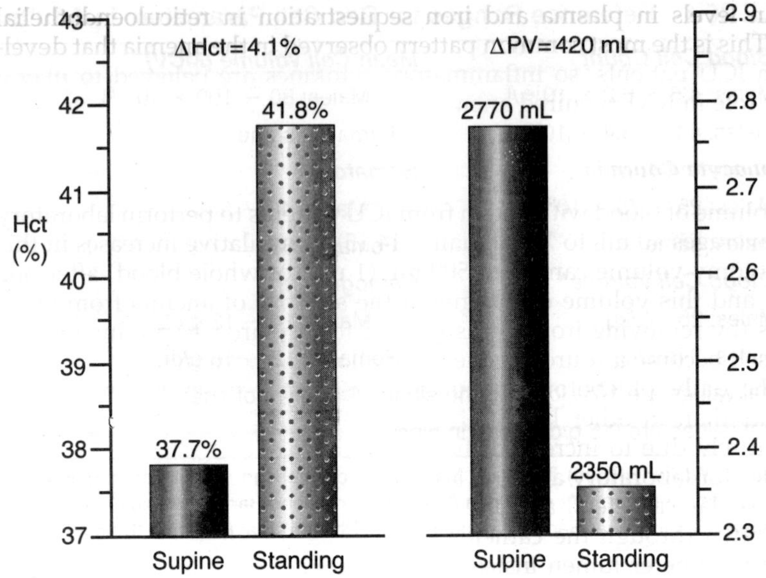

FIGURE 36.2 Postural changes in hematocrit (*Hct*) and plasma volume (*PV*) in a group of healthy adults. The numbers in parenthesis are the mean values of each parameter for the entire study group. (From Jacob G, Raj SR, Ketch T, et al. Postural pseudoanemia: posture-dependent change in hematocrit. Mayo Clin Proc 2005;80:611–614.)

that (0.01 × 30 trillion) **300 *billion* RBCs must be produced daily to maintain a constant pool of circulating erythrocytes**. Failure to meet the energy requirements of this effort could lead to failure of erythropoiesis and subsequent anemia.

This daily production of RBCs (which takes place in the marrow cavities of the axial skeleton in adults) is regulated by *erythropoietin*, a hormone produced in the peritubular capillary endothelium in the kidneys that stimulates erythropoiesis in marrow cavities. The cells that manufacture erythropoietin can respond to decreases in the arterial O_2 content (either hemoglobin or arterial PO_2) by increasing the secretion of erythropoietin. The subsequent actions of erythropoietin on marrow erythropoiesis would then help to correct the deficit in the O_2 content of blood. Interruption of the erythropoietin regulatory system is considered one of the major mechanisms for ICU-acquired anemia (12).

Inflammation and Anemia

Inflammatory cytokines (e.g., tumor necrosis factor) have several effects that can promote anemia, including inhibition of erythropoietin release from the kidneys, reduced marrow responsiveness to erythropoietin, iron sequestration in macrophages, and increased destruction of RBCs (12,13). The anemia associated with inflammation has the same characteristics as the *anemia of chronic disease*: i.e., a decrease in iron, total iron binding capacity, and transferrin levels in plasma, combined with increased ferritin levels in plasma and iron sequestration in reticuloendothelial cells. This is the most common pattern observed in the anemia that develops in ICU patients, so inflammatory cytokines are believed to play a major role in ICU-acquired anemia.

Phlebotomy and Anemia

The volume of blood withdrawn from ICU patients to perform laboratory tests averages 40 mL to 70 mL daily (14,15). Cumulative increases in this phlebotomy volume can reach 500 mL (1 unit of whole blood) after one week, and this volume can augment the severity of anemia from other causes (by removing iron that is needed for erythrocyte production), or can itself become a source of anemia if allowed to continue.

The daily phlebotomy volume is at least 4 times higher in ICU patients than in other hospitalized patients (14), and the difference is not entirely due to increased diagnostic testing in ICU patients. Blood samples for laboratory analysis are usually withdrawn through indwelling vascular catheters, and the initial aliquot of blood (usually 5 mL) withdrawn through the catheter is discarded because it contains fluid from the catheter lumen instead of the bloodstream. Returning the initial aliquot of blood to the patient (using a closed system) reduced the total phlebotomy volume by 50% in one study (16). Of course, decreasing the number of laboratory tests performed daily is always the better choice.

Anemia and Oxygen Transport

The uptake of oxygen into peripheral tissues (VO_2) is described in Chapter 2 using the equation shown below (where Q is cardiac output, Hb is hemoglobin concentration in blood, and $SaO_2 - SvO_2$ is the arteriovenous oxyhemoglobin saturation difference).

$$VO_2 = Q \times 13.4 \times Hb \times (SaO_2 - SvO_2) \tag{36.1}$$

The oxygen transport system operates to maintain a constant VO_2 in the face of changes in any of the variables in Equation 36.1. In the case of anemia, VO_2 remains constant because the decrease in hemoglobin (Hb) is accompanied by increases in both cardiac output (Q) and peripheral O_2 extraction ($SaO_2 - SvO_2$). These compensatory responses to anemia are described next.

Cardiac Output

The influence of anemia on circulatory blood flow is described at the end of Chapter 1. The hematocrit is the principal determinant of blood viscosity (see Table 1.2 in Chapter 1), and thus a decrease in hematocrit will decrease the viscosity of blood. According to the Hagen–Poiseuille equation shown below, a decrease in viscosity (μ) will result in an increase in circulatory blood flow (Q) as long as the pressure gradient along the circulation (ΔP) and the dimensions of the blood vessels (r for radius and L for length) remain constant. (This equation is described in detail in Chapter 1.)

$$Q = \Delta P \times \frac{\pi r^4}{8\mu L} \tag{36.2}$$

A decrease in blood viscosity augments cardiac stroke output by reducing ventricular afterload.

Anemia can also be accompanied by activation of the sympathetic nervous system (4,12), which will augment cardiac output by increases in both myocardial contractility and heart rate. However, this response is not prominent, and thus **tachycardia is not a prominent finding in anemia** (at least at rest) (4).

When considering the isolated effects of anemia on cardiac output, the blood volume should be normal or unchanged (this condition is referred to as *isovolemic anemia*). The changes in cardiac output associated with progressive, isovolemic anemia are shown in Figure 1.8 (Chapter 1). Note that the increase in cardiac output is proportionally much greater than the decrease in hematocrit. This response is attributed to the flow-dependency of blood viscosity; i.e., an increase in blood flow (cardiac output) will decrease blood viscosity. Thus, anemia decreases blood viscosity, which then increases cardiac output, which then decreases blood viscosity, and so on. Ketchup is another fluid with a flow-dependent viscosity, so if you can picture what happens when you pour ketchup (the flow is sluggish at first, then increases as you continue to pour), you will get the idea. Blood viscosity is described at the end of Chapter 1.

In addition to the global changes in cardiac output, anemia can preferentially increase flow in the cardiac and cerebral circulations, and decrease flow in the splanchnic circulation (5). This will have a protective effect on myocardial and cerebral metabolism in the presence of anemia.

Peripheral Oxygen Extraction

The effects of progressive isovolemic anemia on systemic oxygen transport is summarized in the graphs in Figure 36.3 (17). The initial decrease in hematocrit is accompanied by a decrease in systemic oxygen delivery (DO_2), and this is counterbalanced by an increase in O_2 extraction ($SaO_2 - SvO_2$). The reciprocal changes in DO_2 and O_2 extraction keep the VO_2 constant ($VO_2 = DO_2 \times O_2$ extraction). However, when the hematocrit falls below 10%, the increase in O_2 extraction is no longer able to match the decreasing DO_2, and the VO_2 begins to fall. The decrease in VO_2 is a sign of dysoxia (defined in Chapter 2 as oxygen-limited aerobic metabolism), and is accompanied by an increase in lactate production. The point at which the VO_2 begins to fall is thus the threshold for tissue dysoxia, and it usually occurs when the O_2 extraction reaches a maximum level of 50 to 60%. This means that an O_2 extraction ($SaO_2 - SvO_2$) that is 50% or higher is a sign of inadequate tissue oxygenation.

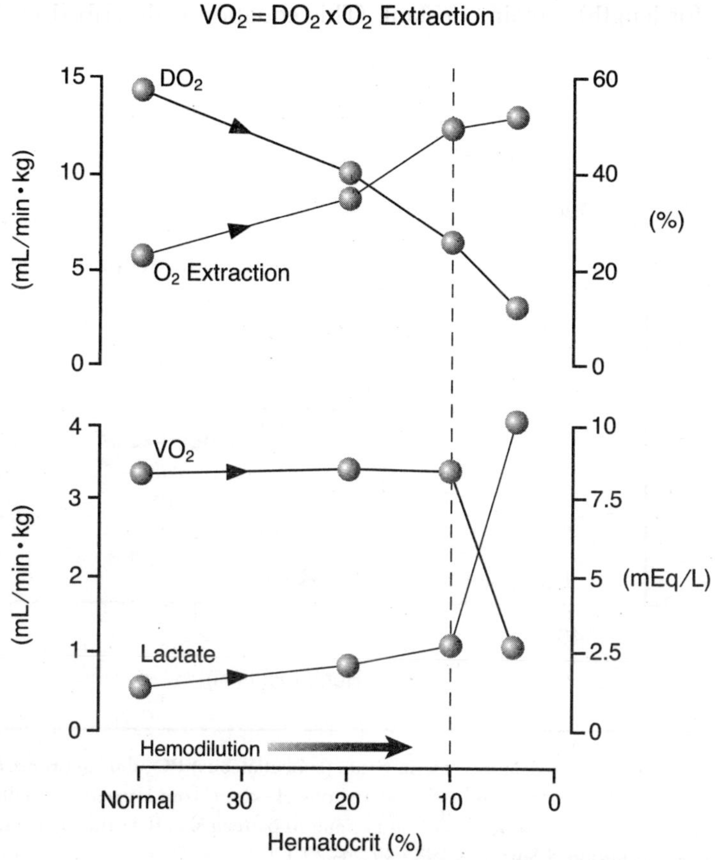

FIGURE 36.3 The effects of progressive isovolemic anemia on oxygen delivery (DO_2), oxygen extraction ratio (O_2ER), oxygen uptake (VO_2), and blood lactate levels in experimental animals. (From Wilkerson DK, Rosen AL, Gould SA, et al. Oxygen extraction ratio: a valid indicator of myocardial metabolism in anemia. J Surg Res 1987;42:629–634.)

Thus, because of the compensatory changes in cardiac output and peripheral O_2 extraction, progressive anemia will not impair tissue oxygenation until the hemoglobin and hematocrit reach dangerously low levels. In the results of the animal study shown in Figure 36.3, the hematocrit had to fall below 10% (corresponding to a hemoglobin concentration of 3 g/dL) before tissue oxygenation was compromised. The experimental animals in this study were anesthetized and breathing pure oxygen (which could favor tolerance to severe anemia), but similar results have been reported in awake animals breathing room air (18). The lowest hemoglobin or hematocrit that is capable of supporting tissue oxygenation in humans in not known, but one study of isovolemic anemia in healthy adults showed that hemoglobin levels of 5 g/dL had no deleterious effects on tissue oxygenation (19).

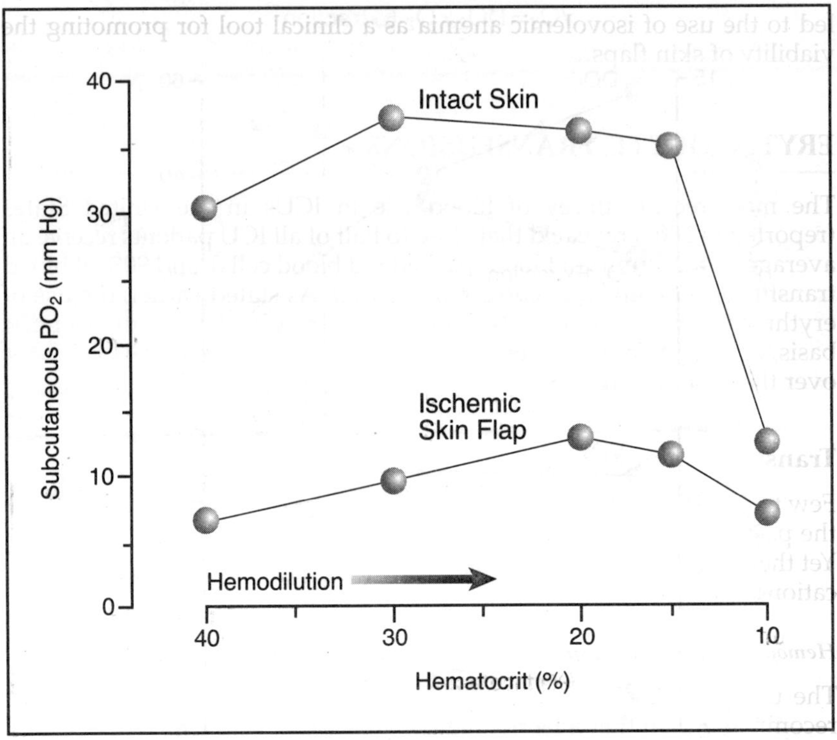

FIGURE 36.4 Paradoxical increase in tissue (subcutaneous) PO_2 during progressive isovolemic anemia in normal and ischemic regions of skin. (From Hansen ES, Gellett S, Kirkegard L, et al. Tissue oxygen tension in random pattern skin flaps during normovolemic hemodilution. J Surg Res 1989;47:24–29.)

Paradoxical Effect

Isovolemic anemia can have a paradoxical effect that *increases* tissue oxygenation. This is shown in Figure 36.4, which is from an animal study that evaluated the effects of isovolemic anemia on skin flaps using a specialized oxygen electrode to measure the PO_2 in subcutaneous tissues below the skin. (20). As indicated in the graph, reductions in hematocrit were associated with increases in the subcutaneous PO_2 in both normal and ischemic skin regions. Furthermore, the increase in tissue PO_2 persisted until the hematocrit fell to 10 to 15% (which is about the same hematocrit where tissue oxygenation became compromised in the study shown in Fig. 36.3).

The improvement in tissue oxygenation shown in Figure 36.4 can be explained if the cardiac output response to anemia is so exaggerated that the oxygen delivery increases despite the decrease in serum hemoglobin. Anemia can preferentially increase flow in certain regional circulations, as mentioned earlier, and the skin may be one of these regions. In fact, the beneficial effects of isovolemic anemia on blood flow to the skin has led to the use of isovolemic anemia as a clinical tool for promoting the viability of skin flaps.

ERYTHROCYTE TRANSFUSIONS

The most recent survey of blood use in ICUs in the United States (reported in 2004) revealed that close to half of all ICU patients receive an average of 4 to 5 units of blood (packed red blood cells), and 90% of blood transfusions are given to correct anemia (2). As stated earlier, the use of erythrocyte transfusions in the ICU is arbitrary and without scientific basis, and the survey just mentioned found no change in this behavior over the past decade.

Transfusion Triggers

Few topics in critical care medicine have received as much attention over the past decade as the use of erythrocyte transfusions to correct anemia. Yet there continues to be no standardized or even appropriate set of indications for these transfusions.

Hemoglobin: Popular but Inappropriate

The use of hemoglobin as a *transfusion trigger* began in 1942 with the recommendation that a hemoglobin of 10 g/dL be used as an indication for erythrocyte transfusions (21). This continues to be the most popular transfusion trigger today. Two clinical trials have shown that a lower hemoglobin of 7 g/dL is safe in most patients (except those with acute myocardial infarction and unstable angina) and also reduces the number of RBC transfusions (22,23). The lower hemoglobin level of 7 g/dL is gaining popularity as a transfusion trigger for all patients who do not have active coronary artery disease, but a recent survey showed that only 25% of RBC transfusions are based on the lower hemoglobin threshold of 7 g/dL (2). This threshold can probably be reduced further because a previously mentioned study has shown that acute isovolemic anemia with hemoglobin levels of 5 g/dL is well tolerated and without adverse consequences (19). This study was conducted in healthy adults, and needs to be repeated using ICU patients as subjects.

The popularity of the hemoglobin level as a transfusion trigger is disturbing because this measurement provides absolutely no information about the state of tissue oxygenation. In fact, according to Figure 36.4, a low serum hemoglobin could be a sign of improved tissue oxygenation in some situations! Furthermore, as mentioned earlier, the hemoglobin is not even an accurate measure of anemia in critically ill patients. An example of the folly of the hemoglobin as a transfusion trigger is shown in the example below.

> A patient is admitted to the ICU with a severe pneumonia and a hemoglobin of 11 g/dL. One week later, when the patient is improved and ready for transfer to the medical floor, the hemoglobin is noted to

be 7 g/dL. There has been no evidence of bleeding, but the patient's weight has increased from 170 to 185 lbs. Does this patient need a blood transfusion?

(I will let you answer the question yourself.) Two practice guidelines published about 15 to 20 years ago recommended abandoning the hemoglobin as a transfusion trigger and adopting more physiologic measures of tissue oxygenation (24,25). Instead of abandoning the hemoglobin, physicians have abandoned the recommendation!

O_2 Extraction: A Better Transfusion Trigger

The graphs in Figure 36.3 (and also in Figs. 2.4 and 11.4) show that the peripheral O_2 extraction, which is equivalent to the (SaO_2 − SvO_2), increases to a maximum level of about 50% in response to a decrease in O_2 delivery (e.g., from anemia), and thus this maximum level of O_2 extraction is a sign of impending or actual tissue dysoxia. This means that **an O_2 extraction, or (SaO_2 − SvO_2), that is 50% or higher can be used as a transfusion trigger** (17,26) because it identifies the threshold for impaired tissue oxygenation. Oxygen extraction can be monitored continuously in the ICU by using pulse oximetry (for arterial O_2 saturation) combined with venous oximetry (for venous O_2 saturation), as described in Chapter 20.

Monitoring the Effects of Erythrocyte Transfusions

The standard end-point of RBC transfusions is an increase in hemoglobin and hematocrit, but these are inappropriate because they provide no information about oxygen transport or tissue oxygenation. The appropriate end-points are an increase in both O_2 delivery and O_2 uptake into tissues.

Cardiac Output

Just as anemia can increase the cardiac output by reducing blood viscosity, infusing red blood cells to increase hematocrit can reduce the cardiac output by increasing blood viscosity (27). The decrease in cardiac output can cancel the benefit of an increased hemoglobin on oxygen transport.

Systemic Oxygenation

Erythrocyte transfusions have a variable effect on systemic oxygenation (28–30). This is demonstrated in Figure 36.5. Each line in this graph shows the effects of erythrocyte transfusions on the hemoglobin concentration and systemic oxygen uptake (VO_2) in individual postoperative patients. The number of units of packed cells transfused in each patient is indicated by the numbers intersecting each line in the graph. Of the six patients who were transfused, all showed an increase in hemoglobin concentration, but only three patients showed an increase in VO_2, while three patients showed a decrease in VO_2. This graph demonstrates that an increase in hemoglobin concentration after erythrocyte transfusions does not necessarily indicate that tissue oxygenation has also improved.

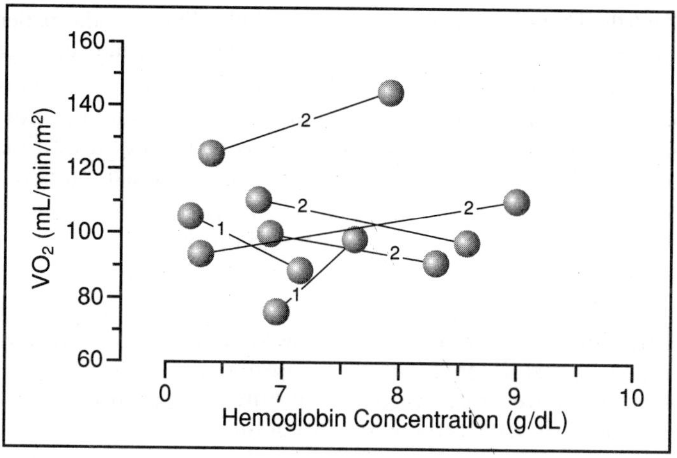

FIGURE 36.5 The effects of erythrocyte transfusions on hemoglobin levels and systemic oxygen uptake (VO_2) in postoperative patients with isovolemic anemia. Each line on the graph represents the changes recorded in a single patient. The numbers that transect each line represent the units of RBCs transfused in each case. (Data from personal observations.)

Erythrocyte Products

All blood products containing erythrocytes are stored at 4°C using a liquid anticoagulant preservative that contains citrate, phosphate, and dextrose (CPD). The citrate binds ionized calcium and acts as an anticoagulant. The phosphate helps retard the breakdown of 2,3-diphosphoglycerate, and the dextrose serves as a fuel source for the erythrocytes. Erythrocytes stored in CPD at 4°C are viable for at least 21 days (10).

Whole Blood

A unit of whole blood contains an average of 510 mL (blood plus CPD solution) (31). Most blood banks will store whole blood only on request. Otherwise, the blood is fractionated into erythrocyte and plasma fractions within a few hours of collection. The separation of whole blood into its component fractions allows more efficient use of blood products to achieve specific transfusion goals.

Packed Red Cells

Erythrocyte concentrates, or *packed red cells,* are prepared by centrifuging whole blood and removing 250 mL of the plasma supernatant (20). Each unit of packed cells contains approximately 200 mL of cells (mostly erythrocytes) and 50 to 100 mL of plasma and CPD solution. The hematocrit is usually between 60 and 80%, and the hemoglobin concentration is between 23 and 27 g/dL (10).

Leukocyte-Poor Red Cells

Removal of the leukocytes in packed red cells is recommended when transfusing patients with a history of febrile, nonhemolytic transfusion reactions (which are caused by antibodies to leukocytes in donor blood) (31). The leukocytes can be separated by centrifugation or filters, but separation is never complete and up to 30% of the leukocytes remain in the sample.

Washed Red Cells

Packed cells can be washed with isotonic saline to remove leukocytes and residual plasma. The removal of plasma helps prevent allergic reactions caused by prior sensitization to plasma proteins in donor blood. Washed red cells are therefore used for transfusing patients with a history of hypersensitivity transfusion reactions.

Infusing Erythrocyte Products

A standard infusion system for transfusing erythrocyte products is shown in Figure 36.6. Each of the numbered components in the system is described briefly in the following paragraphs.

Pressurized Infusions

The gravity-driven flow of whole blood and packed cells is shown in Table 36.2 (32). Because these flow rates do not approach the 250 mL/min or greater flow rates needed for the resuscitation of trauma victims, pressure-generating devices are used to speed infusion rates. The most common device used for this purpose is a standard blood pressure cuff that is wrapped around the collapsible plastic blood containers. When the cuff is inflated to a pressure of 200 mm Hg, the infusion rate of whole blood and packed cells increases approximately threefold, as shown in Table 36.2. Manual hand pumps are also available for increasing infusion rates. These hand pumps are not as effective as the blood pressure cuff (at 200 mm Hg) for infusing whole blood but are equivalent to the pressure cuffs for infusing packed cells (Table 36.2).

Saline Dilution

Packed cells infuse at approximately one-third the rate of whole blood. Special Y-configured tubing in blood infusion sets allows packed cells to be diluted with an equal volume of isotonic saline. When this is done, the infusion rate of packed cells is comparable to that of whole blood. Only isotonic saline should be used as a diluent for packed red cells. Ringer's solutions are not advised for diluting erythrocyte products because the calcium in Ringer's solutions can promote clotting in the blood sample (33).

Blood Filters

Erythrocyte products are infused through filters that trap small clots and other cellular debris (e.g., decomposed platelets and fibrin-coated

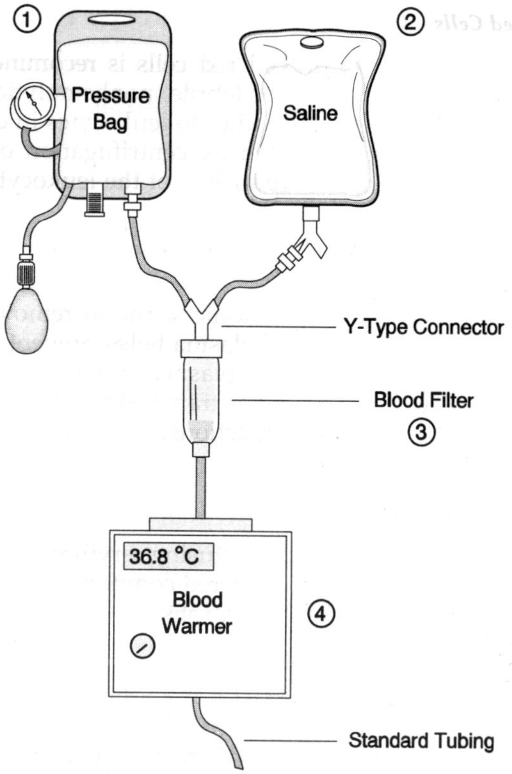

FIGURE 36.6 An infusion system for transfusing erythrocyte products. Each of the numbered components is described in the text.

leukocytes). These filters can become an impediment to flow as they collect trapped debris, and thus they should be replaced periodically (e.g., after every 4 units of blood). The standard filters have a pore size of 170 to 260 microns (23), which allows small fibrin microaggregates to pass freely. These microaggregates can become lodged in the pulmonary capillaries and create abnormalities in gas exchange. Smaller microaggregate filters are available, but their value in preventing pulmonary complications has not been proven (34).

Blood Warmers

Warming reduces the viscosity of refrigerated blood and can increase infusion rates by 30 to 50% (see footnote in Table 36.2). However, the major value of warming blood is considered to be the prevention of hypothermia from rapid transfusions (when 1 unit of blood is transfused every 5 to 10 minutes) (35). The recommended temperature for infused blood is 33° to 35° C (35). Temperatures of 37° C or higher can promote hemolysis.

A simple method for warming blood is to immerse the blood storage bags in hot water before transfusion. However, this rewarming method can take up to 30 minutes, and can produce hemolysis from overheating.

TABLE 36.2 Pressurized Infusion of Erythrocyte Products

Fluid	Catheter Size	Infusion Rate (mL/min)* Gravity Flow	Hand Pump	Pressure Cuff (200 mm Hg)
Tap water	16-gauge 2" length	100	180	285
Whole blood	↓	65	125	185
Packed cells	↓	20	80	70

*Infusion rates for fluids at room temperature. Refrigerated blood products infuse at 30 to 50% slower rates.
Data from Dula DJ et al. Flow rate variance of commonly used IV infusion techniques. J Trauma 1981;21:480–482.

Controlled warming devices that can warm blood to the desired infusion temperatures at flow rates slightly in excess of 100 mL/minute are available (36). However, at the infusion rates often used to resuscitate trauma victims (i.e., greater than 250 mL/minute), blood warming devices are often unable to warm blood to the desired temperature (36).

ADVERSE EFFECTS OF ERYTHROCYTE TRANSFUSIONS

Complications are reported in 2 to 4% of erythrocyte transfusions (2,37). The most notable of these are listed in Table 36.3, along with the frequency of each expressed in relation to the number of units transfused. Note that transfusion errors are much more frequent than transmission of HIV and other infections. The following is a brief description of the acute transfusion reactions (37–41).

TABLE 36.3 Adverse Events Associated with RBC Transfusions (per units transfused)

Immune Reactions	Other Risks
Acute hemolytic reaction (1 per 35,000)	**Infections**
Fatal hemolytic reaction (1 per million)	Bacterial (1 per 500,000)
Acute lung injury (1 per 5,000)	Hepatitis B virus (1 per 220,000)
Allergic reactions	Hepatitis C virus (1 per 1.6 million)
Urticaria (1 per 100)	HIV (1 per 1.9 million)
Anaphylaxis (1 per 1,000)	**Transfusion Errors**
Anaphylactic shock (1 per 50,000)	Wrong person transfused (1 per 15,000)
Non-hemolytic fever (1 per 200)	Incompatable transfusion (1 per 33,000)

From References 37–39.

Acute Hemolytic Reactions

Acute hemolytic reactions are caused by transfusion of ABO-incompatible RBCs, and are usually the result of human error. Fortunately, they are uncommon, and rarely fatal (one fatality per million units transfused). These reactions are the result of antibodies in the recipient binding to ABO surface antigens on donor RBCs. The ensuing lysis of donor RBCs is rapid, and incites a systemic inflammatory response that can be accompanied by hypotension and multiorgan failure.

Clinical Manifestations

Symptoms can appear after infusion of only 5 mL of donor blood (37), and include fever, dyspnea, chest pain, and low back pain. Hypotension can develop suddenly, and may be the only sign of a hemolytic reaction in comatose patients. Severe reactions are accompanied by a consumptive coagulopathy and progressive multiorgan dysfunction.

Bedside Approach

The following approach is recommended for any patient who develops a fever soon after the start of a blood transfusion.

1. ***Stop*** the transfusion immediately. This is imperative because the morbidity and mortality in hemolytic reactions is a function of the volume of incompatible blood transfused (37).
2. Check the blood pressure immediately. If the pressure is dropping, do the following:
   a. Infuse volume (colloids may be preferred because of their ability to rapidly expand the vascular volume).
   b. Start dopamine (at 5 µg/kg/minute). This agent has been preferred for its renal vasodilating effects because renal failure is a poor prognostic sign in hemolytic transfusion reactions (29). However, the relative benefits of dopamine over other pressor agents is unproven.

Once the patient is stabilized, do the following:

3. Obtain a blood sample and inspect the plasma for the pink-to-red hue of hemoglobin.
4. Obtain a freshly voided urine specimen and perform a dipstick test for blood.
5. Send a blood sample for a direct Coomb's test. A positive test confirms a hemolytic transfusion reaction. However, a negative test is possible if most of the donor erythrocytes have already lysed.

Febrile Nonhemolytic Reactions

Fever that is not related to an acute hemolytic reaction occurs in only 0.5% of RBC transfusions (or once per 200 units transfused) (38). This reaction is the result of antibodies in the recipient to leukocytes in donor blood. The antileukocyte antibodies are produced in response to prior transfusions or prior pregnancies, so this type of response is often seen in multiparous women or in patients with a history of prior transfusions. Fever is more of a problem with platelet transfusions, where the incidence of fever is as high as 30% (38).

Clinical Manifestations

The fever usually appears 1 to 6 hours after starting the transfusion (later than the onset of fever associated with hemolytic transfusion reactions), and it is not usually accompanied by signs of systemic illness. However, severe reactions can occur, and patients can have a toxic appearance.

Bedside Approach

The approach to this fever is the same as outlined for hemolytic transfusion reactions, although the transfusion may be completed before the fever appears. The diagnosis of a nonhemolytic febrile reaction is confirmed by excluding the presence of hemolysis with the tests described previously. Bacterial contamination of RBC products is rare (one per 500,000 units), and is much more common in platelet transfusions (one per 2,000 units) (38). The need for routine cultures of donor and recipient blood is usually dictated by local blood bank policies. Many blood banks require cultures for all febrile reactions accompanied by other signs of systemic illness (e.g., rigors, dyspnea). The organism most often isolated in RBC products is *Yersinia enterocolitica,* and transfusions contaminated with this organism are fatal in 60% of cases (38).

Future Transfusions

More than 75% of patients with a nonhemolytic febrile transfusion reaction will not experience a similar reaction during subsequent blood transfusions (38). Therefore, no special precautions are necessary for future transfusions. If a second febrile reaction develops, leukocyte-poor red cell preparations are advised for all further erythrocyte transfusions.

Allergic Reactions

The most common hypersensitivity reaction is urticaria, which is reported in one of every 100 units transfused (39). More severe anaphylactic reactions (e.g., wheezing) are much less common, and anaphylactic shock is rare (1 per 50,000 units) (39). These reactions are the sensitization to plasma proteins in prior transfusions. Patients with IgA deficiency are particularly prone to hypersensitivity reactions, and they do not require prior exposure to plasma products.

Clinical Manifestations

The usual manifestation is mild urticaria that appears during the transfusion and is not accompanied by fever. The sudden onset of wheezing is a clue for anaphylaxis, and sudden hypotension (which is rare) can be mistaken for an acute hemolytic reaction.

Bedside Approach

Mild urticaria without fever does not require interruption of the transfusion. However, the common practice is to stop the transfusion temporarily and administer antihistamines (diphenhydramine, 25 to 50 mg orally or intramuscularly every 6 hours). This practice might provide some symptomatic relief, but is otherwise useless. Transfusion-related anaphylaxis should be managed as described in Chapter 40. Patients who develop anaphylaxis should be tested for an underlying IgA deficiency.

Future Transfusions

Future transfusions should be avoided if possible for all cases of transfusion-associated anaphylaxis. For less severe allergic reactions, washed red cell preparations (plasma removed) are advised for subsequent transfusions. Antihistamine premedication is a popular but unproven practice.

Acute Lung Injury

Transfusion-associated acute lung injury (TRALI) is an inflammatory lung injury that is first apparent during or within 6 hours after the start of transfusion (40). The reported incidence is 1 per 5,000 transfusions (38). The prevailing theory is that antileukocyte antibodies in donor blood bind to circulating granulocytes in the recipient and promote leukocyte sequestration in the pulmonary microcirculation (41). This leads to granulocyte-mediated lung injury, which presents as acute respiratory distress syndrome (ARDS). Although this form of lung injury is fatal in fewer than 10% of patients (40), it is considered the leading cause of death from blood transfusions (37,38).

Clinical Manifestations

Signs of respiratory compromise (dyspnea, hypoxemia) begin to develop during or within a few hours after the transfusion begins. Fever is common, and hypotension has been reported. The chest x-ray film eventually shows diffuse pulmonary infiltrates, and intubation with mechanical ventilation is often necessary. Although the acute syndrome can be severe, the process usually resolves within a week.

Bedside Approach

The transfusion should be stopped (if still running) at the first signs of respiratory compromise. Distinguishing TRALI from hydrostatic pulmonary edema is often mentioned, but this is not necessary because **RBC transfusions are a viscous load, not a fluid load, and they do not produce hydrostatic pulmonary edema** (the RBCs can't get out of the pulmonary capillaries!). Even when combined with an equal volume of isotonic saline, the total volume of exchangeable fluid that is infused (250 mL) is not enough to produce hydrostatic pulmonary edema.

Therefore, what appears to be pulmonary edema shortly after a blood transfusion is ARDS, and the management is similar to that described for ARDS in Chapter 22.

Future Transfusions

There are no firm recommendations regarding future transfusions in patients who develop TRALI. Some recommend using washed RBCs to remove antibodies from the preparation, but the efficacy of this measure is not known.

Transfusion-Associated Immunomodulation

Patients who receive blood transfusions have an increased incidence of nosocomial infections (41), and this, combined with the observation that blood transfusions improve the survival of renal allografts, has led to the proposal that blood transfusions promote immunosuppression in the recipient. The mechanisms for this effect are not known, but one possibility is that antigenic substances or leukocytes in transfused blood persist in the recipient and induce a down-regulation of the recipient's immune system. Removing leukocytes from RBC products is one consideration, but universal leukoreduction for RBC preparations is not currently practiced. Until this problem is resolved, the increased risk of infection associated with RBC transfusions is reason to avoid transfusions whenever possible.

BLOOD CONSERVATION IN THE ICU

A variety of blood conservation strategies have been proposed, but only a few can be applied to patient care in the ICU.

Postoperative Blood Salvage

For surgical procedures involving median sternotomy (such as coronary artery bypass surgery), blood collected from mediastinal drainage tubes can be reinfused (42). Chest tube drainage from the mediastinum is passed through a filter at the bedside to trap large clots and cellular debris, and the filtered blood is then reinfused. Because the blood has undergone endogenous defibrination in the chest, no anticoagulants need to be added. Traumatic disruption of cells is common, and the hematocrit of the reinfused blood is only 15 to 25%. This low hematocrit may explain why reinfusion of shed mediastinal blood does not always reduce the number of homologous transfusions (43).

Erythropoietin

Because the anemia that develops in ICU patients is associated with reduced levels of circulating erythropoietin (as described earlier), exogenously administered erythropoietin has been evaluated as a possible means of reducing RBC transfusions in the ICU. About seven clinical studies have been reported (44), and each shows that patients who receive erythropoietin require fewer RBC transfusions (a subcutaneous dose of 40,000 units once weekly is adequate, and the effects can take 3 weeks to become evident). However, none of the studies have proven that the decreased transfusion requirements from erythropoietin are associated with fewer adverse events or better outcomes. Furthermore, the cost of erythropoietin is a concern: in one analysis, the estimated cost of erythropoietin therapy to prevent one transfusion-related adverse event was $5 million, and the cost of preventing one transfusion-related death was more than $25 million (44). At these prices, erythropoietin will have to do a lot better before it is embraced in the ICU.

A FINAL WORD

The single most important point to remember from this chapter is that anemia is well tolerated as long as intravascular volume is maintained. When blood volume is normal, hemoglobin levels have to drop to 3 g/dL to demonstrate evidence of impaired tissue oxygenation. What this means to me is that cardiac output is more important for tissue oxygenation than the hemoglobin level in blood. The importance of cardiac output over hemoglobin is evident when you consider that hypovolemic shock and cardiogenic shock are recognized entities, while "anemic shock" is not. Since shock is a condition of impaired tissue oxygenation, the fact that anemia is not a recognized cause of shock is proof that anemia does not impair tissue oxygenation (at least not until the anemia reaches dangerously low levels). If this is the case, then most RBC transfusions to correct anemia will not improve tissue oxygenation (and thus are not warranted).

The second point that deserves emphasis is the nonvalue of the hemoglobin for assessing transfusion needs. A better measurement for evaluating systemic oxygenation is the peripheral O_2 extraction, which can be measured as the (SaO_2 − SvO_2) difference. All you need is an indwelling central venous catheter to measure SvO_2, and a pulse oximeter to measure SaO_2. When the (SaO_2 − SvO_2) approaches 50%, and there is no reason to suspect a low cardiac output (which can also increase peripheral O_2 extraction), then transfusion of RBCs is a reasonable consideration.

REFERENCES

Introduction

1. Vincent JL, Baron J-F, Reinhart K, et al. Anemia and blood transfusion in critically ill patients. JAMA 2002;288:1499–1507.
2. Corwin HL, Gettinger A, Pearl R, et al. The CRIT study: anemia and blood transfusion in the critically ill: current clinical practice in the United States. Crit Care Med 2004;32:39–52.

Reviews

3. Ward NS, Levy MM. Blood transfusion practice today. Crit Care Clin 2004; 20:179–186.
4. Hebert PC, Van der Linden P, Biro G, et al. Physiologic aspects of anemia. Crit Care Clin 2004;20:187–212.
5. Hebert PC, McDonald BJ, Tinmouth A. Clinical consequences of anemia and red cell transfusion in the critically ill. Crit Care Clin 2004;20:225–235.
6. Kuriyan M, Carson JL. Blood transfusion risks in the intensive care unit. Crit Care Clin 2004;20:237–253.

Anemia in the ICU

7. Jacob G, Raj SR, Ketch T, et al. Postural pseudoanemia: posture-dependent change in hematocrit. Mayo Clin Proc 2005;80:611–614.
8. Jones JG, Holland BM, Wardrop CAJ. Total circulating red cells versus hematocrit as a primary descriptor of oxygen transport by the blood. Br J Haematol 1990; 76:228–232.
9. Cordts PR, LaMorte WW, Fisher JB, et al. Poor predictive value of hematocrit and hemodynamic parameters for erythrocyte deficits after extensive elective vascular operations. Surg Gynecol Obstet 1992;175:243–248.
10. Walker RH (ed). American Association of Blood Banks technical manual. 10th ed. Arlington, VA: American Association of Blood Banks, 1990:37–58, 635–637, 649–651.
11. Finch CA. Red cell manual. 6th ed. Philadelphia: FA Davis, 1994:30–38.
12. Shander A. Anemia in the critically ill. Crit Care Clin 2004;20:159–178.
13. Stubbs JR. Alternatives to blood product transfusion in the critically ill: erythropoietin. Crit Care Med 2006;34(suppl):S160–S169.
14. Smoller BR, Kruskall MS. Phlebotomy for diagnostic laboratory tests in adults: pattern of use and effect on transfusion requirements. N Engl J Med 1986;314:1233–1235.
15. Corwin HL, Parsonnet KC, Gettinger A, et al. RBC transfusion in the ICU: is there a reason? Chest 1995;108:767–771.
16. Silver MJ, Li Y-H, Gragg LA, et al. Reduction of blood loss from diagnostic sampling in critically ill patients using a blood-conserving arterial line system. Chest 1993;104:1711–1715.
17. Wilkerson DK, Rosen AL, Gould SA, et al. Oxygen extraction ratio: a valid indicator of myocardial metabolism in anemia. J Surg Res 1987;42:629–634.
18. Levine E, Rosen A, Sehgal L, et al. Physiologic effects of acute anemia: implications for a reduced transfusion trigger. Transfusion 1990;30:11–14.
19. Weiskopf RB, Viele M, Feiner J, et al. Human cardiovascular and metabolic response to acute, severe, isovolemic anemia. JAMA 1998;279:217–221.
20. Hansen ES, Gellett S, Kirkegard L, et al. Tissue oxygen tension in random pattern skin flaps during normovolemic hemodilution. J Surg Res 1989; 47:24–29.

Erythrocyte Transfusions

21. Adam RC, Lundy JS. Anesthesia in cases of poor risk: some suggestions for decreasing the risk. Surg Gynecol Obstet 1942:74:1011–1101.

22. Hebert PC, Wells G, Blajchman MA, et al. A multicenter, randomized, controlled clinical trial of transfusion requirements in critical care. N Engl J Med 1999; 340:409–417.
23. Hebert PC, Yetisir E, Martin C, et al. Is a low transfusion threshold safe in critically ill patients with cardiovascular disease? Crit Care Med 2001;29: 227–234.
24. Consensus Conference on Perioperative Red Blood Cell Transfusion. JAMA 1988;260:2700–2702.
25. American College of Physicians. Practice strategies for elective red blood cell transfusion: a clinical practice guideline from the American College of Physicians. Ann Intern Med 1992;116:403–406.
26. Levy PS, Chavez RP, Crystal GJ, et al. Oxygen extraction ratio: a valid indicator of transfusion need in limited coronary vascular reserve? J Trauma 1992;32:769–774.
27. Shah DM, Gottlieb M, Rahm R, et al. Failure of red cell transfusions to increase oxygen transport or mixed venous PO_2 in injured patients. J Trauma 1982; 22:741–746.
28. Silverman H, Tuma P. Gastric tonometry in patients with sepsis: effects of dobutamine and packed red cell transfusions. Chest 1992;102:184–188.
29. Marik PE, Sibbald W. Effect of stored-blood transfusion on oxygen delivery in patients with sepsis. JAMA 1993;269:3024–3029.
30. Robbins JM, Keating K, Orlando R, et al. Effects of blood transfusion on oxygen delivery and consumption in critically ill surgical patients. Contemp Surg 1993;43:281–285.
31. Davies SC. Transfusion of red cells. In: Contreras M, ed. ABCs of transfusion. London: British Medical Journal, 1990:9–13.
32. Dula DJ, Muller A, Donovan SW. Flow rate variance of commonly used IV infusion techniques. J Trauma 1981;21:480–482.
33. Blood Transfusion Practice. In: American Association of Blood Banks technical manual. 10th ed. Arlington, VA: American Association of Blood Banks, 1990:341–375.
34. Kruskall MS, Bergen JJ, Klein HG, et al. Transfusion therapy in emergency medicine. Ann Emerg Med 1988;17:327–335.
35. Iserson KV, Huestis DW. Blood warming: current applications and techniques. Transfusion 1991;31:558–571.
36. Uhl L, Pacini D, Kruskall MS. A comparative study of blood warmer performance. Anesthesiology 1992;77:1022–1028.
37. Kuriyan M, Carson JL. Blood transfusion risks in the intensive care unit. Crit Care Clin 2004;20:237–253.
38. Goodnough LT. Risks of blood transfusion. Crit Care Med 2003;31:S678–S686.
39. Greenberger PA. Plasma anaphylaxis and immediate-type reactions. In: Rossi EC, Simon TL, Moss GS, eds. Principles of transfusion medicine. Philadelphia: Williams & Wilkins, 1991:635–639.
40. Moore SB. Transfusion-related acute lung injury (TRALI): clinical presentation, treatment, and prognosis. Crit Care Med 2006;34(suppl):S114–S117.
41. Curtis BR, McFarland JG. Mechanisms of transfusion-related acute lung injury (TRALI): anti-leukocyte antibodies. Crit Care Med 2006;34(suppl):S118–S123.

42. Vamvakas EC. Pneumonia as a complication of blood product transfusion in the critically ill: transfusion-related immunomodulation (TRM). Crit Care Med 2006;34(suppl):S151–S159.

Blood Conservation in the ICU

43. Ward HB, Smith RR, Landis KP, et al. Prospective, randomized trial of autotransfusion after routine cardiac operations. Ann Thorac Surg 1993;56: 137–141.
44. Roberts SR, Early G, Brown B, et al. Autotransfusion of unwashed mediastinal shed blood fails to decrease banked blood requirements in patients undergoing aortocoronary bypass surgery. Am J Surg 1991;162:477–480.
45. Stubbs JR. Alternatives to blood product transfusion in the critically ill: erythropoietin. Crit Care Med 2006;34(suppl):S160–S169.

Chapter 37

PLATELETS IN CRITICAL ILLNESS

Platelet disorders fall into two categories: those characterized by abnormal numbers of circulating platelets and those characterized by abnormal platelet function. This chapter introduces the common causes of both types of platelet disorders in the ICU population. This is followed by a brief description of the indications, methods, and complications of platelet transfusion therapy (1–3).

PLATELETS AND HEMOSTASIS

Platelets are cytoplasmic remnants of megakaryocytes and are not true cells because they have no nucleus and cannot synthesize proteins. The normal adult has an average of 250 billion platelets per liter of blood. Assuming a normal blood volume of 5.5 L, the total number of platelets in the bloodstream is slightly in excess of 1 trillion. Platelets have a normal life span of 10 days, and each day about 45 billion new platelets must be added to each liter of blood to maintain a constant pool of circulating platelets (4).

Thrombosis

When the vascular endothelium is damaged, platelets adhere to exposed collagen in the subendothelium. The platelets then release calcium, and this activates glycoprotein (IIb-IIIa) receptors on the platelet surface (1). These receptors bind irreversibly to von Willebrand factor in the surrounding endothelium, and this anchors the developing platelet plug. The glycoprotein IIb-IIIa receptors also bind fibrinogen, and fibrinogen bridges between platelets result in platelet aggregation. The released calcium also activates the coagulation cascade, and this results in the production of fibrin strands that form an interlacing meshwork with the platelets to produce a thrombus.

Thrombocytopenia

Thrombocytopenia is defined as a platelet count below 150,000/µL (5), but the ability to form a hemostatic plug is retained until the platelet count falls below 100,000/µL. Therefore, thrombocytopenia that is clinically significant corresponds to a platelet count below 100,000/µL. In this range, the bleeding tendency is determined primarily by the presence or absence of a structural lesion that is prone to bleeding. In the absence of such a lesion, platelet counts down to 5000/µL can be tolerated without evidence of bleeding (6).

Pseudothrombocytopenia

Pseudothrombocytopenia is a condition where the anticoagulant EDTA (used in collection tubes for routine blood counts) promotes clumping of platelets in vitro. The clumped platelets are then misread as leukocytes by automated machines that perform cell counts, and this results in a spuriously low platelet count (2). This phenomenon tends to occur in patients who have antiplatelet antibodies that do cause thrombocytopenia in vivo (e.g., cold agglutinins), and it has been reported in as many as 2% of hospitalized patients (7). The diagnosis can be confirmed by observation of platelet clumps on blood smears obtained with EDTA, or by repeating the platelet counts on blood samples collected with sodium citrate as the anticoagulant (2).

Platelet Adhesion

When the ability of platelets to adhere to the subendothelium is diminished (e.g., as in uremia), the risk of hemorrhage can be increased despite platelet counts that exceed 100,000/µL. Defects in platelet adhesion can be detected by a prolonged bleeding time. However, there is no correlation between the bleeding time and the tendency for bleeding from altered platelet adhesion (8), and thus the bleeding time is not a useful test for detecting clinically significant defects in platelet adhesion. The recognition of abnormal platelet adhesion usually involves simple recognition of conditions that alter platelet adhesiveness in individual patients. These conditions are described later in the chapter.

THROMBOCYTOPENIA IN THE ICU

The incidence of clinically significant thrombocytopenia (<100,000/µL) is 13 to 35% in medical and surgical ICUs (9,10), and the most common predisposing conditions are sepsis and disseminated intravascular coagulation (DIC). The causes of thrombocytopenia most likely to be encountered in the ICU are listed in Table 37.1. The conditions you must be aware of are described next.

Heparin-Induced Thrombocytopenia

Heparin can combine with a heparin-binding protein (platelet factor 4) on platelets to form an antigenic complex that induces the formation of IgG antibodies. These antibodies then bind to platelets and form cross-bridges that result in platelet aggregation. If severe enough, this

TABLE 37.1 Causes of Significant Thrombocytopenia in the ICU

Conditions	Drugs*
Systemic sepsis	Acetaminophen
Disseminated intravascular coagulation	Heparin Quinidine
Thrombotic thrombocytopenia purpura	Rifampin
HELLP syndrome	Trimethoprim-sulfamethoxazole

*Includes only drugs reported to cause bleeding or thrombosis. From Reference 2.

process can result in a consumptive thrombocytopenia and clinically apparent thrombosis (11).

Clinical Features

Heparin-induced thrombocytopenia (HIT) typically appears as a 50% or greater reduction in the platelet count that begins 5 to 10 days after the first exposure to heparin (the onset is earlier in patients with a prior exposure to heparin). Five to ten percent of patients with HIT from subcutaneous heparin will develop erythematous lesions surrounding the injection site, and 25% of patients with HIT from intravenous heparin will develop systemic reactions that include fever, chills, tachypnea, tachycardia and shortness of breath (11).

The major complication of HIT is thrombosis, not bleeding. Approximately **75% of cases of HIT are accompanied by symptomatic thrombosis,** including deep vein thrombosis of the lower extremities (50% of cases) and upper extremities (10% of cases), acute pulmonary embolism (25% of cases), arterial thrombosis involving a limb (5 to 10% of cases, thrombotic stroke (3 to 5% of cases), acute myocardial infarction (3 to 5% of cases), and adrenal vein thrombosis with adrenal hemorrhagic necrosis (3% of cases) (11).

Risk Factors

The risk of HIT is greater with unfractionated heparin (UFH) than with low molecular weight heparin (LMWH). The risk of HIT from UFH is greatest following orthopedic surgery (3 to 5%) and cardiac surgery (1 to 3%), while about 1% of medical patients who receive UFH develop HIT (11). The risk of HIT from LMWH is about 1% in orthopedic surgery cases, and is less than 1% in other clinical settings (11).

One of the important features of HIT is the fact that it can appear with very low doses of heparin. This includes **heparin flushes and** the small amounts on **heparin-coated pulmonary artery catheters, which can induce thrombocytopenia** (12).

Diagnosis

The diagnosis of HIT requires a high-probability clinical scenario (e.g., thrombocytopenia that develops 5 to 10 days after starting heparin and is accompanied by symptomatic thrombosis) combined with serologic evidence of IgG antibodies to the heparin-platelet factor 4 complex (13). The antibody assay measures the release of ^{14}C-labeled serotonin from platelets that are added to a sample of the patient's serum. **A positive**

TABLE 37.2 Anticoagulation with Direct Thrombin Inhibitors

	Lepirudin	Argatroban
Clearance	Renal	Hepatic
Prophylactic Dose	0.10 mg/kg/hr IV or 25 mg SC every 12 h.	———
Therapeutic Dose	0.4 mg/kg IV bolus, then 0.15 mg/kg/hr (max wt = 110 kg). Adjust dose to PTT = 1.5–3 × control.	Start at 2 μg/kg/min & adjust dose to PTT = 1.5–3 × control. Max. rate = 10 μg/kg/min.
Dose Adjustments:		
Renal insufficency	See Appendix 4	No dose adjustment
Liver Failure	No dose adjustment	↓ initial dose rate to 0.5 μg/kg/min

From References 14–16.

antibody assay does not secure the diagnosis of HIT because this assay also detects non-pathogenic IgG antibodies to heparin-platelet-factor-4 complex (13). For this reason, the antibody assay must be combined with a suggestive clinical scenario to make the diagnosis of HIT.

Acute Management

When HIT is first suspected heparin exposure must be discontinued. **Remember to discontinue heparin flushes and remove any heparin-coated intravascular catheters.** If anticoagulation is necessary, two direct thrombin inhibitors are available: lepirudin and argatroban (14–16). These agents inhibit clot-bound thrombin, and they do not cross-react with heparin antibodies. The dose recommendations for each of these agents are shown in Table 37.2.

Lepirudin is a recombinant form of hirudin (a component of leech saliva) that has been used successfully in prophylaxis and treatment of thromboembolism in patients with HIT (14,15). Lepirudin is cleared by the kidneys, and dose adjustments are necessary for renal insufficiency (see Appendix 4 for these dose adjustments). Another thrombin inhibitor, argatroban, may be preferred in renal insufficiency because it does not require dose adjustments (see below).

Argatroban has also been used successfully to treat thromboembolism in patients with HIT (15,16). This drug is cleared by the liver, and dose adjustments are necessary in hepatic insufficiency (see Table 37.2). Lepirudin may be preferred in hepatic insufficiency because it does not require dose adjustments.

Long-Term Management

Heparin antibodies can persist for longer than 100 days after the initial exposure, long after the thrombocytopenia has resolved (15), and heparin should not be re-introduced as long as these antibodies persist in the bloodstream. Coumadin can be used for long-term anticoagulation after the thrombocytopenia has resolved, but **coumadin should never be used during the active phase of HIT because there is an increased risk of limb gangrene** from coumadin (15).

Infections

Thrombocytopenia is almost universal in patients with systemic sepsis, and is presumably due to increased phagocytosis of platelets by macrophages (17). Increased platelet destruction is also responsible for the thrombocytopenia that is reported in 50% of patients with acquired immunodeficiency syndrome (AIDS), but the platelet destruction is immune-mediated in this condition (18). Bleeding is not common in either condition unless the thrombocytopenia is accompanied by other coagulation abnormalities.

Disseminated Intravascular Coagulation

Widespread endothelial damage, as can occur with septicemia or multiple trauma, releases a protein known as *tissue factor* that activates the endogenous coagulation cascade and the fibrinolytic system. This can result in a severe coagulopathy characterized by widespread microvascular thrombosis accompanied by depletion of circulating platelets and procoagulant proteins (18). This condition is called *disseminated intravascular coagulation* (DIC). In addition to sepsis and trauma, the other major causes of DIC are obstetric emergencies (amniotic fluid embolism, abruptio placentae, eclampsia, and retained fetus syndrome).

Clinical Features

The microvascular thrombosis in DIC produces multiorgan dysfunction. The lungs are commonly involved, and the clinical picture is similar to the acute respiratory distress syndrome, which is described in Chapter 22. Advanced cases are accompanied by acute oliguric renal failure and progressive hepatocellular injury. Depletion of platelets and coagulation factors can be accompanied by bleeding from multiple sites, particularly the gastrointestinal tract.

DIC can also be accompanied by symmetrical necrosis and ecchymosis involving the limbs; a condition known as *purpura fulminans*. This condition can develop in any case of overwhelming sepsis, but it is most characteristic of meningococcemia (1).

Diagnosis

The diagnosis of DIC is based on the presence of a predisposing condition (e.g., severe sepsis) combined with laboratory evidence of widespread coagulation deficits. Table 37.3 shows a scoring system for the

TABLE 37.3 Scoring System for Disseminated Intravascular Coagulation*

Points	0	1	2	3
Platelet Count /nL	>100	≥50	<50	
D-dimer (μg/mL)	≤1		1–5	>5
Fibrinogen (g/L)	>1	≤1		
Prothrombin Index (%)	>70	40–70	<40	

*A score of 5 or greater is consistent with the diagnosis of disseminated intravascular coagulation. From Reference 19.

diagnosis of DIC proposed by the International Society on Thrombosis and Haemostasis (19). There are four laboratory abnormalities used in this scoring system. Three of the abnormalities (thrombocytopenia, reduced fibrinogen levels, and prolongation of the prothrombin times) are the result of depletion caused by widespread microvascular thrombosis, and one of the abnormalities (elevated d-dimer levels) is a manifestation of enhanced fibrinolysis. Because the laboratory abnormalities reflect consumption of coagulation factors, DIC is often referred to as a *consumptive coagulopathy*.

Management

Advanced cases of DIC have a mortality rate in excess of 80%, and there is no specific treatment other than that directed against the predisposing conditions. Bleeding often prompts the replacement of platelets and coagulation factors (10 units of cryoprecipitate provides about 2.5 grams of fibrinogen), but this rarely helps, and consumption of the platelets and coagulation proteins can aggravate the microvascular thrombosis. Heparin is usually ineffective in retarding the microvascular thrombosis, probably because of depletion of antithrombin-III (20). Antithrombin-III concentrates can be given with heparin (the AT-III dosage is 90 to 120 Units as a load, then 90 to 120 Units daily for 4 days), but there is no evidence that this practice improves survival (21,22).

Thrombotic Thrombocytopenia Purpura

Thrombotic thrombocytopenia purpura (TTP) is a rare but life-threatening condition caused by immune-mediated platelet aggregation with widespread microvascular thrombosis. Like DIC, it is classified as one of the *thrombotic microangiopathies.*

Clinical Features

TTP often occurs in young adults, particularly women, and usually follows a nonspecific illness like a viral syndrome. The clinical presentation of TTP is characterized by **five clinical features** (pentad): fever, change in mental status, acute renal failure, thrombocytopenia, and microangiopathic hemolytic anemia. All 5 clinical features are required for the diagnosis.

Patients usually experience fever and depressed consciousness that can progress rapidly to coma and generalized seizures. Thrombocytopenia is not associated with other coagulation abnormalities, which distinguishes TTP from DIC. The microangiopathic hemolytic anemia is detected by the presence of schistocytes in the blood smear. Prompt diagnosis is mandatory because the treatment for this condition is most effective early in the course of the illness.

Management

The treatment of choice for TTP is **plasma exchange** (23,24). This can be performed with plasmapheresis equipment that removes blood and separates the plasma from the red cells. The plasma is discarded and the red cells are reinfused with fresh frozen plasma. This is continued until 1.5 times the plasma volume has been exchanged (the normal plasma volume is 40 mL/kg in adult men and 36 mL/kg in adult women). This is repeated daily for approximately 1 week.

If plasmapheresis equipment is unavailable, a "poor man's" plasma exchange can be performed by inserting an arterial catheter into the femoral artery and withdrawing 500 mL aliquots of blood (equivalent to 1 Unit of whole blood) into a blood collection bag. This is then sent to the blood bank for centrifugation to separate the plasma from the blood cells. The cells are then returned to the patient, and one unit of fresh frozen plasma is infused with every unit of packed red blood cells. This is continued until at least one plasma volume has been exchanged.

Acute, fulminant TTP is almost always fatal if untreated. **With prompt use of plasma exchange, as many as 90% of patients can survive** the acute episode (23,24). Platelet transfusions are contraindicated in TTP because they can aggravate the underlying thrombosis.

Blood Transfusions

The viability of platelets in whole blood and erythrocyte concentrates (packed cells) is almost completely lost after 24 hours of storage. Therefore, large-volume transfusions can produce dilutional thrombocytopenia. This effect becomes prominent when the transfusion volume exceeds 1.5 times the blood volume (25).

A rare type of posttransfusion thrombocytopenia appears approximately 1 week after transfusion, usually in multiparous women, and is caused by antiplatelet antibodies. This condition is called *posttransfusion purpura,* and thrombocytopenia is often severe and prolonged (26). Platelet counts can fall to 10,000/µL or lower for as long as 40 days. If hemorrhage ensues, plasma exchange is the treatment of choice.

HELLP Syndrome

HELLP (Hemolysis, Elevated Liver enzymes, Low Platelets) is a thrombotic microangiopathy (like DIC and TTP) that is often associated with preeclampsia. This syndrome is one of the major obstetric emergencies, and develops pre-term in about 80% of cases. The clinical manifestations often include hypertension and abdominal pain (epigastric or right upper quadrant), and the laboratory abnormalities are as indicated by the name of the condition. The management usually involves platelet transfusions to keep the platelet count above 50,000/µL and prompt delivery (see Reference 27 for a more complete description of the management of this condition).

ABNORMAL PLATELET FUNCTION

Renal Failure

Impaired platelet adhesion due to impaired fibrinogen binding to platelets and abnormalities in von Willebrand's factor (which anchors the platelets to damaged endothelium) is a well-described complication of acute and chronic renal failure (28). Bleeding times become prolonged when the serum creatinine climbs above 6 mg/dL. Dialysis corrects the bleeding time in only 30 to 50% of patients (28).

The significance of the impaired platelet adhesion in renal failure is unclear. However, upper gastrointestinal bleeding is the second leading cause of death in acute renal failure (28), so the platelet function abnormality in renal failure should be of some concern. The measures described next may provide some benefit in the renal failure patient who is bleeding.

Desmopressin

Desmopressin is a vasopressin analogue (deamino-arginine vasopressin, or DDAVP) that increases the levels of von Willebrand factor, and can correct the bleeding time in 75% of patients with renal failure (28,29). The recommended dose is **0.3 μg/kg intravenously or subcutaneously, or 30 (μg/kg intranasally** (28,29). The effect lasts only 6 to 8 hours, and repeated dosing leads to tachyphylaxis. Responsiveness is restored if the drug is withheld for 3 to 4 days. Desmopressin does not have the vasoconstrictor actions or antidiuretic effects of vasopressin.

For patients with renal failure who develop significant bleeding, one dose of desmopressin can be given empirically. A second dose can be given 8 to 12 hours later, but repeated dosing for longer than 24 hours is not advisable because of the tachyphylaxis, and also because it is not possible to determine if the drug has a significant effect in individual patients.

Conjugated Estrogens

Conjugated estrogens can also correct the bleeding time in renal failure (mechanism unknown), but the effect lasts for weeks instead of hours. The recommended dose is **0.6 mg/kg IV every day for 5 consecutive days** (1,28,30). The onset of action takes up to one day, but the effect lasts for 2 weeks (30). This regimen has been recommended for patients with recurrent GI bleeding. Conjugated estrogens are not useful for the management of acute bleeding because of the delayed onset of action.

Cardiopulmonary Bypass

Platelet adhesiveness is impaired by unknown mechanisms when blood passes through the oxygenator apparatus used during cardiopulmonary bypass. The severity of the platelet function defect is directly related to the duration of bypass (31). In most cases, the abnormality resolves within a few hours after bypass is completed. However, defects in platelet adhesion may contribute to troublesome mediastinal bleeding in the immediate postoperative period. The management of bleeding in the immediate postop period usually involves reversal of heparin and normalization of all laboratory measurements of coagulation status. There is no proven treatment for impaired platelet adhesion in this situation. Postoperative bleeding after cardiopulmonary bypass often requires reexploration.

Drug-Induced Platelet Defects

A long list of drugs are capable of impairing platelet adhesion, and the ones most likely to be used in the ICU are included in Table 37.4. Clinically significant bleeding is most likely to occur with: 1) aspirin and the other antiplatelet agents, 2) ketorolac when combined with heparin, and 3) the plasma expander hetastarch, when given in a daily volume that exceeds 1.5 liters.

TABLE 37.4 Drugs That Can Cause Platelet Function Abnormalities*

Antiplatelet Agents	*β-Lactam Antibiotics*
Aspirin	Penicillins
Clopidogrel	Cephalosporins
Dipyridamole	
Glycoprotein Inhibitors	*Cardiovascular Drugs*
Ticlodipine	Calcium channel blockers
	Nitroglycerin
Antihistamines	Nitroprusside
Chlorpheniramine	
Diphenhydramine	*Others*
	Dextrans
Antithrombotic Agents	Haloperidol
Alteplase	Hetastarch
Heparin	Ketorolac

*Includes only drugs that are likely to be used in the ICU. From References 1 and 31.

PLATELET TRANSFUSIONS

Random Donor Platelet Concentrates

Platelet concentrates are prepared from fresh whole blood in the following manner (2). First, red blood cells are separated by centrifuging whole blood at low speeds (2,000 rpm). The supernatant, which is called "platelet-rich plasma" is then centrifuged at high speeds (5,000 rpm) to separate the platelets, and the platelet plug is re-suspended in a small volume of plasma. Each platelet concentrate prepared in this fashion contains 50 to 100 billion platelets in 50 mL of plasma (2). These "random donor" platelet concentrates are also rich in leukocytes (10^7 to 10^9 leukocytes per unit), and this is responsible for the high incidence of fever associated with platelet transfusions (see later).

Platelets can be stored for up to 7 days, but viability begins to decline after 3 days. Platelet transfusions are usually given as multiples of 4 to 6 platelet concentrates (units), each one from a different donor. The total volume is 200 to 300 mL.

Effect on Circulating Platelet Counts

In the average-size adult, **each platelet concentrate should raise the circulating platelet count by at least 5,000/μL** (2). For a routine platelet transfusion of 4 to 6 units, the platelet count should increase 20,000/μL to 30,000/μL, respectively. This effect should be apparent one hour after the transfusion, and it should last approximately 8 days.

Reduced Efficacy

Antibodies to ABO antigens on platelets or to leukocyte (HLA) antigens can cause a less-than-expected rise in platelet counts following platelet transfusions, and sensitization to these antigens is responsible for the platelet refractoriness that occurs in 30 to 70% of patients who receive multiple platelet transfusions (2). This problem can be alleviated by transfusing ABO-compatible platelets, removing the leukocytes from platelet concentrates, or using single-donor platelet transfusions.

Complications

Because one platelet transfusion involves platelet concentrates from 4 to 6 individual donors, the infectious risks associated with homologous blood transfusions are four to six times higher with platelet transfusions than with red blood cell transfusions. Febrile nonhemolytic reactions are also more common with platelet transfusions (due to the high leukocyte content of random donor platelet concentrates), and fever has been reported in up to 30% of platelet transfusion recipients (2).

INDICATIONS FOR PLATELET TRANSFUSIONS

Active Bleeding

In the presence of active bleeding other than ecchymoses or petechiae, platelet transfusions are indicated when:

1. The platelet count is below 50,000/µL and there are no contraindications to platelet transfusions (see later).
2. The platelet count is below 100,000/µL and the bleeding is intracranial, or there is a condition that impairs platelet adhesion (e.g., renal failure).

For trauma victims who receive multiple transfusions, the platelet count should be kept above 100,000/µL if there is a risk for intracranial hemorrhage (32).

Prophylactic Platelet Transfusions

When there is no evidence of active bleeding other than ecchymotic or petechial hemorrhages, and there is thrombocytopenia from bone marrow suppression, prophylactic platelet transfusions are indicated when (1–3):

1. The platelet count is below 10,000/µL.
2. The platelet count is below 20,000/µL and there is a risk of hemorrhage (e.g., peptic ulcer disease).
3. The platelet count is below 50,000/µL, and the following procedures are planned: bronchoscopic or endoscopic biopsy, lumbar puncture, percutaneous liver biopsy, and major surgery.

Despite evidence that spontaneous bleeding is uncommon with platelet counts down to 5,000/µL, most of the experts are reluctant to adopt a threshold as low as 5,000/µL for platelet transfusions.

Central Venous Catheterization

Several studies have shown that central venous cannulation can be performed safely in patients with platelet counts down to 10,000/µL (1,33,34), and one study showed that the experience of the operator is more important than the presence of coagulopathy in determining the risk of bleeding with central line placement (34). Therefore, special considerations other than the standard threshold for prophylactic platelet transfusions (i.e., 10,000/µL) are not necessary for central venous catheter placement.

Contraindications to Platelet Transfusions

Platelet transfusions are contraindicated in patients with **thrombotic thrombocytopenia purpura** and **heparin-induced thrombocytopenia** because transfused platelets can aggravate the tendency for thrombosis in these conditions. DIC is not considered a contraindication to platelet transfusions (2), even though transfused platelets can aggravate the microvascular thrombosis in this condition.

FINAL WORD

The following points deserve emphasis regarding platelets in the critically ill patient:

1. Don't forget heparin as source of thrombocytopenia in the ICU, and **don't forget to remove heparin-coated catheters** if heparin-induced thrombocytopenia is a possibility.
2. Central venous catheters can be inserted safely in patients with low platelet counts, but experienced physicians should insert the catheters.

REFERENCES

Reviews

1. DeLoughery TG. Critical care clotting catastrophies. Crit Care Clin 2005;21:531–562.
2. Delinas J-P, Stoddart LV, Snyder EL. Thrombocytopenia and critical care medicine. J Intensive Care Med 2001;16:1–21.
3. Schiffer CA, Anderson KC, Bennett CL, et al. Platelet transfusion for patients with cancer: clinical practice guidelines of the American Society of Clinical Oncology. J Clin Oncol 2001;19:1519–1538.

Platelets and Hemostasis

4. Tomer A, Harker LA. Megakaryocytopoiesis and platelet kinetics. In: Rossi EC, Simon TL, Moss GS, eds. Principles of transfusion therapy. Baltimore: Williams & Wilkins, 1991:167–179.

5. American Association of Blood Banks. Technical Manual, 10th ed. Arlington, VA: American Association of Blood Banks, 1990:649.
6. Slichter SJ, Harker LA. Thrombocytopenia: mechanisms and management of defects in platelet production. Clin Haematol 1978;7:523–527.
7. Payne BA, Pierre RV. Pseudothrombocytopenia: a laboratory artifact with potentially serious consequences. Mayo Clin Proc 1984;59:123–125.
8. Rodgers RP, Levin J. A critical reappraisal of the bleeding time. Semin Thromb Hemost 1990;16:1–20.

Thrombocytopenia

9. Stephan F, Hollande J, Richard O, et al. Thrombocytopenia in a surgical ICU. Chest 1999;115:1363–1379.
10. Strauss R, Wehler M, Mehler K, et al. Thrombocytopenia in patients in the medical intensive care unit: bleeding prevalence, transfusion requirements, and outcome. Crit Care Med 2002;30:1765–1771.
11. Warkentin TE, Cook DJ. Heparin, low molecular weight heparin, and heparin-induced thrombocytopenia in the ICU. Crit Care Clin 2005;21:513–529.
12. Laster J, Silver D. Heparin-coated catheters and heparin-induced thrombocytopenia. J Vasc Surg 1988;7:667–672.
13. Warkentin TE. New approaches to the diagnosis of heparin-induced thrombocytopenia. Chest 2005;127(suppl):35S–45S.
14. Greinacher A, Janssens U, Berg G, et al. Lepirudin (recombinant hirudin) for parenteral anticoagulation in patients with heparin-induced thrombocytopenia. Circulation 1999;100:587–593.
15. Hassell K. The management of patients with heparin-induced thrombocytopenia who require anticoagulant therapy. Chest 2005;127(suppl):1S–8S.
16. Levine RL, Hursting MJ, McCollum D. Argatroban therapy in heparin-induced thrombocytopenia with hepatic dysfunction. Chest 2006;129:1167–1175.
17. Francois B, Trimoreau F, Vignon P, et al. Thrombocytopenia in the sepsis syndrome: role of hemophagocytosis and macrophage colony-stimulating hormone. Am J Med 1997;103:114–120.
18. Doweiko JP, Groopman JE. Hematologic consequences of HIV infection. In: Broder S, Merigan TC, Bolognesi D, eds. Textbook of AIDS medicine. Baltimore: Williams & Wilkins, 1994:617–628.
19. Senno SL, Pechet L, Bick RL. Disseminated intravascular coagulation (DIC): pathophysiology, laboratory diagnosis, and management. J Intensive Care Med 2000;15:144–158.
20. Angstwurm MWA, Dempfle C-E, Spannagl M. New disseminated intravascular coagulation score: a useful tool to predict mortality in comparison with Acute Physiology And Chronic Health Evaluation II And Logistic Organ Dysfunction Scores. Crit Care Med 2006;34:314–320.
21. Clark J, Rubin RN. A practical approach to managing disseminated intravascular coagulation. J Crit Illness 1994;9:265–280.
22. Fourrier F, Chopin C, Huart J-J, et al. Double-blind, placebo-controlled trial of antithrombin III concentrates in septic shock with disseminated intravascular coagulation. Chest 1993;104:882–888.
23. Rock GA, Shumack KH, Buskard NA, et al. Comparison of plasma exchange with plasma infusion in the treatment of thrombotic thrombocytopenia purpura. N Engl J Med 1991;325:393–397.

24. Hayward CP, Sutton DMC, Carter WH Jr, et al. Treatment outcomes in patients with adult thrombotic thrombocytopenic purpura-hemolytic uremic syndrome. Arch Intern Med 1994;154:982–987.
25. Reiner A, Kickler TS, Bell W. How to administer massive transfusions effectively. J Crit Illness 1987;2:15–24.
26. Heffner JE. What caused post-op thrombocytopenia in this 82 year-old man? J Crit Illness 1996;11:666–671.
27. Magann EF, Martin JN. Twelve steps to optimal management of HELLP syndrome. Clin Obstet Gynecol 1999;42:532–550.

Abnormal Platelet Function

28. Salman S. Uremic bleeding: pathophysiology, diagnosis, and management. Hosp Physician 2001;37:45–76.
29. Mannucci PM. Desmopressin (DDAVP) in the treatment of bleeding disorders: the first 20 years. Blood 1997;90:2515–2521.
30. Vigano G, Gaspari F, Locatelli M, et al. Dose-effect and pharmacokinetics of estrogens given to correct bleeding time in uremia. Kidney Int 1988;34:853–858.
31. George JN, Shattil SJ. The clinical importance of acquired abnormalities of platelet function. N Engl J Med 1991;324:27–39.

Platelet Transfusions

32. Lundberg GD. Practice parameter for the use of fresh frozen plasma, cryoprecipitate, and platelets. JAMA 1994;271:777–781.
33. Doerfler ME, Kaufman B, Goldenberg AS. Central venous catheter placement in patients with disorders of hemostasis. Chest 1996;110:185–188.
34. DeLoughery TG, Liebler JM, Simonds V, et al. Invasive line placement in critically ill patients: do hemostatic defects matter? Transfusion 1996;36:827–831.

Section XII

DISORDERS OF BODY TEMPERATURE

As far as organization exists in every system . . the properties of no system can be deduced from a knowledge of its isolated parts.

MAURICE STRAUSS

H
A
I
S

The
eve
of c
tha
ron
pera
the
rise

Hea

The
most
the
with

Mec

Heat
in se

Radi

Radi
tron
from
inten

Chapter 38

HYPERTHERMIA AND HYPOTHERMIA SYNDROMES

The human body is a metabolic furnace that generates enough heat, even at rest, to raise the body temperature by 1°C every hour (1). This, of course, is not allowed to happen thanks to a thermoregulatory system that promotes the transfer of excess body heat to the surrounding environment. This system is so effective that the daily variation in body temperature is only ±0.6°C (2). This chapter describes what happens when the regulation of body temperature is faulty, allowing the temperature to rise or fall to extreme and life-threatening levels.

Heat Exchange through the Skin

The external surface of the body acts like a radiator (with a built-in thermostat) that discharges excess heat into the surroundings. About 90% of the excess heat generated by metabolism is dissipated through the skin, with the remainder being lost in exhaled gas.

Mechanisms of Heat Exchange

Heat exchange between the body and its surroundings is accomplished in several ways, as described next.

Radiation

Radiation refers to the loss of heat via infrared heat rays (a type of electromagnetic wave) that radiate out from the skin. These waves emanate from all objects that exist above absolute zero temperature, and the intensity of radiation increases as the temperature of the object increases.

Under normal conditions, radiation accounts for about 60% of the heat loss from the human body (3).

Conduction

Conduction is the transfer of heat from an object of higher temperature to an object of lower temperature. This is the behavior of heat as kinetic energy, which imparts motion to molecules and results in the transfer of heat from a hotter to a colder object. Heat transfer by conduction alone is responsible for only about 15% of heat loss from the body (2).

Convection

When heat is lost from the skin, it warms the air just above the skin surface. This increase in surface temperature limits the further loss of body heat by conduction. However, when an air current from a fan (or a gust of wind) is passed across the skin, it displaces the warm layer of air above the skin and replaces it with cooler air, and this process facilitates the continued loss of body heat by conduction. The same effect is produced by increases in blood flow just underneath the skin. The action of currents (air and blood) to promote heat loss is known as *convection*.

Evaporation

The transformation of water from liquid to gaseous phase requires heat (called the latent heat of vaporization), and when water or sweat evaporates from the surface of the body, the heat that is utilized is body heat. Normally, evaporation accounts for about 20% of the loss of body heat (mostly as a result of insensible fluid losses from the lungs). Evaporation plays a much greater role in the adaptation to thermal stress (see next).

Response to Thermal Stress

The maintenance of body temperature in conditions of thermal stress (hot weather, strenuous exercise, or both) is primarily achieved by enhanced blood flow to the skin (convective heat loss) and the loss of sweat (evaporative heat loss).

The Role of Sweating

The evaporation of sweat from the skin is responsible for at least 70% of the loss of body heat during periods of thermal stress. The evaporation of one liter of sweat from the skin is accompanied by the loss of 580 kilocalories (kcal) of heat from the body (3). This is about one-quarter of the daily heat production by an average-sized adult at rest. Thermal sweating (as opposed to "nervous sweating") can achieve rates of 1 to 2 liters per hour (3), which means that over 1,000 kcal of heat can be lost hourly during profuse sweating. It is important to emphasize that **sweat must evaporate to ensure loss of body heat**. Wiping sweat off the skin will not result in heat loss, so this practice should be discouraged during strenuous exercise.

Hyperthermia and Fever

The terms *hyperthermia* and *fever* both indicate an elevated body temperature, but hyperthermia is the result of abnormal temperature regulation, while fever is the result of a normal thermoregulatory system operating at a higher set point. In both conditions, extreme elevation in body temperature (>40°C or 104°F) is called *hyperpyrexia*. This chapter will describe specific conditions that result in elevated body temperatures as a result of abnormal thermoregulation (i.e., hyperthermia syndromes). The conditions associated with fever will be described in the next chapter. (Also included in the next chapter is an explanation of how to convert between degrees Celsius and degrees Fahrenheit.)

HEAT-RELATED ILLNESS

Heat-related illnesses are conditions where the thermoregulatory system is no longer able to maintain a constant body temperature in response to thermal stress (from exercise, the environment, or both). There are a number of minor heat-related illnesses, such as heat cramps and heat rash (prickly heat), but the following descriptions are limited to the major heat-related illnesses: *heat exhaustion* and *heat stroke*. The comparative features of these conditions are shown in Table 38.1.

Heat Exhaustion

Heat exhaustion is the most common form of heat-related illness, and is the result of volume depletion. Patients with heat exhaustion experience flu-like symptoms that include hyperthermia (usually below 39°C or 102°F), muscle cramps, nausea, and malaise. The hallmark of this condition is **volume depletion,** which is accompanied by tachycardia but no other signs of hemodynamic compromise. The volume loss can be accompanied by hypernatremia (from net loss of free water) or hyponatremia (usually seen when salt and water losses are replaced with water alone). There is no evidence of significant neurologic impairment.

TABLE 38.1 Comparative Features of Heat Exhaustion and Heat Stroke

Feature	Heat Exhaustion	Heat Stroke
Body Temperature	<39°C	≥41°C
CNS Dysfunction	Mild	Severe
Sweat Production	Yes	Occasionally
Dehydration	Yes	Yes
Multiorgan Dysfunction (e.g., rhabdomyolysis, acute renal failure)	No	Yes

The management of heat exhaustion includes volume repletion and other general supportive measures. Cooling measures to reduce body temperature are not necessary.

Heat Stroke

Heat stroke is a life-threatening condition characterized by extreme elevations in body temperature (≥41°C or 106°F), severe neurologic dysfunction (e.g., delirium, ataxia, coma, and seizures), severe volume depletion with hypotension, and multiorgan involvement that includes rhabdomyolysis (a condition of widespread skeletal muscle injury), acute renal failure, disseminated intravascular coagulopathy (DIC), and marked elevation in serum transaminases (presumably from the liver). The inability to produce sweat (anhidrosis) is a common feature of heat stroke, but it is not frequent enough to be of value in distinguishing heat stroke from heat exhaustion (4). There are two types of heat stroke, one related to environmental temperatures (classic heat stroke) and the other related to strenuous exercise (exertional heat stroke).

Classic heat stroke is the result of exposure to high environmental temperatures, usually in a confined space. This type of heat stroke is usually seem in elderly and debilitated people and in people who are taking psychiatric medications, have a history of alcohol and drug abuse, and have advanced heart failure.

Exertional heat stroke is the result of strenuous physical activity in a hot environment, and is typically seen in athletes and military recruits. Exertional heat stroke tends to be more severe, with a higher incidence of multiorgan dysfunction than seen in classic heat stroke.

Cooling Methods

Immediate cooling to reduce body temperature is essential in heat stroke to reduce the risk of progressive or permanent organ injury (5). External cooling is the easiest and quickest way to reduce the body temperature. This is accomplished by placing ice packs in the groin and axilla, and covering the upper thorax and neck with ice. Cooling blankets are then placed over the entire length of the body. The one drawback with external cooling is the risk of shivering when the skin temperature falls below 30°C (86°F) (5). Shivering is counterproductive because it raises body temperature. If shivering does occur, a switch to one of the internal cooling techniques is indicated.

The most effective external cooling method is **evaporative cooling**, which involves spraying the skin with cool water (at 15°C or 59°F) and then fanning the skin to promote evaporation of the water. This method can reduce the body temperature at a rate of 0.3°C (0.6°F) per minute (6). Evaporative cooling is used mostly in the field, and is particularly effective when the weather is hot and dry (which enhances evaporation from the skin).

Internal cooling can be achieved with a cold-water lavage of the stomach, bladder, or rectum. These methods produce a more rapid reduction in body temperature than external cooling with ice and cooling blankets, but they can be more labor-intensive. Internal cooling is usually reserved for cases where external cooling is ineffective or produces unwanted shivering.

Body cooling should be continued until the body temperature reaches 38°C (100.4°F). While this is taking place, blood samples should be obtained to check for multiorgan dysfunction, including rhabdomyolysis, renal insufficiency, hepatocellular injury, and coagulopathy. Hypovolemia is common in heat stroke, so volume resuscitation is usually necessary.

Rhabdomyolysis

Skeletal muscle seems particularly vulnerable to thermal stress because rhabdomyolysis is a common complication of hyperthermia syndromes, including heat stroke (particularly the exertional type), malignant hyperthermia, and neuroleptic malignant syndrome (the latter two conditions are described later in the chapter). Disruption of myocytes in skeletal muscle leads to the release of creatine kinase (CK) into the bloodstream, and the measurement of CK levels in plasma is used to determine the presence and severity of rhabdomyolysis (7,8). There is no standard CK level for the diagnosis of rhabdomyolysis, but CK levels that are five times higher than normal (or about 1,000 Units/liter) have been used to identify rhabdomyolysis in clinical studies (7). Plasma CK levels above 15,000 Units/L indicate severe rhabdomyolysis and an increased risk of myoglobinuric renal failure (7).

Myoglobinuria and Renal Failure

Acute renal failure occurs in about one-third of patients with rhabdomyolysis (8). The culprit is myoglobin, which is released from injured myocytes and is eventually filtered by the glomeruli in the kidneys. Once in the renal tubules, myoglobin can damage the renal tubular epithelium, particularly when the pH of the fluid in the renal tubules is low (acid pH). The final result can be a condition of acute renal failure that resembles acute tubular necrosis (ATN).

An ordinary urine dipstick test for blood can be used as a simple screening test for myoglobin in the urine. This test uses a colorimetric reaction to detect the iron moiety in myoglobin or hemoglobin. A negative test result is evidence against the presence of myoglobin in the urine. A positive test result is not specific for myoglobin (and could indicate hemoglobin in the urine), and should be combined with urine microscopy to search for red blood cells. **A positive dipstick test for blood in urine *plus* the absence of red blood cells on urine microscopy is evidence of myoglobinuria.**

When myoglobin is detected in the urine, aggressive volume resuscitation is an effective means of preventing or limiting the development of myoglobinuric renal failure. Alkalinizing the urine (with acetazolamide or intravenous bicarbonate infusions) can also reduce the potential for myoglobin to damage the renal tubules, but this measure adds little to the beneficial effects of volume infusion.

DRUG-INDUCED HYPERTHERMIA SYNDROMES

The heat-related illnesses just described are characterized by thermal stress in the environment. The illnesses described in this section are characterized by thermal stress in the interior of the body. The source of the thermal stress in each case is drug-induced increases in metabolic heat production. Three specific hyperthermia syndromes are described: malignant hyperthermia, neuroleptic malignant syndrome, and the serotonin syndrome.

Malignant Hyperthermia

Malignant hyperthermia (MH) is an uncommon disorder that occurs in approximately 1 in 15,000 episodes of general anesthesia and affects approximately 1 in 50,000 adults (9). It is an inherited disorder with an autosomal dominant pattern and it is characterized by excessive release of calcium from the sarcoplasmic reticulum in skeletal muscle in response to halogenated inhalational anesthetic agents (e.g., halothane, isoflurane, servoflurane, and desflurane) and depolarizing neuromuscular blockers (e.g., succinylcholine) (9). The calcium influx into the cell cytoplasm somehow leads to uncoupling of oxidative phosphorylation and a marked rise in metabolic rate.

Clinical Manifestations

The clinical manifestations of MH include muscle rigidity, increased body temperature, depressed consciousness, and autonomic instability. The first sign of MH may be a sudden and unexpected rise in end-tidal PCO_2 (reflecting the underlying hypermetabolism) in the operating room (9,10). This is followed (within minutes to a few hours) by generalized muscle rigidity, which can progress rapidly to widespread myonecrosis (rhabdomyolysis) and subsequent myoglobinuric renal failure. The heat generated by the muscle rigidity is responsible for the marked rise in body temperature (often above 40°C or 104°F) in MH. The altered mental status in MH can range from confusion and agitation to obtundation and coma. Autonomic instability can lead to cardiac arrhythmias, fluctuating blood pressure, or persistent hypotension.

Management

The first suspicion of MH should prompt immediate discontinuation of the offending anesthetic agent. Specific treatment for the muscle rigidity is available with **dantrolene** sodium, a muscle relaxant that blocks the release of calcium from the sarcoplasmic reticulum. When given early in the course of MH, dantrolene can reduce the mortality rate from 70% or higher (in untreated cases) to 10% or less (9,10). The dosing regimen for dantrolene in MH is as follows:

Dose regimen: 1 to 2 mg/kg as IV bolus, and repeat every 15 minutes if needed to a total dose of 10 mg/kg. Follow the initial dosing regimen with a dose of 1 mg/kg IV or 2 mg/kg orally four times daily for 3 days.

Side effects: Muscle weakness, hepatocellular injury.

Treatment is extended to 3 days to prevent recurrences. The most common side effect of dantrolene is muscle weakness, particularly grip strength, which usually resolves in 2 to 4 days after the drug is discontinued (11). The most troublesome side effect of dantrolene is hepatocellular injury, which is more common when the daily dose exceeds 10 mg/kg (9). Active hepatitis and cirrhosis are considered contraindications to dantrolene therapy (11) but, considering the high mortality in MH if left untreated, these contraindications should not be absolute.

All patients who survive an episode of MH should be given a medical bracelet that identifies their susceptibility to MH. In addition, because MH is a genetic disorder with a known inheritance pattern (autosomal dominant), immediate family members should be informed of their possible susceptibility to MH. A test is available to identify the responsible gene for MH in family members (10).

Neuroleptic Malignant Syndrome

The *neuroleptic malignant syndrome* (NMS) is strikingly similar to malignant hyperthermia in that it is a drug-induced disorder characterized by 4 clinical features: increased body temperature, muscle rigidity, altered mental status, and autonomic instability (12). As the name implies, NMS is caused by neuroleptic agents (an alternate term for antipsychotic medications). A list of offending drugs and drug regimens in NMS is shown in Table 38.2. Note that drugs other than neuroleptic agents can trigger NMS, so the name of this syndrome is misleading.

Pathogenesis

The one property shared by all the drugs in Table 38.2 is the ability to influence dopamine-mediated synaptic transmission in the central nervous system. A decrease in dopaminergic neurotransmission in the basal ganglia and hypothalamic-pituitary axis may be responsible for many of the clinical manifestations of NMS (12). As indicated in Table 38.2, there

TABLE 38.2 Drugs Implicated in the Neuroleptic Malignant Syndrome

I. Ongoing Drug Intake	
Antipsychotic agents:	Butyrophenones (eg, haloperidol), phenothiazines, clozapine, olanzapine, respiradone
Antiemetic agents:	Metoclopramide, droperidol, prochlorperazine
CNS stimulants:	Amphetamines, cocaine
Other:	Lithium, overdose with tricyclic antidepressants
II. Discontinued Drug Intake	
Dopaminergic drugs:	Amantidine, bromocriptine, levodopa

are two clinical situations that predispose to NMS: (1) therapy with drugs that inhibit dopaminergic transmission, or (2) discontinuing therapy with drugs that facilitate dopaminergic transmission. Most cases of NMS are triggered by drugs that inhibit dopaminergic neurotransmission, and the ones reported most frequently are **haloperidol** and **fluphenazine** (12). The incidence of NMS during therapy with neuroleptic agents is reported at 0.2% to 1.9% (13).

There is no relationship between the intensity or duration of drug therapy and the risk of NMS (12), so NMS is an idiosyncratic drug reaction and not a manifestation of drug toxicity. There is some evidence of a familial tendency, but a genetic pattern of transmission has not been identified (14).

Clinical Features

Most cases of NMS begin to appear 24 to 72 hours after the onset of drug therapy, and almost all cases are apparent in the first 2 weeks of drug therapy. The onset is usually gradual, and can take days to fully develop. In 80% of cases, the initial manifestation is muscle rigidity or altered mental status (12). The muscle rigidity has been described as *lead-pipe rigidity* to distinguish it from the rigidity associated with tremulousness (cogwheel rigidity). The change in mental status can range from confusion and agitation to obtundation and coma. Hyperthermia (body temperature can exceed 41°C) is required for the diagnosis of NMS (12), but the increase in body temperature can be delayed for 8 to 10 hours after the appearance of muscle rigidity or change in mental status (15). Autonomic instability can produce cardiac arrhythmias, labile blood pressure, or persistent hypotension.

Laboratory Studies

It may be difficult to distinguish the extrapyramidal side effects of neuroleptic agents from the motor effects of NMS. The serum CK level can help in this regard because, although it can rise slightly in dystonic reactions, it should be higher than 1000 Units/L in NMS (13). The leukocyte count in blood can increase to 40,000/μL with a leftward shift in NMS (12), so the clinical presentation of NMS (fever, leukocytosis, altered mental status, hypotension) can be confused with sepsis. The serum CK level will distinguish NMS from sepsis.

Management

The single most important measure in the management of NMS is *immediate* removal of the offending drug. If NMS is caused by discontinuation of dopaminergic therapy, it should be restarted immediately with plans for a gradual reduction in dosage at a later time. General measures, including volume resuscitation and evaluation for multiorgan involvement (e.g., rhabdomyolysis), are the same as described for malignant hyperthermia.

Dantrolene sodium (the same muscle relaxant used in the treatment of MH) can be given intravenously for severe cases of muscle rigidity.

The optimal dose is not clearly defined, but one suggestion is to **start with a single dose of 2–3 mg/kg/day** (12,16), and increase this every few hours if necessary to a total dose of 10 mg/kg/day. Oral dantrolene has also been used successfully in NMS in doses of 50 to 200 mg daily (usually given in divided doses every 6 to 8 hours) (16). In cases of severe muscle rigidity (when the CPK is markedly elevated), the intravenous route seems a better choice, at least in the first few days of treatment. The risk of liver injury should be considered when using dantrolene in NMS because there are alternative treatments.

Bromocriptine mesylate is a dopamine agonist that has been successful in treating NMS when given orally in a dose of 2.5 to 10 mg three times daily (16). Some improvement in muscle rigidity can be seen within hours after the start of therapy, but the full response often takes days to develop. Hypotension is a troublesome side effect. There is no advantage with bromocriptine over dantrolene, except in patients with advanced liver disease (where dantrolene is not advised). Treatment of NMS should continue for about 10 days after clinical resolution because of delayed clearance of many neuroleptics (when depot preparations are implicated, therapy should continue for 2 to 3 weeks after clinical resolution) (12). There is a heightened risk of venous thromboembolism during NMS (12), so heparin prophylaxis is recommended (see Chapter 5). The mortality rate from NMS is about 20% (13), and (surprisingly) it is unclear if specific treatment with dantrolene or bromocriptine has a favorable effect on mortality (12,13).

Serotonin Syndrome

Overstimulation of serotonin receptors in the central nervous system produces a combination of mental status changes, autonomic hyperactivity, and neuromuscular abnormalities that is known as the *serotonin syndrome* (SS) (17). The recent growth in popularity of seritonergic drugs such as selective serotonin reuptake inhibitors (SSRIs) has led to a marked increase in the prevalence of SS in recent years. The severity of illness can vary widely in cases of SS, and the most severe cases can be confused with any of the other hyperthermia syndromes.

Pathogenesis

Serotonin is a neurotransmitter in the central nervous system that participates in neuronal circuits involved in sleep-wakefulness cycles, mood, and thermoregulation. A variety of drugs can enhance serotonin neurotransmission in these circuits, and excessive doses of these *seritonergic* drugs can produce SS. A list of seritonergic drugs that are capable of producing SS is shown in Table 38.3. Many of these drugs work in combination to produce SS, although single-drug therapy can also result in SS. Many of the drugs involved in SS are mood enhancers, including illegal substances. Of particular note is methylenedioxy-methamphetamine or MDMA ("ecstasy"), which has become a favored street drug in recent years and is known for producing severe cases of SS (18). Note also that some of the drugs that can produce SS can also cause NMS (e.g., amphetamines).

TABLE 38.3 Drugs that Can Produce the Serotonin Syndrome*

Mechanism of Action	Related Drugs
Increased serotonin synthesis	L-tryptophan
Decreased serotonin breakdown	MAOIs (including linezolide), ritonavir
Increased serotonin release	Amphetamines, MDMA ("ecstasy"), cocaine, fenfluramine
Decreased serotonin reuptake	SSRIs, TCAs, dextromethorphan, meperidine, fentanyl, tramadol
Serotonin receptor agonists	Lithium, sumitriptan, buspirone, LSD

*See Reference 17 for a comprehensive list of drugs and drug interactions that can produce the serotonin syndrome. Abbreviations: *MAOIs* = monoamine oxidase inhibitors, *MDMA* = methylenedioxy-methamphetamine, *SSRIs* = selective serotonin reuptake inhibitors, *TCAs* = tricyclic antidepressants.

Clinical Manifestations

The onset of SS is usually abrupt (in contrast to NMS, where the full syndrome can take days to develop), and over half of the cases are evident within 6 hours after ingestion of the responsible drug(s) (17). The clinical findings include mental status changes (e.g., confusion, delirium, coma), autonomic hyperactivity (e.g., mydriasis, tachycardia, hypertension, hyperthermia, diaphoresis) and neuromuscular abnormalities (e.g., hyperkinesis, hyperactive deep tendon reflexes, clonus, and muscle rigidity). The clinical presentation can vary markedly (17). Mild cases may include only hyperkinesis, hyperreflexia, tachycardia, diaphoresis, and mydriasis. Moderate cases often have additional findings of hyperthermia (temperature >38°C), clonus, and agitation. The clonus is most obvious in the patellar deep-tendon reflexes, and horizontal ocular clonus may also be present. Severe cases of SS often present with delirium, hyperpyrexia (temperature >40°C), widespread muscle rigidity, and spontaneous clonus. Life-threatening cases are marked by rhabdomyolysis, renal failure, metabolic acidosis, and hypotension.

A useful worksheet for the diagnosis of SS is shown in Table 38.4. The fist step in the diagnostic evaluation is to establish recent ingestion of one or more seritonergic drugs. Although the worksheet in Table 38.4 includes all drug ingestions in the past five weeks, most cases of SS follow within hours of drug ingestion (17). Hyperthermia and muscle rigidity can be absent in mild cases of the illness. **The features that most distinguish SS from other hyperthermia syndromes are hyperkinesis, hyperreflexia and clonus**. However in severe cases of SS, muscle rigidity can mask these clinical findings. Severe cases of SS can be difficult to distinguish from MH and NMS, and the history of drug ingestion is important in these cases (although the same drugs can be implicated in NMS and SS).

Management

As is the case with all drug-induced hyperthermia syndromes, removal of the precipitating drugs is the single most important element in the management of SS. The remainder of the management includes measures to

TABLE 38.4 Diagnostic Worksheet for Serotonin Syndrome*

Answer the following questions:	YES	NO
Has the patient received a seritonergic drug in the past 5 wks?	●	○
If the answer is YES, proceed to the questions below.		
Does the patient have any of the following?	YES	NO
Tremor + hyperreflexia	●	○
Spontaneous clonus	●	○
Rigidity + Temp >38°C + ocular or inducible clonus	●	○
Ocular clonus + agitation or diaphoresis	●	○
Inducible clonus + agitation or diaphoresis	●	○

If the answer is YES to any of the above conditions, then the patient has SEROTONIN SYNDROME

*Adapted from Boyer EW, Shannon M. The serotonin syndrome. N Engl J Med 2005;352:1112.

control agitation and hyperthermia, and the use of serotonin antagonists. Many cases of SS will resolve within 24 hours after initiation of therapy, but seritonergic drugs with long elimination half-lives can produce more prolonged symptomatology.

Benzodiazepines are considered essential for the control of agitation and hyperkinesis in SS. **Physical restraints should be avoided** because they encourage isometric muscle contractions and this can aggravate skeletal muscle injury and promote lactic acidosis (19).

Cyproheptadine is a serotonin antagonist that can be given in severe cases of SS (20). This drug is available for oral administration only, but tablets can be broken up and administered through a nasogastric tube. The recommended **initial dose is 12 mg, followed by 2 mg every 2 hours for persistent symptoms.** The maintenance dose is 8 mg every 6 hours. Cyprohepatidine can be sedating, but this should aid in the control of agitation in SS.

Neuromuscular paralysis may be required in severe cases of SS to control muscle rigidity and extreme elevations of body temperature (>41°C). Nondepolarizing agents (e.g., vecuronium) should be used for muscle paralysis because succinylcholine can aggravate the hyperkalemia that accompanies rhabdomyolysis. Dantrolene is not effective in reducing the muscle rigidity and hyperthermia in SS (17).

HYPOTHERMIA SYNDROMES

Hypothermia, or a decrease in body temperature below 35°C (95°F), can be the result of environmental forces (accidental hypothermia), a primary metabolic disorder (secondary hypothermia) or a therapeutic intervention (induced hypothermia). This section will focus primarily on environmental hypothermia.

Adaptation to Cold

Physiologically, **the human body is much better equipped to survive in hot rather than cold environments**. The physiological response to a decrease in body temperature includes cutaneous vasoconstriction (to reduce convective heat loss) and shivering (which can roughly double metabolic heat production). Unfortunately, these physiological adaptations to cold are protective only in conditions of mild hypothermia (see later), and they must be supplemented by behavioral responses to cold (e.g., wearing warm clothing and seeking shelter from the cold). Because of the importance of behavioral responses, hypothermia is particularly pronounced when behavioral responses are impaired (e.g., in the intoxicated or the elderly) or cannot be carried out (e.g., mountain climbers who are unable to gain shelter from the cold).

Accidental Hypothermia

Environmental hypothermia is most likely to occur in the following situations: (1) prolonged submersion in cold water (the transfer of heat to cold water occurs much more readily than the transfer of heat to cold air), (2) exposure to cold wind (wind promotes heat transfer by convection, as described earlier in the chapter), (3) when the physiological responses to cold are impaired (e.g., alcohol intoxication reduces cutaneous vasoconstriction and shivering in response to cold), and (4) when the behavioral responses to cold are impaired (as described in the last paragraph).

Clinical Features

Most standard thermometers record temperatures down to 34°C (94°F). When hypothermia is suspected, specialized **electronic temperature probes that** can be placed in the bladder, rectum, or esophagus and **can record temperatures down to 25°C** (77°F) **should be used** to record body temperature. The severity of hypothermia can then be classified as shown in Table 38.5.

The clinical manifestations of hypothermia can vary in individual patients, but they generally resemble the patterns shown in Table 38.5.

TABLE 38.5 Manifestations of Hypothermia

Severity	Body Temperature	Clinical Manifestations
Mild	32°C–35°C 90°F–95°F	Confusion, cold, pale skin, shivering, tachycardia
Moderate	28°C–31.8°C 82°F–89°F	Lethargy, reduced or absent shivering, bradycardia, decreased respiratory rate
Severe	<28°C <82°F	Obtundation or coma, no shivering, edematous skin, dilated and fixed pupils, bradycardia, hypotension, oliguria
Life-threatening	<25°C <77°F	Apnea, asystole

In mild hypothermia (32°C to 35°C or 90°F to 95°F), patients are usually confused and show signs of adaptation to cold, which include cold, pale skin (from cutaneous vasoconstriction) and brisk shivering. Shivering may be absent in patients with moderate hypothermia (28°C to 31.8°C or 82°F to 89°F), who instead present with lethargy, sluggish or absent pupillary light reflexes, a decreased heart rate, and hypoventilation. In severe hypothermia (<28°C or <82°F), patients are usually obtunded or comatose with dilated, fixed pupils (which are not a sign of brain death in this situation). Additional findings include hypotension, severe bradycardia, oliguria, and generalized edema. Apnea and asystole are expected at body temperatures below 25°C (77°F).

Laboratory Tests

The laboratory tests of most interest in hypothermia are the arterial blood gases, serum electrolytes (particularly potassium), and tests of coagulation status and renal function. A generalized coagulopathy (with elevation of the INR and prolonged partial thromboplastin times) is common in hypothermia (21), but may not be evident if the coagulation profile is run at normal body temperatures. Arterial blood gases (which should be run at normal body temperatures) can reveal a respiratory acidosis or a metabolic acidosis (21). Serum electrolytes can reveal hyperkalemia, which is presumably due to potassium release by skeletal muscle from shivering or rhabdomyolysis. Serum creatinine levels can be elevated as a result of cold diuresis (which may be the result of diminished tubular responses to antidiuretic hormone), rhabdomyolysis, or acute renal failure.

The Electrocardiogram

About 80% of patients with hypothermia will have prominent J waves at the QRS-ST junction on the electrocardiogram (see Fig. 38.1). These waves, which are called *Osborn waves*, are not specific for hypothermia, and can also occur in association with hypercalcemia, subarachnoid hemorrhage, cerebral injuries, and myocardial ischemia (22). Despite the attention these waves have received, they are merely a curiosity, and have little or no diagnostic or prognostic value in hypothermia (13–21).

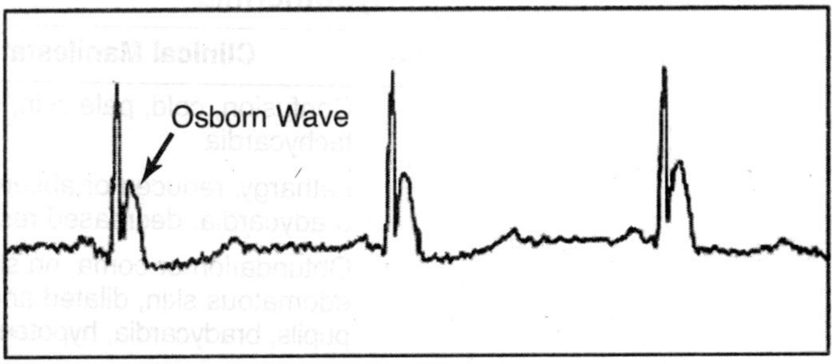

FIGURE 38.1 The (overhyped) Osborn wave.

(Hypothermia should be evident by body temperature measurements before an electrocardiogram is obtained.)

Almost any rhythm disturbance can occur in hypothermia, including first, second, and third-degree heart block, sinus and junctional bradycardia, idioventricular rhythm, premature atrial and ventricular beats, and atrial and ventricular fibrillation (22).

Rewarming

External rewarming (removing wet clothes, covering the patient in blankets, etc.) can increase body temperature at a rate of 1°C to 2°C per hour (21), and **is adequate for most cases of hypothermia** (23). There is a risk of a further decrease in body temperature during external rewarming (called *afterdrop*), which can trigger ventricular fibrillation (24). This phenomenon is attributed to central displacement of cold blood in cutaneous blood vessels. Fortunately, serious cardiac arrhythmias are not common, and do not contribute to mortality, during external rewarming for severe hypothermia (23,24).

There are several methods of internal rewarming, but they are invasive, time-consuming, and are needed only in the most severe cases of hypothermia. The easiest internal warming technique involves increasing the temperature of inhaled gases to 40°C to 45°C (104°F to 113°F), which can raise the core temperature at a rate of 2.5°C per hour in intubated patients (21). Other internal warming techniques include peritoneal lavage with heated fluids (21), extracorporeal blood rewarming (25), and heated intravenous fluids (26). **Warmed gastric lavage is considered ineffective** (21).

Rewarming Shock

Rewarming from moderate-to-severe hypothermia is often accompanied by hypotension (*rewarming shock*) that is attributed to a combination of factors, including hypovolemia (from cold diuresis), myocardial depression, and vasodilation (23,24). Volume infusion can help to alleviate this problem, but the intravenous fluids must be heated because infusion of fluids at room temperature (21°C or 70°F) can aggravate the hypothermia. Vasoactive drugs are required in about half of patients with severe hypothermia, and the need for vasoactive drugs carries a poor prognosis (24).

Induced Hypothermia

External cooling to a body temperature of 32°C to 34°C (89.6°F to 93.2°F) has been shown to improve neurologic outcome in patients who remain comatose after certain types of cardiac arrest. This topic is presented in Chapter 15 (see Table 15.3) and will not be repeated here.

A FINAL WORD

One of the most striking aspects of the disorders in this chapter is how uncommon they are. This is particularly true of the drug-induced hyperthermia syndromes, and is also the case with heat-related illness.

The number of deaths from heat exposure is estimated at only 400 per year in the United States (Morbidity and Mortality Weekly Report 2002;51:567-570). Considering that there are about 6,000 hospitals in the United States, you would have to work in about 15 hospitals per year before you would witness one death from heat exposure. (Presumably, hospitals in urban areas or in the South would be more likely to have deaths from heat exposure, but the number of deaths is still very small.) This suggests a genetic predisposition to hyperthermia, regardless of the cause.

Hypothermia is more prevalent than hyperthermia, but the numbers are still small. In a 20-year survey of a large urban hospital in Paris, France (24), only 0.4% of admissions to the ICU were for severe hypothermia (body temperature <32°C). Presumably, man's tendency to protect himself from the cold (which plays an important role in preventing hypothermia) explains why hypothermia is kept in check.

REFERENCES

Mechanisms of Heat Exchange

1. Keel CA, Neil E, Joels N. Regulation of body temperature in man. In: Samson Wright's applied physiology, 13th ed. New York: Oxford University Press, 1982:346.
2. Guyton AC, Hall JE. Body temperature, temperature regulation, and fever. In: Medical physiology, 10th ed. Philadelphia: WB Saunders, 2000:822–833.

Heat-Related Illness

3. Khosla R, Guntupalli KK. Heat-related illnesses. Crit Care Clin 1999;15:251–263.
4. Lugo-Amador NM, Rothenhaus T, Moyer P. Heat-related illness. Emerg Med Clin North Am 2004;22:315–327.
5. Glazer JL. Management of heat stroke and heat exhaustion. Am Fam Physician 2005;71:2133–2142.
6. Hadad E, Rav-Acha M, Heled Y, et al. Heat stroke: a review of cooling methods. Sports Med 2004;34:501–511.
7. Ward MM. Factors predictive of acute renal failure in rhabdomyolysis. Arch Intern Med 1988;148:1553–1557.
8. Visweswaran P, Guntupalli J. Rhabdomyolysis. Crit Care Clin 1999;15:415–429.

Malignant Hyperthermia

9. Rusyniakn DE, Sprague JE. Toxin-induced hyperthermic syndromes. Med Clin North Am 2005;89:1277–1296.
10. Litman RS, Rosenberg H. Malignant hyperthermia. JAMA 2005;293:2918–2924.
11. McEvoy GK, ed. AHFS Drug Information. Bethesda, MD: American Society of Health-System Pharmacists, 2001:1328–1331.

Neuroleptic Malignant Syndrome

12. Bhanushali NJ, Tuite PJ. The evaluation and management of patients with neuroleptic malignant syndrome. Neurol Clin North Am 2004;22:389–411.
13. Khaldarov V. Benzodiazepines for treatment of neuroleptic malignant syndrome. Hosp Physician 2000;36:51–55.
14. Otani K, Horiuchi M, Kondo T, et al. Is the predisposition to neuroleptic malignant syndrome genetically transmitted? Br J Psychiatry 1991;158:850–853.
15. Lev R, Clark RF. Neuroleptic malignant syndrome presenting without fever: case report and review of the literature. J Emerg Med 1996;12:49–55.
16. Guze BH, Baxter LR. Neuroleptic malignant syndrome. N Engl J Med 1985; 313:163–166.

Serotonin Syndrome

17. Boyer EH, Shannon M. The serotonin syndrome. N Engl J Med 2005;352:1112–1120.
18. Demirkiran M, Jankivic J, Dean JM. Ecstacy intoxication: an overlap between serotonin syndrome and neuroleptic malignant syndrome. Clin Neuropharmacol 1996;19:157–164.
19. Hick JL, Smith SW, Lynch MT. Metabolic acidosis in restraint-associated cardiac arrest. Acad Emerg Med 1999;6:239–245.
20. Graudins A, Stearman A, Chan B. Treatment of serotonin syndrome with cyproheptadine. J Emerg Med 1998;16:615–619.

Hypothermia Syndromes

21. Hanania NA, Zimmerman NA. Accidental hypothermia. Crit Care Clin 1999; 15:235–249.
22. Aslam AF, Aslam AK, Vasavada BC, et al. Hypothermia: evaluation: electrocardiographic manifestations, and management. Am J Med 2006;119: 297–301.
23. Cornell HM. Hot topics in cold medicine: controversies in accidental hypothermia. Clin Pediatr Emerg Med 2001;2:179–191.
24. Vassal T, Bernoit-Gonin B, Carrat F, et al. Severe accidental hypothermia treated in an ICU. Chest 2001;120:1998–2003.
25. Ireland AJ, Pathi VL, Crawford R, et al. Back from the dead: extracorporeal rewarming of severe accidental hypothermia victims in accidental emergency. J Accid Emerg Med 1997;14:255–303.
26. Handrigen MT, Wright RO, Becker BM, et al. Factors and methodology in achieving ideal delivery temperatures for intravenous and lavage fluid in hypothermia. Am J Emerg Med 1997;15:350–359.

Chapter 39

FEVER IN THE ICU

Humanity has but three great enemies:
Fever, famine and war.
Of these, by far the greatest,
By far the most terrible, is fever.

Sir William Osler

Despite Osler's harsh comments about fever, the appearance of fever in an ICU patient is not a sign of impending doom, but it is a sign that requires attention. This chapter describes the conditions that are most often associated with hospital-acquired (nosocomial) fever in the ICU (1,2). Additional considerations in immunocompromised patients are presented in Chapter 43. The final section of the chapter focuses on the practice of suppressing fever and why this practice should be abandoned, particularly in patients with infection.

BODY TEMPERATURE

Two scales (Celsius and Fahrenheit) are used to record body temperature, and the conversion from one scale to the other is shown in Table 39.1. Although readings on the Celsius scale are often called degrees "centigrade," this unit is intended for the degrees on a compass, not for temperatures (3). The appropriate term for temperatures on the Celsius scale is *degrees Celsius*.

Normal Body Temperature

Despite the fact that the body temperature is one of the most common measurements performed in clinical medicine, there is some disagreement about what the normal body temperature is in healthy adults. The following points illustrate some of the confusion regarding the normal body temperature.

TABLE 39.1 Temperature Conversions

Corresponding Scales (°C)	(°F)	Conversion Formulas
100	212	Conversions are based on the corresponding temperatures at the freezing point of water:
41	105.8	
40	104	O°C = 32°F
39	102.2	and the temperture ranges (from freezing point to boiling point of water):
38	100.4	
37	98.6	100°C = 180°F or 5°C = 9°F
36	96.8	The above relationships are then combined to derive the conversion formulas:
35	95	°F = (9/5°C) + 32
34	93.2	°C = 5/9 (°F − 32)
33	91.4	
32	89.6	
31	87.8	
30	86	
0	32	

The traditional norm of 37°C (98.6°F) is a mean value derived from a study of *axillary* temperatures in 25,000 healthy adults, conducted in the late 19th century (4). However, axillary temperatures can vary by as much as 1.0°C (1.8°F) from core body temperatures (5) and, as a result, axillary temperatures are not recommended for recording body temperature in ICU patients (1).

Core body temperature can be 0.5°C (0.9°F) higher than oral temperatures (6), and 0.2°C to 0.3°C lower than rectal temperatures (1).

Elderly subjects have a mean body temperature that is approximately 0.5°C (0.9°F) lower than that of younger adults (4,7).

The normal body temperature has a diurnal variation, with the nadir in the early morning (between 4 and 8 a.m.) and the peak in the late afternoon (between 4 and 6 p.m.). The range of diurnal variation varies in individual subjects, with the highest reported range in an individual subject being 1.3°C (2.4°F) (8).

These observations indicate that the normal body temperature is not a single temperature, but rather is a range of temperatures that is influenced by age, time of day, and measurement site.

Where to Measure Temperature

The consensus view is that the temperatures in the pulmonary artery and the urinary bladder (measured with thermistor-equipped pulmonary artery catheters and bladder catheters, respectively), are the most accurate representations of core body temperature (1). When these temperatures are not available (which is often), infrared probes placed in the external auditory canal to measure "ear canal temperature" (often mistaken as tympanic membrane temperature) can provide suitable measurements when used properly (9–11). Surprisingly, oral temperatures measured in intubated patients can be a close approximation of core body temperature when electronic probes (not mercury thermometers) are placed in the right or left sublingual pockets (10). Finally, rectal temperatures can also provide an accurate reflection of core body temperature (9), but rectal probes are not well tolerated by alert patients.

Definition of Fever

Fever is best defined as a temperature that exceeds the normal daily temperature range for an individual subject. However, this is not a practical definition because the body temperature is not monitored continuously in hospitalized patients, so it is not possible to determine the daily temperature variation for each patient. The Society of Critical Care Medicine, in their practice guideline (1), proposes that **a body temperature above 38.3°C (101°F) represents a fever and deserves further evaluation to search for an infection.** This is more useful as an operational definition that identifies when an elevated body temperature deserves further evaluation.

The Febrile Response

Fever is the result of inflammatory cytokines (called endogenous pyrogens) that act on the hypothalamus to elevate the body temperature. Unlike hyperthermia, which is the result of abnormal temperature regulation in the body (see Chapter 38), fever is a condition where the thermoregulatory system is intact but is operating at a higher set point (12). The elevated body temperatures in fever serve to enhance immune function and inhibit bacterial and viral replication. (The beneficial effects of fever are described in more detail later in the chapter.) Fever is therefore an adaptive response that aids the host in defending against infection and other bodily insults. The following facts about fever deserve mention.

Fever is a sign of inflammation, not infection. Fever is not a specific response to infection, but rather is a response to any form of tissue injury that is sufficient enough to trigger an inflammatory response. This might explain why about 50% of ICU patients with fever have no apparent infection (13,14). The distinction between inflammation and infection is an important one, not only for the evaluation of fever, but also for curtailing the use of antibiotics to treat a fever.

The severity of the fever is not an indication of the presence or severity of infection. High fevers can be associated with noninfectious processes (e.g., drug fever), while fever can be mild or absent in patients with life-threatening infections (2).

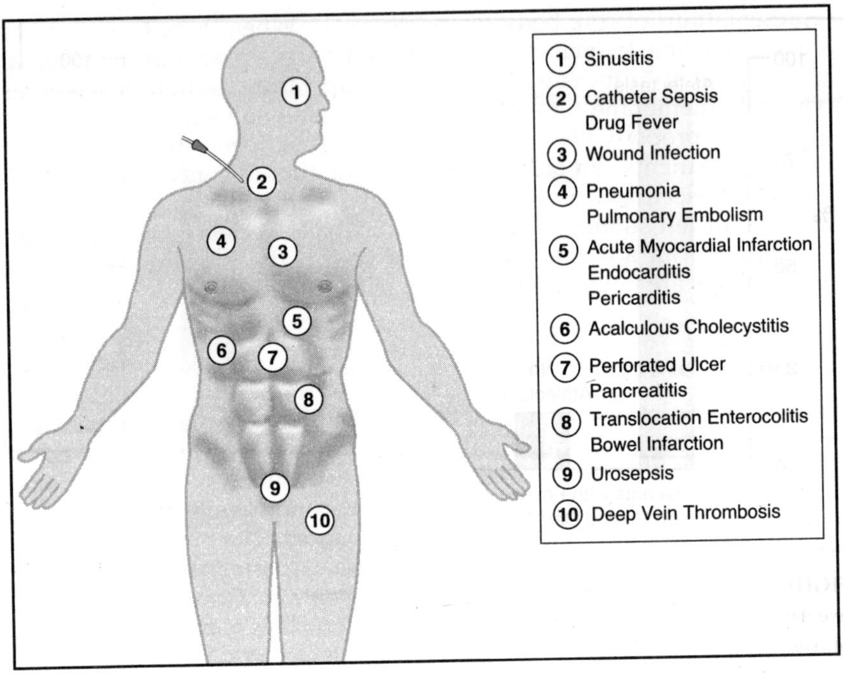

FIGURE 39.1 Common causes of nosocomial fever in the ICU.

Causes of Fever in the ICU

Any condition capable of triggering an immune response is capable of causing a fever. The common conditions associated with hospital-acquired (nosocomial) fever in general medical-surgical ICUs are shown in Fig. 39.1. Most of these conditions are described briefly in this chapter.

Noninfectious Causes of Fever

POSTOPERATIVE FEVER. Surgery always involves some degree of tissue injury, and major surgery can involve considerable tissue injury. (In the words of Dr. John Millili, a surgeon and close friend, major surgery is akin to being *hit with a baseball bat!)* Because inflammation and fever are the normal response to tissue injury, fever is a likely consequence of major surgery. Fever in the first day following major surgery is reported in 15% to 40% of patients (15–17), and in most of these cases, there is no associated infection (15,16). These fevers are short-lived, and usually resolve within 24 to 48 hours.

Atelectasis and Fever There is a longstanding misconception that atelectasis is a common cause of fever in the early postoperative period. One possible source of this misconception is the high incidence of atelectasis in patients who develop a postoperative fever. This is demonstrated in Figure 39.2 (see the graph on the left), which is from a study involving patients who underwent open heart surgery (17). Close to 90% of the patients with a fever on the first postoperative day had radiographic

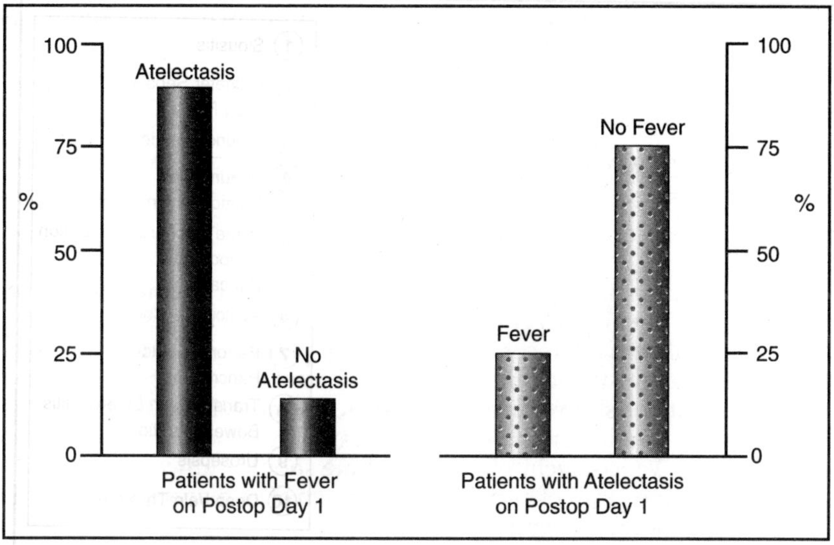

FIGURE 39.2 The relationships between atelectasis and fever on the first postoperative day in 100 consecutive patients who had open heart surgery. (Data from Engoren M. Lack of association between atelectasis and fever. Chest 1995;167:81.)

evidence of atelectasis. This, however, is *not* evidence that the atelectasis is the source of fever. In fact, the graph on the right in Figure 39.2 shows that most (75%) of the patients with atelectasis did not have a fever. The inability of atelectasis to produce fever was demonstrated over 50 years ago in an animal study where lobar atelectasis produced by ligation of a mainstem bronchus was not accompanied by fever (18).

The high incidence of atelectasis in patients with postop fever is explained by the fact that atelectasis is extremely common after major surgery. For example, upper abdominal surgery results in a 40% to 70% decrease in the functional residual capacity (FRC) of the lungs (the volume of air in the lungs at the end of expiration) for up to one week (19). Since atelectasis involves a decrease in FRC, virtually every patient who undergoes upper abdominal surgery is expected to have postop atelectasis. In fact, general anesthesia is accompanied by atelectasis in over 90% of cases (20), so atelectasis is almost a universal consequence of major surgery. Therefore, a high incidence of atelectasis is expected in any group of postop patients, not just those with fever.

Therefore, the available evidence indicates that **atelectasis is very common after major surgery, but is not a common cause of postoperative fever**. Most fevers that appear in the first 24 to 48 hours after surgery are most likely a result of the tissue injury sustained during the procedure.

Malignant Hyperthermia

Another cause of elevated body temperatures in the immediate postoperative period is malignant hyperthermia, an inherited disorder characterized by intense muscle rigidity and hyperthermia in response to halogenated inhalational anesthetics and depolarizing neuromuscular blockers (e.g., succinylcholine). This disorder is described in detail in Chapter 38.

Other Procedures Associated with Fever

The following procedures or interventions can be accompanied by non-infectious fever.

Hemodialysis

Febrile reactions during hemodialysis are attributed to endotoxin contamination of the dialysis equipment, but bacteremia occurs on occasion (21). Blood cultures are recommended for all patients who develop fever during hemodialysis, but the dialysis does not have to be terminated unless the patient shows signs of sepsis (e.g., mental status changes or hypotension). Empiric antibiotics are recommended only for patients who appear septic. Vancomycin plus ceftazidime should suffice pending culture results. (One gram of each antibiotic given after dialysis will provide adequate serum levels pending culture results.)

Bronchoscopy

Fiberoptic bronchoscopy is followed by fever in 5% of cases (22). The fever usually appears 8 to 10 hours after the procedure, and it subsides spontaneously in 24 hours (22). The probable cause is release of endogenous pyrogens from the lung during the procedure. The fever is often associated with leukocytosis (22), but pneumonia and bacteremia are rare (23). There is no need for blood cultures or empiric antimicrobial therapy unless the fever does not subside or the patient shows signs of sepsis (e.g., mental status changes or hypotension).

Blood Transfusions

Febrile reactions occur in as many as 5% of patients receiving blood products. The fever is usually the result of antileukocyte antibodies, and appears during or shortly after the transfusion. For more information on febrile transfusion reactions, see Chapter 36.

Venous Thromboembolism

Several groups of hospitalized patients are at risk for venous thromboembolism (see Table 5.1 and Figure 5.1), but the risk is highest in trauma victims and postoperative patients, particularly following orthopedic procedures involving the hip and knee. Most cases of hospital-acquired deep vein thrombosis are asymptomatic, but acute pulmonary embolism can produce a fever that lasts up to 1 week (24). The diagnostic approach to suspected venous thromboembolism is described in Chapter 5.

Acalculous Cholecystitis

Acalculous cholecystitis is an uncommon but serious disorder reported in up to 1.5% of critically ill patients (25). It is most common in postoperative patients, trauma victims, and patients receiving parenteral nutrition. This condition is believed to be the result of ischemia and stasis within the gallbladder, eventually leading to edema of the cystic duct that blocks drainage of the gallbladder. The resulting clinical syndrome includes fever (70 to 95% of cases) and right upper quadrant tenderness (60 to 100% of cases) (25). Diagnosis is often possible with right upper quadrant ultrasound. Perforation of the gallbladder can occur within 48 hours after onset. The treatment of choice is cholecystectomy, or percutaneous cholecystostomy in patients who are too ill for surgery. (For more information on this disorder, see Chapter 42.)

Pharmaceutical Agents

Drug Fever

Drug-induced fever can be the result of a hypersensitivity reaction, an idiosyncratic reaction, or an infusion-related phlebitis. *Drug fever* is a recognized entity in the ICU, but the significance and prevalence of this entity in the ICU is not known. The therapeutic agents most often implicated in drug fever are listed in Table 39.2.

Drug fever is poorly understood. The onset of the fever varies from a few hours to a few weeks after the onset of drug therapy (2). The fever can appear as an isolated finding or can be accompanied by the other manifestations listed in Table 39.2 (26). Note that about half of patients have rigors, and about 20% develop hypotension, indicating that **patients with a drug fever can appear to be seriously ill**. Evidence of a hypersensitivity reaction (i.e., eosinophilia and rash) is absent in most cases of drug fever.

Suspicion of drug fever usually occurs when there are no other probable sources of fever. In this situation, it is best to discontinue possible offenders. The fever should disappear in 2 to 3 days, but it can take up to 7 days to disappear (27).

Drug-Induced Hyperthermia Syndromes

The drug-induced hyperthermia syndromes include malignant hyperthermia (mentioned earlier), neuroleptic malignant syndrome, and

TABLE 39.2 Drug-Associated Fever in the ICU

Common Offenders	Occasional Offenders	Clinical Findings*
Amphotericin	Cimetidine	Rigors (53%)
Cephalosporins	Carbamazepine	Myalgias (25%)
Penicillins	Hydralazine	Leukocytosis (22%)
Phenytoin	Rifampin	Eosiniphillia (22%)
Procainamide	Streptokinase	Rash (18%)
Quinidine	Vancomycin	Hypotension (18%)

*From Mackowiak and LeMaistre (26).

serotonin syndrome. These disorders are described in detail in Chapter 38. The neuroleptic malignant syndrome may be an important concern in ICUs where haloperidol is used for sedation.

Endocrine Disorders

The endocrine disorders known to produce fever are thyrotoxicosis and adrenal crisis. Thyrotoxicosis is unlikely to appear *de novo* in the ICU, but adrenal crisis due to spontaneous adrenal hemorrhage is a recognized complication of anticoagulant therapy and disseminated intravascular coagulation (DIC). These endocrine disorders are described in Chapter 48.

Infarctions

Ischemic injury in any organ will trigger a local inflammatory response and this can produce a fever. Myocardial and cerebrovascular infarctions are usually heralded by other symptoms, but bowel infarction can be clinically silent in elderly, debilitated patients or patients with depressed consciousness. The only sign of a bowel infarction may be an unexplained fever or metabolic (lactic) acidosis. Unfortunately, there are no reliable diagnostic tests for bowel infarction, and the diagnosis is usually made at laparotomy.

Systemic Inflammatory Response Syndrome

The clinical entity known as *systemic inflammatory response syndrome* (SIRS) is characterized by signs of systemic inflammation (e.g., fever, leukocytosis) without evidence of infection. Possible sources of SIRS include tissue injury from trauma, ischemia, or toxic insults, and translocation of endotoxin and bacterial antigens from the lumen of the gastrointestinal tract. SIRS is often accompanied by inflammatory injury in one or more vital organs (e.g., acute respiratory distress syndrome) (28), and it can progress relentlessly to multiorgan failure and death. This condition is described in more detail in Chapter 40.

Other Causes

Other noninfectious causes of fever in the ICU include toxin-induced organ injury (e.g., alcohol-induced pancreatitis and hepatitis), delirium tremens, and thrombotic thrombocytopenia purpura. In each of these conditions, fever is accompanied by a constellation of clinical findings that, taken together, arouses suspicion of the disorder.

Iatrogenic Fever

Faulty thermal regulators in water mattresses and aerosol humidifiers can cause fever by transference (29). It takes only a minute to check the temperature settings on heated mattresses and ventilators, but it can take far longer to explain why such a simple cause of fever was overlooked.

TABLE 39.3 Nosocomial Infections in Medical and Surgical ICU Patients in the United States*

Nosocomial Infection	% Total Infections: Medical Patients		% Total Infections: Surgical Patients	
Pneumonia	30%	76%	33%	78%
Urinary Tract Infection	30%		18%	
Bloodstream Infection	16%		13%	
Surgical Site Infection	—		14%	
Cardiovascular Infection	5%		4%	
GI Tract Infection	5%		4%	
Ear, Nose & Throat Infection	4%		4%	
Skin & Soft Tissue Infection	3%		3%	
Others	7%		7%	

*From Richards MJ et al. & the National Nosocomial Infections Surveillance System. Nosocomial infections in combined medical-surgical intensive care units in the United States. Infect Control Hosp Epidemiol. 2000;21:510–515.

Common Nosocomial Infections

The National Nosocomial Infections Surveillance System is a government-sponsored program that monitors nosocomial infections in 99 hospitals in the United States, and the results of this survey for medical and surgical ICU patients (over the years 1992 through 1997) is shown in Table 39.3 (30). Four infections account for over three-quarters of the nosocomial infections in these patients: pneumonia, urinary tract infections, bloodstream infections, and surgical site infections. Three of these infections are primarily related to indwelling devices (i.e., 83% of pneumonias occur in intubated patients, 97% of urinary tract infections occur in catheterized patients, and 87% of bloodstream infections originate from intravascular catheters) (30).

The pathogenic organisms isolated in three of the common nosocomial infections are shown in Table 39.4. (31) *Staphylococcus aureus* and *Pseudomonas aeruginosa* are the two most common isolates in pneumonia, *Candida albicans* is the most common isolate in urinary tract infections, and staphylococci are responsible for about half of the bloodstream infections that originate from intravascular catheters. The microbial spectrum of these infections provides a valuable guide for selecting empiric antibiotic regimens.

Pneumonia

Nosocomial pneumonia in the ICU is primarily a disease of ventilator-dependent patients. Pneumonia should be suspected when there is a new infiltrate on chest x-ray and two of the following conditions are present: fever, leukocytosis, and purulent tracheal secretions (32). The diagnosis of pneumonia requires isolation of one or more organisms

TABLE 39.4 Pathogens Involved in Nosocomial Infections*

	% of Infections		
Pathogen	Pneumonia	UTI	Bloodstream Infection
Staphylococcus aureus	20	2	13
Staphylococcus epidermidis	1	2	36
Enterococci	2	14	16
Pseudomonas aeruginosa	21	10	3
Klebsiella pneumoniae	8	6	4
Enterobacter	9	5	3
Escherichia coli	4	14	3
Candida albicans	5	23	6

*From Richards MJ, et al. Nosocomial infections in medical intensive care units in the United States. Crit Care Med 1999;27:887–892.
UTI = urinary tract infection

from the lower respiratory tract. There are a variety of methods for obtaining and culturing respiratory secretions, and these are described in Chapter 41. (For an excellent and up-to-date practice guideline on nosocomial pneumonia, see reference 32.)

Urinary Tract Infections

Urinary tract infection should be suspected as a cause of nosocomial fever in any patient with an indwelling bladder catheter for more than a few days. The diagnosis of urinary tract infection is difficult in chronically catheterized patients because the urine in these patients often contains large numbers of bacteria. Therefore, a positive urine culture is not always evidence of infection in a chronically instrumented patient. The demonstration of pyuria by gram stain or leukocyte esterase dipstick test (for detection of granulocytes in the urine) can help to identify patients with significant bacteriuria. The approach to urinary tract infections in catheterized patients is described in more detail in Chapter 42.

Catheter Sepsis

Infections caused by indwelling vascular catheters should be suspected in any case of unexplained fever when a catheter has been in place for more than 48 hours, or when purulence is found at the catheter insertion site. If the patient appears toxic, or there is purulence at the catheter insertion site, the catheter should be removed and a distal segment of catheter should be sent for *semiquantitative* cultures (see Table 7.4 for the semiquantitative culture technique). This must be combined with a blood culture obtained from a distant venipuncture site. If the patient is not seriously ill and there is no purulence at the catheter insertion site, the catheter can be left in place. In this situation, one blood sample should be withdrawn through the catheter and a second blood sample should be obtained from a distant venipuncture site: both samples should then be submitted for *quantitative* blood cultures (see Table 7.3 for a description of the quantitative culture technique).

Except for the presence of purulent drainage at the catheter insertion site, it is not possible to determine if an intravascular catheter is the source of nosocomial fever without the appropriate culture results. Therefore, the decision to initiate empiric antibiotic therapy will be determined by the clinical condition of the patient. If there are no signs of severe sepsis (e.g., mental status changes or hemodynamic instability) antibiotics can be withheld. If empiric antibiotic therapy is needed, coverage for staphylococci (with vancomycin or a carbepenem) is mandatory. For more information on the diagnosis and treatment of catheter-related sepsis, see Chapter 7.

Wound Infections

Surgical wounds are classified as clean (abdomen and chest unopened), contaminated (abdomen or chest opened), or dirty (direct contact with pus or bowel contents) (33). Wound infections typically appear at 5 to 7 days after surgery. Most infections do not extend beyond the skin and subcutaneous tissues, and can be managed with debridement only. Antimicrobial therapy (to cover streptococcus, staphylococcus, and anaerobes) should be reserved for cases of persistent erythema or for evidence of deep tissue involvement (15). In fever that follows median sternotomy, sternal wound infection with spread to the mediastinum is a prominent concern (34). In this situation, sternal instability can be an early sign of infection.

Necrotizing wound infections are produced by Clostridia or β-hemolytic streptococci. Unlike other wound infections, which appear 5 to 7 days after surgery, necrotizing infections are evident in the first few postoperative days. There is often marked edema around the incision, and the skin may have crepitance and fluid-filled bullae. Spread to deeper structures is rapid and produces progressive rhabdomyolysis and myoglobinuric renal failure. Treatment involves extensive debridement and intravenous penicillin. The mortality is high (above 60%) when treatment is delayed.

LESS COMMON INFECTIONS

Paranasal Sinusitis

Indwelling nasogastric and nasotracheal tubes can block the ostia that drain the paranasal sinuses, leading to accumulation of infected secretions in the sinuses (35,36). The maxillary sinuses are almost always involved, and the resulting acute sinusitis can be an occult source of fever. This complication is reported in 15 to 20% of patients with nasal tubes (35,36) although its significance in many patients is unclear (see later).

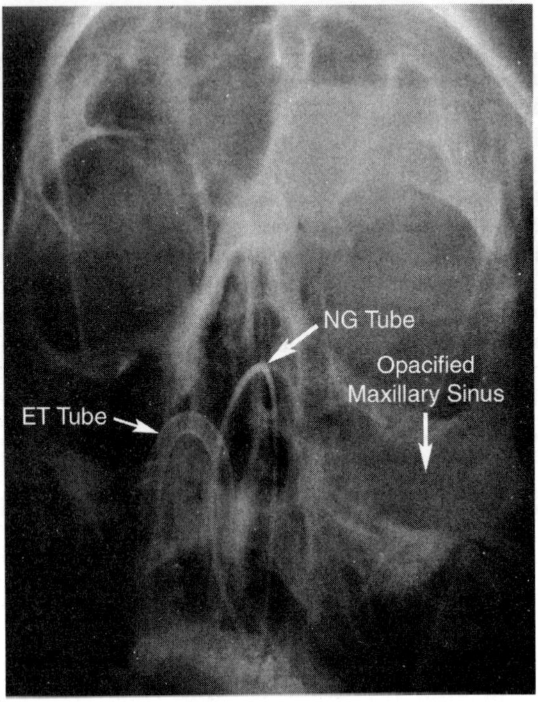

FIGURE 39.3 Portable sinus film showing opacification of the left maxillary and frontal sinuses in a patient with nasotracheal and nasogastric tubes in place. Acute sinusitis was subsequently confirmed by maxillary sinus puncture and quantitative culture of the sinus aspirate, which showed growth of *S epidermidis* at 10^3 CFU/mL.

Diagnosis

Purulent drainage from the nares may be absent, and the diagnosis is suggested by radiographic features of sinusitis (i.e., opacification or air–fluid levels in the involved sinuses). Although CT scans are recommended for the diagnosis of nosocomial sinusitis (35,36), portable sinus films obtained at the bedside can also be revealing, as shown in Figure 39.3. The maxillary sinuses can be viewed with a single "occipitomental view," also called a "Waters view," which can be obtained at the bedside (37). Because CT scans require patient transport out of the ICU, it is convenient to attempt visualization of the maxillary sinuses with portable sinus films. CT scans are then reserved only for cases where the portable sinus films are of poor quality. It is important to emphasize that 30 to 40% of patients with radiographic evidence of sinusitis do not have an infection documented by culture of aspirated material from the involved sinus (35,36). Therefore, **radiographic evidence of sinusitis is not sufficient for the diagnosis of purulent sinusitis**. The diagnosis must be confirmed by sinus puncture and isolation of pathogens by quantitative culture ($\geq 10^3$ colony forming units per milliliter) (35,36).

Treatment

Responsible pathogens include gram-negative bacteria (especially *Pseudomonas aeruginosa*) in 60% of cases, gram-positive bacteria (particularly *Staphylococcus aureus*) in 30% of cases, and yeasts (particularly *Candida albicans*) in 10% of cases (1). Local irrigation of the sinuses with antimicrobial solutions can be effective (36), but a brief course of systemic antibiotics seems wise because invasion of the bloodstream is a recognized risk with nosocomial sinusitis (unlike outpatient sinusitis, where septicemia is rare). When a sinus aspirate is purulent or shows organisms on Gram stain, empiric antimicrobial therapy can be guided by the predominant organism(s) on Gramstain. Nasal tubes should also be removed.

Significance

Despite the recognized potential for harm, nosocomial sinusitis is unproven as an entity that deserves attention in the evaluation of nosocomial fever. The problem is that nosocomial sinusitis occurs in about one-quarter of patients with indwelling nasal tubes, yet sinusitis is often overlooked in the evaluation of nosocomial fever without apparent harm. This issue needs to be resolved before nosocomial sinusitis can gain the respect given to other nosocomial infections.

Pseudomembranous Enterocolitis

Enterocolitis from *Clostridium difficile* should be suspected for cases of nosocomial fever accompanied by diarrhea in patients who have received antibiotics or chemotherapy within 2 weeks prior to the onset of the fever (1). The diagnosis requires documentation of *C. difficile* toxin in stool samples or evidence of pseudomembranes on proctosigmoidoscopy (38). In severe cases of diarrhea, proctosigmoidoscopy is preferred because it allows an immediate diagnosis. Otherwise, a stool sample should be submitted for *C. difficile* toxin assay. If this is negative, a second stool sample should be submitted (1). Empiric antibiotics should not be necessary unless the diarrhea is severe or the patient appears toxic. Therapy can include oral or intravenous metronidazole (500 mg every 6 hours) or oral vancomycin (500 mg orally every 6 hours). This disorder is described in more detail in Chapter 42.

Abdominal Abscess

Abdominal abscesses typically become symptomatic at one to two weeks after laparotomy. Septicemia occurs in approximately 50% of cases (39). Computed tomography of the abdomen will reveal the localized collection in more than 95% of cases (39). Initial antimicrobial therapy should be directed at gram-negative enteric pathogens, including anaerobes (e.g., *Bacteroides fragilis*), but definitive treatment requires surgical or percutaneous drainage.

Other Infections

Other infections that should be considered in selected patient populations are **endocarditis** (in patients with prosthetic valves), **meningitis** (in neurosurgical patients and those with human immunodeficiency virus infection), and **spontaneous bacterial peritonitis** (in patients with cirrhosis and ascites).

EARLY MANAGEMENT DECISIONS

Blood Cultures

Blood cultures should be obtained whenever an infection is suspected as a cause of nosocomial fever. **No more than one set of blood cultures should be obtained from each venipuncture site** (40). The appropriate number of venipuncture sites is determined by the likelihood of bloodstream infection. The following scheme is recommended (40).

1. If the likelihood of septicemia is low (e.g., when pneumonia or urinary tract infection is suspected) no more than two venipuncture sites are required for blood cultures.
2. If the probability of septicemia is high (e.g., when catheter-related sepsis or endocarditis is suspected), at least three venipuncture sites are recommended for blood cultures. If the patient has received antimicrobial agents within the past few weeks, at least four venipuncture sites are recommended.

Volume of Blood

One of the lesser known features of blood cultures is the influence of blood volume on the culture results. In cases of low-level bacteremia, increasing the volume of blood that is cultured will increase the chances of showing growth of the microorganism. Therefore, **to achieve optimal results with blood cultures, a volume of 20 to 30 mL of blood should be withdrawn from each venipuncture site** (40). The volume of blood added to each culture bottle should be kept at the usual 1:5 ratio (blood volume: broth volume).

Empiric Antimicrobial Therapy

Empiric antibiotic therapy is indicated in the following situations:

1. When the likelihood of infection is high.
2. When there is evidence of severe sepsis or severe organ dysfunction (e.g., depressed consciousness, progressive hypoxemia, hypotension, metabolic acidosis, or decreasing urine output).
3. When the patient is immunocompromised (e.g. neutropenia).

Empiric antibiotic therapy should be selected on the basis of antibiotic susceptibility patterns in each ICU. For ICUs with multidrug resistant pathogens (e.g., methicillin-resistant Staphylococcus aureus), empiric coverage for gram-positive infections should include vancomycin or linezolid (the latter agent can be used when vancomycin-resistant enterococci have been encountered in the ICU) and empiric coverage for gram-negative infections can include either a carbepenem (imipenem cilastatin or meropenem), an antipseudomonal cephalosporin (ceftazidime or cefipime) or an antipseudomonal penicillin (ticarcillin clavulnate or pipericillin tazobactam), In immunocompromised patients, an aminoglycoside can be added for gram-negative (particularly pseudomonal) coverage (41), although there is no evidence that this improves outcome.

Antipyretic Therapy

The public perception of fever as a malady that needs to be treated is very much at odds with the emerging concept of fever as an adaptive response that enhances our ability to eradicate infection. The following is a brief description of the benefits derived from fever and the reasons to avoid the urge to suppress fever.

Fever as a Host Defense Mechanism

An increase in body temperature can enhance immune function by increasing the production of antibodies and cytokines, activating T-lymphocytes, facilitating neutrophil chemotaxis, and enhancing phagocytosis by neutrophils and macrophages (2,42,43). In addition, high temperatures inhibit bacterial and viral replication. The effect of body temperature on the growth of bacteria in blood cultures is demonstrated in Figure 39.4.

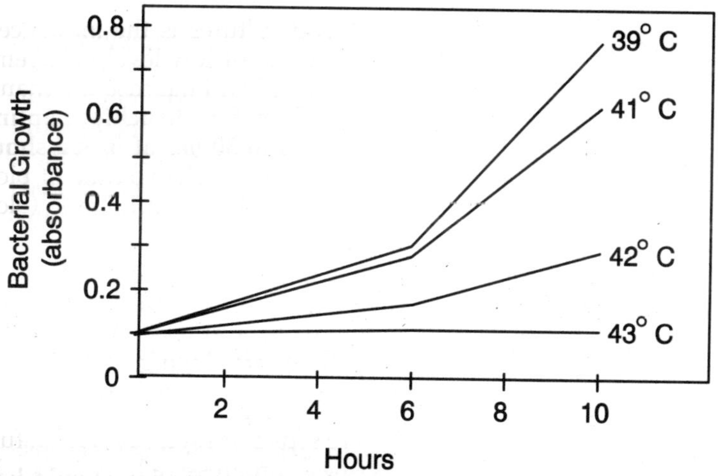

FIGURE 39.4 The influence of body temperature on the growth of *Pasteurella multocida* in the blood of infected laboratory animals. The range of temperatures in the figure is the usual range of febrile temperatures for the study animal (rabbits). (Data from Kluger M, Rothenburg BA. Fever and reduced iron: their interaction as a host defense response to bacterial infection. Science 1979;203:374–376.)

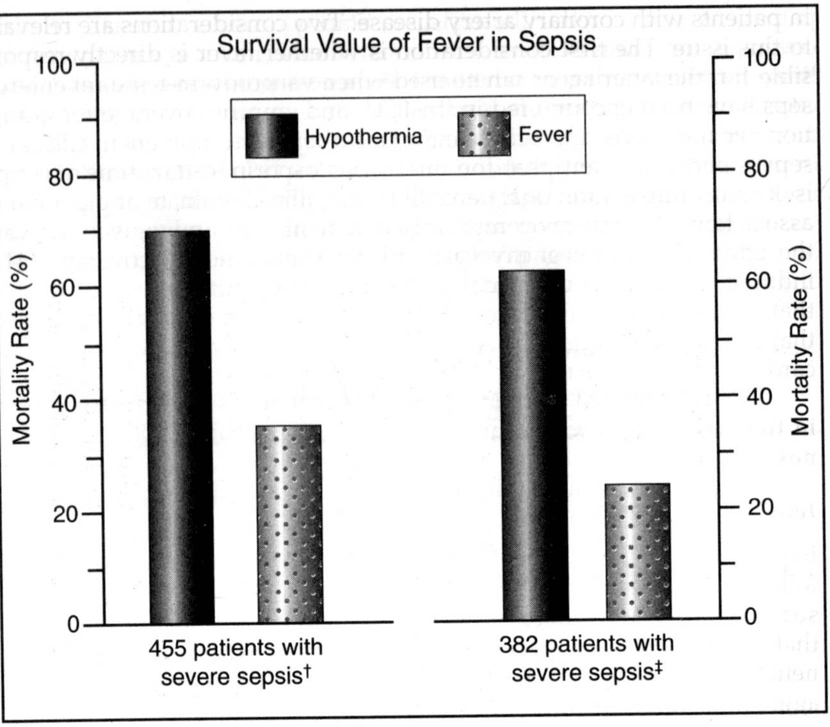

FIGURE 39.5 The influence of body temperature on survival in two cohorts of patients with severe sepsis. †The Ibuprofen in Sepsis Study Group (from Reference 46). ‡The Methylprednisolone Severe Sepsis Study Group (from Reference 45).

Note that an increase in body temperature of 4°C completely suppresses the growth of microorganisms in the blood. This change in body temperature would correspond to an increase in our body temperature from 37°C (98.6°F) to 41°C (105.8°F), thereby showing that increases in body temperature in the same range experienced clinically can halt the growth of microorganisms in blood. A similar ability of increased body temperature to inhibit bacterial growth has been demonstrated in an animal model of pneumococcal meningitis (44).

The beneficial effects of fever on immune function and microbial growth in animal studies is also evident in human studies showing that septic patients who develop hypothermia have at least twice the mortality rate of septic patients who are capable of developing fever (45,46). The results of these studies are shown in Figure 39.5. The apparent survival value of fever in these studies is reason to avoid fever suppression in patients with nosocomial infections. In fact, considering that sepsis is the leading cause of death in most ICUs, **fever suppression should be contraindicated in patients with severe or life-threatening infections.**

Fever and Tachycardia

Tachycardia is considered a consequence of fever, and this is the basis for the claim that fever suppression is necessary to reduce tachycardia in patients with coronary artery disease. Two considerations are relevant to this issue. The first consideration is whether fever is directly responsible for tachycardia, or whether the process producing the fever (e.g., sepsis or inflammation) is responsible for the tachycardia. The association between fever and tachycardia was established in animal models of sepsis, and it is likely that the inflammatory response to sepsis (which is known to include tachycardia) is the real culprit in the apparent association between fever and tachycardia. The second consideration is the pathophysiology of myocardial infarction. The concern that fever-induced tachycardia can trigger a myocardial infarction neglects the fact that acute myocardial infarction is the result of an occlusive blood clot that forms in a coronary artery, and it is unlikely that a fever or a tachycardia will produce such a clot.

The only clinical situation where reduction of a fever is justified is in the early period following ischemic brain injury, which is described next.

Fever and Ischemic Brain Injury

Experimental studies in animals show that increased body temperature following an episode of cerebral ischemia results in more extensive tissue injury (47), and clinical studies in patients with ischemic stroke show that the patients who develop a post-stroke fever have more extensive neurologic deficits and a higher mortality (48). The ability of fever to aggravate ischemic brain injury is presumably related to the increase in cerebral oxygen consumption that accompanies fever. Another possible mechanism is enhanced production of toxic oxygen metabolites, which can be particularly damaging to the brain. Regardless of the mechanism, the consensus of stroke experts is that **antipyretic therapy is mandatory for fever associated with ischemic stroke**. This is similar in principal to the use of therapeutic hypothermia to improve neurologic recovery after cardiac arrest, which is described in Chapter 15.

Antipyretic Drugs

Prostaglandin E is believed to mediate the febrile response to endogenous pyrogens, and drugs that interfere with prostaglandin E synthesis are effective in reducing fever (49). These drugs include aspirin, acetaminophen, and the nonsteroidal anti-inflammatory agents (NSAIDS). Acetaminophen is favored over aspirin and the NSAIDS because of a favorable side effects profile. However, acetaminophen is by no means a benign drug, and life-threatening hepatotoxicity has been reported with doses as low as 4 grams daily (see Chapter 53 for information on acetaminophen toxicity. The usual dose for fever suppression is **325 to 650 mg every 4 to 6 hours,** and the total daily dose should not exceed 4 grams. Acetaminophen is given orally or by rectal suppository, but there is no intravenous preparation of the drug.

Ibuprofen is a popular over-the-counter NSAID that has been given intravenously (in a dose of 10 mg/kg up to 800 mg every 6 hours for 8 doses) to ICU patients with sepsis, and has proven both safe and effective as an antipyretic agent in this patient population (50). Its value as an antipyretic agent in ischemic stroke is unknown. Because ibuprofen (like all NSAIDS), produces a reversible inhibition of platelet adherence, it could pose a risk for the transformation of an ischemic stroke into hemorrhagic stroke.

Cooling Blankets

The use of cooling blankets to reduce fever is inappropriate, and shows a lack of knowledge about the physiology of the febrile response. The febrile response raises the body temperature by promoting cutaneous vasoconstriction and producing a generalized increase in muscle tone. This is what the body normally does in response to a cold environment, so the febrile response mimics the physiological response to cold. Stated another way, **the febrile response makes the body behave like it is wrapped in a cooling blanket**. Adding a cooling blanket will only add to the cold (febrile) response by producing more cutaneous vasoconstriction and a further increases in muscle tone (to the point of shivering). This would explain why cooling blankets are notoriously ineffective in reducing fever.

Cooling blankets are more appropriate for patients with hyperthermia, where the body is trying to give up heat to the environment. However, the tendency for cooling blankets to promote shivering limits their value in hyperthermia syndromes associated with muscle rigidity (e.g., neuroleptic malignant syndrome).

A FINAL WORD

There's a wrong way and a right way to evaluate nosocomial fever. The wrong way is to culture everything in sight, order a barrage of laboratory studies and x-rays, and start antibiotics without hesitation. The right way is to develop a stepwise approach that begins by examining the patient to assess the severity of the condition. Next, consider if anything has been done to the patient in the past 24 to 48 hours (e.g., a procedure or a change in drug therapy). If this is unrevealing, then use the patient's clinical condition to identify possible sources of the fever. (For example, if the patient is on a ventilator, then pneumonia is a consideration.) Remember that you have a 50-50 chance of finding an infection (because infections are present in about 50% of patients with nosocomial fever), so don't start antibiotics unless an infection is apparent or highly suspected, or the patient is immunocompromised. And *please* don't use a cooling blanket!

REFERENCES

Reviews

1. O'Grady NP, Barie PS, Bartlett J, et al. Practice parameters for evaluating new fever in critically ill adult patients. Crit Care Med 1998;26:392–408. (Also available at www.sccm.org/publications/index.asp)
2. Marik PE. Fever in the ICU. Chest 2000;117:855–869.

Body Temperature

3. Stimson HF. Celsius versus centigrade: the nomenclature of the temperature scale of science. Science 1962;136:254–255.
4. Wunderlich CA, Sequine E. Medical thermometry and human temperature. New York: William Wood, 1871.
5. Mellors JW, Horwitz RI, Harvey MR, et al. A simple index to identify occult bacterial infection in adults with acute unexplained fever. Arch Intern Med 1987;147:666–671.
6. Tandberg D, Sklar D. Effect of tachypnea on the estimation of body temperature by an oral thermometer. N Engl J Med 1983;308:945–946.
7. Marion GS, McGann KP, Camp DL. Core body temperature in the elderly and factors which influence its measurement. Gerontology 1991;37:225–232.
8. Mackowiak PA, Wasserman SS, Levine MM. A critical appraisal of 98.6°F, the upper limit of the normal body temperature, and other legacies of Carl Reinhold August Wunderlich. JAMA 1992;268:1578–1580.
9. Amoateng-Adjepong Y, Del Mundo J, Manthous CA. Accuracy of an infrared tympanic thermometer. Chest 1999;115:1002–1005.
10. Giuliano KK, Scott SS, Elliot S, et al. Temperature measurement in critically ill orally intubated adults: a comparison of pulmonary artery core, tympanic, and oral methods. Crit Care Med 1999;27:2188–2193.
11. Erickson RS. The continuing question of how best to measure body temperature. Crit Care Med 1999;27:2307–2310.
12. Saper CB, Breder CB. The neurologic basis of fever. N Engl J Med 1994;330: 1880–1886.
13. Circiumaru B, Baldock G, Cohen J. A prospective study of fever in the intensive care unit. Intensive Care Med 1999;25:668–673.
14. Commichau C, Scarmeas N, Mayer SA. Risk factors for fever in the intensive care unit. Neurology 2003; 60:837–841.

Noninfectious Causes of Fever

15. Fry DE. Postoperative fever. In: Mackowiak PA, ed. Fever: basic mechanisms and management. New York: Raven Press, 1991:243–254.
16. Freischlag J, Busuttil RW. The value of postoperative fever evaluation. Surgery 1983;94:358–363.
17. Engoren M. Lack of association between atelectasis and fever. Chest 1995; 107:81–84.
18. Shelds RT. Pathogenesis of postoperative pulmonary atelectasis: an experimental study. Arch Surg 1949;48:489–503.
19. Meyers JK, Lembeck L, O'Kane H, et al. Changes in functional residual capacity of the lung after operation. Arch Surg 1975;110:576–583.
20. Warlitier DC. Pulmonary atelectasis. Anesthesiology 2005;102:838–854.
21. Pollack VE. Adverse effects and pyrogenic reactions during hemodialysis. JAMA 1988;260:2106–2107.
22. Um SW. Prospective analysis of clinical characteristics and risk factors for postbronchoscopy fever. Chest 2004;125:945–952.
23. Spach DH, Silverstein FE, Stamm WE. Transmission of infection by gastrointestinal endoscopy and bronchoscopy. Ann Intern Med 1993;118:117–128.
24. Murray HW, Ellis GC, Blumenthal DS, et al. Fever and pulmonary thromboembolism. Am J Med 1979;67:232–235.

25. Walden DT, Urrutia F, Soloway RD. Acute acalculous cholecystitis. J Intensive Care Med 1994;9:235–243.
26. Mackowiak PA, LeMaistre CF. Drug fever: a critical appraisal of conventional concepts. Ann Intern Med 1987;106:728–733.
27. Cunha B. Drug fever: the importance of recognition. Postgrad Med 1986;80: 123–129.
28. Rangel-Frausto MS, Pittet D, Costigan M, et al. The natural history of the systemic inflammatory response syndrome (SIRS). JAMA 1995;273:117–123.
29. Gonzalez EB, Suarez L, Magee S. Nosocomial (water bed) fever [Letter]. Arch Intern Med 1990;150:687.

Nosocomial Infections

30. Richards MJ, Edwards JR, Culver DH, et al. The National Nosocomial Infections Surveillance System: nosocomial infections in combined medical-surgical intensive care units in the United States. Infect Control Hosp Epidemiol 2000;21:510–515.
31. Richards MJ, Edwards JR, Culver DH, et al. The National Nosocomial Infection Surveillance System: nosocomial infections in medical intensive care units in the United States. Crit Care Med 1999;27:887–892.
32. American Thoracic Society and the Infectious Disease Society of America. Guidelines for the management of adults with hospital-acquired, ventilator-associated, and healthcare-associated pneumonia. Am J Respir Crit Care Med 2005;171:388–416.
33. Ehrenkranz NJ, Meakins JL. Surgical infections. In: Bennet JV, Brachman PS, eds. Hospital infections, 3rd ed. Boston: Little, Brown, 1992:685–710.
34. Loopp FD, Lytle BW, Cosgrove DM, et al. Sternal wound complications after isolated coronary artery bypass grafting: early and late mortality, morbidity, and cost of care. Ann Thorac Surg 1990;49:179–187.
35. Holzapfel L, Chevret S, Madinier G, et al. Influence of long-term oro- or nasotracheal intubation on nosocomial maxillary sinusitis and pneumonia: results of a prospective, randomized, clinical trial. Crit Care Med 1993;21: 1132–1138.
36. Rouby J-J, Laurent P, Gosnach M, et al. Risk factors and clinical relevance of nosocomial maxillary sinusitis in the critically ill. Am Rev Respir Dis 1994; 150:776–783.
37. Williams JW, Jr., Roberts L, Jr., Distell B, et al. Diagnosing sinusitis by x ray: is a single Waters view adequate? J Gen Intern Med 1992;7:481–485.
38. Roberts DN, Hampal S, East CA, et al. The diagnosis of inflammatory sino-nasal disease. J Laryngol Otol 1995;109:27–30.
38. Kelley CP, Pothoulakis C, Lamont JT. *Clostridium difficile* colitis. N Engl J Med 1994;330:257–262.
39. Stilwell M, Caplan ES. The septic multiple-trauma patient. Crit Care Clin 1988;4:345–373.

Early Management Decisions

40. Aronson MD, Bor DH. Blood cultures. Ann Intern Med 1987;106:246–253.
41. Hughes WH, Armstrong D, Bodey GP, et al. 2002 Guidelines for the use of antimicrobial agents in neutropenic patients with cancer. Clin Infect Dis 2002;34.

42. van Oss CJ, Absolom DR, Moore LL, et al. Effect of temperature on the chemotaxis, phagocytic engulfment, digestion, and O_2 consumption of human polymorphonuclear leukocytes. J Reticuloendothel Soc 1980;27:561–565.
43. Azocar J, Yunis EJ, Essex M. Sensitivity of human natural killer cells to hyperthermia. Lancet 1982;1:16–17.
44. Small PM, Tauber MG, Hackbarth CJ, et al. Influence of body temperature on bacterial growth rates in experimental pneumococcal meningitis in rabbits. Infect Immun 1986;52:484–487.
45. Clemmer TP, Fisher CJ, Bone RC, et al. Hypothermia in the sepsis syndrome and clinical outcome. Crit Care Med 1990;18:801–806.
46. Arons MM, Wheeler AP, Bernard GR, et al. Effects of ibuprofen on the physiology and survival of hypothermic sepsis. Crit Care Med 1999;27:699–707.
47. Kim Y, Busto R, Dietrich WD, et al. Delayed postischemic hyperthermia in awake rats worsens the histopathological outcome of transient focal cerebral ischemia. Stroke 1996;27:2274–2281.
48. Hajat C, Hajat S, Sharma P. Effects of poststroke pyrexia on stroke outcome: a meta-analysis of studies in patients. Stroke 2000;31:410–414.
49. Plaisance KI, Mackowiak PA. Antipyretic therapy: physiologic rationale, diagnostic implications, and clinical consequences. Arch Intern Med 2000;160: 449–456.
50. Bernard GR, Wheeler AP, Russell JA, et al. The effects of ibuprofen on the physiology and survival of patients with sepsis. N Engl J Med 1997;336:912–918.

Section XIII

INFLAMMATION AND INFECTION IN THE ICU

Our arsenals for fighting off bacteria are so powerful . . . that we're in more danger from them than from the invaders..

Lewis Thomas

Chapter 40

INFECTION, INFLAMMATION, AND MULTIORGAN INJURY

Inflammation is not itself considered to be a disease but a salutary operation . . . but when it cannot accomplish that salutary purpose . . . it does mischief.

John Hunter, MD (1728–1793)

The most significant discovery in critical care medicine in the last 20 years is the prominent role played by the inflammatory response in the morbidity and mortality associated with severe sepsis and septic shock. In fact, the tendency for inflammation to "do mischief" that Dr. Hunter described over two centuries ago is probably the leading cause of death in intensive care units. This chapter will describe the relationship between infection, inflammation, and multiorgan failure, and the clinical syndromes that result from this relationship (1–3).

INFLAMMATORY INJURY

The inflammatory response is an extremely complicated process that is triggered by a physical, chemical, or infectious insult to the host. The presumed role of the inflammatory response is to protect the host from the damaging effects of the insult, as illustrated in the panel on the left in Figure 40.1. The inflammatory response generates a variety of noxious substances (e.g., proteolytic enzymes, oxygen metabolites) but, under normal conditions, the host is somehow protected from these substances. However, as shown in the panel on the right in Figure 40.1, when the protective devices of the host are lost, the inflammatory response damages the host organism (4). Inflammatory injury, once it starts, becomes

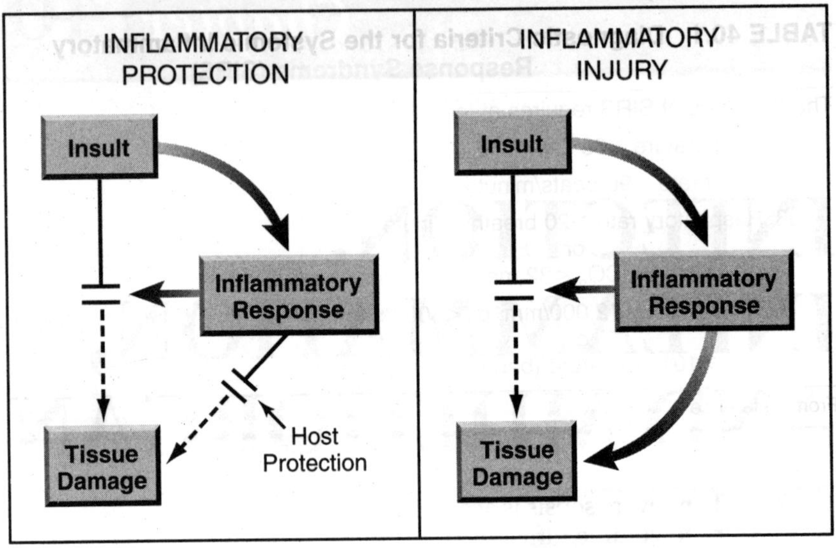

FIGURE 40.1 The dual role of the inflammatory response in protecting and damaging the host organism.

a self-sustaining process, because the tissue damage triggers more inflammation, which produces more tissue damage, and so on. The clinical manifestation of this process is multiorgan dysfunction, which progresses to multiorgan failure (5).

Therefore, when the host is no longer able to protect itself from the damaging effects of inflammation, the inflammatory response become a toxic insult to the host (5). In this situation, the host is defenseless, and inflammation consumes the organs of the host. This process has been called *malignant inflammation* (6).

The role of infection in this scheme is to serve as one of the insults that triggers the inflammatory response. However, inflammation can be triggered by other insults (e.g., trauma, burns), so inflammatory injury can occur without infection.

Clinical Syndromes

The relationships between infection, inflammation, and organ injury just described is the basis for the following nomenclature and abbreviations (3):

1. The condition characterized by signs of systemic inflammation (e.g., fever and leukocytosis) is called the *systemic inflammatory response syndrome* (SIRS).
2. When SIRS is the result of an infection, the condition is called *sepsis*.
3. When sepsis is accompanied by dysfunction in one or more vital organs, the condition is called *severe sepsis*.

TABLE 40.1 Diagnostic Criteria for the Systemic Inflammatory Response Syndrome (SIRS)

The diagnosis of SIRS requires at least 2 of the following:

1. Temperature >38°C or <36°C
2. Heart rate >90 beats/minute
3. Respiratory rate >20 breaths/minute
   or
   Arterial PCO_2 <32 mm Hg
4. WBC count >12,000/mm^3 or <4000/mm^3
   or
   >10% immature (band) forms

From Reference 3.

4. When severe sepsis is accompanied by hypotension that is refractory to volume infusion, the condition is called *septic shock*.
5. Abnormal function in more than one vital organ is called *multiorgan dysfunction syndrome* (MODS), and failure of more than one organ system is called (surprise!) *multiorgan failure* (MOF).

The major value of this nomenclature is to highlight the distinction between inflammation (SIRS) and infection (sepsis).

Systemic Inflammatory Response Syndrome

The diagnostic criteria for SIRS are shown in Table 40.1. Unfortunately, some of the criteria are very non-specific (e.g., an anxiety attack can produce a heart rate above 90 and a respiratory rate above 20, and would thus qualify to be called SIRS). In one survey, 93% of patients in a surgical ICU had SIRS using the criteria in Table 40.1 (7). Infection is identified in only 25 to 50% of patients with SIRS (7,8). Although some patients with SIRS may not be inflamed, these numbers still emphasize the point that **infection and inflammation are distinct entities**.

Multiorgan Dysfunction and Failure

The organs most often injured by sepsis and inflammation are the lungs, kidneys, cardiovascular system, and central nervous system. The clinical syndromes associated with multiorgan failure are shown in Figure 40.2. The most common of these syndromes is the acute respiratory distress syndrome (ARDS), which is associated with 40% of cases of severe sepsis (9). (This condition is described in Chapter 22.)

Mortality Rate

The mortality rate in multiorgan failure is directly related to the number of organ systems that fail. This relationship is shown in Figure 40.3, which includes studies from the United States (9) and Europe (10).

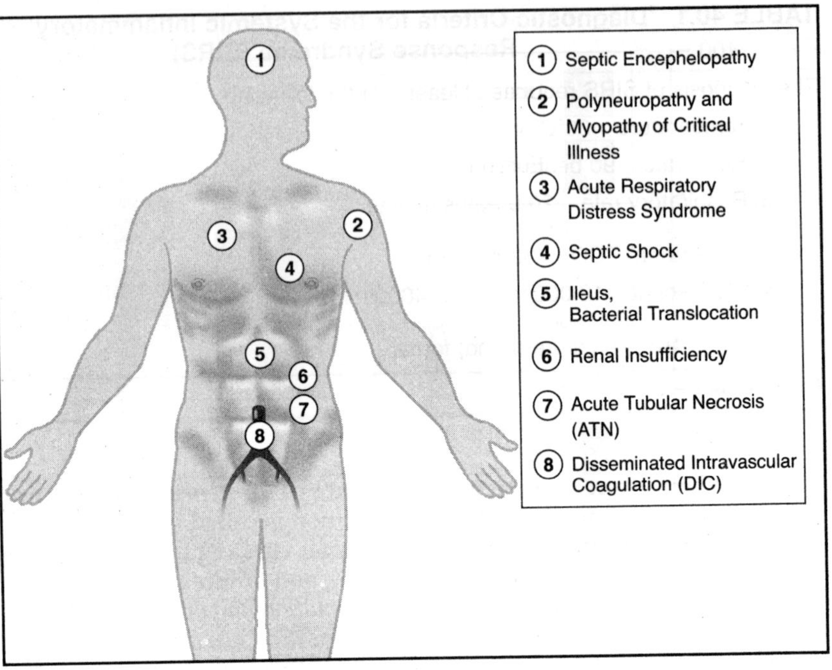

FIGURE 40.2 Components of multiorgan failure. Each of these clinical syndromes is the result of inflammatory injury.

The mortality rate increases steadily as the number of organs fail. This relationship is not surprising, because the chances for survival should diminish as more vital organs fail. In fact, multiorgan failure could be viewed as an expression of the dying process. Death can occur from catastrophic failure of one organ (cardiac arrest), or from a cumulative failure in several organs (multiorgan failure). Why make this point? Because it may not be possible to reverse the dying process, so if multiorgan failure is the dying process, our energies are misplaced because interventions aimed at multiorgan failure will fail (which is the case).

MANAGEMENT OF SEVERE SEPSIS AND SEPTIC SHOCK

The management of patients with severe sepsis and septic shock is almost a daily exercise in most ICUs because septic shock may be the leading cause of death in ICUs (11). Unfortunately, despite all the efforts expended in this area, the mortality in these conditions has changed little over the years (2,12). The following recommendations represent the latest attempt to create a treatment strategy that will have an impact on the outcome of these conditions (2), but there is no "magic bullet" here.

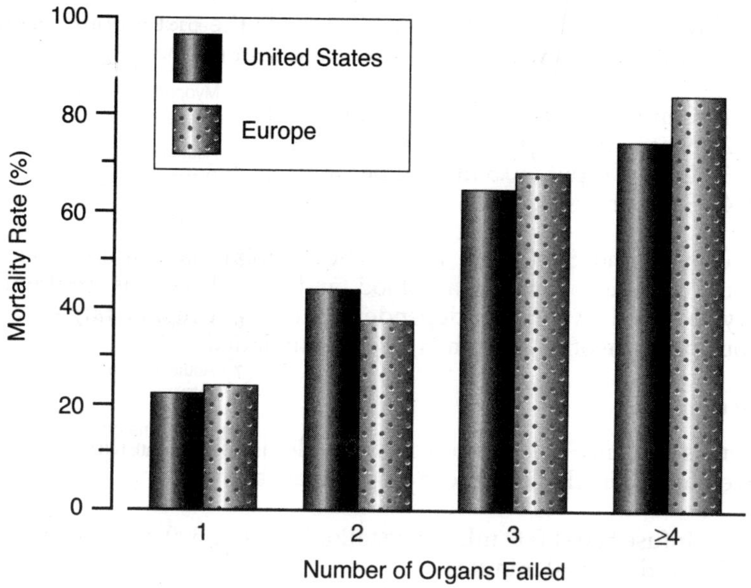

FIGURE 40.3 Relationship between mortality rate and number of organ failures in critically ill patients. (From References 9 and 10).

Tissue Oxygenation Not Impaired in Sepsis

The state of tissue oxygenation in septic shock is described in Chapter 11. To summarize, the prevailing opinion is that the metabolic derangement in severe sepsis and septic shock is not impaired tissue oxygenation, but is a defect in cellular oxygen utilization (13). This condition is called *cytopathic hypoxia* (13), and it explains why **tissue levels of oxygen can be increased in patients with severe sepsis** (14), as shown in Figure 11.3 (see Chapter 11). If this is the case, then efforts to improve tissue oxygenation in septic shock by improving systemic oxygen delivery are misguided.

The VO_2 in Sepsis

Also explained in Chapter 11 is the possibility that the increase in oxygen consumption (VO_2) in sepsis is not related to aerobic metabolism, but is O_2 consumed in the process of neutrophil activation (the respiratory burst) (15). Although this needs further study, it provides another reason to avoid the use of oxygen transport variables for the management of patients with severe sepsis and septic shock.

Initial Resuscitation

The following goals have been established for the first 6 hours of management for patients with severe sepsis and septic shock (1):

1. Central venous pressure 8–12 mm Hg.
2. Mean arterial pressure ≥65 mm Hg.
3. Urine output ≥0.5 mL/kg per hour.
4. SvO_2 or $ScvO_2$ ≥70%

where SvO_2 and $ScvO_2$ are the oxyhemoglobin saturation in central venous (superior vena cava) blood and mixed venous (pulmonary artery) blood. In ventilator-dependent patients, a higher target central venous pressure of 12–15 mm Hg is recommended.

Fluid Challenge

If there is evidence or suspicion of hypovolemia based on the goals listed above, then fluid challenges can be given as follows:

1. Infuse 500–1,000 mL of crystalloid fluid or 300–500 mL of colloid fluid over 30 minutes.
2. Repeat as needed until goals reached or fluid overload imminent.

There is no evidence to favor crystalloid or colloid fluids for volume infusions. Colloid fluids are more likely to expand the plasma volume and less likely to expand the extracellular fluid volume than crystalloid fluids (see Chapter 13). However, because sepsis is often accompanied by hypoalbuminemia (16), initial resuscitation with 5% albumin may be preferred.

Vasopressors

If hypotension persists despite fluid challenges, then vasopressor drug support with either **dopamine or norepinephrine** should be started.

Dopamine: Usual dose range 5–20 μg/kg/min. (See Table 16.3)
Norepinephrine: Effective dose range in sepsis is 0.2–1.3 μg/kg/min (about 1 to 10 μg/min for a 70 kg patient) (17).

Dopamine is more likely to increase cardiac output, while norepinephrine produces vasoconstriction with no change in cardiac output (18). Dopamine can promote tissue acidosis in the splanchnic circulation, while norepinephrine does not have this effect (18), and this might be a reason to prefer norepinephrine. However, the choice of vasopressor is largely one of personal preference.

In cases of hypotension that are refractory to dopamine and norepinephrine, **vasopressin** is a consideration. The recommended **infusion rate is 0.01 to 0.04 units per minute** (1). Vasopressin is a pure vasoconstrictor that will reduce cardiac output (19), so it should be used with caution in patients with a history of heart failure. However, if the patient has refractory hypotension, that is not your major worry.

Empiric Antimicrobial Therapy

Intravenous antibiotics are recommended starting within one hour of recognition of severe sepsis or septic shock (1). Before starting antibiotics, at least 2 sets of blood cultures should be obtained. Remember that the yield from blood cultures is directly dependent on the volume of blood cultured. **For an optimal yield from blood cultures, a volume of 20 to 30 mL of blood should be withdrawn from each venipuncture site** (20).

Unless the patient has an obvious infection, you will start empiric antibiotic coverage. For recommended empiric antibiotic regimens in serious infections, see Table 43.4 (Chapter 43), and for appropriate starting doses of antibiotics, see Table 41.6 (Chapter 41). A simple regimen to remember is **imipenem or meropenem alone** (meropenem has a lower risk of seizures) and, **if there is a risk for methicillin-resistant *Staph aureus* (MRSA), add vancomycin or linezolid**. (For information on linezolid, which may eventually replace vancomycin, see Chapter 44.)

Corticosteroids

Steroids were anathema for septic shock in the 1980s, but based on the results of 3 more recent studies (21–33), they are now **recommended for all patients with septic shock who require vasopressor support** (1). The recommended regimen is shown below (1).

> Hydrocortisone: 200–300 mg IV daily in 2 or 3 divided doses for 7 days.

The benefit from steroids might be the result of adrenal insufficiency, which can occur in patients with severe sepsis and septic shock (see Chapter 48). In one study (21), the patients who showed improvement on steroids had evidence of adrenal insufficiency.

ANAPHYLAXIS

The inflammatory response is also involved in hypersensitivity reactions, and anaphylaxis is the most life-threatening expression of these reactions. Common offenders are antimicrobial agents, anesthetics, radiocontrast dyes, nutrients, and insect venoms (24). Radiocontrast dyes are the most common source of serious anaphylactic reactions, with an incidence of 1 in 1,000 to 14,000 injections (25). About 10% of these reactions are fatal (25).

Clinical Presentation

Anaphylactic reactions vary in presentation and severity. Clinical manifestations appear within minutes to a few hours after exposure to the offending agent. Less serious reactions include flushing, erythematous rashes, urticaria, abdominal cramping, and diarrhea. More severe reactions include **angioedema, laryngeal edema, bronchospasm, and hypotension**. The most life-threatening reaction is a rapid-onset cardiovascular collapse known as *anaphylactic shock*.

Management

The management of anaphylaxis is dictated by the clinical presentation.

Epinephrine

Epinephrine blocks the release of inflammatory mediators from sensitized cells, and it is the drug of choice for severe anaphylactic reactions. Epinephrine is available in strengths of 1:100 (10 mg/mL), 1:1,000 (1 mg/mL), and 1:10,000 (0.1 mg/mL). The usual dose for anaphylactic reactions is 0.3–0.5 mg (or 0.3–0.5 mL of 1:1,000 solution) by deep IM injection in the thigh. Drug absorption is better with IM injection into the thigh instead of the traditional subcutaneous injection (26). Epinephrine can also be nebulized for laryngeal edema: the inhalant is made up of 0.25 mL 1:100 epinephrine added to 2 mL isotonic saline.

For patients being treated with β-blocker drugs, the response to epinephrine may be attenuated, and **glucagon** can be used as a substitute. The glucagon dose is 5–15 μg/min by intravenous infusion.

Second-Line Agents

Histamine blockers have little effect in preventing or treating anaphylaxis, although they can help to relieve pruritis. This lack of efficacy is surprising, considering the presumed importance of histamine in the pathogenesis of anaphylaxis. The histamine H_1 blocker **diphenhydramine** (25–50 mg PO, IM, or IV) and the histamine-H_2 blocker **ranitidine** (50 mg IV or 150 mg PO) should be given together because they are more effective in combination.

Steroids are used primarily to reduce the risk of second-phase symptoms, which appear 1 to 8 hours after the acute episode (24). **Prednisone** (50 mg PO) and **methylprednisolone** (125 mg IV) are equivalent in efficacy. These agents can be given every 6 hours for persistent symptoms.

Albuterol (2.5 mL of 0.5% solution via nebulizer) can be used as an adjunct to epinephrine for persistent bronchospasm.

Anaphylactic Shock

Anaphylactic shock is a life-threatening condition that requires prompt intervention using the following measures:

1. Epinephrine is given intravenously in a dose of 0.3–0.5 mg (3–5 mL of epinephrine 1:10,000). This can be followed by an epinephrine infusion of 2–8 μg/min.
2. Volume resuscitation is very important because anaphylactic shock can be accompanied by profound hypovolemia due to

massive fluid shifts into the interstitium. Colloid fluids may be preferred to crystalloid fluids because they are less likely to escape into the interstitium.

3. Persistent hypotension can be managed with dopamine (5–15 μg/kg/min) or norepinephrine (2–8 μg/min).

A FINAL WORD

The most important message in this chapter is the distinction between inflammation and infection, and the importance of inflammation as a source of lethal injury to the host organism. It is clear that antibiotics provide little benefit to patients with severe sepsis and septic shock (because a majority die despite antibiotic therapy), and now you know why. Because the problem in septic shock and multiorgan failure is not infection, it's inflammation.

REFERENCES

Reviews

1. Dellinger RP, Carlet JM, Masur H, et al. Surviving Sepsis Campaign guidelines for management of severe sepsis and septic shock. Crit Care Med 2004; 32:858–873.
2. Hollenberg SM, Ahrens TS, Annane D, et al. Practice parameters for hemodynamic support of sepsis in adult patients: 2004 update. Crit Care Med 2004;32:1928–1948.
3. American College of Chest Physicians/Society of Critical Care Medicine Consensus Conference Committee. Definitions of sepsis and organ failure and guidelines for the use of innovative therapies in sepsis. Chest 1992;101: 1644–1655.

Inflammatory Injury

4. Fujishima S, Aikawa N. Neutrophil-mediated tissue injury and its modulation. Intensive Care Med 1995;21:277–285.
5. Pinsky MR, Matuschak GM. Multiple systems organ failure: failure of host defense mechanisms. Crit Care Clin 1989;5:199–220.
6. Pinsky MR, Vincent J-L, Deviere J, et al. Serum cytokine levels in human septic shock: relation to multiple-system organ failure and mortality. Chest 1993;103:565–575.
7. Pittet D, Rangel-Frausto S, Li N, et al. Systemic inflammatory response syndrome, sepsis, severe sepsis, and septic shock: incidence, morbidities and outcomes in surgical ICU patients. Intensive Care Med 1995;21:302–309.
8. Rangel-Frausto MS, Pittet D, Costigan M, et al. Natural history of the systemic inflammatory response syndrome (SIRS). JAMA 1995;273:117–123.

9. Angus DC, Linde-Zwirble WT, Lidicker J, et al. Epidemiology of severe sepsis in the United States: analysis of incidence, outcome, and associated costs of care. Crit Care Med 2001;29:1303–1310.
10. Vincent J-L, de Mendonca A, Cantraine F, et al. Use of the SOFA score to assess the incidence of organ dysfunction/failure in intensive care units: results of a multicenter, prospective study. Crit Care Med 1998;26:1793–1800.

Management of Severe Sepsis and Septic Shock

11. Leone M, Bourgoin A, Cambon S, et al. Empirical antimicrobial therapy of septic shock patients: adequacy and impact on the outcome. Crit Care Med 2003;31:462–467.
12. Friedman C, Silva E, Vincent J-L. Has the mortality of septic shock changed with time? Crit Care Med 1998;26:2078–2086.
13. Fink MP. Cytopathic hypoxia: mitochondrial dysfunction as mechanism contributing to organ dysfunction in sepsis. Crit Care Clin 2001;17:219–237.
14. Sair M, Etherington PJ, Winlove CP, et al. Tissue oxygenation and perfusion in patients with systemic sepsis. Crit Care Med 2001;29:1343–1349.
15. Vlessis AA, Goldman RK, Trunkey DD. New concepts in the pathophysiology of oxygen metabolism during sepsis. Br J Surg 1995;82:870–876.
16. Marik PE. The treatment of hypoalbuminemia in the critically ill patient. Heart Lung 1993;22:166–170.
17. Beale RJ, Hollenberg SM, Vincent J-L, et al. Vasopressor and inotropic support in septic shock: an evidence-based review. Crit Care Med 2004; 32(suppl):S455–S465.
18. Marik PE, Mohedin M. The contrasting effects of dopamine and norepinephrine on systemic and splanchnic oxygen utilization in hyperdynamic sepsis. JAMA 1994;272:1354–1357.
19. Holmes CL, Walley KR, Chittock DR, et al. The effects of vasopressin on hemodynamics and renal function in severe septic shock: a case series. Intensive Care Med 2001;27:1416–1421.
20. Aronson MD, Bor DH. Blood cultures. Ann Intern Med 1987;106:246–253.
21. Annane D, Sebille V, Charpentier C, et al. Effect of treatment with low doses of hydrocortisone and fludrocortisone on mortality in patients with septic shock. JAMA 2002;288:862–871.
22. Briegel J, Forst H, Haller M, et al. Stress doses of hydrocortisone reverse hyperdynamic septic shock: a prospective, randomized, double-blind, single-center study. Crit Care Med 1999;27:723–732.
23. Bollaert PE, Charpentier C, Levy B, et al: Reversal of late septic shock with supraphysiologic doses of hydrocortisone. Crit Care Med 1998;26:645–650.

Anaphylaxis

24. Ellis AK, Day JH. Diagnosis and management of anaphylaxis. Can Med Assoc J 2003;169:307–311.

25. Crnkovich DJ, Carlson RW. Anaphylaxis: an organized approach to management and prevention. J Crit Illness 1993;8:332–246.
26. Simons FER, Gu X, Simons KJ. Epinephrine absorption in adults: intramuscular versus subcutaneous injection. J Allergy Clin Immunol 2001;108:871–873.

Chapter 41

PNEUMONIA IN THE ICU

Everything hinges on the matter of evidence.

Carl Sagan

Pneumonias that are acquired in the ICU can be characterized by one word: *problematic*. The diagnosis of ICU-acquired pneumonias is problematic because there is no "gold standard" method for identifying parenchymal lung infections in ICU patients (other than postmortem examination). As a result, the diagnostic approach to ICU-acquired pneumonia is not standardized, and there are at least 6 different diagnostic methods to choose from (qualitative and quantitative cultures of tracheal aspirates, bronchial brushings with and without bronchoscopy, and bronchoalveolar lavage with and without a bronchoscopy). Because of the diagnostic uncertainties, treatment of ICU-acquired pneumonias is also problematic. Deciding whether to start antibiotics or which antibiotics to use is often a matter of speculation because it is unclear in many cases if a pneumonia is actually present. As a result of these problems, the approach to ICU-acquired pneumonias is sometimes more fancy than fact.

This chapter will summarize the current knowledge about pneumonias acquired in the ICU, with emphasis on pneumonias acquired by ventilator-dependent patients. The material in this chapter pertains only to patients who are immunocompetent. Special considerations for nosocomial pneumonia in immunocompromised patients are presented in Chapter 43.

GENERAL FEATURES

The following statements summarize some of the general characteristics of pneumonia acquired in the ICU (1)

1. Pneumonia is considered the most common nosocomial infection in the ICU (see Table 39.3), but the prevalence is overstated

TABLE 41.1 Pathogens Isolated by Bronchoscopy in Ventilator-Associated Pneumonia

Organisms	Frequency
Bacilli	56.5%
Pseudomonas aeruginosa	18.9%
Escherichia coli	9.2%
Hemophilus	7.1%
Enterobacter	3.8%
Proteus	3.8%
Klebsiella	3.2%
Others	10.5%
Cocci	42.1%
Staphylococcus aureus	18.9%
Streptococcus pneumoniae	13.2%
Enterococcus	1.4%
Others	8.6%
Fungi	1.3%

From Chastre J, et al. Comparison of 8 vs 15 days of antibiotic therapy for ventilator-associated pneumonia in adults. JAMA 2003; 290:2558.

because many cases of presumed pneumonia are not corroborated on postmortem exam (see later).

2. Over 90% of ICU-acquired pneumonias occur during mechanical ventilation, and 50% of these *ventilator-associated pneumonias* occur in the first 4 days after intubation (1).
3. The predominant pathogens in ICU-acquired pneumonias are *Staphylococcus aureus, Pseudomonas aeruginosa,* and other gram-negative aerobic bacilli (see Table 41.1). Viruses, fungi, and anaerobes are uncommon isolates.
4. Although the mortality rate in ICU-acquired pneumonia is reported at 30% to 50% (1), some studies show no deaths attributed to this condition (2).

Pathogenesis

Aspiration of pathogenic organisms from the oropharynx is believed to be the inciting event in most cases of hospital-acquired (nosocomial) and ICU-acquired pneumonias (3). The organisms that most often colonize the oropharynx in hospitalized patients are enteric gram-negative bacilli and *Staphylococcus aureus* (see Figure 4.5 in Chapter 4), and this explains the predominance of these pathogens in nosocomial pneumonias. The instances of ventilator-associated pneumonia that appear within 4 days after intubation are most likely caused by microbes that have been dragged into the airways during the intubation procedure. Once the oropharynx is colonized, endotracheal tubes and tracheostomy tubes can

TABLE 41.2 Predictive Value of Clinical Criteria in the Diagnosis of Ventilator-Associated Pneumonia

Study	Clinical Criteria	Likelihood Ratio for Pneumonia on Autopsy*
Fagon et al. (5)	Radiographic infiltrate + purulent sputum + fever or leukocytosis	1.03
Timsit et al. (6)	Radiographic infiltrate + 2 of the following: fever, leukocytosis, or purulent sputum	0.96

*As reported in Reference 4. The likelihood ratio is the likelihood that patients with pneumonia will have the clinical findings compared to the likelihood that patients without pneumonia will have the same clinical findings. A likelihood ratio = 1 indicates that the clinical findings are just as likely to be found in the presence and absence of pneumonia.

serve as a nidus for biofilm formation that protects the colonizing pathogens and allows them to proliferate (1). The frequent passage of suction catheters through these tubes can then introduce the pathogens into the airways. Colonization of the oropharynx and stomach with pathogenic organisms in hospitalized patients is described in detail in Chapter 4.

Clinical Features

Bacterial pneumonias typically present with fever, leukocytosis, purulent sputum production, and a new infiltrate on the chest x-ray. However, these clinical manifestations are nonspecific in ventilator-dependent patients. **In ventilator-dependent patients who are suspected of having pneumonia based on clinical findings** (the presence of a pulmonary infiltrate plus any combination of fever, leukocytosis, or purulent sputum production), **the actual incidence of pneumonia on postmortem exam is only 30% to 40%** (4). The value of clinical findings in the diagnosis of ventilator-associated pneumonia is shown in Table 41.2. This table shows the results of 2 studies that used autopsy evidence of pneumonia to evaluate the premortem diagnosis of ventilator-associated pneumonia based on clinical findings (5,6). In both studies, the clinical criteria for identifying pneumonia were just as likely to occur in the presence and absence of pneumonia. This demonstrates **the diagnosis of pneumonia in ventilator-dependent patients is not possible using clinical criteria alone.**

Sensitivity of Chest Radiography

The definition of pneumonia proposed by the Centers for Disease Control (CDC) requires the presence of a new infiltrate on chest x-ray (7). A patient who presents with fever and purulent sputum production is considered to have a tracheobronchitis (8). However, it seems unlikely that the chest x-ray is always abnormal in the presence of pneumonia (i.e., has a sensitivity of 100%). For example, pulmonary edema is not evident on a chest x-ray until the extravascular lung water has increased 30 to 50% (9), and this lack of sensitivity for pulmonary edema could also apply to parenchymal infections in the lungs.

The traditional teaching is that pneumonia in a dehydrated patient may become radiographically evident only after rehydration. This seems unlikely because it would mean that dehydration can limit or prevent inflammatory infiltration of vital organs. There are few studies that address this question, but one animal study has shown that dehydration does not influence the x-ray appearance of bacterial pneumonia (10).

Specificity of Chest Radiography

Pneumonia accounts for only 1/3 of all pulmonary infiltrates in ICU patients (11,12), which means that **conditions other than pneumonia are the most frequent cause of pulmonary infiltrates in ICU patients.** The noninfectious causes of pulmonary infiltrates in the ICU include pulmonary edema, acute respiratory distress syndrome, and atelectasis. An example of how atelectasis can influence the chest x-ray is shown in Figure 41.1. Both images in this figure were obtained within minutes of each other in the same patient. The image on the left shows a marked reduction in lung volume that occurred when the patient changed from the upright to supine position. Note that the volume loss in the supine position produces an area of crowded lung markings at the base of the right lung (dotted triangle). In a patient with fever, this localized atelectasis could be confused with a pneumonia.

Acute Respiratory Distress Syndrome

The most common noninfectious cause of pulmonary infiltrates in ICU patients is the acute respiratory distress syndrome (ARDS) (12). This

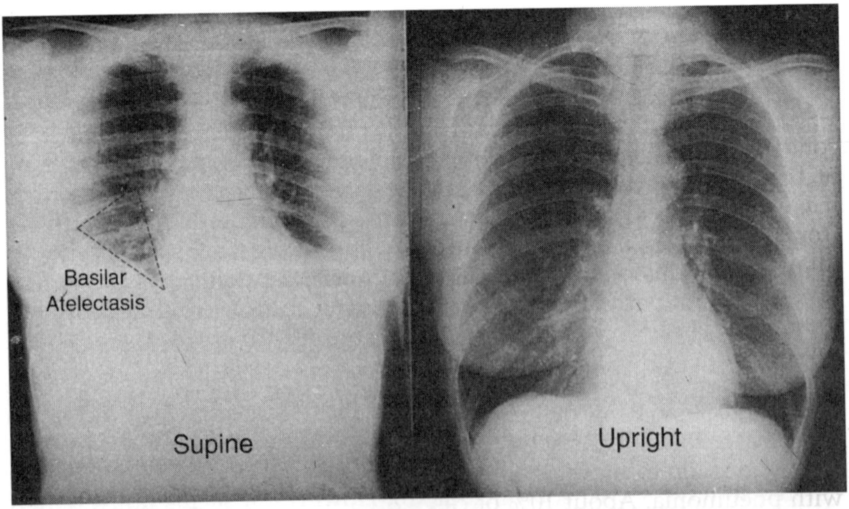

FIGURE 41.1 The effect of body position on the appearance of portable chest x-rays. Both images were obtained within minutes of each other in the same patient. The dotted triangle outlines an area of localized atelectasis that could be misread as a basilar pneumonia. Image on the left digitally enhanced.

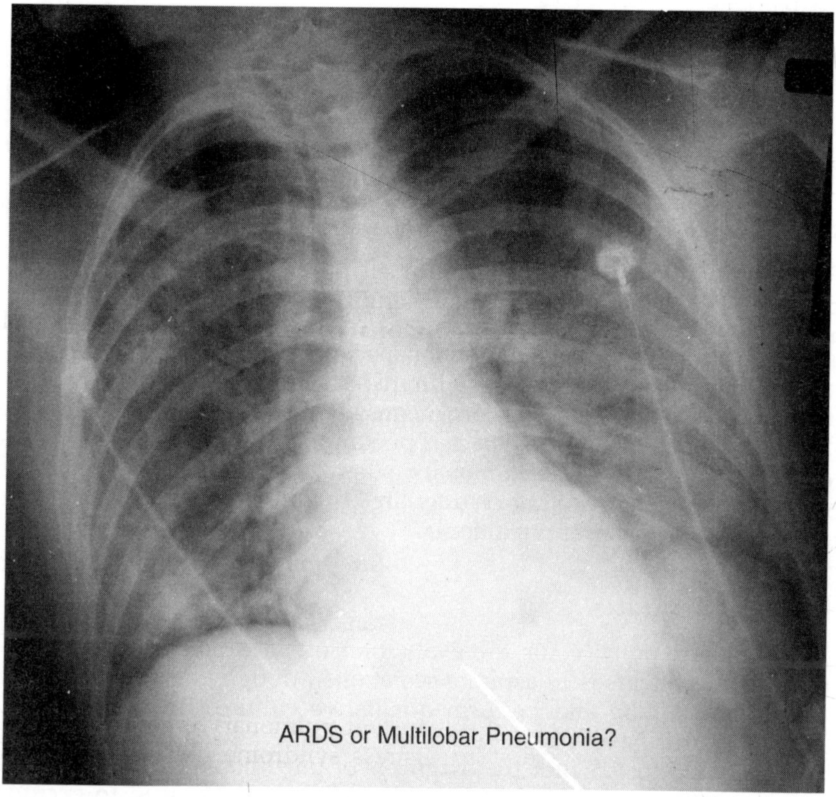

FIGURE 41.2 Chest x-ray from a patient who was admitted to the ICU with fever and respiratory insufficiency. See text for the diagnosis.

condition, which is described in Chapter 22, is an inflammatory disorder of the lungs that produces bilateral infiltrates on chest x-ray. Because it is often accompanied by fever, ARDS can be difficult to distinguish from a multilobar pneumonia. This is illustrated in Figure 41.2. The x-ray image in this figure is from a patient who was admitted to the ICU with fever and respiratory insufficiency. The patient was initially treated for a severe community-acquired pneumonia, but subsequent evaluation revealed *Escherichia coli* in cultures of blood and urine, while cultures taken from the lower respiratory tract (by bronchoscopy) were sterile. The final diagnosis in this case was ARDS secondary to gram-negative septicemia from a urinary tract infection.

In addition to masquerading as pneumonia, ARDS can also co-exist with pneumonia. About 10% of cases of ARDS are the result of a pneumonia, and about 50% of patients with ARDS will develop a pneumonia at some time during their ICU stay (13). The methods used to identify infection in ARDS and other ventilator-dependent patients are described in the next section.

Summary

In summary, the usual clinical criteria for pneumonia (fever, leukocytosis, purulent sputum, and a new infiltrate on chest x-ray) should not be used as evidence of pneumonia in ICU patients, but instead are indications to proceed with the diagnostic evaluation described next to document infection and identify the responsible pathogen.

DIAGNOSTIC EVALUATION

The diagnostic evaluation of suspected pneumonia includes cultures of blood, pleural fluid, and a variety of specimens collected from the respiratory tract. Blood cultures have limited value in the diagnosis of ICU-acquired pneumonia because organisms are isolated from blood in only 25% of ICU patients with suspected pneumonia (1), and these organisms can originate from extrapulmonary sites (14). Cultures of specimens obtained from the respiratory tract are usually required to confirm or exclude the presence of pneumonia.

Tracheal Aspirates

The standard practice for the evaluation of pneumonia in ventilator-dependent patients is to aspirate secretions through an endotracheal or tracheostomy tube and perform qualitative cultures on the aspirates. These cultures have a high sensitivity (usually >90%) but a very low specificity (15 to 40%) for the diagnosis of pneumonia (15). This means that **a negative culture of a tracheal aspirate can be used to exclude the diagnosis of pneumonia, but a positive culture cannot be used to confirm the presence of pneumonia.** The poor predictive value of positive cultures is due to contamination of tracheal aspirates with secretions from the mouth and upper airways. The diagnostic accuracy of tracheal aspirates can be improved by screening the specimens with microscopic visualization to include only specimens originating from the lower airways, and then performing quantitative cultures on the screened specimens. This is explained in the following sections.

Microscopic Analysis

The cells identified in Figure 41.3 can help to determine if aspirated secretions originate in the upper or lower airways, and also if there is evidence of infection. Each type of cell can be identified and interpreted as follows.

The squamous epithelial cells that line the oral cavity are large and flattened with abundant cytoplasm and a small nucleus (see Fig. 41.3). The presence of **more than 25 squamous epithelial cells per low-power field (× 100) indicates that the specimen is contaminated with mouth secretions** (16). If there is evidence of contamination, the specimen should be discarded.

Lung macrophages are large, oval-shaped cells with a granular cytoplasm and a small, eccentric nucleus (Fig. 41.3). The size of the nucleus

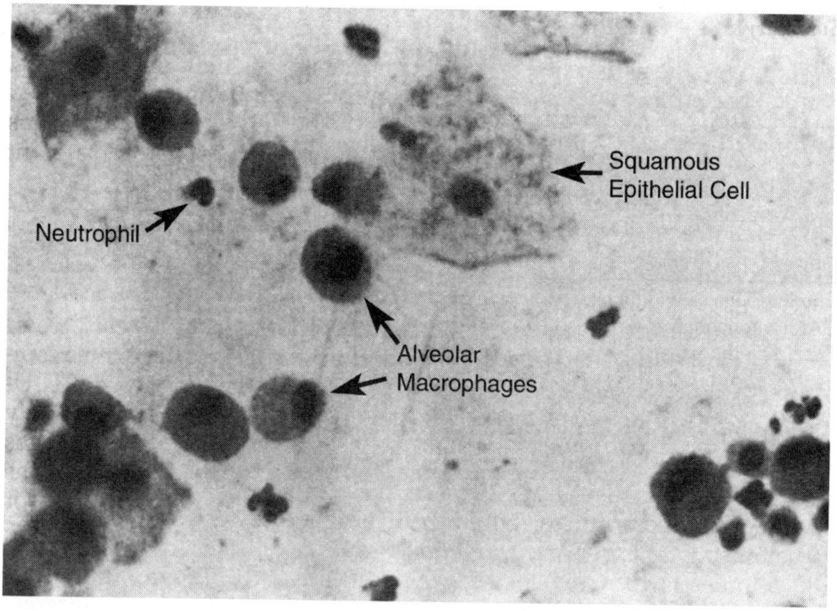

FIGURE 41.3 Microscopic appearance (magnification ×400) of bronchial brushings from a ventilator-dependent patient. The paucity of squamous epithelial cells and the presence of alveolar macrophages both confirm that the specimen is from the distal airways.

in a macrophage is roughly the same size as a neutrophil. Although macrophages can inhabit the airways (17), the predominant home of the macrophage is the distal airspaces. Therefore, **the presence of macrophages, regardless of the number, indicates that the specimen is from the lower respiratory tract.**

The presence of neutrophils in respiratory secretions is not evidence of infection because neutrophils can make up 20% of the cells recovered from a routine mouthwash (17). The neutrophils should be present in abundance to indicate infection. **More than 25 neutrophils per low-power field (× 100) can be used as evidence of infection** (18). When an infection is evident, a search for macrophages and squamous epithelial cells will help to determine if the infection is in the upper airways (tracheobronchitis) or the lower airways (pneumonia). When a tracheal aspirate shows evidence of lower airways infection (i.e., abundant neutrophils and macrophages with few epithelial cells), the specimen is suitable for culture.

Quantitative Cultures

Quantitative cultures of tracheal aspirates produce fewer false-positive results than qualitative cultures. To perform quantitative cultures, the tracheal aspirate should be collected in a sterile trap without adding saline or lidocaine (the latter can inhibit microbial growth). When a volume of at least 1 mL is collected, the specimen is sent to the laboratory

TABLE 41.3 Quantitative Cultures for the Diagnosis of Pneumonia in Ventilator-Dependent Patients

	TA	PSB	BAL
Diagnostic Threshold (CFU/mL)	10^5 to 10^6	10^3	10^4 to 10^5
Sensitivity (mean)	76%	66%	73%
Specificity (mean)	75%	90%	82%
Relative Performance	Most Sensitive	Most Specific	Most Accurate

Abbreviations: *TA* = tracheal aspirates, *PSB* = protected specimen brushings, *BAL* = bronchoalveolar lavage.
From References (1,15,21).

(make sure you specify that you want *quantitative* cultures) where it is vortexed (agitated) in isotonic saline. A sample is then collected with a 0.01mL loop and the sample is placed on a culture plate for incubation. For quantitative cultures, growth on the plate is reported as follows: 10 colonies is reported as 10^3 colony-forming units per mL (CFU/mL), 100 colonies is 10^4 CFU/mL, 1,000 colonies is 10^5 CFU/mL, and more than 1,000 colonies is 10^6 CFU/mL (this technique might vary in different laboratories, but the principle is the same).

For quantitative cultures of tracheal aspirates, the threshold growth for the diagnosis of pneumonia is 10^5 to 10^6 CFU/ per mL (the lower threshold is sometimes used for patients who are on antibiotic therapy when the cultures are performed). Studies using these thresholds have shown a (mean) sensitivity and specificity of 76% and 75%, respectively, for the diagnosis of pneumonia (see Table 41.3) (1,15). Comparing these results to the sensitivity and specificity of qualitative cultures mentioned earlier (i.e., sensitivity >90% and specificity ≤40%) shows that **quantitative cultures of tracheal aspirates are less sensitive but much more specific than qualitative cultures for the diagnosis of pneumonia.**

Protected Specimen Brush

Aspiration of secretions through a bronchoscope produces a high rate of false-positive cultures because the bronchoscope picks up contaminants as it is passes through the upper respiratory tract (19). To eliminate this problem, a specialized brush called a *protected specimen brush* (PSB) was developed to collect uncontaminated secretions from the distal airways. The brush sits in the inner lumen of a catheter-over-catheter device that has a gelatin plug at the distal end. When the device is advanced through the bronchoscope, the gelatin plug protects the brush from contamination with upper airways secretions. When the bronchoscope is advanced into the area of lung infiltration, the entire catheter device is advanced out of the bronchoscope and into the lower airways (see Fig. 41.4). The inner catheter is advanced until it knocks off the gelatin plug (which dissolves without harming the patient), and the brush is then advanced into the distal airways to collect the specimen. After vigorous brushing, the brush is retracted into the inner cannula, the inner cannula is retracted

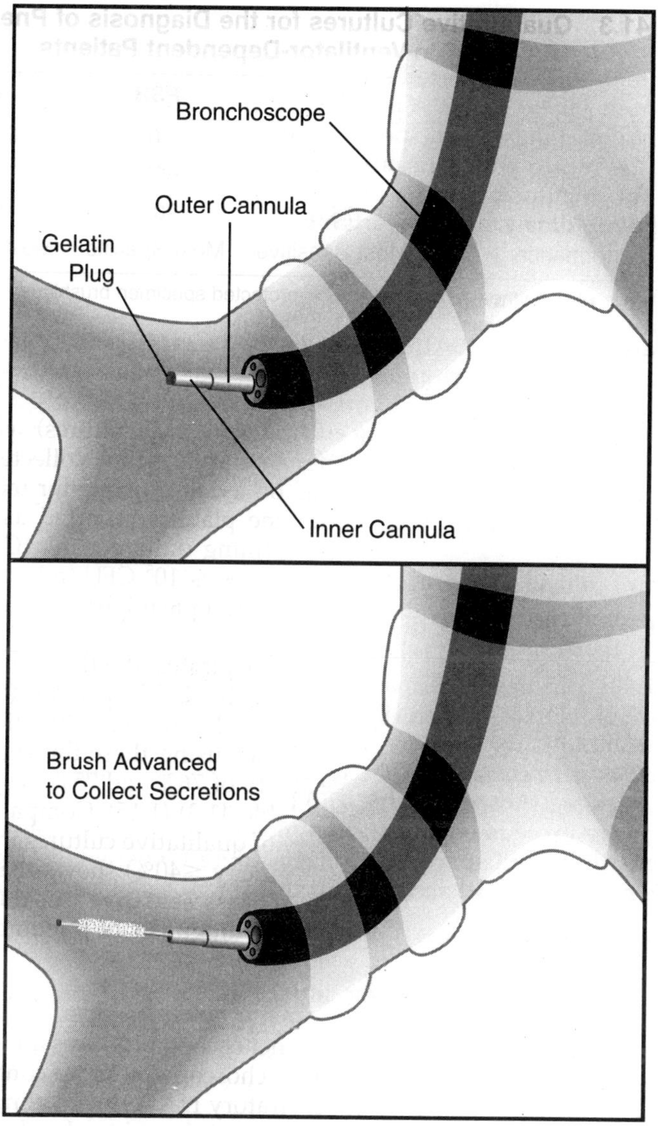

FIGURE 41.4 The protected specimen brush (PSB) technique for obtaining uncontaminated secretions from the lower airways.

into the outer cannula, and the entire device is retracted through the bronchoscope.

Quantitative Cultures

Using sterile technique, the brush is severed from its wire and is placed in 1 mL of transport medium. In the microbiology lab, the brush is vortexed in the transport medium to disperse microorganisms. The specimen is then processed in the same fashion as described for tracheal aspirates. Growth of 10^3 CFU/mL is the threshold for the presence of infection (pneumonia) (1). The reported sensitivity and specificity of PSB cultures are shown in Table 41.3 (1). A positive culture result has a relatively low sensitivity (66%) but a high specificity (90%) for the diagnosis of pneumonia. This means that **a negative PSB culture does not exclude the presence of pneumonia, but a positive PSB culture confirms the presence of pneumonia with 90% certainty.**

Bronchoalveolar Lavage

Bronchoalveolar lavage (BAL) is performed by wedging the bronchoscope in a distal airway and performing a lavage with sterile isotonic saline. A minimum lavage volume of 120 mL is recommended for adequate sampling of the lavaged lung segment (19), and this is achieved by performing a series of 6 lavages using 20 mL for each lavage. The same syringe is used to introduce the fluid and aspirate the lavage specimen (only 25% or less of the volume instilled will be returned via aspiration).

Quantitative Cultures

The first lavage is usually discarded, and the remainder of the lavage fluid is pooled and sent to the microbiology lab, where it is centrifuged and processed in the same manner as described for tracheal aspirates. The threshold for a positive BAL culture is 10^4 to 10^5 CFU/mL (the lower threshold is for patients who are on antibiotic therapy when the procedure is performed) (1). The reported sensitivity and specificity of BAL cultures are shown in Table 41.3 (1,20). Neither the sensitivity nor the specificity exceeds both of the diagnostic methods in Table 41.3, but **when sensitivity and specificity are considered together, BAL cultures have the highest overall accuracy for the diagnosis of pneumonia.**

Intracellular Organisms

Inspection of BAL specimens for intracellular organisms can help in guiding initial antibiotic therapy until culture results are available. **When intracellular organisms are present in more than 3% of the cells in the lavage fluid, the likelihood of pneumonia is over 90%** (21). Unfortunately, this is not done on a routine Gram stain, but requires special processing and staining in the microbiology lab (see references 21 and 22 for the methodology).

BAL without Bronchoscopy

The limited availability of bronchoscopy on a 24-hour basis has led to the introduction of a non-bronchoscopic technique for BAL where specialized catheters are inserted through a tracheal tube and advanced blindly until wedged in the lower airways. A variety of catheters and techniques have been used (for examples of two techniques, see references 23 and 24), and the method has proven safe and effective when performed by respiratory therapists (23). In general, cultures obtained by nonbronchoscopic and bronchoscopic BAL have shown equivalent sensitivities and specificities for the diagnosis of pneumonia (1,25), and there is evidence that nonbronchoscopic BAL is better tolerated than bronchoscopic BAL (24). However, there is concern about adopting nonbronchoscopic procedures to diagnose pneumonia because of the lack of standardization of the techniques in clinical studies (26).

Which Diagnostic Method is Best?

There is little agreement on which method should be preferred for the diagnosis of pneumonia. The following statements include some pertinent observations.

1. The diagnostic yield from all culture methods is adversely affected by ongoing antibiotic therapy (1). Therefore, when possible, cultures should be obtained before antibiotics are started.
2. Tracheal aspirates should be screened by microscopic examination, and the specimens should be discarded if there is evidence of contamination with secretions from the mouth and upper airways.
3. Quantitative cultures of tracheal aspirates are preferred to qualitative cultures because they have a higher specificity, and thus are more likely to identify a pneumonia and the responsible pathogen(s).
4. **Treatment based on cultures of tracheal aspirates will result in excessive use of antibiotics** because cultures of tracheal aspirates are most likely to produce false-positive results (1,27).
5. Most studies show that **the mortality in ventilator-associated pneumonia is not influenced by the diagnostic method** (1,27). In other words, there is no survival benefit with the more invasive methods (protected specimen brushings and bronchoalveolar lavage) compared to the relatively simple method of aspirating secretions through an endotracheal or tracheostomy tube.

Based on the absence of a survival benefit with the invasive diagnostic methods, many prefer tracheal aspirates for the diagnostic approach to pneumonia, even though this practice will result in excessive use of antibiotics (1). Tracheal aspirates should, however, be screened by microscopic inspection and cultured using quantitative techniques. Qualitative cultures of tracheal aspirates are useful only when there is no growth, which can be used to exclude the presence of pneumonia.

Parapneumonic Effusions

Pleural effusions are present in up to 50% of bacterial pneumonias (28), and these *parapneumonic* effusions should be evaluated in the following situations (1): when the pleural effusion is large, when the patient appears toxic, and when the patient is not improving on antibiotic therapy. If the effusion is loculated (i.e., it does not move with change in body position), computed tomography or bedside ultrasound can be

TABLE 41.4 Management of Parapneumonic Effusions

Clinical Finding	Immediate Drainage? Yes	No
Air–fluid level	X	
Hydropneumothorax	X	
Grossly purulent fluid	X	
Pleural fluid pH:		
<7.0	X	
>7.2		X
Pleural fluid glucose:		
<40 mg/dL	X	
>40 mg/dL		X

used to mark the location and depth of the fluid. In addition to Gram stain and culture, the pleural fluid glucose concentration and pH should be measured. Classification of the fluid as a transudate or exudate (by pleural fluid protein and LDH levels) is unnecessary because this does not reliably identify infection.

Indications for Drainage

The indications for immediate drainage of parapneumonic effusions are listed in Table 41.4. The radiographic criteria for drainage include the presence of an air–fluid level in the effusion, or a hydropneumothorax (both are signs of a bronchopleural fistula). Chemical criteria for drainage include a pleural fluid glucose concentration below 40 mg/dL (2.4 μmol/L) or a pleural fluid pH below 7.0 (28). If a patient with a parapneumonic effusion improves clinically on antibiotics, there is little need for further evaluation or drainage of the effusion.

EARLY ANTIMICROBIAL THERAPY

There is a definite tendency to begin antibiotics at the earliest hint of a pneumonia in the ICU. According to one study, **antibiotic treatment for pneumonia accounts for half of all antibiotic use in the ICU**, but 60% of antibiotic use for pneumonias involve suspected pneumonias that are not confirmed by bacteriologic studies (29). The rush to antibiotics in cases of suspected pneumonia is fueled by studies showing that the mortality in ventilator-associated pneumonia is increased when there is a delay in starting appropriate antibiotic therapy (30). However, there are also studies showing that ventilator-associated pneumonia does not increase mortality (2,31,32), so the survival benefit of the rush to antibiotics is not firmly established. (See the last section of this chapter for a comment on this situation.)

Suggested Strategy

One early antibiotic strategy that is appealing is to administer antibiotics immediately (i.e., when pneumonia is first suspected) for patients who are immunocompromised, or have evidence of severe sepsis (i.e., multi-organ dysfunction) or septic shock. Otherwise, hold antibiotics until you collect specimens from the respiratory tract for Gram stain and culture. Then begin antibiotic therapy based on the appearance of the Gram stain, or using recommended empiric regimens (described next) but *stop* the antibiotics in 2 to 3 days if the cultures do not confirm the presence of pneumonia (33). There will be a tendency to continue antibiotics despite sterile cultures in patients with progressive respiratory insufficiency, but these patients are likely to have ARDS and not pneumonia. If respiratory tract cultures are obtained when patients are not receiving antibiotics, continuing antibiotics in the face of sterile cultures is rarely justified.

Empiric Antibiotic Therapy

The choice of empiric antibiotics should be dictated by the likelihood that the patient is colonized with *Staphylococcus aureus* and gram-negative enteric pathogens (the pathogens listed in Table 41.1). The characteristics of patients who are likely and unlikely to be colonized with these pathogens are shown in Table 41.5, along with the recommended empiric antibiotic regimens for each type of patient. The recommended starting doses for each antibiotic are shown in Table 41.6.

Colonization Unlikely

The typical patients who are not colonized by *S. aureus* and gram-negative pathogens have been admitted recently (within 5 days) from home, have no debilitating chronic illness (including renal failure that requires dialysis), and have no other hospital admissions in the past 3 months (1). Patients like this can be treated with a single antibiotic like ceftriaxone or a fluoroquinolone (levofloxacin or moxifloxacin), as shown in Table 41.5. This treatment is primarily directed at pneumococci, including penicillin-resistant strains, and is similar to the treatment of community-acquired pneumonia (34).

Colonization Likely

Colonization with *S. aureus* and gram-negative enteric pathogens is likely when a patient has been in the hospital for 5 days or longer, or when the patient is a nursing home resident, has a chronic debilitating illness, or has had other hospital admissions within the past few months. The empiric antibiotic regimen for these patients, which is shown in Table 41.5, is designed to cover staphylococci and gram-negative enteric pathogens, and is particularly designed for *Pseudomonas aeruginosa* and methicillin-resistant *S. aureus* (MRSA). There is no coverage for fungi, and coverage for anaerobes is not a priority because anaerobes are not considered to be important pathogens in ventilator-associated pneumonia (35). Specific choices of antibiotics will be guided by the profile of nosocomial pathogens and resistance patterns in individual ICUs.

TABLE 41.5 Empiric Treatment for Ventilator-Associated Pneumonia Based on Likelihood of Colonization with Pathogens in Table 41.1†

Colonization Unlikely	Colonization Likely
Type of Patient: • Admitted less than 5 days ago and • Admitted from home, and • No other admissions in past 3 months, and • Not a dialysis patient. *Empiric Antibiotics:* • Ceftriaxone, or • A fluoroquinolone (levofloxacin, moxifloxacin, or ciprofloxacin)	*Type of Patient:* • Admitted more than 5 days ago, or • Admitted from a nursing home, or • Other admissions in the past 3 months, or • A dialysis patient. *Empiric Antibiotics:* • Pipericillin/tazobactam, or • Imipenem or meropenem, or • Ceftazidime or cefepime plus • Ciprofloxacin or levofloxacin*, or • An aminoglycoside* plus • Vancomycin or linezolid‡

*Benefit is questionable (see text).
‡When colonization with methicillin-resistant *S. aureus* is known or likely.
†From the American Thoracic Society and Infectious Disease Society of America: Guidelines for the management of adults with hospital-acquired, ventilator-associated, and healthcare-associated pneumonia. Am J Respir Crit Care Med 2005;171:388–416.

Double Coverage for Pseudomonas?

The empiric regimen for patients likely to be colonized with gram-negative pathogens includes a second antibiotic for gram-negative coverage (a fluoroquinolone or aminoglycoside), which is designed to provide double coverage for pneumonias caused by *Pseudomonas aeruginosa*. This recommendation is questionable and is based on one study that showed improved survival in patients with *Pseudomonas* bacteremia (many of whom did not have pneumonia) when double antibiotic coverage was used instead of monotherapy (36). However, another study shows no difference in survival when double coverage for *Pseudomonas* is compared to single drug therapy in patients with serious gram-negative infections (37). Furthermore, empiric double coverage for *Pseudomonas* pneumonia is not justified based on the following reasoning: (1) pneumonia is expected in only about 30% of ICU patients with suspected pneumonia, (2) in the patients with pneumonia, *Pseudomonas* is expected in only 20% of cases, and (3) in the patients with *Pseudomonas* pneumonia, bacteremia is expected in only about 25% of cases. If these estimates are combined, then *Pseudomonas* bacteremia (the only condition with evidence of benefit from double coverage) is expected in only 1.5% of ICU patients with suspected pneumonia.

TABLE 41.6 Recommended Starting Doses for Empiric Antibiotics†

Antibiotic	Intravenous Dosage*
β-Lactam/β-lactamase inhibitor	
Pipericillin/tazobactam	4.5 grams every 6 hours
Carbepenems	
Imipenem	1 gram every 8 hours
Meropenem	1 gram every 8 hours
Antipseudomonal cephalosporins	
Cefepime	1–2 grams every 8–12 hours
Ceftazidime	2 grams every 8 hours
Antipseudomonal quinolones	
Levofloxacin	750 mg once daily
Ciprofloxacin	400 mg every 8 hours
Aminoglycosides	
Gentamicin	7 mg/kg daily
Tobramycin	7 mg/kg daily
Amikacin	20 mg/kg daily
Antistaphylococcal agents	
Vancomycin	15 mg/kg every 12 hours
Linezolid	600 mg/kg every 12 hours

*For patients with normal renal and hepatic function.
†From the American Thoracic Society and Infectious Disease Society of America: Guidelines for the management of adults with hospital-acquired, ventilator-associated, and healthcare-associated pneumonia. Am J Respir Crit Care Med 2005;171:388–416.

Recommendation

For patients likely to be colonized with *S. aureus* and gram-negative pathogens, empiric antibiotic therapy for most patients will be adequate using **imipenem or imipenem plus vancomycin**. Imipenem has a very broad spectrum of activity, and is active against staphylococci (methicillin-sensitive strains), and gram-negative enteric pathogens, including *Pseudomonas aeruginosa*. The addition of vancomycin is necessary only if methicillin-resistant *Staphylococcus aureus* is a concern. Linezolid is gaining popularity as an alternative to vancomycin because of increasing vancomycin failures for treating MRSA pneumonias (1). The second antipseudomonal antibiotic should not be necessary unless the Gram stain of respiratory secretions shows a preponderance of gram-negative bacilli and the patient is immunocompromised (see Chapter 43 for the management of immunocompromised patients in the ICU).

Duration of Antibiotic Therapy

Empiric antibiotics regimens will be adjusted according to the results of quantitative cultures. For pneumonias documented by culture, the traditional duration of antibiotic therapy has been 14 to 21 days (1). However, one large study (including 50 ICUs) has shown that 8 days of antibiotic therapy for ventilator-associated pneumonia is associated with the same mortality and risk of recurrent infection as 15 days of therapy (38), and the popular opinion at present is that **one week of antibiotic therapy is adequate for most patients with ventilator-associated pneumonia**.

Antibiotic Prophylaxis

Efforts to prevent nosocomial pneumonia continue to be neglected despite evidence that some measures are effective. One of the effective measures involves the topical application of an antimicrobial paste to the oral mucosa to prevent colonization of the oropharynx with pathogenic organisms (39). The preparation most often used is a methylcellulose paste (Orabase, Squibb Pharmaceuticals) containing 2% polymyxin, 2% tobramycin, and 2% amphotericin B, which is applied to the inside of the mouth with a gloved finger every 6 hours (39). As shown in Figure 4.6 (Chapter 4), this regimen of **oral decontamination decreases the incidence of ventilator-associated pneumonia** by about 2/3 (39). Results like this should not be ignored in the approach to pneumonia in the ICU.

A FINAL WORD

Reports that mortality is not increased by ventilator-associated pneumonia (2,31,32) deserve much more attention in discussions of how to manage pneumonia in the ICU. For example, **if mortality is not increased by ventilator-associated pneumonias, then mortality rate should not be used as an end-point for evaluating diagnostic or therapeutic approaches to these pneumonias** (as it often is). It also means that ICU-acquired pneumonia is overhyped as a life-threatening condition that requires immediate and aggressive therapy. Because there is no gold-standard method for identifying ICU-acquired pneumonia other than post-mortem examination (1), it is possible that studies showing a lack of impact on survival included many false-positive diagnoses of pneumonia. However, this observation is still relevant because these studies used methods that we all use to diagnose pneumonia and to justify antibiotic therapy. If what we think is pneumonia has no impact on survival, then the problems mentioned earlier still apply. For now, this is just another problem in a long list of problems associated with pneumonia in the ICU.

REFERENCES

Clinical Practice Guidelines

1. American Thoracic Society and Infectious Disease Society of America. Guidelines for the management of adults with hospital-acquired, ventilator-associated, and healthcare-associated pneumonia. Am J Respir Crit Care Med 2005;171:388–416.

General Features

2. Bregeon F, Cias V, Carret V, et al. Is ventilator-associated pneumonia an independent risk factor for death? Anesthesiology 2001;94:554–560.
3. Estes RJ, Meduri GU. The pathogenesis of ventilator-associated pneumonia, I: mechanisms of bacterial transcolonization and airway inoculation. Intensive Care Med 1995;21:365–383.
4. Wunderink RG. Clinical criteria in the diagnosis of ventilator-associated pneumonia. Chest 2000;117:191S–194S.
5. Fagon JY, Chastre J, Hance AJ, et al. Detection of nosocomial lung infection in ventilated patients: use of a protected specimen brush and quantitative culture techniques in 147 patients. Am Rev Respir Dis 1988;138:110–116.
6. Timsit JF, Misset B, Goldstein FW, et al. Reappraisal of distal diagnostic testing in the diagnosis of ICU-acquired pneumonia. Chest 1995;108:1632–1639.
7. Garner JS, Jarvis WR, Emori TG, et al. CDC definitions for nosocomial infections, 1988. Am J Infect Control 1988;16:128–140.
8. Nsieir S, Di Pompeo C, Pronnier P, et al. Nosocomial tracheobronchitis in mechanically ventilated patients: incidence, aetiology, and outcome. Eur Respir J 2002;20:1483–1489.
9. Pistolesi M, Miniati M, Milne ENC, et al. Measurement of extravascular lung water. Intensive Care World 1991;8:16–21.
10. Caldwell A, Glauser FL, Smith WP, et al. The effects of dehydration on the radiologic and pathologic appearance of experimental canine segmental pneumonia. Am Rev Respir Dis 1975;112:651–659.
11. Louthan FB, Meduri GU. Differential diagnosis of fever and pulmonary densities in mechanically ventilated patients. Semin Resp Infect 1996;11:77–95.
12. Singh N, Falestiny MN, Rogers P, et al. Pulmonary infiltrates in the surgical ICU. Chest 1998;114:1129–1136.
13. Bauer TT, Torres A. Acute respiratory distress syndrome and nosocomial pneumonia. Thorax 1999;54:1036–1040.

Diagnostic Evaluation

14. Luna CM, Videla A, Mattera J, et al. Blood cultures have limited value in predicting severity of illness and as a diagnostic tool in ventilator-associated pneumonia. Chest 1999;116:1075–1084.
15. Cook D, Mandell L. Endotracheal aspiration in the diagnosis of ventilator-associated pneumonia. Chest 2000;117:195S–197S.
16. Washington JA. Techniques for noninvasive diagnosis of respiratory tract infections. J Crit Illness 1996;11:55–62.
17. Rankin JA, Marcy T, Rochester CL, et al. Human airway macrophages. Am Rev Respir Dis 1992;145:928–933.
18. Wong LK, Barry AL, Horgan S. Comparison of six different criteria for judging the acceptability of sputum specimens. J Clin Microbiol 1982;16:627–631.
19. Meduri GU, Chastre J. The standardization of bronchoscopic techniques for ventilator-associated pneumonia. Chest 1992;102:557S–564S.
20. Torres A, El-Ebiary M. Bronchoscopic BAL in the diagnosis of ventilator-associated pneumonia. Chest 2000;117:198S–202S.

21. Veber B, Souweine B, Gachot B, et al. Comparison of direct examination of three types of bronchoscopy specimens used to diagnose nosocomial pneumonia. Crit Care Med 2000;28:962–968.
22. Chastre J, Fagon JY, Domart Y, et al. Diagnosis of nosocomial pneumonia in intensive care unit patients. Eur J Clin Microbiol Infect Dis 1989;8:35–39.
23. Kollef MH, Bock KR, Richards RD, et al. The safety and diagnostic accuracy of minibronchoalveolar lavage in patients with suspected ventilator-associated pneumonia. Ann Intern Med 1995;122:743–748.
24. Perkins GD, Chatterjee S, Giles S, et al. Safety and tolerability of nonbronchoscopic lavage in ARDS. Chest 2005;127:1358–1363.
25. Campbell CD Jr. Blinded invasive diagnostic procedures in ventilator-associated pneumonia. Chest 2000;117:207S–211S.
26. Fujitani S, Yu V. Diagnosis of ventilator-associated pneumonia: focus on nonbronchoscopic techniques (nonbronchoscopic lavage, including mini-BAL, blinded protected specimen brush, and blinded bronchial sampling) and endotracheal aspirates. J Intensive Care Med 2006;21:17–21.
27. Shorr AF, Sherner JH, Jackson WL, et al. Invasive approaches to the diagnosis of ventilator-associated pneumonia: a meta-analysis. Crit Care Med 2005; 33:46–53.
28. Light RW, Meyer RD, Sahn SA, et al. Parapneumonic effusions and empyema. Clin Chest Med 1985;6:55–62.

Early Antimicrobial Therapy

29. Bergmanns DCJJ, Bonten MJM, Gaillard CA, et al. Indications for antibiotic use in ICU patients: a one-year prospective surveillance. J Antimicrob Chemother 1997;111:676–685.
30. Iregui M, Ward S, Sherman G, et al. Clinical importance of delays in the initiation of appropriate antibiotic treatment for ventilator-associated pneumonia. Chest 2002;122:262–268.
31. Rello J, Quintana E, Ausina A, et al. Incidence, etiology, and outcome of nosocomial pneumonia in mechanically ventilated patients. Chest 1991;100:439–444.
32. Papazian L, Bregeon F, Thirion X, et al. Effect of ventilator-associated pneumonia on mortality and morbidity. Am J Respir Crit Care 1996;154:91–97.
33. Singh N, Rogers P, Atwood CW, et al. Short-course empiric antibiotic therapy for patients with pulmonary infiltrates in the intensive care unit. Am J Respir Crit Care Med 2000;162:505–511.
34. American Thoracic Society. Guidelines for the management of adults with community-acquired pneumonia. Am J Respir Crit Care Med 2001;163:1730–1754.
35. Marik P, Careau P. The role of anaerobes in patients with ventilator-associated pneumonia and aspiration pneumonia: a prospective study. Chest 1999;115:178–183.
36. Hilf M, Yu VL, Sharp J, et al. Antibiotic therapy for *Pseudomonas aeruginosa* bacteremia: outcome correlations in a prospective study of 200 patients. Am J Med 1989;87:540–546.
37. Cometta A, Baumgartner JD, Lew D, et al. Prospective, randomized comparison of imipenem monotherapy with imipenem plus netilmicin for treat-

ment of severe infections in nonneutropenic patients. Antimicrob Agents Chemother 1994;38:1309–1313.
38. Chastre J, Wolff M, Fagon J-Y, et al. Comparison of 8 vs 15 days of antibiotic therapy for ventilator-associated pneumonia in adults. JAMA 2003;290:2588–2598.
39. Bergmans C, Bonten M, Gaillard C, et al. Prevention of ventilator-associated pneumonia by oral decontamination. Am J Respir Crit Care Med 2001;164:382–388.

Chapter 42

SEPSIS FROM THE ABDOMEN AND PELVIS

One of the recurring themes in this book is the importance of the gastrointestinal (GI) tract as a source of infection in critically ill patients. This chapter focuses on that theme, and describes the infectious risks at both ends of the GI tract, including the neighboring biliary tree. The last section of this chapter describes nosocomial infections in the urinary tract, with emphasis on infections associated with indwelling urethral catheters.

ACALCULOUS CHOLECYSTITIS

Acalculous cholecystitis is a condition that could be described as an ileus of the gallbladder. Although an uncommon condition, it can be fatal if not recognized and treated promptly (1).

Pathogenesis

There are a number of conditions that predispose to acalculous cholecystitis. Most cases occur in association with multiple trauma and abdominal (nonbiliary) surgery. A number of mechanisms may be involved in the pathogenesis of acalculous cholecystitis, including ischemia (e.g., multiple trauma, shock), stasis (e.g., parenteral nutrition), and reflux of pancreatic secretions (e.g., opioid analgesics). In patients with immunodeficiency virus (HIV) infection, opportunistic pathogens like cytomegalovirus are often found on histologic examination of the gallbladder, but it is unclear if these organisms are the cause or the consequence of the cholecystitis (3).

Clinical Features

The clinical manifestations of acalculous cholecystitis include fever, nausea and vomiting, abdominal pain, and right upper quadrant tenderness

TABLE 42.1 Routine Clinical Evaluation in 143 Patients with Intra-Abdominal Abscesses

Clinical Finding	Frequency (%)
Physical Examination:	
Localized abdominal tenderness	36
Palpable abdominal mass	7
Chest Films:	
Pleural effusion	33
Basilar atelectasis	12
Abdominal Films:	
Extraluminal air or air-fluid level	13
Mechanical bowel obstruction	4

From Fry D. Noninvasive imaging tests in the diagnosis and treatment of intra-abdominal abscesses in the postoperative patient. Surg Clin North Am 1994; 74:693–709.

(Table 42.1). Abdominal findings can be minimal or absent, and fever may be the only presenting manifestation. Elevations in serum bilirubin, alkaline phosphatase, and amylase can occur but are variable (1,2).

Diagnosis

An ultrasound of the right upper quadrant often provides diagnostic information. Gallbladder sludge and distention of the gallbladder are common findings but can be nonspecific. More specific findings include a gallbladder wall thickness of at least 3.5 mm and submucosal edema (1,2). If ultrasound visualization is hampered, computed tomography (CT) scanning can provide useful information (1).

Management

Prompt intervention is necessary to prevent progressive distention and **rupture of the gallbladder.** The latter complication **has been reported in 40% of cases when diagnosis and treatment is delayed for 48 hours** or longer after the onset of symptoms (1). The treatment of choice is cholecystectomy. In patients who are too moribund for surgery, percutaneous cholecystostomy is a suitable alternative. Empiric antibiotics are often recommended, but the value of this practice is unproven.

Colonization of the GI Tract

The GI tract can become a source of sepsis when overgrowth of pathogenic organisms occurs as a result of a change in the normal environment of the bowel lumen. This occurs in the upper GI tract when patients are given acid-suppressing drugs, and occurs in the lower GI tract when patients are given antibiotics. The following is a look at this colonization as a source of sepsis.

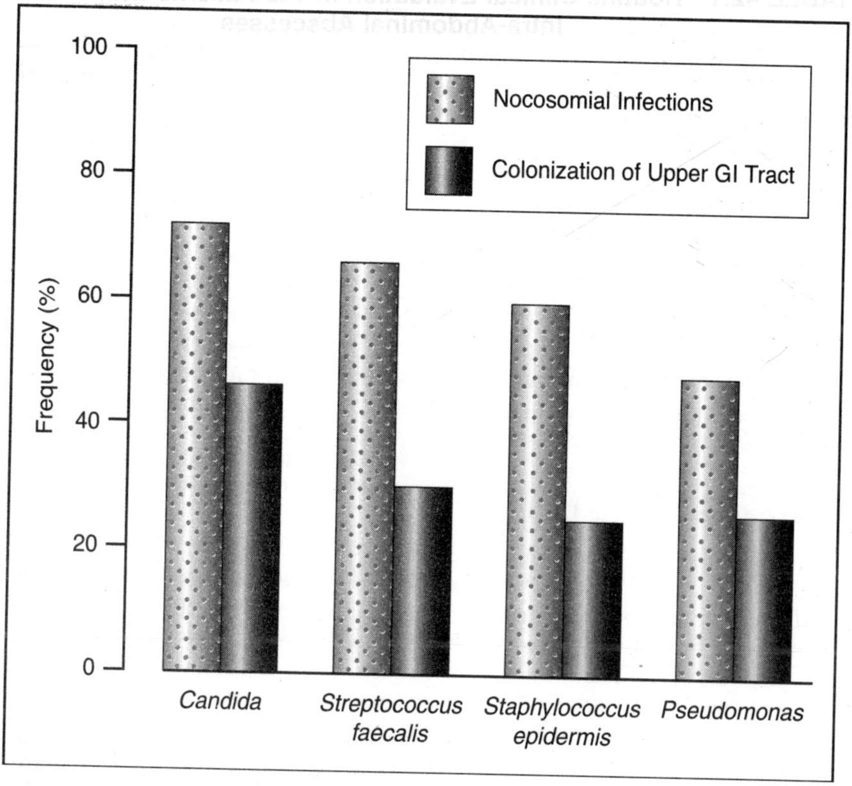

FIGURE 42.1 Correlation between the organisms that most often colonize the upper GI tract and the organisms most often isolated in nosocomial infections in critically ill patients. (Data from Marshall JC, Christou NV, Meakins JL, et al. The gastrointestinal tract: the "undrained abscess" of multiple organ failure. Ann Surg 1993;218:111–119.)

Gastric Colonization

Gastric acid suppression and subsequent colonization of the upper GI tract is discussed in Chapter 4 (see Fig. 4.1 for a demonstration of the bactericidal actions of low pH). The pathogens that commonly colonize the stomach are the same pathogens that are commonly involved in nosocomial infections (4). This correlation is shown in Figure 42.1. Although it does not prove a causal relationship between gastric colonization and nosocomial infections, it does show that the upper GI tract serves as a reservoir for pathogens that are commonly involved in nosocomial sepsis.

Preventive Measures

There are two practices that will reduce colonization of the upper GI tract, and both have proven to reduce the incidence of nosocomial infections. The first practice is to avoid the use of drugs that suppress gastric acidity (i.e., histamine H_2 antagonists and proton pump inhibitors). Prophylaxis for stress ulcer bleeding is not necessary if the patient is eating or receiving enteral tube feedings. If prophylaxis is desired, consider using sucralfate, a cytoprotective agent that does not increase the pH of gastric secretions. The relative advantages and disadvantages of using sucralfate instead of acid-inhibiting drugs are discussed in Chapter 4, and shown in Figure 4.4.

The second practice that impedes colonization is the use of nonabsorbable antibiotics placed in the mouth and stomach. This practice is described in Chapter 4, and the results are shown in Figures 4.6 and 4.7. Despite the obvious benefits for reducing nosocomial infections, this practice is not popular in the United States (see Chapter 4 for more on this topic). However, the success of decontamination practices in reducing nosocomial infections is evidence that the GI tract is indeed an important source of nosocomial sepsis.

Clostridium Difficile Colitis

Colonization with pathogenic organisms can also occur in the lower regions of the GI tract. The most troublesome intruder is *Clostridium difficile,* a spore-forming gram-positive anaerobic bacillus that is not a prominent bowel inhabitant in healthy subjects, but proliferates when the normal microflora of the lower GI tract is altered by antibiotic therapy (5,6). *Clostridium difficile* is not an invasive organism, but it elaborates cytotoxins that incite inflammation in the bowel mucosa. Severe cases of mucosal inflammation are accompanied by raised plaque-like lesions on the mucosal surface called pseudomembranes. These lesions are responsible for the term *pseudomembranous colitis,* which is used to describe advanced cases of *C. difficile* enterocolitis.

Epidemiology

Although *C. difficile* is found in fewer than 5% of healthy adults in the community, it can be seen in as many as 40% of hospitalized patients (7). More than half of the patients who harbor *C. difficile* in their stool are asymptomatic (8). The organism is found primarily in patients receiving ongoing or recent (within 2 weeks) antibiotic therapy and in patients who are in close proximity to other patients who harbor the organism. *C. difficile* is readily transmitted from patient to patient by contact with contaminated objects (e.g., toilet facilities) and by the hands of hospital personnel (8). Strict adherence to the use of disposable gloves can significantly reduce the nosocomial transmission of *C. difficile* (9).

Clinical Manifestations

The most common manifestations of symptomatic *C. difficile* infection are fever, abdominal pain, and watery diarrhea. Bloody diarrhea is seen in 5% to 10% of cases. Rarely, the enterocolitis can progress to toxic megacolon, which presents with abdominal distention, ileus, and clinical shock. This latter complication can be fatal and requires emergent subtotal colectomy (10).

Laboratory Tests

The diagnosis of *C. difficile* enterocolitis requires laboratory tests for the presence of the appropriate toxins in stool. Stool cultures for *C. difficile* are unreliable because they do not distinguish toxigenic from nontoxigenic strains of the organism. Most laboratories use an ELISA (enzyme-linked immunosorbent assay) method to detect the cytotoxins. The sensitivity of this test is about 85% for one stool specimen and up to 95% for 2 stool specimens (5,6,11). Therefore, **the cytotoxin assay will miss 15% of cases of *C. difficile* enterocolitis if one stool specimen is tested, but only misses 5% of cases if two stool specimens are tested.** The specificity of this test is up to 98% (6), so false-positive results are uncommon.

Computed Tomography

Computed tomography (CT) of the abdomen can reveal findings like those shown in Figure 42.2 (12). There is marked thickening in the wall of the colon, which appears as a low density region between the mucosa and serosa. The small bowel is not similarly affected. These findings are characteristic of an inflammatory process involving the large bowel (an enterocolitis), but they are not specific for *C. difficile* enterocolitis.

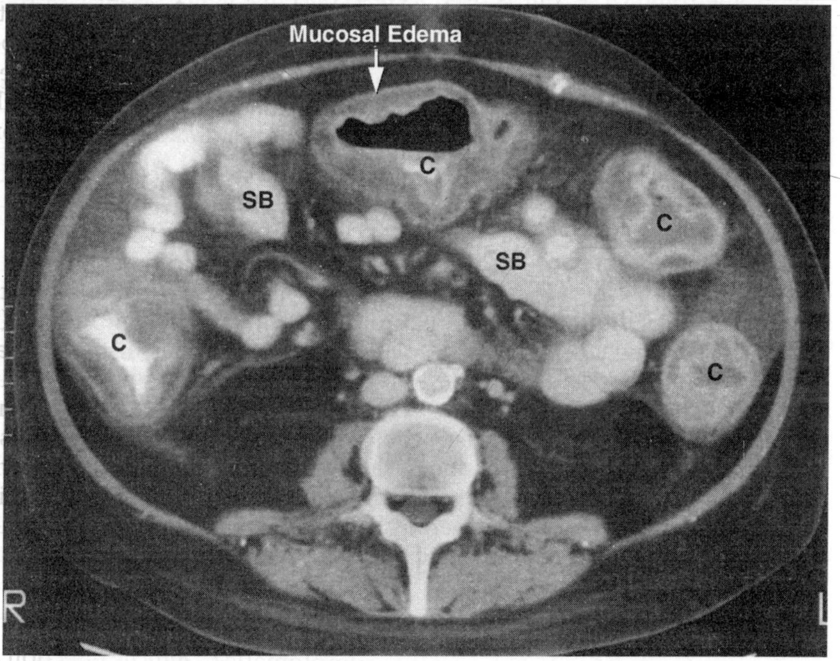

FIGURE 42.2 Contrast-enhanced CT scan of a patient with *C. difficile* enterocolitis. There is marked thickening of the wall of the colon (*C*), but not the small bowel (*SB*). (From Braley SE, Groner TR, Fernandez MU, Moulton JS. Overview of diagnostic imaging in sepsis. New Horiz 1993;1:214–230.) Image digitally enhanced.

Lower GI Endoscopy

Direct visualization of the lower GI mucosa is usually reserved for the few cases where the suspicion of *C. difficile* enterocolitis is high but the toxin assays are negative. The presence of pseudomembranes on the mucosal surface confirms the diagnosis of *C. difficile* enterocolitis. Colonoscopy is preferred to proctosigmoidoscopy for optimal results.

Treatment

The first step in treatment is to discontinue the offending antibiotic(s) if possible, and observe for improvement. Antibiotic therapy to eradicate *C. difficile* is recommended only if the diarrhea is severe and associated with signs of systemic inflammation (fever, leukocytosis, etc.), or if it is not possible to discontinue the offending antibiotic(s) (13). The recommended antibiotic regimens are shown below (5,6,13,14).

1. **Oral or intravenous metronidazole** (500 mg three times daily) is the treatment of choice, and should be continued **for 10 days.** The oral route is preferred, and the intravenous route should be reserved for patients who are unable to receive oral medications. Both routes are equally effective.
2. **Oral vancomycin** (125 mg four times daily) is as effective as metronidazole, but is used as a second-line agent because of the efforts to curtail vancomycin use and limit the spread of vancomycin-resistant enterococci. Vancomycin is preferred for pregnant or lactating females, but is otherwise reserved for cases where metronidazole is ineffective or is not tolerated. Vancomycin is not effective when given intravenously.
3. **Antiperistaltic agents are contraindicated** (5,14) because reduced peristalsis can prolong exposure to the cytotoxins.

The expected response is loss of fever by 24 hours and resolution of diarrhea in 4 to 5 days (5). Most patients show a favorable response, and in the few who do not respond by 3 to 5 days, a switch from metronidazole to vancomycin is indicated. Although rarely necessary, surgical intervention is required when *C. difficile* colitis is associated with progressive sepsis and multiorgan failure, or signs of peritonitis, despite antibiotic therapy (10). The procedure of choice is subtotal colectomy.

Relapses following antibiotic treatment occur in about 25% of cases (5,6,11). Most relapses are evident within 3 weeks after antibiotic therapy is completed. Repeat therapy using the same antibiotic is successful in about 75% of relapses, and another relapse is expected in about 25% of cases (14). As many as 5% of patients experience more than 6 relapses (5).

Probiotic Therapy

Antibiotic therapy for *C. difficile* enterocolitis can itself promote persistence of the organism, and this could explain the high relapse rate. Oral administration of *Saccharomyces boulardii* (lyophilized yeast preparation) or *Lactobacillus* spp. can be used as primary prophylaxis of *C. difficile* enterocolitis, or can be started along with antibiotics and continued to prevent relapses of symptomatic disease. This approach has proven successful in reducing the incidence of *C. difficile* enterocolitis (15,16), but it has not gained favor in the United States.

ABDOMINAL ABSCESS

Abdominal abscesses are an important consideration in septic patients who have sustained blunt abdominal trauma or are recovering from abdominal surgery (17,18).

Clinical Features

Abdominal abscesses are difficult to detect on routine clinical evaluation, as demonstrated in Table 42.1. Note that localized abdominal tenderness is present in only one third of cases, and a palpable abdominal mass is present in fewer than 10% of cases. Note also that routine abdominal films provide valuable information in fewer than 15% of patients.

Computed Tomography

Computed tomography (CT) of the abdomen is the most reliable diagnostic method of detection for intra-abdominal abscesses, with a sensitivity and specificity of 90% or higher (17,18). However, CT imaging in the early postoperative period can be misleading because collections of blood or irrigant solutions in the peritoneal cavity can be misread as an abscess. CT scans are most reliable when performed after the first postoperative week (when peritoneal fluid collections have resorbed) (18). The appearance of an abscess on an abdominal CT scan is demonstrated in Figure 42.3.

Management

Immediate drainage is mandatory for all intra-abdominal abscesses (19). Precise localization with CT scanning allows many abscesses to be drained percutaneously with radiographically-directed drainage catheters. Empiric antibiotic therapy should be started while awaiting the results of abscess fluid cultures. Single drug therapy with ampicillin–sulbactam (Unasyn) or imipenem is as effective as multiple-drug regimens (20).

URINARY TRACT INFECTIONS

Urinary tract infection (UTI) accounts for 30% of all ICU-acquired infections, and 95% of UTIs occur in patients with indwelling urethral catheters (21). The following description is limited to UTIs in the catheterized patient.

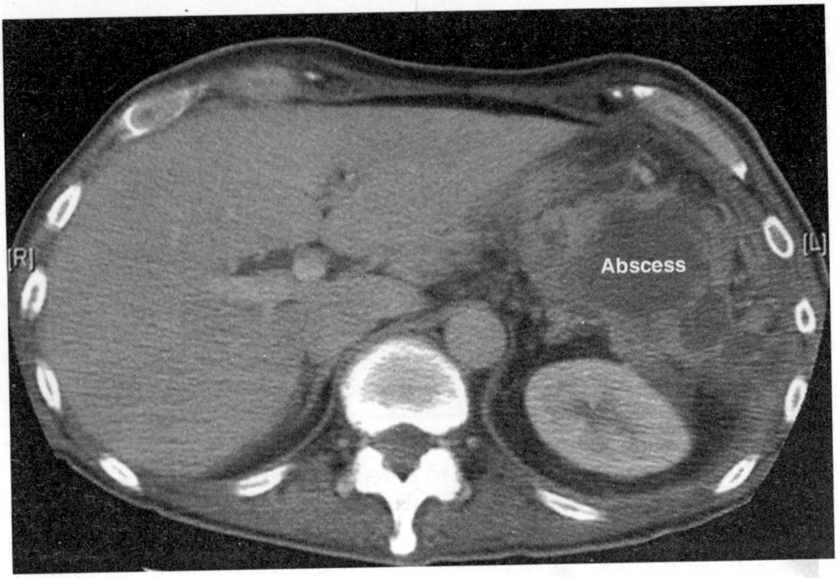

FIGURE 42.3 Abdominal CT scan showing a multiloculated abscess in the left upper quadrant in a post-splenectomy patient. (CT image courtesy of the Loyola University Medical Education Network, www.lumen.luc.edu/lumen)

Pathogenesis

The presence of a bladder drainage catheter in the urethra creates a 4 to 7% risk of developing a UTI *per day* (22). Bacterial migration along the catheter is the presumed mechanism for this risk, but there is more to the puzzle. The question that needs to be answered is why bacteria that migrate up the urethra and into the bladder are not washed out of the bladder by the urine flow. The flushing action of urine is a defense mechanism that protects the bladder from retrograde invasion by skin pathogens. This protective action explains why direct injection of bacteria into the bladder will not produce a UTI in a healthy subject (23).

Bacterial Adherence

The answer to the question posed in the last paragraph is linked to observations regarding bacterial adherence to the bladder epithelium. The epithelial cells of the bladder are normally coated with *Lactobacillus* organisms, as shown in Figure 42.4. These organisms are not pathogenic for man, and their presence on the surface of the epithelial cells prevents organisms that are pathogenic from attaching to the bladder wall. Loss of this protective coating and subsequent colonization of the bladder mucosa with gram-negative pathogens is the critical event that eventually leads to infection in the lower urinary tract (24). This is the same phenomenon that occurs in the oral mucosa in patients who develop nosocomial pneumonias, as described in Chapter 4. The events that link urethral catheterization to bacterial adherence in the bladder are unknown.

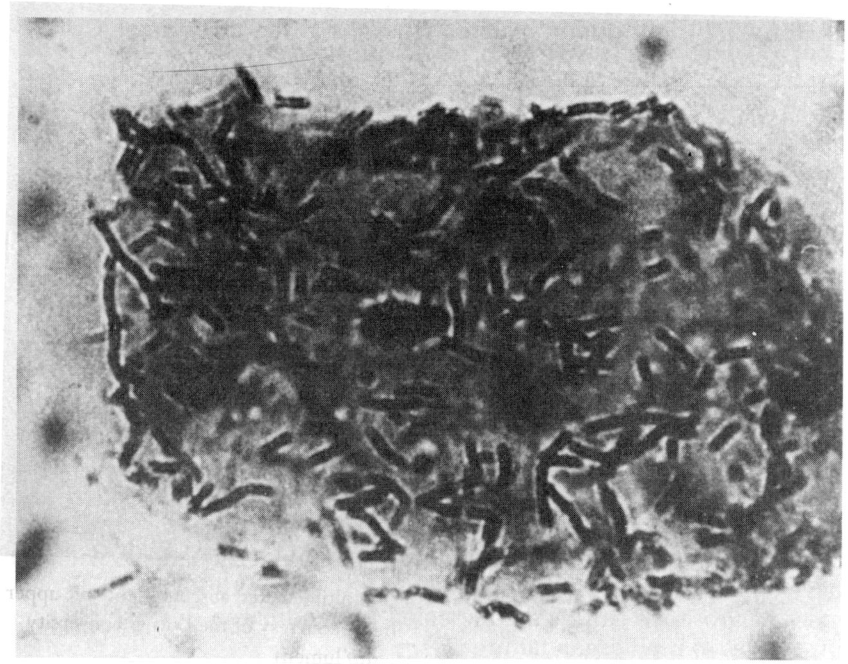

FIGURE 42.4 Photomicrograph showing *Lactobacillus* organisms blanketing a bladder epithelial cell. (From Sobel JD. Pathogenesis of urinary tract infections: host defenses. Infect Dis Clin North Am 1987;1:751–772.)

Microbiology

The common pathogens isolated from urine in medical ICU patients in the United States are listed in Table 42.2. Two surveys are included (21,25) to demonstrate that gram-negative aerobic bacilli are common isolates, but *Candida albicans* has emerged as a prominent isolate. Almost half (46%) of the cases of candiduria are asymptomatic (21) and therefore might not represent infection.

Diagnostic Criteria

The diagnosis of urinary tract infection based on urine cultures alone is misleading in patients with indwelling urethral catheters because half of these patients will have positive urine cultures after 5 days and virtually all patients will have positive urine cultures after 30 days of urethral catheterization (26). The criteria for the diagnosis of urinary tract infection in catheterized patients are shown in Table 42.3. These criteria are from a recent consensus conference on the definition of nosocomial infections (26), and they incorporate criteria proposed by the Centers for Disease Control in 1988 (27). Note that the diagnosis of UTI requires a symptom or sign of infection (fever, etc). Unfortunately, only fever and suprapubic tenderness apply to catheterized patients because indwelling urethral catheters eliminate the discriminating value of urgency,

TABLE 42.2 Pathogens Isolated from the Urine of Medical ICU Patients

Microorganism	Incidence (% total isolates)	
	1990–1992*	1992–1997†
Escherichia coli	31%	14%
Enterococci	15%	14%
Pseudomonas aeruginosa	13%	10%
Klebsiella pneumoniae	8%	6%
Proteus	7%	2%
Staphylococci	6%	6%
Candida albicans	5%	21%

*From Reference 25.
†From Reference 21.

frequency, and dysuria. Approximately 50% of elderly patients will also develop a change in mental status in association with UTIs (28). Severe cases of urosepsis can be accompanied by multiorgan dysfunction that progresses to multiorgan failure (29).

Urine Cultures

The threshold for significant bacteriuria in catheterized patients is 10^5 colony forming units per mL (cfu/mL). However, colony counts as low as 10^2 cfu/mL can represent infection if growth is sustained in more than one urine sample (collected on different days) (30).

Urine Microscopy

Urine microscopy is diagnostic only if an unspun urine specimen shows organisms on Gram stain or at least 3 leukocytes per high-powered field. The common practice of examining spun urine sediments has little value in identifying infection in catheterized patients.

Empiric Antimicrobial Therapy

Empiric antibiotic therapy pending culture results is recommended for patients with suspected UTI who are immunocompromised, have evidence of multiorgan dysfunction, or have a prosthetic or damaged heart valve. The urine Gram stain, if positive, can be used to guide antibiotic selection. The following are some suggestions.

Gram-Negative Bacilli

According to the susceptibility graphs in Chapter 44 (Figs. 44.1 and 44.2), **imipenem** should suffice for empiric coverage of gram-negative bacilli, and **amikacin** could be used for patients who have a prosthetic or damaged heart valve, or are seriously ill (i.e., are hemodynamically unstable or have evidence of multiorgan failure).

TABLE 42.3 Criteria for the Diagnosis of Upper Tract UTI in Patients with Indwelling Urethral Catheters*

I. The presence of one of the following:
- Body temperature >38°C
- Urgency or frequency or dysuria
- Suprapubic tenderness

AND

II. Urine culture growing $\geq 10^5$ CFU/mL of no more than 2 organisms.

OR

III. One of the following is present:
- Positive urine dipstick for leukocyte esterase or nitrates
- $\geq$3 WBCs per high-power field using unspun urine
- Organisms present on Gram stain of unspun urine
- 2 urine cultures with $\geq 10^2$ CFU/mL of the same organism

*Upper tract UTI includes infection involving the kidneys, ureters, bladder, urethra, or tissue surrounding the retroperitoneal or perinephric space.
From Calandra T, Cohen J. The international sepsis forum consensus conference on definitions of infection in the intensive care unit. Crit Care Med 2005; 33:1538.

Gram-Positive Cocci

A preponderance of gram positive cocci on the urine Gram's stain suggests that **enterococcus** is the responsible pathogen because staphylococci are uncommon offenders in nosocomial UTIs. If the patient is not seriously ill, enterococcal UTI can be treated effectively with **ciprofloxacin**. If the patient is seriously ill or has a prosthetic or damaged heart valve, ampicillin or **vancomycin plus gentamicin** is the preferred regimen. Ampicillin resistance is reported in 10 to 15% of nosocomial enterococcal infections (31), so vancomycin may be preferred. If vancomycin-resistant enterococci are a concern, **linezolid** can be used as a substitute for vancomycin (see the very end of Chapter 44 for a description of linezolid).

Candiduria

The presence of *Candida* in the urine often represents colonization, but candiduria can also be a sign of disseminated candidiasis (the candiduria in this case is the result, not the cause, of the disseminated candidiasis). Disseminated candidiasis can be an elusive diagnosis because blood cultures are sterile in more than 50% of cases (32), and candiduria may be the only sign of disseminated disease. The following recommendations are from recent guidelines published by the Infectious Disease Society of America (33).

1. Asymptomatic candiduria in immunocompetent patients does not require antifungal therapy. However, the urinary catheter

should be removed if possible because this can eradicate candiduria in 40% of cases (34).

2. Candiduria should be treated in symptomatic patients (i.e., fever or suprapubic tenderness), and patients with neutropenia or a renal allograft, because candiduria can be a sign of disseminated candidiasis in these patients.
3. Persistent candiduria in immunocompromised patients should prompt further investigation with ultrasonography or CT images of the kidney.

Antifungal Therapy

Bladder irrigation with amphotericin B is not recommended because local recurrence is common (33). For non-neutropenic patients with symptomatic candiduria, **fluconazole** (200 to 400 mg daily) for 7 to 14 days can be effective (33). For patients with renal insufficiency or for infection with species other than *Candida albicans*, the new antifungal agent **capsofungin** (50 mg daily) is a reasonable choice (see Chapter 44 for a description of capsofungin). For all other patients, **amphotericin B** (0.3 to 1 mg/kg daily) for 1 to 7 days can be effective (33).

A FINAL WORD

The unifying feature in infections that involve, or originate from, the gastrointestinal, urinary, and respiratory tracts (see also Chapter 41) is the initial colonization with pathogenic organisms that first takes place. This colonization seems to involve a change in the ability of microorganisms to adhere to epithelial surfaces. In healthy subjects, the epithelial surfaces in the mouth, GI tract, and urinary tract are covered by harmless commensal organisms, but in patients who develop an acute or chronic illness, these surfaces are covered with pathogenic organisms, and this serves as a prelude to nosocomial infections. This repopulation is not just a matter of "territorial imperative" (where one population forces another population to leave), but seems to involve the ability of microorganisms to adhere to the epithelial cells. If this is the case, then we need to study the mechanisms whereby microorganisms adhere to epithelial surfaces in health and disease if we are to effectively deal with the threat of nosocomial infections.

REFERENCES

Acalculous Cholecystitis

1. Walden D, Urrutia F, Soloway RD. Acute acalculous cholecystitis. J Intensive Care Med 1994;9:235–243.
2. Imhof M, Raunest J, Ohmann Ch, Rohrer H-D. Acute acalculous cholecystitis complicating trauma: A prospective sonographic study. World J Surg 1992; 1160–1166.
3. Te HS. Cholestasis in HIV-infected patients. Clin Liver Dis 2004;8:213–228.

Colonization of the GI Tract

4. Marshall JC, Christou NV, Meakins JL. The gastrointestinal tract: the "undrained abscess" of multiple organ failure. Ann Surg 1993;218:111–119.
5. Bartlett JG. Antibiotic-associated diarrhea. N Engl J Med 2002;346:334–339.
6. Mylonakis E, Ryan ET, Calderwood SB. *Clostridium difficile*-associated diarrhea. Arch Intern Med 2001;161:525–533.
7. Fekety R, Kim F H, Brown D, et al. Epidemiology of antibiotic associated colitis. Am J Med 1981;70:906–908.
8. Samore MH, Venkataraman L, DeGirolami, et al. Clinical and molecular epidemiology of sporadic and clustered cases of nosocomial *Clostridium difficile* diarrhea. Am J Med 1996;100:32–40.
9. Johnson S, Gerding DN, Olson MM, et al. Prospective, controlled study of vinyl glove use to interrupt *Clostridium difficile* nosocomial transmission. Am J Med 1990;88:137–140.
10. Lipsett PA, Samantaray DK, Tam ML, et al. Pseudomembranous colitis: a surgical disease? Surgery 1994;116:491–496.
11. Yassin SF, Young-Fadok TM, Zein NN, Pardi DS. *Clostridium difficile*-associated diarrhea and colitis. Mayo Clin Proc 2001;76:725–730.
12. Fishman EK, Kavuru M, Jones B, et al. Pseudomembranous colitis: CT evaluation of 26 cases. Radiology 1991;180:57–60.
13. Guerrant RL, Van Gilder T, Steiner TS, et al. Practice guidelines for the management of infectious diarrhea: Infectious Disease Society of America. Clin Infect Dis 2001;32:331–350.
14. Aslam S, Hamill RJ, Musher DM. Treatment of *Clostridium difficile*-associated disease: Old therapies and new strategies. Lancet Infect Dis 2005;5:549–557.
15. Surawicz C. Prevention of antibiotic-associated diarrhea by *Saccharomyces boulardii:* A prospective study. Gastroenterology 1989;96:981–988.
16. D'Souza AL, Rajkumar C, Cooke J, Bulpitt CJ. Probiotics in prevention of antibiotic-associated diarrhea: Meta-analysis. Br Med J 2002;324:1361–1366.

Abdominal Abscesses

17. Mirvis SE, Shanmuganthan K. Trauma radiology, Part I: Computerized tomographic imaging of abdominal trauma. J Intensive Care Med 1994;9:151–163.
18. Fry DE. Noninvasive imaging tests in the diagnosis and treatment of intra-abdominal abscesses in the postoperative patient. Surg Clin North Am 1994; 74:693–709.
19. Oglevie SB, Casola G, van Sonnenberg E, et al. Percutaneous abscess drainage: Current applications for critically ill patients. J Intensive Care Med 1994; 9:191–206.
20. Mosdell DM, Morris DM, Voltura A, et al. Antibiotic treatment for surgical peritonitis. Ann Surg 1991;214:543–549.

Urinary Tract Infections

21. Richards MJ, Edwards JR, Culver D, Gaynes RP. Nosocomial infections in medical intensive care units in the United States. Crit Care Med 1999;27:887–892.

22. Amin M. Antibacterial prophylaxis in urology: A review. Am J Med 1992;92 (suppl 4A):114–117.
23. Howard RJ. Host defense against infection: Part 1. Curr Probl Surg 1980;27: 267–316.
24. Daifuku R, Stamm WE. Bacterial adherence to bladder uroepithelial cells in catheter-associated urinary tract infection. N Engl J Med 1986;314:1208–1213.
25. Emori TG, Gaynes RP. An overview of nosocomial infections, including the role of the microbiology laboratory. Clin Microbiol Rev 1993;6:428–442.
26. Calandra T, Cohen J, for the International Sepsis Forum Definition of Infection in the ICU Consensus Conference. Crit Care Med 2005;33:1538–1548.
27. Garner JS, Jarvis WR, Emori TG, et al. CDC definitions for nosocomial infections, 1988. Am J Infect Control 1988;16:128–140.
28. McCue JD. How to manage urinary tract infections in the elderly. J Crit Illness 1996;11(suppl):S30–S40.
29. Bone RC, Larson CB. Gram-negative urinary tract infections and the development of SIRS. J Crit Illn 1996;11(suppl):S20–S29.
30. Stamm WE, Hooten TM. Management of urinary tract infection in adults. N Engl J Med 1993;329:1328–1334.
31. Jenkins SG. Changing spectrum of uropathogens: implications for treating complicated UTIs. J Crit Illn 1996;11(suppl):S7–S13.

Candiduria

32. British Society for Antimicrobial Chemotherapy Working Party. Management of deep *Candida* infection in surgical and intensive care unit patients. Intensive Care Med 1994;20:522–528.
33. Pappas PG, Rex JH, Sobel JD, et al..Guidelines for treatment of candidiasis. Clin Infect Dis 2004;38:161–189.
34. Sobel JD, Kauffman CA, McKinsey D, et al. Candiduria: A randomized double-blind study of treatment with fluconazole or placebo. Clin Infect Dis 2000;30:19–24.

Chapter 43

THE IMMUNO-COMPROMISED PATIENT

When you do battle, overcome your opponent by calculation.

Sun Tzu (The Art of War)

The care of critically ill patients is a labor-intensive, time-consuming, and mentally exhausting experience, and each of these aspects of patient care in the ICU reaches its zenith in the care of patients with impaired immune function. This chapter will focus on two patient populations who suffer the consequences of immune suppression: those infected with the human immunodeficiency virus (HIV), and those who develop myelosuppression from cancer chemotherapy. The care of immunocompromised patients like these is a topic of monumental size, and the material in this chapter represents only the tip of the iceberg.

THE HIV-INFECTED PATIENT

The introduction of *highly active antiretroviral therapy* (HAART) in 1996 has changed the character and outlook of patients with HIV infection who are admitted to the ICU. This is demonstrated in Figure 43.1 (1). Prior to HAART, most HIV-related admissions to the ICU were for *Pneumocystis carinii* pneumonia, and about 50% of the patients survived to hospital discharge (1,2). Since the introduction of HAART, the prevalence of pneumocystis pneumonia has decreased considerably, and bacterial pathogens have emerged as the most common etiologic agents in HIV-related pneumonia (1,2). Survival has also improved to the point where three of every four patients admitted to the ICU with an HIV-related disorder can now leave the hospital (1).

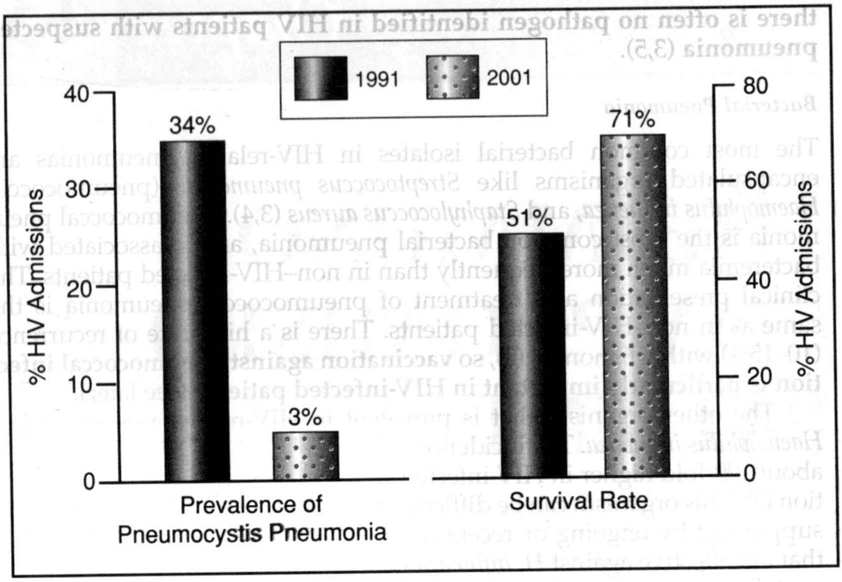

FIGURE 43.1 The change in character of HIV-related ICU admissions after the introduction of highly active antiretroviral therapy (HAART) in the mid-1990s. (Data from Reference 1)

Pneumonia

Pneumonia continues to be the most common cause of HIV-related ICU admissions. The wide spectrum of etiologic agents in HIV-related pneumonias is evident in Table 43.1 (2–5). Bacterial pneumonias are most common, while non-bacterial pneumonias occur more often in the advanced stages of HIV infection (e.g., when CD4-lymphocyte counts are below 200/mL). The shaded box in Table 43.1 highlights the observation that

TABLE 43.1 Causes of Pneumonia in HIV Patients*

Bacterial Pneumonia	Nonbacterial Pneumonia
Streptococcus pneumoniae (15–20%)	*Pneumocystis carinii* (3–15%)
Hemophilus influenza (5–15%)	Fungi (5–10%)
Staphylococcus aureus (3–5%)	*Mycobacterium tuberculosis and Mycobacterium avium* complex (5%)
Pseudomonas aeruginosa (3–6%)	
Other Gram-negative bacilli (3–5%)	Organism never identified (25–60%)
Atypical organisms (1–4%)†	

*From References 1–3. The parentheses show the reported incidence for each microbe.
†Includes *Chlamydia pneumoniae, Legionella spp*, and *Mycoplasma pneumoniae.*

there is often no pathogen identified in HIV patients with suspected pneumonia (3,5).

Bacterial Pneumonia

The most common bacterial isolates in HIV-related pneumonias are encapsulated organisms like *Streptococcus pneumoniae* (pneumococci), *Haemophilus influenza*, and *Staphylococcus aureus* (3,4). Pneumococcal pneumonia is the most common bacterial pneumonia, and is associated with bacteremia much more frequently than in non–HIV-infected patients. The clinical presentation and treatment of pneumococcal pneumonia is the same as in non–HIV-infected patients. There is a high rate of recurrence (10–15%) within 6 months (3), so **vaccination against pneumococcal infection is particularly important in HIV-infected patients** (see later).

The other organism that is prevalent in HIV-related pneumonias is *Haemophilus influenza*. The incidence of *Haemophilus influenza* pneumonia is about 100-fold higher in HIV-infected patients than in the general population (3). This organism can be difficult to isolate because its growth is easily suppressed by ongoing or recent antibiotic treatment (3). The antibiotics that are effective against *H. influenza* include second- and third-generation cephalosporins (e.g., ceftriaxone), azithromycin, and fluoroquinolones.

Pneumocystis Pneumonia

Pneumocystis carinii (renamed *Pneumocystis jurovecii* when it infects humans), is a protozoa-like organism (reclassified as a fungus in 1988) that proliferates in patients who are immunosuppressed. Although declining in frequency, pneumocystis pneumonia is still considered the most common opportunistic infection in HIV-infected patients (6), and it is almost always seen in advanced stages of the disease (e.g., when CD4+ lymphocyte counts are less than 200/mL).

Patients with pneumocystis pneumonia typically present with fever, non-productive cough, and hypoxemia that is out of proportion to the appearance of the chest x-ray. **The initial chest x-ray can be normal in 40% of patients** (7), but as the disease progresses, bilateral infiltrates like those in Figure 43.2 begin to appear. In advanced cases of pneumocystis pneumonia, the bilateral infiltrates coalesce to produce a chest x-ray like the one in Figure 43.3. The radiographic features of severe pneumocystis pneumonia are similar to those of the acute respiratory distress syndrome (ARDS) (see Fig. 22.3).

The diagnosis of pneumocystis pneumonia requires visualization of the organism in specimens obtained from the respiratory tract. The most popular method of detection is the use of monoclonal antibodies directed at pneumocystis antigens (direct fluorescent antibody method), which will detect both trophic and cystic forms of the organism (6). Sputum induction with hypertonic saline has a diagnostic yield of 50 to 90% (3,6), although this varies with the prevalence of HIV infection (and thus the experience of cytopathologists) in individual medical centers. The highest diagnostic yield is provided by bronchoalveolar lavage, which demonstrates the organism in over 90% of cases (3). The treatment of pneumocystis pneumonia is described later in the chapter.

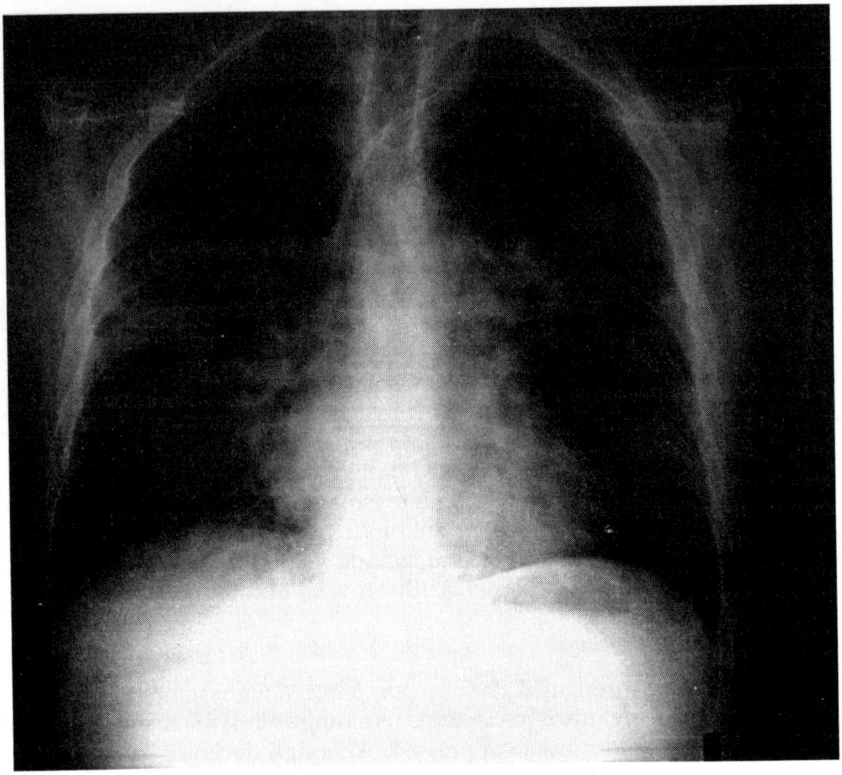

FIGURE 43.2 Portable chest x-ray of an HIV-infected patient who presented with fever, nonproductive cough, and dyspnea. Routine cultures of sputum and blood were unrevealing, but bronchoalveolar lavage showed numerous *Pneumocystis carinii* organisms.

Tuberculosis

As many as 10% of HIV-infected patients who are purified protein derivative (PPD) positive will develop active tuberculosis (TB) each year (3). The radiographic features of pulmonary TB are determined by the CD4+ lymphocyte count in blood. When the CD4+ cell count is above 200/mL, the chest x-ray often shows upper lobe cavitary disease, similar in appearance to active TB in non–HIV-infected patients. However **when the CD4+ cell count is below 200/mL, active TB can be accompanied by non-cavitary infiltrates in the mid-lung fields** (3), and this radiographic appearance **can be confused with a bacterial pneumonia.**

Diagnostic Approaches to Pneumonia

The clinical presentation of HIV-related pneumonia is often nonspecific, and does not allow identification of the responsible pathogen (3,6,7). In particular, **the pattern of infiltration on the chest radiograph is not pathogen specific.** As mentioned earlier, pneumocystis pneumonia can present with a clear chest x-ray or a non-specific radiographic pattern such as the one in

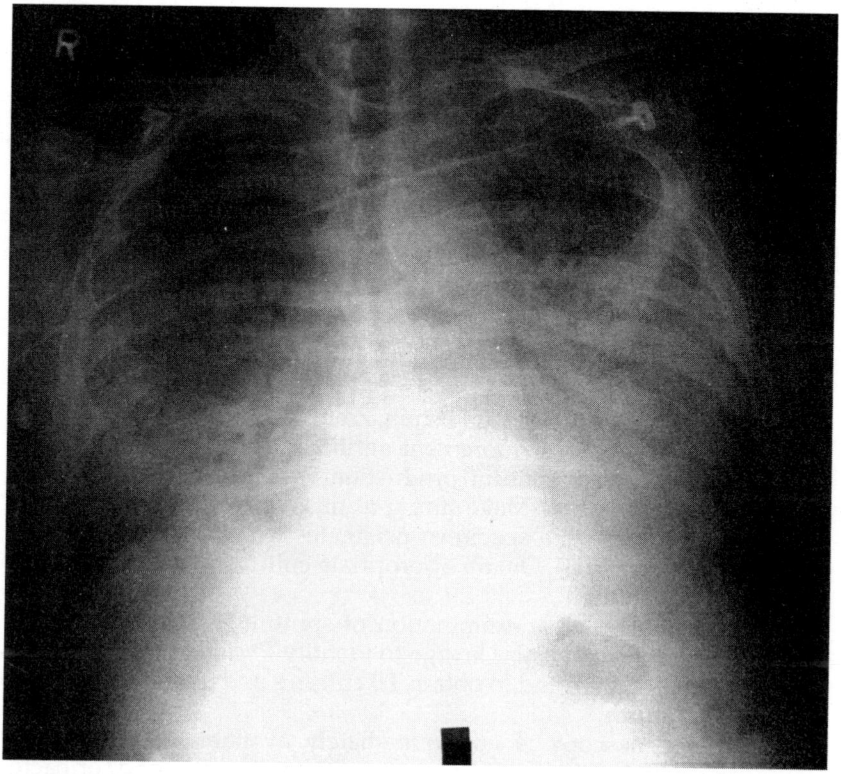

FIGURE 43.3 Radiographic appearance of an advanced case of pneumocystis pneumonia, which is often indistinguishable from the acute respiratory distress syndrome (ARDS).

Figure 43.2, and the typical appearance of advanced pneumocystis pneumonia in Figure 43.3 can also be seen in atypical pneumonias and ARDS. Identification of the etiologic agent requires blood cultures and an evaluation (with histologic examination and cultures) of sputum and bronchoscopic specimens from the lower respiratory tract.

Bronchoscopy

Bronchoscopy is a valuable diagnostic tool in HIV-related pneumonias because specimens obtained from the lower respiratory tract (by bronchial brushing or bronchoalveolar lavage) will identify over 90% of cases of pneumocystis pneumonia and pulmonary TB (3). In addition, quantitative bacterial cultures of bronchial brushings and bronchoalveolar lavage specimens can identify the responsible pathogen(s) in 70 to 80% of bacterial pneumonias (see Table 41.3). The use of bronchoscopy to diagnose bacterial pneumonias is described in Chapter 41. The ability to isolate bacterial pathogens in sputum or bronchoscopic specimens is markedly reduced in patients who are receiving antibiotic treatment. (The ability to identify *Pneumocystis carinii* is not affected by a few days of appropriate antibiotic coverage). Therefore, sputum and bronchoscopic specimens should be collected prior to starting antibiotic therapy, if possible.

An Organized Approach

The initial approach to the HIV-infected patient with pneumonia can be guided by the CD4+ lymphocyte count in blood. If the CD4+ cell count is above 200/mL, then the patient should be evaluated for a bacterial pneumonia as described in Chapter 41. If the CD4+ count is below 200/mL, then the management can proceed as follows:

1. Place the patient in respiratory isolation (because pulmonary TB can have a nonspecific radiographic appearance at reduced CD4+ cell counts).
2. Collect sputum for Gram's stain, Ziehl-Neelson stain (for tubercle bacilli) and direct fluorescent antibody stains (for *Pneumocystis carinii*). Induce sputum production with nebulized hypertonic saline if necessary. Make sure sputum is screened for microscopic evidence that the specimen originates from the lower airways (see Figure 41.3). Obtain appropriate cultures (bacterial and TB) when indicated.
3. If the microscopic examination of sputum is unrevealing, perform bronchoalveolar lavage to identify *Pneumocystis carinii* and tubercle bacilli, and to obtain TB cultures and quantitative bacterial cultures.
4. If bronchoscopy is not immediately available, begin empiric antibiotic treatment for pneumocystis pneumonia and/or bacterial pneumonia based on clinical judgment (e.g., empiric coverage for pneumocystis pneumonia is usually given to patients with respiratory failure or diffuse infiltrates on chest x-ray). Pneumocystis can be demonstrated in the lower respiratory tract for days after starting appropriate antibiotic coverage, so bronchoscopy should be attempted, if possible, in the first few days of empiric antibiotic treatment.
5. Treatment for pulmonary TB is started only if there is evidence of infection on Ziehl-Neelson stains for tubercle bacilli. If there is no evidence of pulmonary TB on two or three sputum samples, respiratory isolation can be discontinued.

Despite its diagnostic value, bronchoscopy is performed on fewer than 50% of patients with the diagnosis of pneumocystis pneumonia (8). Most of these patients are given empiric antibiotic treatment for pneumocystis pneumonia with no attempt to identify the organism. This practice should be discouraged because it mandates three weeks of (possibly unnecessary) antibiotic therapy and the antimicrobial agents are often poorly tolerated (see next).

Treatment for Pneumocystis Pneumonia

Trimethoprim–sulfamethoxazole (TMP–SMX) is the antibiotic of choice for pneumocystis pneumonia. The recommended dose is 20 mg/kg of

TMP and 100 mg/kg of SMX daily, administered in three or four divided doses. Although TMP–SMX can be given orally, intravenous therapy is advised for patients with respiratory failure. A favorable clinical response may not be apparent for 5 to 7 days (9), and there may be an initial period of deterioration. Radiographic improvement lags behind the clinical improvement (9), so the chest x-ray should not be used to evaluate the response to therapy. If a favorable response is not evident after 5 to 7 days, the treatment is considered a failure. If there is improvement in 5 to 7 days, treatment is continued for a total of 3 weeks (3,10).

Adverse reactions to TMP–SMX develop in 30 to 50% of HIV-infected patients (10–14). These reactions usually appear during the second week of treatment, and they are often severe enough to warrant discontinuing the drug. The most common side effects are neutropenia (45 to 50%), fever (45 to 50%), skin rash (35 to 40%), elevated hepatic transaminase enzymes (30 to 35%), hyperkalemia (30%), and thrombocytopenia (10 to 15%). A case of fatal pancreatitis has also been linked to TMP–SMX (14). Only 35 to 45% of patients who receive TMP–SMX are able to complete the full course of therapy. The high incidence of adverse reactions to TMP–SMX is specific for HIV infection. In other groups of patients, adverse reactions to TMP–SMX develop in only 10% of the patients (10).

Pentamidine isothionate is the preferred second-line agent when TMP–SMX fails or is not tolerated. The recommended dose is 4 mg/kg given intravenously as a single daily dose. Intramuscular injection is not recommended because of the risk for sterile abscesses. The response time and duration of therapy are the same as for TMP–SMX. Treatment failures occur in one-third of patients (10).

Adverse reactions are also common with intravenous pentamidine (10,15–17). These side effects include neutropenia (5 to 30%), hyperglycemia and hypoglycemia (10 to 30%), prolonged Q–T interval (3 to 35%), torsade de pointes (up to 20%), renal insufficiency (3 to 5%), and pancreatitis (up to 1%). Almost half of the patients who receive intravenous pentamidine are unable to complete therapy because of adverse reactions (10,15).

In patients who are unable to complete therapy with either TMP–SMX or pentamidine, a variety of other agents (e.g., clindamycin and primaquine) are available. In this situation, leave the decision to an infectious disease specialist.

STEROIDS. A brief course of steroid therapy is standard for cases of pneumocystis pneumonia that result in respiratory failure. When started at the time of antimicrobial therapy, steroid therapy is associated with improved outcomes in pneumocystis pneumonia (18). Most clinical trials used oral prednisone, but intravenous methylprednisolone (40 mg every 6 hours for at least 7 days) has also been recommended (10). Delay of treatment for 72 hours after the start of antimicrobial therapy negates any possible benefit from steroids (18). The response to steroids seems to vary in different clinical reports, and favorable responses can be short-lived (19).

Pneumocystis and Pneumothorax

Pneumothorax is an uncommon (5% of cases) but serious complication of pneumocystis pneumonia (20). When it occurs during mechanical

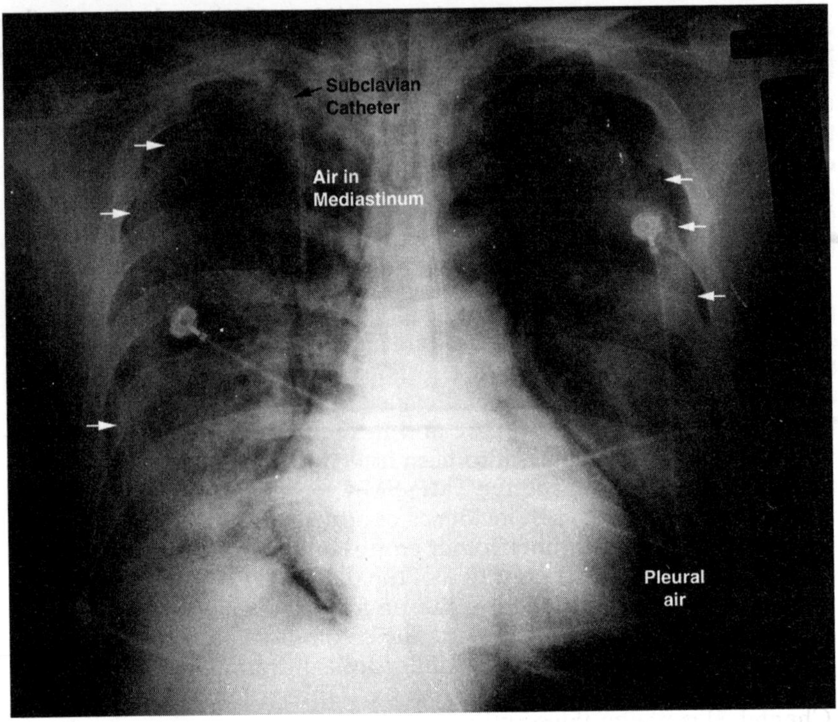

FIGURE 43.4 Portable chest x-ray showing a pneumomediastinum and bilateral pneumothorax in a patient with pneumocystis pneumonia. The white arrows point to the outer edge of the collapsing lungs.

ventilation, as illustrated in Figure 43.4, it is usually a sign of extensive underlying tissue destruction in the lungs, and few patients survive (20). To reduce the risk of this serious complication, it seems wise to adopt the strategy known as "limited-volume" ventilation for patients with pneumocystis pneumonia. This method is designed to limit the inflation volumes during mechanical ventilation, and it is used to prevent lung injury from overdistention in patients with acute respiratory distress syndrome. A description of this method is in Chapter 22 (see Table 22.4).

Cryptococcal Meningitis

Cryptococcal meningitis is the most common life-threatening fungal infection in HIV-infected patients (21,22). It is expected in 10% of patients with HIV infection, and usually appears in the advanced stages of immunosuppression (i.e., when CD4 lymphocyte counts fall below 50/mm^3).

Clinical Features

The most common manifestations are fever and headache, each reported in approximately 85% of cases (21). Other findings include meningeal signs (35 to 40%), altered mental status (10 to 15%), and seizures (less than 10%) (21). Cryptococcal infections at other sites (e.g., pneumonia and skin rash) are seen in 20% of cases (22).

Diagnosis

The diagnosis of cryptococcal meningitis requires lumbar puncture. Standard measurements in cerebrospinal fluid (CSF), such as glucose, protein, and leukocyte count, can be normal in up to 50% of cases (21). The organism can be demonstrated on india ink stains of CSF in 75% of cases (which is higher than the yield from india ink stains in non–HIV-infected patients) (21). CSF cultures and cryptococcal antigen titers are positive in over 90% of cases (21).

Treatment

The recommended treatment for cryptococcal meningitis in HIV-infected patients is shown below (23).

1. Start with **amphotericin B** (0.7–1 mg/kg/day) and **flucytosine** (100 mg/kg/day) for the first 2 weeks.
2. After 2 weeks, switch to oral **fluconazole** (400 mg/day) and continue for a minimum of 10 weeks. Thereafter, the dose of fluconazole is reduced (200 mg/day) and treatment is continued indefinitely.

Chapter 44 contains a description of these antifungal agents. The mortality in this disorder is about 30% despite antifungal therapy (21).

Toxoplasmic Encephalitis

Toxoplasma gondii encephalitis is the most common neurologic disorder in HIV-infected patients. Clinical evidence of toxoplasmic encephalitis is reported in 5 to 15% of HIV-infected patients, and autopsy evidence of the disease is present in up to 30% of patients (21).

Clinical Features

Toxoplasmic encephalitis is characterized by focal brain lesions. Hemiparesis and other focal neurologic deficits are seen in 60% of cases, and seizures are reported in 15 to 30% of patients (21). Other manifestations include fever (5 to 55%), confusion (60 to 65%), and choreiform movements (considered by some to be pathognomonic of toxoplasmic encephalitis) (21). Although extraneural disease is not common, disseminated toxoplasmosis with septic shock has been reported (24).

Diagnosis

Computerized tomography (CT) usually reveals solitary or multiple hypodense, contrast-enhancing lesions in the basal ganglia and frontoparietal regions of the cerebral hemispheres (21). An example of such a lesion is shown in Figure 43.5. Note the hypodense core and the contrast enhancement at the outer edges of the lesion. Because of the radiographic

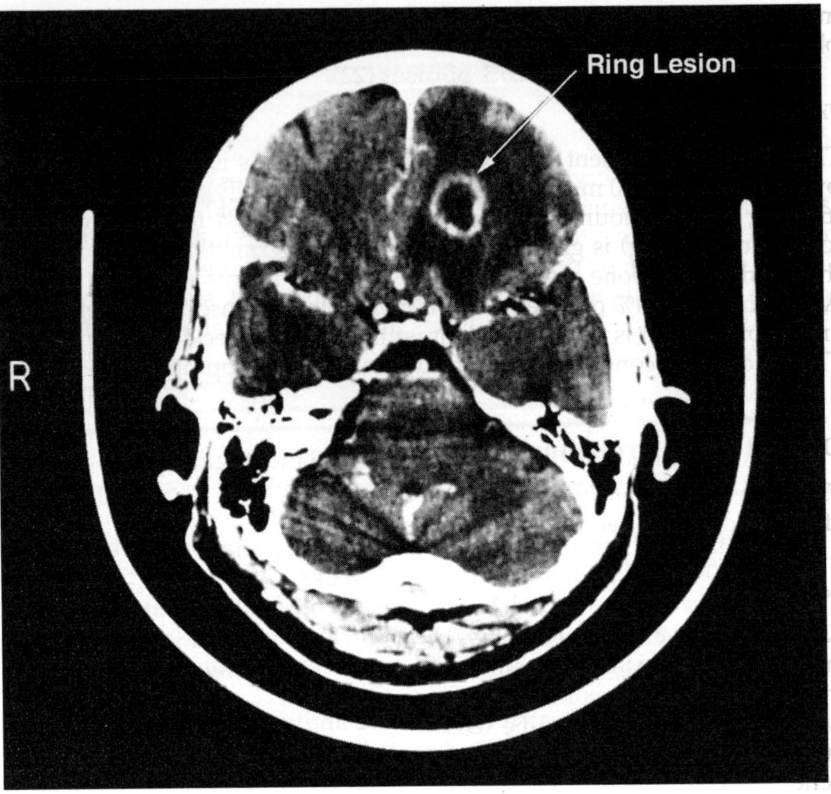

FIGURE 43.5 CT image showing a ring-enhancing lesion in a patient with toxoplasmic encephalitis. The hypodense area surrounding the lesion is evidence of cerebral edema.

appearance, these lesions are sometimes called "ring-enhancing lesions" or "ring lesions." These lesions are not pathognomonic of toxoplasma encephalitis: similar lesions can be found in cases of lymphoma. CT scans can be unrevealing in the early stages of the disease. Magnetic resonance imaging (MRI) is more sensitive than CT scans and can reveal lesions when CT scans are negative (25). Lumbar puncture usually reveals abnormal findings, but these are nonspecific.

The diagnosis of toxoplasma encephalitis can be made with certainty when the organism is identified in excisional brain biopsies using immunoperoxidase staining. (Needle biopsies have a lower diagnostic yield). However, the common practice is to bypass the brain biopsy and rely instead on a presumptive diagnosis of toxoplasmosis based on the presence of characteristic lesions in the brain plus with serologic evidence of recent toxoplasma infection. Over 90% of patients with toxoplasma encephalitis will have anti-toxoplasma antibodies (IgG) in their blood, so a positive antibody titer is a sensitive marker of toxoplasma infection. Unfortunately, 20% of the general population also have these antibodies in their blood (26), so a positive antibody titer lacks specificity for toxoplasma encephalitis.

Treatment

The preferred treatment for toxoplasma encephalitis is a combination of **pyrimethamine** (200 mg loading dose, then 75 mg daily) and **clindamycin** (600 mg every 6 hours). Because pyrimethamine is a folate antagonist, folinic acid (10 mg) is given with each dose of pyrimethamine to reduce the incidence of bone marrow suppression. All agents are given orally. Approximately 70% of cases show a favorable response to this regimen, and improvement is usually evident within the first week of therapy (27). The condition is considered uniformly fatal without appropriate therapy.

Drug-Related Problems

The drugs currently used for antiretroviral therapy have certain adverse effects and drug interactions that deserve mention.

Lactic Acidosis

Nucleoside reverse transcriptase inhibitors can be associated with a lactic acidosis caused by inhibition of mitochondrial enzymes involved in the electron transport chain. This problem is most often associated with danosine and stavudine (28,29). The lactic acidosis can be severe, and a mortality of 77% has been reported (29). Case reports suggest a beneficial response to riboflavin (50 mg daily), thiamine (100 mg daily) and L-carnitine (50 mg/kg) (28), and all three can be given as treatment. The offending drug should, of course, be discontinued.

Drug Interactions

Antiretroviral drugs are sometimes given to patients in the ICU. These drugs have a multitude of potential drug interactions, and the ones most likely to be seen in the ICU are included in Table 43.2. Most of these

TABLE 43.2 Drug Interactions with Antiretroviral Drugs*

Drug	Antiretroviral	Effect
Amiodarone	Ritonavir, Other PIs	Bradycardia, hypotension
Diltiazem	Aprenavir, Atazanavir	Hypotension
Meperidine	Ritonavir	Increased normeperidine
Methadone	PIs, NRTIs, NNRTIs	Opiate withdrawal
Midazolam	PIs, NNRTIs	Enhanced sedation

*From Reference 27.

PI = protease inhibitor, *NRTI* = nucleoside reverse transcriptase inhibitor, *NNRTI* = non-nucleoside reverse transcriptase inhibitor.

interactions are significant enough to recommend avoiding the drug combinations instead of reducing the drug dose.

THE NEUTROPENIC PATIENT

The risk of infection with neutropenia (neutrophil count less than 500/mm^3) depends on the cause, severity, and duration of the neutropenia. Most cases of neutropenia that are complicated by serious infections are persistent (last longer than 10 days) and are caused by bone marrow suppression from chemotherapy (30). Neutropenia from other causes (e.g., viral infections) is rarely associated with an increased risk of infection, particularly if the neutropenia lasts less than 10 days (30). The reason for this discrepancy is not clear, but the propensity for infections in chemotherapy-induced neutropenia may be due to additional immune suppression from the primary disease that requires the chemotherapy (i.e., cancer or organ transplantation).

Febrile Neutropenia

The following statements highlight some of the important observations in patients with neutropenia and fever (30).

1. About two-thirds of patients with fever and neutropenia will not have an apparent infection on the initial evaluation.
2. Gram-positive organisms, especially coagulase-negative staphylococci, are the most frequent causes of bacterial infections in febrile neutropenia.
3. Bacteremia is relatively uncommon, and occurs in only 10 to 15% of patients with neutropenia and fever.

The most likely sites of infection in neutropenic patients are the lungs, urinary tract (in patients with indwelling drainage catheters), central venous catheters, and skin (for transplant patients with surgical wounds). Whether or not there is evidence of infection at these sites, blood cultures should be obtained routinely, prior to starting empiric or directed antibiotic therapy.

Pulmonary Infiltrates

The infectious and noninfectious causes of pulmonary infiltrates in neutropenic patients with fever is shown in Figure 43.6 (31). In this study, fungal pneumonia is the most common lung infection, while bacterial and viral pneumonias are uncommon. The most common cause of fungal pneumonia in this study was *Aspergillus fumigatus*, and the remaining isolates included *Fusarium*, *Histoplasma capsulatum*, and *Candida glabrata*. The bacterial isolates included staphylococci (coagulase positive and negative) and gram-negative enteric organisms, including *Pseudomonas aeruginosa*. The only virus isolated in this study was cytomegalovirus.

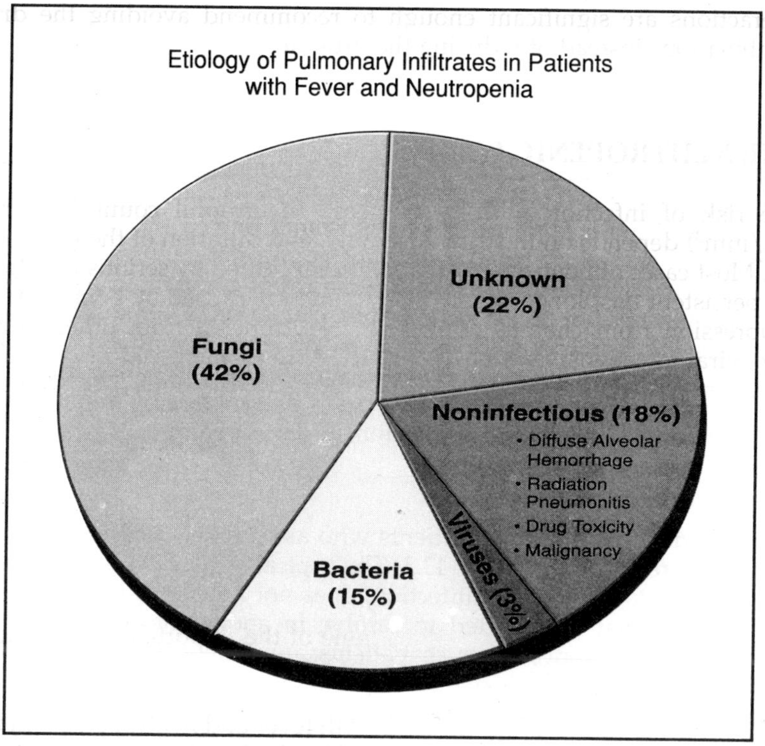

FIGURE 43.6 Pie chart showing the infectious and noninfectious causes of pulmonary infiltrates in neutropenic patients with fever. (Results from Piekert T, et al. Safety, diagnostic yield, and therapeutic implications of flexible bronchoscopy in patients with febrile neutropenia and pulmonary infiltrates. Mayo Clin Proc 2005;80:1414.)

The pie graph in Figure 43.6 also demonstrates that **a considerable proportion of neutropenic patients with suspected fever have no evidence of infection**. Forty percent of the patients in this study had no evidence of infection, and 22% had no identifiable cause for the infiltrates. The noninfectious causes of pulmonary infiltrates are listed in the figure. The most common noninfectious pulmonary disorder is diffuse alveolar hemorrhage.

The prevalence of fungal pneumonias in neutropenic patients highlights the value of bronchoscopy in the diagnostic evaluation of pneumonia in these patients. Sputum is notoriously unreliable for the diagnosis of fungal pneumonia, and demonstration of the organisms deep within the lungs is required. Bronchoscopy can establish the diagnosis of fungal pneumonia with bronchial brushings, bronchoalveolar lavage, or transbronchial lung biopsy (the latter technique is not appropriate for ventilator-dependent patients or patients with thrombocytopenia). In one study that provided the data in Figure 43.6, the results of bronchoscopy resulted in a change in therapy in 50% of the patients. Bronchoscopy also provided the diagnosis in the patient whose chest x-ray is shown in Figure 43.2.

Empiric Antibiotics

Prompt initiation of antibiotic therapy is recommended for all neutropenic patients with fever. This recommendation is based on the observation that patients with gram-negative septicemia due to *Pseudomonas aeruginosa* can deteriorate rapidly without appropriate antibiotic coverage (30). However, pseudomonas bacteremia is not common in neutropenic patients (except following kidney transplantation) (30), so the rush to antibiotics may not be justified in most patients. Regardless of timing, empiric antibiotics are recommended for all patients with neutropenia and fever (32). The choice of antibiotics is determined by the likelihood that the patient has a serious infection, as described next.

Low Risk Patients

The criteria for identifying patients who are unlikely to have a serious infection are shown in Table 43.3. The typical patient who meets these criteria has no evidence of infection, does not appear to be ill, and has neutropenia that is expected to resolve in about one week. The recommended antibiotics for such patients are shown in Table 43.4. The intravenous regimen uses one of three antibiotics: ceftazidime cefepime, or a carbepenem (imipenem or meropenem). These antibiotics provide broad spectrum coverage, but are selected for their activity against *Pseudomonas aeruginosa*. I prefer imipenem because it is active against all possible gram-positive and gram-negative pathogens with the exception of methicillin-resistant *Staph aureus*.

TABLE 43.3 Criteria For a Low Risk of Serious Infection*

History and Physical Exam	X-Ray and Laboratory Tests
• Malignancy in remission. • Neutropenia present <7 days and expected to resolve within 10 days. • Does not appear ill. • Peak temperature <39° C. • No comorbid conditions.† • No abdominal pain or neurologic abnormalities. • No apparent catheter-site infection.	• No infiltrate on chest x-ray. • Neutrophil count ≥100/mm^3. • Monocyte count ≥100/mm^3. • Lab tests of hepatic and renal function close to normal.

*From Hughes WT, et al. 2002 guidelines for the use of antimicrobial agents in neutropenic patients with cancer. Clin Infect Dis 2002; 34:730.

†Includes shock, hypoxia, pneumonia or other deep organ infection, vomiting or diarrhea.

TABLE 43.4 Risk-Based Empiric Antibiotic Therapy*

Low Risk of Serious Infection	High Risk of Serious Infection
Oral Therapy	Vancomycin not Needed
• Ciprofloxacin + amoxicillin clavulenate	• Basic Regimen† or • Aminoglycoside + Basic Regimen†
IV Therapy	Vancomycin Needed
• Basic Regimen†	• Vancomycin + Basic Regimen† ±Aminoglycoside

*For the recommended starting doses of each antibiotic, see Table 41.6.
From Hughes WT, et al. 2002 guidelines for the use of antimicrobial agents in neutropenic patients with cancer. Clin Infect Dis 2002;34:730.
†Basic Regimen = ceftazidine or cefepime or a carbepenem.

High Risk Patients

For patients who do not satisfy the criteria in Table 43.3, the recommended antibiotic regimens are determined by the perceived need for vancomycin. The vancomycin requirement is determined by the likelihood of infection with methicillin-resistant strains of *Staph aureus* (MRSA). The patient who is at risk for MRSA infections will satisfy one or more of the following conditions: (*1*) Has a prior history of colonization or infection with MRSA, (*2*) is a resident of a nursing home, (*3*) has a chronic debilitating illness and has received multiple antibiotics in the past year, or (*4*) is in an ICU where MRSA is prevalent.

All patients in the high risk category will receive one of the drugs in the basic regimen (ceftazidime, cefepime, or a carbepenem). Vancomycin is then added if it is considered necessary. The addition of an aminoglycoside is a consideration in patients who appear seriously ill (e.g., those with septic shock), or if pseudomonas infection is suspected.

Evaluate Response to Therapy

A favorable response is expected within 5 days of starting antibiotics (32). If the fever has resolved and there is no evidence of infection at 3 to 5 days, continued antibiotic therapy for a total of 7 days is still recommended, even when the neutropenia is resolving (32). This practice seems ill-advised, particularly when the bone marrow is recovering and the neutropenia is resolving. The more significant problem is what to do when the fever persists for longer than 5 days on empiric antibiotics and there is no evidence of infection. This situation is considered in the next section.

Persistent Fever

Continued fever after 1 week of empiric antibiotic therapy has several possible explanations (e.g., the fever may be due to a noninfectious process), and one of these is a disseminated fungal infection. Up to one-third of neutropenic patients with persistent fever have a disseminated fungal infection, and most cases involve *Aspergillus* and *Candida* species (32). Because of this possibility, **intravenous amphotericin** (0.5 mg/kg daily) is an appropriate consideration for persistent fever in this setting. The amphotericin trial should probably not exceed 2 weeks (32).

AN OUNCE OF PREVENTION

The Centers for Disease Control and Prevention recommends that pneumococcal polyvalent vaccine should be given to all adults who are immunosuppressed as a result of HIV infection, malignancy (particularly hematologic), chemotherapy, and chronic steroid use (for a complete list of all candidates for vaccination, see reference 33). The vaccine can be administered just prior to discharge from the ICU. Patients who have received the vaccine within the past 5 years do not need revaccination until 5 years have elapsed from the time of initial vaccination. Revaccination is not a universal recommendation, but is advised for patients who are immunosuppressed (33).

Unfortunately, the efficacy of the pneumococcal vaccine is limited in patients who are immunosuppressed. This is not surprising because vaccines require an immune response to confer immunity.

A FINAL WORD

One of the harsh realities in critical care medicine is the realization that antibiotics have had little impact on survival rates in serious, life-threatening infections. This can be explained by the notion that body's immune system and other defenses are the principal deterrents of infection, while antibiotics provide only supplemental aid. Patients who develop serious infections might do so because they have impaired defenses against infection. If this is the case, then antibiotics are expected to have limited efficacy.

The importance of host defenses in the pathogenesis of infection is demonstrated by the colonization of the oropharynx with gram-negative pathogens that occurs in patients who are acutely or chronically ill (see Chapter 4). In this case, a defect in the host's normal defenses allows pathogenic bacteria to adhere to the oral mucosa and proliferate, and this colonization serves as a prelude to nosocomial pneumonia. When a pneumonia does develop, systemic antibiotics might provide some temporary relief, but their impact on the final outcome will be limited as long as the colonization in the mouth is allowed to continue.

The problem of impaired host defenses against infection reaches its pinnacle in the immunocompromised patient, which means that juggling antibiotics to eradicate infections will be particularly futile in this patient population. As Sun Tzu indicates in the opening quote, a more calculated approach than antibiotic therapy is needed to do battle with invading microbes in the immune-impaired patient.

REFERENCES

The HIV-Infected Patient

1. Narashimhan M, Posner AJ, DePalo VA, et al. Intensive care in patients with HIV infection in the era of highly active antiretroviral therapy. Chest 2004; 125:1800–1804.
2. Wolff AJ, O'Donnell AE. Pulmonary manifestations of HIV infection in the era of highly active antiretroviral therapy. Chest 2001;120:1888–1893.
3. Bartlett JG. Pneumonia in the patient with HIV infection. Infect Dis Clin North Am 1998;12:807–820.
4. Afessa B, Green B. Bacterial pneumonia in hospitalized patients with HIV infection. Chest 2000;117:1017–1022.
5. Hirschtick RE, Glassroth J, Jordan MC, et al. Bacterial pneumonia in persons infected with the human immunodeficiency virus. N Engl J Med 1995;333: 845–851.
6. Thomas CF, Limper AH. Pneumocystis pneumonia. N Engl J Med 2004;350: 2487–2498.
7. Opravil M, Marinchek B, Fuchs WA, et al. Shortcomings of chest radiography in detecting *Pneumocystis carinii* pneumonia. J Acquir Immune Defic Syndrome 1994;7:39–45.
8. Uphold CR, Deloria-Knoll M, Parada FJ, et al. U.S. hospital care for patients with HIV infection and pneumonia. Chest 2004;125:548–556.
9. Datta D, Abbas S, Henken EM, et al. *Pneumocystis carinii* pneumonia: the time course of clinical and radiographic improvement. Chest 2003;124:1820–2823.
10. Brooks KR, Ong R, Spector RS, et al. Acute respiratory failure due to *Pneumocystis carinii* pneumonia. Crit Care Clin 1993;9:31–48.
11. Johnson MP, Goodwin D, Shands JW. Trimethoprim-sulfamethoxazole anaphylactoid reactions in patients with AIDS: case reports and literature review. Pharmacotherapy 1990;10:423–426.
12. van der Ven AJAM, Koopmans PP, Vree TB, et al. Adverse reactions to co-trimoxazole in HIV infection. Lancet 1991;338:431–433.
13. Greenberg S, Reiser IW, Chou S-Y, et al. Trimethoprim-sulfamethoxazole induces reversible hyperkalemia. Ann Intern Med 1993;119:291–295.
14. Jost R, Stey C, Salomon F. Fatal drug-induced pancreatitis in HIV. Lancet 1993;341:1412.
15. Dohn MN, Weinberg WG, Torres RA, et al. Oral atovaquone compared with intravenous pentamidine for *Pneumocystis carinii* pneumonia in patients with AIDS. Ann Intern Med 1994;121:174–180.
16. Eisenhauer MD, Eliasson AH, Taylor AJ, et al. Incidence of cardiac arrhythmias during intravenous pentamidine therapy in HIV-infected patients. Chest 1994;105:389–394.
17. Foisey MM, Slayter KL, Morse GD. Pancreatitis during intravenous pentamidine therapy in an AIDS patient with prior exposure to didanosine. Ann Pharmacother 1994;28:1025–1028.
18. National Institutes of Health: University of California Expert Panel for Corticosteroids as Adjunctive Therapy for *Pneumocystis* Pneumonia. Consensus statement on the use of corticosteroids as adjunctive therapy for *Pneumocystis* pneumonia in the acquired immunodeficiency syndrome. N Engl J Med 1990; 323:1500–1504.

19. Schiff MJ, Farber BF, Kaplan MH. Steroids for *Pneumocystis carinii* pneumonia and respiratory failure in the acquired immunodeficiency syndrome. Arch Intern Med 1990;150:1819–1821.
20. Pastores SM, Garay SM, Naidich DP, et al. Review: pneumothorax in patients with AIDS-related *Pneumocystis carinii* pneumonia. Am J Med Sci 1996;312: 229–234.
21. Levy RM, Berger JR. Neurologic critical care in patients with human immunodeficiency virus 1 infection. Clin Crit Care 1993;9:49–72.
22. Ennis DM, Saag MS. Cryptococcal meningitis in AIDS. Hosp Pract 1993;28:99–112.
23. Saag MS, Graybill RJ, Larsen RA, et al. Practice guidelines for the management of cryptococcal diseases: Infectious Disease Society of America. Clin Infect Dis 2000;30:710–718.
24. Lucet J-C, Bailley M-P, Bedos J-P, et al. Septic shock due to toxoplasmosis in patients infected with the human immunodeficiency virus. Chest 1993;104: 1054–1058.
25. Knobel H, Graus F, Miro JM, et al. Toxoplasmic encephalitis with normal CT scan and pathologic MRI. Am J Med 1995;99:220–221.
26. Drew WL. Toxoplasmic encephalitis in HIV patients: how to prevent, how to treat. J Crit Illness 1994;9:223–224.
27. Luft BJ, Hafner R, Korzun AH, et al. Toxoplasmic encephalitis in patients with the acquired immunodeficiency syndrome. N Engl J Med 1993;329:995–1000.
28. Morris A, Masur H, Huang L. Current issues in critical care of the human immunodeficiency virus-infected patient. Crit Care Med 2006;34:42–49.
29. Miller RD, Cameron M, Wood LV, et al. Lactic acidosis and hepatic steatosis associated with the use of stavudine: report of four cases. Ann Intern Med 2000;133:192–196.

The Neutropenic Patient

30. Pizzo PA. Fever in immunocompromised patients. N Engl J Med 1999;341:893–900.
31. Piekert T, Rana S, Edell ES. Safety, diagnostic yield, and therapeutic implications of flexible bronchoscopy in patients with febrile neutropenia and pulmonary infiltrates. Mayo Clin Proc 2005;80:1414–1420.
32. Hughes WT, Armstrong D, Bodey GP, et al. 2002 guidelines for the use of antimicrobial agents in neutropenic patients with cancer. Clin Infect Dis 2002;34:730–751.
33. Centers for Disease Control and Prevention. Prevention of pneumococcal disease: recommendations of the Advisory Committee on Immunization Practices. MMWR 1997;46(RR–8).

Chapter 44

ANTIMICROBIAL THERAPY

The danger with germ-killing drugs is that they may kill the patient as well as the germ.
J.B.S. Haldane

Antibiotic therapy is a way of life in intensive care units. The antibiotics used most often in the ICU are included in the list shown later. Each of these will be presented in alphabetical order as listed.

- Aminoglycosides
- Antifungal agents
- Cephalosporins
- Fluoroquinolones
- Imipenem
- Penicillins
- Vancomycin

AMINOGLYCOSIDES

The aminoglycosides are a group of antibiotics derived from cultures of *Streptomyces* (hence the name streptomycin for the first aminoglycoside). There are eight drugs in this class, but only three are clinically relevant: gentamicin, tobramycin, and amikacin (introduced in 1966, 1975, and 1981, respectively). These drugs were once the darlings of the infectious disease world because of their activity in serious gram-negative infections, but their popularity has waned because of renal toxicity (1).

Activity and Clinical Uses

The aminoglycosides are among the most active antibiotics against aerobic gram-negative bacilli (see Fig. 44.1), including *Pseudomonas aeruginosa* (see Fig. 44.2). Amikacin is the most active of the three aminoglycosides, probably because it has been in clinical use for a shorter period of time

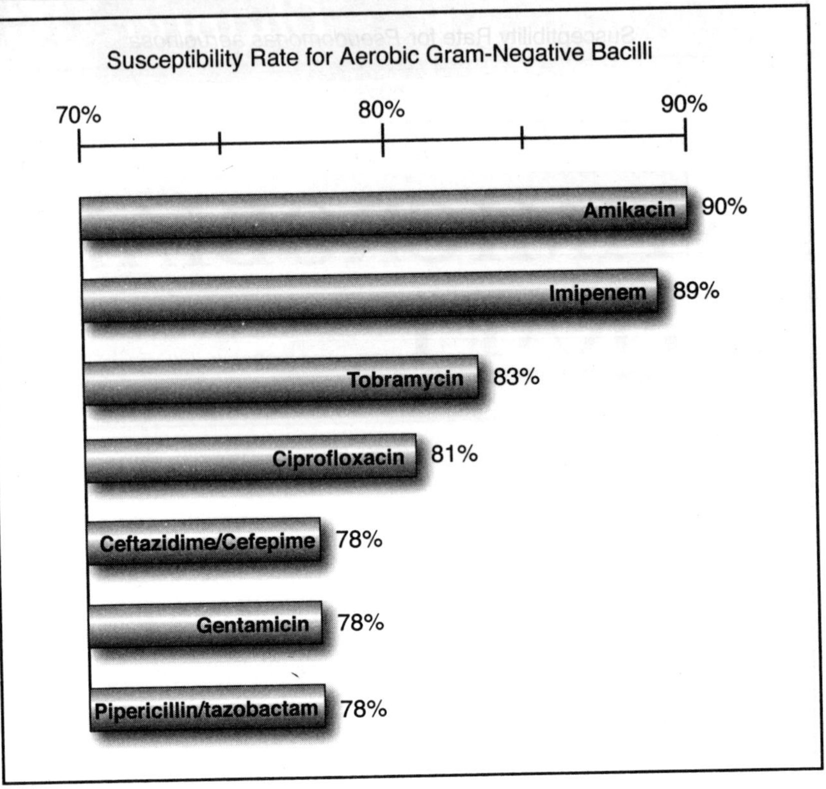

FIGURE 44.1 Susceptibility of gram-negative bacilli to commonly used antibiotics. Data from 35,790 cultures obtained from ICU patients during the years 1994–2000. (From Reference 2).

(giving microbes less time to develop resistance). Aminoglycosides can be used to treat any serious infection caused by gram-negative bacilli, but their use is generally reserved for infections involving *Pseudomonas* species. They are the favored drugs for *Pseudomonas* bacteremia, particularly in immunocompromised patients. Aminoglycosides are also used in empiric antibiotic regimens for neutropenic patients with fever (see Table 43.4).

Dosing

Aminoglycoside dosing is based on body weight, and is influenced by changes in renal function. A dosage chart for the aminoglycosides is shown in Table 44.1.

Dosing by Body Weight

The choice between actual body weight and ideal body weight for aminoglycoside dosing is determined by the weight of the patient. The total

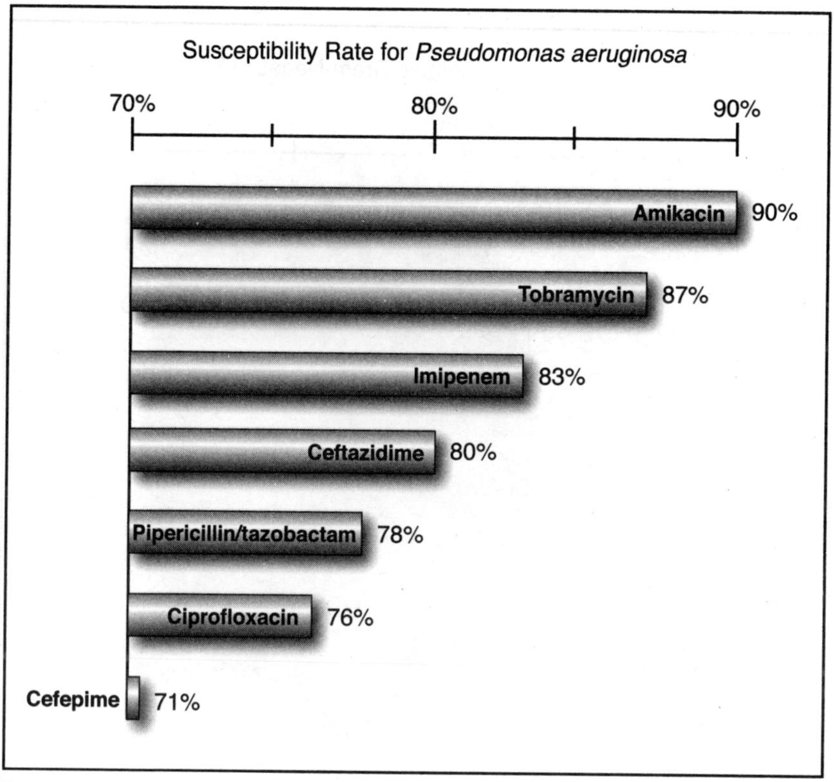

FIGURE 44.2 Susceptibility of *Pseudomonas aeruginosa* to commonly used antibiotics. Data from 8,244 cultures obtained from ICU patients during the years 1994–2000. (From Reference 2).

body distribution of aminoglycosides includes only a small fraction in adipose tissue, so ideal body weight would be appropriate to prevent overdosing in obese patients. However, dosing based on ideal body weight will result in overdosing patients who are underweight, so actual body weight is more appropriate for aminoglycoside dosing in underweight patients. To simplify this situation, you can **compare the ideal and actual body weight of each patient, and use the lower of the two weights to determine the aminoglycoside dose** (1). (Formulas for determining ideal body weight in men and women are in Appendix 2).

Once-Daily Dosing

The bactericidal effect of the aminoglycosides is concentration dependent, so higher drug concentrations in the body will produce more bacterial killing (1). This is the rationale for the popularity of administering aminoglycosides in one daily dose (which produces higher drug concentrations in tissues than divided-dose regimens). The once-daily regimen has not proven more effective than the divided-dose regimens (1).

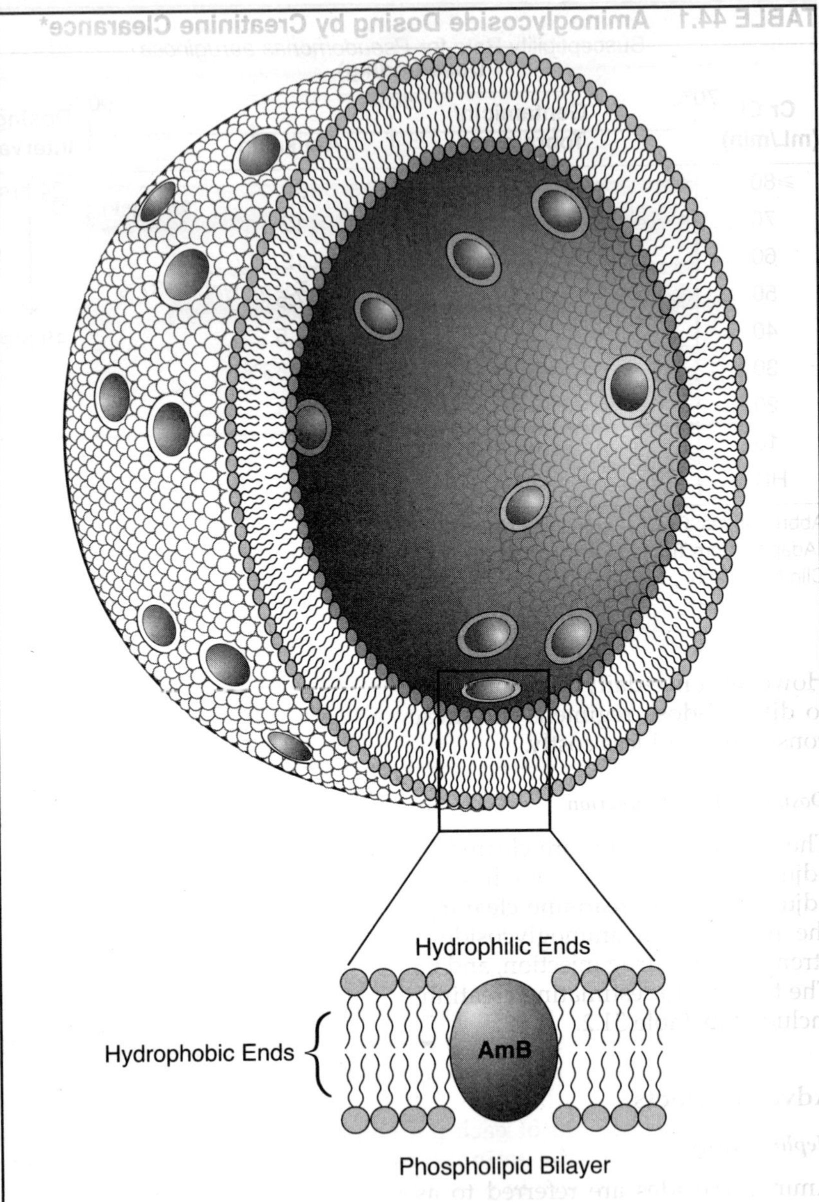

FIGURE 44.3 Schematic view of a liposome shown in cross-section to show the phospholipid bilayer and the amphotericin B (AmB) situated in the bilayer. Scale is in nanometers (nm).

TABLE 44.1 Aminoglycoside Dosing by Creatinine Clearance*

Cr Cl (mL/min)	Dose (mg/kg) Gentamicin/ Tobramycin	Amikacin	Dosing Interval
⩾80	5	15	24 hrs
70	4	12	
60	4	12	
50	3.5	7.5	↓
40	2.5	7.5	48 hrs
30	2.5	4	↓
20	4	7.5	72 hrs
10	3	4	↓
HD	2	5	96 hrs

Abbreviations: Cr Cl = creatinine clearance, HD = hemodialysis.
*Adapted from Turnidge J. Pharmacodynamics and dosing of aminoglycosides. Infect Dis Clin N Am 2003; 17:503–528.

However, once-daily dosing is still preferred because it is equivalent to divided-dose regimens in efficacy and toxicity (1), but is less time-consuming and less costly.

Dosing by Renal Function

The aminoglycosides are cleared by filtration in the kidneys, and dose adjustments are necessary when renal clearance is impaired. The dosing adjustments for creatinine clearance are shown in Table 44.1. Note that the reduction in aminoglycoside dose can involve a decrease in the strength of the drug injection, and increase in the dosing interval, or both. The formula for estimating creatinine clearance based on body weight is included in Table 31.2.

Adverse Effects

Nephrotoxicity

Aminoglycosides are referred to as *obligate nephrotoxins* because renal impairment will eventually develop in all patients if treatment is continued (1). These drugs are capable of provoking oxidative injury in cells lining the proximal tubules, and the risk of renal injury is the same with each of the aminoglycosides. The earliest signs of injury include cylindrical casts in the urine, proteinuria, and inability to concentrate urine (3). The urinary changes appear in the first week of drug treatment, and the serum creatinine begins to rise 5 to 7 days after the start of therapy. The nephrotoxicity is enhanced by hypovolemia, advanced age, preexisting renal impairment, hypokalemia, hypomagnesemia, and concurrent therapy with selected drugs (i.e., loop diuretics, cyclosporin, cisplatin, and vancomycin) (1,3). The renal impairment can progress to acute renal failure, but this is usually reversible.

Other Adverse Effects

Other adverse effects, which include ototoxicity and neuromuscular blockade, are rarely a problem. The ototoxicity can produce irreversible hearing loss and vestibular damage, but these are almost never apparent to the patient (1). Aminoglycosides can block acetylcholine release from presynaptic nerve terminals, but this is never clinically apparent with therapeutic dosing (4). There is a small risk that aminoglycosides will aggravate the neuromuscular blockade associated with myasthenia gravis and nondepolarizing muscle relaxants (1,5), and it is wise to avoid aminoglycosides in these conditions.

Comment

Because of the substantial risk of renal damage, you should **avoid using aminoglycosides** whenever possible. A number of less harmful but equally effective antibiotics are available for treating gram-negative infections. Aminoglycosides should be reserved for immunocompromised or hemodynamically unstable patients with gram-negative bacteremia, particularly when *Pseudomonas* species are involved.

ANTIFUNGAL AGENTS

Amphotericin B

Amphotericin B (AmB) is a naturally occurring antibiotic that is fungicidal for most of the pathogenic fungi in humans (6). It is the most effective antifungal agent in clinical use, but is also the most toxic antifungal agent as well. The adverse effects of AmB include an infusion-related inflammatory response, and nephrotoxicity.

Clinical Uses

AmB is the drug of choice for all life-threatening fungal infections, and for empiric antimicrobial therapy in neutropenic patients with persistent fever. It is gradually being replaced by less toxic agents (described later) for infections caused by *Candida albicans* and *Aspergillus* species.

Dosage and Administration

AmB is available for intravenous use only, and contains a vehicle (sodium deoxycholate) to enhance solubility in plasma. It is given once daily in a dose of 0.5 to 1 mg/kg (higher doses may be required in life-threatening infections). The dose is initially delivered over a 4-hour time period, but this can be reduced to a one-hour infusion if tolerated. Daily infusions are continued until a specified cumulative dose is achieved. The total

AmB dose is determined by the type and severity of the fungal infection: it can be as little as 500 mg (for catheter-related candidemia) or as much as 4 grams (for life-threatening invasive aspergillosis).

INFUSION-RELATED INFLAMMATORY RESPONSE. Infusions of AmB are accompanied by fever, chills, nausea, vomiting, and rigors in about 70% of instances (7). This reaction resembles a systemic inflammatory response, and the presumed culprit is cytokine release from activated monocytes (6). This reaction is most pronounced with the initial infusion, and often diminishes in intensity with repeated infusions. The following measures are used to reduce the intensity of this reaction (7):

1. Thirty minutes before the infusion, give acetaminophen (10 to 15 mg/kg orally) and diphenhydramine (25 mg orally of IV). If rigors are a problem, premedicate with meperidine (25 mg IV).
2. If the premedication regimen does not give full relief, add hydrocortisone to the AmB infusate (0.1 mg/mL).

Central venous cannulation is preferred for AmB infusions to reduce the risk of infusion-related phlebitis, which is common when AmB is infused through peripheral veins (6).

Nephrotoxicity

AmB binds to cholesterol on the surface of renal epithelial cells and produces an injury in the renal tubules that clinically resembles a renal tubular acidosis (distal type), with increased urinary excretion of potassium and magnesium (8). Azotemia is reported in 30% to 40% of patients during daily infusions of AmB (9), and can occasionally progress to acute renal failure that requires hemodialysis (10). The renal impairment from AmB usually stabilizes with continued infusions, and improvement is expected if AmB is discontinued. An increase in the serum creatinine above 3.0 mg/dL should prompt cessation of AmB infusions for a few days (7).

Hypokalemia and hypomagnesemia are common during AmB therapy, and the hypokalemia can be difficult to correct until the magnesium deficits are replaced (the relationship between magnesium and potassium is described in Chapter 34). Because **magnesium depletion is the seminal event** in both electrolyte disorders, oral magnesium supplementation (300 to 600 mg elemental magnesium daily) is recommended if possible during AmB therapy to replace urinary magnesium losses. However, this can result in hypermagnesemia in the presence of renal insufficiency, so magnesium supplementation is not recommended for patients with progressive azotemia.

The nephrotoxic effects of AmB are aggravated by hypovolemia, and by the concurrent use of other nephrotoxic agents (e.g., cyclosporine). The deleterious effects of hypovolemia are explained by the localized vasoconstriction that is observed in AmB nephrotoxicity. Avoiding diuretics and maintaining intravascular volume with isotonic saline infusions is considered essential for reducing the risk of nephrotoxicity.

Liposomal Amphotericin B

Specialized lipid preparations of AmB have been developed to enhance AmB binding to fungal cell membranes and reduce binding to mammalian cells (thereby reducing the risk of renal injury). One of these preparations contains microscopic vesicles like the one depicted in Figure 44.3 to transport amphotericin. These vesicles are made up of phospholipids, and are called *liposomes*. Phospholipid molecules are *amphipathic*; i.e., they have a hydrophilic end and a hydrophobic end. When placed in an aqueous medium, the phospholipid molecules arrange themselves in bilayers so that the hydrophilic ends are on the surface of the bilayer and hydrophobic ends are in the interior. These bilayers then pinch off to form enclosed vesicles,. The phospholipid bilayer becomes a liposomal membrane, and the amphotericin molecules are intercalated in this membrane. This drug preparation is initially kept as a dry powder, and is hydrated just prior to infusion. The hydration triggers the liposome formation.

Clinical trials comparing liposomal AmB (Ambisome) to standard AmB have shown that both are equally effective, but liposomal AmB is associated with fewer infusion-related side effects and a lower incidence of renal dysfunction (6,9,11). The dose of liposomal AmB needed to produce equivalent antifungal effects is 5 times higher than the dose of standard AmB (6).

The major disadvantage of the lipid formulations is the cost. A comparison of the daily cost of treatment with standard AmB and liposomal AmB (Ambisome) for a 70 kg adult is shown below.

	Standard AmB	Liposomal AmB
Avg. Wholesale Price*	$11.54/50 mg	$118.40/50 mg
Daily Dose	1 mg/kg	5 mg/kg
Daily Cost (70 kg)	$16.16	$828.80

*as quoted in Reference 12.

These estimates place the liposomal preparation at about 50 times the cost of standard AmB. However, an occasional episode of renal insufficiency from standard AmB might even the score.

The lipid formulations of AmB are currently approved for the treatment of fungal infections in patients who are intolerant of standard AmB (e.g., those with renal insufficiency). The liposomal formulation is also approved for empiric antifungal coverage in neutropenic patients with persistent fever (6). The future of these compounds will be determined by the availability of other less expensive alternatives to standard AmB (such as the triazoles described next).

Triazoles

The triazoles are synthetic antifungal agents that are less toxic alternatives to AmB for selected fungal infections. There are three drugs in this class currently in use: fluconazole, itraconazole, and voriconazole. Fluconazole has the most applications in the ICU.

Clinical Uses

The major use for fluconazole in the ICU is the treatment of *Candida* septicemia in patients who are hemodynamically stable and are not immunocompromised (13,14). There is some concern that fluconazole does not adequately cover some species other than *Candida albicans*, such as *Candida krusei* (15), but this organism is involved in only 5% to 10% of cases of invasive candidiasis in the ICU (15). In patients with candidemia who are immunocompromised, fluconazole can be used after an initial course of amphotericin (15). Itraconazole is effective for invasive aspergillosis, but is not favored because of multiple drug interactions (16). Voriconazole is effective for aspergillosis, and for emipiric treatment of neutropenic patients with persistent fever (17).

Dosing

Fluconazole can be given orally or intravenously. The usual dose for confirmed infections is 400 to 800 mg daily given as a single dose (the same dose is recommended for oral and intravenous use). The time to reach steady state levels after the start of therapy is 4 to 5 days, and this can be shortened by doubling the initial dose. Adjustments are necessary for renal impairment: if the creatinine clearance is less than 50 mL/min, the dose should be reduced by 50% (6). For the doses of the other triazoles, see reference (6).

Drug Interactions

The triazoles inhibit the cytochrome P450 enzyme system in the liver, and they can potentiate the activity of several drugs. For fluconazole, the significant interactions include phenytoin, cisapride, and the statins (lovastatin, atorvastatin). Fluconazole should not be used with cisapride (Propulsid) or the statins (6). For a list of drug interactions with the other triazoles, see reference (6).

Toxicity

The triazoles are largely devoid of serious toxicity (other than drug interactions). There are rare reports of severe and even fatal hepatic injury associated with fluconazole therapy in HIV patients (18). Asymptomatic elevation of liver enzymes is reported during fluconazole therapy in less than 10% of patients (6).

Echinocandins

The echinocandins are a new class of antifungal agents that are being promoted as a better choice than fluconazole for invasive candidiasis (16). The proposed benefits of these agents include improved coverage for all *Candida* species, less risk of drug interactions, and no dose modification in renal failure. The significance of these advantages is unproven.

Capsofungin

Capsofungin (Cancidas) is the flagship drug in this class. Clinical studies show that capsofungin is comparable to amphotericin for treating

TABLE 44.2 The Generations of Parenteral Cephalosporins

Agent	Generation	Gram⁺ Cocci*	Gram⁻ Bacilli	*P. aeruginosa*	*B. fragilis*	*H. influenza*
Cefazolin (Ancef)	1	++++	++	—	—	++
Cefoxitin (Mefoxin)	2	++	++++	—	++	++
Ceftriaxone (Rocephin)	3	++	++++	—	—	++++
Ceftazidime (Fortaz)	3	—	++++	++++	—	++++
Cefepime (Maxipime)	4	++	++++	++++	—	++++

*Does not include coagulase-negative or methicillin-resistant staphylococci, or enterococci.
Relative antibacterial activity is indicated by number of plus signs.
Adapted from information in References 20 and 21.

invasive candidiasis (19), and for empiric therapy of neutropenic patients with persistent fever (16). For treating invasive candidiasis, the intravenous dose is 70 mg initially, then 50 mg daily thereafter. Although capsofungin is being promoted as an improvement in antifungal therapy (16), the clinical studies so far reveal only that the drug is equivalent in efficacy to the other antifungal agents.

Cephalosporins

After the first cephalosporin (cephalothin) was introduced in 1964, a small army of other cephalosporins followed, and there are now 20 different cephalosporins available for clinical use (20). These agents are divided into *generations,* and some of the parenteral agents in each generation are shown in Table 44.2 (21,22).

The Family of Cephalosporins

The **first-generation** cephalosporins are primarily active against aerobic gram-positive cocci, but are not active against *Staphylococcus epidermidis* or methicillin-resistant strains of *S. aureus.* The popular intravenous agent in this group is cefazolin (Ancef).

The **second-generation** cephalosporins exhibit stronger antibacterial activity against gram-negative aerobic and anaerobic bacilli of enteric origin. The popular parenteral agents in this group are cefoxitin (Mefoxin) and cefamandole (Mandol).

The **third-generation** cephalosporins have greater antibacterial activity against gram-negative aerobic bacilli, including *P. aeruginosa* and *Haemophilus influenzae,* but are less active against aerobic gram-positive

TABLE 44.3 Parenteral Dosing of Cephalosporins

Agent	Dose for Serious Infections	Dose in Renal Failure*
Cefazolin	1 g every 6 h	1 g every 24 h
Ceftriaxone	2 g every 12 h	2 g every 12 h
Ceftazidime	2 g every 8 h	2 g every 48 h
Cefepime	2 g every 8 h	2 g every 24 h

*From Reference 24.

cocci than the first-generation agents. The popular parenteral agents in this group are ceftriaxone (Rocephin), and ceftazidime (Fortaz). Ceftriaxone is popular for the treatment of severe community-acquired pneumonia, and is active against penicillin-resistant pneumococci and *H. influenzae*. Ceftazidime is a popular antipseudomonal antibiotic, particularly because it is devoid of serious adverse effects.

The **fourth-generation** cephalosporins retain activity against gram-negative organisms, but add some gram-positive coverage. The only drug in this generation is cefepime (Maxipime), which has the gram-negative antibacterial spectrum of ceftazidime (i.e., it covers *P. aeruginosa*), but is also active against gram-positive cocci (e.g., streptococci and methicillin-sensitive staphylococci).

Dosing

The doses for the more popular parenteral cephalosporins are shown in Table 44.3, along with dose adjustments for renal failure. Note that the dose in renal failure is adjusted by extending the dosing interval rather than decreasing the amount of drug given with each dose (22). This is done to preserve concentration-dependent bacterial killing. Note also that ceftriaxone requires no dose adjustment in renal failure.

Toxicity

Adverse reactions to cephalosporins are uncommon and nonspecific (e.g., nausea, rash, and diarrhea). There is a 5 to 15% incidence of cross-antigenicity with penicillin (21), which is why cephalosporins should be avoided in patients with a prior anaphylactic reaction to penicillin.

Comment

The popularity of cephalosporins is definitely on the decline (in fact, no new cephalosporin has appeared since 1996, the year cefepime was introduced). The early generation cephalosporins were once unmatched in popularity for gram-positive coverage, but have taken a back seat to vancomycin because of the emergence of methicillin-resistant *S. aureus*. The later generation cephalosporins such as ceftazidime and cefepime are also on the decline because of emerging resistance (see Fig. 44.2).

The only cephalosporin that seems to be holding ground is ceftriaxone, which is a popular agent for severe community-acquired pneumonia.

THE FLUOROQUINOLONES

The fluoroquinolone era began in 1987 with the introduction of ciprofloxacin. This was followed in the mid-1990s by the appearance of the "newer" fluoroquinolones, beginning with levofloxacin (introduced in 1996). These two generations of quinolones differ somewhat in pharmacokinetic properties and spectrum of activity.

Activity and Clinical Use

The early fluoroquinolones (e.g., ciprofloxacin) were active against (methicillin-sensitive) staphylococci and most of the aerobic gram-negative bacilli, including *Pseudomonas aeruginosa* and were less active against streptococci. Rapidly emerging resistance to these antibiotics (caused in part by the excessive use of ciprofloxacin after it was introduced) has reduced their value in treating serious gram-negative infections, particularly those due to *P. aeruginosa* (see Fig. 44.2).

The newer fluoroquinolones (e.g., levofloxacin, gatifloxacin, moxifloxacin) retain the antibacterial spectrum of the early agents (except for reduced activity against *P. aeruginosa*), but provide added coverage for streptococci, pneumococci (including penicillin-resistant strains) and "atypical" organisms like *Mycoplasma pneumoniae* and *Haemophilus influenzae.* The newer fluoroquinolones are used primarily for community-acquired pneumonia, exacerbations of chronic obstructive lung disease, and urinary tract infections. The inability to cover methicillin-resistant staphylococci, and the limited activity against *P. aeruginosa,* limits their value in the ICU.

Dosing

Table 44.4 shows the recommended intravenous doses for four quinolone antibiotics. The newer quinolones have longer half-lives than ciprofloxacin, and require only one dose daily. Dose adjustments are required for all the agents except moxifloxacin, which is metabolized in the liver (23).

TABLE 44.4 Parenteral Dosing of Fluoroquinolones

Agent	Dose for Serious Infections	Dose in Renal Failure*
Ciprofloxacin	400 mg every 8h	400 mg every 18 h
Levofloxacin	500 mg every 24 h	250 mg every 48 h
Gatifloxacin	400 mg every 24 h	200 mg every 24 h
Moxifloxacin	400 mg every 24 h	400 mg every 24 h

*From References 6,22.

DRUG INTERACTIONS

Ciprofloxacin interferes with the hepatic metabolism of theophylline and warfarin and can potentiate the actions of both of these drugs (24,25). Ciprofloxacin causes a 25% increase in serum theophylline levels, and combined therapy has resulted in symptomatic theophylline toxicity (26). Although no dose adjustments are necessary, serum theophylline levels and prothrombin times should be monitored carefully when ciprofloxacin is given in combination with these two agents.

Toxicity

The fluoroquinolones are relatively safe. Neurotoxic reactions (confusion, hallucinations, seizures) can develop days after starting quinolone therapy in 1% to 2% of patients (27). Prolongation of the QT interval and polymorphic ventricular tachycardia (torsades de pointes) have been reported in patients receiving all quinolones except moxifloxacin, but only 25 cases were on record as of 2001 (28).

Comment

The emerging resistance of gram-negative pathogens to ciprofloxacin has diminished the value of fluoroquinolones in the ICU. Ciprofloxacin can no longer be viewed as a first-line drug for *Pseudomonas* infections, and there are better antibiotics available to treat other gram-negative infections (e.g., imipenem or meropenem). The newer agents are popular for community-acquired pneumonia, but are not favored drugs for ventilator-associated pneumonia unless the pneumonia is early-onset (within 5 days of admission) and the patient is in the low risk category for colonization with gram-negative pathogens (see Table 41.5).

IMIPENEM

Imipenem is a member of the carbepenem class of antibiotics (the other drug in the class is meropenem, which is mentioned briefly later), and is distinguished by having **the broadest spectrum of antibacterial activity of any antibiotic currently available** (29).

Activity and Clinical Uses

In short, imipenem is active against all common bacterial pathogens except methicillin-resistant staphylococci. As demonstrated in Figure 44.1 imipenem is one of the most active agents for aerobic gram-negative bacilli, and it is also active against *Pseudomonas aeruginosa* (although less so, as in Fig. 44.2). It provides good coverage for the pneumococcus, methicillin-sensitive staphylococci, and coagulase-negative staphylococci (the latter being a common cause of catheter-related infections). It also proves excellent coverage for anaerobes, and is active against *Bacteroides fragilis* and *Enterococcus faecalis*. Some minor strains of pseudomonads (e.g., *P. cepaciae*) are poorly covered by imipenem, but they are uncommon offenders. There is some acquired resistance by *P. aeruginosa*, but the clinical significance of this is unclear.

Imipenem can be used for virtually any infection that does not involve methicillin-resistant *Staph. aureus*. It is well-suited for mixed aerobic/anaerobic infections such as pelvic and intraabdominal infections. It is also been very effective when used as monotherapy for neutropenic patients with fever (see Table 43.4) (30).

Dosing

Imipenem is inactivated by enzymes on the luminal surface of the proximal renal tubules, so it is impossible to achieve high levels of the drug in urine. To overcome this problem, the commercial preparation of imipenem contains an enzyme inhibitor, cilastatin. The combination imipenem–cilastatin preparation is available as Primaxin. The dose recommendations for imipenem–cilastatin represent the dose of imipenem. The usual intravenous dose in adults is **500 mg every 6 hours.** In suspected *Pseudomonas* infections, the dose is doubled to 1 g every 6 hours. In renal failure, the dose should be reduced by 50 to 75% (22).

Adverse Effects

The major adverse effect associated with imipenem is **generalized seizures,** which occur in 1 to 3% of patients receiving the drug (29). Most patients have a history of a seizure disorder, an intracranial mass, or renal failure. Although this is an uncommon occurrence, a maximum daily dose of 2 g or 25 mg/kg has been recommended (29).

Meropenem

Meropenem is similar to imipenem in its spectrum of antibacterial activity, but does not produce seizures (31). The normal intravenous dose is 1 gram every 8 hours and, in the presence of renal failure, a dose reduction of about 50% is required. Meropenem may, in fact, be slightly superior to imipenem because there is no risk of seizures, but the clinical experience with this drug is limited in comparison to imipenem.

Comment

The ideal antibiotic would be effective against all pathogens and produce no adverse reactions. Imipenem comes closer to this ideal than any antibiotic currently available, with the possible exception of meropenem. This has been my personal favorite for several years because it covers almost everything! The seizure risk is overstated, and is only a concern if you don't adjust the dose in renal failure, or the patient has another reason to have seizures. There is some emerging resistance to imipenem in strains of *P. aeruginosa*, but the significance of this is unclear.

THE PENICILLINS

The penicillin discovered by Alexander Fleming in 1929 is benzylpenicillin, or penicillin G. This substance is active against aerobic streptococci (*S. pneumoniae, S. pyogenes*) and anaerobic mouth flora. The emergence of penicillin-resistant pneumococci in recent years has virtually eliminated penicillin G from the ICU.

Extended-Spectrum Penicillins

The penicillins in this category have an extended antibacterial spectrum that covers aerobic gram-negative bacilli. This category includes the aminopenicillins (ampicillin and amoxicillin), the carboxypenicillins (carbenicillin and ticarcillin), and the ureidopenicillins (azlocillin, mezlocillin, and pipericillin). All groups are active against gram-negative pathogens, but the latter two groups are active against *P. aeruginosa* (32). These agents are also known as *antipseudomonal penicillins*. The most popular drug in this class is pipericillin, which is available in a special combination product (see next).

Pipericillin-Tazobactam

Pipericillin is most often given in combination with tazobactam, a β-lactamase inhibitor that has synergistic activity when combined with pipericillin. The commercial product (Zosyn) contains pipericillin in an 8:1 ratio with tazobactam. The recommended dose of the combination product is 3.375 grams (3 grams pipericillin and 375 mg tazobactam) IV every 4 to 6 hours. In the presence of renal insufficiency, the dose should be changed to 2.25 grams every 8 hours (33).

Pipericillin-tazobactam can be used for empiric therapy of urinary tract infections and intraabdominal sepsis, and it is one of the antibiotics recommended for empiric therapy of neutropenic patients with fever. However, the performance of this preparation in the susceptibility rates in Figures 44.1 and 44.2 indicate that there are better alternatives for the treatment of gram-negative infections in the ICU.

VANCOMYCIN

Vancomycin is one of the staples of antimicrobial therapy in the ICU, but concerns about the emergence of vancomycin-resistant enterococci (VRE) have prompted a general mandate to curtail its use.

Antibacterial Spectrum

Vancomycin is active against all gram-positive cocci, including all strains of *Staphylococcus aureus* (coagulase-positive, coagulase-negative, methicillin-sensitive, methicillin-resistant) as well as aerobic and anaerobic streptococci (including pneumococcus and enterococcus) (34). It is the drug of choice for penicillin-resistant pneumococci, and is one of the most active agents against *Clostridium difficile*, the pathogen responsible for antibiotic-associated pseudomembranous colitis. Enterococcal resistance to vancomycin occurs in 1 to 15% of nosocomial isolates (34), and the prevalence in different hospitals varies widely.

Clinical Use

Vancomycin is the drug of choice for infections caused by methicillin-resistant *Staphylococcus aureus* (MRSA) and *Staphylococcus epidermidis*. However, as much as 2/3 of the vancomycin used in ICUs is not directed at a specific pathogen, but is used for empiric antibiotic coverage in patients with suspected infections (35). The popularity of vancomycin in empiric antibiotic regimens is a reflection of the prominent role played by MRSA and *S. epidermidis* in ICU-related infections.

Dosing

The usual intravenous dose of vancomycin is **1 gram every 12 hours** (34). Each dose must be infused slowly (no faster than 10 mg/min) to prevent infusion reactions (see below). Intermittent dosing is traditional, but continuous infusion also achieves bactericidal drug levels in blood (34). Dose reduction is necessary in renal insufficiency, and is accomplished by increasing the dosing interval. One dose of vancomycin every 4 days is sufficient for hemodialysis patients, and a supplemental dose after dialysis is not required (22).

Serum drug levels are often monitored to limit toxicity and maintain efficacy. Peak levels should be below 40 mg/L to reduce the risk of ototoxicity (for intermittent dosing only), and trough levels should be above 5 mg/L to maintain antibacterial activity (36).

Toxicity

Rapid administration of vancomycin can be accompanied by vasodilation, flushing, and hypotension (*red man syndrome*) as a result of histamine release from mast cells (34). The trigger for this release is unknown, but slowing the infusion rate (to less than 10 mg/minute) usually corrects the problem.

Ototoxicity

Vancomycin can cause reversible hearing loss for high-frequency sounds when serum drug levels exceed 40 mg/L (36). Permanent deafness has been reported when serum levels exceed 80 mg/L (35). Both complications are uncommon, possibly because drug levels are monitored routinely.

Nephrotoxicity

Renal insufficiency of unclear etiology is reported in 5% of patients receiving vancomycin (36). There is no apparent relationship to the dose of vancomycin, but the incidence is higher when aminoglycosides are given concurrently. Renal function usually returns to normal after stopping vancomycin.

Comment

Vancomycin continues to be a solid performer in the ICU. Curtailing its use will be difficult until another antibiotic appears that has the same antibacterial profile as vancomycin. That drug is already here, as described next.

Linezolid

Linezolid (Zyvox) is a synthetic antibiotic that was introduced in 2000 to treat infections caused by resistant gram-positive organisms (37): i.e., MRSA, VRE, and penicillin-resistant pneumococci. Although intended only for cases where vancomycin was ineffective or not tolerated, linezolid is now being considered as a possible replacement for vancomycin. It has the same spectrum of activity, and has proven effective in treating MRSA infections. In fact, one study comparing vancomycin and linezolid for the treatment of MRSA pneumonia showed better results with linezolid (38). Linezolid may be better suited for treating pneumonia because it penetrates into respiratory secretions, while vancomycin does not (34). The recommended intravenous dose of linezolid for serious infections is 600 mg twice daily.

Linezolid is relatively safe when given in short courses. However, prolonged (more than one month) treatment can be associated with thrombocytopenia, peripheral neuropathy, and optic neuropathy (37,39). The optic neuropathy resolves partially, but the peripheral neuropathy is irreversible.

A FINAL WORD

The first rule of antibiotics is try not to use them, and the second rule is try not to use too many of them. If antibiotics are needed pending culture results, the combination of **vancomycin and imipenem** will suffice in most situations. Imipenem covers all of the common bacterial pathogens in the ICU except methicillin-resistant *Staph aureus* (MRSA), hence the vancomycin. If you don't have a problem with MRSA in your ICU, then imipenem alone will suffice. You can then adjust antibiotics according to the culture results. If the cultures are negative and the patient has not improved on antimicrobial therapy, you should stop the antibiotics and rethink your strategy. Remember (from Chapter 40) that fever and leukocytosis are signs of inflammation, not infection, and that about 50% of ICU patients with signs of inflammation will *not* have a documented infection.

REFERENCES

Aminoglycosides

1. Turnidge J. Pharmacodynamics and dosing of aminoglycosides. Infect Dis Clin N Am 2003;17:503–528.
2. Neuhauser MM, Weinstein RA, Rydman R, et al. Antibiotic resistance among gram-negative bacilli in U.S. intensive care units. JAMA 2003;289:885–888.
3. Wilson SE. Aminoglycosides: Assessing the potential for nephrotoxicity. Surg Gynecol Obstet 1986;171(suppl):24–30.
4. Lippmann M, Yang E, Au E, Lee C. Neuromuscular blocking effects of tobramycin, gentamicin, and cefazolin. Anesth Analg 1982;61:767–770.
5. Drachman DB. Myasthenia gravis. N Engl J Med 1994;330:179–180.

Antifungal Agents

6. Groll AH, Gea-Banacloche JC, Glasmacher A, et al. Clinical pharmacology of antifungal compounds. Infect Dis Clin N Am 2003;17:159–191.
7. Bult J, Franklin CM. Using amphotericin B in the critically ill: A new look at an old drug. J Crit Illn 1996;11:577–585.
8. Carlson MA, Condon RE. Nephrotoxicity of amphotericin B. J Am Coll Surg 1994;179:361–381.
9. Walsh TJ, Finberg RW, Arndt C, et al. Liposomal amphotericin B for empirical therapy in patients with persistent fever and neutropenia. N Engl J Med 1999; 340:764–771.
10. Wingard JR, Kublis P, Lee L, et al. Clinical significance of nephrotoxicity in patients treated with amphotericin B for suspected or proven aspergillosis. Clin Infect Dis 1999;29:1402–1407.
11. Hoesly CJ, Dismukes WE. New antifungal agents: Emphasis on lipid formulations of amphotericin B: National Foundation for Infectious Disease, clinical updates: Available at www.nfid.org/publications/clinicalupdates/fungal/ampho.html (Accessed on 5/2006).
12. Red Book, 2005. Montvale, NJ: Thompson PDR, 2005.
13. Rex JH, Bennett JE, Sugar AM, et al. A randomized trial comparing fluconazole with amphotericin B for the treatment of candidemia in patients without neutropenia. N Engl J Med 1994;331:1325–1330.
14. Ostrosky-Zeichner L, Pappas PG. Invasive candidiasis in the intensive care unit. Crit Care Med 2006;34:857–863.
15. Pappas PG, Rex JH, Sobel JD, et al. Guidelines for treatment of candidiasis. Clin Infect Dis 2004;38:161–189.
16. Perfect JR. Management of invasive mycoses in hematology patients: Current approaches. J Crit Illn 2004;19:3–12.
17. Walsh TJ, Pappas P, Winston D, et al. Voriconazole compared with liposomal amphotericin B for empirical antifungal therapy in patients with neutropenia and persistent fever. N Engl J Med 2002;346:225–234.
18. Gearhart MO. Worsening of liver function with fluconazole and a review of azole antifungal hepatotoxicity. Ann Pharmacother 1994;28:1177–1181.
19. Mora-Duarte J, Betts R, Rotstein C, et al. Comparison of capsofungin and amphotericin B for invasive candidiasis. N Engl J Med 2002;347:2020–2029.

Cephalosporins

20. Asbel LE, Levison ME. Cephalosporins, carbapenems, and monobactams. Infect Dis Clin North Am 2000;14:1–10.
21. Gustafferro CA, Steckelberg JM. Cephalosporin antimicrobial agents and related compounds. Mayo Clin Proc 1991;66:1064–1073.
22. Bennett WM, Aronoff GR, Golper TA, et al., eds. Drug prescribing in renal failure. 3rd ed. Philadelphia: American College of Physicians, 1994.

Fluoroquinolones

23. O'Donnell JA, Gelone SP. Fluoroquinolones. Infect Dis Clin North Am 2000;14: 489–513.
24. Walker RC, Wright AJ. The fluoroquinolones. Mayo Clin Proc 1991;66:1249–1259.
25. Robson RA. The effects of quinolones on xanthine pharmacokinetics. Am J Med 1992;92(suppl 4A):22S–26S.
26. Maddix DS. Do we need an intravenous fluoroquinolone? West J Med 1992; 157:55–59.
27. Finch C, Self T. Quinolones: recognizing the potential for neurotoxicity. J Crit Illn 2000;15:656–657.
28. Frothingham R. Rates of torsades de pointes associated with ciprofloxacin, ofloxacin, levofloxacin, gatifloxacin, and moxifloxacin. Pharmacotherapy 2001;21:1468–1472.

Imipenem

29. Hellinger WC, Brewer NS. Imipenem. Mayo Clin Proc 1991;66:1074–1081.
30. Freifield A, Walsh T, Marshall D, et al. Monotherapy for fever and neutropenia in cancer patients: A randomized comparison of ceftazidime versus imipenem. J Clin Oncol 1995;13:165–176.
31. Cunha B. Meropenem for clinicians. Antibiot Clin 2000;4:59–66.

Penicillins

32. Wright AJ. The penicillins. Mayo Clin Proc 1999;74:290–307.
33. McEvoy GK, ed. AHFS drug information, 2001. Bethesda, MD: American Society of Hospital Pharmacists, 2001:419–422.

Vancomycin

34. Lundstrom TS, Sobel R. Antibiotics for gram-positive bacterial infections: Vancomycin, quinapristin-dalfopristin, linezolid, and daptomycin. Infect Dis Clin North Am 2004;18:651–668.
35. Ena J, Dick RW, Jones RN. The epidemiology of intravenous vancomycin usage in a university hospital. JAMA 1993;269:598–605.
36. Saunders NJ. Why monitor peak vancomycin concentrations? Lancet 194; 344:1748–1750.

Linezolid

37. Birmingham MC, Rayner CR, Meagher AK, et al. Linezolid for the treatment of multidrug-resistant gram-positive infections: experience from a compassionate use program. Clin Infect Dis 2003;36:159–164.
38. Wunderink RG, Rello J, Norden C, et al. Linezolid vs. vancomycin: analysis of two double-blind studies of patients with methicillin-resistant *Staphylococcus aureus* pneumonia. Chest 2003;124:1789–1795.
39. Rucker JC, Hamilton SR, Bardenstein D, et al. Linezolid-associated toxic optic neuropathy. Neurology 2006;66:595–598.

Section XIV

NUTRITION AND METABOLISM

The more impure bodies are fed, the more diseased they will become.

HIPPOCRATES

Chapter 45

METABOLIC SUBSTRATE REQUIREMENTS

What is food to one man may be fierce poison to others.

Lucretius

The fundamental goal of nutritional support is to provide individual patients with their daily nutritional requirements. This chapter explains how to determine the nutrient and energy needs of each patient in the ICU (1–6).

OXIDATIVE ENERGY CONVERSION

Oxidative Combustion

According to the Laws of Thermodynamics, energy can neither be produced nor destroyed. Therefore, the only way to obtain energy is to transfer it from an energy source in nature. Natural substances that are rich in stored energy are called *fuels,* and the device that performs the energy transfer is called an *engine.* The process of energy transfer by two types of engines is illustrated in Figure 45.1. The automobile has a mechanical engine that mixes oxygen with a fossil fuel (e.g., gasoline) at high temperatures, and this releases the energy from the fuel that is then used to power the automobile. Likewise, the human body has a biochemical engine (metabolism) that mixes oxygen with an organic fuel (e.g., carbohydrates) at high temperatures, and this releases energy from the fuel that is then used to power the human body. The process that allows the energy to be released from a fuel is called oxidation, or the chemical reaction between oxygen and a fuel. If the oxidation reaction is

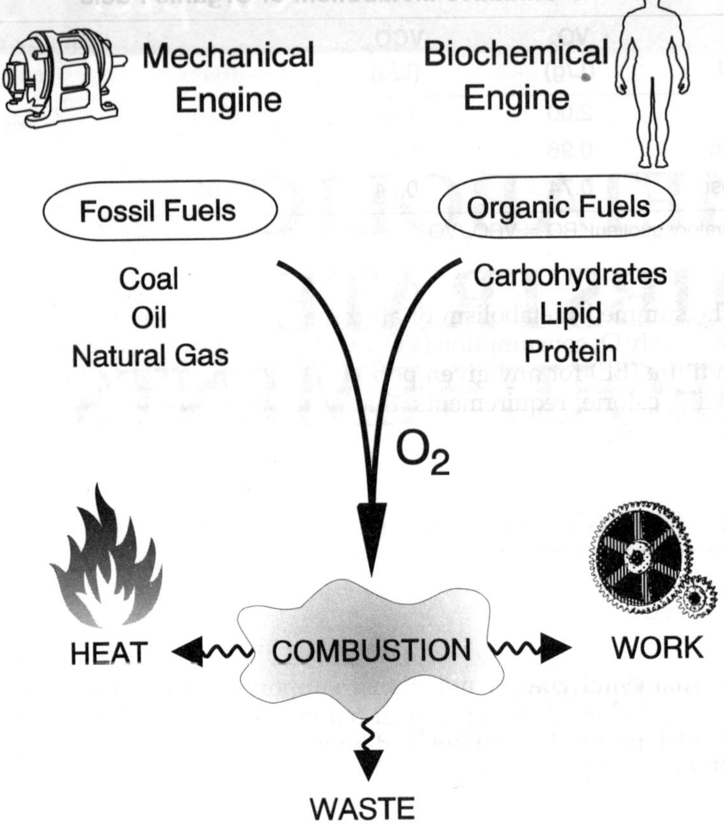

FIGURE 45.1 Energy conversion by two internal combustion engines. One engine is mechanical, and the other is biochemical.

conducted at high temperatures, the energy release from the fuel is more rapid. Such high-temperature oxidation reactions are called *combustion* reactions. Thus, both the automobile engine and oxidative metabolism are internal combustion engines that capture the energy stored in natural fuels.

Organic Fuels

The three organic (carbon-based) fuels used by the human body are carbohydrates, proteins, and lipids. The energy yield from the combustion of these fuels is measured as heat production in kilocalories (kcal) per gram of substrate. The energy yield from the combustion of each of the organic fuels is shown in Table 45.1. The information in this table can be stated as follows:

$$1 \text{ g Glucose} + 0.74 \text{ L of } O_2 \text{ yields } 0.74 \text{ L of } CO_2 + 3.75 \text{ kcal} \quad (45.1)$$

TABLE 45.1 The Oxidative Metabolism of Organic Fuels

Fuel	VO_2 (L/g)	VCO_2 (L/g)	RQ*	Energy Yield (kcal/g)
Lipid	2.00	1.40	0.70	9.1
Protein	0.96	0.78	0.80	4.0
Glucose	0.74	0.74	1.00	3.7

*Respiratory quotient: RQ = VCO_2/VO_2.

The summed metabolism of all three organic substrates determines the total-body O_2 consumption (VO_2), CO_2 production (VCO_2), and energy expenditure (EE) for any given period. The 24-hour EE then determines the daily calorie requirements that must be provided by nutrition support.

DAILY ENERGY EXPENDITURE

The daily energy expenditure of each individual patient can be estimated or measured.

Predictive Equations

In the early part of the twentieth century, the daily energy expenditure of a group of healthy adults (136 men and 103 women) was measured (7). The results of this study were expressed as regression equations for daily energy expenditure based on sex, body weight (in kilograms), and height (in inches). These equations are known as the Harris–Benedict equations (named after the principal investigators in the study), and they are shown in Table 45.2. The daily energy expenditure is expressed as the basal energy expenditure (BEE), which is the heat production of basal metabolism in the resting and fasted state. Because the body weight in the Harris–Benedict equations does not allow for changes in body weight caused by obesity or edema fluid, the ideal body weight should be used in these predictive equations.

Another more simplified predictive equation for the BEE is as follows:

$$\text{BEE (kcal/day)} = 25 \times \text{wt (in kg)} \tag{45.2}$$

This relationship has proven to be equivalent to the more complicated Harris–Benedict equations (8). Although it has not been tested rigorously, this simple relationship provides a "ballpark" estimate of BEE for determining nutritional needs.

Adjustments in BEE

To allow for the thermal effect of food intake, the BEE is multiplied by 1.2 to derive the resting energy expenditure (REE), which is the energy

TABLE 45.2 Methods for Determining Daily Energy Expenditure

Basal Energy Expenditure (BEE):

Men:

$$BEE\ (kcal/24hr) = 66 + (13.7 \times wt) + (5.0 \times ht) - (6.7 \times age)$$

Women:

$$BEE\ (kcal/24hr) = 655 + (9.6 \times wt) + (1.8 \times ht) - (4.7 \times age)$$

(wt = weight in kilograms, ht = height in inches)

Resting Energy Expenditure (REE):

*REE (kcal/24hr) = $[(3.9 \times VO_2) + (1.1 \times VCO_2) - 61] \times 1440$

†REE (kcal/24hr) = BEE $\times$ 1.2

*From Bursztein S, Saphar P, Singer P, et al. A mathematical analysis of indirect calorimetry measurements in acutely ill patients. Am J Clin Nutr 1989;50:227–230. The VO_2 and VCO_2 are measured in mL/min, and the multiplier 1440 is used to convert the time period to 24 hr.

†REE is equivalent to the BEE plus the thermal effect of food.

expenditure of basal metabolism in the resting but not fasted state. Other adjustments in the BEE that allow for enhanced energy expenditure in hypermetabolic conditions are shown below:

Fever: BEE × 1.1 (for each °C above the normal body temperature)
Mild stress: BEE × 1.2
Moderate stress: BEE × 1.4
Severe stress: BEE × 1.6

The actual adjustments for severe illness can vary widely in individual patients (9). Studies comparing predicted and actual energy expenditure in critically ill patients have shown that the predictive equations (with adjustments for degree of stress) overestimate daily energy needs by 20 to 60% (9–12). For this reason, measurements of energy expenditure are more accurate than predictive equations in patients in the ICU.

Indirect Calorimetry

Because it is impossible to measure metabolic heat production in clinical practice, the metabolic energy expenditure is measured indirectly by measuring the whole-body VO_2 and VCO_2. This technique is called indirect calorimetry (2,3). The REE can be derived from the whole-body VO_2 and VCO_2 by using the equation shown in Table 45.2 (13). The original REE equation, which incorporated a measurement of the daily urinary nitrogen excretion, was proposed by the Scottish physiologist J. B. de V. Weir in 1949 (14). A number of adaptations of the original Weir equation have been proposed (15,16), but the REE equations used in the clinical setting do not include the urinary nitrogen excretion.

Method

Indirect calorimetry is performed with specialized instruments called metabolic carts that measure the exchange of O_2 and CO_2 across the lungs. These instruments can be placed at the bedside, and gas exchange measurements are obtained over 15 to 30 minutes. The VO_2 and VCO_2 are then extrapolated to a 24-hour period, and the 24-hour REE is calculated by using an equation similar to the one shown in Table 45.2.

Total Energy Expenditure

The REE obtained from indirect calorimetry is usually measured for 15 to 30 minutes, and then extrapolated to a 24-hour period. The total energy expenditure (TEE), measured over 24 hours, is equivalent to the extrapolated REE in patients who are not hypermetabolic (17), but the TEE can be as much as 40% higher than the extrapolated REE in hypermetabolic septic patients (17). Therefore, the REE measured over limited periods is not necessarily equivalent to the total daily energy expenditure in hypermetabolic patients in the ICU.

Limitations

Indirect calorimetry is the most accurate method for determining the daily energy requirements of individual patients in the ICU. However, several factors limit the popularity of indirect calorimetry in the clinical setting. First and foremost, the technique requires relatively expensive equipment and specially trained personnel, and it is not universally available. In addition, the oxygen sensor in most metabolic carts is not reliable at inspired oxygen levels above 50%, so indirect calorimetry can be unreliable in patients with respiratory failure who require inhaled oxygen concentrations above 50% (2). Because of all these limitations, daily caloric needs are often estimated using predictive formulas such as the Harris–Benedict equations, whereas indirect calorimetry (if available) is reserved for selected patients who require careful titration of daily energy intake (e.g., ventilator-dependent patients).

NONPROTEIN CALORIES

The daily energy requirement should be provided by calories derived from carbohydrates and lipids, and protein intake should be used to maintain the stores of essential enzymatic and structural proteins. The proportion of daily calories that is provided by lipids and carbohydrates is a matter of some debate, but no clear evidence shows one substrate to be superior to the other as a source of calories (2,3).

Carbohydrates

Carbohydrates supply approximately 70% of the nonprotein calories in the average American diet. Because the human body has limited

TABLE 45.3 Endogenous Fuel Stores in Healthy Adults

Fuel Source	Amount (kg)	Energy Yield (kcal)
Adipose tissue fat	15.0	141,000
Muscle protein	6.0	24,000
Total glycogen	0.09	900
		Total:165,900

Data from Cahill GF Jr. N Engl J Med 1970;282:668–675.

carbohydrate stores (Table 45.3), daily intake of carbohydrates is necessary to ensure proper functioning of the central nervous system, which relies heavily on glucose as its principal fuel source. However, excessive intake of carbohydrates can prove detrimental for the following reasons.

1. Carbohydrates stimulate the release of insulin, and insulin inhibits the mobilization of free fatty acids from adipose tissue. Because adipose tissue fat is the major source of endogenous calories (Table 45.3), excessive carbohydrate intake impairs the ability of the body to rely on endogenous fat stores during periods of inadequate nutrition.
2. The oxidative metabolism of glucose produces an abundance of CO_2 relative to the oxygen consumed, as indicated by the respiratory quotients listed in Table 45.1. Furthermore, ingestion of excessive carbohydrates leads to de novo lipogenesis, which has a respiratory quotient of 8.0. Therefore, the ingestion of excessive carbohydrates can be accompanied by an exaggerated production of CO_2 (18), and this could promote hypercapnia in patients with compromised lung function. In fact, excessive calories from any nutrient source can be accompanied by excessive CO_2 production (19).

Lipids

Dietary lipids have the highest energy yield of the three organic fuels (Table 45.1), and lipid stores in adipose tissues represent the major endogenous fuel source in healthy adults (Table 45.3). Most nutritional regimens use exogenous lipids to provide approximately 30% of the daily energy needs.

Linoleic Acid

Dietary lipids are triglycerides, which are composed of a glycerol molecule linked to three fatty acids. The only dietary fatty acid that is considered essential (i.e., must be provided in the diet) is linoleic acid, a long chain, polyunsaturated fatty acid with 18 carbon atoms (20). A deficient intake of this essential fatty acid produces a clinical disorder characterized by a scaly dermopathy, cardiac dysfunction, and increased susceptibility to infections (20). This disorder is prevented by providing 0.5% of the dietary fatty acids as linoleic acid. Safflower oil is used as the source of linoleic acid in most nutritional support regimens.

Protein Requirements

The goal of protein intake is to match the rate of protein catabolism in the individual patient. Protein intake can be estimated by using the following generalized predictions for normal and hypercatabolic patients (21):

Condition	*Daily Protein Intake*
Normal metabolism	0.8 to 1.0 g/kg
Hypercatabolism	1.2 to 1.6 g/kg

The estimated protein intake in hypercatabolic patients is limited by the inability to determine the severity of protein catabolism. A more accurate assessment of daily protein requirements requires some measure of protein catabolism. This measure is the urinary excretion of nitrogen, as described below.

Nitrogen Balance

Two-thirds of the nitrogen derived from protein breakdown is excreted in the urine (21). Because protein is 16% nitrogen, each gram of urinary nitrogen (UN) represents 6.25 g of degraded protein. The total-body nitrogen (N) balance can therefore be determined as follows (22):

$$\text{N Balance (g)} = (\text{Protein intake (g)}/6.25) - (\text{UUN} + 4) \quad (45.3)$$

where UUN is the urinary urea nitrogen excretion (in grams) in 24 hours, and the factor 4 represents the daily nitrogen loss (in grams) other than UUN. If the UUN is greater than 30 (g/24 hours), a factor of 6 is more appropriate for the daily nitrogen losses other than UUN (23). The goal of the nitrogen balance is to maintain a positive balance of 4 to 6 grams.

Total versus Urea Nitrogen

Under normal circumstances, approximately 85% of the nitrogen in the urine is contained in urea and the remainder is contained in ammonia and creatinine. However, in certain groups of patients in the ICU (e.g., postoperative patients), urea may contain less than 50% of the total nitrogen in the urine (24). Therefore, the UUN can underestimate urinary nitrogen losses in patients in the ICU. Measuring the urinary ammonia excretion in addition to the UUN will provide a more accurate assessment of the TUN (total urinary nitrogen) in these patients (25). However, the clinical significance of this added measurement is unknown at present.

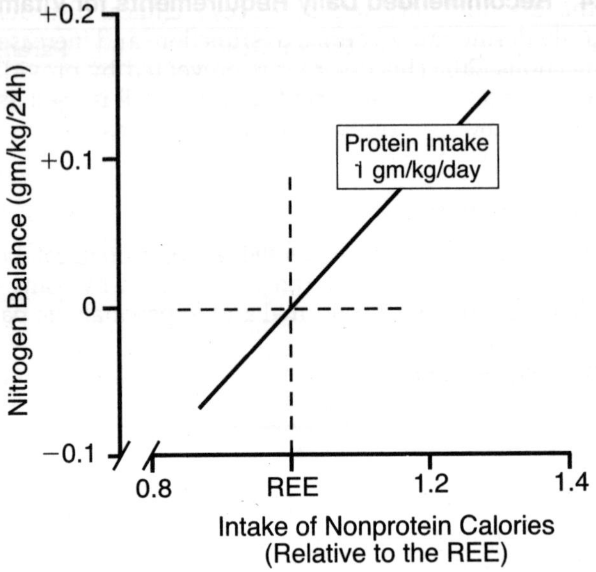

FIGURE 45.2 Graph showing that, when protein intake is constant, the nitrogen balance is directly related to the daily intake of *nonprotein* calories relative to the resting energy expenditure (REE).

Nitrogen Balance and Caloric Intake

The first step in achieving a positive nitrogen balance is to **provide enough nonprotein calories to spare proteins from being degraded to provide energy.** This is demonstrated in Figure 45.2, which shows the relationship between the intake of nonprotein calories and the nitrogen balance. When the daily protein intake is constant, the nitrogen balance becomes positive only when the intake of nonprotein calories is sufficient to meet the daily energy needs (i.e., the REE). If the nonprotein calorie intake is insufficient, some of the protein provided in the diet will be broken down to provide calories, which will produce a negative nitrogen balance. Therefore, when the daily intake of nonprotein calories is insufficient, increasing the protein intake becomes an inefficient method of achieving a positive nitrogen balance.

VITAMIN REQUIREMENTS

Twelve vitamins are considered an essential part of the daily diet. The recommended daily dose of individual vitamins in enteral and parenteral nutritional regimens is shown in Table 45.4 (2,3). It is important to emphasize that the daily vitamin requirements may be much higher than indicated in this table in seriously ill, hypermetabolic patients. In fact, deficiencies in several vitamins have been documented in hospitalized patients, despite the daily provision of vitamins in nutritional support

TABLE 45.4 Recommended Daily Requirements for Vitamins

Vitamin	Enteral Dose	Parenteral Dose
Vitamin A	1000 µg	3300 IU
Vitamin B_{12}	3 µg	5µg
Vitamin C	60 mg	100 mg
Vitamin D	5 µg	200 IU
Vitamin E	10 mg	10 IU
Vitamin K*	100 µg	10 mg
Thiamine (B_1)*	2 mg	3 mg
Riboflavin (B_2)*	2 mg	4 mg
Pyridoxine (B_6)*	2 mg	4 mg
Pantothenic acid*	6 mg	15 mg
Biotin*	150 µg	60 µg
Folate	400 µg	400 µg

Adapted from Dark DS, Pingleton SK. Nutritional support in critically ill patients. Intensive Care Med 1993;8:16–33. Doses for vitamins indicated by asterisks (*) are averaged or rounded off to the nearest whole number.

regimens (26,27). The normal vitamin levels in blood are included in the section on Reference Ranges in the Appendix at the end of this text.

Although it is impossible to comment on the importance of each of the vitamins in ICU patients, the following comments on thiamine and the antioxidant vitamins are deserved.

Thiamine

Thiamine (vitamin B_1) is a component of thiamine pyrophosphate, an essential cofactor in carbohydrate metabolism. Thiamine deficiency is likely to be common in patients in the ICU for the following reasons. First, the normal body content of thiamine is only approximately 30 mg (28), so assuming a daily thiamine requirement of 3 mg in patients in the ICU (Table 45.4), lack of thiamine intake could result in depletion of endogenous thiamine stores after just 10 days. Second, the use of thiamine is increased beyond expected levels in hypercatabolic conditions (29) and may also be increased in patients receiving nutritional support with glucose-rich formulas. Third, urinary thiamine excretion is increased by furosemide (30) which is a commonly used diuretic in the ICU. Finally, magnesium is necessary for the conversion of thiamine into thiamine pyrophosphate, so magnesium depletion (which is common in patients in the ICU) causes a "functional" form of thiamine deficiency (31).

Clinical Features

Four clinical disorders are associated with thiamine deficiency (28,32–34): (*a*) cardiac dysfunction (beriberi heart disease), (*b*) a metabolic (Wernicke's)

TABLE 45.5 Laboratory Evaluation of Thiamine Status

*Plasma Thiamine**

Thiamine Fraction	Normal Range
Total	3.4–4.8 μg/dL
Free	0.8–1.1 μg/dL
Phosphorylated	2.6–3.7 μg/dL

Erythrocyte Transketolase Activity†

Enzyme activity measured in response to thiamine pyrophosphate (TPP).

1. <20% increase in activity after TTP indicates normal thiamine levels.
2. >25% increase in activity after TTP indicates thiamine deficiency.

*From Reference 33.
†From Reference 35.

encephalopathy, (*c*) lactic acidosis (see Chapter 29), and (*d*) a peripheral neuropathy. Similar disorders, such as cardiac dysfunction and metabolic encephalopathy, are common in patients in the ICU, and thiamine deficiency should be considered in each case in which one of these disorders is unexplained.

Diagnosis

The laboratory evaluation of thiamine status is shown in Table 45.5. Although plasma levels of thiamine can be useful in detecting thiamine depletion, the most reliable assay of functional intracellular thiamine stores is the erythrocyte transketolase assay (35). This assay measures the activity of a thiamine pyrophosphate–dependent (transketolase) enzyme in the patient's red blood cells in response to the addition of thiamine pyrophosphate (TPP). An increase in enzyme activity of greater than 25% after the addition of TPP indicates a functional thiamine deficiency. I use the plasma thiamine levels to screen for thiamine depletion and reserve the transketolase assay for determining the end-point of thiamine repletion in patients with documented thiamine deficiency.

Antioxidant Vitamins

Two vitamins serve as important endogenous antioxidants: Vitamin C and Vitamin E. Vitamin E is the major lipid soluble antioxidant in the body, and Vitamin C is water-soluble and serves as one of the major antioxidants in the extracellular fluid. Considering that oxidant-induced cell injury may play an important role in multiorgan failure (see Chapter 40), it is wise to maintain adequate body stores of the antioxidant vitamins in critically ill patients. The increased rates of biological oxidation that are common in critical illness are likely to increase the daily requirements for Vitamin C and Vitamin E far above those listed in Table 45.4. Therefore, it is important to monitor Vitamin C and Vitamin E status carefully in seriously ill patients in the ICU (see the Appendix for the normal plasma levels of Vitamins C and E).

TABLE 45.6 Daily Requirements for Essential Trace Elements

Trace Element	Enteral Dose	Parenteral Dose
Chromium	200 μg	15 μg
Copper	3 mg	1.5 mg
Iodine	150 μg	150 μg
Iron	10 mg	2.5 mg
Manganese	5 mg	100 μg
Selenium	200 μg	70 μg
Zinc	15 mg	4 mg

Doses represent the maximum daily maintenance doses for each element. From Dark DS, Pingleton SK. Nutrition and nutritional support in critically ill patients. Intensive Care Med 1993;8:16–33.

ESSENTIAL TRACE ELEMENTS

A trace element is a substance that is present in the body in amounts less than 50 μg per gram of body tissue (36). Seven trace elements are considered essential in humans (i.e., associated with a deficiency syndrome), and these are listed in Table 45.6 along with their recommended daily maintenance doses (2). As with the vitamin requirements, the trace element requirements in Table 45.6 are for healthy adults; the requirements in hypermetabolic patients in the ICU may be far greater. The following trace elements are mentioned because of their relevance to oxidation-induced cell injury.

Iron

One of the interesting features of iron in the human body is how little is allowed to remain as free, unbound iron. The normal adult has approximately 4.5 g of iron, yet there is virtually no free iron in plasma (37). Most of the iron is bound to hemoglobin, and the remainder is bound to ferritin in tissues and transferrin in plasma. Furthermore, the transferrin in plasma is only approximately 30% saturated with iron, so any increase in plasma iron will be quickly bound by transferrin, thus preventing any rise in plasma free iron.

Iron and Oxidation Injury

One reason why the body may be so concerned with binding iron is the ability of free iron to promote oxidation-induced cell injury (37,38). Iron in the reduced state (Fe-II) promotes the formation of hydroxyl radicals (see Figure 21.5), and hydroxyl radicals are considered the most reactive oxidants known in biochemistry. In this context, the ability to bind and sequester iron has been called the major antioxidant function of blood (38). This might explain why hypoferremia is a common occurrence in patients who have conditions associated with hypermetabolism (39) (because this would limit the destructive effects of hypermetabolism).

In light of this description of iron, **a reduced serum iron level in a critically ill patient should not prompt iron replacement therapy** unless there is evidence of total-body iron deficiency. This latter condition can be detected with a plasma ferritin level; that is, a plasma ferritin below 18 µg/L indicates probable iron deficiency, whereas a plasma ferritin above 100 µg/L means that iron deficiency is unlikely (40).

Selenium

Selenium is an endogenous antioxidant by virtue of its role as a co-factor for glutathione peroxidase, one of the important endogenous antioxidant enzymes (see Chapter 21). Selenium use is increased in acute illness, and plasma selenium levels can fall to subnormal levels within 1 week after the onset of acute illness (41,42). Since selenium supplementation is not routinely included in parenteral nutrition support regimens, prolonged parenteral nutrition is accompanied by selenium deficiency (43,44). The combination of increased selenium use and lack of daily selenium supplementation may make selenium deficiency common in patients in the ICU. Such a condition will promote oxidant cell injury.

The acute selenium status is best monitored by measuring plasma selenium levels. The normal range is 89–113 mg/L (45,46). The minimum daily requirement for selenium is 55 µg (46,47). This requirement is likely to be much higher in hypermetabolic patients in the ICU. The maximum daily dose of selenium that is considered safe is 200 µg, and this dose is probably more appropriate for ICU patients. If needed, selenium can be given intravenously as sodium selenite (200 µg IV daily) (44).

A FINAL WORD (OR TWO)

Before leaving this chapter, it is important to point out that there is a fundamental problem with promoting nutrient intake in critically ill patients. The problem is the fate of administered nutrients in the presence of a serious illness.

Nutrients Won't Correct Malnutrition in the ICU

The goal of nutrient intake in the malnourished patient is to correct the malnourished state. However, the malnutrition that accompanies critical illness is different from the malnutrition that accompanies starvation. Whereas the malnutrition from starvation is due to deficient body stores of essential nutrients, **the malnutrition that accompanies serious illnesses is due to abnormal nutrient processing.** As such, the intake of nutrients will not correct the malnutrition that is associated with serious illnesses until the underlying disease is controlled and the metabolic abnormalities abate. Therefore, the important factor in correcting the malnutrition in critically ill patients is successful treatment of the primary disease process (48), and not the intake of nutrients (48). In fact, in the setting of abnormal nutrient processing, nutrient intake can be used to generate metabolic toxins. This is demonstrated below.

Nutrients as Toxins in the ICU

In healthy subjects, less than 5% of exogenously administered glucose is metabolized to form lactate. However, in acutely ill patients, up to 85% of an exogenous glucose load can be recovered as lactate (49). The graph in Figure 45.3 demonstrates the ability of exogenous glucose to generate lactic acid in acutely stressed patients undergoing major surgery (50). In this case, patients undergoing abdominal aneurysm surgery were given intraoperative fluid therapy with either Ringer's solutions or 5% dextrose solutions. In the patients who received the 5% dextrose solution (total amount of dextrose infused averaged 200 grams), the blood lactate increased by 3 mmol/L, whereas in the patients who received an equivalent volume of the glucose-free (Ringer's) solution, the blood lactate level

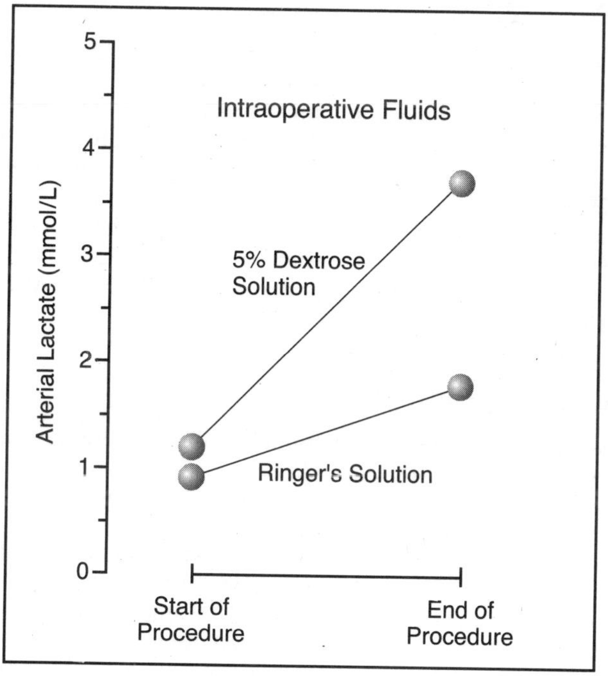

FIGURE 45.3 Effect of carbohydrate infusion on arterial lactate levels during abdominal aortic surgery. Each point represents the mean lactate level for 10 patients receiving Ringer's solution and 10 patients receiving 5% dextrose solution. Total volume infused is equivalent with both fluids. (Data from Degoute CS, Ray MJ, Manchon M, et al. Intraoperative glucose infusion and blood lactate: endocrine and metabolic relationships during abdominal aortic surgery. Anesthesiology 1989;71:355–361.)

increased only 1 mmol/L. Thus an organic nutrient (carbohydrate) can be used to generate a metabolic toxin (lactic acid) when nutrient processing is abnormal (during the stress of abdominal aneurysm surgery).

The study in Figure 45.3 illustrates that nutrient intake can have very different consequences in different subjects, and that *nutrients can become toxins* in the diseased host. Lucretius realized this more than 2000 years ago when he stated, "What is food to one man may be fierce poison to others." For this reason, one should not immediately jump on the bandwagon for aggressive nutritional support in critically ill patients.

REFERENCES

Reviews

1. Mandt J, Teasley-Strausberg K, Shronts E. Nutritional requirements. In: Teasley-Strausberg K, ed. Nutritional support handbook. Cincinnati, OH: Harvey-Whitney Books, 1992:19–36.
2. McClave S, Snider H. Use of indirect calorimety in clinical nutrition. Nutr Clin Pract 1992;7:207–221.
3. Headley JM. Indirect calorimetry: a trend toward continuous metabolic assessment. AACN Clin Issues 2003;14:155–167.
4. Biolo G, Grimble G, Preiser JC, et al. Position paper of the ESICM Working Group on Nutrition and Metabolism: metabolic basis of nutrition in intensive care unit patients: ten critical questions. Intensive Care Med 2002;28:1512–1520.
5. Bistrian BR, McCowen KC. Nutritional and metabolic support in the adult intensive care unit: key controversies. Crit Care Med 2006;34:1525–1531.
6. Sabol VK. Nutrition assessment of the critically ill adult. AACN Clin Issues 2004;15:595–606.

Daily Energy Expenditure

7. Harris JA, Benedict FG. A biometric study of human basal metabolism. Proc Natl Acad Sci U S A 1918;4:370–373.
8. Paauw JD, McCamish MA, Dean RE, et al. Assessment of caloric needs in stressed patients. J Am Coll Nutr 1984;3:51–59.
9. Mann S, Westenskow DR, Houtchens BA. Measured and predicted caloric expenditure in the acutely ill. Crit Care Med 1985;13:173–177.
10. Weissman C, Kemper M, Askanazi J, et al. Resting metabolic rate of the critically ill patient: measured versus predicted. Anesthesiology 1986;64:673–679.
11. Makk LJ, McClave SA, Creech PW, et al. Clinical application of the metabolic cart to the delivery of total parenteral nutrition. Crit Care Med 1990;18:1320–1327.
12. Kan MN, Chang HH, Sheu WF, et al. Estimation of energy requirements for mechanically ventilated, critically ill patients using nutritional status. Crit Care 2003;7:R108–R115.
13. Bursztein S, Saphar P, Singer P, et al. A mathematical analysis of indirect calorimetry measurements in acutely ill patients. Am J Clin Nutr 1989;50:227–230.

14. Weir JB. New methods for calculating metabolic rate with special reference to protein metabolism. J Physiol 1949;109:1–9.
15. Westenskow DR, Schipke CA, Raymond JL, et al. Calculation of metabolic expenditure and substrate utilization from gas exchange measurements. J Parenter Enteral Nutr 1988;12:20–24.
16. Cunningham JJ. Calculation of energy expenditure from indirect calorimetry: assessment of the Weir equation. Nutrition 1990;6:222–223.
17. Koea JB, Wolfe RR, Shaw JH. Total energy expenditure during total parenteral nutrition: ambulatory patients at home versus patients with sepsis in surgical intensive care. Surgery 1995;118:54–62.

Nonprotein Calories

18. Rodriguez JL, Askanazi J, Weissman C, et al. Ventilatory and metabolic effects of glucose infusions. Chest 1985;88:512–518.
19. Talpers SS, Romberger DJ, Bunce SB, et al. Nutritionally associated increased carbon dioxide production: excess total calories vs high proportion of carbohydrate calories. Chest 1992;102:551–555.
20. Jones PJH, Kubow S. Lipids, sterols, and their metabolites. In: Shils ME et al., eds. Modern nutrition in health and disease. 10th ed. Philadelphia: Lippincott Williams & Wilkins, 2006:92–121.

Protein Requirements

21. Matthews DE. Proteins and amino acids. In: Shils ME et al., eds. Modern nutrition in health and disease. 10th ed. Philadelphia: Lippincott Williams & Wilkins, 2006:23–61.
22. Blackburn GL, Bistrian BR, Maini BS, et al. Nutritional and metabolic assessment of the hospitalized patient. J Parenter Enteral Nutr 1977;1:11–22.
23. Velasco N, Long CL, Otto DA, et al. Comparison of three methods for the estimation of total nitrogen losses in hospitalized patients. J Parenter Enteral Nutr 1990;14:517–522.
24. Konstantinides FN, Konstantinides NN, Li JC, et al. Urinary urea nitrogen: too insensitive for calculating nitrogen balance studies in surgical clinical nutrition. J Parenter Enteral Nutr 1991;15:189–193.
25. Burge J, Choban P, McKnight T. Urinary ammonia excretion as an estimate of total urinary nitrogen in patients receiving parenteral nutritional support. J Parenter Enteral Nutr 1993;17:529–531.

Vitamin Requirements

26. Dempsey DT, Mullen JL, Rombeau JL, et al. Treatment effects of parenteral vitamins in total parenteral nutrition patients. J Parenter Enteral Nutr 1987;11:229–237.
27. Beard ME, Hatipov CS, Hamer JW. Acute onset of folate deficiency in patients under intensive care. Crit Care Med 1980;8:500–503.
28. Butterworth RF. Thiamin. In: Shils ME et al., eds. Modern nutrition in health and disease. 10th ed. Philadelphia: Lippincott Williams & Wilkins, 2006:426–433.

29. McConachie I, Haskew A. Thiamine status after major trauma. Intensive Care Med 1988;14:628–631.
30. Seligmann H, Halkin H, Rauchfleisch S, et al. Thiamine deficiency in patients with congestive heart failure receiving long-term furosemide therapy: a pilot study. Am J Med 1991;91:151–155.
31. Dyckner T, Ek B, Nyhlin H, et al. Aggravation of thiamine deficiency by magnesium depletion: a case report. Acta Med Scand 1985;218:129–131.
32. Tan GH, Farnell GF, Hensrud DD, et al. Acute Wernicke's encephalopathy attributable to pure dietary thiamine deficiency. Mayo Clin Proc 1994;69:849–850.
33. Oriot D, Wood C, Gottesman R, et al. Severe lactic acidosis related to acute thiamine deficiency. J Parenter Enteral Nutr 1991;15:105–109.
34. Koike H, Misu K, Hattori N, et al. Postgastrectomy polyneuropathy with thiamine deficiency. J Neurol Neurosurg Psychiatry 2001;71:357–362.
35. Boni L, Kieckens L, Hendrikx A. An evaluation of a modified erythrocyte transketolase assay for assessing thiamine nutritional adequacy. J Nutr Sci Vitaminol (Tokyo) 1980;26:507–514.

Essential Trace Elements

36. Fleming CR. Trace element metabolism in adult patients requiring total parenteral nutrition. Am J Clin Nutr 1989;49:573–579.
37. Halliwell B, Gutteridge JM. Role of free radicals and catalytic metal ions in human disease: an overview. Methods Enzymol 1990;186:1–85.
38. Herbert V, Shaw S, Jayatilleke E, et al. Most free-radical injury is iron-related: it is promoted by iron, hemin, holoferritin and vitamin C, and inhibited by desferoxamine and apoferritin. Stem Cells 1994;12:289–303.
39. Shanbhogue LK, Paterson N. Effect of sepsis and surgery on trace minerals. J Parenter Enteral Nutr 1990;14:287–289.
40. Guyatt GH, Patterson C, Ali M, et al. Diagnosis of iron-deficiency anemia in the elderly. Am J Med 1990;88:205–209.
41. Hawker FH, Stewart PM, Snitch PJ. Effects of acute illness on selenium homeostasis. Crit Care Med 1990;18:442–446.
42. Yusuf SW, Rehman Q, Casscells W. Cardiomyopathy in association with selenium deficiency: a case report. J Parenter Enteral Nutr 2002;26:63–66.
43. Sando K, Hoki M, Nezu R, et al. Platelet glutathione peroxidase activity in long-term total parenteral nutrition with and without selenium supplementation. J Parenter Enteral Nutr 1992;16:54–58.
44. Ishida T, Himeno K, Torigoe Y, et al. Selenium deficiency in a patient with Crohn's disease receiving long-term total parenteral nutrition. Intern Med 2003;42:154–157.
45. Geoghegan M, McAuley D, Eaton S, et al. Selenium in critical illness. Curr Opin Crit Care 2006;12:136–141.
46. Rayman MP. The importance of selenium to human health. Lancet 2000;356:233–241.
47. Food and Nutrition Board IOM. DRI: dietary reference intakes for vitamin C, vitamin E, selenium and carotenoids. Washington, DC: National Academy Press, 2000.

A Final Word

48. Marino PL, Finnegan MJ. Nutrition support is not beneficial and can be harmful in critically ill patients. Crit Care Clin 1996;12:667–676.
49. Gunther B, Jauch KW, Hartl W, et al. Low-dose glucose infusion in patients who have undergone surgery: possible cause of a muscular energy deficit. Arch Surg 1987;122:765–771.
50. Degoute CS, Ray MJ, Manchon M, et al. Intraoperative glucose infusion and blood lactate: endocrine and metabolic relationships during abdominal aortic surgery. Anesthesiology 1989;71:355–361.

Chapter 46

ENTERAL TUBE FEEDING

One of the important features of the gastrointestinal (GI) tract (as described in Chapter 4) is the role of the intestinal epithelium as a barrier to invasion by pathogenic microorganisms. As discussed in this chapter, the barrier function of the bowel mucosa is maintained by the intake and processing of bulk nutrients along the digestive tract. Therefore, providing nutrients via the enteral route not only provides nutritional support for the vital organs, but also supports host defenses against invasive infection (1–3). Several guidelines on the topic of enteral nutrition are included at the end of the chapter (4–6).

TROPHIC EFFECT OF ENTERAL NUTRIENTS

Complete bowel rest is accompanied by progressive atrophy and disruption of the intestinal mucosa (7). This effect becomes evident after just a few days and is not prevented by parenteral (intravenous) nutrition. The influence of luminal nutrients on the morphology of the intestinal mucosa is shown in Figure 46.1 (8,9). The photomicrograph at the top shows the normal appearance of the small bowel mucosa. Note the fingerlike projections (microvilli), which serve to increase the surface area for nutrient absorption. The photomicrograph at the bottom shows the mucosal changes after 1 week of a protein-deficient diet. Note the shortening of the microvillus on the left of the picture and the generalized disruption of the surface architecture. This demonstrates that **depletion of nutrients in the bowel lumen is accompanied by degenerative changes in the bowel mucosa.**

Observations like those in Figure 46.1 indicate that the bowel mucosa relies on nutrients in the bowel lumen to provide its nutritional needs. One of the nutrients that may play an important role in this process is the amino acid glutamine, which is considered the principal metabolic fuel for intestinal epithelial cells (10). The use of glutamine in enteral feedings is discussed later in this chapter.

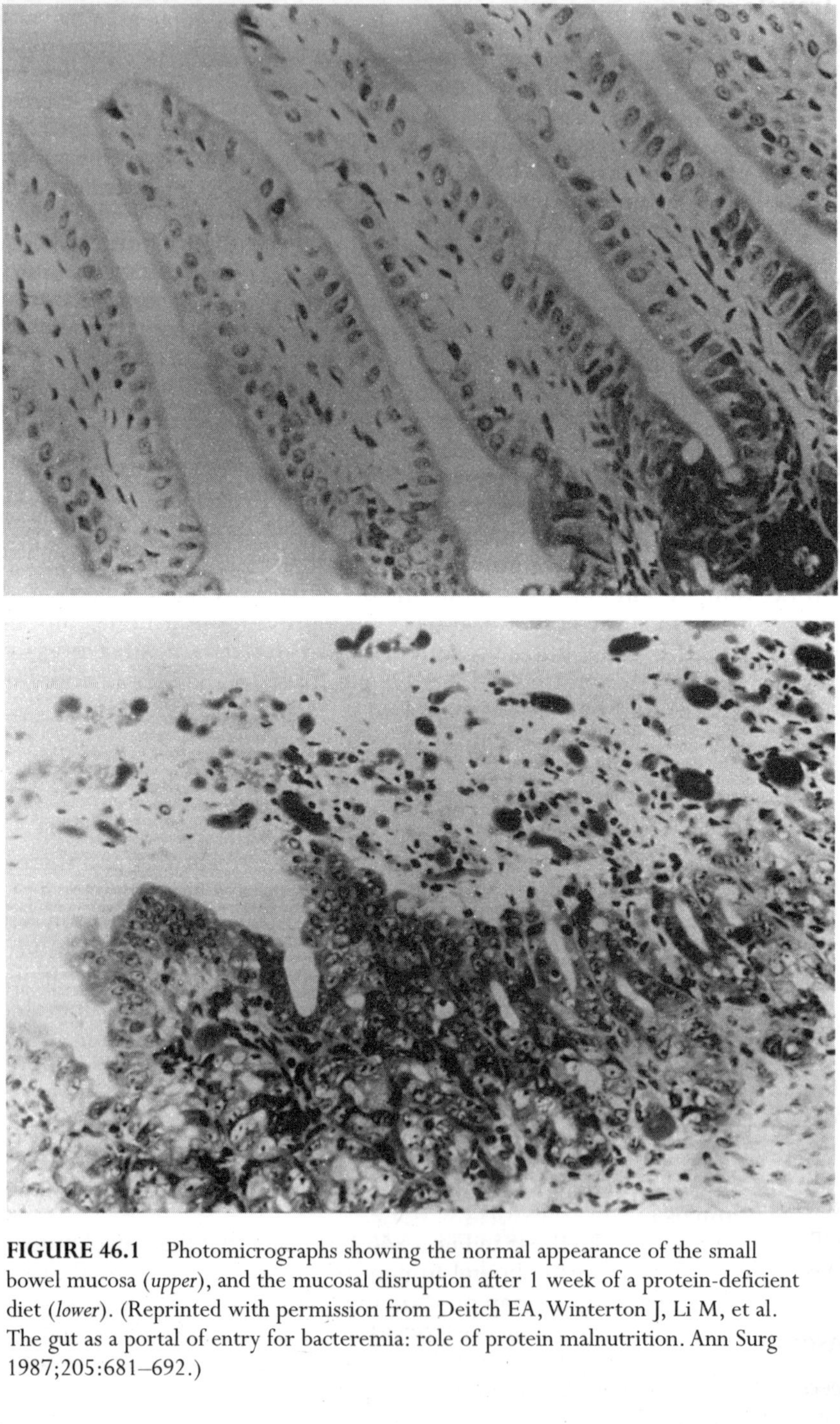

FIGURE 46.1 Photomicrographs showing the normal appearance of the small bowel mucosa (*upper*), and the mucosal disruption after 1 week of a protein-deficient diet (*lower*). (Reprinted with permission from Deitch EA, Winterton J, Li M, et al. The gut as a portal of entry for bacteremia: role of protein malnutrition. Ann Surg 1987;205:681–692.)

Translocation

The process of translocation, where enteric pathogens move across the bowel mucosa and into the systemic circulation, is described in Chapter 4 (see Fig. 4.2). Translocation has been documented during periods of bowel rest in critically ill patients (7,11), and this has been attributed to mucosal disruption from lack of luminal nutrients. This means that enteral nutrition could help prevent translocation and subsequent sepsis by maintaining the functional integrity of the bowel mucosa. The potential for enteral nutrition to prevent sepsis of bowel origin is one of the major reasons why enteral nutrition has become favored over parenteral (intravenous) nutrition in critically ill patients.

PATIENT SELECTION

In the absence of contraindications, enteral tube feedings are indicated when oral nutrient intake has been inadequate for 1–3 days (5,12). In patients who are at risk of bacterial translocation across the bowel (e.g., burn victims), tube feedings should be started as soon as possible after the onset of inadequate nutrient intake (5).

Contraindications

Enteral feedings in any amount are contraindicated in patients with circulatory shock, intestinal ischemia, complete mechanical bowel obstruction, or ileus.

Total enteral nutrition is not advised in patients with the following conditions: partial mechanical bowel obstruction, severe or unrelenting diarrhea, pancreatitis, or high-volume (more than 500 mL daily) enterocutaneous fistulas. Partial (low volume) enteral support is, however, possible in these conditions (13). In the case of pancreatitis, enteral feedings can be delivered into the jejunum (see "Jejunostomy Feedings").

FEEDING TUBES

Standard Salem sump nasogastric tubes (14 to 16 French) are no longer favored for enteral tube feedings because of patient discomfort. Although there has been concern about gastroesophageal reflux with these tubes, clinical studies do not support this concern (14). The feeding tubes that are currently favored are narrower (8 to 10 French) and more flexible than standard nasogastric tubes. Because these tubes are so flexible, a rigid stylet is also provided to facilitate insertion.

Insertion

Feeding tubes are inserted through the nares and advanced into the stomach or duodenum. The distance that the tube must be advanced to reach the stomach can be estimated by measuring the distance from the tip of the nose to the earlobe and then to the xiphoid process (typically 50–60 cm) (4).

Proper placement in the stomach is sometimes possible to determine by measuring the pH (with litmus paper) of a specimen aspirated from the tip of the feeding tube (15). If the specimen has a pH less than 5, the tip of the tube is likely to be in the stomach (15).

Tracheal Intubation

The principal complication of feeding tube placement is accidental tracheal intubation in 1% (16). Because feeding tubes are narrow, they readily pass through the larynx and around the inflated cuffs on tracheal tubes. Accidental **intubation of the trachea is often asymptomatic** (probably because of sedation, depressed consciousness, or an abnormal cough reflex), and in the absence of symptoms, tubes can be advanced into the distal airways. This is illustrated in Figure 46.2, which shows the tip of a small-bore feeding tube in the lower lobe of the right lung. If feeding tubes are advanced too far into the lungs, the rigid stylet makes it easy to puncture the visceral pleura and produce a pneumothorax (16,17).

Because of the risk of asymptomatic intubation of the lungs, a postinsertion chest x-ray is required to evaluate tube placement (unless pH testing confirms gastric placement). **Auscultation of the upper abdomen**

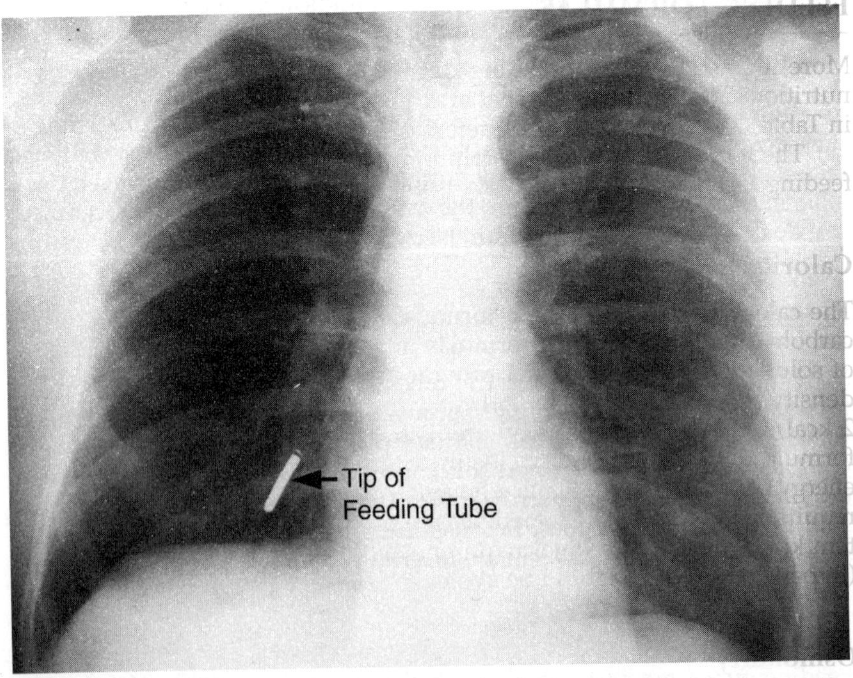

FIGURE 46.2 Routine chest x-ray following insertion of a small bore feeding tube. The tip of the tube is evident in the right lung.

while insufflating air through the tube **is not a reliable method for excluding tube malposition in the lungs** because sounds emanating from a tube in the lower airways can be transmitted into the upper abdomen (17,18).

Duodenal Placement

For those who prefer tube feedings placed in the duodenum instead of the stomach, gastric tubes must be advanced past the pylorus and into the duodenum (5,12). This can be accomplished by specialized bedside maneuvers or may require endoscopic or fluoroscopic guidance (4,16). Tube passage into the duodenum can be confirmed by radiographic localization.

Feeding Site

The proposed advantage of duodenal feedings is a reduced risk of reflux of feeding solution into the esophagus and subsequent pulmonary aspiration (19). However, clinical studies show that **the risk of aspiration in duodenal feedings is the same as that in gastric feedings** (5,20). Therefore, the time and effort devoted to advancing gastric tubes into the duodenum is not justified.

FEEDING FORMULAS

More than 115 liquid feeding formulas are available for enteral nutrition (21). The formulas that are most commonly used are described in Tables 46.1 through 46.5, see reference (22,23).

The following is a brief description of some of the features of enteral feeding formulas.

Caloric Density

The caloric density of feeding formulas is determined primarily by the carbohydrate content. Most formulas provide 1 to 2 kilocalories per liter of solution. The formulas that provide 1 to 1.5 kcal/L (standard caloric density) are listed in Table 46.1, and the formulas that provide 1.5 to 2 kcal/L (high caloric density) are listed in Table 46.2. The energy-rich formulas in Table 46.2 are well-suited for patients with excessive daily energy needs and for patients who are volume-restricted. The nutritional requirements of many ICU patients are met by providing 25–30 nonprotein kcal/kg, but individual requirements vary greatly and overfeeding (hyperalimentation) should be avoided (5).

Osmolality

The osmolality of liquid feeding formulas varies from 280 to 1100 mOsm/kg H_2O. The major determinant of osmolality is the carbohydrate content

TABLE 46.1 Characteristics of Selected Enteral Feeding Formulas

Formula	Caloric Density (kcal/mL)	Protein (g/L)	Osmolarity (mOsm/L)	Volume to Meet US RDA*
Ensure Plus HN	1.5	63	525	1000
Isocal	1.1	34	270	1890
Isocal HN	1.1	44	270	1180
Nutren	1.0	40	315	1500
Osmolite	1.1	37	300	1890
Osmolite HN	1.1	44	300	1320
Peptamen	1.0	40	270	150
Ultracal	1.1	37	500	1180
Vivonex TEN	1.0	38	630	2000
Vital HN	1.0	42	500	1500

*Indicates the volume needed to provide 100% of the recommended daily allowances (RDAs) for vitamins and essential trace elements.

(because this is the most abundant nutrient in most feeding formulas). Because carbohydrates also determine caloric density, osmolality and caloric density are directly related. Formulas with the lowest caloric density (1 kcal/L) have the lowest osmolalities (approximately 300 mOsm/kg H_2O) and are usually isotonic to the body fluids. Formulas with the highest caloric density (2 kcal/L) have the highest osmolalities (1,000 mOsm/kg H_2O) and are markedly hypertonic to the body fluids.

Hypertonic formulas should be infused into the stomach to take advantage of the dilutional effects of the gastric secretions.

Protein

Liquid feeding formulas provide 35 to 40 grams of protein per liter. Although some formulas are designated as being protein-rich (these formulas often have the suffix HN to indicate "high nitrogen"), they provide only 20% more protein than the standard feeding formulas.

TABLE 46.2 Enteral Formulas with a High Caloric Density

Formula	Caloric Density (kcal/mL)	Osmolality (mOsm/Kg)	Volume to Meet US RDA
Nepro	2	665	1000
Novasource Renal	2	700	1000
TwoCal HN	2	725	950

Protein Complexity

Most enteral formulas provide intact proteins that are broken down into amino acids in the upper GI tract. Because small peptides are absorbed more rapidly than amino acids, some feeding formulas contain small peptides instead of intact protein to facilitate absorption. Peptide-based formulas such as Peptamen (Nestlé) and Vital HN (Ross) can be used in patients with impaired intestinal absorption (e.g., from inflammatory bowel disease). These formulas also promote water reabsorption from the bowel, and thus they could prove beneficial in patients with severe or unrelenting diarrhea.

Lipids

The lipid emulsions used in feeding formulas are rich in long-chain triglycerides derived from vegetable oils. These lipids represent a concentrated source of calories, with an energy yield (9 kcal/g) that is almost three times that of carbohydrates (3.4 kcal/g). Because excessive fat ingestion is not well tolerated (i.e., it promotes diarrhea), the lipid content of most feeding formulas is limited to 30% of the total calories. Some formulas with an altered lipid composition are described in the following sections. These formulas are summarized in Table 46.3.

Lipid-Rich Formula

One liquid feeding formula with a high fat content is Pulmocare (Ross), which uses lipids to provide 55% of the total calories. This formula is intended for patients with respiratory failure. The proposed benefit is based on the low rate of CO_2 production relative to O_2 consumption associated with lipid metabolism (see Table 45.1). Thus when lipids replace carbohydrates as the principal nutrient substrate, metabolic CO_2 production will decline and there will be less of a tendency for CO_2 retention in patients with compromised lung function (24).

TABLE 46.3 Feeding Formulas with an Altered Lipid Composition

Formula	Feature	Proposed Benefit
Immun-Aid (McGaw)	Contains omega-3 fatty acids, RNA, arginine, and glutamine.	Enhances immune function, limits inflammatory-mediated tissue injury.
Impact (Novartis)	Contains omega-3 fatty acids, RNA, arginine, and glutamine.	↓
Oxepa (Ross)	Contains omega-3 fatty acids, arginine, antioxidants.	↓
Pulmocare (Ross)	High lipid content. Lipids provide 55% of the calories in the formula.	Limits nutrition-induced CO_2 retention in respiratory failure.

Alternative Lipids

The two feeding formulas described in Table 46.3 contain dietary fat from sources other than vegetable oils. Polyunsaturated fatty acids from vegetable oils can serve as precursors for inflammatory mediators (eicosanoids) that are capable of producing widespread cell injury (1). The omega-3 fatty acids do not promote the production of harmful inflammatory mediators, and these might be preferred to the standard dietary fats to limit the risk of inflammatory-mediated tissue injury.

Several feeding formulas contain omega-3 fatty acids: Oxepa (Ross) (25), Impact (Novartis), and Immun-Aid (McGaw) (see Table 46.3). These formulas are intended for patients with systemic inflammation or acute respiratory distress syndrome who are at risk for inflammatory-mediated tissue injury (1, 26–28).

ADDITIVES

Glutamine

As mentioned earlier, **glutamine is the principal fuel for the bowel mucosa** (10). Therefore, daily supplementation with glutamine seems a reasonable measure for maintaining the functional integrity of the bowel mucosa. Although glutamine is not an essential amino acid (because it is produced in skeletal muscle), tissue glutamine stores decline precipitously in acute, hypercatabolic states. Therefore, glutamine can become an essential nutrient in the hypermetabolic, stressed patient (2,29).

Glutamine-Enriched Formulas

Because glutamine is a natural constituent of proteins, all feeding formulas that contain intact protein will also contain glutamine (30). However, little of this glutamine is in the free or unbound form. The formulas that contain glutamine as a free amino acid are listed in Table 46.4. With the exception of AlitraQ or Impact Glutamine, the glutamine content of enteral feeding formulas is low and may be insufficient to provide a benefit (31–33). In one study of glutamine administration in healthy adults (33), the average glutamine dosage (oral and intravenous) was 0.35 g/kg/day, or 24.5 g/day for a 70-kg subject. Assuming a daily caloric intake of 2,000 kcal, the only feeding formulas in Table 46.4 that will provide a glutamine dosage of 0.35 g/kg/day is AlitraQ or Impact Glutamine. In

TABLE 46.4 Glutamine-Enriched Feeding Formulas

Formula	Manufacturer	Glutamine (g/L)
AlitraQ	Ross	15.5
Impact Glutamine	Novartis	15
Replete	Nestlé	3.3
Vivonex TEN	Novartis	3.3

the setting of hypercatabolism, the glutamine provided by most enteral formulas will be even more inadequate. Therefore, although the use of glutamine-fortified enteral formulas seems reasonable, the amount of glutamine provided by most formulas may be inadequate.

Dietary Fiber

The term *fiber* refers to a group of plant products that are not degradable by human digestive enzymes. These products are classified by their fermentative properties.

FERMENTABLE FIBER (cellulose, pectin, gums) is degraded by intestinal bacteria to form short-chain fatty acids (e.g., acetate), which are used as an energy substrate by the large bowel mucosa. This type of fiber can slow gastric emptying and bind bile salts, and both of these actions can help alleviate diarrhea.

NONFERMENTABLE FIBER (lignins) is not degraded by intestinal bacteria, but it can create an osmotic force that adsorbs water from the bowel lumen. This type of fiber can therefore reduce the tendency for watery diarrhea.

Thus fiber has several actions that can reduce the tendency for diarrhea during enteral feedings. Furthermore, fermentable fiber can serve as a source of metabolic support for the mucosa of the large bowel (34). This latter effect could play an important role in limiting the tendency for translocation across a disrupted large bowel mucosa. Several feeding formulas contain fiber, and they are shown in Table 46.5. The added fiber in all cases is soy polysaccharide, which is a fermentable fiber. Thus there is little difference between the fiber-enriched formulas, either in type or in content of fiber. Fiber-enhanced feedings can also be achieved by adding Metamucil (nonfermentable fiber) or Kaopectate (fermentable fiber) to the feeding regimen.

Performance

The effects of fiber-enriched feedings on the incidence of diarrhea have been inconsistent, with some studies showing a reduced incidence of diarrhea (35,36), and others showing no effect (37). However, relying on fiber to prevent diarrhea neglects the source of the diarrhea; the focus of prevention should be to eliminate or treat the process responsible for the diarrhea.

TABLE 46.5 Fiber-Enriched Enteral Feeding Formulas

Formula	Fiber (g/L)	Formula	Fiber (g/L)
Enrich	14.3	Isosource 1.5 Cal	8
Fibersource	10	Jevity	14.4
Fibersource HN	10	Nutren 1.0 Fiber	14
Glucerna	14.3	Ultracal	14.4

Miscellaneous

Branched Chain Amino Acids

The branched chain amino acids (BCAAs) isoleucine, leucine, and valine are available in feeding formulas intended for trauma victims and patients with hepatic encephalopathy. In trauma victims, the BCAAs can be used as a fuel source in skeletal muscle, thereby sparing the degradation of other muscle proteins to provide energy. In hepatic encephalopathy, the BCAAs can antagonize the uptake of aromatic amino acids (e.g., tryptophan) into the central nervous system, and this helps prevent the subsequent breakdown of the aromatic amino acids to form false neurotransmitters, which have been implicated in the pathogenesis of hepatic encephalopathy (38,39).

Examples of feeding formulas enriched with BCAAs for hepatic encephalopathy include NutriHep (Nestlé) and Hepatic-Aid II (Hormel Health Labs). The benefits of these formulas are unproven.

Carnitine

Carnitine is necessary for the transport of fatty acids into mitochondria for fatty acid oxidation (40). Humans normally synthesize carnitine from lysine and methionine (essential amino acids) in sufficient amounts so that dietary intake is not required (40). Deficiency of carnitine (plasma concentration below 20 μmol/L) can occur in prolonged states of hypercatabolism or during prolonged hemodialysis (40,41). The clinical consequences of carnitine deficiency include cardiomyopathy, skeletal muscle myopathy, and hypoglycemia.

The recommended **daily dose of carnitine is 20–30 mg/kg in adults** (41,42). Enteral formulas that are supplemented with carnitine include Glucerna (Ross), Isocal HN (Novartis), Jevity (Ross), and Peptamen (Nestlé).

FEEDING REGIMEN

Tube feedings are usually infused for 12 to 16 hours in each 24-hour period. Continuous infusion without a period of bowel rest is an unrelenting stress to the bowel mucosa and promotes malabsorption and diarrhea. Intermittent bolus feedings more closely approximate the normal condition, but the volumes required are often too large to be given safely.

Gastric Retention

Before gastric feedings are started, it is necessary to determine how much volume will be retained in the stomach over a 1-hour period because this will determine how fast the feedings can be administered. A volume of water that is equivalent to the desired hourly feeding volume should be infused over 1 hour. After the infusion is complete, the feeding tube should be clamped for 30 minutes. The tube should then be unclamped, and any residual volume should be aspirated from the stomach. If the

4 hour gastric residual volume is less than 200 mL, gastric feeding can proceed (4). If the residual volume is excessively high, duodenal or jejunal feedings may be more appropriate. When the gastric residual volume is measured, it is important not to administer the volume as a bolus because this will produce acute gastric distension and lead to overestimation of the residual volume.

Starter Regimens

The traditional approach to initiating tube feedings is to begin with dilute formulas and a slow infusion rate and gradually advance the formula concentration and infusion rate over the next few days until the desired nutrient intake is achieved. This presumably allows the atrophic bowel mucosa time to regenerate after a period of bowel rest. The drawback with starter regimens is the fact that nutrient intake is inadequate for the time required to advance to full nutritional support. In the malnourished patient, this added period of inadequate nutrition adds to the malnutrition.

Studies involving intragastric feedings show that full feedings can be delivered immediately without troublesome vomiting or diarrhea (43,44). This is presumably due to the ability of gastric secretions to dilute the feeding formula and reduce the osmotic load associated with the feedings. Therefore, **starter regimens are unnecessary for gastric feedings.** Because of the limited reservoir function of the small bowel, starter regimens are usually required for duodenal and jejunal feedings.

COMPLICATIONS

The complications associated with enteral feedings include occlusion of the feeding tube, reflux of gastric contents into the airways, and diarrhea.

Tube Occlusion

Narrow-bore feeding tubes can become occluded by accumulation of residue from the feeding formulas. One important mechanism is the precipitation of proteins in the feeding solution by acidic gastric juice that refluxes up the feeding tubes (45). Standard preventive measures include flushing the feeding tubes with 30 mL of water every 4 hours, and using a 10 mL water flush after medications are instilled (46).

Relieving the Obstruction

If there is still some flow through the tube, warm water should be injected into the tube and agitated with a syringe. This can relieve the obstruction in 30% of cases (47). If this is ineffective, **pancreatic enzyme** can be used as follows (47):

Dissolve 1 tablet of Viokase and 1 tablet of sodium carbonate (324 mg) in 5 mL of water. Inject this mixture into the feeding tube and clamp for 5 minutes. Follow with a warm water flush.

This should relieve the obstruction in approximately 75% of cases (47). If the tube is completely occluded and it is impossible to introduce warm water or pancreatic enzyme, an attempt should be made to insert a flexible wire or a drum cartridge catheter to clear the obstruction.

Aspiration

Retrograde regurgitation of feeding formula is reported in as many as 80% of patients receiving gastric or duodenal feedings (48). As stated earlier, the risk of reflux in gastric feedings is the same as that in duodenal feedings (20,49). Elevating the head of the bed to 30 to 45 degrees can reduce—although not eliminate—the risk of reflux (48,50).

Glucose Reagent Strips

Aspiration of feeding formulas into the airways can be detected by testing tracheal aspirates with glucose oxidase reagent strips. The results are measured with an automated glucose meter. A **glucose concentration greater than 20 mg/dL in tracheal aspirates is evidence of aspiration** (51). Coloring the feeding formulas with food coloring and inspecting the color of the tracheal secretions is an insensitive method for detecting aspiration (51).

Diarrhea

Diarrhea occurs in approximately 30% of patients receiving enteral tube feedings (52). Although the hypertonicity of enteral feeding formulas can induce an osmotic diarrhea, in most cases of diarrhea associated with enteral feedings, the feeding formula is not responsible for the diarrhea (52,53). **The cause of the diarrhea in many cases is a medicinal elixir that contains sorbitol** (an osmotic agent) to improve palatability (52,54). Some of the sorbitol-containing liquid drug preparations are shown in Table 46.6 (54). Also shown is the daily dosage of sorbitol that would accompany each drug when given in the usual therapeutic dosages (54). In most cases, the daily dosage of sorbitol can be enough to induce an osmotic diarrhea. Therefore, a search for sorbitol-containing medicinal elixirs should be the first concern in the evaluation of diarrhea during enteral tube feedings.

Stool Osmolal Gap

Clostridium difficile enterocolitis is also a possible cause of diarrhea during enteral feedings. One method of differentiating the secretory diarrhea caused by *C. difficile* enterocolitis from the osmotic diarrhea caused by hypertonic feedings or medicinal elixirs is to calculate the stool osmolal gap as follows:

$$\text{Osmolal gap} = \text{Measured stool osmolality} - 2 \times (\text{Stool [Na} - \text{Stool [K+]}) \qquad (46.1)$$

TABLE 46.6 Sorbitol-Containing Liquid Drug Preparations

Agent	Preparation	Usual Dosage	Daily Sorbitol Dose (g)
Acetaminophen	Tylenol Elixir	650 mg QID	16
Cimetidine	Tagamet Liquid	300 mg QID	10
Ferrous sulfate	Iberet Liquid	75 mg TID	22
Metoclopramide	Reglan Syrup	10 mg QID	20
Potassium chloride	Kolyum Powder	20 mEq BID	25
Theophylline	Theolar Liquid	200 mg QID	23
Trimethoprim–sulfamethoxazole	Septra Suspension	800/160 mg BID	18

From Cheng EY et al. Unsuspected source of diarrhea in an ICU patient. Clin Intensive Care 1992;3:33–36.

A stool osmolal gap greater than 160 mOsm/kg H_2O suggests an osmotic diarrhea secondary to hypertonic tube feedings or medicinal elixirs, whereas a smaller (or negative) osmolal gap suggests a secretory diarrhea caused by *C. difficile* enterocolitis. (For more information on the diagnosis and treatment of *C. difficile* enterocolitis, see Chapter 42.)

JEJUNOSTOMY FEEDINGS

Although abdominal surgery usually is accompanied by 24 to 48 hours of gastric hypomotility, the motility of the small bowel is often unimpaired (55). Infusion of liquid feeding formulas into the jejunum takes advantage of the continued small bowel motility after abdominal surgery and allows immediate postoperative nutrition. Jejunal feedings can also be performed for nutritional support of patients with pancreatitis.

Needle Catheter Jejunostomy

A feeding jejunostomy can be performed as a "complementary" procedure during laparotomy. A needle catheter jejunostomy is shown in Figure 46.3 (56). A loop of jejunum (15 to 20 cm distal to the ligament of Treitz) is mobilized to the anterior abdominal wall, and a 16-gauge catheter is tunneled through the submucosa of the jejunum for a distance of 30 to 45 cm and then advanced into the bowel lumen. The jejunum is then secured to the peritoneum on the underside of the abdominal wall, and the catheter is secured to the skin.

Feeding Method

As mentioned, the small bowel does not have the reservoir capacity of the stomach, so starter regimens are recommended for jejunal feedings.

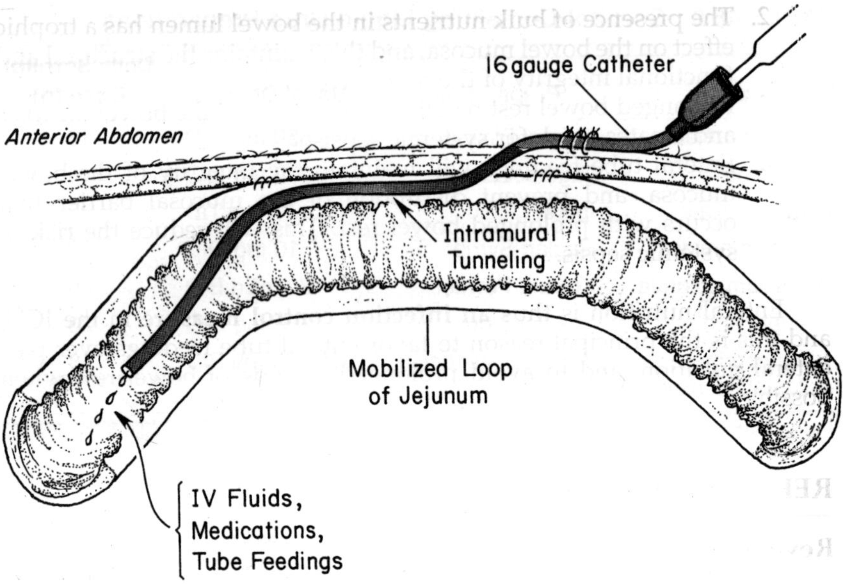

FIGURE 46.3 A needle catheter jejunostomy.

Feedings are usually initiated at a rate of 15 to 25 mL/hour, and the infusion rate is gradually increased over the next few days until full nutritional support is achieved (57). Catheters are flushed with 10 mL of isotonic saline every 6 hours to promote catheter patency.

Complications

The principal complications of needle catheter jejunostomies are diarrhea and occlusion of the narrow feeding catheters (57). Because of the latter complication, needle catheter jejunostomies are used only for temporary nutritional support (approximately 1 week). If more prolonged jejunal feedings are desired, a needle catheter jejunostomy can be converted to a standard jejunostomy (which uses a 12 French feeding tube) using a technique described in Reference 58.

A FINAL WORD

The most important role of enteral tube feedings in the ICU is not directly related to nutrition. This role is reviewed in the sequence of statements listed below.

1. The mucosal lining of the gastrointestinal (GI) tract serves as a barrier to microbial invasion, and disruption of this barrier is an important source of systemic sepsis in critically ill patients.

2. The presence of bulk nutrients in the bowel lumen has a trophic effect on the bowel mucosa, and this maintains the structural and functional integrity of the mucosal barrier.
3. Prolonged bowel rest results in disruption of the bowel mucosa, and creates a risk for systemic sepsis.
4. Enteral tube feedings will maintain the integrity of the bowel mucosa, and prevent disruption of the mucosal barrier that occurs with prolonged bowel rest. This will reduce the risk of systemic sepsis.

Enteral nutrition is thus **an infection control measure** in the ICU, and this is the principal reason to favor enteral tube feedings over parenteral nutrition, and to avoid prolonged periods of bowel rest when possible.

REFERENCES

Reviews

1. Bistrian BR, McCowen KC. Nutritional and metabolic support in the adult intensive care unit: key controversies. Crit Care Med 2006;34:1525–1531.
2. De-Souza DA, Greene LJ. Intestinal permeability and systemic infections in critically ill patients: effect of glutamine. Crit Care Med 2005;33:1125–1135.
3. Wischmeyer PE. The glutamine story: where are we now? Curr Opin Crit Care 2006;12:142–148.

Guidelines

4. Stroud M, Duncan H, Nightingale J. Guidelines for enteral feeding in adult hospital patients. Gut 2003;52(suppl 7):vii1–vii12.
5. Kreymann KG, Berger MM, Deutz NE, et al. ESPEN Guidelines on enteral nutrition: intensive care. Clin Nutr 2006;25:210–223.
6. Lochs H, Allison SP, Meier R, et al. Introductory to the ESPEN guidelines on enteral nutrition: terminology, definitions and general topics. Clin Nutr 2006;25:180–186.

Trophism

7. Alpers DH. Enteral feeding and gut atrophy. Curr Opin Clin Nutr Metab Care 2002;5:679–683.
8. Deitch EA, Winterton J, Li M, et al. The gut as a portal of entry for bacteremia: role of protein malnutrition. Ann Surg 1987;205:681–692.
9. Alverdy JC, Laughlin RS, Wu L. Influence of the critically ill state on host-pathogen interactions within the intestine: gut-derived sepsis redefined. Crit Care Med 2003;31:598–607.
10. Herskowitz K, Souba WW. Intestinal glutamine metabolism during critical illness: a surgical perspective. Nutrition 1990;6:199–206.
11. Wiest R, Rath HC. Gastrointestinal disorders of the critically ill. Bacterial translocation in the gut. Best Pract Res Clin Gastroenterol 2003;17:397–425.

12. Heyland DK, Dhaliwal R, Drover JW, et al. Canadian clinical practice guidelines for nutrition support in mechanically ventilated, critically ill adult patients. J Parenter Enteral Nutr 2003;27:355–373.
13. Meier R, Ockenga J, Pertkiewicz M, et al. ESPEN guidelines on enteral nutrition: pancreas. Clin Nutr 2006;25:275–284.

Feeding Tubes

14. Dotson RG, Robinson RG, Pingleton SK. Gastroesophageal reflux with nasogastric tubes: effect of nasogastric tube size. Am J Respir Crit Care Med 1994;149:1659–1662.
15. Metheny NA, Clouse RE, Clark JM, et al. pH testing of feeding-tube aspirates to determine placement. Nutr Clin Pract 1994;9:185–190.
16. Baskin WN. Acute complications associated with bedside placement of feeding tubes. Nutr Clin Pract 2006;21:40–55.
17. Kolbitsch C, Pomaroli A, Lorenz I, et al. Pneumothorax following nasogastric feeding tube insertion in a tracheostomized patient after bilateral lung transplantation. Intensive Care Med 1997;23:440–442.
18. Fisman DN, Ward ME. Intrapleural placement of a nasogastric tube: an unusual complication of nasotracheal intubation. Can J Anaesth 1996;43:1252–1256.
19. Jabbar A, McClave SA. Pre-pyloric versus post-pyloric feeding. Clin Nutr 2005;24:719–726.
20. Strong RM, Condon SC, Solinger MR, et al. Equal aspiration rates from postpylorus and intragastric-placed small-bore nasoenteric feeding tubes: a randomized, prospective study. J Parenter Enteral Nutr 1992;16:59–63.

Feeding Formulas

21. (NIH/NLM) MP. Enteral Nutrition Formulas (Systemic). 2006 Available at: http://www.nlm.nih.gov/medlineplus/druginfo/uspdi/202673.html (accessed on June 6, 2006).
22. Novartis Medical Nutrition. Product Reference Guide. 2006 Available at: http://www.novartisnutrition.com/pdfs/us/presentations/Source_Chart_04.16400.pdf (accessed on June 7, 2006).
23. Malone A. Enteral formula selection: a review of selected product categories. Pract Gastroenterol 2005;June:44–74.
24. Malone AM. The use of specialized enteral formulas in pulmonary disease. Nutr Clin Pract 2004;19:557–562.
25. Gadek JE, DeMichele SJ, Karlstad MD, et al. Effect of enteral feeding with eicosapentaenoic acid, gamma-linolenic acid, and antioxidants in patients with acute respiratory distress syndrome: Enteral Nutrition in ARDS Study Group. Crit Care Med 1999;27:1409–1420.
26. Zaloga GP, Siddiqui R, Terry C, et al. Arginine: mediator or modulator of sepsis? Nutr Clin Pract 2004;19:201–215.
27. Heyland DK, Dhaliwal R, Suchner U, et al. Antioxidant nutrients: a systematic review of trace elements and vitamins in the critically ill patient. Intensive Care Med 2005;31:327–337.

28. Heyland DK, Novak F, Drover JW, et al. Should immunonutrition become routine in critically ill patients? A systematic review of the evidence. JAMA 2001;286:944–953.

Additives

29. Lacey JM, Wilmore DW. Is glutamine a conditionally essential amino acid? Nutr Rev 1990;48:297–309.
30. Swails WS, Bell SJ, Borlase BC, et al. Glutamine content of whole proteins: implications for enteral formulas. Nutr Clin Pract 1992;7:77–80.
31. Alitra Q. Ross Medical Nutritional Products Pocket Guide. 2005 Ross Laboratories Available at: http://www.ross.com/images/library/Ross_MN_Products_Pocket_Guide.pdf (accessed on June 9, 2006).
32. Garcia-de-Lorenzo A, Zarazaga A, Garcia-Luna PP, et al. Clinical evidence for enteral nutritional support with glutamine: a systematic review. Nutrition 2003;19:809–811.
33. Ziegler TR, Benfell K, Smith RJ, et al. Safety and metabolic effects of L-glutamine administration in humans. J Parenter Enteral Nutr 1990;14:137S–146S.
34. Palacio JC, Rombeau JL. Dietary fiber: a brief review and potential application to enteral nutrition. Nutr Clin Pract 1990;5:99–106.
35. Homann HH, Kemen M, Fuessenich C, et al. Reduction in diarrhea incidence by soluble fiber in patients receiving total or supplemental enteral nutrition. J Parenter Enteral Nutr 1994;18:486–490.
36. Spapen H, Diltoer M, Van Malderen C, et al. Soluble fiber reduces the incidence of diarrhea in septic patients receiving total enteral nutrition: a prospective, double-blind, randomized, and controlled trial. Clin Nutr 2001;20:301–305.
37. Frankenfield DC, Beyer PL. Soy-polysaccharide fiber: effect on diarrhea in tube-fed, head-injured patients. Am J Clin Nutr 1989;50:533–538.
38. Alexander WF, Spindel E, Harty RF, et al. The usefulness of branched chain amino acids in patients with acute or chronic hepatic encephalopathy. Am J Gastroenterol 1989;84:91–96.
39. James JH. Branched chain amino acids in hepatic encephalopathy. Am J Surg 2002;183:424–429.
40. Rebouche CJ. Carnitine. In: Shils ME, et al., eds. Modern nutrition in health and disease. 10th ed. Philadelphia: Lippincott Williams & Wilkins, 2006:537–544.
41. Kazmi WH, Obrador GT, Sternberg M, et al. Carnitine therapy is associated with decreased hospital utilization among hemodialysis patients. Am J Nephrol 2005;25:106–115.
42. Karlic H, Lohninger A. Supplementation of L-carnitine in athletes: does it make sense? Nutrition (Burbank, CA) 2004;20:709–715.

Feeding Regimen

43. Rees RG, Keohane PP, Grimble GK, et al. Elemental diet administered nasogastrically without starter regimens to patients with inflammatory bowel disease. J Parenter Enteral Nutr 1986;10:258–262.

44. Mizock BA. Avoiding common errors in nutritional management. J Crit Illness 1993;10:1116–1127.

Complications

45. Marcuard SP, Perkins AM. Clogging of feeding tubes. J Parenter Enteral Nutr 1988;12:403–405.
46. Benson DW, Griggs BA, Hamilton F, et al. Clogging of feeding tubes: a randomized trial of a newly designed tube. Nutr Clin Pract 1990;5:107–110.
47. Marcuard SP, Stegall KS. Unclogging feeding tubes with pancreatic enzyme. J Parenter Enteral Nutr 1990;14:198–200.
48. Metheny N. Minimizing respiratory complications of nasoenteric tube feedings: state of the science. Heart Lung 1993;22:213–223.
49. Metheny NA. Risk factors for aspiration. J Parenter Enteral Nutr 2002;26: S26–31.
50. Castel H, Tiengou LE, Besancon I, et al. What is the risk of nocturnal supine enteral nutrition? Clin Nutr 2005;24:1014–1018.
51. Potts RG, Zaroukian MH, Guerrero PA, et al. Comparison of blue dye visualization and glucose oxidase test strip methods for detecting pulmonary aspiration of enteral feedings in intubated adults. Chest 1993;103:117–121.
52. Edes TE, Walk BE, Austin JL. Diarrhea in tube-fed patients: feeding formula not necessarily the cause. Am J Med 1990;88:91–93.
53. Eisenberg PG. Causes of diarrhea in tube-fed patients: a comprehensive approach to diagnosis and management. Nutr Clin Pract 1993;8:119–123.
54. Cheng EY, Hennen CR, Nimphius N. Unsuspected source of diarrhea in an ICU patient. Clin Intensive Care 1992;3:33–36.

Jejunostomy Feedings

55. Sagar PM, Kruegener G, MacFie J. Nasogastric intubation and elective abdominal surgery. Br J Surg 1992;79:1127–1131.
56. Nance ML, Gorman RC, Morris JB, et al. Techniques for long-term jejunal access. Contemp Surg 1995;46:21–25.
57. Collier P, Kudsk KA, Glezer J, et al. Fiber-containing formula and needle catheter jejunostomies: a clinical evaluation. Nutr Clin Pract 1994;9:101–103.
58. Antinori CH, Andrew C, Villanueva DT, et al. A technique for converting a needle-catheter jejunostomy into a standard jejunostomy. Am J Surg 1992;164:68–69.

Chapter 47

PARENTERAL NUTRITION

When full nutritional support is not possible with enteral tube feedings, the intravenous delivery of nutrients can be used to supplement or replace enteral nutrition (1,2). This chapter introduces the basic features of intravenous nutritional support (3–6) and explains how to create a total parenteral nutrition (TPN) regimen to meet the needs of individual patients.

INTRAVENOUS NUTRIENT SOLUTIONS

Dextrose Solutions

As mentioned in Chapters 45 and 46, the standard nutritional support regimen uses carbohydrates to supply approximately 70% of the daily (nonprotein) calorie requirements. These are provided by dextrose (glucose) solutions, which are available in the strengths shown in Table 47.1. Because dextrose is not a potent metabolic fuel (see Table 45.1), the dextrose solutions must be concentrated to provide enough calories to satisfy daily requirements. As a result, the dextrose solutions used for TPN are hyperosmolar and should be infused through large central veins.

Amino Acid Solutions

Amino acid solutions are mixed together with the dextrose solutions to provide the daily protein requirements. A variety of amino acid solutions are available for specific clinical settings, as demonstrated in Table 47.2. The standard amino acid solutions contain approximately 50% essential amino acids (N = 9) and 50% nonessential (N = 10) and semiessential (N = 4) amino acids (7). The nitrogen in essential amino acids is partially recycled for the production of nonessential amino acids, so the metabolism of essential amino acids produces less of a rise in the blood urea nitrogen concentration than metabolism of nonessential amino acids. For this reason, amino acid solutions designed for use in renal failure are rich in essential amino acids (see Aminosyn RF in Table 47.2). Finally,

TABLE 47.1 Intravenous Dextrose Solutions

Strength	Concentration (g/L)	Energy Yield* (kcal/L)*	Osmolarity (mOsm/L)
5%	50	170	253
10%	100	340	505
20%	200	680	1010
50%	500	1700	2525
70%	700	2380	3530

*Based on an oxidative energy yield of 3.4 kcal/g for dextrose.

for reasons stated in Chapter 46, nutritional formulas for hypercatabolic conditions (e.g., trauma) and hepatic failure can be supplemented with branched chain amino acids (isoleucine, leucine, and valine), and two specialty amino acid solutions for each of these conditions are included in Table 47.2. It is important to emphasize that none of these specialized nutrient formulas have improved the outcomes in the disorders for which they are designed (8).

Glutamine

As mentioned in Chapter 46, glutamine is the principle metabolic fuel for intestinal epithelial cells, and glutamine-supplemented TPN may play an important role in maintaining the functional integrity of the bowel mucosa and preventing bacterial translocation (9,10). Although glutamine

TABLE 47.2 Standard and Specialty Amino Acid Solutions

Features	Aminosyn 7%, (Abbott)	Aminosyn-HBC 7%, (Abbott)	Aminosyn RF 5.2%, (Abbott)	HepatAmine 8%, (McGaw)
Indication	Standard TPN	Hypercatabolism	Renal Failure	Hepatic Failure
Concentration	70 g/L	70 g/L	52 g/L	80 g/L
Nitrogen Content (g/L)	11	11.2	7.7	12
Essential AAs (% Total)	48%	68%	89%	52%
Branched Chain AAs (% Total)	25%	51%	33%	36%
Osmolarity (mOsm/L)	700	665	475	785

Borgsdorf LR, Cada DJ, Cirigliano M, et al. Drug Facts and Comparisons. 60th ed. St. Louis, MO: Wolters Kluwer, 2006.

TABLE 47.3 Amino Acid Solutions with Glutamic Acid

Preparation	Manufacturer	Glutamate Content (mg/dL)
Aminosyn-PF 7%	Abbott	576
Aminosyn II 10%	Abbott	738
Aminosyn II 15%	Abbott	1107
Novamine 11.4%	Clintec	570
Novamine 15%	Clintec	749

Borgsdorf LR, Cada DJ, Cirigliano M, et al. Drug Facts and Comparisons. 60th ed. St. Louis, MO: Wolters Kluwer, 2006.

is not an essential amino acid (because it is produced in skeletal muscle), glutamine levels in blood and tissues drop precipitously in acute, hypercatabolic conditions (e.g., trauma), so glutamine may be a "conditionally essential" amino acid (9,11). The amino acids that contain glutamic acid are shown in Table 47.3. Glutamine is formed when glutamic acid combines with ammonia in the presence of the enzyme glutamine synthetase, so glutamic acid can be an exogenous source of glutamine.

Available evidence supports the role of glutamate-containing amino acid solutions in reducing infectious complications and mortality in ICU patients (10,12,13). For this reason, glutamine supplementation is recommended (4).

Lipid Emulsions

Intravenous lipid emulsions consist of submicron droplets (≤0.45 mm) of cholesterol and phospholipids surrounding a core of long-chain triglycerides (2). The triglycerides are derived from vegetable oils (safflower or soybean oils) and are rich in linoleic acid, an essential polyunsaturated fatty acid that is not produced by the human body (14). As shown in Table 47.4, lipid emulsions are available in 10% and 20% strengths (the percentage refers to grams of triglyceride per 100 mL of solution). The 10% emulsions provide approximately 1 kcal/mL, and the 20% emulsions provide 2 kcal/mL. Unlike the hypertonic dextrose solutions, lipid emulsions are roughly isotonic to plasma and can be infused through peripheral veins. The lipid emulsions are available in unit volumes of 50 to 500 mL and can be infused separately (at a maximum rate of 50 mL/hour) or added to the dextrose–amino acid mixtures. The triglycerides introduced into the bloodstream are not cleared for 8 to 10 hours, and lipid infusions often produce a transient, lipemic-appearing (whitish) plasma.

Lipid Restriction

Lipids are used to provide up to 30% of the daily (nonprotein) calorie requirements. However, because dietary lipids are oxidation-prone and can promote oxidant-induced cell injury (15), restricting the use of lipids

TABLE 47.4 Intravenous Lipid Emulsions for Clinical Use

Feature	Intralipid* (Clintec)		Liposyn II‡ (Hospira)		Liposyn III* (Hospira)	
	10%	20%	10%	20%	10%	20%
Calories (kcal/mL)	1.1	2	1.1	2	1.1	2
% Calories as EFA (Linoleic acid)†	50%	50%	66%	66%	55%	55%
Cholesterol (mg/dL)	250–300	250–300	13–22	13–22	19–21	19–21
Osmolarity (mOsm/L)	260	260	276	258	284	292
Unit volumes (mL)	50 100 250 500	50 100 250 500	100 200 500	200 500	100 200 500	200 500

*Intralipid and Liposyn III are derived from soybean oil.
‡Liposyn II is derived from soybean oil (50%) and safflower oil (50%).
†The essential fatty acid (EFA) in lipid emulsions is linoleic acid. To prevent EFA deficiency, approximately 4% of the total daily calories should be provided by linoleic acid (Barr LH, Dunn GD, Brennan MF. Essential fatty acid deficiency during total parenteral nutrition. Ann Surg 1981;193:304–311.).
Adapted from: Borgsdorf LR, Cada DJ, Cirigliano M, et al. Drug Facts and Comparisons. 60th ed. St. Louis, MO: Wolters Kluwer, 2006.

in critically ill patients (who often have high oxidation rates) seems wise. Although lipid infusion is necessary to prevent essential fatty acid deficiency (cardiomyopathy, skeletal muscle myopathy), this can be accomplished with minimal amounts of lipid (see footnote in Table 47.4).

ADDITIVES

Commercially available mixtures of electrolytes, vitamins, and trace elements are added directly to the dextrose–amino acid mixtures.

Electrolytes

Most electrolyte mixtures contain sodium, chloride, potassium, and magnesium; they also may contain calcium and phosphorous. The daily requirement for potassium or any specific electrolyte can be specified in the TPN orders. If no electrolyte requirements are specified, the electrolytes are added to replace normal daily electrolyte losses.

TABLE 47.5 Trace Element Preparations and Daily Requirements

Trace Element	Daily Parenteral* Requirement	MTE-5‡ concentrated	MTE-6‡ concentrated
Chromium	10–15 μg	10 μg	10 μg
Copper	300–500 μg	1 mg	1 mg
Iodine	150 μg	———	75 μg
Iron†	2.5–8 mg	———	———
Manganese	60–100 μg	500 μg	500 μg
Selenium	20–60 μg	60 μg	60 μg
Zinc	2.5–5 mg	5 mg	5 mg

*Adapted from: Mirtallo J, Canada T, Johnson D, et al. Safe practices for parenteral nutrition. J Parenter Enteral Nutr 2004;28:S39–70.
‡Borgsdorf LR, Cada DJ, Cirigliano M, et al. Drug Facts and Comparisons. 60th ed. St. Louis, MO: Wolters Kluwer, 2006.
†Iron is not a routine component of premixed element supplements.

Vitamins

Aqueous multivitamin preparations are added to the dextrose–amino acid mixtures. One unit vial of a standard multivitamin preparation will provide the normal daily requirements for most vitamins (see Table 45.4) (16). Enhanced vitamin requirements in hypermetabolic patients in the ICU may not be satisfied. Furthermore, some vitamins are degraded before they are delivered. Some examples are riboflavin and pyridoxine (which are degraded by light) and thiamine (which is degraded by sulfites used as preservatives for amino acid solutions) (17).

Trace Elements

A variety of trace element additives are available, and two commercial mixtures are shown in Table 47.5. Most trace element mixtures contain chromium, copper, manganese, and zinc, but they do not contain iron and iodine. Some mixtures contain selenium, and others do not. Considering the importance of selenium in endogenous antioxidant protection (see Chapter 21), it seems wise to select a trace element additive that contains selenium. Routine administration of iron is not recommended in critically ill patients because of the pro-oxidant actions of iron (see Chapter 21, Fig. 21.5).

CREATING A TPN REGIMEN

The following stepwise approach shows how to create a TPN regimen for an individual patient. The patient in this example is a 70-kg adult who is not nutritionally depleted and has no volume restrictions.

Step 1

The first step is to estimate the daily protein and calorie requirements as described in Chapter 45. For this example, the daily calorie requirement will be 25 kcal/kg, and the daily protein requirement will be 1.4 g/kg. Therefore, for the 70-kg patient, the protein and calorie requirements are as follows:

$$\text{Calorie requirement} = 25\ (\text{kcal/kg}) \times 70\ (\text{kg}) = 1750\ \text{kcal/day}$$

$$\text{Protein requirement} = 1.4\ (\text{g/day}) \times 70\ (\text{kg}) = 98\ \text{g/day} \qquad (47.1)$$

Step 2

The next step is to take a standard mixture of 10% amino acids (500 mL) and 50% dextrose (500 mL) and determine the volume of this mixture that is needed to deliver the estimated daily protein requirement. Although the dextrose–amino acid mixture is referred to as A_{10}–D_{50}, the final mixture actually represents 5% amino acids (50 grams of protein per liter) and 25% dextrose (250 grams dextrose per liter). Therefore, the volume of the A_{10}–D_{50} mixture needed to provide the daily protein requirement is as follows:

$$\text{Volume of } A_{10}\text{–}D_{50} = 98\ (\text{g/day})/50\ (\text{g/L}) = 1.9\ \text{L/day} \qquad (47.2)$$

If this mixture is infused continuously over 24 hours, the infusion rate will be 1900 mL/24 hours = 81 mL/hour (or 81 microdrops/minute).

Step 3

Using the total daily volume of the dextrose–amino acid mixture determined in Step 2, the next step is to determine the total calories that will be provided by the dextrose in the mixture. Using an energy yield of 3.4 kcal/g for dextrose, the total dextrose calories can be determined as follows:

$$\text{Amount of dextrose} = 250\ (\text{g/L}) \times 1.9\ (\text{L/day}) = 475\ \text{g/day}$$

$$\text{Dextrose calories} = 475\ (\text{g/day}) \times 3.4\ (\text{kcal/g}) = 1615\ \text{kcal/day} \qquad (47.3)$$

Because the estimated requirement for calories is 1750 kcal/day, the dextrose will provide all but 135 kcal/day. These remaining calories can be provided by an intravenous lipid emulsion.

Step 4

If a 10% lipid emulsion (1 kcal/mL) is used to provide 135 kcal/day, the daily volume of the lipid emulsion will be 135 mL/day. Because the lipid emulsion is available in unit volumes of 50 mL, the volume can be adjusted to 150 mL/day to avoid wastage. Thus volume can be infused at half the maximum recommended rate (50 mL/hour) to minimize the tendency to develop lipemic serum during the infusion.

Step 5

The daily TPN orders for the previous example can then be written as follows:

1. Provide standard TPN with A_{10}–D_{50} to run at 80 mL/hour.
2. Add standard electrolytes, multivitamins, and trace elements.
3. Give 10% Intralipid: 150 mL to infuse over 6 hours.

TPN orders are rewritten each day. Specific electrolyte, vitamin, and trace element requirements are added to the daily orders as needed.

The example just presented applies to the separate administration of dextrose–amino acid mixtures and lipid emulsions. Another practice that is gaining popularity is to add the nutrient solutions and additives together to form a total nutrient admixture (TNA). Although this simplifies nutrient administration and reduces cost, there are lingering concerns regarding compatibility (e.g., multivitamin preparations may not be compatible with lipid emulsions).

COMPLICATIONS

A multitude of complications are associated with parenteral nutrition (6,18,19). Some of the more prominent ones are mentioned in the following paragraphs.

CATHETER-RELATED COMPLICATIONS

Because the dextrose and amino acid solutions are hyperosmolar (Tables 47.1 and 47.2), TPN is administered through a large central vein, preferably the superior vena cava. The complications associated with central venous catheters are described in Chapters 6 and 7. A misdirected catheter, like the one shown in Figure 47.1, should not be used for the administration of TPN because of the increased risk of venous thrombosis (20). Misdirected catheters can be repositioned over a guidewire as described next.

Catheter Repositioning

When a catheter has been misdirected up into the neck, the patient should be placed in a semirecumbent or upright position if possible and the catheter should be withdrawn until only a few centimeters of the catheter tip remains inserted. A flexible guidewire is then inserted through the catheter and advanced 10 cm. The catheter is removed over the guidewire,

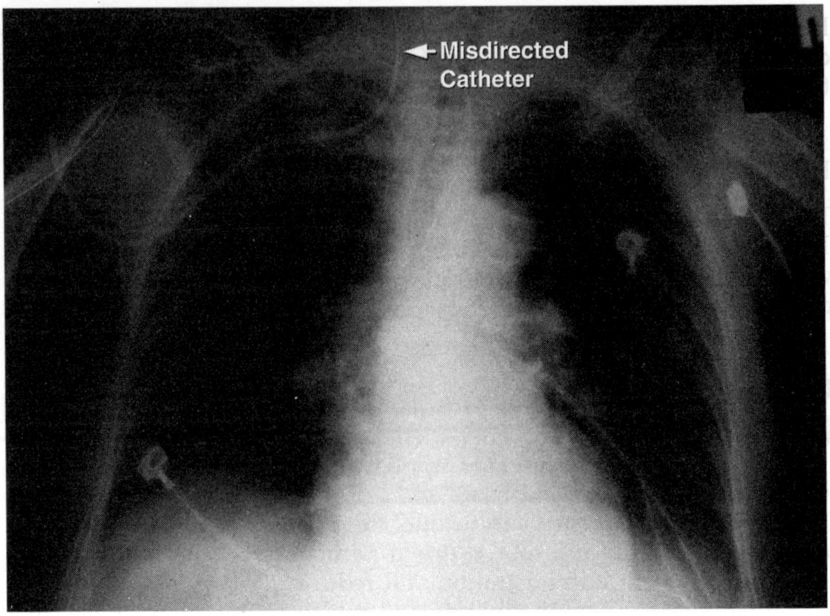

FIGURE 47.1 X-ray showing a central venous catheter misdirected into the neck. Image is digitally enhanced.

and a new catheter is inserted and advanced 15 cm. The guidewire is removed and a Doppler probe (the one used by nurses to detect pedal pulses) is placed over the internal jugular vein in the neck. A bolus of saline is then injected through the catheter. If the catheter has been rethreaded up into the neck, the bolus injection will produce an audible noise from the Doppler probe. If this occurs, a new catheter will need to be inserted into the internal jugular vein on the same side. If no sound is detected, a repeat chest x-ray study should be obtained to determine whether the catheter has been repositioned in the superior vena cava.

CARBOHYDRATE INFUSIONS

Hyperglycemia

Glucose intolerance is one of the most common complications of TPN. Even though this problem can be reduced by providing fewer nonprotein calories as glucose (and more as lipids), persistent hyperglycemia usually requires the addition of insulin to the TPN solutions. It is important to emphasize that **insulin adsorbs to all plastics and glass used in intravenous infusion sets.** The amount lost to adsorption varies with the amount of insulin added, but an average loss of 20 to 30% should be expected (21). Albumin has been used to reduce insulin binding to intravenous infusion sets (21), but this is a costly and unreliable measure.

Instead, the insulin dosage is adjusted to achieve the desired glycemic control. When TPN is discontinued, the insulin requirement will be less than that needed during TPN.

Hypophosphatemia

The effects of TPN on the serum phosphate level is shown in Figure 35.2. This effect is due to enhanced uptake of phosphate into cells associated with glucose entry into cells. The phosphate is then used to form thiamine pyrophosphate, an important cofactor in carbohydrate metabolism.

Fatty Liver

When glucose calories exceed the daily calorie requirements, there is lipogenesis in the liver and this can progress to fatty infiltration of the liver and elevated levels of transaminase enzymes in the blood (19,22). It is unclear whether this process has any pathologic consequences or whether it merely serves as a marker of excess carbohydrate calories.

Hypercapnia

Excess carbohydrates promote CO_2 retention in patients with respiratory insufficiency. Although this has been attributed to the high respiratory quotient associated with carbohydrate metabolism (see Table 45.1), this may be a reflection of overfeeding in general and not specific overfeeding with carbohydrates (23).

LIPID INFUSIONS

One of the major (and often overlooked) toxicities associated with lipid infusions is an **increased risk of oxidation-induced cell injury** (15). Lipid formulations used in TPN are rich in oxidizable lipids, and infusion of such lipids can promote organ injury similar to that seen in critically ill patients. For example, infusion of oleic acid, a fatty acid that is abundant in lipid emulsions used in TPN, is the standard method for producing the acute respiratory distress syndrome (ARDS) in animals (Am Rev Respir Dis 1994;149:245–260), and this might explain why lipid infusions in TPN formulations are associated with impaired oxygenation and prolonged respiratory failure (24,25). The possible role of lipid infusions in promoting oxidant-induced organ injury deserves more attention.

GASTROINTESTINAL COMPLICATIONS

Two indirect complications of TPN are related to the absence of bulk nutrients in the bowel.

Mucosal Atrophy

The absence of bulk nutrients in the bowel produces atrophy and disruption of the bowel mucosa. This is described in Chapter 46 and is illustrated in Figure 46.1. These changes can predispose to translocation of enteric pathogens across the bowel mucosa and subsequent septicemia. Because TPN is usually accompanied by bowel rest, one of the indirect complications of TPN is bacterial translocation and sepsis of bowel origin (9,10). As mentioned earlier, glutamine-supplemented TPN may help reduce the risk of this complication.

Acalculous Cholecystitis

The absence of lipids in the proximal small bowel prevents cholecystokinin-mediated contraction of the gallbladder and the bile stasis that results may promote acalculous cholecystitis (18). This disorder is described in Chapter 42.

PERIPHERAL PARENTERAL NUTRITION

Parenteral nutrition can occasionally be delivered via peripheral veins for short periods. The goal of peripheral parenteral nutrition (PPN) is to provide just enough nonprotein calories to spare the breakdown of proteins to provide energy (i.e., protein-sparing nutritional support). PPN does not create enough of a positive nitrogen balance to build up protein stores, and thus it is not intended for patients who are protein depleted or for patients who are hypercatabolic and at risk of becoming protein depleted.

The osmolality of peripheral vein infusates should be kept below 900 mOsm/L and the pH within the range of 7.2–7.4 to slow the rate of osmotic damage to vessels (26,27). Therefore, PPN must be delivered with dilute amino acid and dextrose solutions. Because lipid emulsions are isotonic to plasma, lipids can be used to provide a significant proportion of the nonprotein calories in PPN.

Method

A common admixture used in PPN is a mixture of 3% amino acids and 20% dextrose. This mixture produces a final concentration of 1.5% amino acids (15 grams of protein per liter) and 10% dextrose (100 grams of dextrose per liter), with an osmolarity of approximately 500 mOsm/L. The dextrose will provide 340 kcal/L, so 2.5 L of the mixture will provide 850 kcal. If 250 mL of 20% Intralipid is added to the regimen (adding 500 kcal), the total nonprotein calories will increase to 1350 kcal/day. This should be close to the nonprotein calorie requirement of an average-size adult at rest (25 kcal/kg/day). In hypermetabolic patients, large volumes of PPN are required to satisfy daily energy requirements.

In summary, peripheral intravenous nutrition can be used as a temporary measure to prevent or limit protein breakdown in patients who are not already protein depleted and are expected to begin oral feedings within a few days. Postoperative patients seem best suited for this form of nutritional support.

A FINAL WORD

The final word on parenteral nutrition is . . *avoid* . . (whenever possible). For an explanation, see the FINAL WORD section of the last chapter.

REFERENCES

Guidelines & Reviews

1. Dudrick SJ. Early developments and clinical applications of total parenteral nutrition. J Parenter Enteral Nutr 2003;27:291–299.
2. Driscoll DF. Compounding TPN admixtures: then and now. J Parenter Enteral Nutr 2003;27:433–438.
3. Mirtallo J, Canada T, Johnson D, et al. Safe practices for parenteral nutrition. J Parenter Enteral Nutr 2004;28:S39–70.
4. Heyland DK, Dhaliwal R, Drover JW, et al. Canadian clinical practice guidelines for nutrition support in mechanically ventilated, critically ill adult patients. J Parenter Enteral Nutr 2003;27:355–373.
5. American Gastroenterological Association. Medical position statement: parenteral nutrition. Gastroenterology 2001;121:966–969.
6. Zaloga GP. Parenteral nutrition in adult inpatients with functioning gastrointestinal tracts: assessment of outcomes. Lancet 2006;367:1101–1111.

Intravenous Nutrient Solutions

7. Borgsdorf LR, Cada DJ, Cirigliano M, et al. Drug facts and comparisons. 60th ed. St. Louis, MO: Wolters Kluwer, 2006.
8. Andris DA, Krzywda EA. Nutrition support in specific diseases: back to basics. Nutr Clin Pract 1994;9:28–32.
9. Souba WW, Klimberg VS, Plumley DA, et al. The role of glutamine in maintaining a healthy gut and supporting the metabolic response to injury and infection. J Surg Res 1990;48:383–391.
10. De-Souza DA, Greene LJ. Intestinal permeability and systemic infections in critically ill patients: effect of glutamine. Crit Care Med 2005;33:1125–1135.
11. Wischmeyer PE. The glutamine story: where are we now? Curr Opin Crit Care 2006;12:142–148.
12. Dechelotte P, Hasselmann M, Cynober L, et al. L-Alanyl-L-glutamine dipeptide-supplemented total parenteral nutrition reduces infectious complications and glucose intolerance in critically ill patients: the French controlled, randomized, double-blind, multicenter study. Crit Care Med 2006;34:598–604.
13. Fuentes-Orozco C, Anaya-Prado R, Gonzalez-Ojeda A, et al. L-Alanyl-L-glutamine-supplemented parenteral nutrition improves infectious morbidity in secondary peritonitis. Clin Nutr 2004;23:13–21.

14. Warshawsky KY. Intravenous fat emulsions in clinical practice. Nutr Clin Pract 1992;7:187–196.
15. Carpentier YA, Dupont IE. Advances in intravenous lipid emulsions. World J Surg 2000;24:1493–1497.
16. Helphingstine CJ, Bistrian BR. New Food and Drug Administration requirements for inclusion of vitamin K in adult parenteral multivitamins. J Parenter Enteral Nutr 2003;27:220–224.
17. Brown RO, Minard G. Parenteral feeding. In: Shils ME, et al., eds. Modern nutrition in health and disease. 10th ed. Philadelphia, PA: Lippincott, Williams & Wilkins, 2006:1567–1597.

COMPLICATIONS

18. Phelps SJ, Brown RO, Helms RA, et al. Toxicities of parenteral nutrition in the critically ill patient. Crit Care Clin 1991;7:725–753.
19. Perry DA, Markin RS, Rose SG, et al. Changes in laboratory values in patients receiving total parenteral nutrition. Lab Med 1990;21:97–102.
20. Padberg FT Jr, Ruggiero J, Blackburn GL, et al. Central venous catheterization for parenteral nutrition. Ann Surg 1981;193:264–270.
21. Trissel LA. Handbook on injectable drugs. 13th ed. Bethesda, MD: American Society Health System Pharmacists, 2005.
22. Freund HR. Abnormalities of liver function and hepatic damage associated with total parenteral nutrition. Nutrition 1991;7:1–5.
23. Talpers SS, Romberger DJ, Bunce SB, et al. Nutritionally associated increased carbon dioxide production: excess total calories vs high proportion of carbohydrate calories. Chest 1992;102:551–555.
24. Suchner U, Katz DP, Furst P, et al. Effects of intravenous fat emulsions on lung function in patients with acute respiratory distress syndrome or sepsis. Crit Care Med 2001;29:1569–1574.
25. Battistella FD, Widergren JT, Anderson JT, et al. A prospective, randomized trial of intravenous fat emulsion administration in trauma victims requiring total parenteral nutrition. J Trauma 1997;43:52–58.

PERIPHERAL PARENTERAL NUTRITION

26. Culebras JM, Martin-Pena G, Garcia-de-Lorenzo A, et al. Practical aspects of peripheral parenteral nutrition. Curr Opin Clin Nutr Metab Care 2004;7:303–307.
27. Anderson AD, Palmer D, MacFie J. Peripheral parenteral nutrition. Br J Surg 2003;90:1048–1054.

Chapter 48

ADRENAL AND THYROID DYSFUNCTION

Endocrine disorders that involve the adrenal and thyroid glands are noted for their ability to act as catalysts for serious, life-threatening conditions while escaping notice themselves. This chapter explains how to unmask an underlying or occult disorder of adrenal or thyroid function and how to treat each disorder appropriately.

ADRENAL INSUFFICIENCY

The adrenal gland plays a major role in the adaptive response to stress. The adrenal cortex releases glucocorticoids and mineralocorticoids that promote glucose availability and maintain extracellular volume, while the adrenal medulla releases catecholamines that support the circulation. Attenuation or loss of this adrenal response leads to hemodynamic instability, volume depletion, and defective energy metabolism. The important feature of adrenal insufficiency is its ability to remain silent until the adrenal gland is called on to respond to a physiologic stress. When this occurs, adrenal insufficiency becomes an occult catalyst that speeds the progression of acute, life-threatening conditions.

Adrenal insufficiency can be a primary (inability of the adrenal gland to elaborate cortisol) or secondary disorder (inability of the hypothalamic–pituitary axis to release ACTH). The description that follows pertains to primary adrenal insufficiency, and how it behaves in the critically ill patient (1–4).

Plasma Cortisol

In healthy subjects, 90% of the cortisol in plasma is bound to corticosteroid-binding globulin and albumin, and only 10% is in the free or biologically active form (1,5). The evaluation of adrenal function is based on a radioimmunoassay that measures total cortisol in plasma (bound and unbound fractions). Unfortunately, this can be misleading in acutely ill patients because the cortisol transport proteins are often decreased in these patients (5). For example, one study of septic patients revealed that total cortisol levels are diminished in 40% of patients, while free cortisol levels are consistently elevated (5). The **inability to measure free cortisol levels in plasma is a major problem** that must be considered in interpreting tests of adrenal function in critically ill patients.

Predisposing Conditions

Several conditions that are common in ICU patients can predispose to primary adrenal insufficiency. These include major surgery, circulatory failure, septic shock, severe coagulopathy, and human immunodeficiency virus (HIV) infections (1,2). In some of these conditions, the adrenal insufficiency is caused by pathologic destruction of the adrenal gland (e.g., coagulopathy with adrenal hemorrhage), while in others, there is diminished adrenal responsiveness (e.g., septic shock). In addition, some of the drugs that are used in critically ill patients can decrease cortisol levels by either inhibiting synthesis (e.g., etomidate and ketoconazole) or accelerating metabolism (e.g., phenytoin or rifampin) (1,2).

Incidence

In surveys of randomly-selected ICU patients, the incidence of adrenal insufficiency is approximately 30% (2). In patients with septic shock, the incidence is higher at 50–60% (2,4). In many of these cases, adrenal insufficiency was not evident clinically but was uncovered by biochemical evidence of abnormal adrenal responsiveness (2,4). In ICU patients with laboratory evidence of adrenal insufficiency, the mortality rate is as much as twice that of patients with normal adrenal responsiveness (6–8).

Clinical Manifestations

In critically ill patients, the most prominent manifestation of adrenal insufficiency is **hypotension that is refractory to vasopressors** (1,2,7,8). Other features of adrenal insufficiency, such as electrolyte abnormalities (hyponatremia, hyperkalemia), weakness, and hyperpigmentation, are either uncommon or not specific enough to suggest the diagnosis in ICU patients.

Hemodynamics

In mild or chronic cases of adrenal insufficiency, the hemodynamic changes are often a reflection of hypovolemia (low filling pressures, low cardiac output, high systemic vascular resistance). In acute adrenal failure, the hemodynamic changes are similar to those of hyperdynamic shock (high cardiac output, low systemic vascular resistance) (1,9). Because many cases of adrenal insufficiency are uncovered in patients with septic shock, where the hemodynamic changes are similar to those of acute adrenal failure (i.e., hyperdynamic shock), it is often impossible to identify adrenal failure based on hemodynamic profiles in critically ill patients.

Clinical Suspicion

Adrenal insufficiency should be suspected in any patient in the ICU who develops an unstable or reduced blood pressure of unclear etiology, or has hypotension that is refractory to fluid resuscitation and vasopressors.

EVALUATION OF ADRENAL FUNCTION

The diagnostic test of choice for primary adrenal insufficiency in ICU patients is the rapid adrenocorticotropic hormone (ACTH) stimulation test (1). This test evaluates the acute adrenal response to a bolus injection of synthetic ACTH (cosyntropin).

Rapid ACTH Stimulation Test

The rapid ACTH stimulation test can be performed at any time of the day or night because it is not influenced by diurnal variations in cortisol secretion (which are often absent in critically ill patients anyway) (2). An initial blood sample is obtained for a plasma cortisol level, and synthetic ACTH (250 μg) is injected intravenously. A post-ACTH plasma cortisol level is then obtained at 30 and 60 minutes after the ACTH injection.

Interpretation

The interpretation of the ACTH stimulation test is outlined in Table 48.1 (1). Both the baseline cortisol level and the increment in cortisol at 30 or 60 minutes (whichever is greater) are used to evaluate adrenal function. A baseline cortisol level that is above 34 μg/dL (940 nmol/L) is evidence of normal or adequate adrenal function, while a baseline cortisol level that is below 15 μg/dL (415 nmol/L) is evidence of adrenal insufficiency. When the baseline cortisol level is between 15 and 34 μg/dL (415 and 940 nmol/L), the increment in plasma cortisol is used in the

TABLE 48.1 Interpretation of the Rapid ACTH Stimulation Test in Critically Ill Patients

Plasma Cortisol in μg/dL*		Probability of
Baseline	Increment	Adrenal Insufficiency
<15	⟶	Very High†
15–34	<9	High†
15–34	>9	Low
>34	⟶	Very Low

*To convert μg/dL to nmol/L, multiply by 27.6.
†Consider corticosteroid replacement therapy.
From Cooper MS, Stewart PM. Corticosteroid insufficiency in critically ill patients. N Engl J Med 2003;348:727–734.

interpretation: an increment that is greater than 9 μg/dL (250 nmol/L) is evidence of normal or adequate adrenal function, while an increment that is less than 9 μg/dL (250 nmol/L) is evidence of adrenal insufficiency.

Steroid Therapy

In patients with suspected adrenal insufficiency who have severe or refractory hypotension, **steroids can be started immediately, before the ACTH stimulation test is performed.** Steroid administration can proceed as follows:

1. Dexamethasone (Decadron) will not interfere with plasma cortisol assay (2) and can be given before or during the ACTH stimulation test. The initial dose should be 2 mg (as an IV bolus), which is equivalent to 270 mg of hydrocortisone (cortisol) (2).
2. After the ACTH stimulation test is completed, empiric therapy can begin with hydrocortisone (Solu-Cortef). The dose is 50 mg IV every 6 hours until the test results are available.
3. If the ACTH stimulation test is normal, the hydrocortisone can be abruptly discontinued, without a taper. If the test reveals primary adrenal insufficiency, the hydrocortisone should be continued at 50 mg IV every 6 hours until the patient is no longer in a stressed condition (1). When this occurs, the daily dose of hydrocortisone should be reduced to 20 mg (which is equivalent to the amount of cortisol secreted daily by the adrenal glands).

Limitations in Adrenal Function Testing

The evaluation of adrenal function is limited in critically ill patients for the following reasons:

1. There is no standard definition of adrenal insufficiency in ICU patients (1,2,6).
2. Cortisol transport proteins in blood are diminished in acutely ill patients, and this invalidates the assessment of adrenal function based on total plasma cortisol (rather than free plasma cortisol) levels.
3. Cytokines released during inflammation can blunt end-organ responsiveness to cortisol (1), which means that blood cortisol levels will underestimate the severity of abnormal adrenal responsiveness in patients with systemic inflammation.
4. The appropriate dose of ACTH to use for the rapid ACTH stimulation test is unclear. The standard dose (250 μg) is 100 times the maximal pituitary output of ACTH, and the excessive adrenal stimulation from this dose could mask a case of adrenal insufficiency that occurs during physiologic conditions of adrenal stimulation (2,6). A small dose of ACTH (1 μg) may be more appropriate for matching the level of adrenal stimulation that occurs during clinical illness (2,6).

5. In cases of vasopressor-dependent septic shock, the ACTH stimulation test does not predict which patients will benefit from corticosteroid supplemenation (10).

Because of these limitations, a clinical suspicion of adrenal insufficiency might be sufficient enough to begin an empiric trial of steroids (e.g., hydrocortisone, 50 mg IV every 6 hours), and then assess the clinical response.

EVALUATION OF THYROID FUNCTION

Laboratory tests of thyroid function can be abnormal in 70% of hospitalized patients and in up to 90% of critically ill patients (11). In most cases, the abnormality represents an adaptive response to non-thyroidal (systemic) illness and is not a sign of pathologic thyroid disease (11,12). This section describes the laboratory evaluation of thyroid function and explains how to determine if a laboratory abnormality represents a true disorder of thyroid function (11–13).

Thyroxine (T_4) and Triiodothyronine (T_3)

Thyroxine (T_4) is the principal hormone secreted by the thyroid gland, but the active form is triiodothyronine (T_3), which is formed by deiodination of thyroxine in extrathyroidal tissues. Both T_3 and T_4 are extensively (>99%) bound to plasma proteins, especially thyroxine-binding globulin. Approximately 0.2% of the total T_3 is in the unbound or physiologically active form. Because of the minor representation of unbound T_3 and T_4 in plasma, and the potential for plasma protein concentrations to vary in ICU patients, **only measurements of free T_3 and T_4 should be performed** in ICU patients.

Thyroid-Stimulating Hormone (TSH)

For patients who have an abnormal level of free T_3 or T_4 in plasma, the thyroid-stimulating hormone (TSH) level in plasma can help to identify those with primary thyroid disorders (hyperthyroidism hypothyroidism), secondary thyroid disorders (hypothalamic-pituitary dysfunction), and non-thyroidal illness. The negative feedback exerted by the thyroid hormones on TSH secretion allows the TSH to distinguish primary from secondary thyroid disorders. For example, in patients with an abnormally low level of free T_4 in plasma, an elevated TSH level is evidence for primary hypothyroidism, while a reduced TSH level is evidence for hypothyroidism secondary to hypothalamic–pituitary dysfunction.

Non-Thyroidal Illness

The TSH level can also help to identify patients with non-thyroidal illness. For example, in patients with a low level of free T_4 in plasma, a normal TSH level is evidence of non-thyroidal illness. The TSH level is

TABLE 48.2 Common Patterns of Thyroid Function Tests in Critically Ill Patients

Condition	Free T_4	Free T_3	TSH
Non-thyroidal illness:			
Early systemic illness	NL	↓	NL
Early critical illness	↓	↓	NL
Chronic critical illness (>2 days)	↓	↓	↓ or NL
Thyroid disease:			
Primary hypothyroidism	↓	↓	↑
Primary hyperthyroidism	↑	↑	↓

Adapted from: Dayan CM. Interpretation of thyroid function tests. Lancet 2001;357:619–624. Peeters RP, Debaveye Y, Fliers E, et al. Changes within the thyroid axis during critical illness. Crit Care Clin 2006;22:41–55.

normal in a majority of patients with non-thyroidal illness, but it can be reduced in 30% and elevated in 10% of these patients (11). TSH secretion can be depressed by sepsis, corticosteroids, diphenylhydantoin, and dopamine infusions (14), and these factors must be considered when interpreting plasma TSH levels.

Patterns of Thyroid Function Abnormalities

The changes in free T_4, free T_3, and TSH levels in both thyroid disease and non-thyroidal illness are shown in Table 48.2.

Non-Thyroidal Illness

Thyroid function abnormalities secondary to systemic illness (e.g., trauma or infection) occur in 70% of hospitalized patients (11,12,15). Within a few hours following the onset of illness, free T_3 is decreased in proportion to illness severity (11). With increasing illness severity, both free T_3 and free T_4 levels are depressed (this pattern occurs in 30 to 50% of ICU patients), and this pattern is associated with an increase in mortality (11,12). After several days of critical illness, there is a further decline in free T_3 levels, and TSH levels may be decreased (11,12). As explained earlier, TSH levels are normal in a majority of patients with non-thyroidal illness.

Thyroid Disorders

Primary thyroid disorders are characterized by changes in both free T_3 and free T_4 levels (increased in hyperthyroidism and decreased in hypothyroidism) with reciprocal changes in the plasma TSH level. Hypothyroidism due to hypothalamic-pituitary dysfunction is characterized by a reduced TSH level, as explained earlier. The salient features of thyroid disorders in critically ill patients are presented next (13).

TABLE 48.3 Manifestations of Thyroid Dysfunction

Hyperthyroidism	Hypothyroidism
Cardiovascular:	Effusions:
Sinus tachycardia	Pericardial effusion
Atrial fibrillation	Pleural effusion
Neurologic:	Miscellaneous:
Agitation	Hyponatremia
Lethargy (elderly)	Skeletal muscle myopathy
Fine tremors	Elevated creatinine
Thyroid Storm:	Myxedema Coma:
Fever	Hypothermia
Hyperdynamic shock	Dermal infiltration
Depressed consciousness	Depressed consciousness

HYPERTHYROIDISM

Most cases of hyperthyroidism are due to primary thyroid disorders (e.g., Grave's disease, autoimmune thyroiditis). Chronic therapy with amiodarone, an iodine-containing antiarrhythmic agent, can also cause hyperthyroidism (16,17).

Clinical Manifestations

Some of the common or characteristic manifestations of hyperthyroidism are listed in Table 48.3. It is important to note that **elderly patients with hyperthyroidism may be lethargic** rather than agitated (apathetic thyrotoxicosis). The combination of lethargy and unexplained atrial fibrillation is characteristic of apathetic thyrotoxicosis in the elderly (18).

Thyroid Storm

An uncommon but severe form of hyperthyroidism known as *thyroid storm* can be precipitated by acute illness or surgery. This condition, characterized by fever, severe agitation, and high-output heart failure, can progress to hypotension and coma (19,20) and is uniformly fatal if overlooked and left untreated.

Diagnosis

As shown in Table 48.2, hyperthyroidism will be accompanied by an elevated free T_4 and free T_3 level, and a reduced TSH level. Because hyperthyroidism is almost always caused by primary thyroid disease, the TSH is not necessary in hyperthyroidism.

Management

β-*Receptor Antagonists*

Immediate management of troublesome tachyarrhythmias can be achieved by administering intravenous propanolol (1 mg every 5 minutes until the desired effect is achieved). Oral maintenance therapy (20 to 120 mg every 6 hours) can be used until antithyroid drug therapy is effective.

Antithyroid Drugs

The two drugs used to suppress thyroxine production are methimazole and propylthiouracil (PTU). Both drugs are given orally. **Methimazole is preferred** to PTU because it causes a more rapid decline in serum thyroxine levels and has a lower incidence of serious side effects (agranulocytosis) (21). The initial dose of methimazole is **10 to 30 mg once a day,** and the initial dose of PTU is 75 to 100 mg three times daily (19,21). The dose of both drugs is reduced by 50% after 4 to 6 weeks of therapy.

Iodide

In severe cases of hyperthyroidism, iodide (which blocks thyroxine release from the thyroid gland) can be added to therapy with PTU. Iodide can be given orally as Lugol's solution (4 drops every 12 hours) or intravenously as sodium iodide (500 to 1,000 mg every 12 hours). If the patient has an iodide allergy, lithium (300 mg orally every 8 hours) can be used as a substitute (20).

Special Concerns in Thyroid Storm

In addition to the above measures, the management of thyroid storm often requires aggressive volume resuscitation to replace fluid losses from vomiting, diarrhea, and heightened insensible fluid loss. Thyroid storm can accelerate glucocorticoid metabolism and create a relative adrenal insufficiency. Therefore, in cases of thyroid storm associated with severe or refractory hypotension, hydrocortisone (300 mg IV as a loading dose, followed by 100 mg IV every 8 hours) may help correct the hypotension. Successful management of thyroid storm also requires treatment of the precipitating event (20,22).

HYPOTHYROIDISM

Hypothyroidism is uncommon in hospitalized patients. When present, most cases represent primary hypothyroidism (23).

Clinical Manifestations

Some of the more common or characteristic manifestations of hypothyroidism are listed in Table 48.3. The most common cardiovascular manifestation is **pericardial effusion** (24), which develops in approximately 30% of cases, and is the most common cause of an enlarged cardiac silhouette in patients with hypothyroidism (24). These effusions usually accumulate slowly and do not cause cardiac compromise. Pleural effusions are also common in hypothyroidism. The pleural and pericardial effusions are due to an increase in capillary permeability and are exudative in quality.

Hypothyroidism can also be associated with hyponatremia and a skeletal muscle myopathy, with elevations in muscle enzymes (creatine phosphokinase, aldolase, lactate dehydrogenase). Enhanced release of creatinine from skeletal muscles can also raise the serum creatinine in the absence of renal dysfunction (25).

Myxedema Coma

Advanced cases of hypothyroidism are accompanied by hypothermia and depressed consciousness. Although this condition is called myxedema coma, frank coma is uncommon (26). The edematous appearance in myxedema is due to intradermal accumulation of proteins (26) and does not represent accumulation of interstitial edema fluid.

Diagnosis

As shown in Table 48.2, the hypothyroid patient will have a decrease in free T_3 and free T_4 levels, and in primary hypothyroidism, the TSH level is elevated. A normal total serum T_4 level will virtually exclude the diagnosis of hypothyroidism.

Thyroid Replacement Therapy

The treatment for mild to moderate hypothyroidism is levothyroxine, which is given orally in a single daily dose of 50 to 200 µg (27). The initial dose is usually 50 µg/day, and this is increased in 50 µg/day increments every 3 to 4 weeks. The optimal replacement dose of levothyroxine is determined by monitoring the serum TSH level. The optimal dose is the lowest dose of levothyroxine that returns the TSH to within the normal range (0.5 to 3.5 mU/L). In 90% of cases, this occurs with a levothyroxine dose of 100 to 200 µg/day (27).

Oral thyroxine therapy can also be effective in severe hypothyroidism, but intravenous therapy is often recommended (at least initially) because of the risk of impaired gastrointestinal motility in severe hypothyroidism. One recommended regimen includes an initial intravenous thyroxine dose of 250 µg, followed on the next day by a dose of 100 µg, and followed thereafter by a daily dose of 50 µg (26).

T Replacement Therapy

Because the conversion of T_4 to T_3 (the active form of thyroid hormone) can be depressed in critically ill patients (26), oral therapy with T_3 can be used to supplement thyroxine replacement therapy. In patients with depressed consciousness, oral T_3 can be given in a dose of 25 µg every 12 hours until the patient awakens (28). However, the benefits of T_3 supplementation are unproven.

A FINAL WORD

Adrenal insufficiency is considered to be common in critically ill patients, but it is difficult to determine how common it is because the rapid ACTH stimulation test is fraught with problems (e.g, which dose of ACTH to use, measuring total cortisol instead of free cortisol, etc). Patients with septic shock, severe coagulopathies, and HIV infection seem to be particularly prone to adrenal insufficiency. When a patient with any of these conditions develops unexplained hypotension or hypotension that is difficult to control with fluids and pressors, adrenal insufficency deserves consideration. You can give steroids first and then do the rapid ACTH stimulation test (don't use hydrocortisone if you are planning to do the test), or just give steroids (hydrocortisone) and see what happens. A response to hydrocortisone should be readily apparent if adrenal insufficency is a problem.

REFERENCES

Reviews: Adrenal Dysfunction

1. Cooper MS, Stewart PM. Corticosteroid insufficiency in acutely ill patients. N Engl J Med 2003;348:727–734.
2. Marik PE, Zaloga GP. Adrenal insufficiency in the critically ill: a new look at an old problem. Chest 2002;122:1784–1796.
3. Prigent H, Maxime V, Annane D. Clinical review: corticotherapy in sepsis. Crit Care 2004;8:122–129.
4. Annane D, Sebille V, Troche G, et al. A 3-level prognostic classification in septic shock based on cortisol levels and cortisol response to corticotropin. JAMA 2000;283:1038–1045.

Adrenal Insufficiency

5. Hamrahian AH, Oseni TS, Arafah BM. Measurements of serum free cortisol in critically ill patients. N Engl J Med 2004;350:1629–1638.
6. Siraux V, De Backer D, Yalavatti G, et al. Relative adrenal insufficiency in patients with septic shock: comparison of low-dose and conventional corticotropin tests. Crit Care Med 2005;33:2479–2486.
7. Rothwell PM, Udwadia ZF, Lawler PG. Cortisol response to corticotropin and survival in septic shock. Lancet 1991;337:582–583.
8. Soni A, Pepper GM, Wyrwinski PM, et al. Adrenal insufficiency occurring during septic shock: incidence, outcome, and relationship to peripheral cytokine levels. Am J Med 1995;98:266–271.
9. Dorin RI, Kearns PJ. High output circulatory failure in acute adrenal insufficiency. Crit Care Med 1988;16:296–297.
10. Morel J, Venet C, Donati Y, et al. Adrenal axis function does not appear to be associated with hemodynamic improvement in septic shock patients systematically receiving glucocorticoid therapy. Intensive Care Med 2006;32:1184–1190.
11. Umpierrez GE. Euthyroid sick syndrome. South Med J 2002;95:506–513.

Evaluation of Thyroid Function

12. Peeters RP, Debaveye Y, Fliers E, et al. Changes within the thyroid axis during critical illness. Crit Care Clin 2006;22:41–55.
13. Dayan CM. Interpretation of thyroid function tests. Lancet 2001;357;619–624.
14. Burman KD, Wartofsky L. Thyroid function in the intensive care unit setting. Crit Care Clin 2001;17:43–57.
15. Fliers E, Alkemade A, Wiersinga WM. The hypothalamic-pituitary-thyroid axis in critical illness. Best Pract Res Clin Endocrinol Metab 2001;15:453–464.

Hyperthyroidism

16. Surks MI, Sievert R. Drugs and thyroid function. N Engl J Med 1995;333:1688–1694.
17. Trip MD, Wiersinga W, Plomp TA. Incidence, predictability, and pathogenesis of amiodarone-induced thyrotoxicosis and hypothyroidism. Am J Med 1991; 91:507–511.
18. Klein I. Thyroid hormone and the cardiovascular system. Am J Med 1990; 88:631–637.
19. Franklyn JA. The management of hyperthyroidism. N Engl J Med 1994;330: 1731–1738.
20. Migneco A, Ojetti V, Testa A, et al. Management of thyrotoxic crisis. Eur Rev Med Pharmacol Sci 2005;9:69–74.
21. Cooper DS. Hyperthyroidism. Lancet 2003;362:459–468.
22. Ehrmann DA, Sarne DH. Early identification of thyroid storm and myxedema coma. Crit Illness 1988;3:111–118.

Hypothyroidism

23. Roberts CG, Ladenson PW. Hypothyroidism. Lancet 2004;363:793–803.
24. Ladenson PW. Recognition and management of cardiovascular disease related to thyroid dysfunction. Am J Med 1990;88:638–641.
25. Lafayette RA, Costa ME, King AJ. Increased serum creatinine in the absence of renal failure in profound hypothyroidism. Am J Med 1994;96:298–299.
26. Myers L, Hays J. Myxedema coma. Crit Care Clin 1991;7:43–56.
27. Toft AD. Thyroxine therapy. N Engl J Med 1994;331:174–180.
28. McCulloch W, Price P, Hinds CJ, et al. Effects of low dose oral triiodothyronine in myxoedema coma. Intensive Care Med 1985;11:259–262.

Section **XV**

CRITICAL CARE NEUROLOGY

There is no delusion more damaging than to get the idea in your head that you understand the functioning of your own brain.

LEWIS THOMAS

Chapter 49

ANALGESIA AND SEDATION

Pain is a more terrible lord of mankind than even death itself.

Albert Schweitzer

Contrary to popular perception, our principal function in patient care is not to save lives (since this is impossible on a consistent basis), but to relieve pain and suffering. And there is no place in the hospital that can match the pain and suffering experienced by patients in the intensive care unit. If you want an idea of how prepared we are to relieve pain and suffering in the ICU, take a look at Figure 49.1.

This chapter focuses on the use of intravenous analgesics and sedatives to achieve patient comfort in the ICU. Several reviews on this topic are included at the end of the chapter (1–5).

PAIN IN THE ICU

Although a majority of ICU patients receive parenteral analgesics routinely (6), 50% of patients discharged from the ICU remember pain as their worst experience while in the ICU (7). This emphasizes the need for effective pain control in the ICU.

Opiophobia

The problem of inadequate pain control is partly due to misconceptions about the addictive potential of opioids, and about the appropriate dose needed to relieve pain (8,9). The following statements are directed at these misconceptions.

1. Opioid use in hospitalized patients does not cause drug addiction (8).

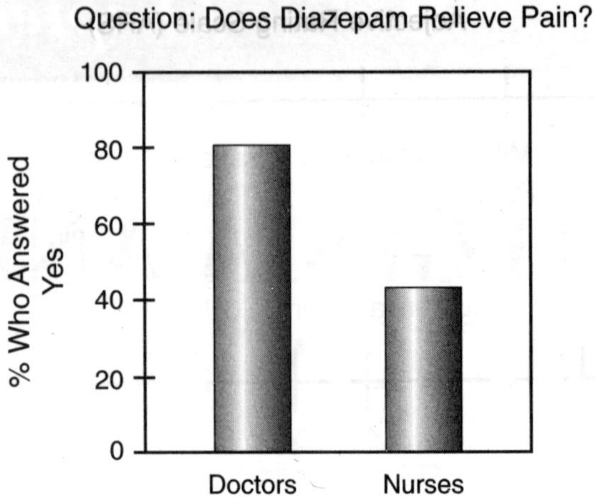

FIGURE 49.1 Percentage of house staff physicians and ICU nurses who answered incorrectly when asked if diazepam (Valium) is an analgesic. (From Loper KA, et al. Paralyzed with pain: the need for education. Pain 1989;37:315.)

2. The effective dose of an opioid should be determined by patient response and not by some predetermined notion of what an effective dose should be (2).

Avoiding irrational fears about opioids (*opiophobia*) is an important step in providing adequate pain relief for your patients.

Monitoring Pain

Pain is a subjective sensation that can be described in terms of intensity, duration, location, and quality (e.g., sharp, dull). Pain intensity is the parameter most often monitored because it best reflects the degree of discomfort. The intensity of pain can be recorded using a variety of scales like the ones shown in Figure 49.2. The uppermost scale (Adjective Rating Scale) uses descriptive terms, the middle scale (Numerical Ranking Scale) uses whole numbers, and the lower scale (Visual Analog Scale) records pain intensity as a discrete point placed along a line between the ends of the pain intensity spectrum.

Pain intensity scales can be used to evaluate the effect of analgesic regimens in individual patients. A numerical score of 3 or less on the Numerical Rating Scale or Visual Analog Scale can be used as evidence of effective analgesia. However, it seems easier to just ask patients if their pain is well controlled. Direct communication with patients is not only the best method of determining comfort needs, it is itself a source of comfort to patients. When critically ill patients are unable to communicate directly about pain intensity, the use of surrogate signs of pain such as physiological parameters (e.g., heart rate) or elicited behaviors (e.g., facial expressions) is an unproven and probably inappropriate practice (2,10).

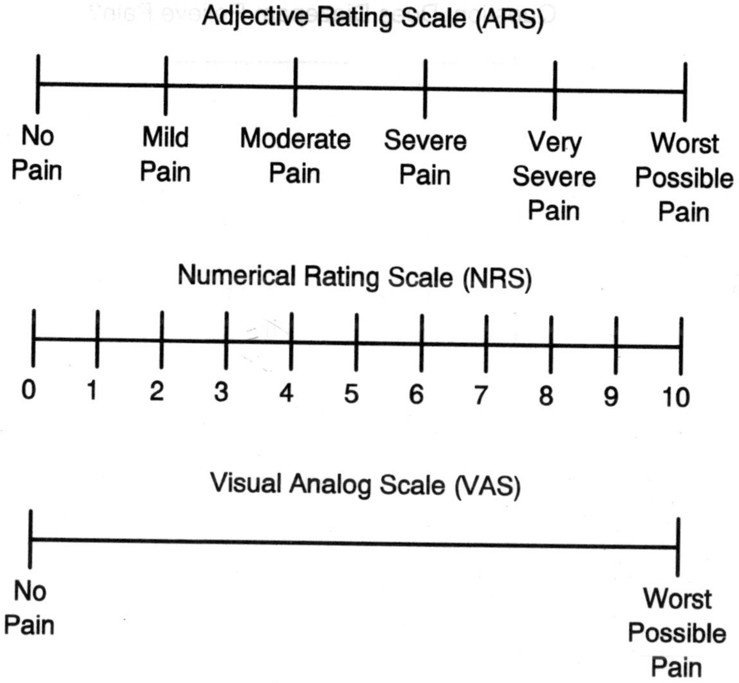

FIGURE 49.2 Three different scales for recording pain intensity. The recommended length for the numeric scales (NRS and VAS) is 10 cm. (For more information on recording pain intensity, see Hamill-Ruth RJ, Marohn ML. Evaluation of pain in the critically ill patient. Crit Care Clin 1999;15: 35.)

OPIOID ANALGESIA

The natural chemical derivatives of opium are called *opiates*. Opiates and other substances that produce their effects by stimulating discrete opioid receptors in the central nervous system are called *opioids*. Stimulation of opioid receptors produces a variety of effects, including analgesia, sedation, euphoria, pupillary constriction, respiratory depression, bradycardia, constipation, nausea, vomiting, urinary retention, and pruritis (11). *Narcotic* (from the Greek *narkotikos*, to benumb) refers to the general class of drugs that blunt sensation and produce euphoria, stupor, or coma.

Opioids are the agents most frequently used for pain relief *and* mild sedation in the ICU (5,6,12). They are most effective for relieving dull tonic pain, less effective for intermittent sharp pain, and relatively ineffective for neuropathic pain. Although opioids cause mild sedation, they do not cause amnesia (unless the patient goes to sleep!) (13).

Intravenous Opioids

The opioids used most often in the ICU are morphine, fentanyl, and hydromorphone (5,6,12). The intravenous administration of these agents

TABLE 49.1 Intravenous Opioid Analgesia

	Morphine	Hydromorphone	Fentanyl
Loading dose	5–10 mg	1–1.5 mg	50–100 μg
Onset of action	10–20 min	5–15 min	1–2 min
Duration (after bolus)	2–3.5 hrs	2–3 hrs	30–60 min
Infusion rate*	1–5 mg/hr	0.2–0.5 mg/hr	50–350 μg/hr
PCA			
demand (bolus)	0.5–3 mg	0.1–0.5 mg	15–75 μg
lockout interval	10–20 min	5–15 min	3–10 min
Potency	x	5x	100x
Lipid solubility	x	0.2x	600x
Active metabolites	Yes	Yes	No
Histamine release	Yes	No	No
Dose adjustment for GFR <10 mL/min	Decrease by 50%	None	Decrease by 0–50%
Cost per 24 hrs†	5 mg/hr: $16	0.75 mg/hr: $10	100 μg/hr: $5.50

*Initial infusion rate. May need further adjustment.
†Based on average wholesale price in 2006.
Adapted from References 1, 2, 14–16.

is described in Table 49.1. The doses shown in this table are the usual effective doses, but individual dose requirements can vary widely. Remember that **the effective dose of an opioid is determined by each patient's response, not by the numeric value of the dose** (2,16). Continued pain relief often requires continued drug administration, either as a continuous infusion or by regularly scheduled drug dosages. Intermittent, **as-needed (PRN) drug administration** is a recipe for inadequate pain control and **is never recommended** (1,2).

Fentanyl versus Morphine

Morphine is the most frequently used opioid in ICUs (12), but fentanyl may be preferred because it is faster acting, devoid of active metabolites, and less likely to decrease blood pressure. Because fentanyl is 600 times more lipid soluble than morphine, it is taken up much more readily into the central nervous system. The result is a quicker onset of action and equivalent analgesia at a fraction (1/100) of the dose of morphine.

Opioids are metabolized primarily in the liver, and the metabolites are excreted in the urine. Morphine has several active metabolites that can accumulate in renal failure. One metabolite (morphine-3-glucuronide) can produce central nervous system excitation with myoclonus and seizures (17), while another metabolite (morphine-6-glucuronide) has more analgesic effect than the parent drug (11). To avoid accumulation of these metabolites, **the maintenance dose of morphine should be reduced by 50% in patients with renal failure** (15). Fentanyl does not have active metabolites, and dose not need dose adjustments in renal failure.

Morphine promotes the release of histamine, which can cause vasodilation and hypotension (18). Fentanyl is devoid of this effect (18), and thus **fentanyl is preferred to morphine for patients with hemodynamic compromise**. Fentanyl also has a faster onset of action, which allows more rapid dose titration.

CAVEAT. Infusions of fentanyl lasting longer than 4 hours can produce prolonged drug effects as a result of drug accumulation in fatty tissue. This effect can be minimized by titrating the dose down to the lowest possible dose that relieves pain.

Patient-Controlled Analgesia

For patients who are awake and capable of drug self-administration, *patient-controlled analgesia* (PCA) can be an effective method of pain control. The PCA method uses an electronic infusion pump that can be activated by the patient. When pain is sensed, the patient presses a button connected to the pump to receive a small intravenous bolus of drug. After each bolus, the pump is disabled for a mandatory time period called the *lockout interval*, to prevent overdosing. The recommended dose regimens for PCA are shown in Table 49.1. The minimum lockout interval is determined by the time required to achieve peak drug effect (14). When writing orders for PCA, you must specify the initial loading dose (if any), the lockout interval, and the repeat bolus dose. PCA can be used alone or in conjunction with a low-dose opioid infusion.

PCA is associated with more effective analgesia, improved patient satisfaction, and fewer side effects than traditional intermittent opioid administration (14). Use of background opioid infusion increases the risk of respiratory depression, especially when combined with sedative drugs (19).

Epidural Opioids

Epidural instillation of opioids is a popular method of pain control following thoracic and abdominal surgery. Epidural catheters are usually placed in the operating room, just before surgery, and are left in place for the first few postoperative days. Drugs administered through the catheter produce a band-like distribution of analgesia extending several dermatomes above and below the catheter tip. Typical dose regimens for epidural analgesia are shown in Table 49.2. Epidural opioids can be given as intermittent boluses, but are more often given as a continuous infusion along with a local anesthetic such as bupivacaine. Adding a local anesthetic increases the analgesic effect of epidural opioids (synergistic effect) and reduces the risk of opioid side effects (20). Epidural instillation of local anesthetics can cause motor weakness and hypotension, and dilute drug solutions are used to avoid these side effects.

Therapeutic and Adverse Effects

Clinical studies comparing epidural and systemic opioid analgesia have been inconsistent, but the general impression is that epidural analgesia is associated with improved analgesia, faster recovery of bowel function, fewer

TABLE 49.2 Epidural Analgesia

Agent	Concentration
Opioids	
Fentanyl	2–5 μg/mL
Morphine	20–100 μg/mL
Dilaudid	0.04 mg/mL
Local Anesthetics	
Bupivacaine	0.06–0.125% (0.6–1.25 mg/mL)
Ropivacaine	0.1–0.2% (1–2 mg/mL)

Note:
1) Typical starting infusion rates are 4 to 8 mL/hr for thoracic epidural and 6 to 12 mL/hr for lumbar epidural. Dilute solutions of opioids and local anesthetics should be used initially for patient age ≥65 yrs.
2) Prolonged infusion of local anesthetics at higher dose ranges can cause hypotension, lower extremity weakness, and urinary retention.

Adapted from Reference 20.

pulmonary complications, and a decreased risk of myocardial infarction (20,21). Epidural analgesia does not reduce postoperative mortality (20).

Adverse effects of epidural analgesia are more common with morphine than fentanyl. Epidural morphine can produce respiratory depression, and the onset can be delayed up to 12 hours (22). **The incidence of respiratory depression is equivalent with epidural and intravenous morphine** (1% and 0.9%, respectively) (20). More frequent side effects of epidural analgesia include pruritis (28–100%), nausea (30–100%), and urinary retention (15–90%) (20). The pruritis from epidural opioids can be treated as described in the next section.

Adverse Effects of Opioids

There is a long list of adverse reactions to opioids; the following ones are of particular concern in the ICU. (For a comprehensive review of opioid side effects, see references 22–24.)

Respiratory Depression

Opioids produce a centrally mediated, dose-dependent decrease in both respiratory rate and tidal volume (23,25), but respiratory depression and hypoxemia are uncommon when opioids are used judiciously (26). High doses of opioids can produce apnea, an effect mediated by peripheral opioid receptors located in the lungs (23). When opioids cause difficulty in arousal, there is almost always an associated respiratory depression with hypercapnia (22). Patients with sleep apnea syndrome or chronic hypercapnia are particularly prone to respiratory depression from opioids, especially when opioids are combined with other respiratory depressant drugs (24).

Cardiovascular Effects

Opioid analgesia is often accompanied by decreases in blood pressure and heart rate, which are the result of decreased sympathetic activity and increased parasympathetic activity. These effects are usually mild and well tolerated, at least in the supine position (24). Decreases in blood pressure can be pronounced in patients with hypovolemia or heart failure (where there is an increased baseline sympathetic tone), or when opioids are given in combination with benzodiazepines (27). Opioid-induced hypotension usually responds to intravenous fluids or small bolus doses of vasopressors.

Intestinal Motility

Opioids are well known for their ability to depress bowel motility, and this effect can be prominent in ICU patients. Oral naloxone in a dose of 4 to 8 mg every 6 hours can antagonize opioid-induced bowel hypomotility without antagonizing the systemic analgesic effect (28). Higher doses will produce systemic opioid antagonism and should be avoided.

Pruritis

A generalized pruritis is reported in 30 to 100% of patients receiving epidural opioids, and in fewer than 10% of patients receiving intravenous opioids (20,28). Symptoms are usually not relieved by antihistamines, but they can be abolished by a low-dose naloxone infusion (0.25–1 μg/kg/hr) without loss of analgesic effects (28).

Nausea and Vomiting

Opioids can promote vomiting via stimulation of the chemoreceptor trigger zone in the lower brainstem (23). All opioids are equivalent in their ability to promote vomiting, but when one agent provokes vomiting, switching to another opioid can sometime provide symptom relief. Antiemetic agents (e.g., ondansetron) and low doses of opioid antagonists can also produce effective symptom relief.

Meperidine

Meperidine (Demerol, Pethidine) is a popular opioid analgesic that can be an excitatory neurotoxin in critically ill patients. Meperidine is metabolized in the liver to form normeperidine, a metabolite that is slowly excreted by the kidneys (elimination half-life is 15–40 hours) (29). Accumulation of normeperidine can produce central nervous system excitation with agitation, tremors, myoclonus, delirium, hallucinations, and tonic–clonic seizures (29). Normeperidine can accumulate with repeated doses of meperidine, and the accumulation is more pronounced when renal function is impaired. Since ICU patients often have impaired renal function, the risk for neurotoxicity from accumulation of normeperidine is high in this patient population.

Because of the risk for neurotoxicity in critically ill patients, meperidine is not advised for pain control in ICU patients. The traditional belief that meperidine is the preferred opioid for pain relief in cholecystitis and pancreatitis is contrary to experimental studies showing that meperidine and morphine are equivalent in their ability to promote spasm of the sphincter of Oddi and increased intrabiliary pressure (29,30). Nonsteroidal antiinflammatory drugs like ketorolac (see later) do not increase intrabiliary pressure (31), and these agents should be used when possible for pancreaticobiliary pain.

Although not advised as an analgesic in the ICU, meperidine continues to be the preferred agent for control of shivering. In postoperative patients, low doses of meperidine (25 mg IV) usually stop shivering due to hypothermia within 5 minutes.

NONOPIOID ANALGESIA

There are few alternatives to the opioids for providing effective analgesia via the parenteral route. In fact, there is only one alternative agent approved for use in the United States: ketorolac.

Ketorolac

Ketorolac is a nonsteroidal antiinflammatory drug (NSAID) introduced in 1990 as a parenteral analgesic for postoperative pain (32, 33). Because ketorolac does not cause sedation or respiratory depression, it was greeted with enthusiasm (34), but its popularity has waned because of the risk for other troublesome side effects.

Analgesic Effects

Ketorolac is a nonspecific inhibitor of cyclooxygenase with strong analgesic activity and moderate antiinflammatory activity (33). On an equal weight basis, it is 350 times more potent than aspirin (33). After intramuscular (IM) injection of ketorolac, analgesia is evident at 1 hour, peaks at 2 hours, and lasts 5–6 hours. The drug is partly metabolized in the liver and excreted in the urine. Elimination is prolonged in renal impairment and old age.

For postoperative analgesia, 30 mg ketorolac IM is equivalent to 10 to 12 mg morphine IM (32). Ketorolac can be given alone, but is often given with an opioid. It has an *opioid sparing effect*, and the opioid dose can often be reduced by 25–50% (32).

Dosing Regimen

Ketorolac can be given orally, intravenously, or by IM injection. For patients under 65 years of age, the initial dose is 30 mg IV or 60 mg IM, followed by 30 mg IM or IV every 6 hours (maximum of 120 mg/day) for up to 5 days. For patients ≥65 years of age, under 50 kg, or with renal dysfunction, the initial dose is 15 mg IV or 30 mg IM, followed by

15 mg IM or IV every 6 hours (maximum of 60 mg/day) for up to 5 days. Because IM injection of ketorolac can cause hematoma formation, IV bolus injection is preferred (35). Ketorolac has also been given by continuous IV infusion (5 mg/hr), resulting in more effective analgesia than intermittent IV doses (35).

Adverse Effects

Like other NSAIDs, ketorolac inhibits platelet aggregation, and it should not be used in patients with a high risk of bleeding (34). When ketorolac is given for more than 5 days, and in doses exceeding 75 mg/day, there is an increased risk of gastrointestinal and operative site bleeding (36). The risk of bleeding is greatest for patients over 65 years old. Ketorolac inhibits renal prostaglandin synthesis and may impair renal function, but the risk of renal toxicity is minimal if drug therapy does not exceed 5 days.

ANXIETY IN THE ICU

Anxiety and related disorders (agitation and delirium) are evident in as many as 85% of patients in the ICU (37). The common denominator in these conditions is the *absence of a sense of well-being*. Anxiety is characterized by exaggerated feelings of fear, nervousness, or apprehension that are sustained more by internal than external events. Agitation is a combination of anxiety and increased motor activity. Delirium is a specific syndrome of altered mental status that may or may not have anxiety as a component. Although delirium is often equated with agitation, there is a hypoactive form of delirium that is characterized by lethargy. The anxiety disorders are described in more detail in Chapter 50.

Sedation

Sedation is the process of establishing a state of calm. Talking to patients and making adjustments in the ICU environment should be the first steps to calm an anxious patient. In the ICU, however, drugs are often needed to calm patients, and as many as 22 different medications are used for this purpose (5). The agents most frequently used are midazolam, propofol, lorazepam, and opioid analgesics (5,6,12).

Monitoring Sedation

Current guidelines recommend routine monitoring of sedation (1), and the use of protocols to guide sedation can decrease the time spent on mechanical ventilation by as much as 50% (38). A number of scoring systems are available for this purpose, but no system has been fully validated (39). Each system evaluates consciousness first by noting spontaneous responsiveness to the observer, and subsequently (if necessary) by noting responses to graded levels of external stimulation (voice or touch). Sedation scores are not intended for patients who are unconscious or receiving a neuromuscular blocking agent.

TABLE 49.3 Ramsay Scale for Scoring Sedation

Score	Description
	Modified Ramsay Scale
1	Anxious and agitated or restless, or both
2	Cooperative, orientated, and tranquil
3	Drowsy, but responds to commands
4	Asleep, brisk response to light glabellar tap or loud auditory stimulus
5	Asleep, sluggish response to light glabellar tap or loud auditory stimulus
6	Asleep and unarousable

Adapted from Reference 39.

The Ramsay scale (see Table 49.3), described in 1974, was the first scoring system for evaluating sedation in mechanically ventilated patients (40). This scale is designed to monitor the level of consciousness more than the degree of agitation because it distinguishes four levels of sedation (score 3 to 6), but only one level of agitation (score = 1). Despite this shortcoming, and a lack of scientific validation, the Ramsay scale is the chosen method of monitoring sedation in more than 75% of ICUs (12).

Other sedation scales are included in the Appendix. The sedation-analgesia scale (SAS) distinguishes three different levels of agitation (41), and the Richmond Agitation Sedation Scale (RASS) offers the advantage of following changes in the level of sedation on consecutive days (42).

The goal of sedation in the ICU is a patient who is calm but easily arousable. The use of a sedation scale will allow you to achieve and maintain this goal with the lowest possible dose of a sedative agent and with the lowest possible risk of harm to your patient.

SEDATION WITH BENZODIAZEPINES

Benzodiazepines are popular sedatives in the ICU because they are generally safe to use, and the sedation is accompanied by amnesia. Of the 13 benzodiazepines available for clinical use, 3 can be given intravenously: midazolam, lorazepam, and diazepam. Table 49.4 presents some pertinent information on the intravenous benzodiazepines, and the following statements summarize some characteristic features of benzodiazepines.

1. All are lipid soluble to some degree, metabolized in the liver, and excreted in the urine.
2. Therapeutic doses of benzodiazepines do not cause respiratory depression in healthy subjects, but this effect can occur in select ICU patients (e.g., those with respiratory insufficiency) (44).
3. The dose of benzodiazepines needed to achieve adequate sedation is lower in elderly patients (45), and in patients with heart failure and hepatic insufficiency, due to a slowing of benzodiazepine metabolism.

TABLE 49.4 Sedation with Intravenous Benzodiazepines

	Midazolam	Lorazepam[1]	Diazepam[2]
Loading dose (IV)	0.02–0.1 mg/kg	0.02–0.06 mg/kg	0.05–0.2 mg/kg
Onset of action	1–5 min	5–20 min	2–5 min
Duration (after bolus)	1–2 hr	2–6 hr	2–4 hr
Maintenance infusion	0.04–0.2 mg/kg/hr	0.01–0.1 mg/kg/hr	Rarely used
Potency	3x	6x	x
Lipid solubility	1.5x	0.5x	x
Active metabolites	Yes	No	Yes
Dose adjustment for GFR <10 mL/min	Decrease 0–50%	None	None
Cost per 24 hours	4 mg/hr: $37	2 mg/hr: $52	8 mg q 4 h: $24

[1] Lorazepam: 2 mg/mL (Abbott Labs, Chicago, IL) contains propylene glycol (830 mg/mL) as solvent.

[2] Diazepam:10 mg/2 mL (Abbott Labs, Chicago, IL) contains propylene glycol (400 mg/mL) as solvent.

Adapted from References 1, 3, 15, 43–45.

4. Even though the elimination half-life of diazepam is 20 to 50 hours versus 2 to 8 hours for midazolam, the clinical recovery time is the same following a single intravenous dose of each drug (46). This discrepancy is explained by the relatively rapid uptake of diazepam from plasma into fatty tissues. Avid uptake by fat is also observed with lorazepam.
5. When an overdose of lorazepam or diazepam is given, the clinical recovery time until the patient is fully awake may be prolonged as a result of drug accumulation.

Drug Comparisons

Midazolam (Versed) is the benzodiazepine of choice for short-term sedation because it has the highest lipid solubility, the fastest onset, and the shortest duration of action of all the intravenous benzodiazepines (43–45). Because of its short duration of action, midazolam is commonly given by continuous infusion. **Infusions of midazolam lasting more than a few hours can produce prolonged sedation** after the drug infusion is stopped. This effects is the result of multiple factors, including (a) drug accumulation in the central nervous system, (b) accumulation of an active metabolite (hydroxymidazolam), especially in renal failure, (c) inhibition of cytochrome P450 (involved in midazolam metabolism) by other medications (Table 49.5), and (4) hepatic insufficiency (1,43,49). To reduce the risk for oversedation, **the infusion rate of midazolam should be determined using ideal body weight** rather than total body weight (43).

Lorazepam (Ativan) has the slowest onset of action of the intravenous benzodiazepines. Because of its long duration of action, lorazepam

TABLE 49.5 Drug Interactions with Benzodiazepines

Drugs	Mechanism	Significance	Recommendations
Interactions that ENHANCE Benzodiazepine Efficacy			
Fluconazole Erythromycin Clarithromycin Diltiazem Verapamil Rifampin Cimetidine Disulfiram Omeprazole	Inhibit cytochrome P-450 to slow hepatic metabolism of diazepam and midazolam.	Interaction between midazolam and erythromycin may be most significant.	Avoid drug combination, or reduce benzodiazepine dose as needed.
Interactions that REDUCE Benzodiazepine Efficacy			
Rifampin	↑ metabolism of diazepam and midazolam.	Significance unclear.	Dosage adjustment when clinically indicated.
Theophylline	Antagonizes benzodiazepine actions by adenosine inhibition.	Significant interaction.	Avoid theophylline.

Adapted from References 43, 47, 48.

is best suited for patients who require prolonged sedation (e.g., ventilator-dependent patients) (1). Lorazepam should not be used when rapid awakening is desired (45).

Diazepam (Valium) is the least favored of the intravenous benzodiazepines because of the risk for oversedation with repeated drug administration. Continuous infusions of diazepam should be avoided because of the risk for prolonged sedation caused by accumulation of parent drug and its active hepatic metabolites (3).

Toxic Effects

Excessive dosing of benzodiazepines can produce hypotension, respiratory depression, and excessive sedation (50). The manifestations and treatment of benzodiazepine toxicity are described in Chapter 53.

Propylene Glycol Toxicity

Intravenous preparations of lorazepam and diazepam contain the solvent propylene glycol to enhance drug solubility in plasma. This solvent can cause local irritation to veins, which is minimized by injecting the drug into a large vein. A bolus of propylene glycol can cause hypotension and bradycardia, and prolonged administration of propylene glycol can cause paradoxical agitation, metabolic acidosis, and a clinical syndrome that mimics severe sepsis. Propylene glycol toxicity is described in more detail in Chapter 29. When propylene glycol toxicity is suspected, it is wise to change to midazolam or propofol for sedation because these drug preparations do not contain this solvent.

Withdrawal Syndrome

Abrupt termination following prolonged benzodiazepine administration can produce a withdrawal syndrome consisting of anxiety, agitation, disorientation, hypertension, tachycardia, hallucinations, and seizures (49). Benzodiazepine withdrawal can also be a cause of unexplained delirium in the first few days after ICU admission (51). The risk of withdrawal is difficult to predict. For patients maintained for several days on a midazolam infusion, transitioning to propofol (mean dose 1.5 mg/kg/hr) 1 day prior to planned tracheal extubation can decrease the incidence of agitation observed after patient extubation (52).

Drug Interactions

Several drugs interfere with hepatic oxidative metabolism of diazepam and midazolam; these are listed in Table 49.5. These interactions do not apply to lorazepam, which is metabolized by glucuronidation (47). The interaction between theophylline and benzodiazepines also deserves mention. Theophylline antagonizes benzodiazepine sedation possibly by inhibiting adenosine, and intravenous aminophylline (110 mg over 5 minutes) has been reported to cause more rapid awakening from benzodiazepine sedation in postoperative patients (48).

OTHER SEDATIVES

Propofol

Propofol (Deprivan) is a rapidly acting sedative agent that is used for induction and maintenance of anesthesia and short-term sedation (<72 hrs). The use of this drug in the ICU should be limited by the risk for adverse reactions (particularly hypotension).

Actions and Uses

Propofol causes sedation and amnesia but has no analgesic activity (53). A single intravenous bolus of propofol produces sedation within 1 minute, and the drug effect lasts 5–8 minutes (53). The properties of this drug are shown in Table 49.6. Due to its short duration of action, propofol is given as a continuous infusion. After discontinuing a propofol infusion, awakening occurs within 10-15 minutes, even after prolonged administration (53).

Propofol can be used for short-term sedation when rapid awakening is desired (e.g., during brief procedures), or during transition from a long-acting sedative during patient recovery (52). Propofol can be useful in neurologic injury because it reduces cerebral oxygen consumption and intracranial pressure (53). Other conditions where propofol has been used include refractory status epilepticus (54) and delirium tremens (55).

TABLE 49.6 Sedation with Alternate Intravenous Agents

	Propofol	Dexmedetomidine
Loading dose	0.25–1 mg/kg	1 μg/kg over 10 min
Onset of action	<1 min	1–3 min
Time to arousal	10–15 min	6–10 min
Maintenance infusion	25–75 μg/kg/min	0.2–0.7 μg/kg/hr
Active metabolites	No	No
Respiratory depression	Yes	No
Side effects	Hypotension	Hypotension
	Hyperlipidemia	Bradycardia
	Contamination/Sepsis	Sympathetic rebound after >24 hr infusion
	Rhabdomyolysis	
	Propofol Infusion Syndrome	
Cost per 24 hrs*	30 μ/kg/min: $303	0.3 μg/kg/hr: $214

*Cost for 70 kg person based on average wholesale price in 2006.
Adapted from References 1, 4, 53.

Preparation and Dosage

Propofol is very lipid soluble, and the drug is suspended in a 10% lipid emulsion to enhance solubility in plasma. This lipid emulsion is almost identical to 10% Intralipid used in parenteral nutrition formulas, and the nutritive content of the emulsion (0.1 mg fat/ml or 1.1 kcal/ml) should be counted as part of the daily nutrient intake. **Propofol is dosed based on ideal rather than actual body weight**, and no dose adjustment is required for renal failure or moderate hepatic insufficiency (53).

Adverse Effects

Propofol is well known for producing pain on injection, respiratory depression, apnea, and hypotension (53). Because of the risk of respiratory depression, infusions of the drug should be used only in patients on controlled ventilation. Decreased blood pressure is frequently observed following a bolus dose of propofol, and significant hypotension is most likely to occur in patients who are elderly or have heart failure (53). Hemorrhagic shock greatly enhances the hypotensive effects of propofol, even after resuscitation with intravenous fluids (56). Propofol should be avoided in patients with hemorrhagic shock. Anaphylactoid reactions to propofol are uncommon but can be severe (53), and green urine is observed occasionally as a result of clinically insignificant phenolic metabolites (53)

The **lipid emulsion** in commercial propofol preparations can be a source of unwanted side effects. Hypertriglyceridemia occurs in up to 10% of patients receiving propofol, especially after 3 days of continuous infusion (57). Serum triglyceride levels should therefore be monitored during prolonged propofol infusions. The lipid emulsion also promotes bacterial growth (53), and improper sterile technique when giving propofol has resulted in an epidemic of hyperthermic reactions and postsurgical wound infections (58). To suppress microbial growth, commercial preparations of propofol contain either disodium edetate (EDTA, AstraZeneca) or sodium metabisulfite (Baxter). EDTA chelates zinc, and zinc supplementation should be considered for propofol infusions lasting longer than 5 days. Allergic reactions to the sulfite preservative are rare but are more common in patients with a history of asthma (1).

Bradycardia—Acidosis (Propofol Infusion Syndrome) is a rare and often lethal idiosyncratic reaction characterized by the abrupt onset of heart failure, bradycardia, lactic acidosis, hyperlipidemia, and rhabdomyolysis (59,60). The underlying mechanism is not clear, but this syndrome is usually associated with prolonged, high-dose propofol infusions (>4–6 mg/kg/hr for longer than 24 to 48 hrs) (59,60). The triad of bradycardia, hyperlipidemia, and rhabdomyolysis are unique features that help to distinguish this syndrome from septic shock. Treatment involves prompt discontinuation of the drug, supportive care, and cardiac pacing when needed. The mortality is high (>80%) despite therapeutic efforts (59). Maintaining propofol infusions below a rate of 4 mg/kg/hr may reduce the risk of this deadly condition (59).

Dexmetomidine

Dexmetomidine was introduced in 1999 as an intravenous sedative that does not produce respiratory depression (61,62).

Actions and Uses

Dexmetomidine is a highly selective α_2-adrenergic agonist that produces sedation, anxiolysis, mild analgesia, and sympatholysis (61). Following a bolus dose of the drug, sedation is evident in a few minutes, and the effect lasts less than 10 minutes. Because of the short duration of action, dexmetomidine is usually given by continuous infusion.

The absence of respiratory depression makes dexmetomidine an appealing sedative for patients who are prone to drug-induced respiratory depression (e.g., patients with sleep apnea or chronic obstructive lung disease), especially when these patients are weaning from mechanical ventilation (62).

Preparation and Dosage

Dexmetomidine is given as a loading dose of 1 μg/kg (infused over 10 minutes), followed by a continuous infusion of 0.2 to 0.7 μg/kg/hr (see Table 49.6). Mild hypertension in response to the loading dose is observed in 15% of patients (due to α-adrenergic stimulation) (61). This effect is usually transient, but it can be minimized by giving the loading dose over 20 minutes. Drug infusions should not be continued for longer than 24 hours (see later), and the dose should be reduced in patients with severe liver dysfunction (61).

Adverse Effects

Adverse effects during dexmetomidine infusion include hypotension (30%) and bradycardia (8%) (61). The latter effect can be severe in patients older than 65, and in the presence of advanced heart block. There is a risk for agitation and "sympathetic rebound" following drug withdrawal (similar to that observed with clonidine). To minimize this risk, **dexmetomidine infusions should not be continued for longer than 24 hours.**

Haloperidol

Haloperidol (Haldol) is an appealing sedative for ICU patients because there is little or no risk of cardiorespiratory depression. Haloperidol is also effective in calming patients with delirium (i.e., agitation or confusional anxiety). The intravenous route has yet to receive approval by the FDA, but intravenous haloperidol has been described in over 700 publications (63) and is supported by the practice guidelines of the Society of Critical Care Medicine (1).

Actions

Haloperidol produces its sedative and antipsychotic effects by blocking dopamine receptors in the central nervous system. Following an intravenous dose of haloperidol, sedation is evident in 10 to 20 minutes, and the effect lasts for hours. The prolonged duration of action makes haloperidol poorly suited for continuous infusion (63). Sedation is not accompanied by respiratory depression, and hypotension is unusual unless the patient is hypovolemic or receiving a β-blocker.

USES. Due to its delayed onset of action, haloperidol is not indicated for immediate control of anxiety. A benzodiazepine (e.g., lorazepam 1 mg) can be added to achieve more rapid sedation (64). Haloperidol is often targeted for the patient with delirium. However, because of the lack of respiratory depression, the drug can be used to sedate ventilator-dependent patients, and to facilitate weaning from mechanical ventilation (63).

DOSAGE. The dose recommendations for intravenous haloperidol are shown in Table 49.7. These doses are higher than the usual intramuscular doses, and amounts up to 1200 mg/day have been well tolerated (63). Individual patients show a wide variation in serum drug levels after a given dose of haloperidol (64). Therefore, if there is no evidence for a sedative response after 10 minutes, the dose should be doubled. If there is a partial response at 10–20 minutes, a second dose can be given along with 1 mg lorazepam (64). Lack of response to a second dose of haloperidol should prompt a switch to another agent.

Adverse Effects

Dopamine antagonism in the basal ganglia can cause extrapyramidal reactions; however, these are uncommon when haloperidol is given intravenously (64). The incidence of extrapyramidal reactions is further decreased when haloperidol is given in combination with a benzodiazepine (64). Halperidol should be avoided in patients with Parkinson's disease.

TABLE 49.7 Intravenous Haloperidol for Sedation

Severity of Anxiety	Dose
Mild	0.5–2 mg
Moderate	5–10 mg
Severe	10–20 mg

1. Administer dose by IV push.
2. Allow 10–20 minutes for response:
   a. If no response, double the drug dose, or
   b. add lorazepam (1 mg)
3. If still no response, switch to another sedative.
4. Give ¼ of the loading dose every 6 hours for maintenance of sedation.

Adapted from References 1, 63.

The most feared adverse effects of haloperidol are the **neuroleptic malignant syndrome** and **torsades de pointes** (polymorphic ventricular tachycardia). The neuroleptic malignant syndrome (described in detail in Chapter 38) is a rare idiosyncratic reaction that presents with hyperthermia, severe muscle rigidity, and rhabdomyolysis, and has been reported in ICU patients receiving intravenous haloperidol (65). Torsades de pointes is a characteristic form of ventricular tachycardia (see Figure 18.7) that is caused by drugs like haloperidol that prolong the QT interval on the electrocardiogram (56). This reaction is reported in up to 3.5% of patients receiving intravenous haloperidol (66) and, for this reason, haloperidol should be avoided in patients with a prolonged QT interval or a prior history of torsades de pointes.

INTERRUPTION OF DRUG INFUSIONS

Prolonged infusions of sedatives and analgesics are accompanied by progressive drug accumulation and persistent sedation after the drug infusion is discontinued. In recovering patients, daily interruption of drug infusions is associated with a shorter duration of mechanical ventilation, a reduced length of ICU stay, and fewer diagnostic tests to evaluate depressed consciousness (67). When patients have been maintained on sedative and analgesic drug infusions for longer than 24 hours and are beginning to recover, daily interruptions of drug infusions for a time period sufficient to allow patient awakening is recommended (67).

AN APPROACH TO THE AGITATED PATIENT

A common scenario in the ICU is a nurse informing you that your patient has suddenly become agitated. The flow diagram in Fig. 49.3 might help in this situation. When you arrive at the bedside, your first priority is to

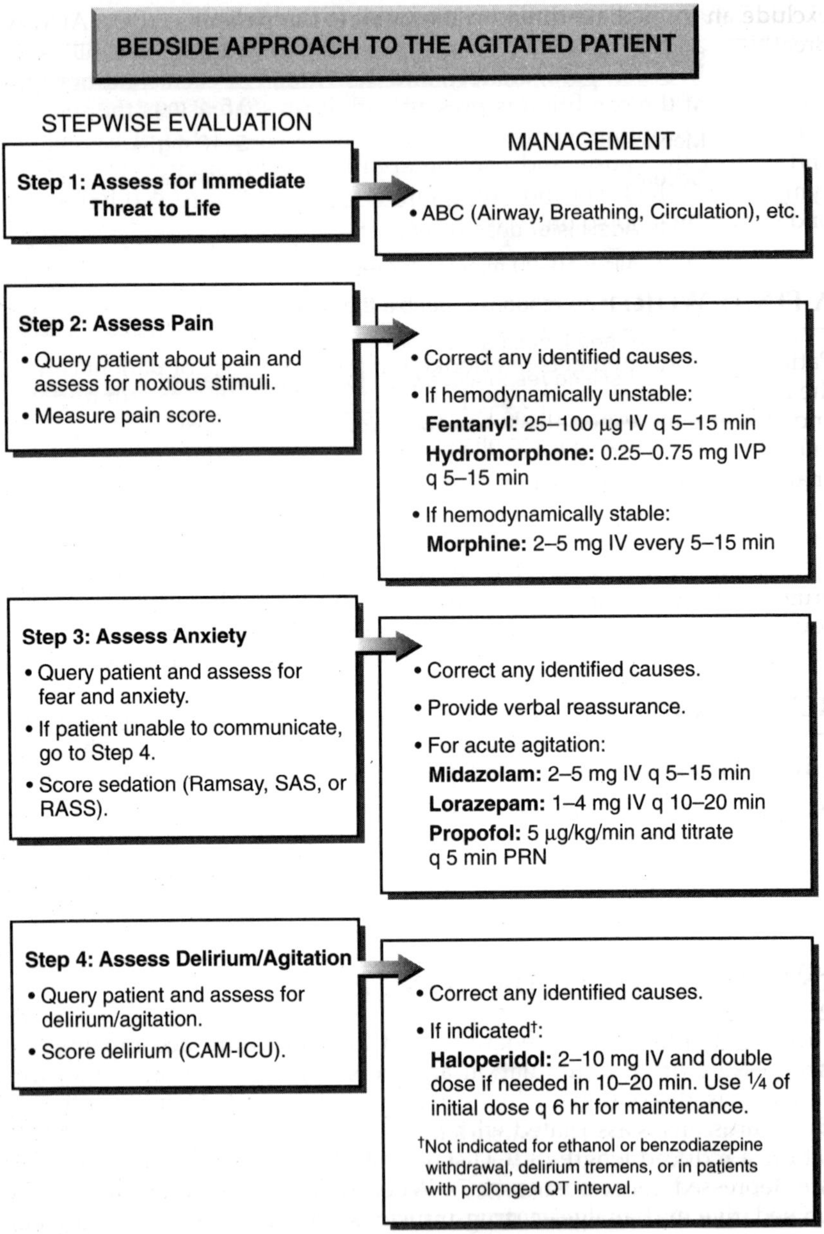

FIGURE 49.3 Bedside approach to the patient with acute agitation. The drug therapy in this figure is intended only for initial patient comfort and should be followed by regular or continuous drug administration to maintain the desired level of comfort. See Appendix for SAS, RASS, and CAM-ICU scoring methods. (Adapted from Jacobi J, et al. Clinical practice guidelines for the sustained use of sedatives and analgesics in the critically ill adult. Crit Care Med 2002;30:119–141.)

exclude an immediate threat to life (review the patient's ABCs, Airway, Breathing, and Circulation). Then proceed by considering the following conditions in order: **pain, anxiety, and delirium**. For each condition, ask the patient if the condition is present and, if present, assess the severity using an appropriate clinical scoring system. Then attempt to identify and correct the cause, and use the appropriate medication to alleviate symptoms. If the first condition (pain) is not present, proceed to the second condition, and so on.

A FINAL WORD

Patient comfort often gets overlooked in the rapid pace of patient care in the ICU. Remember to ask your patients regularly if they are comfortable and free of pain, especially when they're unable to verbalize discomfort due to an endotracheal tube. Also remember that the therapeutic dose of analgesic and sedative drugs differs for each patient, so use the recommended drug doses as a starting point, and titrate the dose as needed until the patient is comfortable. Finally, when the patient begins to recover, start daily wake-up tests to prevent unwanted prolongation of drug effects. These simple measures may be the most important therapy you have to offer your patients during their stay in the ICU.

REFERENCES

Clinical Practice Guidelines

1. Jacobi J, Fraser GL, Coursin DB, et al. Clinical practice guidelines for the sustained use of sedatives and analgesics in the critically ill adult. Crit Care Med 2002;30:119–141. (Available at www.sccm.org.pdf.sedatives.pdf. Accessed 4/2006.)

Reviews

2. Murray MJ, Plevak DJ. Analgesia in the critically ill patient. New Horizons 1994;2:56–63.
3. Young CC, Prielipp RC. Benzodiazepines in the intensive care unit. Crit Care Clin 2001;17:843–862.
4. Angelini G, Ketzler JT, Coursin DB. Use of propofol and other nonbenzodiazepine sedatives in the intensive care unit. Crit Care Clin 2001;17:863–880.
5. Watling SM, Dasta JF, Seidl EC. Sedatives, analgesics, and paralytics in the ICU. Ann Pharmacother 1997;31:148–153.

The Pain Experience

6. Dasta JF, Fuhrman TM, McCandles C. Patterns of prescribing and administering drugs for agitation and pain in patients in a surgical intensive care unit. Crit Care Med 1994;22:974–980.
7. Paiement B, Boulanger M, Jones CW, et al. Intubation and other experiences in cardiac surgery: the consumer's views. Can Anaesth Soc J 1979;26:173–180.

8. Melzack R. The tragedy of needless pain. Sci Am 1990;262:27–33.
9. Zenz M, Willweber-Strumpf A. Opiophobia and cancer pain in Europe. Lancet 1993;341:1075–1076.
10. Hamill-Ruth RJ, Marohn ML. Evaluation of pain in the critically ill patient. Crit Care Clin 1999;15:35–54.

Opioid Analgesia

11. Pasternak GW. Pharmacological mechanisms of opioid analgesics. Clin Neuropharmacol 1993;16:1–18.
12. Soliman HM, Melot C, Vincent JL. Sedative and analgesic practice in the intensive care unit: the results of a European survey. Br J Anaesth 2001;87: 186–192.
13. Veselis RA, Reinsel RA, Feshchenko VA, et al. The comparative amnestic effects of midazolam, propofol, thiopental, and fentanyl at equisedative concentrations. Anesthesiology 1997;87:749–764.
14. White PF. Use of patient-controlled analgesia for management of acute pain. JAMA 1988;259:243–247.
15. Aronoff GR, Berns JS, Brier ME, et al. Drug prescribing in renal failure: dosing guidelines for adults. 4th ed. Philadelphia: American College of Physicians, 1999.
16. Quigley C. A systematic review of hydromorphone in acute and chronic pain. J Pain Symptom Manage 2003;25:169–178.
17. Smith MT. Neuroexcitatory effects of morphine and hydromorphone: evidence implicating the 3-glucuronide metabolites. Clin Exp Pharmacol Physiol 2000;27:524–528.
18. Rosow CE, Moss J, Philbin DM, et al. Histamine release during morphine and fentanyl anesthesia. Anesthesiology 1982;56:93–96.
19. Etches RC. Respiratory depression associated with patient-controlled analgesia: a review of eight cases. Can J Anaesth 1994;41:125–132.
20. Liu S, Carpenter RL, Neal JM. Epidural anesthesia and analgesia: their role in postoperative outcome. Anesthesiology 1995;82:1474–1506.
21. Rodgers A, Walker N, Schug S, et al. Reduction of postoperative mortality and morbidity with epidural or spinal anaesthesia: results from overview of randomised trials. Br Med J 2000;321:1493.
22. Chaney MA. Side effects of intrathecal and epidural opioids. Can J Anaesth 1995;42:891–903.
23. Bowdle TA. Adverse effects of opioid agonists and agonist-antagonists in anaesthesia. Drug Safety 1998;19:173–189.
24. Schug SA, Zech D, Grond S. Adverse effects of systemic opioid analgesics. Drug Safety 1992;7:200–213.
25. Weil JV, McCullough RE, Kline JS, et al. Diminished ventilatory response to hypoxia and hypercapnia after morphine in normal man. N Engl J Med 1975; 292:1103–1106.
26. Bailey PL. The use of opioids in anesthesia is not especially associated with nor predictive of postoperative hypoxemia. Anesthesiology 1992;77:1235.
27. Tomicheck RC, Rosow CE, Philbin DM, et al. Diazepam-fentanyl interaction: hemodynamic and hormonal effects in coronary artery surgery. Anesth Analg 1983;62:881–884.

28. Choi YS, Billings JA. Opioid antagonists: a review of their role in palliative care, focusing on use in opioid-related constipation. J Pain Symptom Manage 2002;24:71–90.
29. Latta KS, Ginsberg B, Barkin RL. Meperidine: a critical review. Am J Ther 2002;9:53–68.
30. Lee F, Cundiff D. Meperidine vs morphine in pancreatitis and cholecystitis. Arch Intern Med 1998;158:2399.
31. Krimmer H, Bullingham RE, Lloyd J, et al. Effects on biliary tract pressure in humans of intravenous ketorolac tromethamine compared with morphine and placebo. Anesth Analg 1992;75:204–207.
32. Gillis JC, Brogden RN. Ketorolac: a reappraisal of its pharmacodynamic and pharmacokinetic properties and therapeutic use in pain management. Drugs 1997;53:139–188.
33. Buckley MM, Brogden RN. Ketorolac: a review of its pharmacodynamic and pharmacokinetic properties, and therapeutic potential. Drugs 1990;39:86–109.
34. Reinhart DI. Minimising the adverse effects of ketorolac. Drug Safety 2000; 22:487–497.
35. Ready LB, Brown CR, Stahlgren LH, et al. Evaluation of intravenous ketorolac administered by bolus or infusion for treatment of postoperative pain: a double-blind, placebo-controlled, multicenter study. Anesthesiology 1994;80: 1277–1286.
36. Strom BL, Berlin JA, Kinman JL, et al. Parenteral ketorolac and risk of gastrointestinal and operative site bleeding: a postmarketing surveillance study. JAMA 1996;275:376–382.

Anxiety in the ICU

37. Ely EW, Inouye SK, Bernard GR, et al. Delirium in mechanically ventilated patients: validity and reliability of the confusion assessment method for the intensive care unit (CAM-ICU). JAMA 2001;286:2703–2710.
38. Brook AD, Ahrens TS, Schaiff R, et al. Effect of a nursing-implemented sedation protocol on the duration of mechanical ventilation. Crit Care Med 1999; 27:2609–2615.
39. De Jonghe B, Cook D, Appere-De-Vecchi C, et al. Using and understanding sedation scoring systems: a systematic review. Intensive Care Med 2000;26: 275–285.
40. Ramsay MA, Savege TM, Simpson BR, et al. Controlled sedation with alphaxalone-alphadolone. Br Med J 1974;2:656–659.
41. Riker RR, Picard JT, Fraser GL. Prospective evaluation of the Sedation-Agitation Scale for adult critically ill patients. Crit Care Med 1999;27:1325–1329.
42. Ely EW, Truman B, Shintani A, et al. Monitoring sedation status over time in ICU patients: reliability and validity of the Richmond Agitation-Sedation Scale (RASS). JAMA 2003;289:2983–2991.
43. Fragen RJ. Pharmacokinetics and pharmacodynamics of midazolam given via continuous intravenous infusion in intensive care units. Clin Ther 1997; 19:405–419.

Sedative Agents

44. Reves JG, Fragen RJ, Vinik HR, et al. Midazolam: pharmacology and uses. Anesthesiology 1985;62:310–324.
45. Barr J, Zomorodi K, Bertaccini EJ, et al. A double-blind, randomized comparison of i.v. lorazepam versus midazolam for sedation of ICU patients via a pharmacologic model. Anesthesiology 2001;95:286–298.
46. Ariano RE, Kassum DA, Aronson KJ. Comparison of sedative recovery time after midazolam versus diazepam administration. Crit Care Med 1994;22: 1492–1496.
47. Dresser GK, Spence JD, Bailey DG. Pharmacokinetic-pharmacodynamic consequences and clinical relevance of cytochrome P450 3A4 inhibition. Clin Pharmacokinet 2000;38:41–57.
48. Hoegholm A, Steptoe P, Fogh B, et al. Benzodiazepine antagonism by aminophylline. Acta Anaesthesiol Scand 1989;33:164–166.
49. Shafer A. Complications of sedation with midazolam in the intensive care unit and a comparison with other sedative regimens. Crit Care Med 1998;26: 947–956.
50. Gaudreault P, Guay J, Thivierge RL, et al. Benzodiazepine poisoning: clinical and pharmacological considerations and treatment. Drug Safety 1991;6:247–265.
51. Moss JH. Sedative and hypnotic withdrawal states in hospitalised patients. Lancet 1991;338:575.
52. Saito M, Terao Y, Fukusaki M, et al. Sequential use of midazolam and propofol for long-term sedation in postoperative mechanically ventilated patients. Anesth Analg 2003;96:834–838.
53. McKeage K, Perry CM. Propofol: a review of its use in intensive care sedation of adults. CNS Drugs 2003;17:235–272.
54. Brown LA, Levin GM. Role of propofol in refractory status epilepticus. Ann Pharmacother 1998;32:1053–1059.
55. McCowan C, Marik P. Refractory delirium tremens treated with propofol: a case series. Crit Care Med 2000;28:1781–1784.
56. Shafer SL. Shock values. Anesthesiology 2004;101:567–568.
57. Riker RR, Fraser GL. Adverse events associated with sedatives, analgesics, and other drugs that provide patient comfort in the intensive care unit. Pharmacotherapy 2005;25:8S–18S.
58. Bennett SN, McNeil MM, Bland LA, et al. Postoperative infections traced to contamination of an intravenous anesthetic, propofol. N Engl J Med 1995;333:147–154.
59. Bray RJ. Propofol infusion syndrome in children. Paediatr Anaesth 1998;8: 491–499.
60. Kang TM. Propofol infusion syndrome in critically ill patients. Ann Pharmacother 2002;36:1453–1456.
61. Bhana N, Goa KL, McClellan KJ. Dexmedetomidine. Drugs 2000;59:263–268.
62. Venn RM, Hell J, Grounds RM. Respiratory effects of dexmedetomidine in the surgical patient requiring intensive care. Crit Care 2000;4:302–308.

Haloperidol

63. Riker RR, Fraser GL, Cox PM. Continuous infusion of haloperidol controls agitation in critically ill patients. Crit Care Med 1994;22:433–440.

64. Sanders KM, Minnema AM, Murray GB. Low incidence of extrapyramidal symptoms in the treatment of delirium with intravenous haloperidol and lorazepam in the intensive care unit. J Intensive Care Med 1989;4:201–204.
65. Sing RF, Branas CC, Marino PL. Neuroleptic malignant syndrome in the intensive care unit. J Am Osteopath Assoc 1993;93:615–618.
66. Sharma ND, Rosman HS, Padhi ID, et al. Torsades de pointes associated with intravenous haloperidol in critically ill patients. Am J Cardiol 1998;81:238–240.

Interruption of Sedative Infusions

67. Kress JP, Pohlman AS, O'Connor MF, et al. Daily interruption of sedative infusions in critically ill patients undergoing mechanical ventilation. N Engl J Med 2000;342:1471–1477.

Chapter 50

DISORDERS OF MENTATION

"If one subject... can be said to be at once well settled and persistently unresolved, it is how to determine that death has occurred."

Alexander Morgan Capron, 2001.

Abnormal mental function is one of the most recognizable signs of serious illness. Disordered mentation occurs in over 80% of ventilator-dependent patients, and is associated with a 3-fold increase in mortality, as well as a longer stay on the ventilator and in the ICU (1,2). Despite its profound significance, mental dysfunction often goes undetected, as will be described.

This chapter begins by focusing on two disorders of mental function that are common in critically ill patients: altered consciousness and delirium. The final section then describes the most severe disorder of mental function that will ever be encountered: brain death (3–7).

MENTAL FUNCTION

The "mental" aspect of brain function is responsible for the manner in which individuals interact with their environment. Mental function is considered normal when all the following mental processes are intact:

1. Awareness of self and surroundings.
2. Ability to accurately perceive what is experienced (sensory input and orientation).
3. Ability to store and retrieve information (memory).
4. Ability to process input data to generate more meaningful information (judgment and reasoning).

The first mental process is known as *consciousness*, while the latter three mental processes make up what is known as *cognition*. The disorders of mental function can therefore be classified as *disorders of consciousness* and *disorders of cognition*.

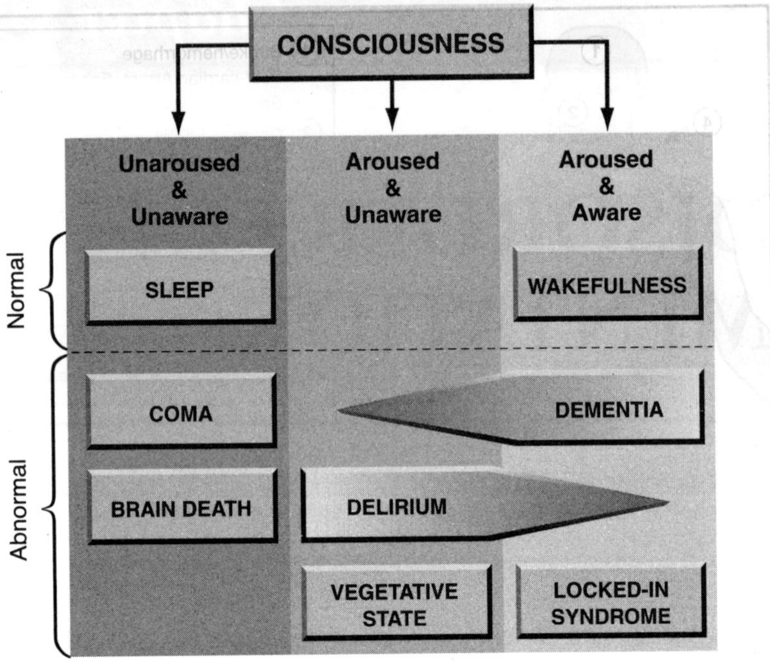

FIGURE 50.1 Diagram depicting states of consciousness.

Disorders of Consciousness

Consciousness has two components: *arousal* (or wakefulness) and *awareness* (or responsiveness). These two components are used to identify the major conditions of normal and abnormal consciousness in Figure 50.1. These conditions are briefly described below.

Normal mentation is characterized by awareness (wakefulness) or arousability (sleep).

Delirium and **dementia** are conditions where arousal is associated with varying degrees of awareness. (The features that distinguish these two conditions are described later in the chapter.)

Vegetative state is characterized by arousal (eyes open) with no awareness (8). Spontaneous movements can occur but are purposeless. After one month, this condition is called a *persistent vegetative state.*

Locked-in state can mimic a vegetative state, but awareness is intact. This disorder is caused by bilateral injury to the motor pathways in the ventral pons disrupting all voluntary movement except for up-down ocular movements and eyelid blinking (9). Function of the cortex and the reticular activating system are unaffected, and the patient is fully awake and aware.

Coma is characterized by the absence of arousal and awareness; i.e., it is a state of *unarousable unawareness.*

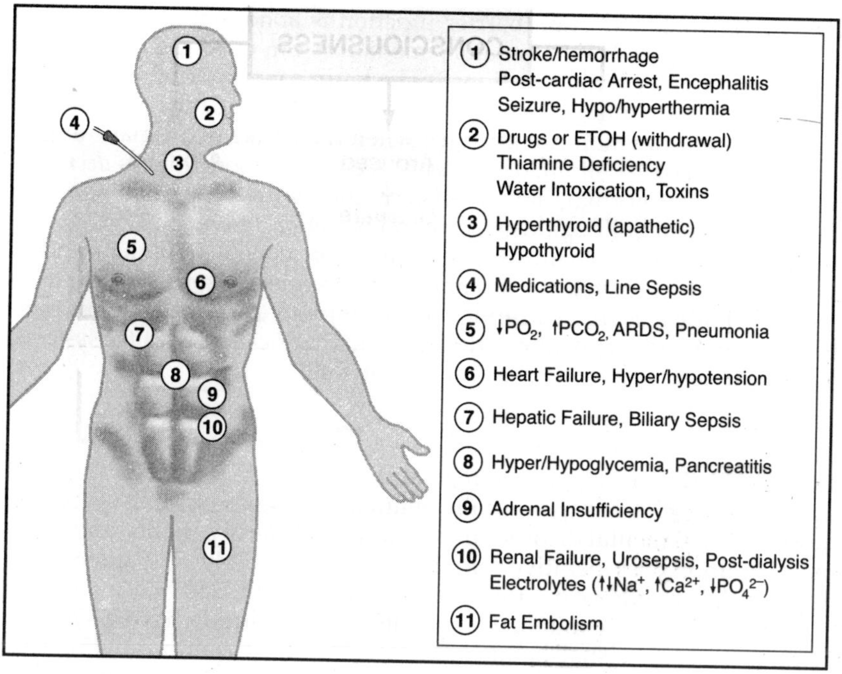

FIGURE 50.2 Possible causes of abnormal mental function.

Brain death is similar to coma in that it is a state of unarousable unawareness. However unlike coma, brain death is irreversible, and is accompanied by cessation of all functions of the brain, including the brainstem (10).

Etiologies of Altered Consciousness

The most common causes of altered consciousness in patients who have not sustained a head injury (nontraumatic) are listed in Figure 50.2. Most of the conditions listed in this figure can be classified as types of *encephalopathies,* which are global brain disorders triggered by factors extrinsic to the central nervous system (e.g., infectious, ischemic, drug-related, or metabolic) (3,11,12). In a prospective survey of neurologic complications in a medical ICU (13), ischemic stroke was the most frequent cause of altered consciousness on admission to the ICU, and septic encephalopathy was the most common cause of altered consciousness that developed *after* admission to the ICU.

Septic Encephalopathy

Septic encephalopathy is the result of infections that originate outside the central nervous system. It is reported in 50–70% of ICU patients with sepsis, and can be an early sign of sepsis, particularly in the elderly (12,13). The encephalopathy can be the result of any of the following processes

(12,14): 1) The blood brain barrier function is abnormal and can result in cerebral edema; 2) Inflammatory mediators can cross the blood brain barrier and impair brain function; 3) The brain concentration of aromatic amino acids and ammonia are increased (similar to hepatic encephalopathy) and brain function can improve when the intake of aromatic amino acids is reduced or eliminated; and 4) Cerebral blood flow is *decreased* to about 60% of normal and, when combined with hyperventilation (in response to metabolic acidosis), cerebral ischemia can result (15).

Although the mechanism is unclear, septic encephalopathy appears to be caused by the systemic inflammatory response to sepsis, rather than the infection itself. In fact, septic encephalopathy can be one manifestation of a more widespread multiorgan injury associated with *the systemic inflammatory response syndrome* (see Chapter 40).

Delirium

Delirium is the most common mental disorder in ICUs, and is reported in as many as 87% of mechanically ventilated patients (2,16). It is also the most common mental disorder in hospitalized elderly patients, and is the most common postoperative complication in the elderly (3). Patients who develop delirium have a 3-fold greater risk of death (2,3).

Over 40% of hospitalized patients with delirium have psychotic symptoms (with visual hallucinations being most common) (17). This condition has been called "ICU psychosis" but a more accurate term is "delirium with psychotic features" (18). Unfortunately, as many as two-thirds of delirium episodes go unnoticed (19).

CLINICAL FEATURES. The clinical features of delirium are summarized in Figure 50.3 (16). Delirium is a cognitive disorder characterized by attention deficits, and either disordered thinking or an altered level of consciousness. The hallmark of delirium (and the feature that distinguishes it from dementia) is its acute onset or fluctuating clinical course.

Hypoactive Delirium

There is a tendency to consider delirium as a state of agitation (as in the delirium tremens syndrome). However, as shown in Figure 50.3, there is also **a hypoactive form of delirium that is characterized by lethargy rather than agitation**. In fact, hypoactive delirium **is the most common form of delirium in the elderly** (2). This is certainly a source of missed diagnoses of delirium in many patients.

Delirium vs. Dementia

Delirium and dementia are distinct mental disorders that are easily confused because of overlapping clinical features (e.g., attention deficits and abnormal thinking) (20). As noted above, the principal features of delirium not present in dementia are its acute onset and/or fluctuating course. As many as two-thirds of hospitalized patients with dementia can have a superimposed delirium (3,20), and the delirium can provoke further mental and functional decline (3).

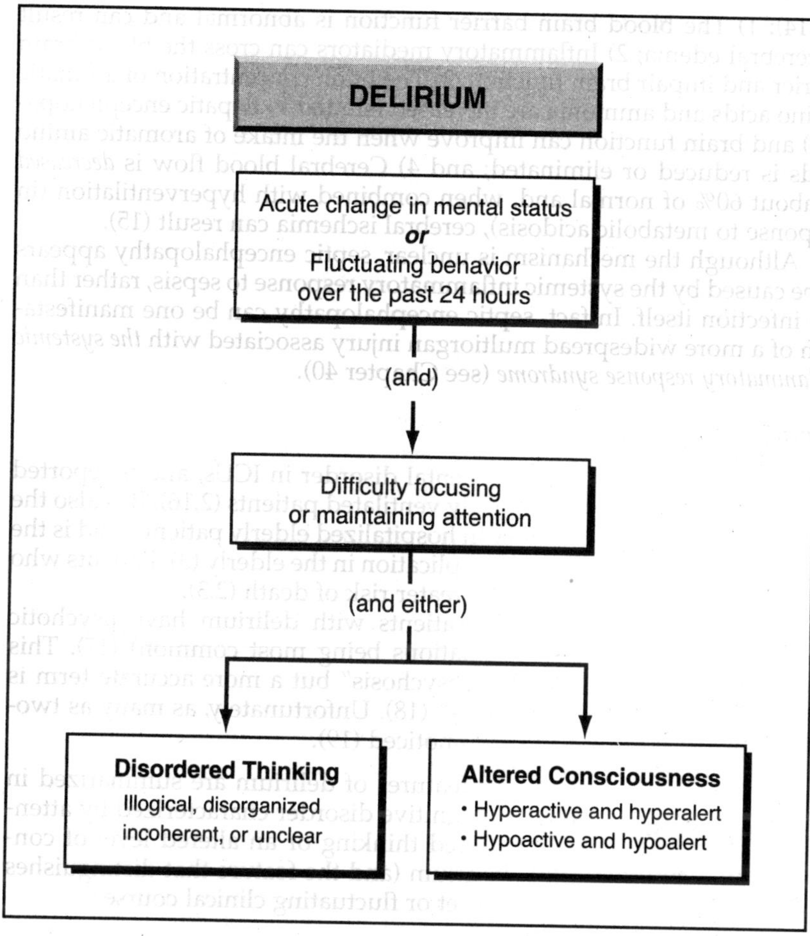

FIGURE 50.3 The clinical features of delirium.

Etiologies

The possible causes of delirium are listed in Figure 50.2. Any type of encephalopathy (i.e., infectious, ischemic, drug-related, or metabolic) can cause a state of delirium. Drugs are implicated as causative or contributory factors in as many as 40% of cases of delirium in the elderly (11). The drugs most likely to be responsible for delirium in ICU patients are listed in Table 50.1 (3,11,18). The principal offenders in this list are alcohol (withdrawal), the long-acting benzodiazepines (lorazepam and diazepam), and opioids.

Management

The management of delirium should focus on identifying and treating the underlying cause of the problem. In addition, the following measures

TABLE 50.1 Medications That Can Cause Delirium in the ICU*

Alcohol (withdrawal)	Corticosteroids (high-dose)
Amphotericin	Digitalis
Aminoglycosides	H_2-Blockers (e.g., cimetidine, ranitidine)
Angiotensin-converting enzyme inhibitors	Isoniazid
Anticholinergics (atropine)	Local anesthetics (lidocaine, bupivacaine)
Anticonvulsants (e.g., phenytoin)	Metoclopramide
Antidysrhythmics (e.g., quinidine, amiodarone)	Metronidazole
Benzodiazepines (e.g., lorazepam)	NSAIDs (e.g., ibuprofen)
β-Blockers	Opioids (especially meperidine)
Cephalosporins	Penicillin (high-dose)
Cocaine	Trimethoprim-sulfamethoxazole

*List is limited to drugs that are likely to be encountered in ICU patients.

may be helpful: provide reassurance and reorientation, assess for and treat pain, maintain normal sleep cycles and avoid sleep interruption, encourage family visitation, place patient in an ICU bed with a window, avoid physical restraints and urinary bladder catheters, and provide patient with eyeglasses and hearing aid (3,11).

Pharmacologic Management

If agitation and disruptive behavior become a problem, the administration of sedatives may be beneficial. The choice of sedative is determined by the cause of the delirium, as described below (3,11,21,22).

1. For ICU-acquired or postoperative delirium, the treatment of choice is **haloperidol** (0.5 to 2 mg PO or IV every 4–6 hours as needed) (3,11). Benzodiazepines should be avoided in these cases because they can aggravate the delirium (3).
2. For delirium that accompanies alcohol withdrawal, **benzodiazepines** are preferred (see Table 49.4 for benzodiazepine dosing recommendations) (21). Haloperidol should be avoided in these cases because it can aggravate the delirium, and it does not prevent seizures (21).
3. If delirium tremens is accompanied by troublesome hypertension, adjunctive therapy with **clonidine** (a centrally-acting alpha-2 agonist) can augment the sedative effect of benzodiazepines while it decreases the blood pressure. Clonidine does not prevent delirium or seizures, and should always be used in combination with a benzodiazepine (21). The dose of clonidine is 0.1 mg orally every 2–4 hours until the pressure is controlled or a cumulative dose of 0.5 mg has been given.

4. The management of cocaine-induced delirium is the same as delirium tremens; i.e., benzodiazepines are preferred, while haloperidol is not advised (22).

COMA

Because of the vast reserves of the brain, persistent unarousability (lasting more than 6 hours) implies extensive brain injury (23). The most common causes of coma in one study were cardiac arrest (31%), and either stroke or intracerebral hemorrhage (36%) (23). The anatomic basis of coma and associated findings are summarized below (7,24):

1. Diffuse and bilateral cerebral damage (brainstem reflexes may remain intact).
2. Unilateral cerebral damage causing midline shift with compression of the contralateral cerebral hemisphere.
3. Supratentorial mass lesion causing transtentorial herniation and brainstem compression (producing ipsilateral third nerve palsy with a fixed dilated pupil and contralateral hemiplegia).
4. Posterior fossa mass lesion causing direct brainstem compression (often associated with the *Cushing reflex* of bradycardia and hypertension).
5. Toxic or metabolic disorders (small or midposition, light-reactive pupils).

Coma is rarely a permanent state, but less than 10% of patients survive coma without significant disability (23). For ICU patients with persistent coma, the outcome is grim. In one study of ICU patients, *all* patients who failed to awaken from coma died after a median duration of 3 days (2).

Bedside Evaluation of Coma

The bedside evaluation of coma must include an assessment of brainstem reflexes, and the following information deserves mention.

Pupils

The conditions that affect pupillary size and light reactivity are shown in Table 50.2 (4,24–26). In the presence of coma, pupillary function may be normal if the brain lesion is above (rostral to) the midbrain (4), or if the patient is receiving neuromuscular blockers (without sedatives) (27).

If the injury is diffuse (e.g., global cerebral anoxia-ischemia), the pupillary abnormality is bilateral. When a brain insult causes cerebral anoxic-ischemia (e.g., cardiac arrest), the pupils become bilaterally dilated and nonreactive, and rapid resuscitation can restore (or even maintain) normal pupil size and light response. When atropine is given in the usual doses during cardiopulmonary resuscitation, the pupils will dilate,

TABLE 50.2 Conditions That Affect Pupillary Size & Reactivity

Pupillary Size	Reactive	Nonreactive	
Dilated	Atropine (low dose) Sympathomimetics	Uncal herniation, (unilateral pupil) Post-CPR Brainstem injury Ocular trauma Hypothermia (<28°C)	Drugs (high dose): Atropine Dopamine Phenylephrine Amphetamine TCA
Midposition	Toxic/metabolic encephalopathy Sedative overdose	Brain death Midbrain lesions Barbiturates (high-dose)	
Constricted	Toxic/metabolic encephalopathy Pontine injury Opioids	Opioids (high-dose) Pilocarpine eye drops	

Abbreviation: TCA: tricyclic antidepressant

but they usually remain reactive to light (25). **If the pupils remain nonreactive for longer than 6–8 hours after resuscitation from cardiac arrest, the prognosis for neurological recovery is generally poor** (28,29).

A unilateral dilated pupil that is unreactive to light, when combined with contralateral hemiplegia, is highly suggestive of unilateral herniation with compression of the third cranial nerve and midbrain (4). This finding should prompt an immediate search for a potentially correctable abnormality (e.g., hemorrhage) because a unilateral herniation can progress rapidly to irreversible injury.

Ocular Motility

Spontaneous eye movements (conjugate or dysconjugate) are a nonspecific sign in comatose patients and can suggest toxic or metabolic etiologies (24). However, a fixed gaze preference involving one or both eyes is highly suggestive of a mass lesion or seizures.

Ocular Reflexes

The ocular reflexes are used to evaluate the functional integrity of the lower brainstem (24). These reflexes are illustrated in Figure 50.4.

The **oculocephalic reflex** is assessed by briskly rotating the head from side-to-side. When the cerebral hemispheres are impaired but the lower brainstem is intact, the eyes will deviate away from the direction of rotation and maintain a forward field of view. When the lower brainstem

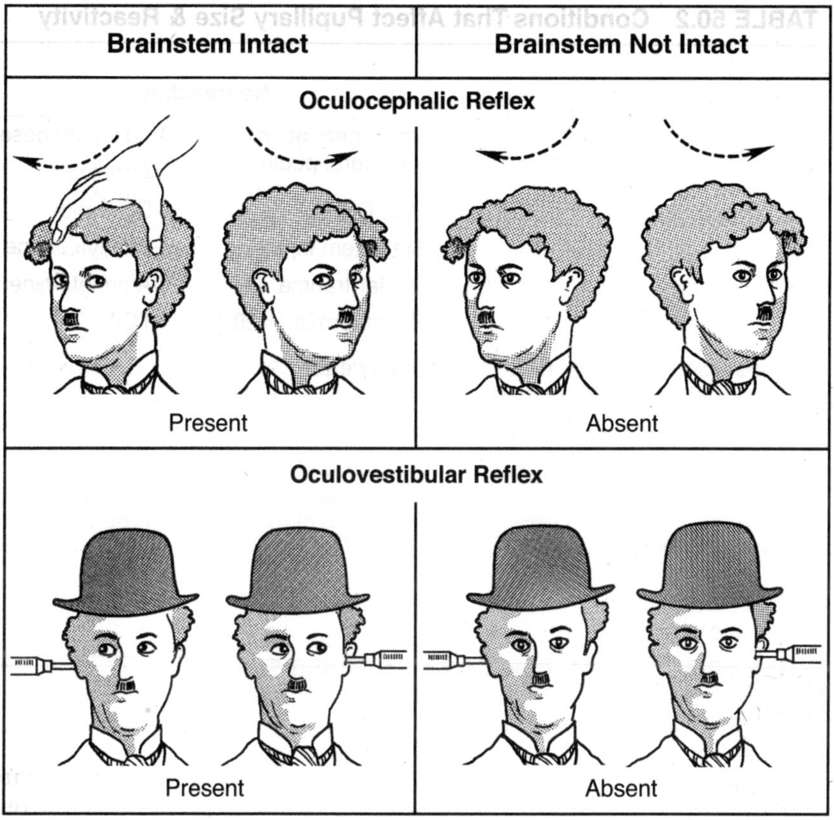

FIGURE 50.4 The ocular reflexes in the evaluation of coma.

is damaged or the patient is awake, the eyes will follow the direction of head rotation. The oculocephalic reflex should *not* be attempted in patients with an unstable cervical spine.

The **oculovestibular reflex** is performed by injecting 50 ml of cold saline in the external auditory canal of each ear (using a 50 ml syringe and a 2-inch soft plastic angiocatheter) (10). Before the test is performed, check to make sure that the tympanic membrane is intact and that nothing is obstructing the ear canal. When brainstem function is intact, both eyes will deviate slowly towards the irrigated ear. This conjugate eye movement is lost when the lower brainstem is damaged. After the test is performed on one side, wait 5 minutes before testing the opposite side.

The Extremities

Clonic involuntary movements elicited by flexion of the hands or feet (asterixis) is a sign of a diffuse metabolic encephalopathy (30). A focal motor or sensory defect in the extremities (e.g., hemiparesis or asymmetric reflexes) is occasionally caused by a diffuse metabolic encephalopathy.

However, the presence of focal neurologic defects should always prompt further investigation (with computed tomography) for a structural brain lesion.

In general, motor responses are characterized as appropriate, posturing, or flaccid. With mild mental clouding, there is no response to verbal command, but painful stimulation elicits a purposeful response to remove the stimulus (localizes to pain). With progressive impairment, there is withdrawal of the extremity that is subjected to painful stimulus. With injury to the thalamus, painful stimuli provoke flexion of the upper extremity; this is called *abnormal flexion* or *decorticate posturing*. With injury to the midbrain and upper pons, the arms and legs extend and pronate in response to pain; this is called *abnormal extension* or *decerebrate posturing*. Finally, with injury that involves the lower brainstem (medulla), the extremities become flaccid.

The Glasgow Coma Scale

The severity of altered consciousness is often evaluated with the Glasgow Coma Scale, which is shown in Table 50.3. The scale consists of three

TABLE 50.3 The Glasgow Coma Scale and Score

	Points	
Eye Opening:		
Spontaneous	4	
To speech	3	
To pain	2	
None	1	☐ Points
Verbal Communication:		
Oriented	5	
Confused conversation	4	
Inappropriate but recognizable words	3	
Incomprehensible sounds	2	
None	1	☐ Points
Motor Response:		
Obeys commands	6	
Localizes to pain	5	
Withdraws to pain	4	
Abnormal flexion (decorticate response)	3	
Abnormal extension (decerebrate response)	2	
No movement	1	☐ Points
Glasgow Coma Score (Total of 3 scales)*		☐ Points

*Worst score is 3 points, and best score is 15 points. With endotracheal intubation, the highest score is 11.

components: 1) eye opening, 2) verbal communication, and 3) motor response to verbal or noxious stimulation (31,32). The **Glasgow Coma Score** is the sum of the three components, and **has a range from 3 to 15** (31,32).

The Glasgow Coma Score can be used as follows (28,32,34).

1. To define coma (GCS ≤8).
2. To stratify the severity of head injury (mild 13–15, moderate 9–12, severe ≤8)
3. To identify candidates for intubation (i.e., patients with GCS ≤8 are usually unable to protect their airway and require endotracheal intubation).
4. As a prognostic marker; e.g., in the initial evaluation of nontraumatic coma, patients with a GCS ≥6 are seven-times more likely to awaken within two weeks than patients with a GCS ≤5 (33).

The verbal communication component of the GCS is a problem in ICU patients who are intubated, since these patients are unable to communicate verbally (34).

Predictive Value

The predictive values of the components of the Glascow Coma Scale are shown in Table 50.4. In this case, the predictive value refers to the chances of a satisfactory neurological recovery in patients who remain comatose after resuscitation from cardiac arrest (28). In patients who show no response to verbal or noxious stimuli at one hour after the cardiac arrest, 70 to 80% will not have a satisfactory neurological recovery. At 24 hours following cardiac arrest, absent pupillary light and corneal reflexes greatly increases the likelihood of an unfavorable outcome (35). If the

TABLE 50.4 Predictive Value of the Pupillary Light Response and the Glasgow Coma Scale Following Cardiac Arrest

	Negative Predictive Value Post-Arrest		
Parameter	1st hour (%)	24 hours (%)	3 days (%)
Absent pupillary response to light	83	93	100
No eye opening to pain	69	92	100
No response to verbal stimuli	67	75	94
No motor response to pain	75	91	100
Glasgow Coma Score less than 6	69	—	100

Data from Edgren E, Hedstrand U, Kelsey S, et al. Assessment of neurological prognosis in comatose survivors of cardiac arrest. Lancet 1994;343:1055–1059.

TABLE 50.5 The Clinical Criteria of Brain Death in Adults

Instructions: When Steps 1, 2, and 3 are confirmed, the patient is declared brain dead.	**Check (✓) Item if Confirmed**	
Step 1: Prerequisite to Exam		
Evaluate and correct potentially reversible causes of the abnormal neurological examination. 1. Hypotension (mean arterial pressure <60 mm Hg, arbitrary) 2. Hypothermia (core temperature <32°C or <90°F) 3. Metabolic disturbances (i.e., glucose, electrolyte, acid-base, or endocrine) 4. Significant drugs or medications 5. Confounding diseases (e.g., locked-in syndrome, Guillain-Barré)	☐	
The cause of coma is known and sufficient to account for irreversible brain and brainstem death. Clinical history and/or neurological imaging are consistent with brain death.	☐	
Step 2: Absence of Brain and Brainstem Function This step involves two exams, usually performed 6 hours apart.	**First Exam**	**Second Exam**
Coma: Absent cerebral motor response in all extremities *and* face to noxious stimuli (nail-bed and supraorbital ridge pressure).	☐	☐
Absent Brainstem Reflexes:		
Pupils		
• Size: midposition to dilated (4 to 9 mm)	☐	☐
• Absent response to bright light	☐	☐
Absent corneal reflex (touch edge of cornea)	☐	☐
Absent gag reflex (stimulate pharynx)	☐	☐
Absent cough response (tracheobronchial suction)	☐	☐
Ocular Movement		
• Absent oculocephalic reflex (perform only if cervical spine is stable)	☐	☐
• Absent deviation of eyes with cold water stimulation of the tympanic membranes	☐	☐
Step 2a: Consider Confirmatory Test* if Steps 1 or 2 cannot be fully performed or adequately interpreted.		
Step 3: Absence of Respiratory Effort†		
Positive Apnea Test: Absent respiratory efforts when the arterial PCO_2 increases by more than 20 mm Hg above the patient's normal baseline.	☐	
Step 3a: Consider Confirmatory Test* if Step 3 cannot be fully performed or adequately interpreted.		

***Confirmatory Testing**

These conditions may warrant confirmatory tests: 1) significant levels of drugs (e.g., sedatives, neuromuscular blocking agents, anticholinergics, organophosphates, tricyclic

(*Continued*)

neurological deficits persist after 3 days following the cardiac arrest, the chances for recovery are practically nil (28).

The data in Table 50-4 also demonstrate that the Glascow Coma Scale does not reach its full predictive power in the first few hours after cardiac arrest. Therefore, **the Glascow Coma Scale should not be used to predict the chances for neurological recovery in the first few hours after cardiac arrest.**

BRAIN DEATH

As mentioned earlier, brain death is a condition of irreversible cessation of function in the entire brain, including the brainstem (10). This condition is most often the result of cardiac arrest, intracerebral hemorrhage or infarction, or trauma. Regardless of the primary event, brain death usually results from widespread brain edema, elevation of intracranial pressure, and irreversible cessation of blood flow to the brain and brainstem (36). Brain death is not a common consequence of the conditions listed in Figure 50.2

Diagnosis

The lack of consensus regarding the diagnosis of brain death makes it impossible to state one unifying set of diagnostic criteria (37). In fact, distinct differences in diagnostic criteria vary by country and even state, and mandate consulting local guidelines. A checklist for the diagnosis of brain death in adults is shown in Table 50.5.

Prior to performing a brain death examination, other confounding conditions (e.g., locked-in syndrome, hypothermia) should be excluded

(*Continued*)

antidepressants, antiepileptic drugs), 2) severe facial trauma, 3) cervical spinal cord injury, 4) preexisting pupillary abnormalities, or 5) severe pulmonary disease and chronic hypercapnia. Confirmatory test options include: cerebral angiography, brain scan with technetium-99m, electroencephalography, transcranial doppler, or somatosensory evoked potentials. (See references for details.)

[†]**Apnea Test**

Prerequisites: 1) Begin test at patient's normal baseline arterial PCO_2 (never less than 40 mm Hg), 2) T ≥36.5°C (97°F), systolic BP ≥90 mm Hg.

Perform test: 1) Preoxygenate with 100% O_2, 2) monitor BP and pulse oximetry, 3) deliver 100% O_2 via canula into the trachea to maintain oxygenation, 4) observe for respiratory movements, 5) measure arterial PO_2, PCO_2, and pH after at least 8 minutes and reconnect the ventilator.

Abort test: Draw blood gas and reconnect ventilator for: 1) spontaneous respirations or movement, 2) systolic BP ≤90 mm Hg, 3) oxygen desaturation, or 4) cardiac dysrhythmias.

Modified from: 1) Practice Parameters for Determining Brain Death in Adults. Neurology, 1995. 45:1012–1014, and 2) Wijdicks EF. The diagnosis of brain death. N Engl J Med 2001;344:1215–1221.

(10). The goal of the brain death determination is to establish: 1) irreversible coma, 2) the absence of brain stem reflexes, and 3) the absence of spontaneous respirations. If the etiology of the coma is unknown, or if part of the clinical examination cannot be performed (e.g., ocular injury), then confirmatory testing (e.g., cerebral blood flow studies) can help make a definitive diagnosis.

Apnea Testing

The hallmark of the brain death examination is the demonstration of the persistent absence of all respiratory efforts in the presence of an acute increase in arterial PCO_2. Because the apnea test can cause hypotension, hypoxemia, and cardiac dysrhythmias, it best to make this the last step in brain death determination. Prior to the test, the patient is preoxygenated with 100% O_2 and minute ventilation is set to the patient's normal baseline arterial PCO_2 (but never less than 40 mm Hg). Next, the patient is separated from the ventilator, oxygen is insufflated into the endotracheal tube (apneic oxygenation helps prevent desaturation), and the PCO_2 rises at about 3 mm Hg per minute. Because hypothermia slows metabolism and the rate of rise of CO_2 in the blood (38), the apnea test should be performed only after normothermia has been established. After 8–10 minutes of apnea, the arterial blood is sampled and the patient should be briefly hyperventilated and then placed back on mechanical ventilation at the pre-test ventilator settings. If apnea persists despite a rise in the arterial $PCO_2 > 20$ mm Hg, the test is positive and consistent with a diagnosis of brain death. If there are complications, hypotension, desaturation, or significant cardiac dysrhythmias, the apnea test is aborted and an arterial blood sample is drawn to determine whether the increase in arterial PCO_2 is adequate to satisfy conditions of the test.

In the absence of normal sympathetic tone, hypercapnia causes a decline in left ventricular function and peripheral vasodilation. Thus, it is not surprising that hypotension is the most commonly observed hemodynamic alteration during an apnea test, with an incidence of 24% (39).

Brain dead patients can exhibit brief, spontaneous movements of the head, torso, or upper extremities (*Lazarus' Sign*), especially after they are removed from the ventilator. These movements are likely due to cervical spinal cord neuronal discharges in response to hypoxemia or mechanical stimulation (40). After the movements cease, the extremities become flaccid.

The Potential Organ Donor

For the potential organ donor, the following measures can be used to enhance organ viability (41).

Hemodynamics

Hypotension (MAP $\leq$60 mm Hg), reduced urinary output (<1 mL/kg per hour), or reduced cardiac output (<2.4 L/min/m_2) should be corrected with fluid resuscitation (to a CVP 6–8 mm Hg or a PCWP 8–12 mm Hg) followed by either dopamine (for hypotension) or dobutamine (for reduced cardiac output) if necessary. The dose of vasopressors should be minimized to help maintain organ perfusion. Pulmonary artery catheterization can be helpful because there may be poor correlation between left and right heart filling pressures (42).

Pituitary Failure

More than half of patients with brain death will develop pituitary failure with **diabetes insipidus** and secondary adrenal insufficiency (43). Both conditions can lead to profound hypovolemia (and reduced organ perfusion) and hypertonic hypernatremia (and cell dehydration). If there is evidence of central diabetes insipidus (i.e., spontaneous diuresis with a urine osmolality below 200 mOsm/L), treatment with **desmopressin**, a vasopressin analog that does not cause vasoconstriction, is advised (44). The usual dose of desmopressin is 0.5 to 2.0 μg IV every 2–3 hours and the dose is titrated to maintain a urine output of about 100–200 ml/hr. Hyperglycemia is also common, especially when dilute dextrose solutions are used to treat hypovolemic hypernatremia, and insulin replacement is required to maintain serum glucose between 80 and 150 mg/dL (41).

Surprisingly, multiple pituitary failure is uncommon in the first few days after brain death, and levels of TSH and ACTH are normal or elevated (45,46). When blood pressure and cardiac function remained depressed despite hemodynamic optimization, hormone replacement therapy (e.g., methylprednisolone and triiodothyronine) can improve organ function and recovery (47,48).

A FINAL WORD

The care of the comatose patient involves as much (if not more) time with families and loved ones, and nothing is more frightening to them than the possible loss of life or independent function on the part of the patient. Be compassionate, but above all, be honest. Avoiding the *conspiracy of silence* (49) is one of the greatest services you can perform as a physician.

REFERENCES

Introduction

1. Ely EW, Gautam S, Margolin R, et al. The impact of delirium in the intensive care unit on hospital length of stay. Intensive Care Med 2001;27:1892–1900.
2. Ely EW, Shintani A, Truman B, et al. Delirium as a predictor of mortality in mechanically ventilated patients in the intensive care unit. JAMA 2004;291: 1753–1762.

Reviews

3. Inouye SK. Delirium in older persons. N Engl J Med 2006;354:1157–1165.
4. Stevens RD, Bhardwaj A. Approach to the comatose patient. Crit Care Med 2006;34:31–41.

5. Wijdicks EFM. Brain death. Oxford: Oxford University Press, 2001.
6. Wijdicks EFM. Neurologic complications of critical illness. 2nd ed. New York: Oxford University Press, 2001.
7. Plum F, Posner JB. The diagnosis of stupor and coma. 3rd ed. Philadelphia: FA Davis, 1982.

Disorders of Consciousness

8. The Multi-Society Task Force on PVS. Medical aspects of the persistent vegetative state (Part 1). N Engl J Med 1994;330:1499–1508.
9. Leon-Carrion J, van Eeckhout P, Dominguez-Morales M del R. The locked-in syndrome: a syndrome looking for a therapy. Brain Injury 2002;16:555–569.
10. The Quality Standards Subcommittee of the American Academy of Neurology. Practice parameters for determining brain death in adults (summary statement). Neurology 1995;45:1012–1014.
11. Brown TM, Boyle MF. Delirium. BMJ 2002;325:644–647.
12. Papadopoulos MC, Davies DC, Moss RF, et al. Pathophysiology of septic encephalopathy: a review. Crit Care Med 2000;28:3019–3024.
13. Bleck TP, Smith MC, Pierre-Louis SJ, et al. Neurologic complications of critical medical illnesses. Crit Care Med 1993;21:98–103.
14. Sprung CL, Cerra FB, Freund HR, et al. Amino acid alterations and encephalopathy in the sepsis syndrome. Crit Care Med 1991;19:753–757.
15. Sari A, Yamashita S, Ohosita S, et al. Cerebrovascular reactivity to CO_2 in patients with hepatic or septic encephalopathy. Resuscitation 1990;19:125–134.

Delirium

16. Ely EW, Margolin R, Francis J, et al. Evaluation of delirium in critically ill patients: validation of the Confusion Assessment Method for the Intensive Care Unit (CAM-ICU). Crit Care Med 2001;29:1370–1379.
17. Webster R, Holroyd S. Prevalence of psychotic symptoms in delirium. Psychosomatics 2000;41:519–522.
18. McGuire BE, Basten CJ, Ryan CJ, et al. Intensive care unit syndrome: a dangerous misnomer. Arch Intern Med 2000;160:906–909.
19. Inouye SK. The dilemma of delirium: clinical and research controversies regarding diagnosis and evaluation of delirium in hospitalized elderly medical patients. Am J Med 1994;97:278–288.
20. Fick DM, Agostini JV, Inouye SK. Delirium superimposed on dementia: a systematic review. J Am Geriatr Soc 2002;50:1723–1732.
21. Kosten TR, O'Connor PG. Management of drug and alcohol withdrawal. N Engl J Med 2003;348:1786–1795.
22. Hoffman RS. An effective strategy for managing cocaine-induced agitated delirium: which therapies improve survival? Which are counterproductive? J Crit Illness 1994;9:139–149.

Coma

23. Hamel MB, Goldman L, Teno J, et al. Identification of comatose patients at high risk for death or severe disability. JAMA 1995;273:1842–1848.

24. Bateman DE. Neurological assessment of coma. J Neurol Neurosurg Psychiatry 2001;71:i13–17.
25. Goetting MG, Contreras E. Systemic atropine administration during cardiac arrest does not cause fixed and dilated pupils. Ann Emerg Med 1991;20: 55–57.
26. Ong GL, Bruning HA. Dilated fixed pupils due to administration of high doses of dopamine hydrochloride. Crit Care Med 1981;9:658–659.
27. Gray AT, Krejci ST, Larson MD. Neuromuscular blocking drugs do not alter the pupillary light reflex of anesthetized humans. Arch Neurol 1997;54:579–584.
28. Edgren E, Hedstrand U, Kelsey S, et al. Assessment of neurological prognosis in comatose survivors of cardiac arrest: BRCT I Study Group. Lancet 1994;343:1055–1059.
29. Zandbergen EG, de Haan RJ, Koelman JH, et al. Prediction of poor outcome in anoxic-ischemic coma. J Clin Neurophysiol 2000;17:498–501.
30. Kunze K. Metabolic encephalopathies. J Neurol 2002;249:1150–1159.
31. Teasdale G, Jennett B. Assessment of coma and impaired consciousness: a practical scale. Lancet 1974;2:81–84.
32. Teasdale G, Jennett B. Assessment and prognosis of coma after head injury. Acta Neurochir (Wien) 1976;34:45–55.
33. Sacco RL, VanGool R, Mohr JP, et al. Nontraumatic coma: Glasgow coma score and coma etiology as predictors of 2-week outcome. Arch Neurol 1990; 47:1181–1184.
34. Sternbach GL. The Glasgow coma scale. J Emerg Med 2000;19:67–71.
35. Booth CM, Boone RH, Tomlinson G, et al. Is this patient dead, vegetative, or severely neurologically impaired? Assessing outcome for comatose survivors of cardiac arrest. JAMA 2004;291:870–879.

Brain Death

36. Smith AJ, Walker AE. Cerebral blood flow and brain metabolism as indicators of cerebral death: a review. Johns Hopkins Med J 1973;133:107–119.
37. Wijdicks EF. Brain death worldwide: accepted fact but no global consensus in diagnostic criteria. Neurology 2002;58:20–25.
38. Dominguez-Roldan JM, Barrera-Chacon JM, Murillo-Cabezas F, et al. Clinical factors influencing the increment of blood carbon dioxide during the apnea test for the diagnosis of brain death. Transplant Proc 1999;31:2599–2600.
39. Goudreau JL, Wijdicks EF, Emery SF. Complications during apnea testing in the determination of brain death: predisposing factors. Neurology 2000; 55:1045–1048.
40. Ropper AH. Unusual spontaneous movements in brain-dead patients. Neurology 1984;34:1089–1092.
41. Wood KE, Becker BN, McCartney JG, et al. Care of the potential organ donor. N Engl J Med 2004;351:2730–2739.
42. Pennefather SH, Bullock RE, Mantle D, et al. Use of low dose arginine vasopressin to support brain-dead organ donors. Transplantation 1995;59:58–62.
43. Detterbeck FC, Mill MR. Organ donation and the management of the multiple organ donor. Contemp Surg 1993;42:281–285.
44. Guesde R, Barrou B, Leblanc I, et al. Administration of desmopressin in brain-dead donors and renal function in kidney recipients. Lancet 1998;352: 1178–1181.

45. Powner DJ, Hendrich A, Lagler RG, et al. Hormonal changes in brain dead patients. Crit Care Med 1990;18:702–708.
46. Gramm HJ, Meinhold H, Bickel U, et al. Acute endocrine failure after brain death? Transplantation 1992;54:851–857.
47. Rosendale JD, Kauffman HM, McBride MA, et al. Hormonal resuscitation yields more transplanted hearts, with improved early function. Transplantation 2003;75:1336–1341.
48. Rosendale JD, Kauffman HM, McBride MA, et al. Aggressive pharmacologic donor management results in more transplanted organs. Transplantation 2003;75:482–487.
49. Fallowfield LJ, Jenkins VA, Beveridge HA. Truth may hurt but deceit hurts more: communication in palliative care. Palliative Med 2002;16:297–303.

Chapter 51

DISORDERS OF MOVEMENT

This chapter focuses on three general types of movement disorders encountered in critically ill patients: (*1*) involuntary movements (seizures), (*2*) weak or ineffective movements (neuromuscular weakness), and (*3*) no movements (neuromuscular blockers).

SEIZURES

Seizures are second only to metabolic encephalopathy as the most common neurological complication following admission to the ICU (1). The incidence of new-onset seizures in ICU patients is 0.8% to 3.5% (1,2).

Definitions

The following definitions will prove helpful in the description, evaluation, and treatment of seizures (3–5).

Types of Movement

Seizures can be accompanied by any of the following patterns of muscular activity: *tonic* contractions (sustained muscle contraction), *atonic* contractions (absence of postural muscle contraction), *clonic* contractions (periodic symmetric body and extremity movements with regular amplitude and frequency), or *myoclonic* contractions (abrupt shock-like muscle contractions with an irregular amplitude and frequency) (5). Seizures can be accompanied by familiar movements known as *automatisms* (e.g., lip smacking or chewing). The *post-ictal* period refers to the time immediately following a seizure and there may be transient impairment of mentation and sensorium.

Generalized Seizures

Generalized seizures arise from symmetric and synchronous electrical discharges involving the entire cerebral cortex. These seizures may or may not be accompanied by muscle contractions. *Atonic seizures* cause a brief loss of motor tone (drop attack) that can cause falling. *Absence seizures* (formerly known as petit-mal seizures) are brief (usually <10 seconds) and are associated with less prominent changes in muscle tone (e.g., tonic, clonic, atonic, or automatisms). *Generalized tonic-clonic seizures* have an initial tonic phase, which is associated with apnea and cyanosis, followed by a clonic phase where respirations become labored (5).

Partial Seizures

Partial seizures originate as abnormal electrical discharges that are confined to a focal or restricted part of the cerebral cortex. They are subdivided into *simple partial seizures* (do not impair consciousness), *complex partial seizures* (cause impaired consciousness) and *partial seizures with secondary generalization* (a partial seizure that evolves into a generalized convulsive seizure). Two types of complex partial seizures that deserve mention are *temporal lobe seizures* (characterized by a motionless stare and automatisms) and *epilepsia partialis continua* (characterized by persistent tonic-clonic movements of the facial and limb muscles on one side of the body).

Status Epilepticus

Status epilepticus is defined as more than 30 minutes of continuous seizure activity, or recurrent seizure activity without an intervening period of consciousness (6). The most common and potentially dangerous forms of status epilepticus are described below.

1. **Generalized convulsive status epilepticus** is the most common form of status epilepticus. Despite treatment, the mortality associated with this type of status epilepticus is 20%–27% (7,8). After about 30 minutes, generalized convulsive status epilepticus can degenerate to non-convulsive status (6).
2. **Non-convulsive generalized status epilepticus** (subtle status epilepticus) is associated with minimal or no motor activity and requires electroencephalography for diagnosis. As many as 25% of cases of status epilepticus are nonconvulsive (6), and this condition is responsible for 8% of cases of unexplained coma (9). In fact, the most common seizure recorded during electroencephalographic monitoring of patients with altered mental status is non-convulsive (10). Non-convulsive seizures are often refractory to therapy, and are associated with a 65% mortality (8).
3. **Refractory status epilepticus** is a seizure that lasts more than 1 or 2 hours or is refractory to therapy with 2 or 3 anticonvulsant agents (11). Almost one-third of cases of status epilepticus are refractory (11).
4. **Myoclonic status epilepticus** can occur in up to one-third of patients with persistent coma following out-of-hospital cardiac arrest. This condition is characterized by sound-induced or spontaneous irregular and repetitive movements of the face and extremities (12). When it persists for 24 hours following resuscitation, myoclonic status is a sign of devastating neurological damage (13).

Etiologies

New-onset seizures can be the result of a drug intoxication (e.g., theophylline), drug withdrawal (e.g., ethanol), infections (e.g., meningoencephalitis, abscess), head trauma, ischemic injury (e.g., focal or diffuse), space-occupying lesions (e.g., tumor of hemorrhage), or systemic metabolic derangements (e.g., hepatic or uremic encephalopathy, sepsis, hypoglycemia, hyponatremia, or hypocalcemia) (4). In one survey of new-onset seizures in ICU patients, the most common causes were sedative or opioid withdrawal (33%), severe metabolic abnormalities (33%), and drug intoxication (15%) (2). The drugs most likely to cause seizures in ICU patients are listed in Table 51.1 (3,4).

Status Epilepticus

In one survey, only 10% of patients who develop seizures in a medical ICU go on to develop status epilepticus (1). The most common causes of status epilepticus are noncompliance with or withdrawal of antiepileptic drug therapy, cerebrovascular disease, and alcohol withdrawal (14).

Evaluation

The evaluation of new-onset seizures should focus on the etiologies previously mentioned. In the absence of an obvious and potentially reversible metabolic or drug-related cause, or when the physical exam reveals a focal abnormality, further evaluation (neuroimaging studies and lumbar puncture) is advised. In ICU patients with depressed mental status or

TABLE 51.1 Drug-Related Seizures in the ICU

Drug Intoxication	Drug Withdrawal
Pharmaceuticals:	Barbiturates
Ciprofloxacin	Benzodiazepines
Imipenem	Ethanol
Isoniazid	Opiates
Lidocaine	
Meperidine	
Penicillins	
Theophylline	
Tricyclics	
Drugs of Abuse:	
Amphetamines	
Cocaine	
Phencyclidine	

Adapted from Delanty N, Vaughan CJ, French JA. Medical causes of seizures. Lancet 1998;352:383–390.

following an episode of status epilepticus, electroencephalography is necessary to detect non-convulsive seizures, which are the most common type of seizures observed when EEG monitoring is used (10).

Complications

The adverse effects of generalized seizures include hypertension, lactic acidosis, hyperthermia, respiratory compromise, pulmonary aspiration or edema, rhabdomyolysis, self-injury, and irreversible neurological damage (when seizures persist for longer than 30 minutes) (6).

Management

If the seizure stops and the immediate cause is corrected, anti-epileptic medication may not be necessary. Seizures that persist for longer than 5–10 minutes should be treated urgently because of the risk for permanent neurological injury, and also because seizures become refractory to therapy the longer they persist (15). The acute drug management of convulsive seizures is summarized in Figure 51.1 (7,8,15-17). Most neurologists concur regarding the drug management indicated in Steps 1 and 2, and opinions vary regarding agents to be used in Step 3.

Benzodiazepines

Intravenous benzodiazepines will terminate 65–80% of convulsive seizures within 2 to 3 minutes (8,15). Lorazepam (Ativan) in a dose of 0.1 mg/kg IV or diazepam (Valium) in a dose of 0.15 mg/kg IV is equally effective in aborting a generalized seizure (7,15). However, the anticonvulsant effects of lorazepam lasts longer than those of diazepam (12–24 hours vs. 15–30 minutes, respectively), so recurrent seizures are less likely following lorazepam (7,15). Because of its prolonged effect, lorazepam is the initial agent of choice for treatment of convulsive seizures. If diazepam is used, it should be followed immediately by phenytoin to prevent seizure recurrence.

Phenytoins

Intravenous phenytoin has been widely used to treat seizures since 1956. The standard intravenous dose is 20 mg/kg in adults; a smaller dose of 15 mg/kg is recommended in the elderly (16). A maximum infusion rate of 50 mg/min is advised to reduce the risk for cardiovascular depression (which is due to the drug itself and the propylene glycol diluent used in intravenous preparations) (15). If the initial dose of phenytoin is unsuccessful, additional doses can be given to a total cumulative dose of 30 mg/kg (15). The therapeutic serum level for phenytoin is 10 to 20 μg/mL. Phenytoin should not be given in dextrose-containing solutions because it can precipitate (18), and tissue extravasation must be avoided because the highly alkaline pH of 12 can cause tissue necrosis.

Fosphenytoin (Cerebyx) is a prodrug that may be preferred to phenytoin because: 1) it can be infused faster than phenytoin, 2) it does not

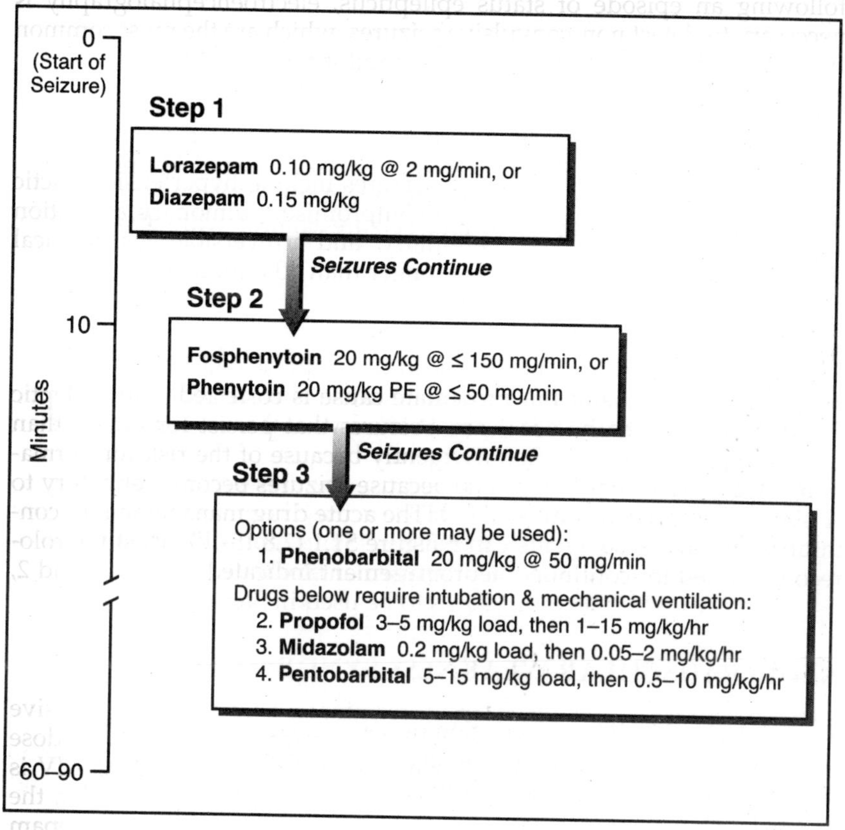

FIGURE 51.1 Intravenous drug therapy for convulsive seizures in the ICU. PE = phenytoin equivalents.

contain propylene glycol (which contributes to cardiovascular depression), 3) it is compatible with dextrose-containing solutions, and 4) drug extravasation does not cause skin necrosis (18). Fosphenytoin is rapidly converted to phenytoin (half life is 7–15 minutes), and the therapeutic doses are the same as those recommended for phenytoin (18). However, the maximum allowable infusion rate for fosphenytoin is 150 mg/min, which is three times faster than phenytoin, so fosphenytoin could produce more rapid suppression of seizures than phenytoin.

Phenobarbital

The combination of benzodiazepines and phenytoin will control seizures in 60–90% of cases of convulsive status epilepticus (11). In refractory cases, intravenous phenobarbital can be effective when given in a dose of 50–75 mg/min until seizures are controlled or a maximum of 20 mg/kg is achieved. The therapeutic serum level for phenobarbital is 20 to 40 µg/mL. Common side effects include hypotension (usually responsive to IV fluids), respiratory depression, and prolonged sedation (at the higher dose range). Phenobarbital is also the most effective agent available for the initial treatment of nonconvulsive seizures (8).

Anticonvulsant hypersensitivity syndrome is an uncommon (incidence 1:1,000 to 1:10,000) idiosyncratic reaction to phenytoin or phenobarbital (cross-reactivity is 50%) associated with the triad of fever, rash, and lymphadenopathy (19). Elevated liver enzymes and lymphocytosis occur in up to two-thirds of cases. Treatment involves immediate withdrawal of the offending agent and seizure control with diazepam at 0.05–0.4 mg/kg/hr (20).

Refractory Status Epilepticus

Status epilepticus that is refractory to first and second line agents can be treated with infusions of propofol, midazolam, or pentobarbital (see Figure 51.1). Pentobarbital is the most effective of these agents but it often causes hypotension (21). Refractory cases require endotracheal intubation, mechanical ventilation, and electroencephalographic monitoring. A single dose of neuromuscular blocker may be required to facilitate intubation, but these agents can mask seizures, and EEG monitoring is recommended for continued neuromuscular blockade.

NEUROMUSCULAR WEAKNESS SYNDROMES

The following is a brief description of neuromuscular disorders that can produce severe and life-threatening neuromuscular weakness. Some comparative features of these disorders are included in Tables 51.2 and 51.3 (22–24).

Myasthenia Gravis

Myasthenia gravis is an autoimmune disease that is characterized by antibody-mediated destruction of acetylcholine receptors located at the postsynaptic side of neuromuscular junctions. This condition is uncommon, and affects about 1 in every 100,000 adults (25).

TABLE 51.2 Comparative Features of Myasthenia Gravis and Guillain-Barré Syndrome

Features	Myasthenia Gravis	Guillain-Barré Syndrome
Ocular findings	Yes	No
Fluctuating weakness	Yes	No
Bulbar weakness	Yes	Yes
Deep tendon reflexes	Intact	Depressed
Autonomic instability	No	Yes
Nerve conduction	Normal	Slowed

TABLE 51.3 Comparative Features of Conditions Associated with ICU-Acquired Neuromuscular Weakness

	Critical Illness Polyneuropathy	Residual Neuromuscular Block	Critical Illness Myopathy
Sensory	Moderate to severe	Normal	Normal
Motor	Symmetric weakness, respiratory failure	Symmetric weakness, respiratory failure	Symmetric weakness, respiratory failure
Creatine Kinase	Normal	Normal	Mild elevation in 50%
Electrodiagnostic Studies	Motor & sensory axonal degeneration, normal conduction velocity	Fatigue at neuromuscular junction	Myopathic changes, normal conduction velocity
Muscle Biopsy	Denervation atrophy	Normal	Muscle atrophy, loss of thick (myosin) filaments

Clinical Features

The weakness in myasthenia gravis worsens with repeated activity and improves with rest (25). Signs of weakness are usually first evident in the eyelids and extraocular muscles, and generalized weakness of the limbs follows in 85% of cases (26). The proximal limb muscles are often affected, and weakness can involve the diaphragm and thoracic musculature. Weakness of pharyngeal muscles can impair swallowing and predispose to pulmonary aspiration. Rapid progression to respiratory failure and ventilator dependence, called *myasthenic crisis,* occurs in 15–20% of patients (27). The deficit in myasthenia is purely motor, with no sensory involvement. Deep tendon reflexes are usually preserved.

In addition to concurrent illness and surgery, several medications can precipitate or aggravate the myasthenic syndrome. The principle offenders are antibiotics (e.g., aminoglycosides, ciprofloxacin), cardiac drugs (e.g., beta-adrenergic blockers, lidocaine, procainamide, quinidine), and magnesium (28). Magnesium blocks the presynaptic release of acetylcholine, and can be particularly detrimental in myasthenic patients.

Diagnosis

The diagnosis of myasthenia gravis is based on the characteristic pattern of muscle weakness (e.g., eyelid or extraocular muscle weakness, worse with activity) and the finding of increased muscle strength after the administration of **edrophonium** (Tensilon), an acetylcholinesterase inhibitor. Acetylcholine receptor antibodies can be demonstrated in the blood (by radioimmunoassay) in 85% of cases, and presence of antibodies confirms the diagnosis (25). Once the diagnosis is confirmed, a search for associated conditions such as thymic tumors (10–20% of cases) and hyperthyroidism (5% of cases) is advised.

Treatment

The first line of therapy in myasthenia gravis is the administration of acetylcholinesterase inhibitors like **pyridostigmine** (Mestinon), which is started at an oral dose of 60 mg every 6 hours and is increased if necessary to a maximum dose of 120 mg every 6 hours. Pyridostigmine can be given intravenously to treat myasthenic crisis (the IV dose is 1/30 of the oral dose) (27,29). **Immunotherapy** is added if needed using either prednisone (1–1.5 mg/kg/day), azathioprine (1 to 3 mg/kg/day), or cyclosporine (2.5 mg/kg twice per day) (29).

In advanced cases requiring mechanical ventilation, **plasmapheresis** (to remove anti-acetylcholine receptor antibodies) is often effective in producing short-term improvement (29). **Intravenous immunoglobulin G** (0.4 to 2 g/kg/day for 2 to 5 days) to neutralize pathogenic antibodies is also effective (26,29). Both therapies are equally effective; however, plasmapharesis may produce a more rapid response (29). Surgical thymectomy is often advised in patients under 60 years of age to reduce the need for immunosuppressive therapy (29).

Guillain-Barré Syndrome

The Guillain-Barré syndrome is an acute inflammatory demyelinating polyneuropathy that follows an acute infectious illness (by 1 to 3 weeks) in two-thirds of cases (30,31). The infectious agents most often associated with this disorder are *Campylobacter jejuni* and cytomegalovirus (30). An immune etiology is suspected, and some patients have circulating antibodies to gangliosides in peripheral nerves (30).

Clinical Features

The clinical presentation is marked by paresthesias, diminished reflexes, and symmetric limb weakness that evolve over a period of a few days to a few weeks. Symptoms of a preceding infection usually subside before the weakness becomes apparent. Approximately 25% of cases show progression to respiratory failure requiring mechanical ventilation (30). Advanced cases can also be associated with autonomic instability and bulbar paralysis (30,32,33). The condition resolves spontaneously in approximately 80% of cases; however, residual neurological deficits are common (30).

Diagnosis and Therapy

The diagnosis is based on the clinical presentation (progressive symmetric limb weakness following an acute infectious illness), the results of nerve conduction studies (slowing of nerve conduction due to demyelination), and cerebrospinal fluid analysis (elevated protein content in 80%) (30).

The treatment of Guillain-Barré syndrome mostly involves supportive care. In severe cases requiring mechanical ventilation, **plasmapheresis or intravenous immunoglobulin G** (0.4 g/kg/day for 5 days) **are equally effective in producing short-term improvement.** Immunoglobulin G is often preferred because it is easiest to administer (30). Since this disorder resolves spontaneously in most cases, careful attention to the potential complications (e.g., pneumonia, thromboembolism) is mandatory for optimal patient outcome. The respiratory management of this disorder is described later in the chapter.

Critical Illness Polyneuropathy and Myopathy

Critical illness polyneuropathy and myopathy are complications of clinical disorders that are associated with progressive and uncontrolled systemic inflammation. These conditions, which are described in Chapter 40, include the systemic inflammatory response syndrome (SIRS), severe sepsis, and multiorgan failure. Although common, these neuromuscular complications often go undetected because they are overshadowed by the more prominent clinical manifestations of the inciting conditions (34).

Clinical Features

As many as 70% of patients with SIRS or sepsis and multiple organ failure will have evidence of polyneuropathy or myopathy, and both disorders can occur in the same patient (22). Although there may be severe limb and truncal involvement, the weakness usually becomes apparent only after the underlying illness begins to resolve. In many cases, the weakness is first discovered when a patient is unable to wean from mechanical ventilation. Persistent weakness after discontinuing treatment with a neuromuscular blocking agent is another way these conditions can become apparent.

Critical Illness Polyneuropathy

Critical illness polyneuropathy is a diffuse sensory and motor axonal neuropathy that is reported in 50–70% of patients with SIRS (22,35). It is often preceded by septic encephalopathy, and the two occur together in 70% of patients (22). Bulbar weakness is uncommon and autonomic function is preserved, which helps to distinguish this condition from the Guillain-Barré syndrome (36). The onset of polyneuropathy is variable, occurring from 2 days to a few weeks after the onset of the inciting illness (37–39).

Electrodiagnostic testing (with nerve conduction studies and electromyograms) is necessary to establish the diagnosis. There is no specific treatment for this disorder, and prevention (by prompt treatment of the predisposing condition) is currently the only option. One study has shown that intensive insulin therapy (to achieve tight control of blood glucose) can reduce the incidence of critical illness polyneuropathy by 44% (40). Complete recovery is expected in 50% of cases (36). In mild cases of polyneuropathy, recovery can be complete within a few weeks, but in severe cases, recovery can take months.

Critical Illness Myopathy

Critical illness myopathy is a spectrum of muscle disorders that present with diffuse weakness, depressed deep tendon reflexes, and mildly elevated creatine kinase levels (in 50% of cases) (24). Electrodiagnostic testing reveals a myopathy, and muscle biopsy reveals atrophy and loss of thick (myosin) filaments (24). Critical illness myopathy is observed in about one-third of patients with status asthmaticus, (particularly those receiving high-dose corticosteroids) (24). This myopathy is also more prevalent with prolonged use of corticosteroids and neuromuscular blocking agents (22,24). Like the polyneuropathy, there is no specific treatment for critical illness myopathy. Most patients with isolated critical illness myopathy make a full recovery in a few months (24).

Pulmonary Complications

The pulmonary consequences of progressive neuromuscular weakness are summarized in Table 51.4. Respiratory muscle strength must decrease considerably before pulmonary complications appear. The earliest complication is a depressed cough with difficulty clearing secretions. This can lead to aspiration and retained secretions with infection and airway obstruction. When patients are unable to swallow or clear secretions adequately, tracheal intubation is warranted. As the neuromuscular weakness progresses, atelectasis and hypoxemia become prominent, followed by alveolar hypoventilation and progressive CO_2 retention. Hypoxemia is often a late finding, especially when patients are breathing supplemental oxygen.

One of the important points to note in Table 51.4 is the recommendation for early tracheal intubation and mechanical ventilation before

TABLE 51.4 Respiratory Consequences of Neuromuscular Weakness

Vital Capacity (mL/kg)	Consequences	Management
70	Normal respiratory muscle strength	Observe
30	Impaired cough with difficulty clearing secretions	Chest physiotherapy
25	Accumulation of secretions, with risk of infection and airways obstruction	Tracheal intubation
20	Atelectasis and progressive hypoxemia	Supplemental oxygen
10	Alveolar hypoventilation and hypercapnia	Mechanical ventilation

the appearance of respiratory failure (31,41). This is necessary in cases of neuromuscular weakness to prevent complications arising from the inability to clear respiratory secretions. The most sensitive measure of respiratory muscle strength in this situation is the maximum inspiratory pressure (PImax) (42), which is described in Chapter 27. A PImax <30 cm H_2O is evidence of severe respiratory muscle weakness, and is an indication for tracheal intubation and assisted ventilation.

NEUROMUSCULAR BLOCKERS

Drug-induced neuromuscular blockade is sometimes needed to manage ventilator-dependent patients who are agitated and difficult to ventilate. However, this practice has serious potential drawbacks (43,44), as described later. Overall, less than 10% of ICU patients receive these agents (45). The clinical practice guidelines for the sustained use of neuromuscular blockers in the ICU are listed in the bibliography at the end of the chapter (46,47).

Mechanisms

Neuromuscular blocking agents act by binding to nicotinic acetylcholine receptors on the postsynaptic side of the neuromuscular junction. Once bound, there are two different modes of action. The *depolarizing agents* act like acetylcholine, producing a sustained depolarization of the postsynaptic membrane that blocks subsequent muscle contraction. The *nondepolarizing agents* act by competitively inhibiting acetylcholine-induced depolarization of the post-synaptic membrane.

Neuromuscular Blockers

The neuromuscular blocking drugs that are most frequently used in the ICU are shown in Table 51.5 (46,48). All three agents in this table are nondepolarizing blockers.

Pancuronium (Pavulon) is a relatively long-acting neuromuscular blocker that was introduced for clinical use in 1972. The initial popularity of this agent has dwindled because of its long duration of action (tendency to accumulate with prolonged use) and vagolytic effect (which causes an increase in heart rate) (49). Although pancuronium can be given by continuous infusion, it is usually given as intermittent bolus doses to decrease the risk of drug accumulation. About 60% of pancuronium is excreted unchanged by the kidneys, and dosage reduction is therefore necessary in renal failure. When hepatic and renal function are intact, pancuronium is the preferred agent in the ICU (46,47).

Rocuronium (Zemuron) is a newer drug that produces a rapid onset of block and is devoid of cardiovascular side effects. Rocuronium is eliminated mostly in the bile and the dosage must be reduced in liver failure.

Cisatracurium (Nimbex) consists of a single potent isomer of its parent drug, atracurium (which consists of 10 isomers). While atracurium

TABLE 51.5 Pharmacology of Selected Nondepolarizing Neuromuscular Blockers

	Pancuronium (Pavulon)	Rocuronium (Zemuron)	Cisatracurium (Nimbex)
Initial Dose (mg/kg)	0.1	0.6–1.0	0.1–2.0
Duration (min)	60–100	30–40	35–50
Infusion (μg/kg/min)	1–2	10–12	2.5–3
Effect on Heart Rate	Tachycardia	Mild increase at high dose	None
Active Metabolite	Yes	No	Yes
Effect of Renal Failure	Prolongs effect of drug & metabolite	Minimally prolonged	None
Effect of Hepatic Failure	Mildly prolonged	Prolonged	None

can be used in the ICU, cisatracurium is preferred because: 1) it does not cause histamine release, 2) it does not cause cardiac depression, and 3) it generates less laudanosine, a metabolite that may cause neuroexcitation (50). Cisatracurium is rapidly degraded in the plasma, and it must be given by continuous infusion. The clinical effect is not prolonged by liver or kidney failure (51).

Succinylcholine (Anectine) is the only approved *depolarizing* neuromuscular blocker, and it is not included in Table 51.5 because it is used infrequently in the ICU. This agent is ultra-short acting, and is used only to facilitate endotracheal intubation. An intravenous dose of 1–2 mg/kg produces paralysis within 60 seconds, and the effect lasts for about 5 minutes. The depolarization of muscles cells produced by this agent is accompanied by potassium efflux out of muscle cells, and this can transiently raise the serum potassium by about 0.5 mEq/L (52). Life-threatening increases in serum potassium can occur when succinylcholine is given in the presence of denervation injury (e.g., head or spinal cord injury), rhabdomyolysis, hemorrhagic shock, thermal injury, and chronic immobility. Because these conditions are prevalent in ICU patients, it is wise to avoid succinylcholine in the ICU (53).

Monitoring

The standard method of monitoring drug-induced neuromuscular blockade is to apply a series of four low-frequency (2 Hz) electrical pulses (current strength 50 to 90 milliamps) to the ulnar nerve at the forearm, and observe for adduction of the thumb. Total absence of thumb adduction is evidence of excessive block. The desired goal is 1 or 2 perceptible twitches, and the drug infusion is adjusted to achieve that end-point (46,54).

Disadvantages

The following risks of neuromuscular paralysis are considerable enough to avoid this practice whenever possible. With the aggressive use of sedation and analgesia, use of neuromuscular blockers can often be avoided.

Inadequate Sedation

Neuromuscular blocking drugs do not produce analgesia or sedation and, because paralysis is an extremely frightening and even painful experience, it is imperative to establish the desired levels of sedation and analgesia *before* initiating drug-induced paralysis (44,46). Once the patient is paralyzed, liberal use of sedatives is advised to minimize the risk of awakening.

Prolonged Weakness

Neuromuscular blocking drugs can be associated with prolonged periods of muscle weakness after the drugs are discontinued. There are several possible reasons for this, including residual drug effect, and the presence of an underlying condition that predispose to neuromuscular weakness (46). Because of the risk for prolonged weakness, neuromuscular blocking drugs should be avoided (if possible) in any patient with a condition that predisposes to neuromuscular weakness (e.g., prolonged corticosteroid therapy).

Hypostatic Pneumonia

The absence of coughing during paralysis impairs the clearance of respiratory secretions. Endotracheal suction catheters are unable to reach the distal airways and prevent pooling of secretions in dependent lung regions. This can lead to *hypostatic pneumonia*.

Venous Thromboembolism

Loss of the milking action of muscle contraction on the venous return from the legs predisposes to venous thrombosis during neuromuscular paralysis. Therefore, prophylaxis for venous thrombosis (as described in Chapter 5) is mandatory during neuromuscular paralysis.

A FINAL WORD

Critical illness polyneuropathy and myopathy are common in conditions like severe sepsis that are associated with inflammatory injury to major organs. In fact, these neuromuscular disorders are probably the result of inflammatory injury involving peripheral nerves and skeletal muscle, which means they are probably part of the multiorgan failure that develops in patients with uncontrolled systemic inflammation (see Chapter 40). Like the other forms of inflammatory organ injury (e.g., acute respiratory distress syndrome) in the multiorgan failure syndrome, critical illness polyneuropathy and myopathy remain untreatable conditions that can add considerably to the morbidity and mortality of the ICU stay.

REFERENCES

Seizures

1. Bleck TP, Smith MC, Pierre-Louis SJ, et al. Neurologic complications of critical medical illnesses. Crit Care Med 1993;21:98–103.
2. Wijdicks EF, Sharbrough FW. New-onset seizures in critically ill patients. Neurology 1993;43:1042–1044.
3. Varelas PN, Mirski MA. Seizures in the adult intensive care unit. J Neurosurg Anesthesiol 2001;13:163–175.
4. Delanty N, Vaughan CJ, French JA. Medical causes of seizures. Lancet 1998;352:383–390.
5. Chabolla DR. Characteristics of the epilepsies. Mayo Clin Proc 2002;77:981–990.

Status Epilepticus

6. Marik PE, Varon J. The management of status epilepticus. Chest 2004;126:582–591.
7. Manno EM. New management strategies in the treatment of status epilepticus. Mayo Clin Proc 2003;78:508–518.
8. Treiman DM, Meyers PD, Walton NY, et al. A comparison of four treatments for generalized convulsive status epilepticus: Veterans Affairs Status Epilepticus Cooperative Study Group. N Engl J Med 1998;339:792–798.
9. Towne AR, Waterhouse EJ, Boggs JG, et al. Prevalence of nonconvulsive status epilepticus in comatose patients. Neurology 2000;54:340–345.
10. Claassen J, Mayer SA, Kowalski RG, et al. Detection of electrographic seizures with continuous EEG monitoring in critically ill patients. Neurology 2004;62:1743–1748.
11. Mayer SA, Claassen J, Lokin J, et al. Refractory status epilepticus: frequency, risk factors, and impact on outcome. Arch Neurol 2002;59:205–210.
12. Wijdicks EF, Parisi JE, Sharbrough FW. Prognostic value of myoclonus status in comatose survivors of cardiac arrest. Ann Neurol 1994;35:239–243.
13. Morris HR, Howard RS, Brown P. Early myoclonic status and outcome after cardiorespiratory arrest. J Neurol Neurosurg Psychiatry 1998;64:267–268.
14. Bassin S, Smith TL, Bleck TP. Clinical review: status epilepticus. Crit Care 2002;6:137–142.
15. Lowenstein DH, Alldredge BK. Status epilepticus. N Engl J Med 1998;338:970–976.
16. Epilepsy Foundation of America's Working Group on Status Epilepticus. Treatment of convulsive status epilepticus: recommendations of the Epilepsy Foundation of America's Working Group on Status Epilepticus. JAMA 1993;270:854–859.
17. Claassen J, Hirsch LJ, Mayer SA. Treatment of status epilepticus: a survey of neurologists. J Neurol Sci 2003;211:37–41.

18. Fischer JH, Patel TV, Fischer PA. Fosphenytoin: clinical pharmacokinetics and comparative advantages in the acute treatment of seizures. Clin Pharmacokinet 2003;42:33–58.
19. Morkunas AR, Miller MB. Anticonvulsant hypersensitivity syndrome. Crit Care Clin 1997;13:727–739.
20. Bertz RJ, Howrie DL. Diazepam by continuous intravenous infusion for status epilepticus in anticonvulsant hypersensitivity syndrome. Ann Pharmacother 1993;27:298–301.
21. Claassen J, Hirsch LJ, Emerson RG, et al. Treatment of refractory status epilepticus with pentobarbital, propofol, or midazolam: a systematic review. Epilepsia 2002;43:146–153.

Weakness in the ICU

22. Bolton CF. Neuromuscular manifestations of critical illness. Muscle Nerve 2005;32:140–163.
23. Hund E. Neurological complications of sepsis: critical illness polyneuropathy and myopathy. J Neurol 2001;248:929–934.
24. Lacomis D. Critical illness myopathy. Curr Rheumatol Rep 2002;4:403–408.

Myasthenia Gravis

25. Vincent A, Palace J, Hilton-Jones D. Myasthenia gravis. Lancet 2001;357:2122–2128.
26. Drachman DB. Myasthenia gravis. N Engl J Med 1994;330:1797–1810.
27. Berrouschot J, Baumann I, Kalischewski P, et al. Therapy of myasthenic crisis. Crit Care Med 1997;25:1228–1235.
28. Wittbrodt ET. Drugs and myasthenia gravis. An update. Arch Intern Med 1997;157:399–408.
29. Saperstein DS, Barohn RJ. Management of myasthenia gravis. Semin Neurol 2004;24:41–48.

Guillain-Barré Syndrome

30. Hughes RA, Cornblath DR. Guillain-Barre syndrome. Lancet 2005;366:1653–1666.
31. Hund EF, Borel CO, Cornblath DR, et al. Intensive management and treatment of severe Guillain-Barre syndrome. Crit Care Med 1993;21:433–446.
32. Pfeiffer G, Schiller B, Kruse J, et al. Indicators of dysautonomia in severe Guillain-Barre syndrome. J Neurol 1999;246:1015–1022.
33. Hughes R, McGuire G. Neurologic disease and the determination of brain death: the importance of a diagnosis. Crit Care Med 1997;25:1923–1924.

Critical Illness Polyneuropathy and Myopathy

34. Hudson LD, Lee CM. Neuromuscular sequelae of critical illness. N Engl J Med 2003;348:745–747.
35. Hund E. Critical illness polyneuropathy. Curr Opin Neurol 2001;14:649–653.
36. van Mook WN, Hulsewe-Evers RP. Critical illness polyneuropathy. Curr Opin Crit Care 2002;8:302–310.

37. Tennila A, Salmi T, Pettila V, et al. Early signs of critical illness polyneuropathy in ICU patients with systemic inflammatory response syndrome or sepsis. Intensive Care Med 2000;26:1360–1363.
38. Bolton CF. Neuromuscular complications of sepsis. Intensive Care Med 1993;19(suppl 2):S58–S63.
39. Bolton CF, Gilbert JJ, Hahn AF, et al. Polyneuropathy in critically ill patients. J Neurol Neurosurg Psychiatry 1984;47:1223–1231.
40. van den Berghe G, Wouters P, Weekers F, et al. Intensive insulin therapy in the critically ill patients. N Engl J Med 2001;345:1359–1367.
41. Newton-John H. Prevention of pulmonary complications in severe Guillain-Barre syndrome by early assisted ventilation. Med J Aust 1985;142:444–445.
42. Mier-Jedrzejowicz AK, Brophy C, Green M. Respiratory muscle function in myasthenia gravis. Am Rev Respir Dis 1988;138:867–873.
43. Hansen-Flaschen J, Cowen J, Raps EC. Neuromuscular blockade in the intensive care unit: more than we bargained for. Am Rev Respir Dis 1993;147:234–236.
44. Parker MM, Schubert W, Shelhamer JH, et al. Perceptions of a critically ill patient experiencing therapeutic paralysis in an ICU. Crit Care Med 1984;12:69–71.
45. Watling SM, Dasta JF, Seidl EC. Sedatives, analgesics, and paralytics in the ICU. Ann Pharmacother 1997;31:148–153.
46. Murray MJ, Cowen J, DeBlock H, et al. Clinical practice guidelines for sustained neuromuscular blockade in the adult critically ill patient. Crit Care Med 2002;30:142–156.
47. Vender JS, Szokol JW, Murphy GS, et al. Sedation, analgesia, and neuromuscular blockade in sepsis: an evidence-based review. Crit Care Med 2004;32:S554–S561.
48. Coursin DB, Prielipp RC. Use of neuromuscular blocking drugs in the critically ill patient. Crit Care Clin 1995;11:957–981.
49. Murray MJ, Coursin DB, Scuderi PE, et al. Double-blind, randomized, multicenter study of doxacurium vs. pancuronium in intensive care unit patients who require neuromuscular-blocking agents. Crit Care Med 1995;23:450–458.
50. Fodale V, Santamaria LB. Laudanosine, an atracurium and cisatracurium metabolite. Eur J Anaesthesiol 2002;19:466–473.
51. Kisor DF, Schmith VD. Clinical pharmacokinetics of cisatracurium besilate. Clin Pharmacokinet 1999;36:27–40.
52. Koide M, Waud BE. Serum potassium concentrations after succinylcholine in patients with renal failure. Anesthesiology 1972;36:142–145.
53. Gronert GA. Cardiac arrest after succinylcholine: mortality greater with rhabdomyolysis than receptor upregulation. Anesthesiology 2001;94:523–529.
54. Rudis MI, Guslits BG, Zarowitz BJ. Technical and interpretive problems of peripheral nerve stimulation in monitoring neuromuscular blockade in the intensive care unit. Ann Pharmacother 1996;30:165–172.

Chapter 52

STROKE AND RELATED DISORDERS

The principal focus of this chapter is a cerebrovascular disorder that was first described over 2,400 years ago, and since then has suffered through a variety of poorly descriptive names like apoplexy, stroke, cerebrovascular accident (what accident?), and brain attack. Considering that this disorder is the third leading cause of death in the United States, and the number one cause of long-term disability (1,2), it deserves a more appropriate name.

This chapter is devoted to the clinical presentation and early management of patients with stroke and other life-threatening cerebrovascular disorders. Several reviews on this topic are included at the end of the chapter (2–4).

DEFINITIONS

The following definitions and classifications are from the National Institute of Neurological Disorders and Stroke (5).

Stroke

Stroke is an **acute** brain disorder of **vascular** origin accompanied by **neurological dysfunction** that persists for **longer than 24 hours** (5). The neurological dysfunction is usually **focal** (which is typical of vascular occlusion), however, global dysfunction can occur when vascular rupture leads to hemorrhage and mass effect.

Classification of Stroke

Stroke can be classified according to its cause, as *ischemic* or *hemorrhagic* (citations specify the treatment guidelines) (1,3,5).

1. **Ischemic stroke** accounts for 80 to 88% of all strokes (6–9).
   a. **Thrombotic stroke** accounts for 80% of ischemic strokes and is caused by atherosclerotic disease (3).
   b. **Embolic stroke** accounts for 20% of ischemic strokes. Most emboli originate from thrombi in the left atrium (from atrial fibrillation) or left ventricle (from acute MI), but some originate from venous thrombi in the legs that reach the brain through a patent foramen ovale (10).
2. **Hemorrhagic stroke** accounts for 12–20% of all strokes.
   a. **Intracerebral hemorrhage** makes up 75% of hemorrhagic strokes, and is due to rupture of a blood vessel located within the brain parenchyma (11).
   b. **Subarachnoid hemorrhage** makes up 25% of hemorrhagic strokes, and is due to rupture of a blood vessel (often a saccular aneurysm) into the subarachnoid (cerebrospinal fluid) space (12,13).

Epidural and subdural hematomas are not considered to be strokes (5), and are not described in this chapter.

Transient Ischemic Attack

A *transient ischemic attack* (TIA) is an acute episode of focal loss of brain function due to ischemia that lasts less than 24 hours (5,14). **The one feature that distinguishes TIA from stroke is the reversibility of clinical symptoms.** Reversibility of cerebral injury is not a distinguishing feature because one-third of TIAs are associated with cerebral infarction (detected by magnetic resonance imaging) (9,15).

BEDSIDE EVALUATION

Acute stroke is a condition of ongoing ischemic injury that should be approached as a medical emergency. Each minute of ischemic stroke causes the destruction of 1.9 million neurons, 14 billion synapses, and 7.5 miles of myelinated nerves (16). In light of these numbers, the popular saying *time is brain*, should be upgraded to state *time is a lot of brain!*

Stroke is primarily a clinical diagnosis (17). The presentation is characterized by one or more focal neurological deficits corresponding to the region(s) of the brain that is ischemic (4). The clinical findings and corresponding regions of ischemic brain injury are shown in Figure 52.1 (6). The following is a summary of the pertinent clinical features of acute stroke (18).

Consciousness

Most cerebral infarctions are unilateral, and thus loss of consciousness is not a common finding (19,20). The causes of altered consciousness are

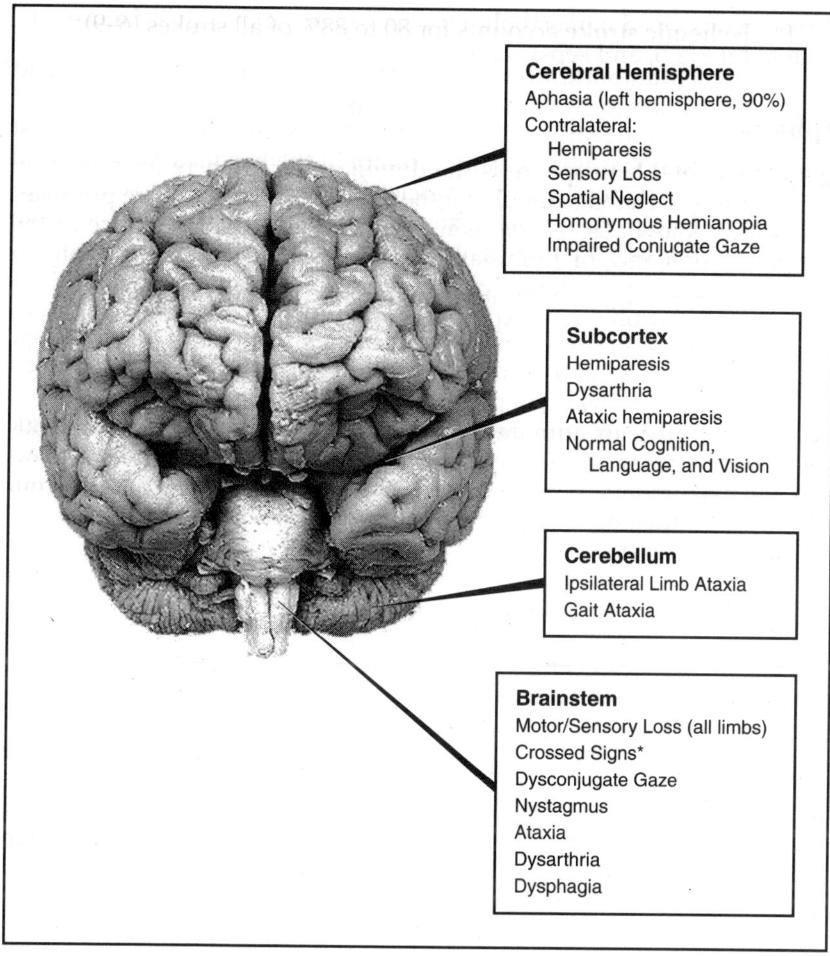

FIGURE 52.1 Neurological abnormalities and corresponding areas of ischemic brain injury. *Signs on same side of face and other side of body.

described in Chapter 50). When focal neurological deficits are accompanied by altered consciousness or coma, the most likely diagnoses are intracerebral hemorrhage, massive cerebral infarction with cerebral edema, brainstem infarction, or seizures (nonconvulsive seizures or post-ictal state).

Sensorimotor Function

The hallmark of ischemic or hemorrhagic injury involving the cerebral hemispheres is motor weakness and sensory loss on the contralateral side of the face and body. The presence of hemiparesis supports the diagnosis of TIA or stroke, but is not specific for these conditions. Hemiparesis has also been described in metabolic encephalopathy due to liver failure (21), renal failure (22), and sepsis (23).

Aphasia

The left cerebral hemisphere is the dominant hemisphere for speech in 90% of subjects. Damage involving the left cerebral hemisphere produces a condition known as *aphasia,* which is defined as a disturbance in the comprehension and/or formulation of language. Patients with aphasia can have difficulty in verbal comprehension (receptive aphasia), difficulty in verbal expression (expressive aphasia), or both (global aphasia).

Dysphagia

Up to half of patients admitted to the hospital for stroke will have swallowing dysfunction (3). These patients are at risk for pulmonary aspiration and pneumonia. Because of this, these patients might benefit from oral decontamination as a preventive measure for nosocomial pneumonia (see Chapter 4).

Fever

Fever ($T > 37.5°C$) develops in 40% of cases of acute stroke, and usually appears in the first 24 hours after symptom onset (24,25). The severity of the fever usually correlates with severity of the stroke (25–27).

Seizures

Seizures are uncommon (5%) in the first 2 weeks after ischemic stroke (28). They often occur as a single event in the first day after stroke onset. Partial seizures are most common. (28). Primary generalized convulsive seizures and recurrent seizures (2.5%) are uncommon after stroke or TIA (28).

DIAGNOSTIC EVALUATION

Once a stroke is suspected, candidates for thrombolytic therapy must be identified, and they must be identified *quickly* because the benefit of thrombolytic therapy in ischemic stroke is confined to the first 3 hours after symptom onset (see Table 52.1) (6). The checklist in Table 52.1 contains all the elements of the evaluation for thrombolytic therapy in individual patients. Most of the evaluation involves a search for hemorrhage and other contraindications to thrombolytic therapy. The search for intracranial hemorrhage requires neuroimaging studies.

Computed Tomography

The principal role of head CT imaging in suspected stroke is to identify hemorrhage, which is an absolute contraindication to thrombolytic

TABLE 52.1 Checklist for Thrombolytic Therapy

1. *Check the* ***indications*** *below that apply:*

- [x] Patient is 18 years of age or older
- [x] Time of symptom onset can be identified accurately
- [x] Thrombolytic therapy can be started within 3 hours of symptom onset

2. *If all the boxes in Step 1 are checked, then review the* ***absolute contraindications*** *below and check the ones that apply:*

- [ ] Head CT scan today shows intracranial bleeding
- [ ] Head CT scan today shows no intracranial bleeding but the clinical presentation is suspicious for subarachnoid hemorrhage
- [ ] Head CT scan today shows multilobar infarction (hypodense area $>$ one-third the area of the cerebral hemisphere)
- [ ] Any of the following within the past 3 months: intracranial or intraspinal surgery, serious head trauma, or a witnessed seizure
- [ ] Witnessed seizure since the onset of symptoms
- [ ] Blood pressure $>$ 185 mm Hg (systolic) or $>$ 110 mm Hg (diastolic)
- [ ] Arterial puncture at non-compressible site within past 7 days

Risk of hemorrhage:

- [ ] Evidence of active internal bleeding
- [ ] Patient has an arteriovenous malformation, aneurysm, or neoplasm
- [ ] Prior history of intracranial bleeding
- [ ] Laboratory evidence of a coagulopathy (e.g., platelet count $<$100,000/μL)
- [ ] Patient on coumadin and INR $\geq$ 1.7, or patient received heparin in past 48 hr and aPTT above normal range

3. *If none of the boxes in Step 2 are checked, review the* ***relative contraindications*** *below and check any that are considered an unacceptable risk:*

- [ ] Major surgery or serious trauma in past 14 days
- [ ] Gastrointestinal or urinary tract bleeding within past 21 days
- [ ] Acute MI in past 3 months or post-MI pericarditis
- [ ] Blood glucose $<$ 50 mg/dL or $>$ 400 mg/dL

If all boxes in step 1 are checked, and no boxes in steps 2 and 3 are checked, then give thrombolytic therapy.

From the 2005 American Heart Association Guidelines for Cardiopulmonary Resuscitation and Emergency Cardiovascular Care. Part 9, Adult Stroke. Circulation 2005;112:IV111–120.

therapy. The sensitivity of CT scans for intracerebral hemorrhage is almost 100%, and the sensitivity for subarachnoid hemorrhage is 90 to 95% (9). Computed tomography will also identify the occasional case of a space-occupying lesion (e.g., epidural or subdural hematoma, tumor, or abscess) (6,9).

The diagnostic yield of CT imaging is much less for infarction. One-half of cerebral infarcts are not apparent on CT scan (3), and the diagnostic yield is even less in the first 24 hours after symptom onset (9). An example of the influence of timing on the diagnostic yield from CT scans is illustrated in Figure 52.2 (29). Therefore, a negative CT scan, especially when performed within 24 hours after symptom onset, does not rule out the presence of cerebral infarction.

Magnetic Resonance Imaging

Magnetic resonance imaging (MRI) can detect 90% of strokes in the first 24 hours after symptom onset (9). The value of MRI in suspected stroke is illustrated by the case in Figure 52.3. The MRI in this figure is from a previously healthy 39-year-old woman who presented with acute onset of right arm and leg weakness. The initial CT scan was unrevealing, but the MRI reveals multiple (hyperdense) infarctions along the course of the left middle cerebral artery (infarctions are hypodense on CT scans, and

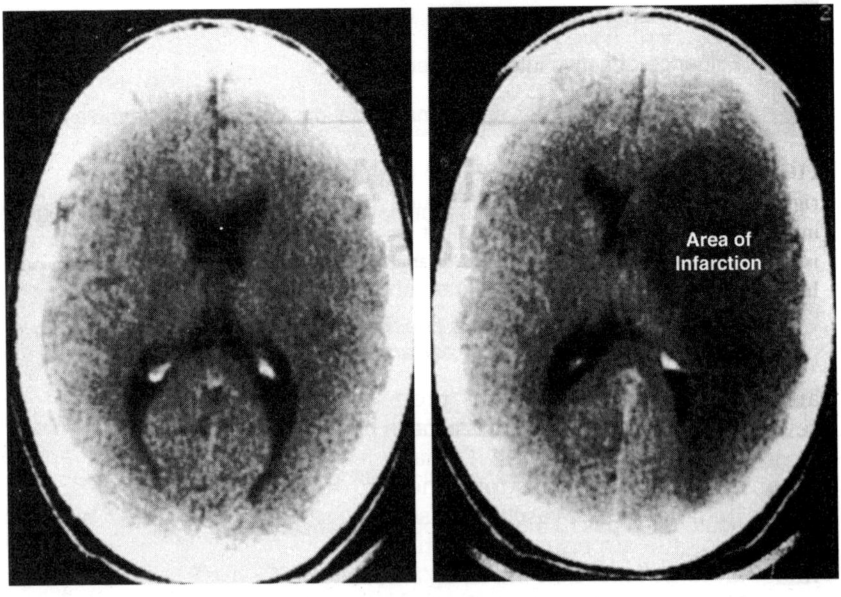

FIGURE 52.2 The influence of timing on the yield from CT scans. Both CT scans are from the same patient. The scan on the left was obtained within 24 hours after the onset of symptoms, and is unrevealing. The scan on the right was obtained 3 days later, and shows a large hypodense area on the left cerebral hemisphere. Reproduced with permission from (29). Images are digitally enhanced.

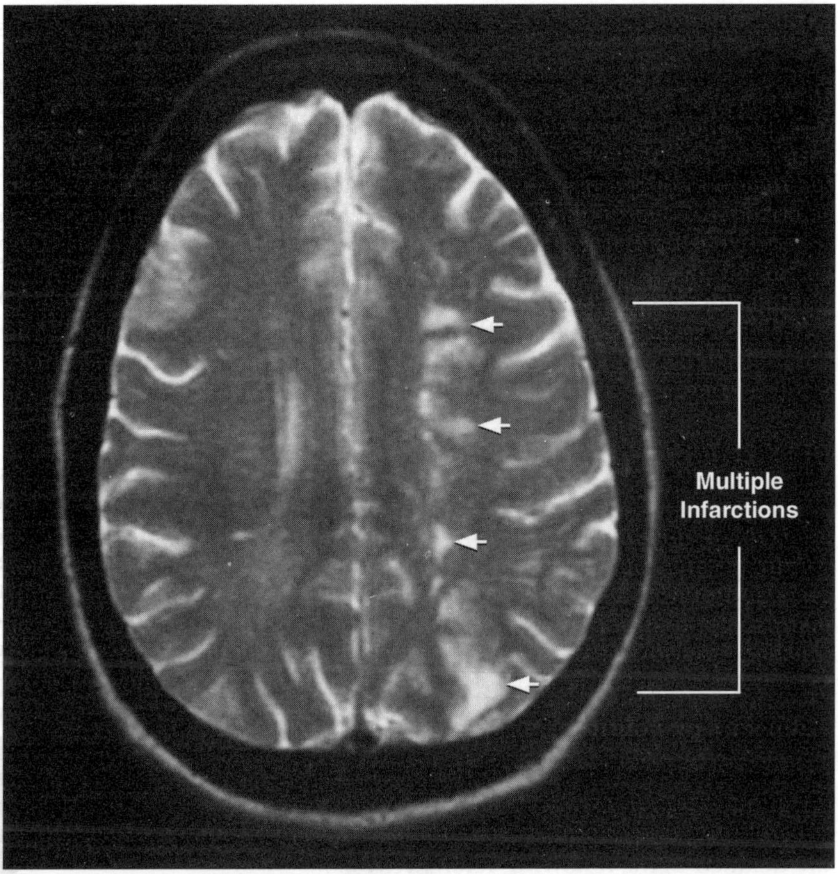

FIGURE 52.3 A T_2-weighted MRI from a 39-year-old woman with acute onset of right-sided weakness and a normal CT scan. The arrows point to hyperdense areas of infarction along the distribution of the left middle cerebral artery. Cerebral angiography revealed probable vasculitis. Case history and MRI courtesy of Dr. Sami Khella, M.D. Image digitally enhanced for clarity.

are hyperdense on MRI). This prompted a cerebral angiogram, which revealed probable vasculitis as a cause of the cerebral infarction.

MRI is also superior to CT imaging for detecting the following conditions: hemorrhage, subdural hematoma, aneurysms, arteriovenous malformations, microvascular disease, and venous sinus thrombosis. Because of the superior diagnostic yield, MRI is likely to replace CT imaging in the future for the early evaluation of stroke.

Because MRI uses magnetic pulses, it is contraindicated in patients with implanted pacemakers and cardioverter/defibrillators, as well as ferromagnetic implants, (e.g., some aneurysm clips, prosthetic joints, and cochlear implants). Intracoronary stents are not a contraindication to MRI imaging (30).

Other Diagnostic Tests

The following tests are appropriate for the indications cited.

1. **Lumbar puncture** is not indicated in most patients with suspected stroke. It can be useful when the CT scan reveals subarachnoid hemorrhage, or to exclude meningitis.
2. **Echocardiography** is indicated when stroke is associated with atrial fibrillation, acute MI, or left-sided endocarditis. It may also be indicated in stroke of undetermined etiology, and to identify a patent foramen ovale (and possible paradoxical cerebral embolism).
3. **Electroencephalography** is indicated in cases where seizures are suspected as the cause of the neurological deficits.

THROMBOLYTIC THERAPY

The popularity of thrombolytic therapy for ischemic stroke is based on a single (albeit multicenter) study showing that treatment with tissue plasminogen activator (0.9 mg/kg infused over 1 hr, max = 90 mg) improved neurological outcome if therapy was started within 3 hours after symptom onset (31). Mortality was unaffected, and the incidence of intracerebral hemorrhage associated with lytic therapy was 6.4% (10-fold greater than in the control group) (31,32). Despite the lack of survival benefit and the increased risk of intracranial hemorrhage, **the Food and Drug Administration (in 1996) approved the use of tissue plasminogen activator (tPA) for acute, ischemic stroke in the first 3 hours after symptom onset.** The drug approval is limited to strokes involving the anterior cerebral circulation only. The guidelines for patient management are detailed in the following references (6,7).

Where's the Beef?

The approval of thrombolytic therapy for acute stroke was heralded as a "breakthrough" in the treatment of stroke. However, the eligibility criteria for thrombolytic therapy (e.g., therapy must begin within 3 hours after symptom onset) are restrictive and, as a result, **only 1–2% of patients with acute stroke** (and 3–4% of patients that reach the hospital) **receive tissue plasminogen activator** (33,34).

The number of people who benefit from thrombolytic therapy each year can be estimated as follows (see Fig. 52.4). There are an estimated 700,000 acute strokes each year in the United States (1), and up to 88% (616,000) are ischemic strokes (1). Of these 616,000 ischemic strokes, a maximum of 2% get lytic therapy (12,320 patients) (34) (Fig. 52.4). At least nine patients need to be treated in order to produce one beneficial neurological outcome (that would not have occurred without therapy) (32). This means that for the maximum 12,320 patients that get tPA yearly, **only 1,369 patients (0.2% of all cases of ischemic stroke) will benefit from therapy each year.**

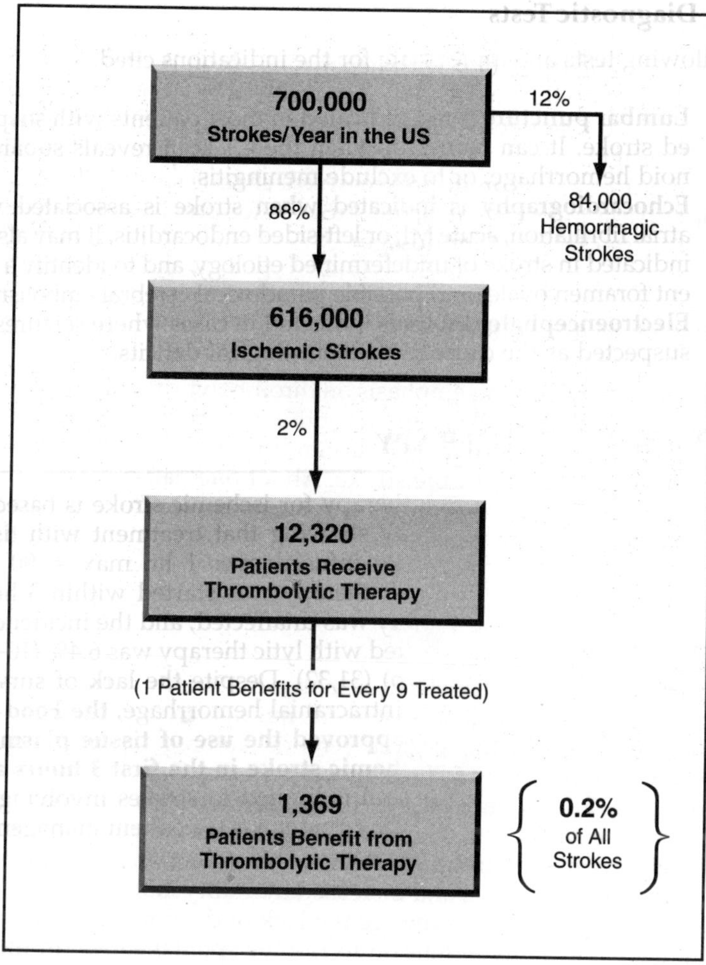

FIGURE 52.4 Impact of thrombolytic therapy in the United States each year.

ANTITHROMBOTIC THERAPY

Aspirin

Aspirin has been shown to reduce the recurrence of ischemic stroke and to reduce the mortality and long-term disability by 1% (3,35,36). Therefore, aspirin is recommended for all cases of acute ischemic stroke (3,35,36). When thrombolytic therapy is given, aspirin should be started on the following day, otherwise the first dose of aspirin should be given after intracranial hemorrhage is ruled out by neuroimaging. The recommended dose is 160–300 mg initially (orally or per rectum) and followed by 75–150 mg daily.

Heparin

Therapeutic anticoagulation with heparin has been the traditional practice for patients with progressive ischemic stroke (37). Although early studies showed a possible benefit from this practice, these studies were not well designed, and more recent studies reveal **little or no benefit from full anticoagulation in progressive ischemic stroke** (37). The only role for heparin following an acute stroke is for prevention of deep vein thrombosis (see Table 5.4 for dosage).

MEDICAL MANAGEMENT

Despite the overwhelming emphasis on thrombolytic therapy in the early management of acute stroke, patients with acute stroke who are admitted to the hospital are more likely to succumb from medical complications than from complications of the stroke. About one-half of deaths following stroke are related to medical complications (2). The following is a brief description of the most troublesome medical problems in stroke victims.

Hypertension

Hypertension may be a beneficial response that helps to maintain blood flow to borderline tissue that is ischemic but not irreversibly injured (*the ischemic penumbra*). In this region, cerebral autoregulation is impaired and blood flow passively follows blood pressure (38). This dependence on blood pressure is verified by clinical studies showing that systolic blood pressure <130 mm Hg or acute lowering of blood pressure in hypertensive ischemic stroke victims is often accompanied by worsening of the neurological deficits and increased mortality (38). Other reasons to avoid antihypertensive therapy are the lack of documented benefit, and the tendency for the hypertension to resolve spontaneously in the days following an acute ischemic stroke (6,39).

Despite a lack of experimental validation, the American Stroke Association recommends antihypertensive treatment if the systolic pressure rises above 220 mm Hg or if the diastolic blood pressure rises above 140 mm Hg (6). In the setting of an acute ischemic stroke, the reduction in blood pressure should not exceed 10–15%. For intravenous therapy, labetalol (10–20 mg) and nicardipine (5 mg/hr) are preferred because they preserve cerebral blood flow (6). Sublingual nifedipine should be avoided because it may cause a rapid fall in blood pressure.

Hyperglycemia

Hyperglycemia is common in severe stroke and is associated with a poor neurological outcome (6,40). Despite the association between hyperglycemia and poor outcome, a causal relationship is unproven (6,40). Current guidelines recommend that blood glucose be maintained below 300 mg/dL (6). Tighter glycemic control has been advocated (41); but has unproven benefits and there is a risk for hypoglycemia. Hypoglycemia can aggravate the neurological outcome and should be avoided (6).

Fever

Patients who develop a fever following an ischemic stroke have more extensive neurological deficits and a higher mortality (26). Although a causal relationship between fever and neurological outcome is unproven, the guidelines of the American Stroke Association recommend antipyretic therapy (acetaminophen) for all patients with post-stroke fever (6,42). Fever that follows acute stroke can be infectious in origin, so a search for infection is warranted,

SUBARACHNOID HEMORRHAGE

Subarachnoid hemorrhage (SAH) is usually the result of aneurysmal rupture (43,44). Aneurysmal subarachnoid hemorrhage has a mortality rate of 50%, and one-third of survivors become functionally dependent (43,44). Although classified as a type of stroke, SAH can differ from the other types of stroke in both presentation and management (12,45,46).

Clinical Presentation

The hallmark of the clinical presentation of SAH is the acute onset of an excruciating headache. The full-blown syndrome is preceded 40% of the time by a severe but self-limited headache, called a *sentinel headache* (44), which is presumably due to aneurysm dilation or a small hemorrhagic leak. The headache of SAH is usually abrupt in onset, progressive, and worse with exertion. Other manifestations can include: nausea and vomiting, altered mental status, meningismus, focal neurological signs (especially, oculomotor or abducens nerve palsy), hemiparesis, aphasia, or leg weakness. Because of its variable clinical presentation, one-half of the cases of SAH are misdiagnosed (44).

Diagnostic Evaluation

Computer tomography (CT) of the head (unenhanced) has a 90–95% sensitivity for the detection of a SAH, and is the initial diagnostic test of choice for suspected SAH (12,43). The shortcoming of CT imaging is that it may fail to detect cases of SAH that are small or confined to the posterior fossa (where the brainstem and cerebellum are located).

The image in Figure 52.5 is an MRI from a 30 year old woman with severe and persistent headache who had a normal CT scan of the head. The MRI shows a hyperdense area (indicated by the arrows) just ventral to the pons, which represents a SAH. Thus, even though CT scans have a high sensitivity for SAH, a negative CT scan does not eliminate the possibility for SAH.

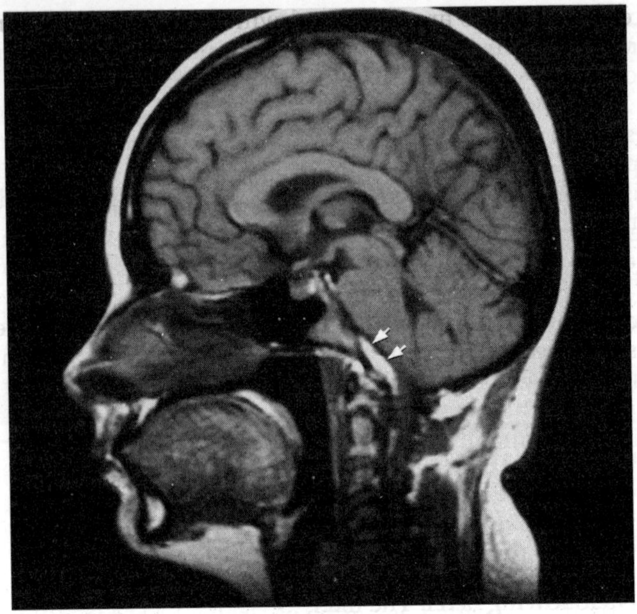

FIGURE 52.5 An MRI performed on a 30-year-old woman with severe, persistent headache and a normal CT scan of the head. Note the arrows pointing to a hyperdense area ventral to the brainstem. This represents a *prepontine subarachnoid hemorrhage*. Lumbar puncture confirmed the presence of blood in the subarachnoid space. Case history and MRI courtesy of Dr. Sami Khella, M.D.

In cases where neuroimaging is equivocal and there is a high clinical suspicion for SAH, a lumbar puncture should be performed (44).

Cerebral angiography is the gold standard for identifying the vascular lesion that is responsible for SAH. Results of angiography are needed to determine the appropriate management strategy (e.g., surgical clipping or endovascular coiling) (12).

Complications

The complications following SAH can be classified as medical, cardiac and neurological.

The most troublesome medical complications include pulmonary edema (13–23%), hyponatremia (due to SIADH or cerebral salt-wasting) (44,47,48), and deep vein thrombosis (requires prophylaxis).

The most common cardiac condition following SAH is EKG abnormalities which occur in 50–90% of cases. These abnormalities include elevation or depression of RST segment, prolongation of the QT interval, inversion of the T wave, or appearance of a U wave (49). These EKG changes can occur in the absence of coronary artery disease, and may be associated with cardiac dysfunction and release of cardiac enzymes (suggesting myocardial injury or infarction) (49). For patients who have EKG changes following SAH, cardiac troponin I levels should be measured because elevated levels are associated with cardiac dysfunction (49). In patients without coronary artery disease, cardiac dysfunction is transient and almost always returns to baseline (49).

The neurological complications after SAH are related to three processes: recurrent hemorrhage (7%), cerebral vasospasm (46%), and hydrocephalus (20%) (44). Hydrocephalus is usually diagnosed by head CT and is treated by ventricular drainage of cerebrospinal fluid with an indwelling catheter.

Recurrent Subarachnoid Hemorrhage

In most cases of SAH, the bleeding has stopped long before the time of diagnosis. Rebleeding from an aneurysm usually occurs within the first few days and is associated with a 50% mortality (44). To prevent rebleeding, aneurysm repair is usually done in the first few days by open surgical clipping or minimally invasive endovascular coiling (50).

Cerebral Vasospasm

Spasm of the cerebral blood vessels is common following SAH and can promote cerebral ischemia or infarction. The peak incidence occurs from 4 to 12 days following SAH. The likely source of vasospasm is inflammatory mediators in subarachnoid blood (44).

NIMODIPINE. The calcium channel blocker, nimodipine, improves neurological outcome following SAH (51,52). The recommended dose is 60 mg orally every 4 hours for 21 days (44). The shortcoming with nimodipine is the "number needed to treat"; i.e., an average of 20 patients must be treated to produce one case of improved neurological outcome (53).

HYPERVOLEMIA-HYPERTENSION. Promoting cerebral blood flow is an important management goal in vasospasm following SAH. This is the basis for the traditional therapy involving induction of hypervolemia (with colloid infusion) and induced hypertension (by infusing vasoconstrictors, e.g., phenylephrine) (44,45). This therapy does not necessarily increase cerebral perfusion or reverse the signs of cerebral ischemia and it is associated with potential complications (e.g., heart failure or pulmonary edema) (45). **The most important goals of therapy are to prevent hypovolemia and to maintain or augment systemic cardiac output** (e.g., with dobutamine infusion).

A FINAL WORD

About 10 to 15 years ago, someone decided that myocardial infarction and cerebral infarction were similar disease processes directed at different organs. The term *brain attack* was introduced to acknowledge the similarities between cerebral infarction and myocardial infarction, and specialized *stroke units* were created to provide the same type of specialized care provided in coronary care units. The success of thrombolytic therapy in acute coronary syndromes prompted an evaluation of lytic therapy in ischemic stroke. The results of this study did not match the success of thrombolytic therapy in acute coronary syndromes. Despite equivocal evidence of benefit, thrombolytic therapy was approved for use in acute ischemic stroke in the mid 1990s. There was, however, one catch—the treatment had to be given within three hours after the onset of symptoms. This restriction essentially eliminated any chance of a large-scale impact of thrombolytic therapy on stroke.

A decade has now passed and, as demonstrated in Figure 52.4, thrombolytic therapy has added only a sliver of light to the world of stroke victims. The 3-hour time restriction is blamed for the disappointing results with thrombolytic therapy, but these drugs have never shown dramatic results in the treatment of acute stroke. In fact, aspirin is more likely to produce a favorable outcome than thrombolytic therapy. The different response to thrombolytic therapy in ischemic stroke could indicate that coronary artery disease and cerebrovascular disease are not as related as presumed.

So, after all the fuss about thrombolytic therapy, it seems that the best treatment for patients with ischemic stroke is general critical care support. Just as it should be.

REFERENCES

Reviews

1. Thom T, Haase N, Rosamond W, et al. Heart disease and stroke statistics: 2006 update: a report from the American Heart Association Statistics Committee and Stroke Statistics Subcommittee. Circulation 2006;113:85–151.
2. Brott T, Bogousslavsky J. Treatment of acute ischemic stroke. N Engl J Med 2000;343:710–722.
3. Warlow C, Sudlow C, Dennis M, et al. Stroke. Lancet 2003;362:1211–1224.
4. Goldstein LB, Simel DL. Is this patient having a stroke? JAMA 2005;293:2391–2402.
5. Special report from the National Institute of Neurological Disorders and Stroke. Classification of cerebrovascular diseases III. Stroke 1990;21:637–676.

Guidelines

6. Adams HP, Jr., Adams RJ, Brott T, et al. Guidelines for the early management of patients with ischemic stroke: a scientific statement from the Stroke Council of the American Stroke Association. Stroke 2003;34:1056–1083.
7. Adams H, Adams R, Del Zoppo G, et al. Guidelines for the early management of patients with ischemic stroke: 2005 guidelines update a scientific statement from the Stroke Council of the American Heart Association/American Stroke Association. Stroke 2005;36:916–923.
8. Sacco RL, Adams R, Albers G, et al. Guidelines for prevention of stroke in patients with ischemic stroke or transient ischemic attack: a statement for healthcare professionals from the American Heart Association/American Stroke Association Council on Stroke: co-sponsored by the Council on Cardiovascular Radiology and Intervention: the American Academy of Neurology affirms the value of this guideline. Stroke 2006;37:577–617.

9. Culebras A, Kase CS, Masdeu JC, et al. Practice guidelines for the use of imaging in transient ischemic attacks and acute stroke: a report of the Stroke Council, American Heart Association. Stroke 1997;28:1480–1497.
10. Kizer JR, Devereux RB. Clinical practice: patent foramen ovale in young adults with unexplained stroke. N Engl J Med 2005;353:2361–2372.
11. Broderick JP, Adams HP Jr, Barsan W, et al. Guidelines for the management of spontaneous intracerebral hemorrhage: a statement for healthcare professionals from a special writing group of the Stroke Council, American Heart Association. Stroke 1999;30:905–915.
12. Mayberg MR, Batjer HH, Dacey R, et al. Guidelines for the management of aneurysmal subarachnoid hemorrhage: a statement for healthcare professionals from a special writing group of the Stroke Council, American Heart Association. Stroke 1994;25:2315–2328.
13. Bederson JB, Awad IA, Wiebers DO, et al. Recommendations for the management of patients with unruptured intracranial aneurysms: a statement for healthcare professionals from the Stroke Council of the American Heart Association. Stroke 2000;31:2742–2750.
14. Albers GW, Hart RG, Lutsep HL, et al. AHA Scientific Statement: supplement to the guidelines for the management of transient ischemic attacks: A statement from the Ad Hoc Committee on Guidelines for the Management of Transient Ischemic Attacks, Stroke Council, American Heart Association. Stroke 1999;30:2502–2511.
15. Ovbiagele B, Kidwell CS, Saver JL. Epidemiological impact in the United States of a tissue-based definition of transient ischemic attack. Stroke 2003;34:919–924.

Evaluation

16. Saver JL. Time is brain-quantified. Stroke 2006;37:263–266.
17. Hand PJ, Kwan J, Lindley RI, et al. Distinguishing between stroke and mimic at the bedside: the brain attack study. Stroke 2006;37:769–775.
18. Goldstein LB, Matchar DB. The rational clinical examination: clinical assessment of stroke. JAMA 1994;271:1114–1120.
19. Adams HP Jr, Brott TG, Crowell RM, et al. Guidelines for the management of patients with acute ischemic stroke: a statement for healthcare professionals from a special writing group of the Stroke Council, American Heart Association. Circulation 1994;90:1588–1601.
20. Bamford J. Clinical examination in diagnosis and subclassification of stroke. Lancet 1992;339:400–402.
21. Atchison JW, Pellegrino M, Herbers P, et al. Hepatic encephalopathy mimicking stroke: a case report. Am J Phys Med Rehabil 1992;71:114–118.
22. Palmer CA. Neurologic manifestations of renal disease. Neurol Clin 2002;20:23–34.
23. Maher J, Young GB. Septic encephalopathy. Intensive Care Med 1993;8:177–187.
24. Georgilis K, Plomaritoglou A, Dafni U, et al. Aetiology of fever in patients with acute stroke. J Intern Med 1999;246:203–209.
25. Boysen G, Christensen H. Stroke severity determines body temperature in acute stroke. Stroke 2001;32:413–417.

26. Reith J, Jorgensen HS, Pedersen PM, et al. Body temperature in acute stroke: relation to stroke severity, infarct size, mortality, and outcome. Lancet 1996; 347:422–425.
27. Hajat C, Hajat S, Sharma P. Effects of poststroke pyrexia on stroke outcome: a meta-analysis of studies in patients. Stroke 2000;31:410–414.
28. Bladin CF, Alexandrov AV, Bellavance A, et al. Seizures after stroke: a prospective multicenter study. Arch Neurol 2000;57:1617–1622.
29. Graves VB, Partington VB. Imaging evaluation of acute neurologic disease. In: Goodman LR Putman CE, eds. Critical care imaging. 3rd ed. Philadelphia: WB Saunders, 1993:391–409.

Thrombolytic Therapy

30. Gerber TC, Fasseas P, Lennon RJ, et al. Clinical safety of magnetic resonance imaging early after coronary artery stent placement. J Am Coll Cardiol 2003; 42:1295–1298.
31. NINDS. Tissue plasminogen activator for acute ischemic stroke: The National Institute of Neurological Disorders and Stroke rt-PA Stroke Study Group. N Engl J Med 1995;333:1581–1587.
32. Kwiatkowski TG, Libman RB, Frankel M, et al. Effects of tissue plasminogen activator for acute ischemic stroke at one year: National Institute of Neurological Disorders and Stroke Recombinant Tissue Plasminogen Activator Stroke Study Group. N Engl J Med 1999;340:1781–1787.
33. Reeves MJ, Arora S, Broderick JP, et al. Acute stroke care in the US: results from 4 pilot prototypes of the Paul Coverdell National Acute Stroke Registry. Stroke 2005;36:1232–1240.
34. Caplan LR. Thrombolysis 2004: the good, the bad, and the ugly. Rev Neurol Dis 2004;1:16–26.

Antithrombotic Therapy

35. CAST: randomised placebo-controlled trial of early aspirin use in 20,000 patients with acute ischaemic stroke. CAST (Chinese Acute Stroke Trial) Collaborative Group. Lancet 1997;349:1641–1649.
36. The International Stroke Trial (IST). A randomised trial of aspirin, subcutaneous heparin, both, or neither among 19435 patients with acute ischaemic stroke. International Stroke Trial Collaborative Group. Lancet 1997;349: 1569–1581.

Medical Management

37. Rothrock JF, Hart RG. Antithrombotic therapy in cerebrovascular disease. Ann Intern Med 1991;115:885–895.
38. Mistri AK, Robinson TG, Potter JF. Pressor therapy in acute ischemic stroke: systematic review. Stroke 2006;37:1565–1571.
39. Semplicini A, Maresca A, Boscolo G, et al. Hypertension in acute ischemic stroke: a compensatory mechanism or an additional damaging factor? Arch Intern Med 2003;163:211–216.
40. Bruno A, Levine SR, Frankel MR, et al. Admission glucose level and clinical outcomes in the NINDS rt-PA Stroke Trial. Neurology 2002;59:669–674.

41. Bruno A, Williams LS, Kent TA. How important is hyperglycemia during acute brain infarction? Neurologist 2004;10:195–200.

Subarachnoid Hemorrhage

42. Dippel DW, van Breda EJ, van Gemert HM, et al. Effect of paracetamol (acetaminophen) on body temperature in acute ischemic stroke: a double-blind, randomized phase II clinical trial. Stroke 2001;32:1607–1612.
43. Schievink WI. Intracranial aneurysms. N Engl J Med 1997;336:28–40.
44. Suarez JI, Tarr RW, Selman WR. Aneurysmal subarachnoid hemorrhage. N Engl J Med 2006;354:387–396.
45. Naval NS, Stevens RD, Mirski MA, et al. Controversies in the management of aneurysmal subarachnoid hemorrhage. Crit Care Med 2006;34:511–524.
46. Wijdicks EF, Kallmes DF, Manno EM, et al. Subarachnoid hemorrhage: neurointensive care and aneurysm repair. Mayo Clin Proc 2005;80:550–559.
47. Diringer MN, Zazulia AR. Hyponatremia in neurologic patients: consequences and approaches to treatment. Neurologist 2006;12:117–126.
48. Wartenberg KE, Schmidt JM, Claassen J, et al. Impact of medical complications on outcome after subarachnoid hemorrhage. Crit Care Med 2006;34: 617–623.
49. Deibert E, Barzilai B, Braverman AC, et al. Clinical significance of elevated troponin I levels in patients with nontraumatic subarachnoid hemorrhage. J Neurosurg 2003;98:741–746.
50. Molyneux A, Kerr R, Stratton I, et al. International Subarachnoid Aneurysm Trial (ISAT) of neurosurgical clipping versus endovascular coiling in 2143 patients with ruptured intracranial aneurysms: a randomised trial. Lancet 2002;360:1267–1274.
51. Allen GS, Ahn HS, Preziosi TJ, et al. Cerebral arterial spasm: a controlled trial of nimodipine in patients with subarachnoid hemorrhage. N Engl J Med 1983;308:619–624.
52. Petruk KC, West M, Mohr G, et al. Nimodipine treatment in poor-grade aneurysm patients: results of a multicenter double-blind placebo-controlled trial. J Neurosurg 1988;68:505–517.
53. Barker FG 2nd, Ogilvy CS. Efficacy of prophylactic nimodipine for delayed ischemic deficit after subarachnoid hemorrhage: a meta-analysis. J Neurosurg 1996;84:405–414.

Section **XVI**

TOXIC INGESTIONS

Poisons and medicines are often the same substance given with different intents.

PETER LATHAM *(1865)*

Chapter 53

PHARMACEUTICAL TOXINS & ANTIDOTES

There is little doubt that pharmaceutical mishaps are a source of considerable morbidity and even mortality. Adverse drug reactions are responsible for up to 7% of hospital admissions, and 20% of ICU admissions (1,2). Once in the hospital, 7% of patients experience a severe adverse drug reaction (3). The average ICU patient receives 6 to 9 different medications daily and 8 to 12 different medications during the ICU stay (4). Therefore, the ICU is a fertile environment for pharmaceutical misadventures.

This chapter describes the clinical toxicity associated with the pharmaceutical agents listed below, and the treatment of each with specific antidotes (shown in parentheses). Included are toxic drug ingestions that prompt admission to the ICU and toxic drug reactions that surface after admission to the ICU.

Acetaminophen (N-acetylcysteine)
Benzodiazepines (flumazenil)
β-Blockers (glucagon)
Calcium antagonists (calcium, glucagon)
Opioids (naloxone)

ACETAMINOPHEN

Acetaminophen is a ubiquitous analgesic-antipyretic agent that is included in over 600 commercial drug preparations. It is also a hepatotoxin, and is the **leading cause of toxic drug ingestion and acute liver failure in**

the United States (5,6). The general public seems unaware of acetaminophen's toxic potential, and almost one-third of overdoses are unintentional, occurring in people who are using the drug for pain relief (7).

Toxic Mechanism

The toxicity of acetaminophen is related to its metabolism, which is shown in Figure 53.1. The bulk of acetaminophen metabolism involves the formation of sulfate and glucuronide conjugates in the liver, which are then excreted in the urine (8,9). Approximately 5 to 15% of the metabolism involves formation of a highly reactive intermediate that promotes oxidant injury in hepatic parenchymal cells. This toxic metabolite is normally removed by conjugation with glutathione, an intracellular antioxidant. Large doses of acetaminophen saturate the conjugation pathways and spill over into the glutathione pathway to deplete glutathione reserves. When hepatic glutathione stores fall to 30% of normal, the toxic

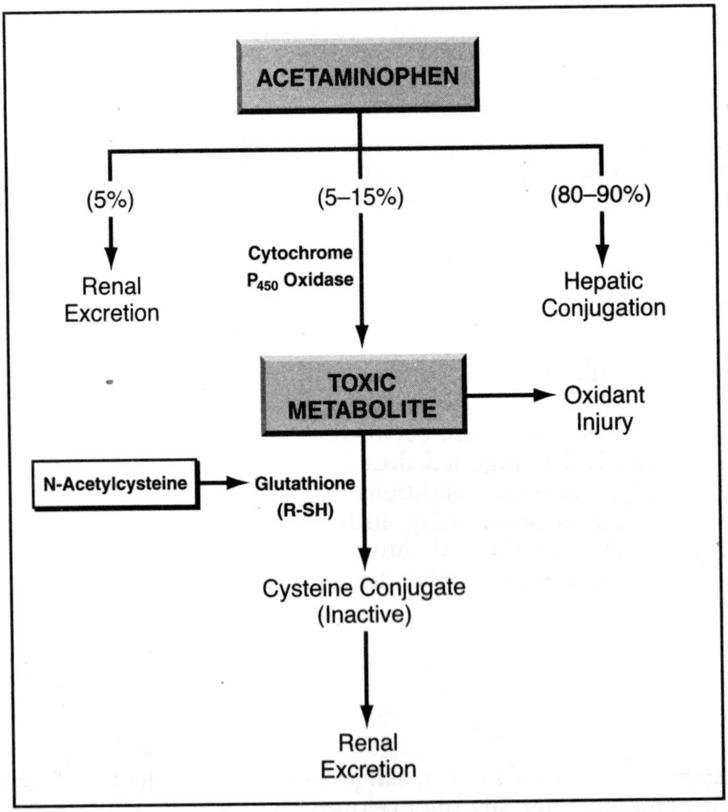

FIGURE 53.1 The hepatic metabolism of acetaminophen and the mechanism of action of N-acetylcysteine.

acetaminophen metabolite can accumulate and promote widespread hepatocellular damage (9).

Clinical Presentation

The period following acetaminophen overdose is divided into four stages of toxicity (8,10,11). In the initial stage (the first 24 hours), symptoms are either absent or non-specific (e.g., nausea), and no laboratory evidence of hepatic injury exists. In patients who develop hepatotoxicity, a second stage (24–72 hours after drug ingestion) occurs where clinical manifestations continue to be minimal or absent, but laboratory evidence of hepatic injury begins to appear. Elevated aspartate aminotranferase (AST) is the most sensitive marker of acetaminophen toxicity; the rise of AST precedes the hepatic dysfunction, and peak levels are reached at 72–96 hours. In advanced cases of hepatic injury, a third stage follows (after 72–96 hours) that is characterized by clinical and laboratory evidence of progressive hepatic injury and hepatic insufficiency (e.g., encephalopathy, coagulopathy) occasionally combined with renal insufficiency. Death from hepatic injury usually occurs within 3 to 5 days. Patients who survive often recover completely, although recovery can be prolonged.

Diagnosis

In most cases of acetaminophen overdose, the initial presentation occurs within 24 hours after drug ingestion, when there are no manifestations of hepatic injury. The principal task at this time is to identify those who are likely to develop hepatotoxicity. Two variables can have prognostic value.

Ingested Dose

Determining the risk of hepatotoxicity from the ingested dose is problematic because: 1) The minimum toxic dose can vary in individual patients, and is somewhere between 7.5–15 grams in an average sized adult (8–10), 2) The ingested dose is often difficult to determine accurately, and 3) Several conditions can increase the susceptibility to acetaminophen hepatotoxicity, including: glutathione depletion (e.g., malnutrition), isoniazid, and chronic ethanol ingestion (6,7,9). For these reasons, plasma acetaminophen levels should be used to assess the risk of hepatotoxicity.

Plasma Drug Levels

Plasma acetaminophen levels obtained from 4 to 24 hours after drug ingestion can be used to predict the risk of hepatotoxicity using the nomogram in Figure 53.2 (9). If the plasma level is in the high-risk region of the nomogram, the risk of developing hepatotoxicity is 60% or higher, and antidote therapy is warranted. The risk of hepatotoxicity is only 1 to 3% in the low-risk region of the nomogram, and this does not warrant antidote therapy (9).

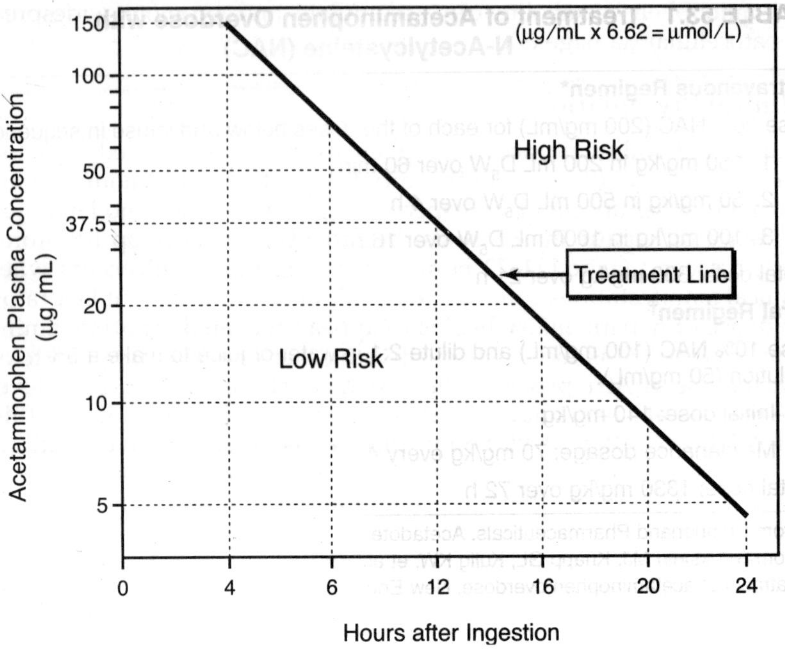

FIGURE 53.2 Nomogram for predicting the risk of hepatotoxicity using plasma acetaminophen levels obtained between 4 and 24 hours after ingestion. A plasma level that falls on or above the treatment line is an indication to begin antidotal therapy with N-acetylcysteine. From Rumack BH. Acetaminophen hepatotoxicity: the first 35 years. J Toxicol Clin Toxicol 2002;40:3–20.

N-Acetylcysteine

The goal of antidote therapy for acetaminophen overdose is to limit accumulation of the toxic metabolite and prevent hepatocellular damage. Since glutathione does not readily cross cell membranes, the administration of exogenous glutathione is not well suited for this task. N-acetylcysteine (NAC) is a glutathione analogue that can cross cell membranes and act as an intracellular glutathione surrogate (12). As shown in Figure 53.1, NAC contains a sulfhydryl group that allows it to act as a reducing agent and inactivate the toxic acetaminophen metabolite.

Timing

NAC is indicated only when therapy can be started within 24 hours after acetaminophen overdose (13). Protection is most effective when NAC is started in the first 8 hours after ingestion (8,10,14,15), so avoiding treatment delays is necessary to ensuring optimal protection. In some circumstances, NAC can be protective when given 24–36 hours after drug ingestion (16), but consensus opinion is not to extend the 24 hour treatment window.

TABLE 53.1 Treatment of Acetaminophen Overdose with N-Acetylcysteine (NAC)

Intravenous Regimen*

Use 20% NAC (200 mg/mL) for each of the doses below and infuse in sequence:

1. 150 mg/kg in 200 mL D_5W over 60 min
2. 50 mg/kg in 500 mL D_5W over 4 h
3. 100 mg/kg in 1000 mL D_5W over 16 h

Total dose: 300 mg/kg over 21 h

Oral Regimen†

Use 10% NAC (100 mg/mL) and dilute 2:1 in water or juice to make a 5% solution (50 mg/mL).

Initial dose: 140 mg/kg

Maintenance dosage: 70 mg/kg every 4 h for 17 doses

Total dose: 1330 mg/kg over 72 h

*From Cumberland Pharmaceuticals. Acetadote Package Insert. 2006.
†From Smilkstein MJ, Knapp GL, Kulig KW, et al. Efficacy of oral N-acetylcysteine in the treatment of acetaminophen overdose. New Engl J Med 1988;319:1557–1562.

Therapeutic Regimens

NAC can be given intravenously or orally using the dosing regimens shown in Table 53.1. Even though there is no direct comparison of these two approaches, they are considered equally effective (17,18). The intravenous route is preferred because it is the most reliable mode of drug delivery, and because oral ingestion of NAC can be problematic (see next section). (15).

Adverse Reactions

Intravenous NAC can cause troublesome anaphylactoid reactions, which are uncommon but can be severe (in 1% of treatments) (19,20). The sulfur content of NAC gives the liquid drug preparation a very disagreeable taste (often described as rotten eggs). As a result, oral administration of NAC frequently incites vomiting, and a nasogastric tube is sometimes required to administer therapy. The oral regimen of NAC is also associated with a dose-dependent diarrhea that appears in about half the patients who complete the 72-hr regimen (21). This resolves with continued therapy in over 90% of cases.

Activated Charcoal

Acetaminophen is completely absorbed from the gastrointestinal tract in the first few hours after drug ingestion (10). Therefore, activated charcoal (1 g/kg body weight) is recommended only in the first 4 hours after acetaminophen overdose (10,22). Although charcoal can also adsorb N-acetylcysteine, this interaction is probably not significant (10).

BENZODIAZEPINES

Benzodiazepines are the second most frequently overdosed prescription drugs in the United States, and are second only to analgesics as the leading cause of medication-related death (5). Benzodiazepine-related fatalities almost always involve other respiratory depressants (23). Admissions for drug overdose are not the only source of benzodiazepine toxicity in the ICU. Surveys reveal that roughly 50% of ICU patients receive benzodiazepines for sedation (24), and adverse reactions to benzodiazepine sedation is likely to be a significant source of clinical toxicity. The use of benzodiazepines for sedation in the ICU is described in Chapter 49.

Clinical Toxicity

Benzodiazepines produce a dose-dependent depression in the level of consciousness, but there is usually no respiratory or cardiovascular depression. However, there are several factors in the ICU that predispose to respiratory and cardiovascular depression from benzodiazepines. These include advanced age of the patients, combined therapy with opioid analgesics, and drug accumulation from prolonged drug therapy (see Chapter 49 for a description of benzodiazepine accumulation).

Flumazenil

Flumazenil is a benzodiazepine antagonist that binds to benzodiazepine receptors in the central nervous system but does not exert any agonist actions (25,26). This agent is most effective in reversing the sedative effects of the benzodiazepines, but is inconsistent in reversing benzodiazepine-induced respiratory depression (27,28). Flumazenil can also improve the sensorium in hepatic encephalopathy (29) and ethanol intoxication (30), but the doses required are large (5 mg) and potentially hazardous.

Drug Administration

Flumazenil is given as an intravenous bolus. The initial dose is 0.2 mg, and this can be repeated at 1 to 6 minute intervals if necessary to a cumulative dose of 1.0 mg. The response is rapid, with onset in 1–2 minutes, peak effect at 6–10 minutes, and duration of approximately one hour (25, 31). Since flumazenil has a shorter duration of action than the benzodiazepines, resedation is common after 30–60 minutes. Because of the risk for resedation, the initial bolus dose of flumazenil is often followed by a continuous infusion at 0.3–0.4 mg/hr (31).

Adverse Reactions

Flumazenil produces few undesirable side effects (25,26,32,33). It can precipitate a benzodiazepine withdrawal syndrome in patients with a long-standing history of benzodiazepine use, but this is uncommon (32). Flumazenil can also precipitate seizures in patients receiving benzodiazepines for seizure control, and in mixed overdoses involving tricyclic antidepressants (34).

Clinical Uses

Because of the benign nature of benzodiazepine toxicity, flumazenil is a treatment in search of an illness. The principal use of flumazenil is in patients with known or suspected benzodiazepine overdose, but only when a mixed overdose involving tricyclic antidepressants is not suspected, and only in patients who are not receiving benzodiazepines for control of seizures. Flumazenil has even fewer uses in the ICU. Although flumazenil can reverse oversedation with benzodiazepines in ventilator-dependent patients (31), the hazards of oversedation are minimal in patients receiving ventilatory support. Flumazenil has been reported to hasten weaning from mechanical ventilation (35), but this application seems limited by the lack of respiratory depression when the benzodiazepine dose is not excessive.

β-RECEPTOR ANTAGONISTS

According to the 2004 annual report of the Toxic Exposure Surveillance System, there were 8,186 β-blocker overdoses treated in a health care facility resulting in 481 major adverse outcomes and 25 mortalities (5). Intentional overdose is not the only source of β-blocker toxicity in the ICU. At present, 15 different β-blockers are approved for use in the United States (36). β-Blockers are used to manage several conditions in the ICU, including hypertension, narrow-complex tachycardias, unstable angina, and acute myocardial infarction, and these uses create an additional source of β-blocker toxicity. The β-receptor antagonists used most frequently in the ICU are shown in Table 53.2.

Clinical Toxicity

The manifestations of β-receptor blockade arise primarily from the cardiovascular system and the central nervous system (36–38).

TABLE 53.2 Comparison of Intravenous β-Receptor Antagonists

Antagonist	Target Receptors	Relative Potency	Intravenous Dosage	Lipid Solubility	Metabolism
Propranolol	All β	1	1–10 mg	+++	Hepatic
Metoprolol	β_1	1	5–15 mg	+	Hepatic
Atenolol	β_1	1	5–10 mg	0	Renal
Timolol	All β	6	0.3–1 mg	+	Hepatic/Renal
Labetalol	α, all β	0.3	2 mg/kg 0.5–1 mg/kg	++	Renal
Esmolol	All β	0.06	0.1–0.3 mg/kg/min	0	Plasma

Cardiovascular Toxicity

The most common manifestations of β-blocker toxicity are **bradycardia** and **hypotension** (36–38). The bradycardia is usually sinus in origin, and is well tolerated. The hypotension can be due to peripheral vasodilatation (renin blockade), or a decrease in cardiac output (β_1 receptor blockade). Hypotension that is sudden in onset is usually a reflection of a decrease in cardiac output and is an ominous sign.

Especially in overdose, the β-blockers can exert a membrane-stabilizing (quinidine-like) effect that inhibits fast sodium channels, prolongs atrioventricular (AV) conduction (causing **heart block**), and can impair myocardial contractility (causing **refractory hypotension**) (39,40). Membrane-stabilizing activity is greatest for propranolol, less for metoprolol and labetalol, and is not important for timolol and atenolol (39). When a lipophilic agent with membrane stabilizing properties (e.g., propranolol) crosses the blood brain barrier, neurotoxicity can be especially severe (36).

Neurotoxicity

Most β-blockers are lipid soluble to some degree and thus have a tendency to accumulate in lipid-rich organs like the central nervous system. As a result, β-blocker overdose is often accompanied by lethargy, **depressed consciousness**, and **generalized seizures**. The latter manifestation is more prevalent than suspected, and has been reported in 60% of overdoses with propranolol (38). Like the prolonged AV conduction, the neurological manifestations are not the result of β-receptor blockade and are likely related to membrane stabilizing activity. Thus, seizures are most frequently observed in association with propranolol overdose (usually in excess of 1.5 grams) (41).

Glucagon

The cardiovascular depression from β-receptor blockade (especially those agents with intrinsic membrane stabilizing effects) can be resistant to conventional therapy with atropine (1 mg IV), isoproterenol (0.1–0.2 mg/min titrated to effect), and transvenous ventricular pacing (37,42). The regulatory hormone glucagon is the agent of choice for reversing the cardiovascular depression in β-receptor blockade. The actions of glucagon in β-blocker overdose are explained below.

Mechanism of Action

The diagram in Figure 53.3 shows the chain of events responsible for the positive inotropic actions of β_1 receptor activation in the heart. The β-receptor is functionally linked (via specialized G proteins) to the adenyl cyclase enzyme on the inner surface of the cell membrane. Activation of the receptor-enzyme complex results in the hydrolysis of adenosine triphosphate (ATP) to form cyclic adenosine monophosphate (cyclic AMP). The cyclic AMP then activates a protein kinase that promotes the inward movement of calcium through the cell membrane. The influx of

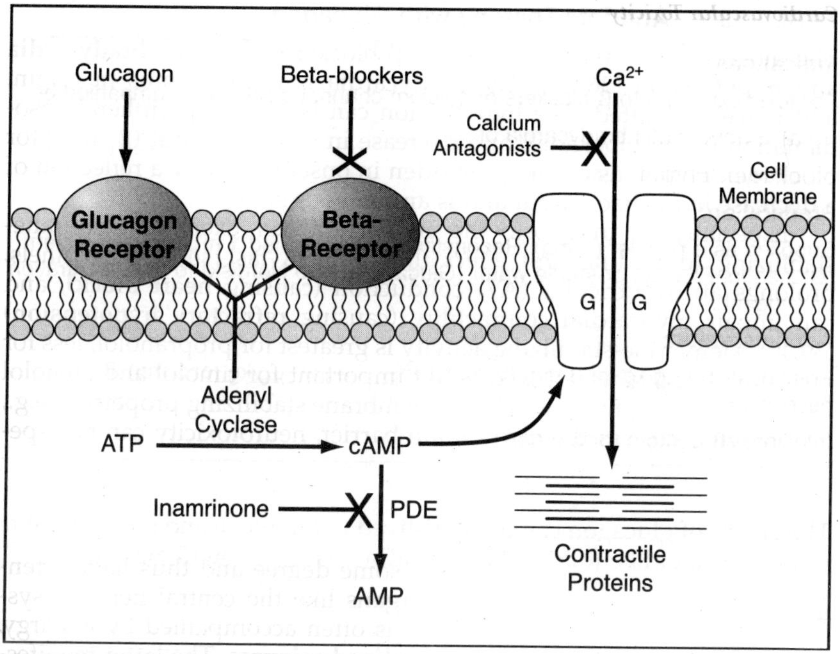

FIGURE 53.3 The mechanism of action of drugs that affect the strength of cardiac contraction. Abbreviations: ATP: adenosine triphosphate, cAMP: cyclic adenosine monophosphate, PDE: phosphodiesterase, AMP: adenosine monophosphate.

calcium promotes interactions between contractile proteins and thereby augments the strength of cardiac contraction.

The diagram in Figure 53.3 also shows that glucagon can activate adenyl cyclase through a membrane receptor that is distinct from the β-receptor. This allows glucagon to mimic the positive inotropic effects of β-receptor activation when the β-receptors are quiescent.

Indications

Glucagon is indicated for the treatment of hypotension and *symptomatic* bradycardia associated with toxic exposure to β-blockers (see Table 53.3). When used in the appropriate doses, glucagon will elicit a favorable response in 90% of patients (37). Glucagon is *not* indicated for reversing the prolonged AV conduction or neurological abnormalities in β-blocker overdose because these effects are not mediated by β-receptor blockade.

Dosage Recommendations

The effective dose of glucagon can vary in individual patients, but **a bolus dose of 3 to 5 mg IV should be effective in most adults** (37,38,43). The initial dose is 3 mg (or 0.05 mg/kg), and this can be followed by a second dose of 5 mg (or 0.07 mg/kg) if necessary. The response to glucagon is most pronounced when the plasma ionized calcium is normal (44).

TABLE 53.3 Antidote Therapy with Glucagon

Indications:

For toxic exposure to β-blockers or calcium channel blockers accompanied by

a) Symptomatic bradycardia or

b) Hypotension

Preparation:

Supplied as a powder (1 mg). Reconstitute with supplied 1 mL bottle of diluent (Glucagon, Eli Lilly) or sterile water (Glucagen Novo Nordisk) to a concentration of 1 mg/mL.

Administration:

Initial dose: 50 μg/kg (or 3 mg) IV over 1 min, then 70 μg/kg (or 5 mg) if necessary.

Infusion: 70 μg/kg/h (or 5 mg/h)

The effects of glucagon can be short-lived (5 minutes), and so a favorable response should be followed by a continuous infusion (5 mg/hr).

Adverse Effects

Nausea and vomiting are common at glucagon doses above 5 mg/hr. Mild hyperglycemia is common, and is due to glucagon-induced glycogenolysis and gluconeogenesis. The insulin response to the hyperglycemia can drive potassium into cells and promote hypokalemia. Finally, glucagon stimulates catecholamine release from the adrenal medulla, and this can raise the blood pressure in hypertensive patients. This hypertensive response is exaggerated in pheochromocytoma, so glucagon is contraindicated in patients with pheochromocytoma.

CALCIUM ANTAGONISTS

Calcium blockers are among the five most frequently reported (and most lethal) toxic ingestions in the United States in 2004 (5,45). At present, 10 different calcium channel blockers are available in the US (36); however, the three original calcium antagonists (verapamil, nifedipine, and diltiazem) are responsible for most of the clinical experience with calcium antagonist toxicity.

Mechanisms

Calcium

Calcium has a profound influence on the electrical and mechanical performance of smooth muscle. Its role in the contraction of cardiac smooth muscle is shown in Figure 53.3. The inward movement of calcium across the cell membrane (triggered by depolarization of the cell membrane or by activation of the cyclic AMP pathway) promotes the interaction between contractile proteins that ultimately determines the strength of muscle contraction. Although not shown in the figure, calcium influx triggers calcium release from the sarcoplasmic reticulum, which is the primary source of calcium that produces muscle contraction). This process from membrane depolarization to muscle contraction is called excitation-contraction coupling (46).

Calcium also participates in the propagation of electrical impulses in smooth muscle. The depolarization-triggered inward movement of calcium facilitates the propagation of electrical impulses in cardiac muscle, and speeds conduction through the atrioventricular (AV) node.

The calcium antagonists block the inward movement of calcium across smooth muscle membranes, but not across the sarcoplasmic reticulum. This can result in any of the following: negative inotropic and chronotropic effects, prolonged atrioventricular conduction (negative dromotropic effect), decreased arrhythmogenicity, vascular dilatation, and bronchial dilatation. The individual calcium antagonists differ in their ability to elicit these responses, as described below.

Clinical Toxicity

The toxic manifestations of the three most popular calcium antagonists (verapamil, nifedipine, and diltiazem) are shown in Table 53.4 (47). Verapamil is most likely to produce hypotension and prolonged AV conduction. Verapamil is only a weak vasodilator and the hypotension is due to a decrease in cardiac output (negative inotropic effect) without compensatory vasoconstriction. Nifedipine is predominantly a vasodilator (hence the high incidence of reflex tachycardia) and has little influence on AV conduction. Diltiazem is similar to verapamil in its ability to prolong AV conduction, but it causes less cardiac depression than verapamil and less vasodilatation than nifedipine.

Noncardiovascular manifestations of calcium blocker toxicity include lethargy and depressed consciousness (most common), generalized seizures, and hyperglycemia (caused by inhibition of insulin release, which is calcium-dependent) (47,48).

TABLE 53.4 Clinical Features Associated with Overdose of Specific Calcium Antagonists

	Incidence (%)		
Clinical Manifestation	**Verapamil**	**Nifedipine**	**Diltiazem**
Hypotension	53	32	38
Sinus tachycardia	23	57	26
Sinus bradycardia	29	14	29
Prolonged AV condition	55	18	29

From Ramoska EA, Spiller HA, Winter M, et al. A one-year evaluation of calcium channel blocker overdoses: toxicity and treatment. Ann Emerg Med 1993;22:196–200.

TABLE 53.5 Antidote Therapy with Intravenous Calcium

Characteristics	10% Calcium Chloride	10% Calcium Gluconate
Unit volume	10 mL per ampule	10 mL per ampule
Calcium content	1.36 mEq/mL	0.46 mEq/mL
Dose to prevent calcium channel blockage	3 mL	10 mL
Dose to reverse calcium channel blockage	13.6 mEq (10 mL)	13.8 mEq (30 mL)

Treatment

There are two approaches to calcium channel blockade (37). The first involves the administration of calcium to antagonize the blockade on the outer surface of the cell membrane. The second involves the use of drugs that activate the cyclic AMP pathway, which antagonizes the blockade from the inner surface of the cell membrane.

Intravenous Calcium

Intravenous calcium is the traditional first-line therapy for reversing calcium channel blockade, and elicits favorable responses in 35 to 75% of cases (47–49) resulting in improved inotropy, conduction disorders, and hypotension (45). As described in Chapter 35, there are two calcium salts for intravenous use (calcium chloride and calcium gluconate), and equivalent weights of each salt do not contain equivalent amounts of elemental calcium. This is shown in Table 53.5. One gram of 10% calcium chloride contains roughly three times more elemental calcium than one gram of 10% calcium gluconate. Therefore, ordering calcium without identifying the calcium salt, is inappropriate.

Although the calcium dose varies widely in clinical reports, calcium is most effective when given in doses that will increase the serum calcium level (48). The dose of calcium for reversing calcium channel blockade shown in Table 53.5 should raise the serum calcium level. The response to calcium may last only 10 to 15 minutes, so the initial response to calcium should be followed by a continuous infusion at 0.3 to 0.7 mEq/kg/hr (37,45). Calcium infusions are *not* recommended for patients being treated with digitalis.

Atropine

Atropine is the agent of choice to reverse significant bradycardia due to calcium channel blocker overdose, but it is not effective in severe cases of toxicity. The effect of atropine is enhanced by prior administration of calcium; therefore, calcium should be given before atropine (50). The dose of atropine is 0.5–1 mg given intravenously every 2–3 minutes up to a maximum of 3 mg (45).

Catecholamines

A variety of catecholamines have been used clinically to antagonize calcium channel blockade (e.g., epinephrine, norepinephrine, dopamine) but no single agent has proven to be effective on a consistent basis and the dosage requirements may be in the high range (45).

Preventive Therapy

Hypotension is a common complication of therapy with intravenous verapamil for supraventricular tachyarrhythmias. Pretreatment with 3 mL of 10% calcium chloride or 10 mL of 10% calcium gluconate (4.6 mEq calcium) is effective in preventing verapamil-induced hypotension in most cases (see Table 53.5) (49).

OPIOIDS

The opioids are common offenders in overdoses involving illicit street drugs, and the opioid analgesic morphine is the most common cause of toxic drug reactions in hospitalized patients (51). The adverse side effects of the opioid analgesics are described in Chapter 49. The following description will focus on the treatment of opioid intoxication with the opioid antagonist naloxone.

Naloxone

Naloxone is a pure opioid antagonist that binds to endogenous opioid receptors but does not elicit any agonist responses. It is most effective in blocking μ-receptors (primarily responsible for analgesia, sedation, and respiratory depression) and less effective in blocking κ-receptors and δ-receptors (52,53).

Routes of Administration

Naloxone (0.4 mg/ml or 1 mg/ml) is usually given intravenously (onset 2–3 minutes) or intramuscularly (onset 15 minutes) (52, 54), but can also be given endotracheally (55), or by intralingual injection (56, 57).

Dosing Recommendations

In opioid overdose, reversal of the sedation usually requires smaller doses of naloxone than reversal of the respiratory depression.

DEPRESSED MENTAL STATE. For patients with a depressed sensorium but no respiratory depression, the initial dose of naloxone should be 0.4 mg IV push. This can be repeated in 2 minutes, if necessary. A total dose of 0.8 mg should be effective if the mental status changes are caused by an opioid derivative (32). In patients with known opioid dependency, the bolus dose of naloxone should be reduced to 0.1 or 0.2 mg (32).

RESPIRATORY DEPRESSION. For patients who have evidence of respiratory depression (e.g., respiratory rate less than 12 breaths/min), the initial dose of naloxone should be 2 mg IV push. This dose is repeated every 2 minutes if necessary, to a total dose of 10 mg (32).

The effects of naloxone last about 60 to 90 minutes, which is less than the duration of action of most opioids. Therefore, a favorable response to naloxone should be followed by repeat doses at one-hour intervals, or by a continuous infusion. For a **continuous naloxone infusion,** the hourly dose of naloxone should be two-thirds of the effective bolus dose (diluted in 250 or 500 mL of isotonic saline and infused over 6 hours) (58). To achieve steady-state drug levels in the early infusion period, a second bolus of naloxone (at one-half the original bolus dose) is given 30 minutes after the infusion is started. The duration of treatment varies (according to the drug and the dose ingested), but averages 10 hours (32).

Empiric Therapy

Patients with a depressed mental state of undetermined etiology are often given naloxone (0.8–2 mg IV push) as empiric therapy. This practice has been questioned, because it elicits a favorable response in fewer than 5% of cases (59). An alternative approach has been proposed where **empiric naloxone is indicated only for patients with pinpoint pupils who have circumstantial evidence of opioid abuse** (e.g., needle tracks) (32,59). When naloxone is used in this manner, a favorable response is expected in approximately 90% of the patients (59).

Adverse Reactions

Naloxone has few side effects. The most common adverse reaction is the opioid withdrawal syndrome (anxiety, abdominal cramps, vomiting, and piloerection). There are case reports of acute pulmonary edema (most in the early postoperative period) and generalized seizures following naloxone administration (32), but these complications are rare.

A FINAL WORD

The drug that deserves the most attention in this chapter is acetaminophen, which is now the leading cause of acute liver failure in the United States and Great Britain (where it is called paracetamol). The general public seems unaware of the toxic potential of this drug, which is why one of every three overdoses is unintentional. When presented with a possible acetaminophen overdose, remember that the effectiveness of the antidote, N-acetylcysteine (NAC), is time-dependent, even within the 24-hour treatment window, so don't delay in starting therapy when it is indicated by the nomogram in Figure 53.2. The recent approval of the intravenous NAC regimen represents a real advance in treatment because patient compliance with the oral regimen is poor due to the foul taste of NAC.

Acetaminophen became popular in the 1970s because of concerns about the toxicity of aspirin, and it looks like we replaced a mouse with a gorilla.

REFERENCES

Introduction

1. Bond CA, Raehl CL. Adverse drug reactions in United States hospitals. Pharmacotherapy 2006;26:601–608.
2. Trunet P, Borda IT, Rouget AV, et al. The role of drug-induced illness in admissions to an intensive care unit. Intensive Care Med 1986;12:43–46.
3. Lazarou J, Pomeranz BH, Corey PN. Incidence of adverse drug reactions in hospitalized patients: a meta-analysis of prospective studies. JAMA 1998; 279:1200–1205.
4. Dasta JF. Drug prescribing issues in the intensive care unit: finding answers to common questions. Crit Care Med 1994;22:909–912.

Acetaminophen

5. Watson WA, Litovitz TL, Rodgers GC Jr, et al. 2004 Annual report of the American Association of Poison Control Centers Toxic Exposure Surveillance System. Am J Emerg Med 2005;23:589–666.
6. Larson AM, Polson J, Fontana RJ, et al. Acetaminophen-induced acute liver failure: results of a United States multicenter, prospective study. Hepatology (Baltimore) 2005;42:1364–1372.
7. Schiodt FV, Rochling FA, Casey DL, et al. Acetaminophen toxicity in an urban county hospital. N Engl J Med 1997;337:1112–1117.
8. Hendrickson RG, Bizovi KE. Acetaminophen. In: Flomenbaum NE, Goldfranck LR, Hoffman RS, et al., eds. Goldfrank's toxicologic emergencies. 8th ed. New York: McGraw-Hill, 2006:523–543.
9. Rumack BH. Acetaminophen hepatotoxicity: the first 35 years. J Toxicol Clin Toxicol 2002;40:3–20.
10. Anker AL, Smilkstein MJ. Acetaminophen: concepts and controversies. Emerg Med Clin North Am 1994;12:335–349.

N-acetylcysteine

11. Rumack BH, Peterson RC, Koch GG, et al. Acetaminophen overdose: 662 cases with evaluation of oral acetylcysteine treatment. Arch Intern Med 1981; 141:380–385.
12. Holdiness MR. Clinical pharmacokinetics of N-acetylcysteine. Clin Pharmacokinet 1991;20:123–134.
13. Cumberland Pharmaceuticals. Acetadote Package Insert. 2006.
14. Janes J, Routledge PA. Recent developments in the management of paracetamol (acetaminophen) poisoning. Drug Saf 1992;7:170–177.
15. Smilkstein MJ, Knapp GL, Kulig KW, et al. Efficacy of oral N-acetylcysteine in the treatment of acetaminophen overdose: analysis of the national multicenter study (1976 to 1985). N Engl J Med 1988;319:1557–1562.
16. Harrison PM, Keays R, Bray GP, et al. Improved outcome of paracetamol-induced fulminant hepatic failure by late administration of acetylcysteine. Lancet 1990;335:1572–1573.
17. Howland MA. N-Acetylcysteine. In: Flomenbaum NE, Goldfranck LR, Hoffman RS, et al., eds. Goldfrank's toxicologic emergencies. 8th ed. New York: McGraw-Hill, 2006: 544–549.

18. Buckley NA, Whyte IM, O'Connell DL, et al. Oral or intravenous N-acetylcysteine: which is the treatment of choice for acetaminophen (paracetamol) poisoning? J Toxicol Clin Toxicol 1999;37:759–767.
19. Sunman W, Hughes AD, Sever PS. Anaphylactoid response to intravenous acetylcysteine. Lancet 1992;339:1231–1232.
20. Appelboam AV, Dargan PI, Knighton J. Fatal anaphylactoid reaction to N-acetylcysteine: caution in patients with asthma. Emerg Med J 2002;19:594–595.
21. Miller LF, Rumack BH. Clinical safety of high oral doses of acetylcysteine. Semin Oncol 1983;10:76–85.
22. Spiller HA, Krenzelok EP, Grande GA, et al. A prospective evaluation of the effect of activated charcoal before oral N-acetylcysteine in acetaminophen overdose. Ann Emerg Med 1994;23:519–523.

Benzodiazepines

23. Lee DC. Sedative-hypnotics. In: Flomenbaum NE, Goldfranck LR, Hoffman RS, et al., eds. Goldfrank's toxicologic emergencies. 8th ed. New York: McGraw-Hill, 2006:1098–1111.
24. Dasta JF, Fuhrman TM, McCandles C. Patterns of prescribing and administering drugs for agitation and pain in patients in a surgical intensive care unit. Crit Care Med 1994;22:974–980.

Flumazenil

25. Roche Laboratories. Romazicon (flumazenil) package insert. 2004.
26. Howland MA. Flumazenil. In: Flomenbaum NE, Goldfranck LR, Hoffman RS, et al., eds. Goldfrank's toxicologic emergencies. 8th ed. New York: McGraw-Hill, 2006:1112–1117.
27. Gross JB, Weller RS, Conard P. Flumazenil antagonism of midazolam-induced ventilatory depression. Anesthesiology 1991;75:179–185.
28. Shalansky SJ, Naumann TL, Englander FA. Effect of flumazenil on benzodiazepine-induced respiratory depression. Clin Pharmacol 1993;12:483–487.
29. Grimm G, Ferenci P, Katzenschlager R, et al. Improvement of hepatic encephalopathy treated with flumazenil. Lancet 1988;2:1392–1394.
30. Martens F, Koppel C, Ibe K, et al. Clinical experience with the benzodiazepine antagonist flumazenil in suspected benzodiazepine or ethanol poisoning. J Toxicol Clin Toxicol 1990;28:341–356.
31. Bodenham A, Park GR. Reversal of prolonged sedation using flumazenil in critically ill patients. Anaesthesia 1989;44:603–605.
32. Doyon S, Roberts JR. Reappraisal of the "coma cocktail": dextrose, flumazenil, naloxone, and thiamine. Emerg Med Clin North Am 1994;12:301–316.
33. Chern TL, Hu SC, Lee CH, et al. Diagnostic and therapeutic utility of flumazenil in comatose patients with drug overdose. Am J Emerg Med 1993;11: 122–124.
34. Haverkos GP, DiSalvo RP, Imhoff TE. Fatal seizures after flumazenil administration in a patient with mixed overdose. Ann Pharmacother 1994;28:1347–1349.
35. Pepperman ML. Double-blind study of the reversal of midazolam-induced sedation in the intensive care unit with flumazenil (Ro 15-1788): effect on weaning from ventilation. Anaesth Intensive Care 1990;18:38–44.

β-Receptor Antagonists

36. Newton CR, Delgado JH, Gomez HF. Calcium and beta receptor antagonist overdose: a review and update of pharmacological principles and management. Semin Respir Crit Care Med 2002;23:19–25.
37. Kerns W, 2nd, Kline J, Ford MD. Beta-blocker and calcium channel blocker toxicity. Emerg Med Clin North Am 1994;12:365–390.
38. Weinstein RS. Recognition and management of poisoning with beta-adrenergic blocking agents. Ann Emerg Med 1984;13:1123–1131.
39. Henry JA, Cassidy SL. Membrane stabilising activity: a major cause of fatal poisoning. Lancet 1986;1:1414–1417.
40. Lane AS, Woodward AC, Goldman MR. Massive propranolol overdose poorly responsive to pharmacologic therapy: use of the intra-aortic balloon pump. Ann Emerg Med 1987;16:1381–1383.
41. Reith DM, Dawson AH, Epid D, et al. Relative toxicity of beta blockers in overdose. J Toxicol Clin Toxicol 1996;34:273–278.
42. Brubacher J. β-Adrenergic antagonists. In: Flomenbaum NE, Goldfranck LR, Hoffman RS, et al., eds. Goldfrank's toxicologic emergencies. 8th ed. New York: McGraw-Hill, 2006: 924–941.
43. Howland MA. Glucagon. In: Flomenbaum NE, Goldfranck LR, Hoffman RS, et al., eds. Goldfrank's toxicologic emergencies. 8th ed. New York: McGraw-Hill, 2006:942–945.
44. Chernow B, Zaloga GP, Malcolm D, et al. Glucagon's chronotropic action is calcium dependent. J Pharmacol Exp Ther 1987;241:833–837.

Calcium Antagonists

45. DeRoos F. Calcium Channel Blockers. In: Flomenbaum NE, Goldfranck LR, Hoffman RS, et al. eds. Goldfrank's toxicologic emergencies. 8th ed. New York: McGraw-Hill, 2006: 911–923.
46. Lucchesi BR. Role of calcium on excitation-contraction coupling in cardiac and vascular smooth muscle. Circulation 1989;80:IV1–IV13.
47. Ramoska EA, Spiller HA, Winter M, et al. A one-year evaluation of calcium channel blocker overdoses: toxicity and treatment. Ann Emerg Med 1993;22: 196–200.
48. Ramoska EA, Spiller HA, Myers A. Calcium channel blocker toxicity. Ann Emerg Med 1990;19:649–653.
49. Jameson SJ, Hargarten SW. Calcium pretreatment to prevent verapamil-induced hypotension in patients with SVT. Ann Emerg Med 1992;21:68.

Opioids

50. Howarth DM, Dawson AH, Smith AJ, et al. Calcium channel blocking drug overdose: an Australian series. Hum Exp Toxicol 1994;13:161–166.
51. Evans RS, Pestotnik SL, Classen DC, et al. Preventing adverse drug events in hospitalized patients. Ann Pharmacother 1994;28:523–527.
52. Handal KA, Schauben JL, Salamone FR, et al. Ann Emerg Med 1983;12:438–445.
53. Howland MA. Opioid antagonists. In: Flomenbaum NE, Goldfranck LR, Hoffman RS, et al. eds. Goldfrank's toxicologic emergencies. 8th ed. New York: McGraw-Hill, 2006:614–619.

54. Naloxone hydrochloride. In: McEvoy GK, Litvak K, eds. AHFS Drug Information. Bethesda, MD: American Society of Hospital Systems Pharmacists, 1995:1418–1420.
55. Tandberg D, Abercrombie D. Treatment of heroin overdose with endotracheal naloxone. Ann Emerg Med 1982;11:443–445.
56. Maio RF, Gaukel B, Freeman B. Intralingual naloxone injection for narcotic-induced respiratory depression. Ann Emerg Med 1987;16:572–573.
57. Salvucci AA Jr, Eckstein M, Iscovich AL. Submental injection of naloxone. Ann Emerg Med 1995;25:719–720.
58. Goldfrank L, Weisman RS, Errick JK, et al. A dosing nomogram for continuous infusion intravenous naloxone. Ann Emerg Med 1986;15:566–570.
59. Hoffman JR, Schriger DL, Luo JS. The empiric use of naloxone in patients with altered mental status: a reappraisal. Ann Emerg Med 1991;20:246–252.

Section XVII

APPENDICES

When you're through learning, you're through.

VERNON LAW

Appendix 1

UNITS AND CONVERSIONS

The units of measurements in the medical sciences are taken from the metric system (centimeter, gram, second) and the Anglo-Saxon system (foot, pound, second). The metric units were introduced during the French Revolution and were revised in 1960. The revised units are called Système International (SI) units and are currently the worldwide standard. The United States initially refrained from adopting the SI units, but this position has softened in recent years.

Units of Measurement in the Système International (SI)

Parameter	Dimensions	Basic SI Unit (Symbol)	Equivalences
Length	L	Meter (m)	1 inch = 2.54 cm
Area	L^2	Square meter (m^2)	1 square centimeter (cm^2) = 10^4 m^2
Volume	L^3	Cubic meter (m^3)	1 liter (L) = 0.001 m^3 1 milliliter (ml) = 1 cubic centimeter (cm^3)
Mass	M	Kilogram (kg)	1 pound (lb) = 453.5 g 1 kg = 2.2 lbs
Density	M/L^3	Kilogram per cubic meter (kg/m^3)	1 kg/m^3 = 0.001 kg/dm^3 Density of water = 1.0 kg/dm^3 Density of mercury = 13.6 kg/dm^3
Velocity	L/T	Meters per second (m/sec)	1 mile per hour (mph) = 0.4 m/sec
Acceleration	L/T^2	Meters per second squared (m/sec^2)	1 ft/sec^2 = 0.03 m/sec^2

(Continued)

Units of Measurement in the Système International (SI) (*Continued*)

Parameter	Dimensions	Basic SI Unit (Symbol)	Equivalences
Force	$M \times (L/T^2)$	Newton (N) = kg × (m/sec^2)	1 dyne = 10^{-5} N
Pressure	$\frac{M \times (L/T^2)}{L^2}$	Pascal (Pa) = N/m^2	1 kPa = 7.5 mm Hg = 10.2 cm H_2O 1 mm Hg = 1.00000014 torr (See conversion table for kPa and mmHg)
Heat	$M \times (L/T^2) \times L$	Joule (J) = N × m	1 kilocalorie (kcal) = 4184 J
Temperature	None	Kelvin (K)	0° C = −273 K (See conversion table for °C and °F)
Viscosity	M, 1/L, 1/T	Newton × second per square meter ($N \cdot sec/m^2$)	Centipoise (cP) = 10^{-3} $N \cdot sec/m^2$
Amount of a substance	N	Mole (mol) = molecular weight in grams	Equivalent (Eq) = mol × valence
Concentration	N/L^3	mol/m^3 = Molarity	Ionic strength = mol/kg
	N/M	mol/kg = Molality	

Temperature Conversions

(°C)	(°F)
100	212
41	105.8
40	104
39	102.2
38	100.4
37	98.6
36	96.8
35	95
34	93.2
33	91.4
32	89.6
31	87.8
30	86
0	32

°F = (9/5 °C) + 32
°C = 5/9 (°F − 32)

Apothecary and Household Conversions

Apothecary	Household
1 grain = 60 mg	1 teaspoonful = 5 mL
1 ounce = 30 g	1 dessertspoonful = 10 mL
1 fluid ounce = 30 mL	1 tablespoonful = 15 mL
1 pint = 500 mL	1 wineglassful = 60 mL
1 quart = 947 mL	1 teacupful = 120 mL
	1 tumblerful = 240 mL
	1 petroleum barrel = 42 gal

Pressure Conversions

mm Hg	kPa	mm Hg	kPa	mm Hg	kPa
41	5.45	61	8.11	81	10.77
42	5.59	62	8.25	82	10.91
43	5.72	63	8.38	83	11.04
44	5.85	64	8.51	84	11.17
45	5.99	65	8.65	85	11.31
46	6.12	66	8.78	86	11.44
47	6.25	67	8.91	87	11.57
48	6.38	68	9.04	88	11.70
49	6.52	69	9.18	89	11.84
50	6.65	70	9.31	90	11.97
51	6.78	71	9.44	91	12.10
52	6.92	72	9.58	92	12.24
53	7.05	73	9.71	93	12.37
54	7.18	74	9.84	94	12.50
55	7.32	75	9.98	95	12.64
56	7.45	76	10.11	96	12.77
57	7.58	77	10.24	97	12.90
58	7.71	78	10.37	98	13.03
59	7.85	79	10.51	79	13.17
60	7.98	80	10.64	100	13.90

Kilopascal (kPa) = 0.133 × mmHg
mm Hg = 7.50 × kPa

pH and Hydrogen Ion Concentration

pH	$[H^+]$ (nEq/L)
6.8	160
6.9	125
7.0	100
7.1	80
7.2	63
7.3	50
7.4	40
7.5	32
7.6	26
7.7	20
7.8	16

Sizes of Plastic Tube Devices

French	Outside Diameter*		
Size	Inches	mm	Device
1	0.01	0.3	Vascular catheters
4	0.05	1.3	
8	0.10	2.6	Small-bore feeding tubes
10	0.13	3.3	
12	0.16	4.0	
14	0.18	4.6	Nasogastric tubes
16	0.21	5.3	
18	0.23	6.0	
20	0.26	6.6	Chest tubes
22	0.28	7.3	
24	0.31	8.0	
26	0.34	8.6	
28	0.36	9.3	
30	0.39	10.0	
32	0.41	10.6	
34	0.44	11.3	
36	0.47	12.0	
38	0.50	12.6	

*Diameters can vary with manufactures. However, a useful rule of thumb is OD (mm) × 3 = French size.

Sizes of Intravascular Catheters

	Outside Diameter*		
Gauge	Inches	mm	Type of Catheter
26	0.018	0.45	Butterfly devices
25	0.020	0.50	
24	0.022	0.56	
23	0.024	0.61	
22	0.028	0.71	Peripheral vascular catheters
21	0.032	0.81	
20	0.036	0.91	
19	0.040	1.02	
18	0.048	1.22	Central venous catheters
16	0.064	1.62	
14	0.080	2.03	Introducer catheters
12	0.104	2.64	
10	0.128	3.25	

*Diameters can vary with manufacturers.

Appendix 2

SELECTED REFERENCE RANGES

Reference Ranges for Selected Clinical Laboratory Tests

Substance	Fluid*	Traditional Units	×	k	=	SI Units
Acetoacetate	P, S	0.3–3.0 mg/dL		97.95		3–30 μmol/L
Alanine aminotransferase (SGPT)	S	0–35 U/L		0.016		0–0.58 μkat/L
Albumin	S CSF	4–6 g/dL 11–48 mg/dL		10 0.01		40–60 g/L 0.11–0.48 g/L
Aldolase	S	0–6 U/L		16.6		0–100 nkat/L
Alkaline phosphatase	S	(F)30–100 U/L (M)45–115 U/L		0.016		0.5–1.67 μkat/L 0.75–1.92 μkat/L
Ammonia	P	10–80 μg/dL		0.587		5–50 μmol/L
Amylase	S	0–130 U/L		0.016		0–2.17 μkat/L
Aspartate aminotransferase (SGOT)	S	0–35 U/L		0.016		0–0.58 μkat/L
β-Hydroxybutyrate	S	<1.0 mg/dL		96.05		<100 μmol/L
Bicarbonate	S	22–26 mEq/L		1		22–26 mmol/L
Bilirubin: Total Conjugated	S S	0.1–1.0 mg/dL ≤0.2 mg/dL		17.1		2–18 μmol/L ≤4 μmol/L
Blood urea nitrogen (BUN)	P, S	8–18 mg/dL		0.367		3.0–6.5 mmol/L

(*Continued*)

Reference Ranges for Selected Clinical Laboratory Tests (*Continued*)

Substance	Fluid*	Traditional Units	× k	= SI Units
Calcium: Total	S	8.5–10.5 mg/dL	0.26	2.2–2.6 mmol/L
Ionized	P	2.2–2.3 mEq/L	0.49	1.10–1.15 mmol/L
Chloride	P, S	95–105 mEq/L	1	95–105 mmol/L
	CSF	120–130 mEq/L		120–130 mmol/L
	U	10–200 mEq/L		10–200 mmol/L
Creatinine	S	0.6–1.5 mg/dL	0.09	0.05–0.13 mmol/L
	U	15–25 mg/kg/24 hr	0.009	0.13–0.22 mmol/kg/24 h
Cyanide: Nontoxic	WB	<5 μg/dL	3.8	<19 μmol/L
Lethal		>30 μg/dL		>114 μmol/L
Fibrinogen	P	150–350 mg/dL	0.01	1.5–3.5 g/L
Fibrin split products	S	<10 μg/mL	1	<10 mg/L
Glucose (fasting)	P	70–100 mg/dL	0.06	3.9–6.1 mmol/L
	CSF	50–80 mg/dL		2.8–4.4 mmol/L
Lactate: Resting	P	<2.0 mEq/L	1	<2 mmol/L
Exercise		<4.0 mEq/L		<4 mmol/L
Lactate dehydrogenase (LDH)	S	50–150 U/L	0.017	0.82–2.66 μkat/L
Lipase	S	0–160 U/L	0.017	0–2.66 μkat/L
Magnesium	P, S	1.8–3.0 mg/dL	0.41	0.8–1.2 mmol/L
		1.5–2.4 mEq/L	0.5	0.8–1.2 mmol/L
Osmolality	S	280–296 mOsm/kg	1	280–96 mmol/kg
Phosphate	S	2.5–5.0 mg/dL	0.32	0.80–1.60 mmol/L
Potassium	P, S	3.5–5.0 mEq/L	1	3.5–5.0 mmol/L
Total protein	P, S	6.0–8.0 g/dL	10	60–80 g/L
	CSF	<40 mg/dL	0.01	<0.40 g/L
	U	<150 mg/24 hr	0.01	<1.5 g/24 hr
Sodium	P, S	135–147 mEq/L	1	135–147 mmol/L
Thyroxine: Total	S	4–11 μg/dL	12.9	51–142 nmol/L
Free		0.8–2.8 ng/dL		10–36 pmol/L
Triiodothyronine (T_3)	S	75–220 ng/dL	0.015	12–3.4 nmol/L

**P* = Plasma, *S* = serum, *U* = urine, *WB* = whole blood, *CSF* = cerebrospinal fluid, *RBC* = red blood cell.

Adapted from the New England Journal of Medicine SI Unit Conversion Guide. Waltham, MA: Massachusetts Medical Society, 1992.

Reference Ranges for Vitamins and Trace Elements

Substance	Fluid*	Traditional unit ×	k =	SI Units
Chromium	S	0.14–0.15 ng/mL	17.85	2.5–2.7 nmol/L
Copper	S	70–140 μg/dL	0.16	11–22 μmol/L
Folate	RBC	140–960 ng/mL	2.26	317–2169 nmol/L
Iron	S	(M)80–180 μg/dL (F)60–160 μg/dL	0.18	(M)14–32 μmol/L (F)11–29 μmol/L
Ferritin	P, S	(M)20–250 ng/mL (F)10–120 ng/mL	1	(M)20–250 μg/L (F)10–120 μg/L
Manganese	WB	0.4–2.0 μg/dL	0.018	0.7–3.6 μmol/L
Pyridoxine	P	20–90 ng/mL	5.98	120–540 nmol/L
Riboflavin	S	2.6–3.7 μg/dL	26.57	70–100 nmol/L
Selenium	WB	58–234 μg/dL	0.012	0.7–2.5 μmol/L
Thiamine (total)	P	3.4–4.8 μg/dL	0.003	98.6–139 μmol/L
Vitamin A	P, S	10–50 μg/dL	0.349	0.35–1.75 μmol/L
Vitamin B_{12}	S	200–1000 pg/mL	0.737	150–750 pmol/L
Vitamin C	S	0.6–2 mg/dL	56.78	30–100 μmol/L
Vitamin D	S	24–40 ng/mL	2.599	60–105 nmol/L
Vitamin E	P, S	0.78–1.25 mg/dL	23.22	18–29 μmol/L
Zinc	S	70–120 μg/dL	0.153	11.5–18.5 μmol/L

**P* = plasma, *S* = serum, *WB* = whole blood, *RBC* = red blood cell.
Adapted from the New England Journal of Medicine SI Unit Conversion Guide, Waltham, MA: Massachusetts Medical Society, 1992.

Laboratory Measurements Influenced by Body Position

Measurement	% Decrease When Upright	
	Average	Range
Hemoglobin	5	3–7
Hematocrit	6	4–9
Serum calcium	4	2–6
Total protein	9	7–10
Serum albumin	9	6–14
Cholesterol	9	5–15
Alkaline phosphatase	9	5–11
Alanine aminotransferase	7	4–14

From Ravel R. Clinical laboratory medicine, Chicago: Yearbook Medical Publishing, 1989;4.

Volume Used by Automated Analyzers in the Clinical Laboratory

Laboratory Test	Instrument Volume (mL)
Arterial blood gases	1.0
Electrolyte panel	0.15
Complete blood cell count	0.125
Glucose	0.04

For serum assays, the volume of whole blood to be withdrawn is:

$$\text{Whole blood volume} = \frac{\text{Serum volume}}{1 - \text{Hematocrit}}$$

From Mayo Clin Proc 1993;68:255.

Desirable Weights for Adults*

Height		Males		
Feet	Inches	Small Frame	Medium Frame	Large Frame
5	2	128–134	131–141	138–150
5	3	130–136	133–143	140–153
5	4	132–138	135–145	142–156
5	5	134–140	137–148	144–160
5	6	136–142	139–151	146–164
5	7	138–145	142–154	149–168
5	8	140–148	145–157	152–172
5	9	142–151	148–160	155–176
5	10	144–154	151–163	158–180
5	11	146–157	154–166	161–184
6	0	149–160	157–170	164–188
6	1	152–164	160–174	168–192
6	2	155–168	164–178	172–197
6	3	158–172	167–182	172–202
6	4	162–176	171–187	181–207
		Females		
4	10	102–111	109–121	112–131
4	11	103–113	111–123	120–134
5	0	104–115	113–126	122–137
5	1	106–118	115–129	125–140
5	2	108–121	118–132	128–143

Desirable Weights for Adults* (*Continued*)

Height		Males		
Feet	Inches	Small Frame	Medium Frame	Large Frame
5	3	111–124	121–135	131–147
5	4	114–127	124–138	134–151
5	5	117–130	127–141	137–155
5	6	120–133	130–144	140–159
5	7	123–136	133–147	143–163
5	8	126–139	136–150	146–167
5	9	129–142	139–153	149–170
5	10	132–145	142–156	152–173
5	11	135–148	145–159	155–176
6	0	138–151	148–162	158–179

*Unclothed weights associated with the longest life expectancies. From the statistics bureau of the Metropolitan Life Insurance Company, 1983.

Basal Metabolic Rates

	kcal/24 hours	
Body Weight (kg)	Male	Female
40	1340	1241
50	1485	1399
52	1505	1429
54	1555	1458
56	1580	1487
58	1600	1516
60	1630	1544
62	1660	1572
64	1690	1599
66	1725	1626
68	1765	1653
70	1785	1679
72	1815	1705
74	1845	1731
76	1870	1756
78	1900	1781
80	—	1805

From Talbot FB. Am J Dis Child 1938;5:455–459.

Determinations of Body Size

Ideal Body Weight*

Males: IBW (kg) = 50 + 2.3 (Ht in inches − 60)

Females: IBW (kg) = 45.5 + 2.3 (Ht in inches − 60)

Body Mass Index†

$$BMI = \frac{\text{Wt (in lbs)}}{\text{Ht (in inches)}^2 \times 703}$$

Body Surface Area

Dubois Formula‡

$$BSA\ (m^2) = \text{Ht (in cm)}^{0.725} \times \text{Wt (in kg)}^{0.425} \times 0.007184$$

Jacobson Formula§

$$BSA\ (m^2) = \frac{\text{Ht (in cm)} + \text{Wt (in kg)} - 60}{100}$$

*Devine BJ. Drug Intell Clin Pharm 1974;8:650.
†Matz R. Ann Intern Med 1993;118:232.
‡Dubois EF. Basal metabolism in health and disease. Philadelphia: Lea & Febiger, 1936.
§Jacobson B. Medicine and clinical engineering. Englewood Cliffs, NJ: Prentice-Hall, 1977.

Body Build and Blood Volume in Adults

	Average Blood Volume (mL/kg)	
Body Build	**Males**	**Females**
Thin	65	60
Normal	70	65
Muscular	75	70
Obese	60	55

From Documenta Geigy Scientific Tables. 7th ed. Basel, Switzerland: JR Geigy, SA, 1970;528.

Blood Volumes in the Elderly

Volume(mL)	Elderly Men	Elderly Women
Whole blood	(3809 × BSA) − 2362	(1591 × BSA) + 889
Plasma	(1,995 × BSA) − 667	(925 × BSA) + 802
Erythrocytes	(1761 × BSA) − 1609	(716 × BSA) + 14

From Cordtes PR et al. Surg Gynecol Obstet 1992;175:243–248.

Body Fluid Distribution in Healthy Adults

Parameter	Derivation	Males	Female
Total body water	0.55 × body wt (kg)	600 mL/kg	500 mL/kg
Interstitial fluid	0.16 × body wt (kg)	160 mL/kg	160 mL/kg
Blood volume (BV)	0.065 × body wt (kg)	70 mL/kg	65 mL/kg
Erythrocyte volume (EV)	EV = BV × Hct	33 mL/kg	27 mL/kg
Plasma volume (PV)	PV = BV − EV	37 mL/kg	38 mL/kg
Hematocrit (Hct)	EV/BV × 100	47% (mean) 40–54% (range)	42% (mean) 37–47% (range)

From Documenta Geigy Scientific Tables. 7th ed. Basel, Switzerland: JR Geigy SA, 1970.

Peak Expiratory Flow Rates for Healthy Males

	Average Peak Flow (L/min)			
Age (yr)	Ht: 60"	65"	70"	75"
20	602	649	693	740
25	590	636	679	725
30	577	622	664	710
35	565	609	651	695
40	552	596	636	680
45	540	583	622	665
50	527	569	607	649
55	515	556	593	634
60	502	542	578	618
65	490	529	564	603
70	477	515	550	587

Peak Flow (L/min) = [3.95 − (0.0151 × Age)] × Ht (cm)
Regression equation from Leiner GC et al. Am Rev Respir Dis 1963;88:646.

Peak Expiratory Flow Rates for Healthy Females

		Average Peak Flow (L/min)			
Age (yr)	**Ht:**	**55"**	**60"**	**65"**	**70"**
20		309	423	460	496
25		385	418	454	490
30		380	413	448	483
35		375	408	442	476
40		370	402	436	470
45		365	397	430	464
50		360	391	424	457
55		355	386	418	451
60		350	380	412	445
65		345	375	406	439
70		340	369	400	432

Peak Flow (L/min) = [2.93 − (0.0072 × Age)] × Ht (cm)
Regression equation from Leiner GC et al. Am Rev Respir Dis 1963;88:647.

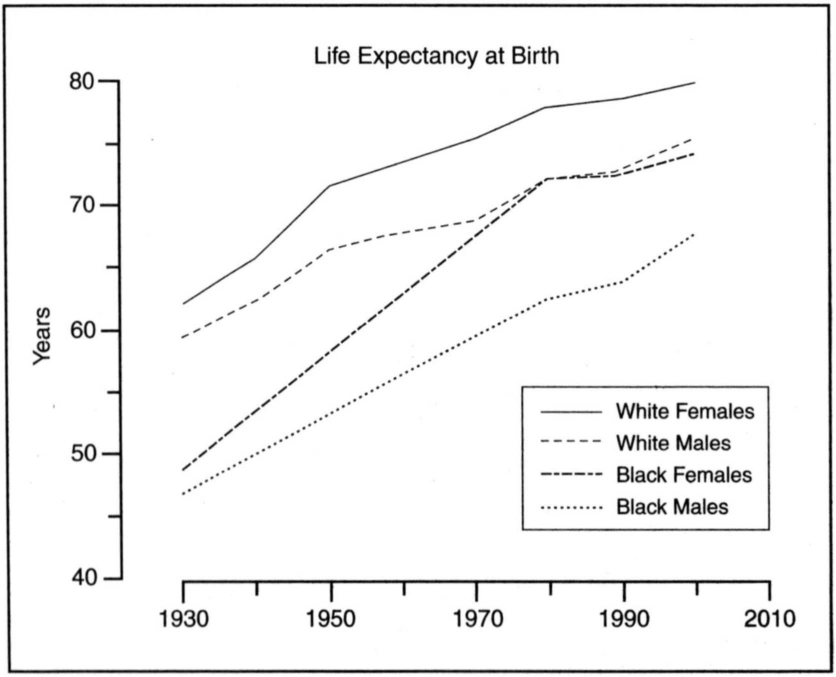

National Vital Statistics Reports, Sept. 18, 2003; 53(3).

Appendix 3

CLINICAL SCORING SYSTEMS

APACHE II SCORING SYSTEM

The APACHE (Acute Physiology and Chronic Health Evaluation) scoring system was developed to provide an objective assessment of severity of illness in patients in the ICU. The scoring system is not meant for burn patients or post–cardiopulmonary bypass patients. Although there are limitations in predicting mortality in individual patients in the ICU, the APACHE scoring system is widely used in clinical studies to provide some measure of disease severity in the study patients. The following pages demonstrate how to generate an APACHE II score (1). Although there is an APACHE III scoring system (2), the APACHE II score is more widely used.

The APACHE II score is made up of three components:

1. **Acute Physiology Score (APS).** The largest component of the APACHE II score is derived from 12 clinical measurements that are obtained within 24 hours after admission to the ICU. The *most abnormal measurement* is selected to generate the APS component of the APACHE II score. If a variable has not been measured, it is assigned zero points.
2. **Age Adjustment.** From one to six points is added for patients older than 44 years of age.
3. **Chronic Health Evaluation.** An additional adjustment is made for patients with severe and chronic organ failure involving the heart, lungs, kidneys, liver, and immune system.

Acute Physiology Score

Points:	+4	+3	+2	+1	0	+1	+2	+3	+4
Temperature (°C)	≥41	39–40.9		38.5–38.9	36–38.4	34–35.9	32–33.9	30–31.9	≤29.9
Mean arterial pressure	≥160	130–159	110–129		70–109		50–69		≤49
Heart rate	≥180	140–179	110–139		70–109		55–69	40–54	≤39
Respiratory rate	≥50	35–49		25–34	12–24	10–11	6–9		≤5
[1]A-aPo$_2$	≥500	350–499	200–349		<200				
[2]PAO$_2$					>70	61–70		55–60	<55
Arterial pH	≥7.7	7.6–7.69		7.5–7.59	7.33–7.49		7.25–7.32	7.15–7.24	<7.15
[3]Serum bicarbonate (mEq/L)	≥52	41–51.9		32–40.9	23–31.9		18–21.9	15–17.9	<15
Serum sodium (mEq/L)	≥180		160–179	155–159	150–154	130–149	120–129	111–119	≤110
Serum potassium (mEq/L)	≥7	6–6.9		5.5–5.9	3.5–5.4	3–3.4	2.5–2.9		<2.5
Serum creatinine (mg/dL)	≥3.5	2–3.4	1.5–1.9		0.6–1.4		<0.6		
Hematocrit	≥60		50–59.9	46–49.9	30–45.9		20–29.9		<20
WBC count	≥40		20–39.9	15–19.9	3–14.9		1–2.9		<1
[4]15 − (Glasgow Coma Score) =									

1. If FiO$_2$ >50%. 2. If FiO$_2$ <50%. 3. Use only if no ABGs.

Scoring Method

1. Select the *most abnormal measurement* for each parameter in the first 24 hours after ICU admission.
2. If a parameter has not been measured, assign it zero points.
3. Add the corresponding points for all 12 parameters to obtain the Acute Physiology Score.
4. Glasgow Coma Scale follows.

The Glasgow Coma Scale*

Eye Opening:	Points	
Spontaneous	4	
To Speech	3	
To Pain	2	
None	1	☐ Points
Verbal Communication†:		
Oriented	5	
Confused conversation	4	
Inappropriate words	3	
Incomprehensible sounds	2	
None	1	☐ Points
Motor Response:		
Obeys commands	6	
Localizes to pain	5	
Withdraws to pain	4	
Abnormal flexion	3	
Abnormal extension	2	
None	1	☐ Points
	Total Points‡	☐

*Adapted from Teasdale G, Jennet B. Assessment of coma and impaired consciousness. A practical approach. Lancet 1974;2:81–86.
†For intubated patients, assign a score of 1 for verbal communication.
‡Best score is 15 points; worst score is 3 points.

Age Adjustment

Age (yr)	Points
<44	0
45–54	2
55–64	3
65–74	5
>75	6

Chronic Health Adjustment

For any of the following:

1. Biopsy proven cirrhosis.
2. Heart failure: NYHA Class IV
3. Severe COPD (hypercapnia, home oxygen)
4. Chronic dialysis
5. Immunocompromised

Add 2 points for elective surgery or neurosurgery, 5 points for emergency surgery.

Total APACHE II Score

APS score	________
Age adjustment	________
Chronic health adjustment	________
Total APACHE II score	________

APACHE II Score and Mortality in 5,185 ICU Patients

	Hospital Mortality (%)	
APACHE II Score	**Nonoperative**	**Postoperative**
0–4	4	1
5–9	6	3
10–14	12	6
15–19	22	11
20–24	40	29
25–29	51	37
30–34	71	71
≥35	82	87

Data from Knaus WA et al. Crit Care Med 1985;13:818–829.

Limitations

The following limitations of the APACHE II score deserve mention.

1. The APS score has no adjustments for measurements obtained in the presence of interventions such as hemodynamic support drugs, mechanical ventilation, or antipyretic therapy.
2. There is an exaggerated penalty for old age. For example, age greater than 65 years adds more points than an A-a Po_2 gradient above 500 mm Hg (6 points versus 4 points, respectively).
3. There is no consideration for malnutrition or cachexia in the chronic health evaluation.

SEQUENTIAL ORGAN FAILURE ASSESSMENT (SOFA) SCORE

The Sequential Organ Failure Assessment (SOFA) score is designed to evaluate the function of six major organ systems (i.e., cardiovascular, respiratory, renal, hepatic, central nervous system, and coagulation) over time. The score is obtained on the day of admission and each of the following days in the ICU. Because the SOFA score monitors daily changes in organ function, it can evaluate the patient's response to treatment, and sequential changes in the SOFA score (e.g., increasing or decreasing) can predict the eventual outcome of the ICU stay.

The SOFA score differs from the APACHE II score in the following ways: (1) The APACHE II score is performed only on the day of admission, and does not monitor the clinical course of the patient, and (2) The APACHE II score has no adjustment for the use of hemodynamic support drugs, and the SOFA score does.

The Sequential Organ Failure Assessment (SOFA) Score

	Points				
Variables	**0**	**1**	**2**	**3**	**4**
PaO_2/FiO_2 (mmHg)	>400	≤400	≤300	≤200*	≤100*
Platelets (10^3/μL)	>150	≤150	≤100	≤50	≤20
Billrubin (mg/dL)	<1.2	1.2–1.9	2.0–5.9	6.0–11.9	≥12
Creatinine (mg/dL) or Urine Output (mL/day)	<1.2	1.2–1.9	2.0–3.4	3.5–4.9 or <500	>5.0 or <200
Glasgow Coma Score†	15	13–14	10–12	6–9	<6
Hypotension	None	Mean BP <70 mmHg	Dopa ≤5 or Dobu (any dose)‡	Dopa >5 or Epi ≤0.1 or Norepi ≤0.1‡	Dop >15 or Epi >0.1 or Norepi >0.1‡

*Values obtained during respiratory support.

†In patients who are sedated, use the best estimate of what the GCS would be without sedation.

‡Adrenergic agents administered for at least one hour. Doses expressed in μg/kg/min.
Dopa = Dopamine, Dobu = dobutamine, Epi = epinephrine, Norepi = norepinephrine.

Scoring Method:

1. Use the *most abnormal value* for each variable in a 24-hour period.
2. If a single value is missing, use the mean value of the sum of the results immediately preceding and following the missing value.
3. Add the corresponding points for all 6 parameters to obtain the final score (range = 0–24).

From Ferreira FL, et al. Serial evaluation of the SOFA score to predict outcome in critically ill patients. JAMA 2001; 286:1754–1758.

SOFA Score and Mortality*

Initial Score	Mortality Rate	Highest Score	Mortality Rate
0–1	0	0–1	0
2–3	7%	2–3	2%
4–5	20%	4–5	7%
6–7	22%	6–7	18%
8–9	33%	8–9	26%
10–11	50%	10–11	46%
>11	95%	>11	86%

*SOFA scores obtained on admission and every 48 hrs until discharge in 352 consecutive patients admitted to a medicosurgical ICU. Data from Ferreira et al. JAMA 2001; 286:1754.

The Richmond Agitation Sedation Scale (RASS)

Score	Term	Description
+4	Combative	Overly combative or violent; immediate danger to staff.
+3	Very agitated	Pulls on or removes tube(s)/catheter(s), or aggressive behavior.
+2	Agitated	Frequent non-purposeful movement or patient-ventilator asynchrony.
+1	Restless	Anxious or apprehensive but movements not aggressive or vigorous.
0	Alert & calm	
−1	Drowsy	Not fully alert, but awakens for >10 sec, with eye contact, to voice.
−2	Light sedation	Briefly awakens (<10 sec), with eye contact, to voice.
−3	Moderate sedation	Any movement (but no eye contact) to voice.
−4	Deep sedation	No response to voice, but movement to physical stimulation.
−5	Unarousable	No response to voice or physical stimulation.

To determine the RASS, proceed as follows:

Step 1. **Observation:** Observe the patient without interaction. If patient is alert, assign the appropriate score (0 to +4). If patient is not alert, go to Step 2.

Step 2. **Verbal Stimulation:** Address patient by name in a loud voice and ask the patient to look at you. Can repeat once if necessary. If patient responds to voice, assign the appropriate score (−1 to −3). If there is no response, go to Step 3.

Step 3. **Physical Stimulation:** Shake the patient's shoulder. If there is no response, rub the sternum vigorously. Assign the appropriate score (−4 to −5).

From Sessler CN, Gosnell MS, Grap MJ, et al. The Richmond Agitation-Sedation Scale: validity and reliability in adult intensive care unit patients. Am J Respir Crit Care Med 2002; 166:1338–1344.

THE CONFUSION ASSESSMENT METHOD FOR THE ICU

The Confusion Assessment Method for the ICU (CAM-ICU) was developed by Dr. Wes Ely at Vanderbilt University (and is reproduced here with his kind permisison). The CAM-ICU is a validated scale that can be used to evaluate and serially monitor delirium (both hyperactive and hypoactive forms) in critically ill patients, including nonverbal patients and patients with coexisting dementia. Performing the test requires under 2 minutes.

The Confusion Assessment Method for the Intensive Care Unit (CAM-ICU)

Feature 1: Acute Onset or Fluctuating Course Positive if you answer "yes" to either 1A or 1B.	**Positive**	**Negative**
1A: Is the pt different than his/her baseline mental status?	**Yes**	**No**
Or		
1B: Has the patient had any fluctuation in mental status in the past 24 hours as evidenced by fluctuation on a sedation scale (e.g., RASS), GCS, or previous delirium assessment?		
Feature 2: Inattention	**Positive**	**Negative**
Positive if either score for 2A <u>or</u> 2B is less than 8. Attempt the ASE letters first. If pt is able to perform this test and the score is clear, record this score and move to Feature 3. If pt is unable to perform this test <u>or</u> the score is unclear, then perform the ASE Pictures. If you perform both tests, use the ASE Pictures' results to score the Feature.		
2A: ASE Letters: record score (enter NT for not tested)	**Score (out of 10):** ___	
Directions: Say to the patient, *"I am going to read you a series of 10 letters. Whenever you hear the letter 'A,' indicate by squeezing my hand."* Read letters from the following letter list in a normal tone.		
S A V E A H A A R T		
Scoring: Errors are counted when patient fails to squeeze on the letter "A" and when the patient squeezes on any letter other than "A."		
2B: ASE Pictures: record score (enter NT for not tested)	**Score (out of 10):** ___	
Directions are included on the picture packets.		

The Confusion Assessment Method for the Intensive Care Unit (CAM-ICU)

Feature 3: Disorganized Thinking **Positive** **Negative**

Positive if the combined score is less than 4

Combined Score (3A+3B): ___ (out of 5)

3A: Yes/No Questions

(Use either Set A or Set B, alternate on consecutive days if necessary):

Set A	Set B
1. Will a stone float on water?	1. Will a leaf float on water?
2. Are there fish in the sea?	2. Are there elephants in the sea?
3. Does one pound weigh more than two pounds?	3. Do two pounds weigh more than one pound?
4. Can you use a hammer to pound a nail?	4. Can you use a hammer to cut wood?

Score ___ (Patient earns 1 point for each correct answer out of 4)

3B: Command

Say to patient: *"Hold up this many fingers"* (Examiner holds two fingers in front of patient) *"Now do the same thing with the other hand"* (Not repeating the number of fingers).

*If pt is unable to move both arms, for the second part of the command ask patient *"Add one more finger."*

Score___ (Patient earns 1 point if able to successfully complete the entire command)

Feature 4: Altered Level of Consciousness **Positive** **Negative**

Positive if the RASS score is anything other than "0" (zero)

Overall CAM-ICU (Features 1 and 2 and either Feature 3 or 4) **Positive** **Negative**

From Ely EW, Margolin R, Francis J, et al. Evaluation of delirium in critically ill patients: validation of the Confusion Assessment Method for the Intensive Care Unit (CAM-ICU). Crit Care Med 2001; 29:1370–1379. Further details available @ www.icudelirium.org/delirium.

Index

Page numbers set in *italics* denote figures; those followed by a *t* denote tables.

R